Breast Cancer

Breast Cancer

Second Edition

Daniel F. Roses, MD
Jules Leonard Whitehill Professor of Surgery and Oncology
New York University School of Medicine
Senior Attending Surgeon
New York University Medical Center
New York, New York

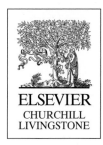

ELSEVIER
CHURCHILL
LIVINGSTONE

ELSEVIER
CHURCHILL
LIVINGSTONE

1600 John F. Kennedy Blvd.
Ste 1800
Philadelphia, PA 19103-2899

BREAST CANCER   ISBN   0-443-06634-5
Copyright © 2005, 1999 by Elsevier Inc.

Notice

Library of Congress Cataloging-in-Publication Data

Breast cancer / [edited by] Daniel F. Roses.—2nd ed.
        p. ; cm.
    Includes bibliographical references and index.
    ISBN 0-443-06634-5
    1. Breast–Cancer.   I. Roses, Daniel F.
    [DNLM: 1. Breast Neoplasms. WP 870 B821135 2005]
RC280.B8B66554 2005
616.99'449—dc22   2004063454

Publishing Director: Judith Fletcher
Senior Developmental Editor: Jennifer Ehlers
Publishing Services Manager: Tina Rebane
Project Manager: Amy Norwitz
Design Director: Steven Stave
Cover Art: Michelangelo (1475–1564). The Libyan Sibyl. Detail of the Sistine ceiling. Sistine Chapel, Vatican Palace, Vatican State. Scala/Art Resource, NY

Printed in the United States of America

Last digit is the print number: 9 8 7 6 5 4 3 2 1

Contributors

Barbara Baskin, MD
Associate Clinical Professor of Pathology
Mount Sinai School of Medicine and Medical Center
Associate Radiologist
Murrary Hill Radiology and Mammography
New York, New York
Sonographic Diagnosis of Breast Cancer

Anthony Berson, MD
Associate Professor of Clinical Radiation Medicine
New York Medical College
Valhalla, New York
Chairman, Department of Radiation Oncology
St. Vincent's Comprehensive Cancer Center
New York, New York
Management of Metastatic Breast Cancer: Radiation Therapy for Metastatic Breast Cancer

Ira J. Bleiweiss, MD
Professor of Pathology
Mount Sinai School of Medicine
Director of Surgical Pathology
Director, Division of Breast Pathology
Attending Pathologist
Mount Sinai Medical Center
New York, New York
Pathology of Invasive Breast Cancer

Patrick I. Borgen, MD
Associate Professor of Surgery
Weill Medical College of Cornell University
Head, Breast Cancer Research Laboratory
Chief, Breast Service
Director, Breast Cancer Disease Management Team
Attending Surgeon
Memorial Sloan-Kettering Cancer Center
New York, New York
Treatment of Male Breast Cancer

Stephen R. Colen, MD
Associate Professor of Plastic Surgery
New York University School of Medicine
Chairman, Department of Plastic Surgery
Hackensack University Medical Center
Hackensack, New Jersey
Reconstruction Following Surgery for Breast Cancer

Paul R. Cooper, MD
Attilio and Olympia Ricciardi Professor of Neurosurgery
New York University School of Medicine
Attending Neurosurgeon
New York University Medical Center and Bellevue
    Hospital
New York, New York
Management of Metastatic Breast Cancer: Spinal Column Metastases from Breast Cancer

Pamela Cowin, PhD
Professor of Cell Biology and Dermatology
New York University School of Medicine
New York, New York
Molecular, Cellular, and Developmental Biology of Breast Cancer

John Curtin, MD, MBA
Professor and Chair, Department of Obstetrics and
    Gynecology
New York University School of Medicine
New York, New York
Gynecologic Management of the Woman with Breast Cancer

Hakan Demirci, MD
Lecturer
Kellogg Eye Center
University of Michigan
Ann Arbor, Michigan
Management of Metastatic Breast Cancer: Ocular Metastases from Breast Cancer

Andrea F. Douglas, MD
Chief Resident in Neurosurgery
New York University Medical Center and Bellevue
    Hospital
New York, New York
Management of Metastatic Breast Cancer: Spinal Column Metastases from Breast Cancer

Stephen B. Edge, MD
Professor of Surgery
State University of New York at Buffalo School of
    Medicine and Biomedical Sciences
Chair, Department of Breast and Soft Tissue Surgery
Roswell Park Cancer Institute
Buffalo, New York
Surveillance Following Breast Cancer Treatment

Alison Estabrook, MD
Professor of Clinical Surgery
Columbia University College of Physicians and Surgeons
Chief of Breast Surgery
St. Luke's–Roosevelt Hospital
New York, New York
Treatment of Unusual Malignant Neoplasias and Clinical Presentations

Polly R. Etkind, PhD
Associate Professor of Medicine and of Microbiology and Immunology
New York Medical College
Valhalla, New York
Associate Professor
Comprehensive Care Center
Our Lady of Mercy Medical Center
Bronx, New York
Prevention of Breast Cancer

Stephen A. Feig, MD
Professor of Radiology
University of California, Irvine, School of Medicine
Director of Breast Imaging
University of California, Irvine, Medical Center
Orange, California
Surveillance Strategy for Detection of Breast Cancer

Silvia Formenti, MD
Sandra and Edward H. Meyer Professor and Chairman, Department of Radiation Oncology
New York University School of Medicine
Chairman, Department of Radiation Oncology
New York University Medical Center
New York, New York
Treatment of Locally Advanced Breast Cancer

Gladys Giron, MD
Medical Director, Taylor Breast Center
Jackson Memorial Hospital
Miami, Florida
Treatment of Unusual Malignant Neoplasias and Clinical Presentations

Armando E. Giuliano, MD
Clinical Professor of Surgery
David Geffen School of Medicine at UCLA
Los Angeles, California
Chief of Surgical Oncology
John Wayne Cancer Institute
Santa Monica, California
Surgery for Breast Cancer

Lawrence R. Glassman, MD
Chief, Division of Thoracic Surgery
North Shore University Hospital
Manhasset, New York
Management of Metastatic Breast Cancer: Thoracic Metastases from Breast Cancer

Steven R. Goldstein, MD
Professor of Obstetrics and Gynecology
New York University School of Medicine
Director, Gynecologic Ultrasound
Co-Director, Bone Densitometry
New York University Medical Center
New York, New York
Gynecologic Management of the Woman with Breast Cancer

Orna Hadar, MD
Associate Clinical Professor of Pathology
Mount Sinai School of Medicine
Associate Radiologist
Murray Hill Radiology and Mammography
New York, New York
Sonographic Diagnosis of Breast Cancer

Matthew N. Harris, MD
Professor of Surgery
New York University School of Medicine
Attending Surgeon
New York University Medical Center
New York, New York
Clinical Assessment of Breast Cancer and Benign Breast Disease

Sarah Hatsell, PhD
Research Assistant, Department of Cell Biology
New York University School of Medicine
New York, New York
Molecular, Cellular, and Developmental Biology of Breast Cancer

Minoti Hiremath, MBBS
Graduate Assistant, Department of Cell Biology
New York University School of Medicine
New York, New York
Molecular, Cellular, and Developmental Biology of Breast Cancer

Clifford A. Hudis, MD
Associate Professor of Medicine
Weill Medical College of Cornell University
Chief, Breast Cancer Medicine Service
Associate Attending
Memorial Sloan-Kettering Cancer Center
New York, New York
Systemic Treatment for Stage I and Stage II Breast Cancer

Tara L. Huston, MD
Clinical Fellow, Department of Surgery
Weill Medical College of Cornell University
Resident in General Surgery
New York-Presbyterian Hospital
New York, New York
Evaluating and Staging the Patient with Breast Cancer
Emerging Local Treatment Modalities for Breast Cancer

Giorgio Inghirami, MD
Associate Professor of Pathology
New York University School of Medicine
New York, New York
Molecular Pathology Assays for Breast Cancer

Shabnam Jaffer, MD
Assistant Professor of Pathology
Mount Sinai School of Medicine
New York, New York
Pathology of Invasive Breast Cancer
Pathology of Special Forms of Breast Cancer

Peter R. Jochimsen, MD
Professor Emeritus, Department of Surgery
University of Iowa College of Medicine
Iowa City, Iowa
Treatment of the Pregnant Patient with Breast Cancer

Andrew I. Kaplan, JD
Partner
Aaronson, Rappaport, Feinstein and Deutsch, LLP
New York, New York
Medicolegal Issues in Breast Cancer Diagnosis and Treatment

Nolan S. Karp, MD
Assistant Professor of Plastic Surgery
New York University School of Medicine
New York, New York
Reconstruction Following Surgery for Breast Cancer

Patrick J. Kelly, MD
Joseph Ransohoff Professor and Chairman, Department of
  Neurosurgery
New York University School of Medicine
New York, New York
Management of Metastatic Breast Cancer: Brain Metastases from Breast Cancer

Savitri Krishnamurthy, MD
Associate Professor of Pathology
University of Texas M. D. Anderson Cancer Center
Houston, Texas
Pathology of Regional Lymph Nodes

Michael D. Lagios, MD
Clinical Associate Professor in Pathology
Stanford University School of Medicine
Stanford, California
Associate Clinical Professor in Pathology
University of California, San Francisco, School of Medicine
San Francisco, California
Medical Director, Breast Cancer Consultation Service
St. Mary's Medical Center
Tiburon, California
Pathology of In Situ Breast Cancer

Justin G. Lamont, MD
Clinical Associate Professor of Orthopedic Surgery
New York University School of Medicine
New York, New York
Management of Metastatic Breast Cancer: Metastases from Breast Cancer

Jane Lincoln, MSW
Senior Associate and Writer
Healthmark Multimedia, LLC
Washington, DC
Needs of Breast Cancer Patients and Their Families: Psychosocial Adaptation

Allan Lipton, MD
Professor of Medicine and Oncology
Pennsylvania State University College of Medicine
Attending
Division of Hematology/Oncology
Milton S. Hershey Medical Center
Hershey, Pennsylvania
Hormonal Influences on Oncogenesis and Growth of Breast Cancer

Joseph Lowy, MD
Associate Professor of Clinical Medicine
New York University School of Medicine
New York, New York
Management of Metastatic Breast Cancer: Management of Pain for Metastatic Breast Cancer and Management of the Terminal Patient

Jean Lynn, RN, MPH, OCN
Adjunct Assistant Professor
Health Care Sciences, Surgery and Health Policy
George Washington University School of Medicine and
  Health Sciences
Washington, DC
Rehabilitation and Nursing Care

Kelsey Menehan, BA, MS, MSW
Faculty, Center for Mind-Body Medicine
Associate, Healthmark Multimedia, LLC
Washington, DC
Needs of Breast Cancer Patients and Their Families: Psychosocial Adaptation

Julie Mitnick, MD
Associate Professor of Clinical Radiology
New York University School of Medicine
President
Murray Hill Radiology and Mammography
New York, New York
Mammographic Diagnosis of Breast Cancer

Elizabeth A. Morris, MD
Associate Professor of Radiology
Weill Medical College of Cornell University
Director of Breast MRI
Associate Attending, Radiology
Memorial Sloan-Kettering Cancer Center
New York, New York
  Advanced Techology and Diagnostic Strategy for Breast Cancer

Shalini Mulaparthi, MD
Fellow in Oncology
New York University Medical Center
Medical Staff Attending
Orange Regional Medical Center
Middletown, New York
  *Management of Metastatic Breast Cancer: Chemotherapy for
    Metastatic Breast Cancer*

Colleen D. Murphy, MD
Fellow, Department of Breast Surgery
Memorial Sloan-Kettering Cancer Center
New York, New York
  Treatment of Male Breast Cancer

John E. Niederhuber, MD
Professor of Surgery and Oncology
University of Wisconsin-Madison Medical School
University of Wisconsin Hospital and Clinics
Madison, Wisconsin
  Multimodality Treatment of Breast Cancer

Larry Norton, MD
Professor of Medicine
Weill Medical College of Cornell University
Deputy Physician-in-Chief for Breast Cancer Programs
Attending Physician
Memorial Sloan-Kettering Cancer Center
New York, New York
  Systemic Treatment for Stage I and Stage II Breast Cancer

Tracey O'Connor, MD
Assistant Professor of Medicine
State University of New York at Buffalo School of
    Medicine and Biomedical Sciences
Assistant Professor of Medicine/Breast Program
Roswell Park Cancer Institute
Buffalo, New York
  Surveillance Following Breast Cancer Treatment

Ruth Oratz, MD
Associate Professor of Clinical Medicine
New York University School of Medicine
Attending Physician
New York University Medical Center
New York, New York
  *Management of Metastatic Breast Cancer: Introduction and
    Principles of Treatment; Hormonal and Biologic Therapy for
    Metastatic Breast Cancer; Hypercalcemia from Metastatic
    Breast Cancer*

Michael P. Osborne, MD
Professor of Surgery
Weill Medical College of Cornell University
Chief, Breast Service
New York-Presbyterian Hospital
President, Strang Cancer Prevention Center
New York, New York
  Evaluating and Staging the Patient with Breast Cancer

Harry Ostrer, MD
Professor of Pediatrics, Pathology, and Medicine
New York University School of Medicine
Attending Physician
New York University Medical Center
New York, New York
  *Genetic Counseling for Patients with Breast Cancer and
    Their Families*

David L. Page, MD
Professor of Pathology and Epidemiology
Vanderbilt University School of Medicine
Nashville, Tennessee
  *Pathologic Evolution of Preinvasive Breast Cancer: The Atypical
    Hyperplasias*

Erik C. Parker, MD
Clinical Assistant Professor, Department of Neurosurgery
New York University School of Medicine
New York University Medical Center
New York, New York
  *Management of Metastatic Breast Cancer: Brain Metastases from
    Breast Cancer*

Ramon Parsons, MD, PhD
Avon Foundation Associate Professor of Pathology and
    Medicine
Columbia University College of Physicians and Surgeons
New York, New York
  The Oncogenetic Basis of Breast Cancer

Malcolm C. Pike, PhD
Flora L. Thornton Professor and Chairman, Department of
    Preventive Medicine
University of Southern California Keck School of Medicine
Norris Comprehensive Cancer Center
Los Angeles, California
  Risk Factors for Development of Breast Cancer

Mary Politi, MPhil
Behavioral Medicine Predoctoral Intern
Brown University
Providence, Rhode Island
  *Needs of Breast Cancer Patients and Their Families: Psychosocial
    Adaptation*

Elisa Rush Port, MD
Assistant Professor of Surgery
Weill Medical College of Cornell University
Assistant Attending Surgeon
Memorial Sloan-Kettering Cancer Center
New York, New York
Advanced Techology and Diagnostic Strategy for Breast Cancer

Peter I. Pressman, MD
Clinical Professor of Surgery
Weill Medical College of Cornell University
New York, New York
Treatment of Bilateral Breast Cancer

Jay A. Rapaport, JD
Senior Partner
Aaronson, Rappaport, Feinstein and Deutsch, LLP
New York, New York
Medicolegal Issues in Breast Cancer Diagnosis and Treatment

Elsa Reich, MS
Professor of Pediatrics
New York University School of Medicine
New York, New York
*Genetic Counseling for Patients with Breast Cancer and
Their Families*

John Rescigno, MD
Assistant Professor of Clinical Radiation Medicine
New York Medical College
Valhalla, New York
Associate Attending, Department of Radiation Oncology
St. Vincent's Comprehensive Cancer Center
New York, New York
*Management of Metastatic Breast Cancer: Radiation Therapy for
Metastatic Breast Cancer*

Daniel F. Roses, MD
Jules Leonard Whitehill Professor of Surgery and Oncology
New York University School of Medicine
Senior Attending Surgeon
New York University Medical Center
New York, New York
*Development of Modern Breast Cancer Treatment
Surgery for Breast Cancer*

Freya R. Schnabel, MD
Associate Professor of Clinical Surgery
Columbia University College of Physicians and Surgeons
Chief, Section of Breast Surgery
Columbia University Medical Center
New York-Presbyterian Hospital
New York, New York
Surgical Treatment of Patients at High Risk of Breast Cancer

Gordon Francis Schwartz, MD, MBA
Professor of Surgery
Jefferson Medical College
Attending Surgeon
Thomas Jefferson University Hospital
Consulting Surgeon
Pennsylvania Hospital
Philadelphia, Pennsylvania
Treatment of In Situ Breast Cancer

Carol E. H. Scott-Conner, MD, PhD
Professor, Departments of Surgery and Anatomy and
Cell Biology
University of Iowa College of Medicine
Staff Surgeon
University of Iowa Hospitals and Clinics
Iowa City, Iowa
Treatment of the Pregnant Patient with Breast Cancer

Peter Shamamian, MD
Associate Professor of Surgery
New York University School of Medicine
New York, New York
Molecular, Cellular, and Developmental Biology of Breast Cancer

Jason P. Shaw, MD
Chief Resident, Department of Surgery
North Shore University Hospital
Manhasset, New York
*Management of Metastatic Breast Cancer: Thoracic Metastases
from Breast Cancer*

Carol L. Shields, MD
Professor of Ophthalmology
Jefferson Medical College
Co-Director and Attending Surgeon, Oncology Service
Wills Eye Hospital
Philadelphia, Pennsylvania
*Management of Metastatic Breast Cancer: Ocular Metastases
from Breast Cancer*

Jerry A. Shields, MD
Professor of Ophthalmology
Jefferson Medical College
Director, Oncology Service
Wills Eye Hospital
Philadelphia, Pennsylvania
*Management of Metastatic Breast Cancer: Ocular Metastases
from Breast Cancer*

Roy E. Shore, PhD, DrPH
Professor of Environmental Medicine
New York University School of Medicine
New York, New York
Epidemiology of Breast Cancer

Rache M. Simmons, MD
Associate Professor of Surgery
Weill Medical College of Cornell University
Associate Attending Surgeon
New York-Presbyterian Hospital
New York, New York
  Emerging Local Treatment Modalities for Breast Cancer

Joel I. Sorosky, MD
Chief, Department of OB-GYN
Co-Director, Women's Health Services
Hartford Hospital
Hartford, Connecticut
  Treatment of the Pregnant Patient with Breast Cancer

Joseph A. Sparano, MD
Professor of Medicine
Albert Einstein College of Medicine of Yeshiva University
Director, Breast Evaluation Center
Montefiore-Einstein Cancer Center
Bronx, New York
  Prevention of Breast Cancer

Darcy V. Spicer, MD
Associate Professor of Clinical Medicine
University of Southern California Keck School of
  Medicine
Norris Comprehensive Cancer Center
Los Angeles, California
  Risk Factors for Development of Breast Cancer

Randy E. Stevens, MD
Director, Radiation Oncology
Dickstein Cancer Treatment Center
White Plains Hospital Center
White Plains, New York
  Radiotherapy for In Situ, Stage I, and Stage II Breast Cancer

Alexander J. Swistel, MD
Associate Professor of Clinical Surgery
Weill Medical College of Cornell University
Associate Attending, Surgery
Director, Weill Cornell Breast Center
New York-Presbyterian Hospital
New York, New York
  Treatment of Bilateral Breast Cancer

W. Fraser Symmans, MD, ChB
Associate Professor of Pathology
University of Texas M. D. Anderson Cancer Center
Houston, Texas
  Molecular Pathology Assays for Breast Cancer

Stacey Tashman, MD
Associate Clinical Professor of Pathology
Mount Sinai School of Medicine
Associate Radiologist
Murray Hill Radiology and Mammography
New York, New York
  Sonographic Diagnosis of Breast Cancer

Amy D. Tiersten, MD
Associate Professor of Medicine
New York University School of Medicine
New York, New York
  *Management of Metastatic Breast Cancer: Chemotherapy for
  Metastatic Breast Cancer*

Madeline F. Vazquez, MD
Associate Professor of Clinical Pathology
Chief of Cytopathology
Weill Medical College of Cornell University
Associate Attending Pathologist
New York-Presbyterian Hospital
New York, New York
  Needle Biopsy Diagnosis of Breast Cancer

Stacey Vitiello, MD
Associate Radiologist
Murray Hill Radiology and Mammography
New York, New York
  Sonographic Diagnosis of Breast Cancer

Matthew Volm, MD
Assistant Professor of Medicine
New York University School of Medicine
New York, New York
  Treatment of Locally Advanced Breast Cancer

Karen L. Weihs, MD
Associate Professor of Psychiatry
University of Arizona College of Medicine
Tucson, Arizona
  *Needs of Breast Cancer Patients and Their Families: Psychosocial
  Adaptation*

James C. Wittig, MD
Assistant Professor of Orthopedic Surgery
New York University School of Medicine
New York University Medical Center
New York, New York
  *Management of Metastatic Breast Cancer: Bone Metastases from
  Breast Cancer*

Stefanie Zalasin, MD
Associate Clinical Professor of Pathology
Mount Sinai School of Medicine
Associate Radiologist
Murray Hill Radiology and Mammography
New York, New York
  Sonographic Diagnosis of Breast Cancer

Anne Zeleniuch-Jacquotte, MD
Associate Professor of Environmental Medicine
New York University School of Medicine
New York, New York
  Epidemiology of Breast Cancer

Preface

Perhaps no malignant disease has so attracted the attention of physicians and patients, as well as the general public, as cancer of the breast. Since the publication of the first edition of *Breast Cancer* in 1999, public attention has justifiably remained riveted to this subject. The annual incidence of invasive breast cancer remains at 200,000, but increasingly diagnosed noninvasive cancers add to this statistic, broadening the concerns of an ever-expanding patient population. Even more so than when the first edition was published, century-old dogmas on pathophysiology and treatment continue to undergo critical scrutiny, while diagnostic advances and a broadened spectrum of therapeutic options continue to proliferate. The role of physicians in multiple disciplines continues to expand, while patients and their families rightfully are enlarging their own roles in ensuring optimal care, increasingly asserting their determination to participate in diagnostic and therapeutic decision-making and more openly conveying their concerns related to quality-of-life issues. Furthermore, decisions that were once based on relatively straightforward perceptions of pathology and surgery now involve increasingly complex issues of molecular biology and genetics, epidemiology, radiology, cytology, histopathology, and a spectrum of multidisciplinary treatment options, along with even greater sensitivity to cosmetic, emotional, economic, and social concerns, all requiring the coordination of radiologists, pathologists, surgical oncologists, medical oncologists, radiation oncologists, reconstructive surgeons, gynecologists, primary care physicians, and genetics counselors, nurses, and psychosocial support professionals. Decision-making increasingly requires a familiarity with issues in basic research that have refined and even redefined our concepts of the pathophysiology of breast cancer.

More than ever, brief information sources for physicians may be inadequate in the face of the expanding complexity of issues and controversies and the growing empowerment of patients in the decision-making process. Conversely, encyclopedic sources may not fulfill the needs of physicians seeking cogent and tangible information on which to base recommendations for patients, particularly as specialists are expected to bring to their discussion with patients and colleagues a degree of knowledge of other disciplines not previously envisioned. For example, increasingly, medical oncologists are expected to be articulate in discussing issues of oncogenesis and surgery; similarly, surgeons must be able to understand and communicate a greater knowledge with pathologists as well as with medical and radiation oncologists, and they must be able to discuss with patients and families the broadened basis for prognostication and recommendations for additional nonsurgical therapy. At the same time, the abundance of excellent publications written for patients, along with the ever-increasing media saturation and Internet resources on the subject of breast cancer, have elevated the level of information that patients bring to discussions with physicians. Disparate sources of information may give patients unrealistically simple impressions of the issues, which may contradict data presented by the physician. Furthermore, new technologies, as well as pharmacologic and biologic therapies, while often untested, are presented to physicians and the public almost daily through the media.

It is the object of *Breast Cancer* to present the issues in the diagnosis and management of breast cancer, based on clinically relevant information ranging from the basic mechanisms of oncogenesis and pathophysiology to psychosocial support, and to present evidence-based recommendations to help readers determine which diagnostic and therapeutic strategies are established, which are worthy of continued consideration and scrutiny although not established, and which are clearly unproven. Authors were asked to make their contributions understandable to physicians of all disciplines, not only their own. Our goal was to achieve a uniform level of discussion for physicians who are increasingly called upon to be knowledgeable about these issues of concern expressed by patients that relate to their problems, even if these issues are far afield from the physician's usual research and practice. To achieve the objectives of clarity and clinical relevance, the text is structured to answer questions that are focused and that reflect, as often as possible, those that a patient might ask.

In any multiauthor text, repetition of certain material and even divergence of opinion are inevitable. This is particularly so when issues are covered in the context of differing broad disciplines, such as those directed at research goals as opposed to current treatment recommendations. The reader should appreciate the context in which information is provided when such repetition or differences occur.

I hope that we have achieved the goal of providing lucid information that enables all specialists caring for the breast cancer patient to communicate clearly with one another and with the patient, through a basic understanding of the breadth of issues that have an impact on the treatment of this disease.

I wish to extend my deepest gratitude to my distinguished colleagues who contributed so generously and enthusiastically of their knowledge and experience to this volume. I am also most grateful to the staff of Elsevier, Inc., and in particular I wish to acknowledge the calm encouragement and patient support of Jennifer Ehlers and the work of Amy Norwitz, Judith Fletcher, Ryan Creed, and Steven Stave. I am grateful to Lydia Kibiuk, our illustrator, for her skill, collegiality, and professionalism. Special appreciation goes to Nancy Ehrlich Lapid, who was invaluable in assisting me in reviewing the contributions. A special thanks again to my wife, Helene, who, as always, continues to be extraordinary in her support and encouragement.

Daniel F. Roses, MD

Contents

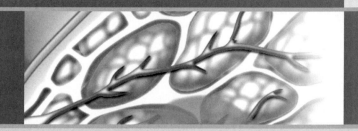

SECTION I

MOLECULAR AND EPIDEMIOLOGIC ISSUES

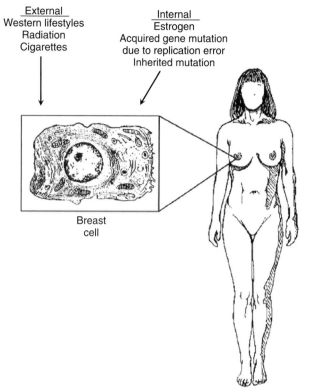

Figure 2–1   External and internal agents affecting tumor formation. External agents include radiation exposure, cigarette smoke, and a Western lifestyle. Internal agents include estrogen, acquired mutations due to replication errors, and inherited mutations. These agents slowly lead to the accumulation of genetic damage that may eventually result in a tumor.

What is an oncogene?

The word "oncogene" is derived from two Greek words: *onkos* for mass and *gignesthai* for birth, which is the etymologic root for the word "gene." An oncogene has a more specific meaning than its name implies, however. Oncogenes are a class of genes that cause tumor growth when activated.[2] These genes behave dominantly because they promote tumor enlargement.

Oncogenes were first found to reside within retroviruses. The first example of such a retrovirus was discovered by Peyton Rous near the turn of the century.[17] This virus was capable of causing tumors in chickens and is known as Rous sarcoma virus (RSV). Over 20 years ago, the *src* gene, which is the gene in RSV that is responsible for its tumorigenic activity, was found to be an activated form of a gene that is normally found in chickens.[18] In effect, the virus had taken the *src* gene from the cell and modified it to produce tumors.

How are oncogenes activated?

In humans, oncogenes are rarely activated by viruses. Instead, the activation is typically triggered by mutation of the gene, usually by one of three major mechanisms (Fig. 2–2). The first mechanism of activation was identified in the *ras* family of oncogenes; these genes are mutated in a variety of human tumors.[19] A single amino acid alteration activates the ras protein product to continuously signal the cell to divide.[20] The *k-ras* gene is mutated in about half of all colon cancers.[21]

The second mechanism of oncogene activation occurs through chromosomal translocation, which was first observed

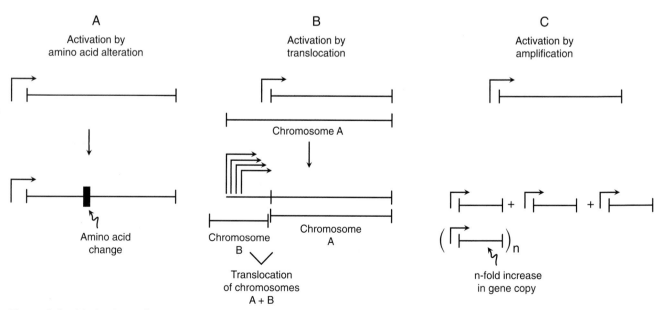

Figure 2–2   Mechanisms of oncogene activation. The three mechanisms of oncogene activation are depicted: amino acid alteration, translocation, and amplification. The level of transcription from their promoters is indicated by the 90-degree angle arrows to the left of each gene. More arrows indicate increased levels of transcription. *A*, Activation by point mutation leading to a new amino acid. *B*, Activation by translocation. The normal promoter of a gene is replaced by a very active promoter from another chromosome, which induces overexpression. *C*, Amplification. Multiple copies are present in tandem, each with a functional promoter. The level of amplification can be anywhere from 5-fold to 100–fold, as indicated by the symbol + $(gene)_n$.

in chronic myelogenous leukemia.[22] The end result of a translocation is the overexpression of a protein that either stimulates cell division or prevents cellular death.[23] In the case of chronic myelogenous leukemia, the translocation of chromosomes 9 and 22 leads to the overexpression of the bcr-abl fusion protein, which is an active tyrosine kinase that signals the cell to divide.[24] Another important example is the translocation of chromosomes 14 and 18, which is found in follicular lymphomas.[25] This translocation leads to the overexpression of the *bcl-2* oncogene, which functions to prevent cell death. In general, by placing a strong promoter of gene transcription near an oncogene, translocations lead to gene overexpression and tumor growth.

The third mechanism of activation of oncogenes is amplification, in which multiple copies of a gene are reproduced in a single chromosome.[26] By increasing the gene dosage, the protein product of the gene is overexpressed within the cell. Genes activated in this way in breast cancer include the epidermal growth factor (EGF) receptor, *erbB-2/HER-2/neu*, *c-myc*, and *cyclin D1*, all of which stimulate cell division.[27–30] Each of these genes is amplified in breast cancer; hence, amplification is the major mechanism of oncogene activation in breast cancer.[31]

How do oncogenes function in the cell?

Oncogenes can either stimulate cellular division or prevent cell death (Fig. 2–3). All of the genes that stimulate division have a role in transmitting a signal from a growth factor receptor to the nucleus to initiate cellular replication. Oncogenes of this type vary in their specific functions, whether they are receptors, guanosine triphosphate (GTP)-binding proteins, kinases, or transcription factors, but all stimulate the cell to leave a resting state (G_0) and enter the DNA synthesis (S) phase of the cell cycle.[20] *Bcl-2* and its homologues stimulate tumor growth by a completely different mechanism. These genes function to inhibit apoptosis or programmed cell death.[32] Less is known about the cell death pathways, but they clearly function through a protease cascade to cleave nuclear DNA and destroy the nuclear and plasma membranes.[25]

What is a tumor suppressor gene?

The concept of tumor suppressors is the result of two different branches of cancer research: studies of tumor cells in vitro and studies of families with a hereditary predisposition to cancer. The original in vitro studies of tumor suppression were derived from the observation that when a tumor cell was fused with a nontumor cell, the resulting fused cell lost its tumor characteristics.[33] These experiments were further refined by the observation that a single normal chromosome, when introduced into a tumor cell, could suppress the growth of the tumor cell. The interpretation of these findings was that normal cells have tumor suppressor genes that are inactivated in the tumor. A similar model of tumor suppressors was developed by Knudson for explaining the mechanism of inheriting a predisposition to retinoblastoma.[34] This model is based on the concept that with the exception of the sex chromosomes, people normally have two functional alleles

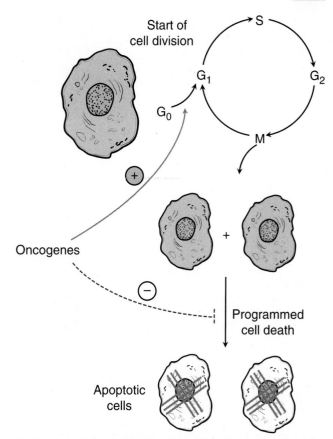

Figure 2–3 Mechanism of oncogenic stimulation of tumor growth. Oncogenes are depicted to signal (+) the cell to leave G_0 and commit to mitosis. In addition, they also inhibit (–) the induction of the cell death pathway (apoptosis).

(copies) of every gene. For a tumor to develop, both alleles of a specific gene must be inactivated.

What is Knudson's hypothesis for tumor suppressor genes?

By comparing rates of retinoblastoma in predisposed families and the general population, Alfred Knudson proposed his "two-hit" model, in which both alleles of a gene must be inactivated before tumor formation can occur[34] (Fig. 2–4). In his model of tumor suppression, he proposed that the early-onset and multiple tumors found in familial forms of cancer could be accounted for by the inheritance of one defective allele. His insight was to realize that this inherited mutation was not sufficient alone for the formation of a tumor. He hypothesized that inactivation of the second healthy allele of the same gene was also necessary and could thus explain the dominant inheritance pattern found in families. Thus, both alleles are altered in the tumor. This is a paradox of genetics in which the mutated gene behaves dominantly during transmission in families but behaves recessively during tumorigenesis within the cell. With the prominent exception of the germline mutation of the *c-ret* oncogene in multiple endocrine neoplasia syndrome,[35] Knudson's tumor suppressor hypothesis for retinoblastoma has proved to be broadly applicable to all of the tumor predisposition syndromes characterized to date.[36]

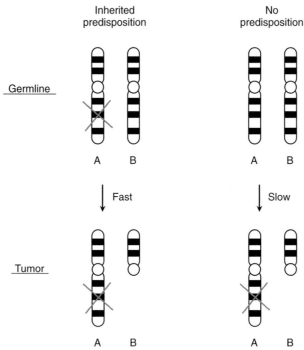

Figure 2–4 Knudson's model of tumor suppressors. A pair of autosomal alleles (A and B) is indicated for individuals with (*left*) and without (*right*) an inherited germline mutation of a tumor suppressor gene. The inherited mutation is indicated by an X on allele A of the predisposed individual. Tumor establishment occurs much faster in an individual who is predisposed because only one further copy need be inactivated. In the individual without predisposition (wild type), the inactivation of both alleles is a rare event. The large deletion seen on the B allele is an example of loss of heterozygosity (LOH).

How are tumor suppressor genes inactivated?

Genes have now been identified not only for retinoblastoma but also for inherited predispositions to a variety of tumors, including those of the breast (see below), ovary, kidney, colon, skin, lymphocytes, and peripheral nerves.[37–48] In all cases, one defective copy is inherited and the second copy is altered in the tumor. Many of these genes are also inactivated in sporadic tumors of people who inherit two functional alleles. Because mutation of both copies of the gene must occur somatically, sporadic tumors occur later in life and in a smaller proportion of nonpredisposed individuals. However, because sporadic tumors are much more common than familial tumors, somatic mutation is the most common form of tumor suppressor inactivation.

What is loss of heterozygosity?

In familial cancer syndromes, the mechanism of inactivation of the normal copy of a tumor suppressor usually occurs through loss of heterozygosity (LOH), which is due to the deletion of a large chromosomal region containing the wild-type tumor suppressor allele (see Fig. 2–4). In sporadic cancer, LOH may be the first or second event in the inactivation of a tumor suppressor.

How commonly are tumor suppressors inactivated in sporadic tumors?

Mutation of tumor suppressor genes is by far the most common genetic alteration found in the tumors of nonpredisposed individuals. A handful of tumor suppressors are inactivated in a large fraction of nearly all invasive cancers regardless of organ of origin. The *p53* tumor suppressor is the most commonly mutated cancer gene.[49] The *p16/CDKN2/ARF* and *PTEN* tumor suppressor loci vie for second place.[50,51]

Why are tumors clonal?

Unlike a model based on the relative simplicity of inheriting a single mutation in a tumor suppressor gene, Peter Nowell's model for the development of a solid tumor depends on the mutation of many genes.[52] The model is based on two principles: (1) the principle of clonal expansion, in which a mutant cell with a selective advantage for growth will outgrow its neighbors; and (2) the principle that expansions occur in consecutive waves that result in the accumulation of multiple genetic alterations within the evolving tumor. Somatic mutations that take place with each advancing wave of tumor expansion occur in both tumor suppressor genes and oncogenes. In the case of tumor suppressors, both alleles must be inactivated during tumor development. For oncogenes, point mutations, amplifications, and translocations lead to activation. For a tumor to evolve, several distinct regulatory pathways must be compromised, including those regulating the cell cycle, apoptosis, and genomic stability. The clonal nature of a tumor allows for the accumulation of multiple growth disruptions within one cell. Because multiple independent mutations must accumulate within a single clone, the evolution of a tumor occurs over years to decades.

What is genomic instability?

In general, the rate of mutation is low within genes (for any given gene, mutations occur once in every 1×10^6 cell divisions).[53] Based on the low frequency of mutations in the genes of a normal cell, tumor formation should be an extremely rare event because it would require occurrence of several rare events within a single cell during the course of a lifetime. Because tumor formation is a common occurrence, however, it is believed that the rate of gene mutations must be increased during the clonal expansion of a tumor. This increase in the rate of mutation is known as genomic instability.

A great deal of evidence currently supports the theory that tumors become genomically unstable during their development.[54] Tumor cells inactivate pathways that normally ensure that errors in the genetic code are repaired. Thus, the frequency of genetic alterations increases in the tumor cell. The result of this increased genetic instability is that cells within a tumor acquire mutations that allow them to outgrow their neighbors.

What causes genomic instability?

Three major systems are involved in preserving the integrity of the genome during each replication cycle. The first major system depends on the cell's various biochemical mechanisms for replicating and dividing (the cell cycle system).[50] The coordination of the different phases of the cell cycle—G_1, S (synthesis), G_2, and M (mitosis)—is orchestrated by a variety of gene products, which include the cyclins (A, B, D, and E) and their respective cyclin-dependent kinases (CDKs) (Fig. 2–5A). Aberrant overexpression of cyclin E has been shown to increase genomic instability.[55] CDKs are regulated by CDK inhibitors, which are capable of blocking the cell's progress through the cell cycle in response to signals from within and without the cell. Also included in the cell cycle system are the various replication enzymes and the mitotic spindles that function to reproduce a daughter genome and separate the two genomes into daughter cells. Mistakes or inappropriate signals in any of these pathways can lead to genetic damage.

The second major system is composed of the various repair pathways that fix genetic alterations once they are detected (the DNA repair system). These include the ultraviolet (UV) excision repair system and the double-strand break repair system, which repair external DNA damage, and the mismatch repair system, which repairs mismatches generated during DNA replication.[56–58]

The third major system comprises the checkpoint control pathways of the cell (the checkpoint system)[59] (Fig. 2–5B). These pathways monitor the genome for alterations that affect its integrity and can regulate the cell cycle and DNA repair systems. Alterations can be due to external mutations from ionizing radiation or from errors in replication during S phase or the separation of chromosomes during mitosis. Checkpoint pathways respond to these alterations by inhibiting the cell's progress through the cell cycle and coordinating the assembly of the proper DNA repair machinery. In effect, these pathways stall the cell to give it an opportunity to repair itself before proceeding to the next phase of the cycle.

The best characterized checkpoint pathway in humans is induced by ionizing radiation. The *ATM* gene encodes a protein kinase that senses genetic damage and transmits this information to other checkpoint proteins in the cell by phosphorylating them.[60,61] *ATM* is able to activate a large number of different checkpoint and repair pathways. In one of these pathways, *ATM* transmits a signal to *p53*, a transcription factor and tumor suppressor, to induce the expression of the CDK inhibitor *p21*, which arrests the cell in the G_1 phase of the cell cycle.[62] In the absence of functional *ATM* or *p53*, the arrest in response to DNA damage is impaired. Alternatively, DNA damage can induce programmed cell death (apoptosis), a process that is *p53* dependent.[25] In addition, the *ATM–p53* pathway appears to regulate checkpoint controls in other phases of the cell cycle. In particular, *p53* has a role in monitoring the fidelity of mitosis.[63] In the absence of *p53*, chromosomes segregate aberrantly, and cells soon become polyploid.[64] Another branch of the *ATM* pathway regulates the cell cycle without the help of *p53*. In this branch, DNA damage activates *ATM*, which phosphorylates the checkpoint kinases (*CHK1* and *CHK2*), key kinases that in turn

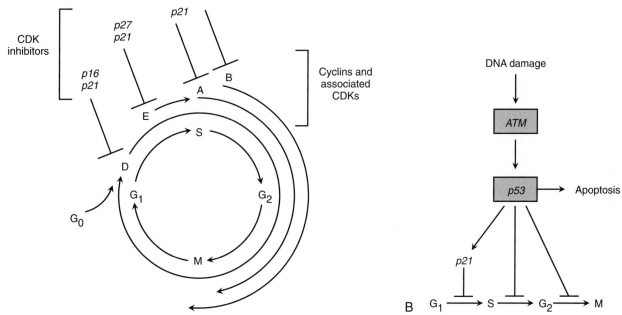

Figure 2–5 Regulation of the cell cycle and its checkpoints. *A*, The phases of the cell cycle G_1, S, G_2, and M are regulated by a series of cyclin protein–cyclin-dependent kinase (CDK) complexes that are synthesized and degraded at discrete times. The D cyclins are induced by mitogenic stimuli and remain elevated as long as the cell is cycling. They are potently inhibited by the CDK inhibitors *p16* and *p21*. Cyclin E is the critical cyclin for entry into S phase and is tightly regulated by *p27*, a CDK inhibitor, and also responds to *p21*. Cyclins A and B are involved in shepherding the cell through S phase, G_2, and mitosis when they are degraded. *B*, The best understood checkpoint in the mammalian cell cycle is the response to high-energy radiation. The ensuing DNA damage is detected by the *ATM* gene, which signals *p53* to induce *p21* and arrest the cell in G_1, induces arrest in S and G_2, or by a different pathway signals the cell to undergo apoptosis; *p53* is clearly a nodal point in the cell's response to DNA damage.

phosphorylate the *CDC25* tyrosine phosphatases to induce their inactivation.[65] After their inhibition due to *CHK1*, *CDC25* tyrosine phosphatases no longer remove a critical phosphate residue from CDKs to activate cyclin–CDK complexes in different phases of the cell cycle. Yet another branch of the *ATM* pathway mediates the repair of double-strand DNA breaks. To respond to DNA damage, this branch depends on the *BRCA1* protein.[66]

Genes involved in the regulation of the cell cycle, checkpoint, and DNA repair systems frequently behave as either tumor suppressor genes or oncogenes when mutated. Alterations of these genes lead to an increase in genomic instability. These include *cyclin D, p53, ATM,* and the mismatch repair genes *hMSH2* and *hMLH1.*[59,67] Cells with aberrations of either *p53* or cyclin D are permissive for gene amplification of other genes.[50] Cells with inactive *hMSH2* or *hMLH1* have an increased frequency of point and frameshift mutations.[43,67] Finally, as mentioned above, a cell deficient for *ATM* or *p53* is unable to properly repair DNA damaged by ionizing radiation.[62] All of these genes are components of one of the major cellular systems for preventing genetic damage.

What are the different forms of familial breast cancer?

There are several forms of familial breast cancer.[15] Familial early-onset breast-ovarian cancer is an autosomal dominant disease that usually affects those at risk before 50 years of age and is typically due to *BRCA1* mutation. Breast cancer without ovarian cancer can be seen in families as well and is associated with either *BRCA1* or *BRCA2* mutations. This form of disease also has an early onset and is associated with male breast cancer in families with *BRCA2* mutations.

How were the *BRCA1* and *BRCA2* genes discovered?

Large extended families with autosomal dominant patterns of inheritance of breast cancer risk were the impetus for genome-wide scans to find breast cancer susceptibility genes. Because no knowledge of the function or location for such a hypothesized gene existed, DNA was collected from the blood of as many family members as possible and subjected to linkage analysis. With linkage analysis, the DNA from both affected and unaffected individuals is characterized to determine the size of polymorphic alleles at known chromosomal locations distributed throughout the entire genome. Polymorphic alleles that are shared among affected family members are linked to the disease (Fig. 2–6). However, alleles may be shared due to random clustering because each offspring of an affected carrier has a 50% chance of coinheritance of breast cancer susceptibility along with one of any two alleles throughout the 22 autosomal chromosomes. As the size of the family under study increases, the likelihood that polymorphic alleles are linked to disease and are not merely chance clusterings increases as well. This approach led to the identification of polymorphic markers on chromosome 17q21 and on chromosome 13q12 that were highly linked to breast cancer in specific families.[68,69] A search for genes within these regions uncovered *BRCA1* and *BRCA2* on chromosomes 17 and 13, respectively.[38,39] These two genes were definitively identified as the causative lesions within these families by virtue of the mutations found in their DNA sequence that segregated with affected family members. Mutations of both of these genes usually disrupt the open reading frame, leading to a truncated protein product. Moreover, in the tumors of these patients, the remaining functional allele of the gene is also mutated somatically in most cases.

Who is at risk for inheriting mutations of *BRCA1* and *BRCA2*?

Individuals at risk are obviously those with a family history of breast cancer. In families with an identified mutation, the risk for being a carrier is 50%. In addition, about 10% of women without a family history but with a breast cancer diagnosis before 35 years of age are born with a mutation of *BRCA1*.[70] Perhaps the largest population of women at risk for harboring germline mutations can be found among Ashkenazi Jews of Eastern European descent. The combined frequency of germline mutation of *BRCA1* and *BRCA2* among these women is about 2%.[71,72] Patients with these mutations frequently lack a family history of breast cancer.[73]

How does the *BRCA1* gene function in the body to prevent breast cancer?

A clue to identifying the regions of the gene that are functionally important may be gained from analyzing the *BRCA1* gene in other species. A homologue of *BRCA1* is present in the mouse, and only two domains show significant areas of conservation of the amino acid code.[74] One of these is a ring-finger domain near the amino terminus of the protein.[38] Ring fingers are zinc-binding protein motifs. The other conserved domain is at the carboxyl terminus of the protein (Fig. 2–7). This domain has been shown to activate transcription when fused to the DNA-binding domain of *GAL4*, a yeast transcription factor.[75] These data suggest that *BRCA1* may be involved in the regulation of transcription. Interestingly, point mutations (mutations that change only a single amino acid) of *BRCA1* that disrupt the zinc-binding amino acids or disrupt the activation of transcription are found in breast cancer families.[75,76] Mutation of the mouse *BRCAl* gene in mammary tissue predisposes these animals to a high rate of mammary tumors.[77] Other early studies of *BRCA1* indicate that it is capable of slowing cellular proliferation and inhibits tumor growth in vitro.[78] The gene may be exerting its effects during G_1 and S phases of the cell cycle when *BRCA1* is most expressed.[79]

Several genetic and biochemical facts have emerged that are leading to a better understanding of the function of *BRCA1*. After DNA damage, *BRCA1* is recruited to sites of double-strand DNA breaks.[80] Recruitment appears to be important because mutation of *BRCA1* in cells leads to increased susceptibility to DNA damage.[81] *BRCA1* is an integral part of the *ATM* pathway because it is phosphorylated by *ATM* after DNA damage at the sight of DNA breaks.[66] Moreover, disruption of

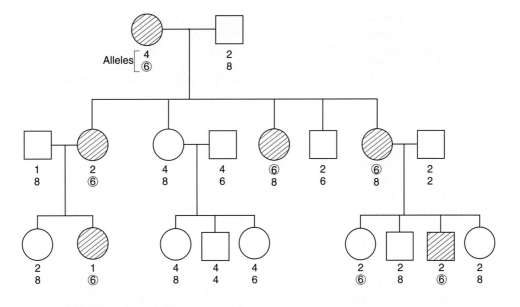

Number identifies different alleles that differ based on their size.

○ Female

□ Male

▨ or ⬚ affected with breast cancer

Figure 2–6 Segregation of a polymorphic marker in a family with hereditary breast cancer. A family affected by six cases of breast cancer over three generations is depicted. The numbers below each individual indicate the alleles that each has inherited for a specific marker located very close to the *BRCA1* gene. The numbers refer to the size of the allele, with 1 being the smallest and 8 being the largest allele. This allele is highly polymorphic because nearly all cases have alleles of two different sizes. In cases with two alleles of differing size, the marker is said to be informative because one is able to trace the origin of the alleles in the parents. The circled allele 6 has the same pattern of inheritance as breast cancer and appears at first glance to be linked. In one case in the third generation, the disease has not become penetrant. To test this hypothesis, one must compare the observed results with the likelihood of a similar segregation pattern of a marker far from the diseased locus.

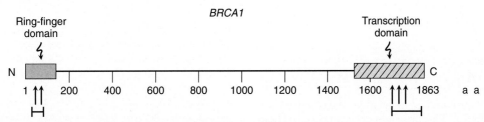

Figure 2–7 Functional domains of human *BRCA1*. The ring-finger domain is a putative zinc-binding domain that may be involved in ubiquitin ligation of proteins (minimally amino acids 25–64). The transcription transactivating domain is at the carboxyl terminus from amino acids 1528 to 1863. *Arrows* below the gene indicate amino acid point mutations that are associated with early-onset breast cancer. Mutations of the ring finger would disrupt zinc, whereas mutations of the transactivation domain are known to disrupt transactivation.

BRCA1 in cells interrupts DNA repair signals downstream of *ATM*. BRCA1 exists in a heterodimer with another ring-finger protein, BARD1.[82] Together, BRCA1 and BARD1 form a potent ubiquitin ligase enzyme complex that is able to conjugate chains of ubiquitin onto other proteins. The nature of these substrates is currently unknown. Presumably, *BRCA1* is involved in the regulation of repair proteins through ubiquitination.

How does the *BRCA2* gene function?

Like *BRCA1*, mutation of mouse *BRCA2* predisposed animals to mammary cancer.[83] Cells lacking *BRCA2* are highly sensitive to DNA damage and display marked genetic instability.[84] Analysis of Fanconi anemia patient samples, which are highly sensitive to DNA damage, has demonstrated that two of the

Fanconi anemia complementation groups are due to biallelic mutation of *BRCA2*.[85] Biochemical analysis of the BRCA2 protein has demonstrated that it is part of the homologous recombination DNA repair complex that repairs double-strand breaks.[84]

Are there other genes that cause a predisposition to breast cancer?

More than half of the families with early-onset breast cancer in the absence of ovarian cancer (breast site–specific families) have no identified mutation of either *BRCA1* or *BRCA2*.[86] This information suggests that an unidentified gene exists that also increases susceptibility to breast cancer. Two rare syndromes, Li-Fraumeni and Reifenstein syndromes, occasionally lead to breast cancer as well. They are caused by genetic lesions in *p53* and the androgen receptor, respectively.[46,87] In addition, heterozygote carriers of ataxia-telangiectasia, who harbor *ATM* mutations, as well as patients with Cowden syndrome who are born with *PTEN* mutations, are at increased risk for breast cancer.[88,89]

What is the difference between sporadic breast cancer and familial breast cancer?

Sporadic breast cancer is defined as breast cancer that occurs without an identifiable inherited risk. The risk for breast cancer over a lifetime is about 13%.[90] In contrast, familial breast cancer is an autosomally dominant inherited predisposition to breast cancer. The lifetime risk for breast cancer for carriers in these families is about 80%. This increased risk is due to the inherited mutation of *BRCA1* or *BRCA2* or perhaps other genes.

How is the estrogen receptor altered in breast cancer?

The first gene product studied in detail for breast cancer was the estrogen receptor.[91] This protein is not expressed in about 40% of both ductal carcinoma in situ (CIS) and invasive breast cancers.[91–93] Because the proportion of tumors lacking estrogen receptor does not change during the transition from CIS to invasive breast cancer, one interpretation is that loss of the receptor influences CIS development but not the transition to invasive cancer. Even though tumor progression appears to be influenced by the loss of estrogen receptor expression, this gene does not behave as a typical tumor suppressor. In particular, the lack of expression in tumors is not associated with mutation of the gene or loss of heterozygosity. Rather, loss of expression appears to be due to repression of transcription through hypermethylation of nearby CpG islands, which are found in the transcriptional control region (promoter) of a gene.[94] This form of down-regulation of gene expression inactivates tumor suppressors, such as *p16*, in a variety of tumors.[95]

Which oncogenes are altered in breast cancer?

The early analysis of genetic alterations in sporadic breast cancer focused on oncogenes. The two oncogenes that are commonly altered are the *erbB-2/HER-2/neu* oncogene and *cyclin D* oncogenes.[96,97] These genes are overexpressed in both CIS and invasive carcinoma of the breast.[98–100] The basis for overexpression is often amplification of the gene; however, overexpression is often seen in the absence of gene amplification. Other oncogenes are also altered by amplification in invasive breast cancer. They include *EGFR*, *c-myc*, and *IGFIR*.

What tumor suppressors are altered in breast cancer?

The most commonly mutated tumor suppressor in breast cancer is *p53*.[31] Although an inherited mutation of *p53* is a rare cause of cancer, *p53* is mutated in nearly half of all invasive breast tumors.[31,46] Immunohistochemical analysis of *p53* in ductal CIS also indicates a similar proportion of altered tumors.[101,102] Of course, *BRCA1* and *BRCA2* are mutated in tumors of patients who inherited a defective copy of one of these genes, but these two genes are not mutated in sporadic breast cancer.[103,104] However, silencing of *BRCA1* transcription due to methylation of the *BRCA1* promoter is detected in about 10% of unselected cancers and is particularly prevalent in medullary and mucinous carcinomas.[105] E-cadherin is mutated in a high fraction of lobular carcinomas and is methylated and silenced in a large proportion of ductal carcinomas.[106,107] PTEN protein expression is not detected in about one third of sporadic carcinomas.[108] In addition, the tumor suppressors *Rb* and *p16* are rarely mutated.[109,110]

How do these oncogenes and tumor suppressors normally function in the cell?

The oncogenes that are altered in breast cancer and some of the tumor suppressors all share one major feature. They are key components of signal transduction pathways that regulate the cell cycle by controlling the entrance into S phase[20,50] (Fig. 2–8). In particular, *erbB-2/HER-2/neu*, *EGFR*, *c-myc*, *cyclin D*, *Rb*, and *p16* are all part of a pathway that responds to EGF (as well as other growth factors), which stimulates the cell to divide. PTEN is a negative regulator of signals that emerge from cell surface receptors.

How does *p53* normally function?

The function of *p53* is quite distinct from the other oncogenes and tumor suppressors. Instead of regulating the cell cycle, this gene appears to monitor and preserve genomic integrity.[62] Cells lacking *p53* become genomically unstable and quickly lose the ability to maintain the correct number of chromosomes.[63] The *p53* gene responds to genetic damage by stalling the cell in G_1, S, or G_2 phase of the cell cycle to prevent mitosis before repairs on the damaged DNA can be made[59] (see Fig. 2–5B). Alternatively, after sensing damage, *p53* can induce the cell to undergo apoptosis.[25]

How do genetic changes correlate with breast cancer development?

Breast cancer evolves over many years and is likely to involve the mutation of many genes. The natural history of the disease is unclear but may occur as follows: a normal breast epithelial cell acquires genetic damage that leads to a clonal proliferation of cells that eventually evolves into a CIS. The in situ lesion then matures to an invasive carcinoma, which in turn metastasizes to the lymph nodes and other organs[111] (Fig. 2–9). Current models of tumor progression for colon cancer correlate alterations of genes with the different phases of tumor development.[112] The simplistic model of breast tumor progression presented here (see Fig. 2–9) attempts to integrate much of the molecular information attained to date.

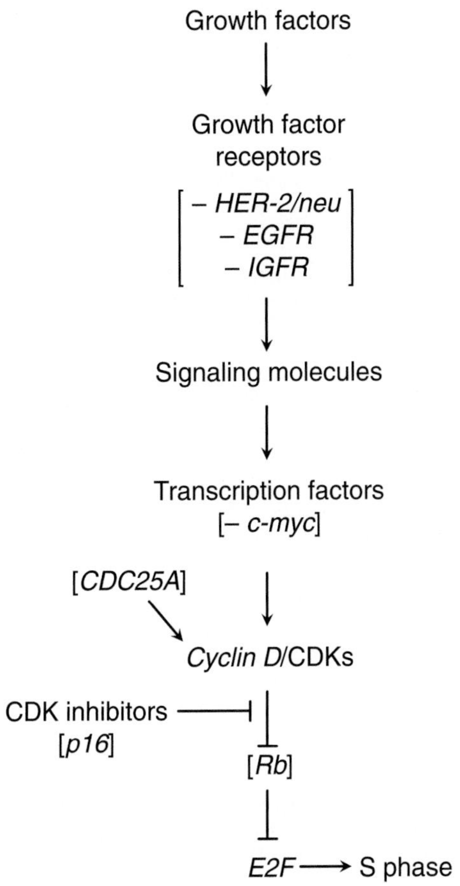

What is the earliest point in tumor development associated with genetic alterations?

The earliest genetic alterations have been observed in morphologically normal breast lobules and ducts near the site of a primary tumor[113] (see Fig. 2–9). Similar structures distant from the tumor have no genetic changes. The alterations observed are large chromosomal deletions (LOH). These normal-appearing breast cells may be precursors of the nearby tumor because identical losses are seen in the more advanced lesion. These foci of histologically normal cells may have been the direct precursor of an invasive breast cancer or may have passed through the intermediate step of CIS. Nevertheless, no genes that are necessary for the early steps in tumor development have been identified.

What genetic changes are associated with carcinoma in situ?

Many genetic alterations have occurred by the time CIS has developed. These include alterations of the estrogen receptor, p53, erb-2/HER-2/neu, and cyclin D.[31] In addition, CIS is usually genetically unstable, as evidenced by the high frequency of aneuploidy and alteration of both p53 and cyclin D.[100–102] These data have three important implications. First, the many mutations seen at this stage of development indicate that these lesions have gone through many rounds of clonal selection and are many steps away from their normal epithelial precursors. Second, the level of genetic instability seen in these lesions implies that selective pressure for the tumor to invade the basement membrane is likely to ultimately allow for the emergence of an invasive clone. Third, the frequency of alterations of estrogen receptor, p53, erb-2/HER-2/neu, and cyclin

Figure 2–8   Mitogenic pathways and their relationship to breast cancer. Mitogenic pathways that stimulate cell division are affected in multiple ways in breast cancer.

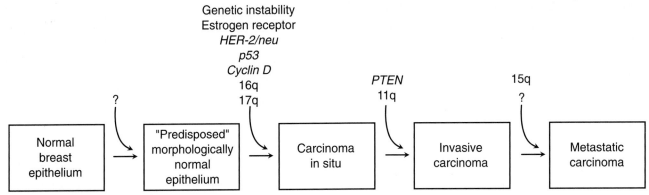

Figure 2–9   Model of breast cancer progression from normal epithelium to metastatic tumor. A possible pathway of tumor progression is shown. A *question mark* indicates that at present no gene has been identified that is altered specifically at the indicated transition point. Although many alterations have been observed in invasive breast cancer, they are also shared by carcinoma in situ.

D apparently peaks with CIS, which implies that most of the genetic steps in the tumor's development occur before invasion. On the other hand, although CIS differs tremendously from normal breast epithelial cells, CIS apparently differs little from invasive breast cancer.

What are the genetic changes associated with invasive and metastatic breast cancer?

Little is known about what genetically distinguishes CIS from invasive breast cancer. One clue is that loss of *PTEN* expression appears to occur in carcinomas and is rarely seen in CIS. Similarly, no genetic lesions have been identified that mark the transition to metastasis. However, a distinct gene expression pattern is associated with tumors that are destined to become metastatic.[114] This suggests that one or more programs of gene expression are altered in tumor to favor metastasis.

Are there other genes altered in breast cancer?

Our understanding of the genetic basis for the pathogenesis of breast cancer is incomplete. In the past 15 years, great strides have been made to delineate some of the pathways targeted for mutation. Most of these alterations seem to occur in pathways affecting proliferation and genomic stability. Nothing is known of the initiating events in sporadic breast cancer, nor has the actual chain of genetic events been determined for familial tumorigenesis involving *BRCA1* or *BRCA2*. Identification of a breast stem cell population should lead to a better understanding of breast epithelial development. Aberrant expansion of breast stem cells may provide the basis for tumor initiation and expansion.[115,116] Furthermore, no genes that are responsible for the transition from CIS to invasive carcinoma have been identified, although one locus has been implicated in this transition. Finally, the transition from locally invasive to metastatic disease is also likely to be associated with specific genetic alterations. Characterization of these genetic events will define the pathogenesis of breast cancer and hopefully produce the rational targets for drug therapy that are needed to improve patient care.

REFERENCES

1. Weinstein IB. The origins of human cancer: Molecular mechanisms of carcinogenesis and their implications for cancer prevention and treatment—twenty-seventh G.H.A. Clowes Memorial Award Lecture. Cancer Res 1988;48:4135–4143.
2. Weinberg RA. Oncogenes and antioncogenes, and the molecular basis of multistep carcinogenesis. Cancer Res 1989;49:3713–3721.
3. Cohen SM, Ellwein LB. Cell proliferation in carcinogenesis. Science 1990;249:1007–1011.
4. Ames BN, Gold LS, Willett WC. The causes and prevention of cancer. Proc Natl Acad Sci U S A 1995;92:5258–5265.
5. Loeb LA. Mutator phenotype may be required for multistage carcinogenesis. Cancer Res 1991;51:3075–3079.
6. Bhatia S, Robison LL, Oberlin O, et al. Breast cancer and other second neoplasms after childhood Hodgkin's disease. N Engl J Med 1996;334:745–751.
7. Tokunaga M, Land CE, Yamamoto T, et al. Incidence of female breast cancer among atomic bomb survivors: Hiroshima and Nagasaki, 1950–1980. Radiat Res 1987;112:243–272.
8. Ambrosone CB, Freudenheim JL, Graham S, et al. Cigarette smoking, N-acetyltransferase 2 genetic polymorphisms, and breast cancer risk. JAMA 1996;276:1494–1501.
9. Muir C, Waterhouse J, Mack T, et al. Cancer Incidence in the Five Continents, vol. 5. Lyon, France, International Agency for Research on Cancer, 1987.
10. Kelsey JL, Horn-Ross PL. Breast cancer: Magnitude of the problem and descriptive epidemiology. Epidemiol Rev 1993;15:7–16.
11. McMichael AJ, Giles GG. Cancer in migrants to Australia: Extending the descriptive epidemiological data. Cancer Res 1988;48:751–756.
12. Kelsey JL, Bernstein L. Epidemiology and prevention of breast cancer. Ann Rev Pub Health 1996;17:47–67.
13. Nandi S, Guzman RC, Yang J. Hormones and mammary carcinogenesis in mice, rats, and humans: A unifying hypothesis. Proc Natl Acad Sci U S A 1995;92:3650–3657.
14. Strauss BS. The origin of point mutations in human tumor cells. Cancer Res 1992;52:249–253.
15. Szabo CI, King MC. Inherited breast and ovarian cancer. Hum Mole Genet 1995;4:1811–1817.
16. Easton DF, Bishop DT, Ford D, et al. Genetic linkage analysis in familial breast and ovarian cancer: Results from 214 families. Am J Hum Genet 1993;52:678–701.
17. Rous P. The challenge to man of the neoplastic cell. Science 1967;157:24–28.
18. Stehelin D, Varmus HE, Bishop JM, Vogt PK. DNA related to the transforming gene(s) of avian sarcoma viruses is present in normal avian DNA. Nature 1976;260:170–173.
19. Barbacid M. ras Genes. Ann Rev Biochem 1987;56:779–827.
20. Schlessinger J, Bar-Sagi D. Activation of ras and other signaling pathways by receptor tyrosine kinases. Cold Spring Harbor Symp Quant Biol 1994;LIX:173–179.
21. Vogelstein B, Fearon ER, Hamilton SR, et al. Genetic alterations during colorectal-tumor development. N Engl J Med 1988;319:525–532.
22. Rowley JD. A new consistent chromosomal abnormality in chronic myelogenous leukemia identified by quinacrine fluorescence and Giemsa staining. Nature 1973;243:290–293.
23. Rabbitts TH. Chromosomal translocations in human cancer. Nature 1994;372:143–149.
24. McLaughlin J, Chianese W, Witte ON. Alternative forms of the BCR-ABL oncogene have quantitatively different potencies for stimulation of immature lymphoid cells. Mol Cell Biol 1989;9:1866–1874.
25. White E. Life, death, and the pursuit of apoptosis. Genes Dev 1996;10:1–15.
26. Roberts JM, Buck LB, Axel R. A structure for amplified DNA. Cell 1983;33:53–59.
27. Lin CR, Chen WS, Kruiger W, et al. Expression cloning of human EGF receptor complementary DNA: Gene amplification and three related messenger RNA products in A431 cells. Science 1984;224:843–848.
28. Semba K, Kamata N, Toyoshima K, et al. A v-erbB-related protooncogene, c-erbB-2, is distinct from the c-erbB-1/epidermal growth factor-receptor gene and is amplified in a human salivary gland adenocarcinoma. Proc Natl Acad Sci U S A 1985;82:6497–6501.
29. Collins S, Groudine M. Amplification of endogenous myc related DNA sequences in a human myeloid leukemia cell line. Nature 1982;298:670–681.
30. Jiang W, Kahn SM, Tomita N, et al. Amplification and expression of the human cyclin D gene in esophageal cancer. Cancer Res 1992;52:2980–2983.
31. Devilee P, Schuuring E, van de Vijver MJ, et al. Recent developments in the molecular genetic understanding of breast cancer. Crit Rev Oncogenesis 1994;5:247–270.
32. Fraser A, Evan G. A license to kill. Cell 1996;85:781–784.
33. Stanbridge EJ. Suppression of malignancy in human cells. Nature 1976;260:17–20.
34. Knudson AG. Mutation and cancer: Statistical study of retinoblastoma. Proc Nat Acad Sci U S A 1971;68:820–823.
35. Mulligan LM, Kwok JBJ, Healey CS, et al. Germ-line mutations of the RET protooncogene in multiple endocrine neoplasia type 2A. Nature 1993;263:458–460.
36. Knudson AG. Hereditary cancer, oncogenes, and antioncogenes. Cancer Res 1985;45:1437–1443.
37. Friend SH, Bernards R, Rogelj S, et al. A human DNA segment with properties of the gene that predisposes to retinoblastoma and osteosarcoma. Nature 1986;323:643–646.

38. Miki Y, Swensen J, Shattuck-Eidens D, et al. A strong candidate for the breast and ovarian cancer susceptibility gene BRCA1. Science 1994;266:66–71.
39. Wooster R, Bignell G, Lancaster J, et al. Identification of the breast cancer susceptibility gene BRCA2. Nature 1995;378:789–792.
40. Latif F, Tory K, Gnarra J, et al. Identification of the von Hippel-Lindau disease tumor suppressor gene. Science 1993;260:1317–1320
41. Kinzler KW, Nilbert MC, Su L, et al. Identification of the FAP locus genes from chromosome 5q21. Science 1991;253:661–669.
42. Groden J, Thliveris A, Samowitz W, et al. Identification and characterization of the familial adenomatous polyposis coli gene. Cell 1991;66:589–600.
43. Fishel R, Lescoe MK, Rao MRS, et al. The human mutator gene homolog MSH2 and its association with hereditary nonpolyposis colon cancer. Cell 1993;75:1027–1038.
44. Leach FS, Nicolaides NC, Papadopoulos N, et al. Mutations of a MutS homolog in hereditary nonpolyposis colorectal cancer. Cell 1993;75:1215–1225.
45. Kamb A, Gruis NA, Weaver-Feldhaus J, et al. A cell cycle regulator potentially involved in genesis of many tumor types. Science 1994;264:436–440.
46. Malkin D, Li FP, Strong LC, et al. Germ line p53 mutations in a familial syndrome of breast cancer, sarcomas and other neoplasms. Science 1990;250:1233–1236.
47. Wallace MR, Marchuk DA, Andersen LB, et al. Type I neurofibromatosis gene: Identification of a large transcript disrupted in three patients. Science 1990;249:181–186.
48. Rouleau GA, Merel P, Lutchman M, et al. Alteration of a new gene encoding a putative membrane-organizing protein causes neurofibromatosis type 2. Nature 1993;363:515–521.
49. Hollstein M, Sidransky D, Vogelstein B, Harris CC. p53 Mutations in human cancers. Science 1991;253:49–53.
50. Sherr CJ. Cancer cell cycles. Science 1996;274:1672–1677.
51. Parsons R. Human cancer, PTEN and the PI-3 kinase pathway. Semin Cell Dev Biol 2004;15(2):171–176.
52. Nowell PC. The clonal evolution of tumor cell populations. Science 1976;194:23–27.
53. Strauss BS. The origin of point mutations in human tumor cells. Cancer Res 1992;52:249–253.
54. Hartwell LH, Kastan MB. Cell cycle control and cancer. Science 1994;266:1821–1828.
55. Spruck CH, Won KA, Reed SI. Deregulated cyclin E induces chromosome instability. Nature 1999;401:297–300.
56. Cleaver JE. It was a very good year for DNA repair. Cell 1994;76:1–4.
57. Symington LS. Role of RAD52 epistasis group genes in homologous recombination and double-strand break repair. Microbiol Mol Biol Rev 2002;66(4):630–670.
58. Petrini JH. The Mre11 complex and ATM: Collaborating to navigate S phase. Curr Opin Cell Biol 2000;12:293–296.
59. Elledge SJ. Cell cycle checkpoints: Preventing an identity crisis. Science 1996;274:1664–1671.
60. Savitsky K, Bar-Shira A, Gilad S, et al. A single ataxia telangiectasia gene with a product similar to PI-3 kinase. Science 1995;268:1749–1753.
61. Bakkenist CJ, Kastan MB. Initiating cellular stress responses. Cell 2004;118:9–17.
62. Kastan MB, Canman CE, Leonard CJ. p53, Cell cycle control and apoptosis: Implications for cancer. Cancer Metastasis Rev 1995;14:3–15.
63. Cross SM, Sanchez CA, Morgan CA, et al. A p53-dependent mouse spindle checkpoint. Science 1995;267:1353–1356.
64. Fukasawa K, Choi T, Kuriyama R, et al. Abnormal centrosome amplification in the absence of p53. Science 1996;271:1744–1747.
65. Sorensen CS, Syljuasen RG, Falck J, et al. Chk1 regulates the S phase checkpoint by coupling the physiological turnover and ionizing radiation-induced accelerated proteolysis of Cdc25A. Cancer Cell 2003;3:247–258.
66. Cortez D, Wang Y, Qin J, Elledge SJ. Requirement of ATM-dependent phosphorylation of brca1 in the DNA damage response to double-strand breaks. Science 1999;286(5442):1162–1166.
67. Parsons R, Li G-M, Longley MJ, et al. Hypermutability and mismatch repair deficiency in RER+ tumor cells. Cell 1993;75:1227–1236.
68. Hall JM, Lee MK, Newman B, et al. Linkage of early-onset familial breast cancer to chromosome 17q21. Science 1990;250:1684–1689.
69. Wooster R, Neuhausen SL, Mangion J, et al. Localization of a breast cancer susceptibility gene, BRCA2, to chromosome 13q12–13. Science 1994;265:1088–1090.
70. Langston AA, Malone KE, Thompson JD, et al. BRCA1 mutations in a population-based sample of young women with breast cancer. N Engl J Med 1996;334:137–142.
71. Struewing JP, Abeliovich D, Peretz T, et al. The carrier frequency of the BRCA1 185delAG mutation is approximately 1% in Ashkenazi Jewish individuals. Nature Genet 1995;11:198–200.
72. Oddoux C, Struewing JP, Clayton CM, et al. The carrier frequency of the BRCA2 6174delT mutation among Ashkenazi Jewish individuals is approximately 1%. Nature Genet 1996;14:188–190.
73. FitzGerald MG, MacDonald DJ, Krainer M, et al. Germ-line BRCA1 mutations in Jewish and non-Jewish women with early-onset breast cancer. N Engl J Med 1996;334:143–149.
74. Abel KJ, Xy J, Yin GY, et al. Mouse Brc1: Localization sequence analysis and identification of evolutionary conserved domains. Hum Mol Genet 1995;4:2265–2273.
75. Chapman MS, Verma IM. Transcriptional activation by BRCA1. Nature 1996;382:678–679.
76. Shattuck-Eidens D, McLure M, Simard J, et al. A collaborative survey of 80 mutations in the BRCA1 breast and ovarian cancer susceptibility gene. JAMA 1995;273:535–541.
77. Xu X, Wagner KU, Larson D, et al. Conditional mutation of BRCA1 in mammary epithelial cells results in blunted ductal morphogenesis and tumour formation. Nat Genet 1999;22(1):37–43.
78. Holt JT, Thompson ME, Szabo C, et al. Growth retardation and inhibition by BRCA1. Nat Genet 1996;12:298–302.
79. Chen Y, Farmer AA, Chen CF, et al. BRCA1 is a 220-kDa nuclear phosphoprotein that is expressed and phosphorylated in a cell cycle-dependent manner. Cancer Res 1996;56:3168–3172.
80. Scully R, Chen J, Ochs RL, et al. Dynamic changes of BRCA1 subnuclear location and phosphorylation state are initiated by DNA damage. Cell. 1997;90(3):425–435.
81. Scully R, Ganesan S, Vlasakova K, et al. Genetic analysis of BRCA1 function in a defined tumor cell line. Mol Cell 1999;4(6):1093–1099.
82. Baer R, Ludwig T. The BRCA1/BARD1 heterodimer, a tumor suppressor complex with ubiquitin E3 ligase activity. Curr Opin Genet Dev 2002;12(1):86–91.
83. Ludwig T, Fisher P, Murty V, Efstratiadis A. Development of mammary adenocarcinomas by tissue-specific knockout of BRCA2 in mice. Oncogene 2001;20(30):3937–3948.
84. Sharan SK, Morimatsu M, Albrecht U, et al. Embryonic lethality and radiation hypersensitivity mediated by Rad51 in mice lacking BRCA2. Nature 1997;386:804–810.
85. Howlett NG, Taniguchi T, Olson S, et al. Biallelic inactivation of BRCA2 in Fanconi anemia. Science 2002;297(5581):606–609.
86. Phelan CM, Lanchaster JM, Tonin P, et al. Mutation of the BRCA2 gene in 49 site-specific breast cancer families. Nat Genet 1996;13:120–122.
87. Wooster R, Mangion J, Eeles R, et al. A germline mutation in the androgen receptor gene in two brothers with breast cancer and Reifenstein syndrome. Nat Genet 1992;2:132–134.
88. Swift M, Morrell D, Massey RB, et al. Incidence of cancer in 161 families affected by ataxia-telangiectasia. N Engl J Med 1991;325:1831–1836.
89. Liaw D, Marsh DJ, Li J, et al. Germline mutations of the PTEN gene in Cowden disease, an inherited breast and thyroid cancer syndrome. Nat Genet 1997;16:64–67.
90. Breast Cancer Facts and Figures: 2003–2004. Atlanta, American Cancer Society, 2004.
91. Folca PJ, Glascock RF, Irvine WT. Studies with tritium labeled hexoestrol in advanced breast cancer. Lancet 1961;11:796.
92. Giri D, Dundas S, Nottingham J, et al. Oestrogen receptors in benign epithelial lesions and intraduct carcinomas of the breast: An immunohistological study. Histopathology 1989;15:575–584.
93. Bur M, Zimarowski M, Schnitt S, et al. Estrogen receptor immunohistochemistry in carcinoma in situ of the breast. Cancer 1992;69:1174–1181.
94. Ottaviano YL, Issa JP, Parl FF, et al. Methylation of the estrogen receptor gene CpG island marks loss of estrogen receptor expression in human breast cancer cells. Cancer Res 1994;54:2552–2555.
95. Herman JG, Merlo A, Mao L, et al. Inactivation of the CDKN2/p16/MTS 1 gene is frequently associated with aberrant DNA methylation in all common human cancers. Cancer Res 1995;55:4525–4530.
96. Slamon DJ, Clark GM, Wong SG, et al. Correlation of relapse and survival with amplification of the HER-2/neu oncogene. Science 1987;235:177–182.

97. Keyomarsi K, Pardee AB. Redundant cyclin overexpression and gene amplification in breast cancer cells. Proc Natl Acad Sci U S A 1993; 90:1112–1116.

98. Van de Vijver MJ, Peterse JL, Moor WJ, et al. Neu protein overexpression in breast cancer. Association with comedo-type ductal carcinoma in situ and limited prognostic value in stage II breast cancer. N Engl J Med 1988;319:1239–1245.

99. Ramachandra S, Machin L, Ashley S, et al. Immunohistochemical distribution of c-erbB-2 in in situ breast carcinoma—a detailed morphological analysis. J Pathol 1990;161:7–14.

100. Weinstat-Saslow D, Merino MJ, Manrow RE, et al. Overexpression of cyclin DmRNA distinguishes invasive and in situ breast carcinomas from non-malignant lesions. Nat Med 1995;1:1257–1260.

101. Poller D, Roberts E, Bell J, et al. p53 Protein expression in mammary ductal carcinoma in situ: Relationship to immunohistochemical expression of estrogen receptor and erbB-2 protein. Hum Pathol 1993;24:463–468.

102. Leal CB, Schmitt FC, Bento MJ, et al. Ductal carcinoma in situ of the breast. Histologic categorization and its relationship to ploidy and immunohistochemical expression of hormone receptors, p53, and c-erbB-2 protein. Cancer 1995;75:2123–2131.

103. Futreal PA, Liu Q, Shattuck-Eidens D, et al. BRCA1 mutations in primary breast and ovarian carcinomas. Science 1994;266:120–122.

104. Teng D, Bogden R, Mitchell J, et al. Low incidence of BRCA2 mutations in breast carcinoma and other cancers. Nature 1996;13:241–244.

105. Esteller M, Silva JM, Dominguez G, et al. Promoter hypermethylation and BRCA1 inactivation in sporadic breast and ovarian tumors. J Natl Cancer Inst 2000;92(7):564–569.

106. Berx G, Cleton-Jansen AM, Nollet F, et al. E-cadherin is a tumour/invasion suppressor gene mutated in human lobular breast cancers. EMBO J 1995;14(24):6107–6115.

107. Graff JR, Herman JG, Lapidus RG, et al. E-cadherin expression is silenced by DNA hypermethylation in human breast and prostate carcinomas. Cancer Res 1995;55:5195–5199.

108. Bose S, Crane A, Hibshoosh H, et al. Reduced expression of PTEN correlates with breast cancer progression. Hum Pathol 2002;33:405–409.

109. Lee EY, To H, Shew JY, et al. Inactivation of the retinoblastoma susceptibility gene in human breast cancers. Science 1988;241:218–221.

110. Brenner AJ, Aldaz CM. Chromosome 9p allelic loss and p16/CDKN2 in breast cancer and evidence of p16 inactivation in immortal breast epithelial cells. Cancer Res 1995;55:2892–2895.

111. Page DL, Anderson TJ. Diagnostic Histopathology of the Breast. Edinburgh, Churchill-Livingstone, 1987.

112. Fearon ER, Vogelstein B. A genetic model for colorectal tumorigenesis. Cell 1990;61:759–767.

113. Deng G, Lu Y, Zlotnikov G, et al. Loss of heterozygosity in normal tissue adjacent to breast carcinomas. Science 1996;274:2057–2059.

114. van't Veer LJ, Dai H, van de Vijver MJ, et al. Gene expression profiling predicts clinical outcome of breast cancer. Nature 2002;415:530–536.

115. Dontu G, Abdallah WM, Foley JM, et al. In vitro propagation and transcriptional profiling of human mammary stem/progenitor cells. Genes Dev 2003;17(10):1253–1270.

116. Al-Hajj M, Wicha MS, Benito-Hernandez A, et al. Prospective identification of tumorigenic breast cancer cells. Proc Natl Acad Sci U S A 2003;100(7):3983–3988.

CHAPTER 3

Molecular, Cellular, and Developmental Biology of Breast Cancer

Sarah Hatsell, Minoti Hiremath, Peter Shamamian, and Pamela Cowin

Breast is a dynamic gland that undergoes considerable postnatal development and dramatic, cyclic morphologic changes throughout a woman's reproductive life. The temporal and spatial synchronization of these events requires endocrine and paracrine signals as well as a host of self-regulatory constraints. The chain of command begins with temporal signals from globally dispersed hormones. These are sensed by cells, discretely positioned throughout the breast, expressing hormone receptors. Hormone receptor–positive cells respond to hormones by producing highly localized growth factors that activate their receptors on neighboring cells. This in turn generates intracellular signals that produce the expression of cytoskeletal, adhesion, and extracellular matrix proteins as well as protein involved in tissue remodeling, cell cycle, and apoptosis.

Cancer research has approached breast biology with two major goals: to identify proteins that could serve as prognostic indicators or tumor cell markers and to curb breast cell proliferative pathways. Yet breast tumors grow slowly, developing with long latency, and mortality from breast cancer relates principally to metastatic spread and high rates of tumor recurrence. Cancers arise from inherited or acquired mutations. An increasing number of genetic mouse models, which provide powerful and incisive tools to dissect the consequences of such mutations, have suggested links between normal development and pathology of mammary gland. Moreover, a recent focus on stem cell biology has highlighted potential connections between normal breast stem-progenitor cells and cancer stem cells that are thought to be responsible for tumor recurrence. This chapter focuses on a selection of proteins and processes implicated in breast cancer viewed through the lens of their normal role in breast development and function.

Does the evolution of mammary glands suggest a mechanism for breast cancer metastases to bone?

Mammary glands are epidermal appendages that likely evolved from hair-associated apocrine glands.[1] Evidence for this may be found in a number of living species. For example, duck-billed platypuses have mammo-pilo-sebaceous units, which secrete milk that is lapped by their hatchlings from the ends of specialized hairs; koala bears form vestigal mammary hairs that regress as nipples form; and squirrels show bilateral development of sensory hairs and nipples from the same original epidermal anlage.[1] Molecular evidence suggests that lactation evolved from cutaneous secretions serving as antimicrobial protectants and as egg supplements.[1] Prolactin, the hormone that stimulates milk protein expression, belongs to the inflammatory cytokine gene family, and the α-lactalbumin subunit of the lactose synthetase enzyme resembles lysozyme, an antimicrobial component of egg yolk.

The ability of the mammary gland to promote bone resorption is thought to have evolved from ancient mechanisms involving estrogenic mobilization and transfer of maternal skeletal calcium reserves to eggshell in birds and to egg vitellogenin in freshwater fish.[2] Mammary glands mobilize bone calcium by secreting parathyroid hormone–related protein (PTHrP). This protein was discovered as a tumor product that induced humoral hypercalcemia of malignancy (HHM), a metabolic complication of many cancers. Expression of PTHrP within primary breast tumors is predictive of bone metastases. PTHrP is proposed to promote osteotropism by enabling breast cancer metastases to carve a foothold and simultaneously release growth factors from bone. Thus, bone tropism of breast cancer metastases may be considered an unintended consequence of a physiologic mechanism that evolved to trigger bone resorption for the purpose of lactation.[2]

How do mammary glands develop in the embryo?

PTHrP is essential for the earliest stages of embryonic mammary development. Mammary glands form during early embryonic development as bilateral epidermal placodes that coalesce and invaginate to form mammary buds (Fig. 3–1). Epithelial cells within the mammary buds secrete PTHrP,

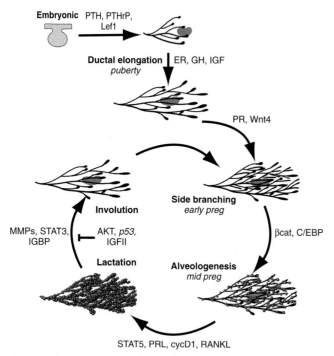

Figure 3–1 Diagram of the development of the mammary gland during puberty and pregnancy indicating some of the major signaling proteins involved. The mammary bud forms on about embryonic day 13 when epithelium, under the control of parathyroid hormone–related protein (PTHrP) and lymphoid-enhancer binder factor 1 (Lef1), grows down into the mammary mesenchyme and branches to form the small ductal structure present at birth. The gland stays quiescent until puberty, when estrogen receptor (ER), growth hormone (GH), and insulin-like growth factor (IGF) induce ductal elongation. In early pregnancy, progesterone receptor (PR) and Wnt4 stimulate side branching. Alveologenesis occurs in mid to late pregnancy and is controlled by β-catenin (βcat), CCAAT-enhancer binding protein beta (C/EBP), STAT5 (Signal transducer and activator of transcription), prolactin (PRL), cyclin D1 (cycD1), and receptor activator of NF-Kappa B ligand (RANKL). At the cessation of lactation, involution is mediated by matrix metalloproteinases (MMPs), STAT3, and IGF-binding protein (IGBP), where the gland undergoes remodeling to resemble a virgin gland.

which induces underlying stromal cells to become mammary mesenchyme.[3] Mammary mesenchymal cells signal back, inducing the epidermis to form nipple skin and suppress hair follicle formation.[3] PTHrP induces mesenchymal expression of androgen receptor (AR) and the transcription factor Lef-1, which is critical for elongation and formation of the rudimentary mammary tree.[3] Male fetal androgens stimulate mammary mesenchymal cells to constrict around the mammary bud, leading to its degeneration. PTHrP[-/-] and Lef-1[-/-] mice fail to specify the mammary mesenchyme, extend the mammary ductal tree, or show sexual dimorphism.[3,4] This phenotype is seen in Blomstrand chondroplasia, a form of human dwarfism resulting from mutations in the *PTHrP* gene.[5] During embryogenesis in females, the mammary bud elongates and branches to form a rudimentary mammary tree that remains quiescent until puberty.

What are the normal roles of estrogen, growth hormone, and insulin-like growth factor in pubertal mammary development?

Pituitary and ovarian hormones produced during puberty induce proliferation of cap cells occupying multilayered club-shaped structures known as terminal end buds (TEBs) (Fig. 3–2). This results in rapid ductal elongation and progressive branching[6] (see Fig. 3–1). Both estrogen and growth hormone (GH) are required for this to occur.[7] These hormones act synergistically on stromal cells to induce insulin-like growth factor-1 (IGF-1).[8] This protein appears to be the critical paracrine effector because ductal extension does not proceed in the absence of IGF-1, even when estrogens and GH are present.[7] At the end of puberty, TEBs disappear, and the gland again becomes dormant.

What are the contributions of estrogen to breast cancer?

Alveola-like eruptions appear transiently in response to hormonal surges in estrogen and progesterone accompanying estrus or ovulation. The number of ovulatory cycles is a significant risk factor in breast cancer, suggesting that such transient hyperplasia could be important in the etiology of breast tumors. However, because epithelial estrogen receptor (ER) is required for progesterone receptor (PR) expression, it is presently unclear whether ovulation-induced hyperplasia is stimulated by estrogen or progesterone.[9] Estrogen's role in breast cancer was first noted when oophorectomy in premenopausal women resulted in tumor regression.[10] The role of estrogen in breast cancer was further supported by the observation of enhanced risk for breast cancer associated with early menarche, late first full-term pregnancy, late menopause, or oral contraceptive use. This has been interpreted as resulting from increased lifetime exposure to estrogen. However, the finding of the Women's Health Initiative Trial that estrogen-only hormone replacement therapy does not increase the risk for breast cancer suggests that these earlier epidemiologic data need re-evaluation regarding the potential detrimental role of progesterone in these processes.[11]

Estrogen's biologic activities are mediated through ER, which occurs in α and β isoforms. In normal breast, ER-positive cells are seldom associated with markers of proliferation. Estrogen is thought to exercise its mitogenic effects by stimulating further paracrine signals.[12] In breast cancer, ER expression and proliferative markers overlap. About 70% of breast cancers express ER, and ER-positive breast tumors proliferate in response to estrogen when implanted into athymic nude mice.[12] The acquisition of proliferative capacity by ER-positive cells occurs at the earliest stages of tumorigenesis and therefore appears to contribute to breast tumor formation.[12]

In the absence of estrogen, ER is complexed with chaperone proteins (Hsp90, p23, Cyp-40, and FKBP52) that modulate ER DNA binding abilities. In the presence of estrogen, ER dissociates from chaperone proteins that bind to estrogen response elements (EREs) in the 5′-flanking regions of estrogen-responsive genes and initiates transcription in conjunction with coactivators (SRC-1, GRIP1, AIB1). ER

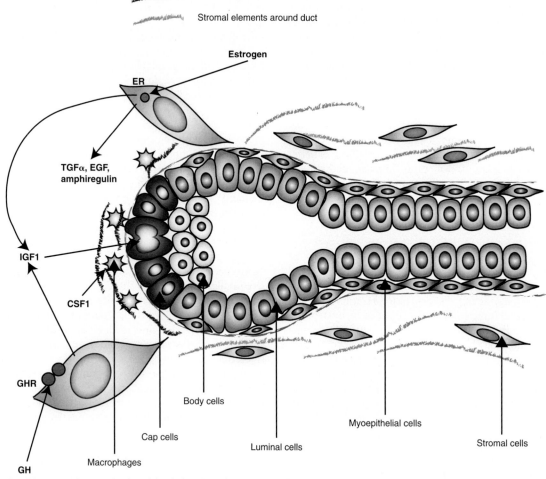

Figure 3–2 Diagram of a terminal end bud showing the major pathways involved in ductal extension during puberty. Estrogen and growth hormone (GH) promote ductal extension by stimulating estrogen receptor (ER)- and growth hormone receptor (GHR)-positive stromal cells surrounding the terminal end bud to produce insulin-like growth factor-1 (IGF1). IGF induces the proliferation of the cap cells, which differentiate and move to the more proximal part of the duct to become myoepithelial cells. The body cells divide and differentiate into luminal cells. Macrophages stimulated by colony-stimulating factor-1 (CSF1) are required for ductal elongation. EGF, epidermal growth factor; TGFα, transforming growth factor-α.

coactivators function by recruiting a histone acetyltransferase (CBP/p300) and basal transcription machinery (RNA polymerase, TBP, TFIIB). EREs are found in many promoters, and a large number of estrogen-responsive genes have been described (*http://research.i2r.a-star.edu.sg/promoter/Ergdb-v11/index.htm*). Genes encoding growth factors, such as IGF-1, and cell cycle regulators *cyclin D1* and *c-myc* are important transcriptional targets in the mitogenic response of breast to estrogen. In addition to its transcriptional targets, ER may also affect growth through "nongenomic activity." An alternative plasma membrane–associated ER is proposed to stimulate growth through activation of the mitogen-activated protein kinase (MAPK) pathway by forming complexes with the MNAR scaffold protein and src, or with shc.[13] Despite the demonstrated mitogenic effects of estrogen, ER-positive tumors are associated with better clinical outcome than ER-negative tumors, likely because ER also stimulates breast differentiation and contributes to epithelial stability and architecture by indir-ectly regulating expression of the E-cadherin breast tumor suppressor gene (discussed subsequently).

ER expression predicts tumor responsiveness to selective estrogen receptor modifiers (SERMs) such as tamoxifen and a related drug, raloxifene. SERMs have been used successfully as anti-cancer adjuvant therapies against hormone-responsive breast cancer.[10] They compete with estrogen for ER binding and act in a tissue-specific manner as estrogen agonists or antagonists. ER crystal structures indicate that the receptor adopts different conformations when bound to specific ligands (estrogen, tamoxifen, and raloxifene).[14,15] The type of steroid receptor coregulator in the tissue determines the effects of the ligand. For example, in the breast cancer cell line MCF7, both tamoxifen and raloxifene recruit corepressors and histone deacetylases (HDACs) to inhibit transcription of estrogen-stimulated genes, such as *c-myc* and *IGF-1*. However, in the uterus, tamoxifen, but not raloxifene, recruits the *SRC-1* coactivator and promotes transcription of these genes.[16] This explains the observations of the STAR (Study of Tamoxifen and Raloxifene) trial in which tamoxifen, but not raloxifene, increased the risk for uterine cancer in breast cancer patients treated with these drugs. Although SERMs are effective adjuvant therapies, reducing the incidence of ER-positive breast cancer and significantly prolonging survival, the benefits of these drugs are complicated by significant increases in gynecologic cancer and in cardiovascular deaths. In addition, most patients who show an initial response to SERMs eventually develop resistance to the treatment. Alternatively, aromatase inhibitors, such as anastrozole, which inhibits estrogen production rather than selectively modulating ER activity, have been effective. The ATAC (Arimidex, Tamoxifen, Alone or in Combination) trial has shown that anastrozole is superior to tamoxifen in reducing the incidence of contralateral invasive breast cancers. Anastrozole is better tolerated and induces fewer cardiovascular events and endometrial carcinomas. Side effects include bone loss from estrogen deprivation.[17]

What are the connections between cell–cell adhesion proteins and breast cancer?

Mammary ductal and alveolar epithelia are arranged in two layers (Fig. 3–3). Epithelial cells (expressing keratins 8, 18, and 19) line the central lumen and are surrounded by myoepithelial cells (expressing keratins 5 and 14) that directly contact the basal lamina. Cells in both layers are connected by cadherins (calcium-dependent cell–cell adhesion proteins). These proteins are essential for cell adhesion and exert profound effects on cell polarity, growth factor–mediated cell survival, and cell migration. Luminal cells adhere to one another by E-cadherin, and myoepithelial cell adhesion is mediated by P-

cadherin.[18,19] Luminal and myoepithelial layers interconnect through the desmosomal cadherins, desmogleins (Dsg 2/3), and desmocollins (Dsc 2/3). Each of these proteins has a documented role in mammary development and breast cancer.

E-cadherin, the best characterized breast tumor suppressor protein, mediates luminal cell–cell adhesion.[20] It also stabilizes growth factor receptors, sustains survival signals, and is required for the formation of tight junctions, which maintain cell polarity and seal the alveolar lumen during lactation.[21] Loss of E-cadherin$^{-/-}$ in the mouse mammary gland causes precocious apoptosis and involution during late pregnancy.[22] Germline mutations in the E-cadherin gene, *CDH1*, mildly predispose individuals to breast cancer. Loss of heterozygosity (LOH) of 16q22.1, which contains *CDH1*, is the second most frequent somatic genetic event in sporadic breast cancer, occurring in both lobular breast cancer and ductal carcinoma in situ (DCIS).[23] LOH with subsequent inactivating mutations in *CDH1* occurs in 50% of lobular breast cancers and is used as a diagnostic indicator of this type of tumor. LOH also occurs early in the more common grade 1 DCIS and preinvasive lobular carcinoma in situ (LCIS) but is not accompanied by further *CDH1* inactivating mutation.[23–28]

Abundant evidence links poor E-cadherin expression with tumor invasion and metastasis, which has been correlated with metastasis and poor prognosis.[23] Increasing E-cadherin expression reduces the invasive capacities of cells in vitro by restoring cell–cell adhesion, sequestering the β-catenin proto-oncogene, and elevating expression of the *p27* cell cycle inhibitor. However, several studies of human breast cancer cell lines have shown that decreased E-cadherin

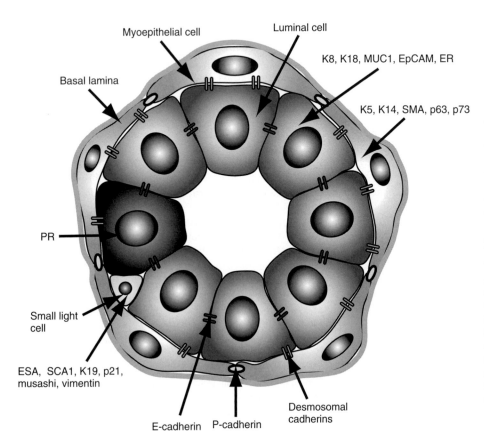

Figure 3–3 Diagram of a cross-section through mammary duct showing expression of markers commonly used to distinguish myoepithelial and luminal cell populations. Adherens junctions contain P-cadherin between myoepithelial cells and E-cadherin between luminal epithelial cells. Desmosomal cadherins link the two cell types. Progesterone receptor (PR) is expressed nonuniformly along the duct in mature virgins, where it is involved through the paracrine action of Wnt4 in side branching. The small light cell population is thought to comprise the stem and progenitor cells of the mammary gland. This cell population shows expression of several putative stem cell markers, including epithelium-specific antigen (ESA), K19, p21, stem cell antigen-1 (SCA1), and musashi. EpCAM, epithelial cell adhesion molecule; ER, estrogen receptor; SMA, smooth muscle actin.

Myoepithelial cell Luminal cell

Basal lamina

K8, K18, MUC1, EpCAM, ER

K5, K14, SMA, p63, p73

PR

Small light cell

ESA, SCA1, K19, p21, musashi, vimentin

E-cadherin   P-cadherin   Desmosomal cadherins

expression level is not an absolute predictor of tumor invasive and metastatic behavior and that derivative metastases frequently show strong E-cadherin expression.[29–31] In contrast, increased expression of other cadherins, N-, P-, and OB- (osteoblast cadherin 11), correlates with experimental parameters of invasion and metastasis. Little is known about expression patterns of these cadherins in normal breast, but they have been noted in several invasive breast cancer cell lines.[29–32] P-cadherin[−/−] mice show precocious mammary development, suggesting that loosening of myoepithelial cell junctions may be a key event precipitating alveologenesis.[18] P-cadherin expression is associated with high histologic grade of ER-negative DCIS and invasive carcinomas.[19] N-cadherin is proposed to enhance motility and epithelial-to-mesenchymal transition (EMT) by stabilizing the surface expression of the fibroblast growth factor receptor-1 (FGFR-1), enhancing its responsiveness to fibroblast growth factor-2 (FGF-2), and sustaining activation of the MAPK pathway.[33] This, in turn, increases expression of matrix remodeling agents, such as matrix metalloproteinase-9 (MMP-9).[33]

The intracellular domain of cadherins associates with catenins.[26] α-Catenin, which connects the adhesion complex to the actin cytoskeleton, is down-regulated in breast cancer.[31] β-Catenin, which forms a modulatable link between cadherins and α-catenin, shows aberrant expression and phosphorylation in human breast cancer and induces mouse mammary adenocarcinomas.[34–37] Reduction in cell adhesion due to down-regulation of the desmosomal cadherin, Dsc 3, or the desmosomal plaque proteins desmoplakin and plakoglobin has been reported in poorly differentiated and invasive ductal carcinomas.[36,38]

What do slug and snail transcription factors have to do with metastasis? Is estrogen good or bad?

Studies have suggested that estrogen regulates epithelial architecture through modulating E-cadherin.[39,40] Estrogen-activated ER indirectly stimulates expression of *MTA3*, a component of Mi-2/NuRD, nucleosome-remodeling complex.[39] This represses expression of snail, a transcription factor and master regulator of epithelial-to-mesenchymal transition. Snail, like its related transcription factors slug and SIP, represses transcription from the E-cadherin promoter.[41] Snail expression correlates with infiltration by ductal carcinomas and down-regulation of the aromatase gene.[42] Slug expression correlates with lack of E-cadherin transcripts in breast cancer cell lines.[43,44] Estrogen is hypothesized to maintain epithelial architecture by constraining these transcriptional repressors of E-cadherin expression.[39,40] Studies in *Drosophila* species have also identified genetic connections between *taiman*, the homologue of the estrogen coactivator amplified in breast cancer (*AIB1*), cadherin expression, and cell migration.[45–47] Thus, evidence is accumulating that estrogens, ER, and estrogen coactivators function to regulate cell morphology and migration in addition to proliferation. Each of these factors likely functions in the continual remodeling that is required of normal breast throughout the mammary cycle, but when dysregulated, each promotes invasion and metastasis, which lie at the root of breast cancer mortality.

What are the contributions of growth hormone and insulin-like growth factor to breast cancer?

IGF-1 is a potent mitogen that is essential during puberty for ductal proliferation and extension. Estrogens induce IGF-1, its receptor IGFR-1, and the downstream signaling molecules insulin receptor substrate-1 (IRS-1) and IRS-2, leading to enhanced epithelial survival in response to IGF-1.[48] IGF-1 is also a key survival factor for the breast epithelium during lactation.[49] Involution, following cessation of lactation, is triggered by STAT3–induced expression of an IGF-binding protein (IGF-BP), which provokes breast epithelial apoptosis by sequestering the IGF survival factor.[50] High IGF-BP levels have been associated with both increased and decreased risk for premenopausal breast cancer.[51] Increased levels of GH and IGF-1 are found in premenopausal breast cancer, and IGFRs are increased 40-fold.[51,52] IGFR-1 represses apoptosis that would result from the unbridled activity of other oncoproteins.[53] Its antiapoptotic effects may also negatively affect therapies dependent on radiation-induced cell death and underlie resistance to *HER-2* inhibitors, such as trastuzumab (Herceptin), that develop under selective pressure of breast cancer treatment.[52]

What is the role of the *HER* family in mammary development and breast cancer?

All four members (*HER-1–4*) of the *HER/erbB/EGFR* gene family are expressed in breast.[54] The *HER* genes encode transmembrane receptors that bind growth factors and initiate internal mitogenic signal transduction pathways through their tyrosine-kinase domains. Although they are potent breast mitogens, they can also stimulate apoptosis when overexpressed.[53] *HER-1* binds epidermal growth factor (EGF), transforming growth factor-α (TGF-α), and amphiregulin. *HER-1* and *HER-4* bind betacellulin, epiregulin, and HBEGF. *HER-3* and *HER-4* bind neuregulins 1 to 4.[55] Many of these ligands are lipid bound in precursor form to the surface of the cells that produce them. Their polarized expression, cleavage, binding to heparin sulphate proteoglycans, and subsequent receptor internalization are important points of regulation that affect the initiation and duration of their signals. *HER-2* and *HER-3* are unusual in that so far no *HER-2* ligand has been identified and *HER-3* lacks intrinsic kinase activity.[54]

On binding to ligand, members of the *HER* receptor family dimerize and phosphorylate specific tyrosine residues within their cytoplasmic domains. Each receptor contains specific phosphorylation sites that form binding sites for different downstream signaling molecules. Phosphorylation can lead to the association of Src-homology 2 proteins (SH2) and phosphotyrosine-binding domain proteins (PTBs), such as Src, PLCγ, and PI3K, and to adaptor proteins, such as Shc, Grb2, Grb7, and Nck.[54] These proteins link to intracellular signaling pathways, including the MAPK/ERK1. Downstream mediators also provide ample opportunity for integration with TGF-β and BMP2 signaling through MAPK-mediated phosphorylation of the Smad pathway.

The complexities introduced by receptor dimerization, ligand redundancy, and multiple levels of signal regulation make defining the roles of individual HER proteins in breast biology challenging. This remains a work in progress. However, the following generalizations may be made. Epithelial amphiregulin and stromal HER-1/2 heterodimers play significant roles in ductal extension and maintain the survival of periductal stromal cells. During pregnancy, HER-1 TGF-α heterodimers affect side branching and alveologenesis. The naturally occurring HER-1 hypomorph, *waved-2* mouse, shows impaired lactation. HER-3 and the neuregulins play a major role in proliferation and differentiation, and HER-4 is critical for lactation.[55]

Deregulated expression of *HER-1* and *HER-2* occurs frequently in breast cancer and may provide routes to estrogen-independent growth. *HER-2* is amplified in 30% of breast cancers, and this overexpression results in ligand-independent activation of its kinase domain.[56] Expression of activated or wild-type *HER-2* under the control of the MMTV promoter in mice causes tumors, supporting the hypothesis that *HER-2* is important in tumorigenesis.[57,58] *MMTV-HER-2* tumors form with long latency, resemble human comedocarcinomas, and can develop metastasis to the lung.[58]

HER-2 is the preferred dimerization partner for other family members and is required for activating downstream signaling of the kinase-dead *HER-3* receptor. High levels of phosphorylated *HER-3* are frequently found in tumors overexpressing *HER-2*, and this particular heterodimer appears to be the most potent.[58] Activation of *HER-2/3* recruits PI3K, which promotes the antiapoptotic AKT/PKB survival pathway and stimulates proliferation through effects on *cyclin D3* and *p27* elements of the cell cycle machinery. These observations have led to the use of antibodies directed against *HER-1* (C225), *HER-2* (Herceptin), and the *HER-2/3* heterodimer (2C4) and to the development of small molecule inhibitors of *HER-1* ZD1839 (Iressa) and OSI774.[59]

Overexpression of *HER-2* also promotes invasion and metastasis. It may achieve this either by inhibiting E-cadherin transcription or by sequestering β-catenin.[25,60] *HER-2* may also increase invasiveness by associating with ASGP2, the transmembrane component of MUC4, a protein that sterically hinders cadherin-mediated cell adhesion.[61] *HER-2* has been proposed to increase cell motility by stimulating expression of MMP-9, uPA, and uPAR through MAPK pathways.

What changes take place in mammary glands during pregnancy? What are the roles of progesterone receptor and its paracrine pathways in breast cancer?

During pregnancy, mammary glands undergo extensive ductal side branching followed by alveolar development. These morphologic changes are accompanied by sequential expression of the milk proteins: WDNM1, casein, whey acid protein (WAP), and α-lactalbumin. Genetically engineered mice have provided definitive evidence of signaling pathways regulating these proliferative and differentiating processes as well as increased risk of cancer. Mice lacking progesterone receptor (PR[−/−]) or Wnt-4[−/−] show impaired ductal side branching, whereas those overexpressing Wnt-1 show increased branching.[62,63] This form of increased branching is a premalignant condition. P-cadherin[−/−] mice or those overexpressing β-catenin, cyclin D1, or one of several MMPs show precocious

alveolar development, again a premalignant condition.[18,35,64-66] In contrast, mice expressing β-catenin suppressors or lacking cyclin D1, RANKL/osteoprotegerin (OPGL), or the transcription factor C/EBP-β are impaired in alveologenesis.[67-71] Mice lacking prolactin receptor (PrlR[−/−]) or STAT5a[−/−] show impaired development and milk synthesis.[72-74] The fact that several of these mice develop tumors suggests links between activation of developmental pathways and breast cancer.[35,65,66,75,76]

Hormone receptors (ER, PR, and PrlR) are expressed uniformly in virgin epithelial cells but adopt an intermittent expression pattern in adults.[77] This change is critical for proliferation and further development and is dependent on the transcription factor C/EBP-β.[71,78,79] Proliferative cells lack steroid hormone receptors but reside near hormone-responsive cells.[12,80,81] Thus, steroid receptor–positive cells may represent a stem-progenitor cell or a niche that acts as a sensor to influence the activity of nearby steroid receptor–negative stem or progenitor division-competent cells.[82] An increased incidence of breast cancer in postmenopausal women receiving combined hormone replacement therapy (estrogen plus progesterone), compared with those receiving estrogen only, suggests that prolonged stimulation of PR may predispose to breast cancer.[11] Tumors that are positive for PR, however, have a better prognosis because they must also express ER and are therefore likely to respond to SERMs. In the current model of breast development, receipt of progesterone by PR-positive cells stimulates release of paracrine growth factor survival signals, including IGF-II, RANKL, and Wnt-4.[83,84] These factors are prime candidates to mediate hormone-independent proliferation of tumors. IGF-II expression is responsive to hormone stimulation and is constitutively expressed in estrogen-independent MDA-MB-231 breast cancer cells. RANKL, a key osteoclast differentiation or activation factor that is essential for bone remodeling, is secreted by breast during pregnancy.[70] RANKL interaction with its receptor RANK results in activation of NFκ-B and up-regulation of cyclin D1, both of which are highly expressed in many breast tumors.[84] Ectopic expression of Wnt-1, which is presumed to mimic the endogenous *Wnt-4* gene, rescues the PR[−/−] block in side-branching and induces mammary adenocarcinomas.[63,85]

What is the evidence that cancer stem cells are central to breast cancer development and progression?

The long time lag (up to 30 years) in breast cancer incidence following radiation exposure in atomic bomb victims has strongly suggested that long-lived and possibly immortal stem-progenitor cells are targets for transformation. Further circumstantial evidence in support of this concept comes from high rates of breast cancer in women exposed to radiation during adolescence, a time when stem cells reside close to the surface of the epidermis and hence are more exposed to damage. The concept that breast tumors arise from transformation of stem cells, or from transformation of differentiated cells that revert to stem cell–like behavior, is of paramount importance for the design of therapeutic strategies.[86,87] Current radiotherapy and chemotherapies target rapidly dividing cells, and their effectiveness is measured by their ability to reduce tumor mass and induce tumor regression by apoptosis. As such, they effectively kill the differentiated and harmless progeny of stem cells, which form the tumor bulk, and quickly become limited in their effectiveness by the emergence of therapy-resistant cancer cells. Similarly, adjuvant therapies such as tamoxifen are directed at the ER-positive or *HER-2*-positive differentiated cells. They are not tailored to target stem cells, which by their nature are slowly dividing and resistant to apoptosis owing to higher levels of expression of the antiapoptotic factor *BCL-2* and of multidrug resistance channels, such as breast cancer–related protein-1 (BCRP1), which efficiently export chemotherapeutic agents.[86–91] Stem cells therefore remain, causing tumor recurrence. Tumors contain heterogenous mixtures of different cell types. However, studies in mouse models of breast cancer have shown that all cells within a tumor contain the same genetic mutational fingerprint, supporting their origin from a common precursor.[92] Nevertheless, very few of these cells are capable of reforming tumors.[93,94] Such a subset of cells may be considered "tumor stem cells" that produce heterogenous progeny, of limited tumorigenic capacity, that form the tumor bulk.[86,87,93,94] Studies have shown that epithelial-specific antigen (ESA-positive, CD44-positive, CD24-negative, lineage marker-negative) cells, isolated from nine different human breast tumors, are enriched 50-fold in their ability to form xenografted tumors compared with unsorted cells. Significantly, these cells are perpetuated within serial transplants and reproduce the heterogenous complexity of the original tumor, suggesting that they possess the twin stem cell capabilities of self-renewal and the ability to generate differentiated progeny.[94]

Where are mammary stem cells and their cancer-prone progenitors?

The relationship between tumor stem cells and normal stem cells is implied but not proven. Identification of mammary stem cells has been approached from many angles. Transplantation studies established that stem cells, dispersed throughout the mammary epithelial tree, are capable of regenerating an entire gland.[95,96] The presence of "small light cells" (SLCs), which occupy a niche intermediate between luminal and myoepithelial cell layers (see Fig. 3–3), correlates with regenerative capacity of such serial transplants.[97] These cells are capable of mitosis but are generally quiescent and display other stem cell–like features, including undifferentiated ultrastructural characteristics; an ability to retain BrdU label (indicating a low proliferative rate); expression of putative stem cell markers, such as Sca-1, p21, a6-integrin, ESA, cytokeratin 19, telomerase, and musashi; and lack of differentiation markers.[98,99] Recent work has applied the Hoechst dye–effluxing technique to the mammary gland. This approach led to isolation of hematopoietic stem cells by fluorescence-activated cell sorting into a side population (SP). Mammary SP overlaps with SLCs and label-retaining cells.[99,100] A further approach has been to analyze cells capable of perpetuating three-dimensional mammosphere cultures, a technique that is proposed to select for stem cells. Gene expression profiles of such cells have revealed the presence of many proteins common to hemopoietic, neural, and embryonic stem cells.[101]

It is currently a matter of debate as to whether mammary stem cells are ER positive or ER negative.[12,80,81] In addition to stem cells, the mammary gland appears to regenerate itself through a hierarchy of progenitors, which may also be targets for oncogenic transformation. Mammary gland contains three types of lineage-limited progenitor cells. In serial transplantation studies, these give rise to outgrowths composed of ducts, alveoli, or both, the latter case indicating the presence of a common bipotent progenitor for ductal and alveolar structures.[96] In each case, outgrowths contain both luminal and myoepithelial cells. Wnts and their downstream signal transducer β-catenin play key roles in expanding specific mammary stem-progenitor populations.[26,35,82,92,102] β-catenin expands an alveolar progenitor population and induces tumors when ectopically expressed in mammary gland.[35,82] Inactivating mutations or down-regulation of Wnt and β-catenin suppressors, such as FRP, AXIN, and APC, and high levels of expression of β-catenin target genes, such as *cyclin D1* and *c-myc*, have been reported in a significant proportion of human breast tumors.[26] These studies suggest a connection between mammary stem-progenitor cell expansion and cancer susceptibility.

What is the involvement of cell cycle proteins in breast cancer?

An alternative view is that breast cancer is a disease of abnormal or uncontrolled proliferation resulting from deregulated growth factor signaling or aberrations in cell cycle control machinery. Thus, a great deal of interest has focused on the potential role of cell cycle elements in breast cancer. The cell cycle (Fig. 3–4) comprises four phases: G_1(gap 1), S (DNA

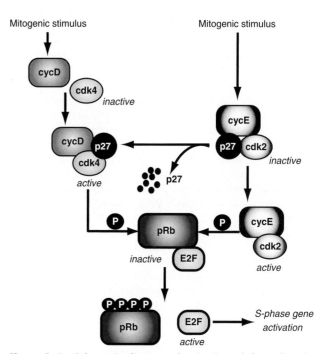

Figure 3–4 Schematic diagram of activation of the cell cycle. Mitogenic stimuli cause the sequestration of p27 from its complex with cyclin-dependent kinase-2 (cdk2) and cyclin E (cycE) into a complex with cyclin D (cycD) and cyclin-dependent kinase-4 (cdk4). This activates both cyclin-dependent kinases to phosphorylate Rb, resulting in the dissociation of E2F, which activates expression of S-phase genes.

synthesis), G_2, and M (mitosis), in which cells duplicate their chromosomes and divide in two. Progression through this cycle is promoted by cyclin-dependent kinases (CDKs), which are positively regulated by cyclins and negatively regulated by CDK inhibitors. Cyclins are synthesized at different times in the cell cycle and are rapidly degraded by protein complexes that target them for proteasomal destruction. D-type cyclins provide a fundamental link between mitogens such as erbB-2 and ras, which activates the MAPK cascade, and the cell cycle machinery. D-type cyclins interact with CDK4 and CDK6 to drive the progression of a cell through early and mid G_1 phase. They promote the activity of cyclin E–CDK2, which forms an active complex in late G_1 and directs entry into S phase, by sequestering the p21 and p27 inhibitors. Both cyclin D–CDK4 and cyclin E–CDK2 phosphorylate Rb, leading to the dissociation of E2F transcription factor from the pRb–E2F complex. E2F activates genes necessary for further cell cycle progression. S-phase progression to G_2 is directed by the cyclin A–CDK2 and cyclin A–CDK1 complexes. Lastly, cyclin B–CDK1 complex is necessary for the entry into mitosis.

Cyclin D1 is the most studied cell cycle protein in breast cancer. Cyclin D1 serves an essential role in alveologenesis, as demonstrated by the failure of alveoli to expand during late pregnancy in *cyclin D1*[−/−] mice.[69,103] The *cyclin D1* gene is amplified in 10% of breast cancers, and cyclin D1 protein is elevated in a further 40%.[104] The significance of these correlative findings in humans is bolstered by the observation that MMTV–cyclin D1 mice develop tumors, albeit with long latency and at low frequency.[64] Mammary glands of *cyclin D1*[−/−] mice are resistant to transformation by oncogenic *ras* and *HER-2/neu*.[105] Thus, *ras* and *HER-2* signal exclusively through cyclin D1 to provoke hyperplasia and tumors. In contrast, although cyclin D1 is up-regulated in human tumors displaying nuclear β-catenin and in MMTV–Wnt-1 and β-catenin mouse tumors, the latter form tumors in the absence of cyclin D1 and indeed are suppressed to some extent by its presence.[82,105] The involvement of cyclin D1 in tumor formation or promotion is currently a matter of debate. The partial rescue of the cyclin D1[−/−] phenotype by placing the *cyclin E* gene under the control of the *cyclin D1* promoter or by loss of the *p27* cell cycle inhibitor gene has suggested that cyclin D1 functions solely to advance the cell cycle. However, recent data have shown that cyclin D1 has additional roles in differentiation.[106,107] Indeed, patients with tumors expressing high levels of cyclin D1 generally have a better outcome. Cyclin D1 can act as a transcriptional coactivator of estrogen receptor and associate with and antagonize the transcriptional functions of C/EBP-β.[106] Statistical investigation of a large panel of human tumors shows a tight association of cyclin D1 up-regulation with a set of C/EBP-β–regulated genes, suggesting that this function contributes significantly to tumor progression.[106] C/EBP-β has several different isoforms. Cyclin D1 antagonizes the full-length form, LAP, which acts as a constitutive repressor of *cyclin D1* target genes. A shorter dominant negative isoform of C/EBP-β, LIP, mimics the effects of cyclin D1 on these transcriptional targets. The LAP/LIP ratio is tightly regulated and increases during terminal differentiation. This ratio is decreased markedly in breast tumors owing to increased levels of LIP.[108]

Cell cycle inhibitors, such as *p27* and *p21*, have also received attention as potential prognostic indicators. Their expression has been correlated with proliferation and differentiation.

Thus, p27 and p21 inhibit cyclin E–CDK-2 and arrest the cell cycle by halting G_1 progression. However, they facilitate the formation and action of cyclin D1–CDK-4, promoting differentiation. The p27[−/−] mice show multiorgan hyperplasia. In addition, *p27* is rarely mutated in breast cancer, but the cell cycle inhibitory action of this protein is often impaired through accelerated degradation, sequestration by cyclin D–CDK complexes and mislocalization. Reduction of p27 does not alone cause cancer but accelerates tumor formation by tumor promoters. Many studies have suggested that loss of *p27*, or cytoplasmic p27, is a strong independent predictor of decreased disease-free survival and correlates with ER-positive status and high cyclin D1 expression.[109] However, others have suggested that p27 has no prognostic value.[109] Increased cytosolic *p21* is associated with poor prognosis and is an early event in many neoplasias.[110] It is highly expressed in stem cells and is responsible for maintaining them quiescent.[98] Furthermore, p21 arrests growth after DNA damage to allow repair. Thus, *p21*-deficient tumors are sensitive to radiation. Attenuating *p21* in tumor cells can lead to an increased susceptibility to currently used DNA-damaging therapeutic agents, suggesting this may be a viable target for cancer therapy.

What role do apoptotic and survival pathways play in involution and breast cancer?

After weaning, the mammary alveolar epithelium undergoes apoptosis, causing the mammary gland to involute, resuming an appearance similar to that of the pubertal ductal tree.[6] Studies in mice have shown that proteins that play a normal physiologic role as survival signals for the breast epithelium during lactation or as apoptotic or adipogenic signals during involution play significant roles in human breast cancer.

The p53[−/−] mice fail to induce p21 at the end of lactation, resulting in a reduced apoptotic response and delayed involution.[111] Sixty percent of p53[−/+] mice produce significant numbers of mammary tumors after about 50 weeks, and mammary epithelial cells derived from p53[−/−] mice produce mammary tumors when transplanted into wild-type fat-pads.[111] The long latency with which these tumors develop indicates the need for other genetic events. Inactivating mutations in *p53* are the most common mutation of sporadic breast cancer, being present in about 60% of tumors.[112] Germline mutation of *p53* is found in less than 1% of breast cancers and is not accompanied by LOH.[112] Thus, p53 deficiency promotes mammary tumors in mice and humans, and loss of one allele is sufficient to increase risk. Germline mutations in *p53* are present in Li-Fraumeni syndrome, which is characterized by an increased risk for many cancers, including an 18-fold higher risk for developing breast cancer before the age of 45 years.[113]

In addition, p53 forms a tetrameric transcription factor that plays important tumor suppressor roles guarding the integrity of the genome. Its levels are tightly regulated by a complex feedback mechanism involving its transcriptional target mdm2, which binds to p53 and facilitates its ubiquitination and hence proteolysis (Fig. 3–5). Although p53 levels are kept low by this mechanism, p53 is stabilized and activated in response to stressful stimuli such as DNA damage or hypoxia. It induces cell cycle arrest and apoptosis in response

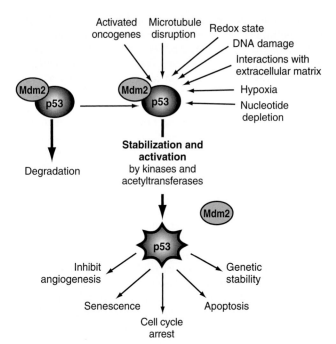

Figure 3–5 In unstimulated cells, p53 levels are kept low by rapid degradation by Mdm2. Large numbers of signals lead to the modification of p53 by various kinases and acetyltransferases, resulting in the detachment of Mdm2, stabilization, and activation, causing a number of downstream effects.

to these stresses by regulating expression of *p21* and *Bax*, respectively. In addition, p53 has 3′, 5′ exonuclease activity that contributes to fidelity of DNA replication. Thus, in the absence of functional p53, cells are retained that are genetically damaged and genomically unstable.[112]

The observation that p53[+/−] mice replicate Li-Fraumeni syndrome only when bred onto a BALB/c background indicates the importance of modifier genes that cooperate in tumor progression. Cooperativity between *p53* and *BRCA1* and *BRCA2* in the rate of tumor incidence has been demonstrated by crossing mice deficient for these genes. Inactivation of *p53* is seen in less than 90% of *BRCA*-mediated breast cancers. Crosses between mice depleted in *p53* and those overexpressing *HER-2/neu*, *ras*, and *Wnt-1* show accelerated tumor incidence.[111]

Mice with targeted deletion of STAT3 within the mammary gland show reduced expression of IGF-binding proteins, reduced apoptosis, and delayed involution.[114] Thus, the physiologic role of STAT3 within the mammary gland is to regulate the early apoptotic stage of involution through inhibition of IGF-1 survival signals. STAT3 transcriptionally regulates genes involved in both apoptosis and the cell cycle and therefore can function as an oncogene or tumor suppressor depending on the cellular context. Cytoplasmic expression of STAT3 and phosphorylated (Tyr705) STAT3 is seen in a large number of breast cancers but does not correlate with survival. However, activated nuclear STAT3 (23% of tumors) and phospho-STAT3 (45% of tumors) predicts significantly improved survival.[115] These observations support the possibility that STAT3 acts as a tumor suppressor in breast, consistent with its physiologic role in the gland in promoting apoptosis and involution.

Mice expressing constitutively activated AKT under the MMTV promoter show delayed involution and apoptosis. AKT lies downstream of *PTEN* and *HER* signaling through the PI3K survival pathway and therefore is activated in many breast cancers. Activated AKT phosphorylates *p27*, preventing nuclear import and cyclin–CDK complex formation, thereby leading to tumor progression.[116]

What is the involvement of DNA repair genes in breast cancer?

Germline mutations in several DNA repair genes have been linked to inherited predisposition to breast cancer. The *BRCA1* gene (17q21), isolated in 1994, accounts for almost 95% of familial breast and ovarian cancer but for less than 5% of all breast cancers. Somatic mutations are rare, but promoter hypermethylation is thought to occur in a significant proportion of sporadic breast cancers, and loss of the BRCA1 protein is reported in high-grade ductal carcinomas. BRCA1 serves multiple roles as a tumor suppressor in breast cancer tumorigenesis by coordinating multiple processes required for the maintenance of genomic integrity during DNA replication. It interacts directly and indirectly with many proteins, including DNA repair components (RAD50 and RAD51, BRCA2, p53, ATR and ATM, and BRCA1-associated surveillance complex [BASC]) and a large number of cell cycle and checkpoint control proteins (Rb, Esf1 E2F, c-Myc, and p53).[117] Loss of *BRCA1* function is associated with defects in S-phase checkpoint and G₂-to-M transition. BRCA1-deficient cells are radiation sensitive and defective in the rate of homologous recombination.[118] In addition, BRCA1 forms complexes with transcriptional activators and repressors, participates in chromatin remodeling (RNA polymerase II, RHA, HDAC complex, and CtIP), and may function in ubiquitination.[119,120] *BRCA2* (13q12-13), discovered in 1995, bears no resemblance to *BRCA1*.[121] It functions exclusively in DNA repair by homologous recombination through interaction with RAD51, a key component of the double-strand break repair pathway. BRCA2 is proposed to sequester RAD51 in an inactive state and to facilitate RAD51 binding to single-stranded DNA at double-strand breaks. In the absence of BRCA2, critical events in the initiation of homologous recombination are impaired, and repair and replication errors accrue with each cell cycle. BRCA1[−/−] mice die embryonically (~E8) with severe growth deficit and elevation of p21. Mice with conditional knockout of the *BRCA1* or *BRCA2* gene in mammary gland fail to differentiate properly and develop tumors with long latency (1.6 years).[122,123]

What other genes and gene expression profiles are associated with breast cancer?

In addition to *BRCA1* and *BRCA2*, other breast cancer susceptibility genes are proposed to exist on 8p11-21 and 13q21.[124] Several rare genetic syndromes account for about 1% of familial breast cancer. The *PTEN* gene is mutated in 80% of patients with Cowden syndrome, and truncating mutations confer a 25% to 50% increased lifetime breast cancer risk. Germline and somatic mutations in PTEN are rare in the general population, but LOH occurs in 11% to 40% of sporadic breast cancers. Truncating mutations in the *LKB1* gene, found in Peutz-Jeghers syndrome, confer increased breast cancer risk on patients with this syndrome. Mutations in the *APC* gene confer increased risk for developing breast cancer in patients with familial adenopolyposis coli, in the *Min* mouse model of this disease, and are found in a small percentage of sporadic breast tumors. A number of polymorphisms increase breast cancer susceptibility. These include polymorphisms in the *p53* and *mdm2* genes that increase and decrease susceptibility and rare alleles of HRAS: cytochrome P-450 genes *CYP1A1, CYP2D6,* and *CYP19*; vitamin D receptor; and glutathione-S-transferase genes *GSTM1* and *GSTP1*.[125] These low penetrance genes add incrementally to breast cancer risk.

Microarray technology has been deployed to classify breast cancer into subtypes with specific gene expression profiles.[126–131] Botstein and colleagues have classified breast tumors into five subsets based on a marker profile indicative of a predominant cell type: luminal type A, luminal type B, basal epithelial, HER-2–positive, and "normal."[127] Their findings support the concept that tumors arise from different breast cell types. The luminal group had improved survival rates, whereas the basal and HER-2–positive subtypes had the worst survival rates. Basal cells have been proposed to represent bipotent stem-progenitor cells that give rise to both luminal and myoepithelial lineages. BRCA1 tumors display basal cell phenotypes. HER-2–positive cells are usually ER negative, a known indicator of poor survival.[130,131] This report also noted that gene expression patterns do not change substantially between early DCIS and later stages, indicating that the various molecular events in breast tumor progression occur before metastasis.[129] A second study by van't Veer and colleagues identified a set of 70 genes that together form a "poor prognosis signature."[128] These include cell cycle, invasion, metastatic, and angiogenic markers. Patients with the poor prognosis signature had almost half the likelihood of remaining free of metastases or of surviving 10 years compared with those of the "good prognosis" category. This gene expression signature predicts disease outcome with 83% accuracy, performing better than St. Gallen's and National Institutes of Health's (NIH) standards, which use histologic and clinical criteria.[132] However, the false-negative rate with this profile would result in undertreatment for 9% of patients and therefore requires further refinement before it can be used within a clinical setting. Several studies have evaluated the prognostic and predictive value of gene expression profiles found within early-stage breast cancer. Currently, issues of lack of validation of gene sets across platforms point to the need for further investigation and refinement of this otherwise promising approach.

What other cells promote tumorigenesis?

Although 90% of tumors are epithelial in origin, communication between different cell types within breast can contribute to tumor progression and metastasis. Myoepithelial cells modify the behavior and organization of epithelial cells.[133] For example, mammary epithelial cells plated onto plastic fail to differentiate. Addition of myoepithelial cells to the culture leads to correct apical polarization, tight junction formation, and differentiation.[134–136] Myoepithelial cells are thought to achieve this by secreting basement lamina components, such as laminin, and by regulating the access of luminal cells to these proteins. Normal myoepithelial cells have been proposed to act as natural tumor suppressors. Myoepithelial cells from human breast tumors fail to interact with epithelial cells and induce epithelial organization and show impaired laminin production capabilities.[137] Cells attach to proteins of the basal lamina, including collagens, fibronectin, and laminins, through members of the integrin family of cell surface receptors that are composed of α and β subunits. Integrin engagement by the ECM conveys critical survival and differentiating signals to epithelial cells.[138] They achieve these effects by synergizing with growth factors to cause sustained elevation of signaling pathways, including MAPK, GSK-3β, and PI3-K. The repertoire of integrins changes when cells become invasive. The importance of integrin-mediated survival signals has been vividly demonstrated in mice expressing MMTV-polyoma middle-T antigen. Inactivation of β_1-integrin induced apoptosis and inhibited metastasis.

Stromal cells surrounding the epithelial ducts and macrophages clustered in front of growing terminal end buds promote proliferation of epithelial cells by secreting growth factors, such as IGF-1, FGF-7, and CSF-1.[139] In addition, stromal cells can secrete proteins, such as scatter factor and hepatocyte growth factor, which induce changes in cell shape and motility, referred to as epithelial-to-mesenchymal transitions (EMTs), which induce migration.[140] Stromal cells further facilitate the processes of cell migration, extravasation, and metastasis by secreting proteases that degrade and compromise the basement membrane, remodel the extracellular matrix, and release and activate ECM-bound growth factors. Epithelial tumor cells stimulate stromal cells to secrete MMPs, a large family of ECM-degrading proteins that include collagenases, stromelysins, membrane-type MMPs, and gelatinases.[141] Many are secreted in latent precursor forms that are activated in a cascade fashion by other members of the family. MMP-3 and MMP-7 give rise to preneoplastic and malignant mammary tumors, respectively, in mice, and MMP-3$^{-/-}$ mice show decreased incidence of chemically induced tumorigenesis.[66,142,143] MMP-2, MMP-9, and MMP-11 are more highly expressed in invasive breast cancer than in premalignant and normal breast, and a higher ratio of activated to latent forms is present in breast cancer samples.[144] MT-MMP, MMP-2, and MMP-11 are secreted in the stromal compartment around tumors. MMP activity is regulated by a family of three tissue inhibitors of metalloproteinase (TIMPs), and the balance between MMPs and TIMPs likely regulates many aspects of invasive and metastatic phenotype. Paradoxically, high levels of TIMP-1 and TIMP-2 in breast tumors predict adverse outcome for patients.[144] The extracellular matrix surrounding tumors is remodeled by the action of MMPs in a unique fashion that exposes "tumor-specific" collagen epitopes.[145] The exposure of such cryptic epitopes assists migration and metastasis and promotes the formation of new blood vessels, a process known as angiogenesis.

What is the role of angiogenesis in breast cancer development and metastasis?

For tumors to grow to more than a few millimeters, an extensive neovasculature must develop to supply the tumor with oxygen and nutrients. A consistent body of experimental and clinical evidence has demonstrated the necessity of angiogenesis for the growth of solid tumors, including breast carcinoma.[146,147] Angiogenesis is observed in all phases of breast cancer from benign hyperplastic breast lesions to DCIS and invasive ductal cancers.[148,149] Tumor-associated angiogenesis is a complex process dependent on a variety of growth factors that are also associated with non-neoplastic vascularization seen in wound healing, ischemic tissue, reproduction, and development.[150,151] Non-neoplastic vascularization is a tightly regulated process balanced by angiogenesis activators (vascular endothelial growth factor [VEGF], FGF-2, platelet-derived growth factor [PDGF]) and inhibitors (thrombospondin-1, angiostatin, endostatin). In the developing tumor bed, angiogenesis occurs when the balance of regulators favors angiogenesis activators, which allows tumors to grow and metastasize to the detriment of the host.[152] The tumor vascular network is derived from two sources: sprouting of capillaries from preexisting blood vessels and endothelial progenitor cells (EPCs) that are mobilized from the bone marrow (BM).[153] Successful metastasis of a tumor is dependent on angiogenesis at both primary and metastatic sites. In order for a tumor cell to metastasize, it must gain access to the vasculature. In highly angiogenic tumors, multiple contact points between tumor cells and endothelial cells facilitates tumor cell entry into the circulation.[154]

What initiates angiogenesis?

There have been several proangiogenic factors described, the most potent of which is VEGF. Up-regulation of VEGF by a tumor will result in stimulation of local endothelial ingrowth into the tumor bed and recruitment of EPC to traffic from the BM to the tumor bed. There are several potential mechanisms for VEGF up-regulation in breast cancer. In the developing tumor bed as the mass of rapidly dividing cells enlarges, oxygen diffusion is limited, resulting in local hypoxia. Hypoxia is a potent angiogenic stimulus that triggers vessel growth through hypoxia-inducible transcription factor (HIF). HIF induces expression of the potent proangiogenic growth factor VEGF and its receptor VEGF receptor-1 (VEGFR-1). Higher levels of HIF are associated with more advanced pathologic stage in breast cancer and are higher in poorly differentiated tumors. Increased levels of HIF-1 are also associated with increased expression of VEGF, suggesting that increased levels of HIF-1 are potentially associated with more aggressive breast cancers.[155] HER-2/neu contributes to angiogenesis by up-regulating VEGF expression.[156] Breast cancer overexpression of MMP-9 promotes the release of sequestered VEGF from the extracellular matrix.[157] The net result of these early local factors is up-regulation of VEGF production, which can be found even in noninvasive high-grade DCIS.[158]

What factors are required for angiogenesis to progress?

The previous section should not be taken to suggest that VEGF is the lone growth factor responsible for angiogenesis; it merely outlines the most convincing data on the initiation of angiogenesis in breast cancer. Once angiogenesis is initiat-

ed and the tumor begins rapid growth, a host of additional factors, including FGF-2, Ang1, and placenta growth factor (PlGF), act in concert to maintain the developing vascular network. It is not clear why the balance favors proangiogenic factors over angiogenesis inhibitors such as angiostatin, endostatin, or thrombospondin-1. The new developing vascular channels are leaky in response to VEGF and allow extravasation of plasma proteins to provide a new matrix for endothelial cell migration. EPCs are recruited from the bone marrow by a complex sequence of events, whereby MMP-9 releases membrane-bound Kit ligand (mKitL), allowing soluble Kit ligand (sKitL) to induce trafficking of cKit-positive EPCs from the BM to the tumor.[159,160]

What is the effect of neovascularization on prognosis?

Several methods have been proposed to measure tumor angiogenesis.[161,162] Microvessel density has been accepted as the standard to evaluate the angiogenic potential of a tumor.[163] Using this technique, several studies have demonstrated an inverse relationship between survival of patients with breast cancer and angiogenesis measured by microvessel density.[147,164,165] The recognition that the level of tumor angiogenesis may predict a poor outcome in invasive cancer is valid for several solid malignancies. A unique finding in noninvasive breast cancer was that high-grade DCIS with increased vascularity, measured by microvascular density, was more likely to recur following resection.[149] In another series, inflammatory breast cancers expressed higher levels of proangiogenic mRNA (VEGF, flt-1, Ang1/2, Tie2) than noninflammatory breast cancers.[166]

An alternative measure of tumor angiogenic potential is the number of circulating endothelial progenitors (CEPs) in the peripheral circulation. CEPs are bone marrow–derived EPCs that are found in the peripheral circulation, in transit from the bone marrow as they traffic to the neovasculature of the tumor bed.[167,168] Resting and activated CEPs were found to be significantly increased in the peripheral blood of patients with breast cancer. CEPs decreased to healthy control levels following curative surgical resection.[167] Breast cancer patients have been found to have a fivefold increase in these cells when compared with non–tumor-bearing individuals. This observation was confirmed in another study that found CECs to be increased in cancer patients, including breast cancer patients, with progressive disease when compared with patients with stable disease.[169] These data would suggest that breast cancer is angiogenesis dependent even at the earliest stage and that the switch to an angiogenic phenotype is associated with more aggressive tumors.

What are the therapeutic implications of angiogenesis in breast cancer?

The ability to develop antiangiogenic strategies would be an important new weapon to treat breast cancer. Agents that inhibit angiogenesis have been shown to block tumor growth and promote tumor regression in animal models.[170,171] The translation of laboratory observations that inhibition of angiogenesis can block tumor growth and metastasis is now clinically applicable because angiogenesis inhibitors are being used to treat cancer patients.[172] One approach to breast cancer treatment is to target the potent proangiogenic growth factor VEGF. High tumor levels of VEGF have been associated with recurrence of node-negative breast cancer and resistance to radiation and systemic chemotherapy.[173–175]

Clinical trials of bevacizumab, a humanized monoclonal anti-VEGF antibody (Avastin), suggest that inhibition of angiogenesis is beneficial to patients with breast, renal cell, and colorectal cancer, although this agent is presently only approved for patients with colorectal cancer.[176–178] As the clinical experience with angiogenesis inhibitors grows, synergy between angiogenesis inhibitors and conventional chemotherapy may be exploited.[178] This is certainly one of the more exciting areas in anticancer therapy and will likely affect treatment in the near future.

REFERENCES

1. Oftedal OT. The origin of lactation as a water source for parchment-shelled eggs. J Mammary Gland Biol Neoplasia 2002;7:253–266.
2. Wysolmerski JJ. The evolutionary origins of maternal calcium and bone metabolism during lactation. J Mammary Gland Biol Neoplasia 2002;7:267–276.
3. Foley J, Dann P, Hong J, et al. Parathyroid hormone-related protein maintains mammary epithelial fate and triggers nipple skin differentiation during embryonic breast development. Development 2001;128:513–525.
4. van Genderen C, Okamura RM, Farinas I, et al. Development of several organs that require inductive epithelial-mesenchymal interactions is impaired in Lef-1 deficient mice. Genes Dev 1994;8:2691–2704.
5. Wysolmerski JJ, Cormier S, Philbrick WM, et al. Absence of functional type 1 parathyroid hormone (PTH)/PTH-related protein receptors in humans is associated with abnormal breast development and tooth impaction. J Clin Endocrinol Metab 2001;86:1788–1794.
6. Daniel CW, Silberstein GB. Postnatal development of the rodent mammary gland. In Neville MC, Daniel CW (eds). The Mammary Gland. New York, Plenum, 1987, pp 3–31.
7. Kleinberg DL, Feldman M, Ruan W. IGF-I: An essential factor in terminal end bud formation and ductal morphogenesis. J Mammary Gland Biol Neoplasia 2000;5:7–17.
8. Cunha GR, Young P, Hom YK, et al. Elucidation of a role for stromal steroid hormone receptors in mammary gland growth and development using tissue recombinants. J Mammary Gland Biol Neoplasia 1997;2:393–402.
9. Couse JF, Korach KS. Estrogen receptor null mice: What have we learned and where will they lead us? Endocr Rev 1999;20:358–417.
10. Park WC, Jordan VC. Selective estrogen receptor modulators (SERMS) and their roles in breast cancer prevention. Trends Mol Med 2002;8:82–88.
11. Luukkainen T. Issues to debate on the Women's Health Initiative: Failure of estrogen plus progestin therapy for prevention of breast cancer risk. Hum Reprod 2003;18:1559–1561.
12. Anderson E. The role of oestrogen and progesterone receptors in human mammary development and tumorigenesis. Breast Cancer Res 2002;4:197–201.
13. Wong CW, McNally C, Nickbarg E, et al. Estrogen receptor-interacting protein that modulates its nongenomic activity-crosstalk with Src/Erk phosphorylation cascade. Proc Natl Acad Sci U S A 2002;99:14783–14788.
14. Brzozowski AM, Pike AC, Dauter Z, et al. Molecular basis of agonism and antagonism in the oestrogen receptor. Nature 1997;389:753–758.
15. Lewis DF, Parker MG, King RJ. Molecular modelling of the human estrogen receptor and ligand interactions based on site-directed mutagenesis and amino acid sequence homology. J Steroid Biochem Mol Biol 1995;52:55–65.
16. Shang Y, Brown M. Molecular determinants for the tissue specificity of SERMs. Science 2002;295:2465–2468.
17. Baum M. Has tamoxifen had its day? Breast Cancer Res 2002;4:213–217.
18. Radice G, Ferreira-Cornwall C, Robinson SD, et al. Precocious mammary gland development in P-cadherin-deficient mice. J Cell Biol 1997;139:1025–1032.
19. Paredes J, Milanezi F, Reis-Filho JS, et al. Aberrant P-cadherin expression: Is it associated with estrogen-independent growth in breast cancer? Pathol Res Pract 2002;198:795–801.
20. Berx G, Cleton-Jansen AM, Nollet F, et al. E-cadherin is a tumour/invasion suppressor gene mutated in human lobular breast cancers. EMBO J 1995;14:6107–6115.
21. Eelkema R, Cowin P. General themes in cell-cell junctions and adhesion. In Cereijido M, Anderson J (eds). Tight Junctions. Boca Raton, FL, CRC Press, 2001, pp 121–145.
22. Boussadia O, Kutsch S, Hierholzer A, et al. E-cadherin is a survival factor for the lactating mouse mammary gland. Mech Dev 2002;115:53–62.
23. Berx G, Van Roy F. The E-cadherin/catenin complex: An important gatekeeper in breast cancer tumorigenesis and malignant progression. Breast Cancer Res 2001;3:289–293.
24. Hoschuetzky H, Aberle H, Kemler R. Beta-catenin mediates the interaction of the cadherin-catenin complex with epidermal growth factor receptor. J Cell Biol 1994;127:1375–1381.
25. D'Souza B, Taylor-Papadimitriou J. Overexpression of ERBB2 in human mammary epithelial cells signals inhibition of transcription of the E-cadherin gene. Proc Natl Acad Sci U S A 1994;91:7202–7206.
26. Hatsell S, Rowlands TR, Hiremath M, et al. The role of beta-catenin and Tcfs in mammary development and neoplasia. J Mammary Gland Biol Cancer 2003;8:143–156.
27. Litvinov SV, Balzar M, Winter MJ, et al. Epithelial cell adhesion molecule (Ep-CAM) modulates cell-cell interactions mediated by classic cadherins. J Cell Biol 1997;139:1337–1348.
28. Gastl G, Spizzo G, Obrist P, et al. Ep-CAM overexpression in breast cancer as a predictor of survival. Lancet 2000;356:1981–1982.
29. Nieman MT, Prdoff RS, Johnson KR, et al. N-cadherin promotes motility in human breast cancer cells regardless of their E-cadherin expression. J Cell Biol 2000;147:631–643.
30. Hazan RB, Phillips GR, Qiao RF, et al. Exogenous expression of N-cadherin in breast cancer cells induces cell migration, invasion and metastasis. J Cell Biol 2000;148:779–790.
31. Rimm DL, Sinard JH, Morrow JS. Reduced alpha-catenin and E-cadherin expression in breast cancer. Lab Invest 1995;72:506–512.
32. Pishvaian MJ, Feltes CM, Thompson P, et al. Cadherin-11 is expressed in invasive breast cancer cell lines. Cancer Res 1999;59:947–952.
33. Suyama K, Shapiro I, Guttman M, et al. A signaling pathway leading to metastasis is controlled by N-cadherin and the FGF receptor. Cancer Cell 2002;2:301–314.
34. Chung GG, Zerkowski MP, Ocal IT, et al. beta-Catenin and p53 analyses of a breast carcinoma tissue microarray. Cancer 2004;100:2084–2092.
35. Imbert A, Eelkema R, Jordan S, et al. ΔN89ß-catenin induces precocious development, differentiation, and neoplasia in mammary gland. J Cell Biol 2001;153:555–568.
36. Sommers CL, Gelmann EL, Kemler R, et al. Alterations in beta-catenin phosphorylation and plakoglobin expression in human breast cancer cells. Cancer Res 1994;54:3544–3552.
37. Lin SY, Xia W, Wang JC, et al. Beta-catenin, a novel prognostic marker for breast cancer: Its roles in cyclin D1 expression and cancer progression. Proc Natl Acad Sci U S A 2000;97:4262–4266.
38. Klus GT, Rokaeus N, Bittner ML, et al. Down-regulation of the desmosomal cadherin desmocollin 3 in human breast cancer. Int J Oncol 2001;19:169–174.
39. Fujita N, Jaye DL, Kajita M, et al. MTA3, a Mi-2/NuRD complex subunit, regulates an invasive growth pathway in breast cancer. Cell 2003;113:207–219.
40. Fearon ER. Connecting estrogen receptor function, transcriptional repression, and E-cadherin expression in breast cancer. Cancer Cell 2003;3:307–310.
41. Cano A, Perez-Moreno MA, Rodrigo I, et al. The transcription factor snail controls epithelial-mesenchymal transitions by repressing E-cadherin expression. Nat Cell Biol 2000;2:76–83.
42. Chen S, Itoh T, Wu K, et al. Transcriptional regulation of aromatase expression in human breast tissue. J Steroid Biochem Mol Biol 2002;83:93–99.

43. Hajra KM, Chen DY, Fearon ER. The SLUG zinc-finger protein represses E-cadherin in breast cancer. Cancer Res 2002;62:1613–1618.

44. Blanco MJ, Moreno-Bueno G, Sarrio D, et al. Correlation of snail expression with histological grade and lymph node status in breast carcinomas. Oncogene 2002;21:3241–3246.

45. Bai J, Uehara Y, Montell DJ. Regulation of invasive cell behavior by taiman, a Drosophila protein related to AIB1, a steroid receptor coactivator amplified in breast cancer. Cell 2000;103:1047–1058.

46. Montell DJ. Command and control: Regulatory pathways controlling invasive behavior of the border cells. Mech Dev 2001;105:19–25.

47. Neubauer BL, Best KL, Counts DF, et al. Raloxifene (LY156758) produces antimetastatic responses and extends survival in the PAIII rat prostatic adenocarcinoma model. Prostate 1995;27:220–229.

48. Lee AV, Jackson JG, Gooch JL, et al. Enhancement of insulin-like growth factor signaling in human breast cancer: Estrogen regulation of insulin receptor substrate-1 expression in vitro and in vivo. Mol Endocrinol 1999;13:787–796.

49. Hadsell DL, Bonnette SG. IGF and insulin action in the mammary gland: lessons from transgenic and knockout models. J Mammary Gland Biol Neoplasia 2000;5:19–30.

50. Watson CJ. Stat transcription factors in mammary gland development and tumorigenesis. J Mammary Gland Biol Neoplasia 2001;6:115–127.

51. Renehan AG, Zwahlen M, Minder C, et al. Insulin-like growth factor (IGF)-I, IGF binding protein-3, and cancer risk: Systematic review and meta-regression analysis. Lancet 2004;363:1346–1353.

52. Laban C, Bustin SA, Jenkins PJ. The GH-IGF-I axis and breast cancer. Trends Endocrinol Metab 2003;14:28–34.

53. Hynes NE. Tyrosine kinase signalling in breast cancer. Breast Cancer Res 2000;2:154–157.

54. Hackel PO, Zwick E, Prenzel N, et al. Epidermal growth factor receptors: Critical mediators of multiple receptor pathways. Curr Opin Cell Biol 1999;11:184–189.

55. Stern DF. ErbBs in mammary development. Exp Cell Res 2003;284:89–98.

56. Slamon DJ, Clark GM, Wong SG, et al. Human breast cancer: Correlation of relapse and survival with amplification of the HER-2/neu oncogene. Science 1987;235:177–182.

57. Muller WJ, Sinn E, Pattengale PK, et al. Single-step induction of mammary adenocarcinoma in transgenic mice bearing the activated c-neu oncogene. Cell 1988;54:105–115.

58. Guy CT, Webster MA, Schaller M, et al. Expression of the neu protooncogene in the mammary epithelium of transgenic mice induces metastatic disease. Proc Natl Acad Sci U S A 1992;89:10578–10582.

59. Arteaga CL. Trastuzumab, an appropriate first-line single-agent therapy for HER2-overexpressing metastatic breast cancer. Breast Cancer Res 2003;5:96–100.

60. Schroeder JA, Adriance MC, McConnell EJ, et al. ErbB-beta-catenin complexes are associated with human infiltrating ductal breast and murine mammary tumor virus (MMTV)-Wnt-1 and MMTV-c-Neu transgenic carcinomas. J Biol Chem 2002;277:22692–22698.

61. Ramsauer VP, Carraway CA, Salas PJ, et al. Muc4/sialomucin complex, the intramembrane ErbB2 ligand, translocates ErbB2 to the apical surface in polarized epithelial cells. J Biol Chem 2003;278:30142–30147.

62. Lydon JP, DeMayo FJ, Funk CR, et al. Mice lacking progesterone receptor exhibit pleiotropic reproductive abnormalities. Genes Dev 1995;9:2266–2278.

63. Brisken C, Heineman A, Chavarra T, et al. Essential function of Wnt-4 in mammary gland development downstream of progesterone signaling. Genes Dev 2000;14:650–654.

64. Wang TC, Cardiff RD, Zukerberg L, et al. Mammary hyperplasia and carcinoma in MMTV-cyclin D1 transgenic mice. Nature 1994;369:669–671.

65. Witty JP, Wright JH, Matrisian LM. Matrix metalloproteinases are expressed during ductal and alveolar mammary morphogenesis, and misregulation of stromelysin-1 in transgenic mice induces unscheduled alveolar development. Mol Biol Cell 1995;6:1287–1303.

66. Rudolph-Owen LA, Matrisian LM. Matrix metalloproteinases in remodeling of the normal and neoplastic mammary gland. J Mammary Gland Biol Neoplasia 1998;3:177–189.

67. Hsu W, Shakya R, Costantini F. Impaired mammary gland and lymphoid development caused by inducible expression of Axin in transgenic mice. J Cell Biol 2001;155:1055–1064.

68. Tepera SB, McCrea PD, Rosen JM. A beta-catenin survival signal is required for normal lobular development in the mammary gland. J Cell Sci 2003;116:1137–1149.

69. Fantl V, Stamp G, Andrews A, et al. Mice lacking cyclin D1 are small and show defects in eye and mammary gland development. Genes Dev 1995;9:2364–2372.

70. Fata JE, Kong YY, Li J, et al. The osteoclast differentiation factor osteoprotegerin-ligand is essential for mammary gland development. Cell 2000;103:41–50.

71. Seagroves TN, Krnacik S, Raught B, et al. C/EBPbeta, but not C/EBPalpha, is essential for ductal morphogenesis, lobuloalveolar proliferation, and functional differentiation in the mouse mammary gland. Genes Dev 1998;12:1917–1928.

72. Ormandy CJ, Camus A, Barra J, et al. Null mutation of the prolactin receptor gene produces multiple reproductive defects in the mouse. Genes Dev 1997;11:167–178.

73. Kelly PA, Bachelot A, Kedzia C, et al. The role of prolactin and growth hormone in mammary gland development. Mol Cell Endocrinol 2002;197:127–131.

74. Liu X, Robinson GW, Wagner KU, et al. Stat5a is mandatory for adult mammary gland development and lactogenesis. Genes Dev 1997;11:179–186.

75. Sympson CJ, Talhouk RS, Alexander CM, et al. Targeted expression of stromelysin-1 in mammary gland provides evidence for a role of proteinases in branching morphogenesis and the requirement for an intact basement membrane for tissue-specific gene expression. J Cell Biol 1994;125:681–693.

76. Sympson CJ, Bissell MJ, Werb Z. Mammary gland tumor formation in transgenic mice overexpressing stromelysin-1. Semin Cancer Biol 1995;6:159–163.

77. Ismail PM, Li J, DeMayo FJ, et al. A novel LacZ reporter mouse reveals complex regulation of the progesterone receptor promoter during mammary gland development. Mol Endocrinol 2002;16:2475–2489.

78. Grimm SL, Seagroves TN, Kabotyanski EB, et al. Disruption of steroid and prolactin receptor patterning in the mammary gland correlates with a block in lobuloalveolar development. Mol Endocrinol 2002;16:2675–2691.

79. Grimm SL, Rosen JM. The role of C/EBPbeta in mammary gland development and breast cancer. J Mammary Gland Biol Cancer 2003;8:191–204.

80. Anderson E, Clarke R, Howell A. Estrogen responsiveness and control of normal human breast proliferation. J Mammary Gland Biol Neoplasia 1998;3:23–35.

81. Anderson E, Clarke RB. Epithelial stem cells in the mammary gland: Casting light into dark corners. Breast Cancer Res 1999;1:11–13.

82. Rowlands TR, Pechenkina I, Hatsell SJ, et al. Dissecting the roles of beta-catenin and cyclin D1 during mammary development and neoplasia. Proc Nat Acad Sci U S A 2003;100:11400–11405.

83. Brisken C, Park S, Vass T, et al. A paracrine role for the epithelial progesterone receptor in mammary gland development. Proc Natl Acad Sci U S A 1998;95:5076–5081.

84. Mulac-Jericevic B, Lydon JP, DeMayo FJ, et al. Defective mammary gland morphogenesis in mice lacking the progesterone receptor B isoform. Proc Natl Acad Sci U S A 2003;100:9744–9749.

85. Tsukamoto A, Grosschedl R, Guzman R, et al. Expression of the int-1 gene in transgenic mice is associated with mammary gland hyperplasia and adenocarcinomas in male and female mice. Cell 1988;55:619–625.

86. Reya T, Morrison SJ, Clarke MF, et al. Stem cells, cancer, and cancer stem cells. Nature 2001;414:105–111.

87. Waterworth A. Introducing the concept of breast cancer stem cells. Breast Cancer Res 2004;6:53–54.

88. Goodell MA. Multipotential stem cells and "side population" cells. Cytotherapy 2002;4:507–508.

89. Domen J, Cheshier SH, Weissman IL. The role of apoptosis in the regulation of hematopoietic stem cells: Overexpression of Bcl-2 increases both their number and repopulation potential. J Exp Med 2000;191:253–264.

90. Zhou S, Morris JJ, Barnes Y, et al. Bcrp1 gene expression is required for normal numbers of side population stem cells in mice, and confers relative protection to mitoxantrone in hematopoietic cells in vivo. Proc Natl Acad Sci U S A 2002;99:12339–12344.

91. Zhou S, Schuetz JD, Bunting KD, et al. The ABC transporter Bcrp1/ABCG2 is expressed in a wide variety of stem cells and is a molecular determinant of the side-population phenotype. Nat Med 2001;7:1028–1034.

92. Li Y, Welm B, Podsypanina K, et al. Evidence that transgenes encoding components of the Wnt signaling pathway preferentially induce

mammary cancers from progenitor cells. Proc Natl Acad Sci U S A 2003;100:15853–15858.

93. Al-Hajj M, Becker MW, Wicha M, et al. Therapeutic implications of cancer stem cells. Curr Opin Genet Dev 2004;14:43–47.

94. Al-Hajj M, Wicha MS, Benito-Hernandez A, et al. Prospective identification of tumorigenic breast cancer cells. Proc Natl Acad Sci U S A 2003;100:3983–3988.

95. Smith GH. Experimental mammary epithelial morphogenesis in an in vivo model: Evidence for distinct cellular progenitors of the ductal and lobular phenotype. Breast Cancer Res Treat 1996;39:21–31.

96. Smith GH, Boulanger CA. Mammary epithelial stem cells: transplantation and self-renewal analysis. Cell Prolif 2003;36(Suppl 1):3–15.

97. Chepko G, Smith GH. Three division-competent, structurally-distinct cell populations contribute to murine mammary epithelial renewal. Tissue Cell 1997;29:239–253.

98. Smalley M, Ashworth A. Stem cell and breast cancer: A field study. Nat Rev Cancer 2003;3:832–844.

99. Welm BE, Tepera SB, Venezia T, et al. Sca-1(pos) cells in the mouse mammary gland represent an enriched progenitor cell population. Dev Biol 2002;245:42–56.

100. Alvi AJ, Clayton H, Joshi C, et al. Functional and molecular characterisation of mammary side population cells. Breast Cancer Res 2003;5:R1–8.

101. Dontu G, Al-Hajj M, Abdallah WM, et al. Stem cells in normal breast development and breast cancer. Cell Prolif 2003;36(Suppl 1):59–72.

102. Liu BY, McDermott SP, Khwaja SS, et al. The transforming activity of Wnt effectors correlates with their ability to induce the accumulation of mammary progenitor cells. Proc Natl Acad Sci U S A 2004;101:4158–4163.

103. Sicinski P, Donaher JL, Parker SB, et al. Cyclin D1 provides a link between development and oncogenesis in the retina and breast. Cell 1995;82:621–630.

104. Dickson C, Fantl V, Gillett C, et al. Amplification of chromosome band 11q13 and a role for cyclin D1 in human breast cancer. Cancer Lett 1995;90:43–50.

105. Yu Q, Geng Y, Sicinski P. Specific protection against breast cancers by cyclin D1 ablation. Nature 2001;411:1017–1021.

106. Lamb J, Ramaswamy S, Ford H, et al. A mechanism of cyclin D1 action encoded in the patterns of gene expression in human cancer. Cell 2003;114:323–334.

107. Rowlands TM, Pechenkina IV, Hatsell S, et al. Beta-catenin and cyclin D1: Connecting development to breast cancer. Cell Cycle 2004;3:145–148.

108. Rosen JM. Striking it rich by data mining. Cell 2003;114:271–272.

109. Chiarle R, Pagano M, Inghirami G. The cyclin dependent kinase inhibitor p27 and its prognostic role in breast cancer. Breast Cancer Res 2001;3:91–94.

110. Winters ZE, Hunt NC, Bradburn MJ, et al. Subcellular localisation of cyclin B, Cdc2 and p21(WAF1/CIP1) in breast cancer. Association with prognosis. Eur J Cancer 2001;37:2405–2412.

111. Blackburn AC, Jerry DJ. Knockout and transgenic mice of Trp53: What have we learned about p53 in breast cancer? Breast Cancer Res 2002;4:101–111.

112. Gasco M, Shami S, Crook T. The p53 pathway in breast cancer. Breast Cancer Res 2002;4:70–76.

113. Varley JM, Evans DG, Birch JM. Li-Fraumeni syndrome—a molecular and clinical review. Br J Cancer 1997;76:1–14.

114. Chapman RS, Lourenco PC, Tonner E, et al. Suppression of epithelial apoptosis and delayed mammary gland involution in mice with a conditional knockout of Stat3. Genes Dev 1999;13:2604–2616.

115. Dolled-Filhart M, Camp RL, Kowalski DP, et al. Tissue microarray analysis of signal transducers and activators of transcription 3 (Stat3) and phospho-Stat3 (Tyr705) in node-negative breast cancer shows nuclear localization is associated with a better prognosis. Clin Cancer Res 2003;9:594–600.

116. Clarke RB, Howell A, Potten CS, et al. P27(KIP1) expression indicates that steroid receptor-positive cells are a non-proliferating, differentiated subpopulation of the normal human breast epithelium. Eur J Cancer 2000;36(Suppl 4):S28–29.

117. Deng CX, Brodie SG. Roles of BRCA1 and its interacting proteins. Bioessays 2000;22:728–737.

118. Snouwaert JN, Gowen LC, Latour AM, et al. BRCA1 deficient embryonic stem cells display a decreased homologous recombination frequency and an increased frequency of non-homologous recombination that is corrected by expression of a brca1 transgene. Oncogene 1999;18:7900–7907.

119. Fan S, Wang J, Yuan R, et al. BRCA1 inhibition of estrogen receptor signaling in transfected cells. Science 1999;284:1354–1356.

120. Hashizume R, Fukuda M, Maeda I, et al. The RING heterodimer BRCA1-BARD1 is a ubiquitin ligase inactivated by a breast cancer-derived mutation. J Biol Chem 2001;276:14537–14540.

121. Wooster R, Bignell G, Lancaster J, et al. Identification of the breast cancer susceptibility gene BRCA2. Nature 1995;378:789–792.

122. Xu X, Wagner KU, Larson D, et al. Conditional mutation of Brca1 in mammary epithelial cells results in blunted ductal morphogenesis and tumour formation. Nat Genet 1999;22:37–43.

123. Cheung AM, Elia A, Tsao MS, et al. Brca2 deficiency does not impair mammary epithelium development but promotes mammary adenocarcinoma formation in p53(+/−) mutant mice. Cancer Res 2004;64:1959–1965.

124. Nathanson KL, Weber BL. "Other" breast cancer susceptibility genes: Searching for more holy grail. Hum Mol Genet 2001;10:715–720.

125. de Jong MM, Nolte IM, Meerman GJ, et al. Genes other than BRCA1 and BRCA2 involved in breast cancer susceptibility. J Med Genet 2002;39:225–242.

126. Zhao H, Langerod A, Ji Y, et al. Different gene expression patterns in invasive lobular and ductal carcinomas of the breast. Mol Biol Cell 2004;15:2523–2536.

127. Sorlie T, Tibshirani R, Parker J, et al. Repeated observation of breast tumor subtypes in independent gene expression data sets. Proc Natl Acad Sci U S A 2003;100:8418–8423.

128. van't Veer LJ, Dai H, van de Vijver MJ, et al. Gene expression profiling predicts clinical outcome of breast cancer. Nature 2002;415:530–536.

129. Perou CM, Sorlie T, Eisen MB, et al. Molecular portraits of human breast tumours. Nature 2000;406:747–752.

130. Bertucci F, Eisinger F, Houlgatte R, et al. Gene-expression profiling and identification of patients at high risk of breast cancer. Lancet 2002;360:173–174.

131. Bertucci F, Houlgatte R, Granjeaud S, et al. Prognosis of breast cancer and gene expression profiling using DNA arrays. Ann N Y Acad Sci 2002;975:217–231.

132. van de Vijver MJ, He YD, van't Veer LJ, et al. A gene-expression signature as a predictor of survival in breast cancer. N Engl J Med 2002;347:1999–2009.

133. Deugnier MA, Teuliere J, Faraldo MM, et al. The importance of being a myoepithelial cell. Breast Cancer Res 2002;4:224–230.

134. Streuli CH, Schmidhauser C, Bailey N, et al. Laminin mediates tissue-specific gene expression in mammary epithelia. J Cell Biol 1995;129:591–603.

135. Gudjonsson T, Ronnov-Jessen L, Villadsen R, et al. To create the correct microenvironment: Three-dimensional heterotypic collagen assays for human breast epithelial morphogenesis and neoplasia. Methods 2003;30:247–255.

136. Runswick SK, O'Hare MJ, Jones L, et al. Desmosomal adhesion regulates epithelial morphogenesis and cell positioning. Nat Cell Biol 2001;3:823–830.

137. Gudjonsson T, Ronnov-Jessen L, Villadsen R, et al. Normal and tumor-derived myoepithelial cells differ in their ability to interact with luminal breast epithelial cells for polarity and basement membrane deposition. J Cell Sci 2002;115:39–50.

138. Deugnier MA, Faraldo MM, Rousselle P, et al. Cell-extracellular matrix interactions and EGF are important regulators of the basal mammary epithelial cell phenotype. J Cell Sci 1999;112(Pt 7):1035–1044.

139. Lin EY, Pollard JW. Macrophages: Modulators of breast cancer progression. Novartis Found Symp 2004;256:158–172, 259–269.

140. Rosario M, Birchmeier W. How to make tubes: Signaling by the Met receptor tyrosine kinase. Trends Cell Biol 2003;13:328–335.

141. Fata JE, Werb Z, Bissell MJ. Regulation of mammary gland branching morphogenesis by the extracellular matrix and its remodeling enzymes. Breast Cancer Res 2004;6:1–11.

142. Sternlicht MD, Lochter A, Sympson CJ, et al. The stromal proteinase MMP3/stromelysin-1 promotes mammary carcinogenesis. Cell 1999;98:137–146.

143. Masson R, Lefebvre O, Noel A, et al. In vivo evidence that the stromelysin-3 metalloproteinase contributes in a paracrine manner to epithelial cell malignancy. J Cell Biol 1998;140:1535–1541.

144. Duffy MJ, Maguire TM, Hill A, et al. Metalloproteinases: Role in breast carcinogenesis, invasion and metastasis. Breast Cancer Res 2000;2:252–257.

145. Hangai M, Kitaya N, Xu J, et al. Matrix metalloproteinase-9-dependent exposure of a cryptic migratory control site in collagen is

required before retinal angiogenesis. Am J Pathol 2002;161:1429–1437.

146. Hanahan D, Folkman J. Patterns and emerging mechanisms of the angiogenic switch during tumorigenesis. Cell 1996;86:353–364.

147. Uzzan B, Nicolas P, Cucherat M, et al. Microvessel density as a prognostic factor in women with breast cancer: A systematic review of the literature and meta-analysis. Cancer Res 2004;64:2941–2955.

148. Brem SS, Jensen HM, Gullino PM. Angiogenesis as a marker of preneoplastic lesions of the human breast. Cancer 1978;41:239–244.

149. Engels K, Fox SB, Whitehouse RM, et al. Distinct angiogenic patterns are associated with high-grade in situ ductal carcinomas of the breast. J Pathol 1997;181:207–212.

150. Asahara T, Masuda H, Takahashi T, et al. Bone marrow origin of endothelial progenitor cells responsible for postnatal vasculogenesis in physiological and pathological neovascularization. Circ Res 1999;85:221–228.

151. Luttun A, Tjwa M, Moons L, et al. Revascularization of ischemic tissues by PlGF treatment, and inhibition of tumor angiogenesis, arthritis and atherosclerosis by anti-Flt1. Nat Med 2002;8:831–840.

152. Baillie CT, Winslet MC, Bradley NJ. Tumour vasculature: A potential therapeutic target. Br J Cancer 1995;72:257–267.

153. Yancopoulos GD, Klagsbrun M, Folkman J. Vasculogenesis, angiogenesis, and growth factors: Ephrins enter the fray at the border. Cell 1998;93:661–664.

154. Takeda A, Stoeltzing O, Ahmad SA, et al. Role of angiogenesis in the development and growth of liver metastasis. Ann Surg Oncol 2002;9:610–616.

155. Bos R, Zhong H, Hanrahan CF, et al. Levels of hypoxia-inducible factor-1 alpha during breast carcinogenesis. J Natl Cancer Inst 2001;93:309–314.

156. Petit AM, Rak J, Hung MC, et al. Neutralizing antibodies against epidermal growth factor and ErbB-2/neu receptor tyrosine kinases down-regulate vascular endothelial growth factor production by tumor cells in vitro and in vivo: Angiogenic implications for signal transduction therapy of solid tumors. Am J Pathol 1997;151:1523–1530.

157. Bergers G, Brekken R, McMahon G, et al. Matrix metalloproteinase-9 triggers the angiogenic switch during carcinogenesis. Nat Cell Biol 2000;2:737–744.

158. Guidi AJ, Schnitt SJ, Fischer L, et al. Vascular permeability factor (vascular endothelial growth factor) expression and angiogenesis in patients with ductal carcinoma in situ of the breast. Cancer 1997;80:1945–1953.

159. Heissig B, Hattori K, Dias S, et al. Recruitment of stem and progenitor cells from the bone marrow niche requires MMP-9 mediated release of kit-ligand. Cell 2002;109:625–637.

160. Heissig B, Hattori K, Friedrich M, et al. Angiogenesis: Vascular remodeling of the extracellular matrix involves metalloproteinases. Curr Opin Hematol 2003;10:136–141.

161. Brower V. Evidence of efficacy: Researchers investigating markers for angiogenesis inhibitors. J Natl Cancer Inst 2003;95:1425–1427.

162. Davis DW, McConkey DJ, Abbruzzese JL, et al. Surrogate markers in antiangiogenesis clinical trials. Br J Cancer 2003;89:8–14.

163. Willett CG, Boucher Y, di Tomaso E, et al. Direct evidence that the VEGF-specific antibody bevacizumab has antivascular effects in human rectal cancer. Nat Med 2004;10:145–147.

164. Weidner N, Folkman J, Pozza F, et al. Tumor angiogenesis: A new significant and independent prognostic indicator in early-stage breast carcinoma. J Natl Cancer Inst 1992;84:1875–1887.

165. Weidner N, Semple JP, Welch WR, et al. Tumor angiogenesis and metastasis—correlation in invasive breast carcinoma. N Engl J Med 1991;324:1–8.

166. Shirakawa K, Kobayashi H, Heike Y, et al. Hemodynamics in vasculogenic mimicry and angiogenesis of inflammatory breast cancer xenograft. Cancer Res 2002;62:560–566.

167. Mancuso P, Burlini A, Pruneri G, et al. Resting and activated endothelial cells are increased in the peripheral blood of cancer patients. Blood 2001;97:3658–3661.

168. Mancuso P, Calleri A, Cassi C, et al. Circulating endothelial cells as a novel marker of angiogenesis. Adv Exp Med Biol 2003;522:83–97.

169. Beerepoot LV, Mehra N, Vermaat JSP, et al. Increased levels of viable circulating endothelial cells are an indicator of progressive disease in cancer patients. Ann Oncol 2004;15:139–145.

170. O'Reilly MS, Holmgren L, Chen C, et al. Angiostatin induces and sustains dormancy of human primary tumors in mice. Nat Med 1996;2:689–692.

171. Parangi S, O'Reilly M, Christofori G, et al. Antiangiogenic therapy of transgenic mice impairs de novo tumor growth. Proc Natl Acad Sci U S A 1996;93:2002–2007.

172. Davis DW, McConkey DJ, Zhang W, et al. Antiangiogenic tumor therapy. Biotechniques 2003;34:1048.

173. Gasparini G, Toi M, Gion M, et al. Prognostic significance of vascular endothelial growth factor protein in node-negative breast carcinoma. J Natl Cancer Inst 1997;89:139–147.

174. Foekens JA, Peters HA, Grebenchtchikov N, et al. High tumor levels of vascular endothelial growth factor predict poor response to systemic therapy in advanced breast cancer. Cancer Res 2001;61:5407–5414.

175. Manders P, Sweep FC, Tjan–Heijnen VC, et al. Vascular endothelial growth factor independently predicts the efficacy of postoperative radiotherapy in node-negative breast cancer patients. Clin Cancer Res 2003;9:6363–6370.

176. Rugo HS. Bevacizumab in the treatment of breast cancer: Rationale and current data. Oncologist 2004;9(Suppl 1):43–49.

177. Yang JC, Haworth L, Sherry RM, et al. A randomized trial of bevacizumab, an anti-vascular endothelial growth factor antibody, for metastatic renal cancer. N Engl J Med 2003;349:427–434.

178. Kabbinavar F, Hurwitz HI, Fehrenbacher L, et al. Phase II, randomized trial comparing bevacizumab plus fluorouracil (FU)/leucovorin (LV) with FU/LV alone in patients with metastatic colorectal cancer. J Clin Oncol 2003;21:60–65.

Alterations in hormone levels are thought to influence breast carcinogenesis through several mechanisms. One hypothesis is that the total number of ovulatory cycles, and thus exposure to higher estrogen levels, is the principal factor contributing to the risk for breast cancer.[28,29] Estrogen exposure may contribute to carcinogenesis by increasing the rate of cell division and proliferation, thereby allowing for an increase in the accumulation of random genetic errors.[29,30] Another hypothesis is that the continued cell division and proliferation resulting from multiple ovulatory cycles, principally between menarche and first birth, increases the susceptibility of breast tissue to carcinogenic environmental insults.[31] The duration of exposure to both endogenous and exogenous estrogens is directly related to the risk for developing breast cancer. The role of prolactin in breast cancer development has been clearly established in the rat, but no clearcut role for prolactin has yet been established in humans.

What menstrual and reproductive factors influence breast cancer risks?

1. *Age at menarche.* One of the most significant associations established to date is age at menarche and subsequent development of breast cancer. Early age at menarche has been demonstrated as a risk factor for breast cancer in most case-control studies. Each earlier year of onset of menarche appears to add about 4% to 5% to the risk for breast cancer.[28,32] Women with early menarche (≤12 years of age) and rapid establishment of regular cycles have an almost fourfold greater risk for breast cancer than women with late menarche (≥13 years of age) and long duration of irregular cycles.[33,34]

2. *Age at menopause.* Age at menopause is another factor in breast cancer risk. Premenopausal women who undergo oophorectomy dramatically lower their risk for breast cancer. As mentioned earlier, bilateral oophorectomy before the age of 40 years reduces breast cancer risk by at least 50%.[27] In similar fashion, women who experience natural menopause (defined as cessation of periods) before age 45 years have only half the breast cancer risk of those in whom

menopause occurs after age 55 years.[35] Each additional year until menopause adds a risk of about 4%.[35] The influences of menarcheal and menopausal age may partly explain some of the geographic variance in breast cancer incidence around the world.[36] For example, in Asian countries, the age at menarche is later and menopause occurs earlier than in the United States. The expected lower breast cancer incidence is observed in Asian women.

3. *Age at first term pregnancy.* Parity and age at first birth are other endogenous hormonal factors that influence breast cancer risk. Nulliparous women are at greater risk for the development of breast cancer than parous women, with a relative risk of 1.4.[37] The age at first birth is extremely important for subsequent development of breast cancer. Age younger than 20 years at first childbirth can reduce breast cancer risk by about 50%, compared with first birth beyond age 35 years.[37–39] Abortion, whether spontaneous or induced, before full-term pregnancy has no protective effect and has been shown to increase breast cancer risk.[40] Breast-feeding, once thought to decrease the risk for breast cancer and then abandoned as a factor in decreasing breast cancer risk, has been restudied and does appear to have a small protective effect.[41]

Does the use of oral contraceptives predispose to the development of breast cancer?

Oral contraceptives were introduced in the 1960s and each year are taken by millions of women. On the basis of proposed hypotheses of breast carcinogenesis, a role for exogenous hormones, such as oral contraceptives and hormone replacement therapy, might be expected. Numerous studies examining the association between exogenous hormones and the risk for breast cancer have been published. The results are conflicting and difficult to interpret because of changes in dose of hormones over time and in methods of delivery (e.g., sequential versus combination).

When the overall risk for breast cancer in birth control pill users has been studied in large populations, no increased risk has been seen (Fig. 4–4). Despite this, there is continuing

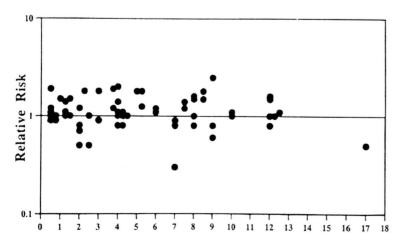

Figure 4–4 The relative risk for being diagnosed with breast cancer as a function of years of birth control pill (BCP) usage (summary of 17 studies). Almost all studies cluster around a relative risk of 1, indicating no influence of birth control pills on the occurrence of breast cancer. (Data from Abeloff MD, Lichter AS, Niederhuber JE, et al. Breast. In Abeloff MD, Armitage JO, Lichter AS, et al. [eds]. Clinical Oncology. New York, Churchill Livingstone, 1995, p 1626; adapted from Schlesselman JJ. Cancer of the breast and reproductive tract in relation to use of oral contraceptives. Contraception 1989;40:1–39.)

Years of BCP Use

concern about the potential risks in several subgroups. Several studies have demonstrated an increased risk for breast cancer in long-term users of oral contraceptives. Risk estimates range from 1.7 for use longer than 8 years to 4.1 for use for 10 or more years.[42-46] One of the largest case-control studies, the Cancer and Steroid Hormone Study,[47] found no association between breast cancer and oral contraceptive use for women up to the age of 54 years. A risk was again found only among a subgroup of women, that is, those who experienced menarche before age 13 years and who had used oral contraceptives for at least 10 years before the birth of their first child.[48] At present, oral contraceptive use appears to be safe and beneficial to women, especially women older than 25 years and women who have already had their first pregnancy.

Are replacement estrogens safe for postmenopausal women?

Many studies and meta-analyses have examined the possible relation between estrogen replacement therapy and breast cancer. Most studies have found no association between breast cancer and short-term use of replacement estrogens (5 years or less).[49-52] Several meta-analyses have discovered an increase in relative risk for development of breast cancer for each year after 5 years of estrogen use.[53-55] The highest risk calculated was 1.3 (95% confidence interval, 1.2–1.6) for more than 15 years of use.[51]

Hormone use has dropped sharply since July 2002, when a large study in the United States called the Women's Health Initiative was stopped ahead of schedule because it detected an increased risk for breast cancer in women who took Prempro, a widely used hormone combination.[56] The Women's Health Initiative included 16,608 postmenopausal women aged 50 to 79 years with an intact uterus at baseline recruited by 40 U.S. clinical centers from 1993 to 1998. Participants received conjugated equine estrogens, 0.625 mg/day, plus medroxyprogesterone acetate, 2.5 mg/day in one tablet (n = 8506) or placebo (n = 8102). On May 31, 2002, after a mean of 5.2 years of follow-up, the Data and Safety monitoring board recommended stopping the trial because the test statistic for invasive breast cancer exceeded the stopping boundary. The hazard ratio for breast cancer in the patients who received hormone replacement therapy was 1.26 (166 invasive cancers on Prempro versus 124 on placebo). The 26% excess of breast cancer is consistent with estimates from pooled epidemiologic data, which reported a 15% increase for estrogen plus progestin use for less than 5 years and a 53% increase for use for more than 5 years. In summary, overall health risks exceeded benefit from use of combined estrogen plus progestin for an average 5.2-year follow-up among healthy postmenopausal U.S. women.

Does a family history of breast cancer affect other risk factors for this disease?

Older studies suggest that the use of estrogen replacement therapy by postmenopausal women with a positive family history of breast cancer has been associated with an elevated risk for breast cancer.[57-60] In similar fashion, estrogen use in women with benign breast disease has been associated with an increased risk for the development of breast cancer.[61,62]

Recently, a large prospective study was performed to determine the effect of a family history of breast cancer on other risk factors for this disease. A cohort of 89,132 women aged 30 to 55 years was followed for 14 years (1.1 million person-years of follow-up). Reproductive factors were associated with different degrees of risk in women with and without a family history of breast cancer.[63] In women with a family history of breast cancer, there was little protection from later age at menarche; no protection from multiple births when compared with nulliparity; and no protection from early, as compared with later, age at first birth. The most significant finding was a consistent increase in risk for breast cancer among women with a mother or sister with a history of the disease that was exacerbated by first pregnancy. This adverse effect of pregnancy persisted to age 70 years. In contrast, among women with no family history of breast cancer, first pregnancy was associated with a smaller risk. The greater magnitude of the adverse effect of first pregnancy among women with a positive family history of breast cancer is consistent with the hypothesis that a subset of these women inherit genetic changes that are multiplied during cell proliferation of first pregnancy. History of benign breast disease, past use of oral contraceptives, and use of postmenopausal hormones showed relative risks that did not differ between women with a family history and those without a family history of the disease. In summary, among women with a family history of breast cancer, many of the traditional reproductive risk factors should not be used to predict risk for breast cancer.

Should women with a personal history of breast cancer receive hormone replacement therapy after menopause?

With more widespread use of mammography over the past decade, more women are being diagnosed with very-early-stage breast cancer. In addition, as adjuvant chemotherapy and hormone therapy are employed more commonly in premenopausal women, increasing numbers of young women will undergo premature menopause. These women will live longer and be at greater risk for the complications of menopause. Should they receive estrogen replacement therapy?

Relatively few studies have been performed examining the risk for administration of estrogen replacement therapy to women with a history of breast cancer. Most studies are nonrandomized and of small size and have a short duration of follow-up.[64-69] A large study of breast cancer survivors in Sweden was conducted.[70] Patients were randomized to hormone therapy for menopausal symptoms or placebo. The study was halted when an increase in recurrent breast cancer was detected in the women receiving hormone therapy. Thus, women who have had breast cancer should avoid hormones and find other ways to treat menopause. Bisphosphonate treatment is one such alternative therapy. Bisphosphonates such as Actonel and Fosamax can retard the rate of bone loss and development of fractures in postmenopausal women.

Is pregnancy advisable after a diagnosis of breast cancer?

This question is frequently asked by patients because adjuvant oophorectomy in the surgical management of breast cancer is not common, and women are bearing children in later years. About 7% of women who are fertile after mastectomy have one or more pregnancies, and 70% of these pregnancies occur within the first 5 years.[71]

Several studies have examined the influence of pregnancy before, during, or after a diagnosis of breast cancer, but in each study, the number of women was relatively small. In these studies, there was no adverse effect on relapse rate or survival associated with subsequent pregnancy.[72–77] In fact, in one recent study, there is a suggestion of a decreased incidence of distant metastases in women who became pregnant after their breast cancer.[78]

When counseling women about becoming pregnant after breast cancer, the clinician needs to consider that the reports of the effect of pregnancy on breast cancer prognosis are of limited sample size and include select populations. We cannot, at this time, be certain about the effect of pregnancy. Most women are advised to wait 2 to 3 years before becoming pregnant to allow aggressive disease to become manifest. Despite these limitations, the consistent lack of an adverse influence of pregnancy on breast cancer prognosis should reassure young women with breast cancer who want to have children.

What effect do growth factors have on breast cancer?

About two thirds of breast malignancies are dependent on estrogens for growth, but not all breast cancers that express the ER respond to hormone manipulation. Furthermore, many breast cancers that initially express ER gradually become hormone independent and capable of sustaining themselves without the need for estrogenic stimulation. What, then, promotes the growth of the estrogen-independent breast cancer cell?

Growth factors are polypeptides that regulate cell growth by binding to specific receptor molecules in the plasma membrane and stimulating receptor-mediated activation of intracellular signal transduction pathways. More than 60 growth factors have been described. The main group of non-hematopoietic growth factors mediate their effects by means of receptors containing an intrinsic protein, tyrosine kinase. Growth factor receptors are transmembrane glycoproteins. They have an extracellular ligand-binding domain, a transmembrane portion, and an intracellular tyrosine kinase domain; these domains mediate signal transduction into growth regulatory pathways. The binding of ligand alters the state of the receptor (monomeric to oligomeric), and this stimulates the internal tyrosine kinase domain to carry out transphosphorylation of other cell proteins. This results in activation of a cascade of biochemical reactions collectively referred to as the *signal transduction pathways*. These pathways initiate cell cycle traversal and differentiation (Fig. 4–5).

Growth factors are found in all tissues of the body. Simultaneous production of a growth factor and expression of

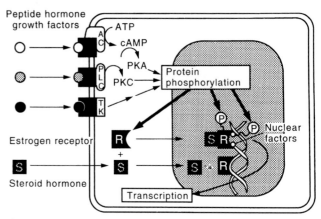

Figure 4–5   Model depicting protein kinase and estrogen receptor transcriptional synergism. AC, adenylate cyclase; ATP, adenosine triphosphate; cAMP, cyclic adenosine monophosphate; P, phosphorus; PKA, protein kinase A; PKC, protein kinase C; PLC, phospholipase C; R, receptor; S, steroid; TK, tyrosine kinase. (From Katzenellenbogen BS, Montano MM, LeGoff P, et al. Antiestrogens: Mechanisms and actions in target cells. J Steroid Biochem Mol Biol 1995;53:390.)

its specific receptor by the same cell is called *autocrine growth*. When the growth factor for a particular cell is produced by a neighboring cell, this is called *paracrine growth*. This latter type of interaction can be between cells of the same or different histologic type. For example, breast cancer cell lines can be stimulated by insulin-like growth factor-2 (IGF-2), which is produced by fibroblasts in adjacent normal tissues. Platelet-derived growth factor (PDGF) produced by breast cancer cells can in turn activate the fibroblasts, which bear PDGF receptors, but not breast cancer cells, because they do not express PDGF receptors.

Many primary human tumors and human tumor cell lines express high levels of growth factor receptors and are capable of producing the relevant growth factors, thus establishing conditions necessary for autocrine or paracrine growth stimulation. Membrane receptors for prolactin, insulin, IGF-1, epidermal growth factor (EGF), and transforming growth factor-β (TGF-β) have been identified in cultured human breast cancer cell lines and also in human breast cancer biopsy specimens. Expression of high levels of growth factor receptors in primary human tumor specimens correlates with a poor clinical outcome for these patients. For example, high epidermal growth factor receptor (EGFR) levels predict a poor prognosis in adenocarcinoma of the breast, transitional bladder cancer, and squamous cell lung carcinoma.[79–82] In similar fashion, increased expression of *HER-2/neu/c-erbB-2* (a shortened molecule similar to EGFR) is associated with a worse prognosis in breast and ovarian cancer.[83–85]

What is the significance of *HER-2/neu* in breast cancer?

About one fourth of primary or metastatic breast cancers overexpress *HER-2/neu*. As a result, some breast cancers that are ER positive also are *HER-2/neu* positive. They have an intact mechanism to be stimulated by either an estrogen or a growth factor pathway. Recent observations have demonstrated that ER-positive, *HER-2/neu*-positive metastatic human breast cancers are less likely to respond to hormone therapy than are cancers that are only ER postive.[86,87] This is consistent with the in vitro observation that MCF-7 cells (ER positive) become resistant to tamoxifen after they are transfected with the *HER-2/neu* oncogene.[88] Recent biochemical evidence suggests that *HER-2/neu* activation can result in an alteration of the ER. Treatment of cells that overexpress *HER-2/neu* with estrogen decreases *HER-2/neu* mRNA, as well as down-regulating the *HER-2/neu* product.[89] Conversely, treatment of ER-positive cells with *HER-2/neu* ligand leads to decreased ER expression.[90,91] This crosstalk between a polypeptide growth factor receptor–activated pathway and a hormone receptor pathway appears to be a mechanism by which the cell can become hormone independent. Preliminary experiments suggest that blocking both pathways may result in an enhanced antiproliferative effect.[92]

REFERENCES

1. Cooper AP. The Principles and Practice of Surgery. London, Cox, 1836, pp 333–336.
2. Beatson GT. On the treatment of inoperable cases of carcinoma of the mamma: Suggestions for a new method of treatment with illustrative cases. Lancet 1896;2:104.
3. Huggins C, Bergenstal DM. Inhibition of mammary and prostatic cancer by adrenalectomy. Cancer Res 1952;12:134.
4. Pearson OH, Ray BS. Results of hypophysectomy in the treatment of metastatic mammary carcinoma. Cancer 1959;12:85.
5. Cash R, Brough AJ, Cohen MNP, et al. Aminoglutethimide (Elipten-CIBA) as an inhibitor of adrenal steroidogenesis. Mechanism of action and therapeutic trial. J Clin Endocrinol Metab 1967;27:1239.
6. Lipton A, Santen RJ. Medical adrenalectomy using aminoglutethimide and dexamethasone in advanced breast cancer. Cancer 1974;33:503–512.
7. Jensen EV, DeSombre ER. Estrogen-receptor interaction. Science 1973;182:126.
8. Jensen EV, DeSombre ER. The diagnostic implications of steroid binding in malignant tissues. Adv Clin Chem 1977;19:57.
9. Kumar V, Green S, Staub A, et al. Localization of the oestradiol-binding and putative DNA-binding domains of the human oestrogen receptor. EMBO J 1986;5:2231–2236.
10. Beato M. Gene regulation by steroid hormones. Cell 1989;56:335–344.
11. Evans RM. The steroid and thyroid hormone receptor superfamily. Science 1988;240:889–895.
12. Carson-Jurica MA, Schrader W, O'Malley B. Steroid receptor family: Structure and functions. Endocr Rev 1990;11:201–220.
13. Green S, Chambon P. The oestrogen receptor: From perception to mechanism. In Parker M (ed). Nuclear Hormone Receptors. New York, Academic Press, 1991, pp 15–38.
14. Ryffel GU, Klein-Hitpass L, Druege P, et al. The estrogen-responsive DNA-element: Structure and interaction with the estrogen receptor. J Steroid Biochem 1988;35:219–222.
15. Kumar V, Chambon P. The estrogen receptor binds tightly to its responsive element as a ligand-induced homodimer. Cell 1988;55:145–156.
16. Meyer ME, Gronemeyer H, Turcotte B, et al. Steroid hormone receptors compete for factors that mediate their enhancer function. Cell 1989;57:433–442.
17. Katzenellenbogen BS, Miller MA, Mullick A, et al. Antiestrogen action in breast cancer cells: Modulation, proliferation and protein synthesis, and interaction with estrogen receptors and additional antiestrogen binding sites. Breast Cancer Res Treat 1985;5:213–243.
18. Jordan VC, Murphy CS. Endocrine pharmacology of antiestrogens as antitumor agents. Endocr Rev 1990;11:578–610.
19. Folca PJ, Glascock RF, Irvine WT. Studies with tritium-labelled hexoestrol in advanced breast cancer. Comparison of tissue accumulation of hexoestrol with response to bilateral adrenalectomy and oophorectomy. Lancet 1961;2:796.
20. Walt AJ, Singhakowinta A, Brooks SC, et al. The surgical implications of estrophile protein estimations in carcinoma of the breast. Surgery 1976;80:506.
21. Knight WA III, Livingston RB, Gregory EJ, et al. Estrogen receptor as an independent prognostic factor for early recurrence in breast cancer. Cancer Res 1977;37:4669.
22. McGuire WL, Horwitz KB, Pearson OH, et al. Current status of estrogen and progesterone receptors in breast cancer. Cancer 1977;39:2934.
23. Bryan RM, Mercer RJ, Bennett RC, et al. Androgen receptors in breast cancer. Cancer 1984;54:2436.
24. Ochi H, Hayashi T, Nakao K, et al. Estrogen, progesterone, and androgen receptors in breast cancer in the Japanese: Brief communication. J Natl Cancer Inst 1978;60:291.
25. Teulings FAG, Van Gilse HA. Demonstration of glucocorticoid receptors in human mammary carcinoma. Horm Res 1977;8:107.
26. Bulbrook RD, Hayward IL, Spicer CC, et al. Abnormal excretion of urinary steroids by women with early breast cancer. Lancet 1962;2:1238.
27. Adami H-O, Adams G, Boyle P, et al. Breast cancer etiology. Int J Cancer Suppl 1990;55:22039.
28. Henderson BE, Ross R, Bernstein L. Estrogens as a cause of human cancer: The Richard and Hinda Rosenthal Foundation Award Lecture. Cancer Res 1988;48:246–253.
29. Henderson BE, Ross RK, Pike MC. Hormonal chemoprevention of cancer in women. Science 1993;259:633–638.
30. Preston-Martin S, Pike MC, Ross RK, et al. Epidemiologic evidence for the increased cell proliferation model of carcinogenesis. Prog Clin Biol Res 1991;369:21–24.
31. DeWaard F. Prevention intervention in breast cancer, but when? Eur J Cancer Prev 1992;1:395–399.
32. Henderson BE, Pike MC, Casagrande JT. Breast cancer and the estrogen window hypothesis. Lancet 1981;2:363.
33. Henderson BE, Ross RK, Judd HL, et al. Do regular ovulatory cycles increase breast cancer risk? Cancer 1985;56:1206.
34. Henderson BE, Gerkins V, Rosario I, et al. Elevated serum levels of estrogen and prolactin in daughters of patients with breast cancer. N Engl J Med 1975;293:790.
35. Trichopoulos D, MacMahon B, Cole P. The menopause and breast cancer risk. J Natl Cancer Inst 1972;48:605.
36. Kvale G, Heuch I, Eide GE. A prospective study of reproductive factors and breast cancer. I. Parity. Am J Epidemiol 1987;126:831–840.
37. MacMahon B, Cole P, Lin TM, et al. Age at first birth and breast cancer risk. Bull WHO 1970;43:209–221.
38. Ewertz M, Duffy S, Adami HO, et al. Age at first birth, parity and risk of cancer: A meta-analysis of 8 studies from the Nordic countries. Int J Cancer 1990;46:597–603.
39. Leon DA. A prospective study of the independent effects of parity and age at first birth on breast cancer incidence in England and Wales. Int J Cancer 1989;43:986–991.
40. Hadjimichael OC, Boyle CA, Miegs JW. Abortion before first live birth and risk of breast cancer. Br J Cancer 1986;53:281.
41. Newcomb PA, Storer BE, Longnecker MP, et al. Lactation and a reduced risk of premenopausal breast cancer. N Engl J Med 1994;330:81–87.
42. Miller D, Rosenberg L, Kaufman D. Breast cancer before age 45 and oral contraceptive use: New findings. Am J Epidemiol 1989;129:269–280.
43. Bernstein L, Pike M, Krailo M, et al. Update of the Los Angeles study of oral contraceptives and breast cancer. In Mann R (ed). Oral Contraceptives and Breast Cancer. London, Parthenon, 1990, p 169.
44. Meirik O, Lund E, Adami H. Oral contraceptive use and breast cancer in young women. Lancet 1986;2:650–653.
45. McPherson K, Vessey M, Neil A. Early oral contraceptive use and breast cancer. Results of another case-control study. Br J Cancer 1987;56:653–660.
46. The Centers for Disease Control Cancer and Steroid Hormone Study. Long-term oral contraceptive use and the risk of breast cancer. JAMA 1983;259:1591–1595.
47. Cancer and Steroid Hormone Study of the Centers for Disease Control and the National Institute of Child Health and Human Development. Oral contraceptive use and the risk of breast cancer. N Engl J Med 1986;315:405–411.
48. Schlesselman JJ. Cancer of the breast and reproductive tract in relation to use of oral contraceptives. Contraception 1989;40:1–38.
49. Colditz GA, Stampfer MT, Willet AC, et al. Prospective study of oestrogen replacement therapy and risk of breast cancer in postmenopausal women. JAMA 1990;264:2648–2653.

50. Schairer C. Risk of breast cancer after menopausal estrogen: A meta-analysis of the published literature to examine the effect of method of classification. Cancer Detect Prev 1992;16:67–72.

51. Steinberg KK, Thacker SB, Smith SJ, et al. A meta-analysis of the effect of estrogen replacement therapy on the risk of breast cancer. JAMA 1991;265:1985–1990.

52. Colditz GA, Egan KM, Stampfer MJ. Hormone replacement therapy and risk of breast cancer: Results from epidemiologic studies. Am J Obstet Gynecol 1993;168:1473–1480.

53. Armstrong BK. Oestrogen therapy after the menopause–boon or bane? Med J Aust 1988;148:213–214.

54. Dupont WD, Page DL. Menopausal estrogen replacement therapy and breast cancer. Arch Intern Med 1991;151:67–72.

55. Sillero-Arenas M, Delgado-Rodriguez M, Rodrigues-Canteras R, et al. Menopausal hormone replacement therapy and breast cancer: A meta-analysis. Obstet Gynecol 1992;79:286–294.

56. Writing Group for the Women's Health Initiative Investigators: Risks and benefits of estrogen plus progestin in healthy postmenopausal women. JAMA 2002;288:321–333.

57. Hoover R, Glass A, Finkle WD, et al. Conjugated estrogens and breast cancer risk in women. J Natl Cancer Inst 1981;67:815.

58. Hulka BS, Chambless LE, Deubner DC, et al. Breast cancer and estrogen replacement therapy. Am J Obstet Gynecol 1982;143:638.

59. Nomura AMY, Kolonel LN, Hirohata T, et al. The association of replacement estrogens with breast cancer. Int J Cancer 1986;37:49.

60. Wingo PA, Layde PM, Lee NC, et al. The risk of breast cancer in postmenopausal women who have used estrogen replacement therapy. JAMA 1987;257:209.

61. Hoover R, Gray LA, Cole P, et al. Menopausal estrogens and breast cancer. N Engl J Med 1976;295:401.

62. Ross RK, Paganini-Hill A, Gerkins VR, et al. A case-control study of menopausal estrogen therapy and breast cancer. JAMA 1980;243:1635.

63. Colditz GA, Rosner BA, Speizer FE. Risk factors for breast cancer according to family history of breast cancer. J Natl Cancer Inst 1996;88:365.

64. Stoll BA. Hormone replacement therapy in women treated for breast cancer. Eur J Cancer Clin Oncol 1989;25:1909–1913.

65. DiSaia PJ, Odicino F, Grosen EA, et al. Hormone-replacement therapy in breast cancer. Lancet 1993;342:1232.

66. Powles TJ, Hickish T, Casey S, et al. Hormone replacement after breast cancer. Lancet 1993;342:60–61.

67. Wile AG, Opfel RW, Margileth DA, et al. Hormone replacement therapy does not affect breast cancer outcome [abstract]. Proc Am Soc Clin Oncol 1991;10:58.

68. Cobleigh MA, Berris RF, Bush T, et al. Estrogen replacement therapy in breast cancer survivors. A time for change. JAMA 1994;272:540–545.

69. Eden J, Bush T, Nand S, et al. The Royal Hospital for Women Breast Cancer Study: A case-controlled study of combined continuous hormone replacement therapy amongst women with a personal history of breast cancer. North Am Menopause Soc 1995;2:66–72.

70. Holmberg L, Anderson H: HABITS (hormonal replacement therapy after breast cancer—is it safe?), a randomised comparison: Trial stopped. Lancet 2004;363:453–455.

71. Donegan WL. Pregnancy and breast cancer. Obstet Gynecol 1977;50:244–251.

72. Harvey JC, Rosen PP, Ashikari R, et al. The effect of pregnancy on the prognosis of carcinoma of the breast following mastectomy. Surg Gynecol Obstet 1981;153:723–725.

73. Rissanen PM. Pregnancy following treatment of mammary carcinoma. Acta Radiol Ther 1968;8:415–422.

74. Holleb AL, Farrow JH. The relation of carcinoma of the breast and pregnancy in 283 patients. Surg Gynecol Obstet 1962;115:65–71.

75. Sutton R, Buzdar AU, Hortobagyi GN. Pregnancy and offspring after adjuvant chemotherapy in breast cancer patients. Cancer 1990;65:847–850.

76. Cooper DR, Butterfield J. Pregnancy subsequent to mastectomy for cancer of the breast. Ann Surg 1970;171:429–433.

77. Ariel IM, Kempner R. The prognosis of patients who become pregnant after mastectomy for breast cancer. Int Surg 1989;74:185–187.

78. Von Schoultz E, Johannsson H, Wilking N, et al. Influence of prior and subsequent pregnancy on breast cancer prognosis. J Clin Oncol 1995;13:430–434.

79. Harris AL, Nicholson S, Sainsbury JRC. Epidermal growth factor receptor: A marker of early relapse in breast cancer and tumor stage progression in bladder cancer interactions with NEU. In Furth M, Greaves M (eds). The Molecular Diagnostics of Human Cancer, vol 7. Cold Spring Harbor, NY, Cold Spring Harbor Laboratory Press, 1989, pp 353–357.

80. Sainsbury JRC, Malcolm AJ, Appleton DR, et al. Presence of epidermal growth factor receptor as an indicator of poor prognosis in patients with breast cancer. J Clin Pathol 1985;38:1225–1228.

81. Neal DE, Bennett MK, Hall RR, et al. Epidermal growth factor receptors in human bladder cancer: Comparison of invasive and superficial tumors. Lancet 1985;1:366–368.

82. Hendler F, Shum-Siui A, Nanu L, et al. Increased EGF receptors and the absence of an alveolar differentiation marker predict a poor survival in lung cancer [abstract]. Proc Am Soc Clin Oncol 1989;8:223.

83. Slamon DJ, Godolphin W, Jones LA, et al. Studies of the HER-2/NEU proto-oncogene in human breast and ovarian cancer. Science 1989;244:707–712.

84. Wright C, Angus B, Nicholson S, et al. Expression of c-erbB-2 oncoprotein: A prognostic indicator in human breast cancer. Cancer Res 1989;49:2087–2090.

85. Gullick WJ. The role of the epidermal growth factor receptor and the c-erbB-2 protein in breast cancer. Int J Cancer 1990;5S:55–61.

86. Wright C, Nicholson S, Angus B, et al. Relationship between c-erbB-2 protein product expression and response to endocrine therapy in advanced breast cancer. Br J Cancer 1992;65:118–121.

87. Leitzel K, Teramoto Y, Konrad K, et al. Elevated serum c-erbB-2 antigen levels and decreased response to hormone therapy of breast cancer. J Clin Oncol 1995;13:1129–1135.

88. Benz CC, Scott GK, Sarup JC, et al. Estrogen-dependent, tamoxifen-resistant tumorigenic growth of MCF-7 cells transfected with HER2/neu. Breast Cancer Res Treat 1992;24:85–95.

89. Read LD, Keith D Jr, Slamon DJ, et al. Hormonal modulation of HER-2/neu proto-oncogene messenger ribonucleic acid and p185 protein expression in human breast cancer cell lines. Cancer Res 1990;50:3947–3951.

90. Pietras RJ, Arboleda J, Reese DM, et al. HER-2 tyrosine kinase pathway targets estrogen receptor and promotes hormone-independent growth in human breast cancer cells. Oncogene 1995;10:2435–2446.

91. Kumar R, Mandal M, Ratzlain B, et al. NDF induces expression of a novel 46 kD protein in estrogen receptor positive breast cancer cells. J Cell Biochem 1996;62:102–112.

92. Witters L, Kumar R, Chinchilli V, et al. Enhanced anti-proliferative activity of the combination of tamoxifen plus HER-2/neu antibody. Breast Cancer Res Treat 1997;42:1–5.

CHAPTER 5

Risk Factors for Development of Breast Cancer

Darcy V. Spicer and Malcolm C. Pike

Epidemiologic research has clearly identified important reproductive risk factors for breast cancer, including age at menarche, age at menopause, and age at first-term pregnancy (Table 5–1). These provide important clues to the hormonal origin of this disease. The widespread use of exogenous sex steroids as contraceptive agents by premenopausal women and as hormone replacement therapy (HRT) by postmenopausal women has provided a unique opportunity for epidemiologists to further understand the role of sex steroids in the genesis of breast cancer, and recent randomized clinical trials testing the impact of HRT have provided important insights into their effects on breast cancer (and other diseases). As we will show, the effects of sex steroids on the normal breast in women are increasingly well understood—estrogen induces some breast epithelial cell proliferation, but estrogen plus progesterone produces much greater cell proliferation.[1] Proliferating cell populations are more susceptible to carcinogenic effects, and the rise in cancer risk associated with cell proliferation is secondary to an increased chance of mutation.[2–6] Thus, breast cancer risk would be predicted to increase to the greatest extent during periods of exposure to both estrogen and progestin, as in the premenopausal period or in women receiving oral contraceptives; to be less during periods of estrogen-only exposure, as in postmenopausal women receiving estrogen replacement therapy (ERT) or in obese postmenopausal women; and to be least during periods of exposure to neither hormone, as in slender postmenopausal Asian women. These predictions fit very well with epidemiologic observations. The more complex effects of term pregnancy on breast cancer risk are discussed below.

Is age a risk factor for breast cancer?

It is essential to understand the relationship of breast cancer incidence to age (i.e., the risk for breast cancer diagnosis during a 1-year period at different ages). Although breast cancer risk rises throughout life in almost all populations (although not after menopause in some "traditional" Asian populations),[7] the rate at which risk rises declines significantly around age 50 years. Most common non–hormone-dependent adult cancers increase in incidence with advancing age; when age and incidence are plotted logarithmically, a straight line is seen, as in Figure 5–1 for colorectal cancer in white U.S. women.[8] The incidence of these common non–hormone-dependent cancers rises continuously and increasingly rapidly with age. The incidence at age t, $I(t)$, of such a cancer rises as the k power of age and can be written as $I(t) = constant \times t^k$.[9] This pattern is consistent with such cancers arising from a multistage process in which the stochastic rate of change from stage to stage is relatively independent of age,[10] consistent with modern molecular biology concepts of cancer as a multistep process.

A similar logarithmic plot of age and breast cancer incidence is shown in Figure 5–2[8]; in contrast to non–hormone-dependent cancers, this curve is best described as two straight lines—a steeply sloped line until about age 50 years, followed by a second line with a more gentle slope after this age. The implication of this observation is that elements important in the genesis of breast cancer decline at about 50 years of age. Ovarian and endometrial cancers have the same complex relationship between age and incidence.[11]

Is age at menopause a risk factor for breast cancer?

Early natural menopause substantially reduces breast cancer risk.[12,13] Similarly, early bilateral oophorectomy reduces breast cancer risk, an observation that effectively proves a cause-and-effect relationship between ovarian function and breast cancer risk. Menopause is the proximate cause of the complex relationship between age and breast cancer risk. If menopause did not occur, then the age-incidence curve for breast cancer would in all likelihood be similar to that for other adult malignancies.

The data from the large case-control study of Trichopoulos and colleagues[14] are given in Table 5–2, whereby artificial menopause before age 35 years is associated with a breast cancer relative risk of 0.36 (a 64% reduction). Feinleib[15] noted in his large cohort study that among 1278 women with artificial menopause before age 40 years, 6 had breast cancer, as compared with an expected incidence of 24.0—a 75% reduction. The epidemiologic study of breast cancer by Hirayama

26. Coleman S, Daniel CW. Inhibition of mouse mammary ductal morphogenesis and down-regulation of the EGF receptor by epidermal growth factor. Dev Biol 1990;137:425–433.

27. Haslam SZ, Counterman LJ, Nummy KA. Effects of epidermal growth factor, estrogen and progestin on DNA synthesis in mammary cells in vivo are determined by the developmental state of the gland. J Cell Physiol 1993;155:72–78.

28. Haslam SZ, Counterman LJ, Nummy KA. EGF receptor regulation in normal mouse mammary gland. J Cell Physiol 1992;152:553–557.

29. Silberstein GB, Flanders KC, Roberts AB, Daniel CV. Regulation of mammary morphogenesis: Evidence for extracellular matrix-mediated inhibition of ductal budding by transforming growth factor beta1. Dev Biol 1992;152:354–362.

30. Meyer JS, Connor RE. Cell proliferation in fibrocystic disease and postmenopausal breast ducts measured by thymidine labeling. Cancer 1982;50:746–751.

31. Henderson BE, Ross RK, Judd HL, et al. Do regular ovulatory cycles increase breast cancer risk? Cancer 1985;56:1206–1208.

32. Collaborative Group on Hormonal Factors in Breast Cancer. Breast cancer and breastfeeding: Collaborative reanalysis of individual data from 47 epidemiological studies in 30 countries, including 50 302 women with breast cancer and 96 973 women without the disease. Lancet 2002;360:187–195.

33. Russo J, Tay L, Russo I. Differentiation of the mammary gland and susceptibility to carcinogenesis. Breast Cancer Res Treat 1982;2:5–73.

34. Bernstein L, Pike MC, Ross R, et al. Estrogen and sex hormone-binding globulin levels in nulliparous and parous women. J Natl Cancer Inst 1985;74:741–745.

35. Yu MC, Gerkins VR, Henderson BE, et al. Elevated levels of prolactin in nulliparous women. Br J Cancer 1981;43:826–831.

36. Battersby A, Anderson TJ. Proliferative and secretory activity in the pregnant and lactating human breast. Virchows Arch Pathol Anat 1988;413:189–196.

37. Medina D, Sivaraman L, Hilsenbeck SG, et al. Mechanisms of hormonal prevention of breast cancer. Ann N Y Acad Sci 2001;952:23–35.

38. Master SR, Chodosh LA. Evolving views of involution. Breast Cancer Res 2004;6:89–92.

39. Rajkumar L, Guzman RC, Yang J, et al. Prevention of mammary carcinogenesis by short-term estrogen and progestin treatments. Breast Cancer Res 2004;6:31–37.

40. Michels KB, Willett WC, Rosner A, et al. Prospective and secretory activity in the pregnant and lactating human breast. Virchows Archiv A Pathol Anat 1996;413:189–196.

41. Tao S, Yu M, Ross M, et al. Risk factors for breast cancer in Chinese women in Beijing. Int J Cancer 1988;42:459–598.

42. Hunter DJ, Willett WC. Diet, body size, and breast cancer. Epidemiol Rev 1993;15:110–132.

43. Zumoff B. Relationship of obesity to blood estrogens. Cancer Res 1982;42:3289s–3294s.

44. Shoupe D. Effect of body weight on reproductive function. In Mishell DR, Davajan V, Lobo RA (eds). Infertility, Contraception and Reproductive Endocrinology, 3rd ed. Boston, Blackwell Scientific Publications, 1991, pp 288–316.

45. Blankenstein MA, van de Ven J, Maitimu-Smeele I, et al. Intratumoral levels of estrogen in the breast. J Steroid Biochem Mol Biol 1999;69:293–297.

46. Friedenreich CM. Physical activity and cancer prevention: From observational to intervention research. Cancer Epidemiol Biomark Prev 2001;10:287–301.

47. Bernstein L, Henderson BE, Hanisch R, et al. Physical exercise and reduced risk of breast cancer in young women. J Natl Cancer Inst 1994;86:1403–1408.

48. Patel AV, Calle EE, Bernstein L, et al. Recreational physical activity and risk of postmenopausal breast cancer in a large cohort of US women. Cancer Causes Control 2003;14:519–529.

49. Bernstein L, Ross RK, Lobo R, et al. The effects of moderate physical activity on menstrual cycle patterns in adolescence: Implications for breast cancer prevention. Br J Cancer 1987;55:681–685.

50. MacMahon B, Cole P, Brown JB, et al. Urine estrogen profiles of Asian and North American Women. Int J Cancer 1974;14:161–167.

51. Goldin BR, Adlercreutz H, Gorbach SL, et al. The relationship between estrogen levels and diets of Caucasian American and Oriental immigrant women. Am J Clin Nutr 1986;44:945–953.

52. Bernstein L, Yuan J-M, Ross RK, et al. Serum hormone levels in premenopausal Chinese women in Shanghai and white women in Los Angeles: Results from two breast cancer case-control studies. Cancer Causes Control 1990;1:51–58.

53. Key TJA, Chen J, Wang DY, et al. Sex hormones in women in rural China and in Britain. Br J Cancer 1990;62:631–636.

54. Ursin G, Bernstein L, Pike MC. Breast cancer. In Doll R, Fraumeni J, Muir CS (eds). Cancer Surveys: Trends in Cancer Incidence and Mortality, vol. 19/20, 1994, pp 241–264.

55. Pike MC, Kolonel LN, Henderson BE, et al. Breast cancer in a multiethnic cohort in Hawaii and Los Angeles: Risk factors–adjusted incidence in Japanese equals and in Hawaiians exceeds that in Whites. Cancer Epidemiol Biomark Prev 2002;11:795–800.

56. Zeigler R, Hoover R, Pike MC, et al. Migration patterns and breast cancer risk in Asian-American women. J Natl Cancer Inst 1993;85:1819–1827.

57. Ponder B. An overview of genetic predisposition and the search for predisposing genes for breast cancer. In Hormones, Genes and Cancer. New York, Oxford University Press, 2003, pp 157–168.

58. Venkitaraman AR. Cancer susceptibility and the functions of BRCA1 and BRCA2. Cell 2002;108:171–182.

59. Fitzgibbons PL, Henson DE, Hutter RVP. Benign breast changes and the risk for subsequent breast cancer: An update of the 1985 consensus statement. Arch Pathol Lab Med 1998;122:1053–1055.

60. Fabian CJ, Kimler BF, Zalles CM, et al. Short-term breast cancer prediction by random periareolar fine-needle aspiration cytology and the Fail risk model. J Natl Cancer Inst 2000;92:1217–1227.

61. Wrensch MR, Petrakis NL, Miike R et al. Breast cancer incidence in women with abnormal cytology in nipple aspirates of breast fluid. J Natl Cancer Inst 2001;93:1791–1798.

62. Oza AM, Boyd NF. Mammographic parenchymal patterns: a marker of breast cancer risk. Epidemiol Rev 1993;15:196–208.

63. Boyd NF, Jensen HM, Cooke G, et al. Mammographic densities and the prevalence and incidence of histological types of benign breast disease. Eur J Cancer Prev 2000;9:15–24.

64. Boyd NF, Dite GS, Stone J, et al. Heritability of mammographic density, a risk factor for breast cancer. N Engl J Med 2002;347:886–894.

65. Spicer DV, Ursin G, Parisky YR, et al. Changes in mammographic densities induced by a hormonal contraceptive designed to reduce breast cancer risk. J Natl Cancer Inst 1994;86:431–436.

66. Greendale GA, Reboussin BA, Slone S, et al. Postmenopausal hormone therapy and change in mammographic density. J Natl Cancer Inst 2003;95:30–37.

67. Gram IT, Ursin G, Spicer DV, et al. Reversal of gonadotropin-releasing hormone agonist induced reductions in mammographic densities on stopping treatment. Cancer Epidemiol Biomark Prev 2001;10:1117–1120.

68. Dickey RP, Stone SC. Progestational potency of oral contraceptives. Obstet Gynecol 1976;47:106–112.

69. Back DJ, Bates M, Breckenridge AM, et al. The pharmacokinetics of levonorgestrel and ethynylestradiol in women—studies with Ovran and Ovranette. Contraception 1981;23:229–239.

70. Collaborative Group on Hormonal Factors in Breast Cancer. Breast cancer and hormonal contraceptives: Collaborative reanalysis of individual data on 53 297 women with breast cancer and 100 239 women without breast cancer from 54 epidemiological studies. Lancet 1996;347:1713–1727.

71. Marchbanks PA, McDonald JA, Wilson HG, et al. Oral contraceptives and the risk of breast cancer. N Engl J Med 2002;346:2025–2032.

72. Mishell DR, Kharma KM, Thorneycroft IH, et al. Estrogenic activity in women receiving an injectable progestogen for contraception. Am J Obstet Gynecol 1972;113:372–376.

73. Jeppsson S, Johansson EDB, Ljungberg O, et al. Endometrial histology and circulating levels of medroxyprogesterone acetate (MPA): Estradiol, FSH and LH in women with MPA induced amenorrhoea compared with women with secondary amenorrhoea. Acta Obstet Gynecol Scand 1977;56:43–48.

74. Lee NC, Rosero-Bixby L, Oberle MW, et al. A case-control study of breast cancer and hormonal contraception in Costa Rica. J Natl Cancer Inst 1987;79:1247–1254.

75. Paul C, Skegg DCG, Spears GFS. Depot medroxyprogesterone (Depo-Provera) and risk of breast cancer. BMJ 1989;299:759–762.

76. Hofseth LJ, Raafat AM, Osuch JR, et al. Hormone replacement therapy with estrogen or estrogen plus medroxyprogesterone acetate is associated with increased epithelial proliferation in the normal postmenopausal breast. J Clin Endocrinol Metab 1999;84:4559–4565.

77. Pike MC, Ross RK, Spicer DV. Problems involved in including women with simple hysterectomy in epidemiologic studies measuring the effects of hormone replacement therapy on breast cancer risk. Am J Epidemiol 1998;147:718–721.

78. Collaborative Group on Hormonal Factors in Breast Cancer. Breast cancer and hormone replacement therapy: Collaborative reanalysis of individual data from 51 epidemiological studies on 53 705 women with breast cancer and 108 411 women without breast cancer. Lancet 1997;350:1047–1059.

79. Selby PL, Peacock M. Dose dependent response of symptoms, pituitary, and bone to transdermal estrogen in postmenopausal women. BMJ 1986;293:137–1339.

80. Anderson GL, Limacher M, Assaf AR, et al. Effects of conjugated equine estrogen in postmenopausal women with hysterectomy: The Women's Health Initiative randomized controlled trial. JAMA 2004;291:1701–1712.

81. Ross RK, Paganini-Hill A, Wan PC, et al. Effect of hormone replacement therapy on breast cancer risk: Estrogen versus estrogen plus progestin. J Natl Cancer Inst 2000;92:328–332.

82. Schairer C, Lubin J, Troisi R, et al. Estrogen-progestin replacement and risk of breast cancer. JAMA 2000;284:691–694.

83. Magnusson C, Baron JA, Correia N, et al. Breast-cancer risk following long-term oestrogen- and oestrogen-progestin-replacement therapy. Int J Cancer 1999;81:339–344.

84. Hulley S, Grady D, Bush T, et al. Randomized trial of estrogen plus progestin for secondary prevention of coronary heart disease in postmenopausal women. JAMA 1998;280:605–613.

85. Rossouw JE, Anderson GL, Prentice RL, et al. Risks and benefits of estrogen plus progestin in healthy postmenopausal women: principal results from the Women's Health Initiative randomized controlled trial. JAMA 2002;288:321–333.

86. Chlebowski RT, Hendrix SL, Langer RD, et al. Influence of estrogen plus progestin on breast cancer and mammography in healthy postmenopausal women: the Women's Health Initiative Randomized Trial. JAMA 2003;289:3243–3253.

87. Greendale GA, Reboussin GA, Slone S, et al. Postmenopausal hormone therapy and change in mammographic density. J Natl Cancer Inst 2003; 95:30–37.

88. Lee S, Ross RK, Pike MC. An overview of postmenopausal estrogen-progestin hormone therapy and breast cancer risk. (Submitted for publication.)

CHAPTER 6

Prevention of Breast Cancer

Polly R. Etkind and Joseph A. Sparano

The potential benefits of a disease prevention strategy depend on the incidence of the disease in the population and the associated morbidity and mortality. Breast cancer is very common in North America and Western Europe. For the average white American woman, there is a 1 in 8 lifetime risk of developing breast cancer, and a nearly 1 in 28 chance of dying of breast cancer.[1] Furthermore, breast cancer results in substantial cost and morbidity because of the need for screening, surgery, adjuvant local or systemic therapy, and follow-up. It is clearly reasonable, therefore, to consider breast cancer prevention in healthy populations, particularly in those that have a high incidence of the disease.

PREVENTION STRATEGIES

What populations should be targeted for prevention?

The likelihood of benefit from prevention is increased by targeting high-risk populations for prevention, although this assumes that the intervention strategy is equally effective in such targeted populations. A germline mutation in the tumor suppressor gene *BRCA1* or *BRCA2* is the most reliable predictive factor because it is associated with up to an 80% lifetime risk for developing breast cancer as well as about a 20% to 40% lifetime risk for ovarian cancer.[2] However, it is estimated that *BRCA1* gene mutations account for only 5% of all breast cancers.[2] Age is perhaps the next most important factor: the incidence of the disease increases with each decade of life.[3] Other factors are outlined in Table 6–1 and include family history,[4] reproductive factors, and exogenous hormone use (as reviewed in Chapter 4). Although there are many risk factors, nearly one half of patients with the disease have no identifiable risk factor.[5]

What factors should be considered in selecting a prevention strategy?

The characteristics of a sound prevention strategy include a substantial reduction in risk, a reasonable likelihood of deriving benefit, absence of any short-term or long-term deleterious effects, feasibility of implementation, and reasonable cost. The appeal of a prevention strategy would be greatly strengthened by secondary benefits in reducing other major causes of morbidity or mortality, such as other malignancies and cardiovascular disease.

What prevention strategies are available or under investigation?

Potential strategies for breast cancer prevention include modification of reproductive factors and hormone use (e.g., early pregnancy, lactation, prophylactic oophorectomy), modification of lifestyle (e.g., diet, exercise), chemoprevention (e.g., tamoxifen), and removal of the target organ (e.g., prophylactic mastectomy).

MODIFICATION OF REPRODUCTIVE FACTORS AND EXOGENOUS HORMONE USE

What role do steroid hormones play in the pathogenesis of breast cancer?

Although the pathogenesis of breast cancer is not completely understood, a popular theory is that mutagenesis and mitogenesis are important factors.[6] Sex steroid hormones have potent mitogenic effects and also increase the susceptibility of breast epithelia to mutagens. Breast epithelial cells undergo cycles of cell proliferation and cell loss in response to ovarian production of estrogen and luteal production of progesterone. The cells of the terminal duct lobular units increase in number in response to progesterone during the luteal phase and stop dividing and enter apoptosis when progesterone production wanes. Such proliferating cells are more susceptible to mutagens and are more likely to develop somatic mutations. Numerous clinical observations support the importance of hormones in the pathogenesis of breast cancer; they have been reviewed in Chapter 4. The role of hormones is believed to be manifested in a protective effect of early menopause,[7] the steeper age-related increase in breast cancer incidence that occurs in premenopausal compared with postmenopausal women,[1] the multifactorial effects of pregnancy on breast cancer risk,[8] the association between more prolonged ovarian cycling (i.e., early menarche, late menopause) and increased breast cancer risk,[9] and the association between relatively high circulating estrogen levels and breast cancer in postmenopausal women.[10] Factors supporting a mutagenic role for hormones include the increased incidence of oxidative

Table 6–1 Classification of Breast Cancer Risk

Group	Lifetime Risk for Breast Cancer (%)	Risk Factors
Average risk	11–12	No family history or reproductive factors*
Increased risk	10–20	No family history but at least two reproductive factors Atypical hyperplasia without a family history Weak family history (no more than two second-degree or more distant relatives with breast cancer)
High risk	>20	Atypical hyperplasia with a family history Lobular carcinoma in situ Strong family history (any first-degree relative, any second-degree relative with onset <40 yr, or 3 or more family members with breast cancer)
Very high risk	Up to 85	Breast cancer susceptibility gene (BRCA1, BRCA2, or other cancer susceptibility syndromes)

*Reproductive factors include (1) menarche ≤11 years of age, (2) menopause ≥55 years of age, (3) nulliparity, (4) first pregnancy after age 30 years, (5) current use of hormone replacement therapy.

DNA damage in the peripheral blood and breast tissue of women with breast cancer.[11,12]

What is the relationship between pregnancy and breast cancer?

Pregnancy is associated with a short-term increase in breast cancer risk followed by a long-term protective effect. Lambe and colleagues[8] reported a case-control study involving 12,666 patients with breast cancer and 62,121 age-matched residents of Sweden. Uniparous women had a higher risk for breast cancer than nulliparous women for up to 15 years following delivery. For women aged 25 to 35 years at the time of delivery, the risk steadily declined over 10 to 15 years following delivery until a protective effect began to be evident. For women aged 20 years at first delivery, long-term reduction in breast cancer occurred without a short-term increase. Having a second delivery at 30 years old or younger also had a protective effect without a short-term increase. This study provides explanations of why nulliparous women have reduced breast cancer risk during the childbearing years despite having a higher lifetime breast cancer risk, why the average age at diagnosis of breast cancer is younger in parous compared with nulliparous women, and why previous studies that did not consider the potential interaction among age at delivery, age at breast cancer diagnosis, and parity demonstrated conflicting results.[13] A plausible biologic interpretation is that pregnancy increases the short-term risk for breast cancer by stimulating the growth of cells that have undergone the early stages of malignant transformation, but confers long-term protection by inducing the differentiation of normal mammary stem cells, which, when undifferentiated, have a greater potential for neoplastic change.

The Russos and their colleagues[14] have proposed a biologic model that provides an explanation for these clinical observations. They have shown that in rats, pregnancy results in complete differentiation of terminal end buds to lobules and renders the mammary gland relatively resistant to malignant transformation. In humans, the Russos[15] have identified four distinct lobular structures in the breast, each representing sequential developmental stages in mammary development. Type 1 lobules are the most undifferentiated and are most prevalent in the immature female breast before menarche. Type 2 lobules arise from type 1 and have a more complex morphology. Type 3 lobules are seen during pregnancy. Type 4 lobules are present only during the lactation period and are considered the most differentiated lobules. Type 1 lobules are postulated to give rise to invasive and noninvasive ductal carcinomas. Pregnancy between the ages of 14 and 20 years results in an increase in type 3 lobules that persists until the age of 40 years, when the lobules involute. It has been postulated that the artificial induction of a pregnancy-like state in the late teens could theoretically reduce breast cancer incidence by about one third.[15] Although the timing of such an intervention and the optimal hormonal differentiation-producing combination are under intense investigation, there are considerable research and ethical hurdles to clear before any clinical applications of this idea are possible.

What is the relationship between lactation and breast cancer?

Most epidemiologic studies demonstrate that lactation is associated with a small but significant reduction in breast cancer risk, although its protective effect is observed only in premenopausal women and only after relatively long periods of lactation.[16,17] Newcomb and colleagues[16] studied 5878 women who had nursed their offspring and 8216 parous women who had not nursed offspring. All of these women were homemakers whose duration or extent of lactation was not limited by a return to employment. The relative risk for developing breast cancer in women who had ever nursed a child was 0.72 for premenopausal women and 1.04 for postmenopausal women. Increasing duration of lactation was associated with significantly more protection for premenopausal women, with a significant protective effect observed for women who lactated for at least 4 months after one pregnancy. Younger age at first lactation was associated with significantly lower breast cancer risk, although protection was observed for patients who initiated lactation up to 29 years of age. In contrast to previous data suggesting that insufficient milk production was associated with increased breast cancer risk, the authors found no difference in breast cancer risk whether insufficient milk production or other reasons were the cause of a short (less than 4 months) period of lactation. The use of hormones to discontinue milk flow was reported by an equal proportion in the case-control group and had no effect on breast cancer risk. A similar, more recent study involving 110,604 premenopausal Korean women provided additional empirical evidence that lactation decreases the risk for breast cancer among premenopausal women.[18] Lactation may be protective against breast cancer by modifying pituitary and ovarian hormone production, thereby resulting in more anovulatory cycles.[19] In mice, lactation also results in relative resistance to chemical carcinogens, lowers the rate of epithelial proliferation, and allows the elimination of carcinogen through the mammary gland.[20]

Can modification of endogenous steroid hormone production protect against breast cancer?

For women seeking contraception, Spicer and Pike[6] have proposed that a combination of a gonadotropin-releasing hormone agonist (to suppress ovarian function) and low-dose hormone replacement therapy (with exogenous synthetic estrogen and progestogen) can produce effective contraception and reduce breast cancer risk. This treatment results in hormone levels that are insufficient to promote ovulation or stimulation of breast epithelium but sufficient to prevent vasomotor symptoms, urogenital atrophy, atherosclerosis, and osteoporosis. It has been estimated that this method can reduce lifetime breast cancer risk by 50% if used for 10 years and by as much as 70% if used for 15 years. This strategy also results in a significant reduction in mammographic density at 1 year in premenopausal women.[21] Increased mammographic density is associated with increased breast cancer risk for both premenopausal and postmenopausal women and is independent of other recognized variables.[22] This strategy has not been tested in large-scale trials.

Therefore, for women seeking to have children, pregnancy at a young age, multiple pregnancies, and lactation at an early age can all have a substantial protective effect. On the other hand, education, employment, and other societal factors may make this approach impractical for many women.

What is the role of prophylactic oophorectomy in reducing breast cancer risk?

Observational studies have suggested that bilateral oophorectomy performed before menopause is associated with a reduced breast cancer risk.[23,24] Although prophylactic oophorectomy may be impractical to consider in average-risk women, it may be a reasonable option for women with a heritable predisposition to breast cancer. Because mutations in the BRCA1 and BRCA2 genes are associated with an increased risk for not only breast cancer but also ovarian cancer, it is logical to consider this procedure for women with mutations in these genes. Kauff and colleagues enrolled 170 premenopausal women at least 35 years of age who had BRCA1 or BRCA2 mutations and had not yet developed breast or ovarian cancer.[25] All were offered risk-reducing salpingo-oophorectomy, of whom 98 chose surgery and 72 chose surveillance. After a mean follow-up of 2 years, there were 3 cases of breast cancer and 1 case of peritoneal cancer among the 98 women in a surgery group, compared with 8 cases of breast cancer, 4 cases of ovarian cancer, and 1 case of peritoneal cancer among the 72 patients in the surveillance group. The hazard rate for a breast or gynecologic cancer among patients who chose risk-reducing salpingo-oophorectomy was significantly reduced (hazard ratio, 0.25%; 95% confidence interval [CI], 0.08%–0.74%). Risk-reducing salpingo-oophorectomy may therefore be a reasonable option for premenopausal women known to have BRCA1 or BRCA2 mutations and who have completed childbearing. The procedure may also have a role in postmenopausal women, although when used in that setting it would not likely have a protective effect in reducing breast cancer risk.

Would avoidance of oral contraceptives help in breast cancer prevention?

In the past, some studies have suggested increased risk for breast cancer with the use of oral contraceptives (OCs),[26–29] whereas others have shown no association.[30,31] Most studies do not show a consistent effect of various OC formulations and risk, although some studies have found a higher breast cancer risk among patients who took OCs containing high-risk progestins,[32] perhaps owing to progestin-related increases in breast epithelial replication.[33] Recent studies suggest that newer low-potency/low-estrogen-dose contraceptives may impart a lower risk for breast cancer than those associated with earlier high-potency/high-dose preparations.[34] An exhaustive analysis representing about 90% of all worldwide epidemiologic evidence on breast cancer risk and birth control pills has concluded that there is no evidence of an increase in risk for having breast cancer diagnosed 10 or more years after cessation of use.[35] This meta-analysis did report that women who are currently using combined OCs or have used them in the past 10 years are at a slightly increased risk for having breast cancer diagnosed, although the cancers diagnosed in these women tend to be localized to the breast.

Is hormone replacement therapy associated with an increase in breast cancer risk?

Hormone replacement therapy (HRT) became a popular treatment for postmenopausal women because it effectively relieves vasomotor symptoms and urogenital atrophy and was thought to protect against bone fractures and cardiovascular disease based on case-control retrospective studies. The Women's Health Initiative[36,37] prospectively evaluated the health effects of conjugated equine estrogens (0.625 mg daily) plus medroxyprogesterone acetate (2.5 mg daily) in 16,608 postmenopausal women who had a uterus, and estrogen alone in those who had prior hysterectomy. The trial was halted by the data and safety monitoring board when it was determined that HRT increased the risk for cardiovascular disease (nonfatal myocardial infarction or death due to coronary heart disease), which was the primary efficacy outcome; after a mean follow-up of 5.2 years (planned duration, 8.5 years), HRT was associated with about a 25% increase in this end point. The incidence of breast cancer was also increased in the HRT group compared with placebo (hazard ratio, 1.24%; $P < .001$). The invasive breast cancers diagnosed in the HRT group were at a more advanced stage (regional/metastatic 25.4% vs. 16.0%, respectively; $P = .04$), although they did not differ in histology or grade. The percentage of women with abnormal mammograms was significantly higher at 1 year in the HRT group (9.4% vs. 5.4%; $P < .001$). The study also included women without a uterus receiving estrogen alone, and that part of the study remains in blinded follow-up with no evidence of increased risk for cardiovascular disease or breast cancer for estrogen alone.

LIFESTYLE MODIFICATION

Is there a role for exercise in breast cancer prevention?

Recreational physical activity appears to be inversely related to risk for breast cancer,[38,39] yet some results remain inconsistent.[40,41] Bernstein and associates[38] reported a case-control study involving personal interviews with a total of 545 women (aged 40 years and younger at diagnosis) who had been newly diagnosed with invasive or in situ carcinoma and 545 control subjects matched for age, race, parity, and neighborhood of residence. Lifetime histories of participants in physical exercise activities on a regular basis were obtained during the interview. After adjustment for potential confounding factors, the average number of hours spent in physical exercise activities per week from menarche to 1 year before diagnosis was a significant predictor of reduced breast cancer risk during the reproductive years. More recently, Dirx and colleagues[39] reported on their findings from the Netherlands Cohort Study on diet and breast cancer in which exercise information was collected by questionnaire from 62,537 women aged 55 to 69 years at baseline. After 7.3 years of follow-up, 1208 incident breast carcinoma cases were available for case-cohort analysis. A summed total of baseline exercise showed an inverse association between exercise and breast carcinoma for postmenopausal women.

Although physical activity in untrained women results in acute increases in estradiol and progesterone levels,[42] with continued physical activity performed on a regular basis, there is a reduction in the length of the luteal phase and in luteal phase progesterone levels.[43] Strenuous activity may even result in secondary amenorrhea during adolescence.[44] This may explain why menarche is delayed in premenarcheal girls who engage in regular exercise and why physical activity may result in anovulatory cycles in adolescent girls.[45] It is unclear whether the protective effect of exercise, however, is due to reduction in ovulatory cycles, later menarche, earlier menopause, or other factors that tend to be associated with exercise, such as leaner body weight, reduced fat consumption, or other unrecognized factors. The etiologic window in a woman's life for a protective effect of physical activity on breast cancer prevention has not been determined. Given the other known benefits of regular exercise, however, including its effects in reducing the risk for atherosclerotic heart disease, diabetes mellitus, osteoporosis, and colon and endometrial carcinoma, it seems justified to advise regular exercise beginning early in life, specifically during puberty, and continuing into adulthood.[46-48]

Is there a role for dietary modification in breast cancer prevention?

Epidemiologic studies have consistently noted a lower risk for breast cancer, gastrointestinal cancers, and cardiovascular disease among persons whose diets include relatively large amounts of fruits and vegetables.[49,50] Ecologic studies have also noted a positive correlation between national per capita fat consumption and breast cancer[51] and an inverse correlation between soy consumption and both breast cancer and cardiovascular disease.[52-54]

Does dietary fat have any effect on breast cancer development?

Dietary experiments in rats and mice demonstrate a mammary tumor–promoting effect of diets high in total fat (approximately 35% to 40% fat in calories, which is similar to the typical American diet) as compared with diets low in total fat (approximately 10% fat in calories, which is similar to the Japanese diet). Moreover, diets with a greater proportion of unsaturated fats (specifically corn oil) were more effective than diets rich in saturated fats in increasing the mammary tumor incidence or reducing the latent period of mammary tumor appearance.[55-59] Monounsaturated fat (e.g., olive oil), on the other hand, appears either to act as a poor promoter or to have a protective effect.[59] In humans, ingestion of a low-fat diet reduces endogenous estradiol and estrone levels without affecting ovulation.[60]

Hunter and colleagues[61] reported a meta-analysis of seven prospective cohort studies that included 4980 breast cancer cases among 337,819 women in four countries: the United States, Canada, Sweden, and the Netherlands. When women in the highest quartile of energy-adjusted total fat intake were compared with women in the lowest quartile, there was no significant difference in breast cancer risk when adjusted for other factors. There was also no association when intakes of cholesterol, saturated fat, monounsaturated fat, and polyunsaturated fat were considered individually. In contrast, Howe and colleagues[62] in a meta-analysis of 12 case-control studies that included 4427 breast cancer cases and 6095 controls, revealed a highly significant positive association between saturated fat intake and breast cancer risk in postmenopausal women. The relative risk for the highest to lowest quintile was 1.46. Cho and associates reported a slight increased risk for dietary fat and breast cancer for premenopausal women.[63] In this study, dietary fat and breast cancer risk were assessed among 90,655 premenopausal women in the Nurses' Health Study II. During the 8 years of follow-up, 714 women developed incident breast cancer. The relative risk for the highest to lowest quintile was 1.25. The increase was associated with intake of animal fat but not of vegetable fat. Among food groups contributing to animal fat, red meat and high-fat dairy foods each was associated with an increased risk for breast cancer.

Changing one's dietary habits to protect against breast cancer may mean lowering fat levels far below what the average American woman consumes. In addition, the times of consumption of dietary fat such as during childhood and adolescence may play an important role in prevention.

Do dietary monounsaturated fats protect against breast cancer?

Some evidence suggests a protective effect from monounsaturated fats. Although corn oil, a polyunsaturated fat, promotes mammary cancer in animal models, olive oil, a monounsaturated fat, either acts as a poor promoter or has a protective effect.[59] Furthermore, Greek women have a substantially lower breast cancer mortality than American women despite their higher relative energy intake from fat.[64] Three case-control studies have evaluated the effect of monounsaturated fats in the form of olive oil consumption on breast cancer risk in Greece, Italy, and Spain, all of which have high per capita consumption of olive oil.[65–67] Two of the studies (performed in Greece and Spain) demonstrated a protective effect for relatively high olive oil consumption. A protective effect for monounsaturated fat was not found in the pooled analysis of cohort studies reported by Hunter and colleagues,[61] although none of the cohort studies included in this analysis were performed in countries with high consumption of olive oil. Cho and associates reported that both saturated and monounsaturated fat were related to modestly elevated breast cancer risk.[63]

Is there a role for soy or soy derivatives in breast cancer prevention?

Soybeans and soy-based products and derivatives of soy-based products, such as genistein and daidzein, contain isoflavonoids, which are naturally occurring phytoestrogens that inhibit carcinogen-induced mammary tumors in animals.[68] The isoflavonoids are weak estrogen agonists and may interfere with the promoting effects of physiologic concentrations of estrogens. Soy-based products are also rich in protease inhibitors, which also inhibit carcinogen-induced mammary tumors. Although there are epidemiologic data that demonstrate an inverse correlation between soy consumption and breast cancer risk,[69] other studies have not been consistent in this correlation.[70,71] Also, there is no evidence that supplementation of a typical Western diet with soy-based products modifies breast cancer risk.

Does obesity control play a role in breast cancer prevention?

Obesity is associated with an increased risk for breast cancer, specifically in postmenopausal women.[72,73] Obesity is also associated with a higher recurrence rate and poorer survival in women with breast cancer.[74] In a prospectively studied population of more than 900,000 U.S. adults who were free of cancer at enrollment and followed for up to 16 years, there was a positive association between high body mass index (BMI—weight in kilograms divided by the square of the height in meters) and breast cancer mortality. In addition, there was a linear association between increasing BMI and breast cancer mortality; the relative risk (RR) was 1.34% for a BMI between 25 and 29.9, 1.63% for a BMI between 30 and 34.9, 1.70% for a BMI between 35 and 39.9, and 2.12% (1.41%–3.19%) for a BMI of 40 or more ($P < .001$ for trend).[75] Avoidance of weight gain during adulthood has many benefits that are likely to include reduction in risk for postmenopausal breast cancer.[76]

What role does fiber play in breast cancer prevention?

Fiber ingestion inhibits the intestinal resorption of estrogens in humans and reduces mammary cancer incidence in animals.[60,77] Asian women eating a traditional low-fat, high-fiber diet have lower estrogen levels before and after menopause and have a lower breast cancer risk compared with Western populations.[78] Ingestion of a low-fat (less than 10% of calories), high-fiber (35 to 45 g/day) diet by white women significantly reduces serum estrone and estradiol levels during the early follicular and late luteal phases of the menstrual cycle without affecting ovulation.[79] In another study, however, ingestion of pure fiber (20 g of α-cellulose daily) without modification of fat intake had no effect on estrogen metabolism.[80]

Despite a strong biologic rationale, epidemiologic data do not demonstrate a consistent benefit for fiber. Howe[51] reported a meta-analysis of 12 case-control studies in which the relative risk for breast cancer was 0.85 for subjects who consumed more fiber. Other studies employing prospective cohort methodology observed no effect or a marginally significant effect of fiber ingestion.[81–83]

What role do vitamins play in breast cancer prevention?

There has been increasing scientific and public interest in supplemental vitamin ingestion to reduce cancer risk, including breast cancer risk. Observational studies had suggested that people who consume more fruits and vegetables containing the antioxidant vitamins A, C, and E have somewhat lower risks for cancer.[49,50,84] Vitamin A reduces the proliferative capacity and promotes the differentiation of primary human mammary epithelial cells.[85] The antioxidant vitamins may prevent cancer-causing DNA damage and inhibit atherogenesis by their ability to scavenge free radicals, the byproducts of normal metabolism.[86,87] In order to assess the impact of vitamin ingestion on cancer risk, Hunter and colleagues[88] prospectively studied 89,494 women aged 34 to 59 years in 1980 who did not have cancer, assessing their intakes of vitamins C, E, and A at baseline and 4 years later with a validated semiquantitative food frequency questionnaire. During the 8-year follow-up period, large intakes of vitamins C and E were not protective against breast cancer. A low intake of vitamin A from food was associated with increased breast cancer risk; this was reduced by ingestion of vitamin A supplements. Similar results were recently published by Michels and coworkers[89] based on a large population-based prospective cohort study in Sweden. This study comprised 59,036 women, 40 to 76 years of age, who were free of breast cancer at baseline and 1271 of these women who later developed breast cancer. Trials are underway to determine whether the retinoids, which include vitamin A and its synthetic analogues (i.e., fenretidine), may play a role in breast cancer prevention.

There has also been interest in a possible relationship between calcium and vitamin D intake and breast cancer. There is an inverse correlation between sunlight exposure (as a source of vitamin D) and breast cancer.[90] The promoting activity of high dietary fat in animals is enhanced by low intake of calcium and vitamin D and can be inhibited by increased calcium (and probably vitamin D) supplementation.[91] Vitamin D and its synthetic analogues have been shown to promote the death of breast cancer cells grown in the laboratory.[92] Vitamin D and calcium intake is well below the recommended daily allowance in American women in all age groups, but especially in elderly people.[93] Breast cancer prevention, and simultaneous prevention of osteoporosis, might be achieved by increasing dietary intake of calcium and vitamin D to recommended dietary allowance (RDA) levels. This may be particularly applicable to females during puberty and adolescence. There is currently no proof, however, that calcium or vitamin D supplements are protective against breast cancer development.

Can consumption of no alcohol or decreased consumption of alcohol be associated with breast cancer prevention?

The available evidence from more than 50 epidemiologic studies, as well as numerous meta-analyses involving cohort and case control studies, indicates that alcohol consumption (i.e., beer, wine, and spirits) is associated with a moderate increase in breast cancer risk.[94,95] Data indicate a modest positive association between alcohol and breast cancer (an approximately 25% increase in risk with daily intake of the equivalent of two drinks) and a dose-response relation.[94] The biologic basis for the effect of alcohol is unclear, although some data suggest that alcohol may augment gonadotropin-induced increases in serum estradiol levels.[96] The alcohol–breast cancer hypothesis is important because alcohol consumption is common and drinking is a potentially modifiable behavior for a motivated individual. In one survey, 61% of women reported being "current drinkers" (at least 12 drinks yearly). Of the current drinkers, 39% were light drinkers (up to 3 drinks weekly), 27% were moderate drinkers (4 to 13 drinks weekly), and 9% were heavy drinkers (14 or more drinks weekly).[94]

MODIFICATION OF EXPOSURE TO ENVIRONMENTAL FACTORS

What role does radiation exposure play in breast cancer development?

The risk for breast cancer is increased in women exposed to relatively high doses of ionizing irradiation, such as in therapeutic use (for postpartum mastitis, thymic enlargement, and Hodgkin's disease) and after inadvertent or accidental exposure (fluoroscopy for tuberculosis or nuclear fallout from an atomic bomb).[97–100] Exposure during puberty or earlier is associated with a substantially greater risk for breast cancer than comparable exposure at an older age, and thus the benefit of using diagnostic radiation, particularly in women younger than 20 years, should be considered carefully. The low irradiation dose employed in a routine mammogram (0.15 cGy to each breast) and chest film (0.002 cGy to each breast) and the relatively advanced age during which these modalities are employed make it extremely unlikely that they in any way contribute to breast cancer risk. Furthermore, annual screening mammography clearly reduces breast cancer mortality in women 50 years or older, indicating that the benefits far outweigh any risks that may be involved.[101]

Exposure to diagnostic radiation may be associated with increased breast cancer risk, however, in patients who are heterozygotes for the ataxia-telangiectasia (*AT*) gene, a group that makes up about 1.4% of the general population.[102] *AT* heterozygotes are healthy persons, whereas homozygotes have a characteristic disorder including cerebellar ataxia, oculocutaneous telangiectases, endocrine disorders, and humoral and cellular immune defects. The homozygotes have a markedly increased risk for developing lymphoid and epithelial neoplasms, and they exhibit tissue necrosis after exposure to therapeutic irradiation, effects that are due to an inherent deficiency in repairing damaged DNA.[103] Evidence suggests that *AT* heterozygotes have a fivefold increased risk for breast cancer and that exposure to diagnostic irradiation (in the form of fluoroscopic examination of the chest, back, or abdomen) contributes to this increased risk.[104,105] Although screening of the general population for the *AT* gene is not yet practical, it may be prudent to screen relatives of *AT* homozygotes. It appears that special measures involving low-dose radiation exposure could help prevent breast cancer development in these persons and others who are heterozygous for familial and chromosomal breakage syndromes.

Is electromagnetic radiation exposure associated with breast cancer?

Increased breast cancer risk has been reported in female and male electrical workers.[106,107] In contrast, others have found no association between low-frequency field exposure in the workplace and breast cancer risk.[108–110] A recent study of the effect of exposure of magnetic fields to female residents of Los Angeles county, California (743 breast cancer cases and 699 controls) suggest that residential magnetic field exposure did not influence risk for breast cancer.[111] Similarly, a case-control study of the relationship between electromagnetic fields and breast cancer on Long Island (the Electromagnetic Field Breast Cancer Long Island Study, or EBCLIS) reported no association between breast cancer and residential electromagnetic field exposures.[112]

CHEMOPREVENTION

What is the rationale for chemoprevention with tamoxifen and other selective estrogen modulators?

The selective estrogen receptor modulators (SERMs) are chemically diverse compounds that lack the steroid structure of estrogen yet bind to the estrogen receptor (ER) and mediate antagonist or agonist effects, depending on the conformation of the SERM, differing level of ER expression in the target tissue, and differing expression and binding of coregulatory proteins.[113] Both tamoxifen and raloxifene are SERMs that have many attributes of a good chemoprevention agent. Both are taken once daily, are commonly prescribed for other conditions, and are generally safe and well tolerated. Furthermore, substantial preclinical and clinical evidence has demonstrated potential chemopreventive effects for these agents. Tamoxifen has been approved for many years for the treatment of early-stage and advanced breast cancer in both premenopausal and postmenopausal women, whereas raloxifene is approved for the treatment and prevention of osteoporosis in postmenopausal women.[114] Tamoxifen significantly reduces the risk for contralateral breast cancer in patients with a prior history of breast cancer. In the meta-analysis performed by the Early Breast Cancer Trialists' Collaborative Group, tamoxifen reduced the rate of contralateral breast cancer by 47%.[115] Raloxifene has likewise been associated with a reduced breast cancer risk in patients with osteopenia or osteoporosis. The Multiple Outcomes of Raloxifene Evaluation (MORE) Trial included 7704 healthy postmenopausal subjects with osteoporosis up to 80 years of age who were randomized to receive either raloxifene (60 or 120 mg daily) or a placebo.[116] Although raloxifene was also associated with an increased risk for thromboembolic disease comparable to tamoxifen, it was not associated with an increased risk for endometrial cancer. Although these studies would seem to indicate that these drugs have equivalent chemopreventive effects, there were important differences between the study populations. Tamoxifen was evaluated in both premenopausal and postmenopausal patients with a previous diagnosis of breast cancer, a condition known to be associated with an increased risk for breast cancer. Raloxifene was evaluated only in postmenopausal patients with osteoporosis, a condition known to be associated with reduced breast cancer risk.[117] These findings have prompted the evaluation of SERMs as chemopreventive agents.

Does tamoxifen reduce the risk for developing breast cancer?

The National Surgical Adjuvant Breast and Bowel Project (NSABP) performed a trial that included 13,388 healthy female subjects who had an elevated risk for developing breast cancer (P-1 trial). Selection criteria included prior diagnosis of lobular carcinoma in situ of any age, age of at least 60 years, or age between 35 and 59 years with a 5-year risk for developing breast cancer as estimated by the Gail model to be at least equivalent to that of a 60-year-old woman (at least 1.66%).[118] Seventy-seven percent had at least one first-degree relative with breast cancer, and the age distribution was fairly evenly balanced between older women (30% older than 60 years), middle-aged women (31% between 50 and 60 years), and younger women (39% between 35 and 49 years). All women were followed with annual physical examination and mammography. After a median follow-up of 3.5 years, the Data Monitoring Committee recommended unblinding the treatment arms because of a 49% reduction in the risk for developing breast cancer (both invasive and noninvasive cancer) in

the tamoxifen arm compared with the placebo arm. Other noteworthy findings included the following: (1) about 4% of women in the placebo arm developed invasive breast cancer during the course of the study, indicating that the eligibility criteria used were successful in selecting a group at elevated risk for developing breast cancer; (2) tamoxifen reduced the risk for estrogen receptor (ER)–positive breast cancers but had no effect on the development of ER-negative breast cancers; (3) there was a reduction in the risk for both invasive and in situ carcinoma; and (4) tamoxifen reduced the risk for breast cancer in all age groups, in patients with a family history, and in patients with lobular carcinoma in situ (LCIS) or atypical hyperplasia. Tamoxifen had no effect on survival, although a beneficial effect on survival was not expected.

On the basis of these findings, the U.S. Food and Drug Administration approved tamoxifen for reducing the risk for breast cancer in women at high risk for developing the disease. Three other trials evaluating tamoxifen were ongoing at the time that these findings were initially reported, prompting early reporting of the trials. The results of these trials are contrasted with the P-1 trial in Table 6–2.[119-121] The trials varied in their sample size, selection criteria, and other factors, including the use of concurrent hormone replacement therapy in 20% to 40% of patients in these trials. Only IBIS-I trial demonstrated that tamoxifen significantly reduced the risk for breast cancer by 33%. A meta-analysis that included these four trials confirmed a significant reduction in breast cancer risk of 38% (95% CI, 28%–46%; $P < .0001$) for tamoxifen, with no significant reduction in the risk of ER-negative breast cancer but a 48% reduction (95% CI, 36%–58%; $P < .0001$) in the risk for ER-positive breast cancer.[122] It also confirmed that tamoxifen was associated with an increased risk for endometrial cancer (RR 2.4%; 95% CI, 1.5%–4.0%; $P = .0005$), an effect that was not seen with raloxifene. Both tamoxifen and raloxifene were associated with an increased risk for thromboembolic events (RR, 1.9%; 95% CI, 1.4%–2.6%; $P < .0001$). The American Society of Clinical Oncology Technology Assessment Panel[123] concluded, "For women with a defined five year projected breast cancer risk of > 1.66%, tamoxifen (at 20 mg/day for 5 years) may be offered to reduce their risk." The panel did not recommend against the use of raloxifene, aromatase inhibitors, or retinoids for prevention. Other expert panels, including the Canadian Task Force on Preventive Health Care[124] and the National Comprehensive Cancer Network,[125] came to similar conclusions.

How should subjects be selected for tamoxifen prevention therapy?

Healthy subjects were selected for participation in the P-1 trial. Ideally, an individual should not have a significant comorbid condition or history of or known predisposition to thromboembolic disease. Individuals were selected by the Gail model, which includes the following factors in estimating risk: (1) current age, (2) age at menarche, (3) age at first live birth [nulliparous, <20, 20–24, 25–29, >29, unknown], (4) number of first-degree relatives with breast cancer [0, 1, 2 or more, unknown], (5) number of prior breast biopsies [0, 1, 2 or more, unknown], (6) did any prior biopsy show atypical hyperplasia [yes, no, unknown], and (7) race [white, black, Hispanic].[126-128] The model calculates a 5-year risk and a

Table 6–2   Phase III Trials Comparing Tamoxifen with Placebo in Healthy Female Subjects

	NSABP P-1	Royal Marsden	Italian Trial	IBIS-I
Reference (no.)	Fisher et al., 1998 (118)	Powles et al., 1998 (119)	Veronesi et al., 1998 (120)	IBIS, 2002 (121)
No. of subjects	13,388	2494	5408	7410
Selection	5-year risk ≥ 1.66% due to age (≥60 yr), Gail model, or LCIS	Age 30–70 yr and family history	Age 35–70 yr and prior hysterectomy	Age 35–70 yr with family history, LCIS, or atypia
Family history	77%	96%	18%	97%
Age ≥ 50 yr	61%	39%	62%	<50%
Concurrent HRT use	None	42%	19%	40%
Mean follow-up	55 mo	70 mo	46 mo	50 mo
Risk reduction (RR)	49%	NS	NS	33%

NS, not significant; HRT, hormone replacement therapy; LCIS, lobular carcinoma in situ; RR, risk reduction includes both invasive and noninvasive breast cancer.

lifetime risk for the individual, and a comparison risk of a woman having the same current age but with average risk factors. Individuals were required to have an estimated 5-year risk of at least 1.66% to be eligible for the P-1 trial. The Gail model is appropriate for women without prior breast cancer and those who are not known to have or to be at increased risk for having a *BRCA1* or *BRCA2* mutation. In addition, for women who have family members with breast cancer diagnosed before the age of 50 years, the Claus model may be preferable.[129]

A version of the Gail Model may be found on the National Cancer Institute website (*http://bcra.nci.nih.gov/brc*).

What are the side effects of tamoxifen therapy when used for risk reduction?

The NSABP trial demonstrated that tamoxifen has a 2.5-fold elevation in the risk for uterine carcinoma and a nearly 2-fold elevation in the risk for thromboembolic disease in women 50 years of age or older, but not in younger women. Women taking tamoxifen were also slightly more likely to be diagnosed with cataracts and to require cataract surgery. There was no significant difference in the risk for bone fracture, and there was no difference in mortality between the tamoxifen and placebo groups. There was an increased prevalence of bothersome symptoms (described as extremely bothersome or quite a bit bothersome), including hot flashes (46% vs. 29%) and vaginal discharge (13% vs. 3%).[118] There was no difference found in the health-related quality-of-life measures (including depression and physical well-being). Patients taking tamoxifen reported problems with sexual function at a definite or serious level, although the overall rates of sexual activity in the two groups were not different.[130]

Does the risk-to-benefit ratio favor taking tamoxifen?

A key question for an individual considering tamoxifen for risk reduction is whether the benefits of tamoxifen outweigh

the risk. The risk-to-benefit ratio is therefore dependent not only on the subject's underlying risk for developing breast cancer but also on the subject's likelihood of developing serious problems such as thromboembolic disease or uterine carcinoma. Gail and colleagues[131] have developed models for estimating risk-to-benefit ratio for individuals considering tamoxifen for risk reduction. The models are based on assumptions regarding underlying risks for uterine cancer, thromboembolic disease, fractures, and cataracts in the general population, factors that vary by race. In general, women who are younger, who have a higher risk for breast cancer, and who have had a prior hysterectomy are more likely to have a favorable risk-to-benefit ratio. For example, the risk-to-benefit ratio using this model does not favor use of tamoxifen for any white or black women with a uterus who is 60 years of age or older. For women between the ages of 50 and 59 years, the risk-to-benefit ratio is favorable only for white women who have a 5-year breast cancer risk exceeding 4%, or black women who have a 5-year risk exceeding 6.5%. For women 49 years or younger, the risk-to-benefit ratio is favorable for both black and white women of all risk groups. For women who have had a prior hysterectomy, the risk-to-benefit ratio becomes favorable for white women between 50 and 59 years, and between 60 and 69 years if their risk exceeds 3.5%, but is generally not favorable for black women of the same age. Subjects considering tamoxifen prophylaxis should be routinely counseled regarding their risk-to-benefit ratio.

Is tamoxifen beneficial in women with hereditary breast cancer?

Tamoxifen is clearly effective in reducing the risk for breast cancer in women who have at least one first-degree relative with the disease. There is less information regarding its effectiveness in subjects with known heritable mutations predisposing to breast cancer, such as *BRCA1* or *BRCA2*. Because about 80% of breast cancers in women with *BRCA1* mutations are ER negative, there is concern that tamoxifen may not be effective in such women; on the other hand, risk-reducing salpingo-oophorectomy seems to reduce breast cancer risk in this setting. King and associates reported on a subset of 288 women participating in the P-1 trial who developed breast cancer, of whom only 8 had *BRCA1* mutations and 11 had *BRCA2* mutations.[132] Because of the relatively small sample size and relative wide confidence intervals, firm conclusions could not be drawn. However, a case-control study demonstrated a protective effect of tamoxifen against contralateral breast cancer for women with *BRCA1* mutations but not *BRCA2* mutations.[133] There is currently a need for additional information concerning the use of tamoxifen in women with *BRCA1* or *BRCA2* mutations.

Are there alternatives to tamoxifen?

No drug other than tamoxifen has been proven to reduce the risk for breast cancer in women at elevated risk for developing the disease, but other agents are currently being evaluated in ongoing clinical trials, including retinoids, other SERMs, and aromatase inhibitors. Raloxifene is being evaluated as an alternative to tamoxifen because it does not seem to be associated with an increased risk for uterine cancer. Aromatase inhibitors offer a promising route of chemoprevention through suppression of estrogen formation within the breast tissue. Aromatase converts androgens to estrogen and is expressed at a higher level in breast tissue than in the surrounding tissue. Aromatase inhibitors (e.g., anastrozole, letrozole, exemestane) are being evaluated based on sound preclinical and clinical rationale,[134] a position that is supported by several recently reported trials in women with early-stage breast cancer. For example, the risk for contralateral breast cancer was reduced by about 60% in women treated with anastrozole compared with tamoxifen in the ATAC trial.[135] In addition, letrozole reduced the risk for contralateral breast cancer by approximately 45% when used following 5 years of tamoxifen therapy.[136] Ongoing trials evaluating these agents are summarized in Table 6–3.[136–140]

The studies evaluating SERMs and aromatase inhibitors outlined above are generally being performed in patients with either natural or induced menopause, either because of the lack of safety information in premenopausal women (i.e., raloxifene) or because the drug requires a menopausal state to

be effective (i.e., aromatase inhibitors). Veronesi evaluated the synthetic retinoid fenretinide (200 mg daily) compared with a placebo for 5 years in 2972 women with early-stage breast carcinoma. Although there was no effect in reducing contralateral breast cancer in the entire study population, there was a significant reduction in contralateral breast cancer in premenopausal women.[141] There is insufficient evidence, however, to recommend retinoids for this indication. Recently, grapes and red wine have been shown to contain the compound resveratrol that inhibits aromatase. Resveratrol has been shown to inhibit the development of preneoplastic lesions in mouse mammary tumor cells and human cancer cells grown in the laboratory.[142]

What other candidate chemopreventive agents may be considered in the future?

There are numerous additional agents that are currently under active evaluation as potential chemopreventive agents. In addition, recent studies suggest that protocols based on combinations of chemopreventive agents should be the focus of future investigations. A few of the more promising compounds under evaluation are reviewed here.

Nonsteroidal anti-inflammatory agents (NSAIDs), including inhibitors of cyclo-oxygenase-2 (COX-2), have received much attention as potential chemopreventive agents.[143] For example, regular NSAID use (2 or more tablets/week) for 10 or more years was associated with a 28% reduction in the incidence of breast cancer (RR, 0.72; 95% CI, 0.56%–0.91%) in the Women's Health Initiative, and there was a statistically significant inverse linear trend of breast cancer incidence with the duration of NSAID use ($P < .01$).[144] Regular use of acetaminophen (an analgesic agent with little or no anti-inflammatory activity) or low-dose aspirin (<100 mg) was unrelated to the incidence of breast cancer. The inducible prostaglandin synthetase COX-2 is normally expressed predominantly in kidney and brain. COX-2 overexpression has been described in numerous human cancers, and recently COX-2 has been shown to be present in approximately 40% of invasive breast cancers, particularly those that overexpress *HER-2/neu*. There is an increasing body of evidence supporting a role for COX-2 in breast cancer development and pro-

Table 6–3   Summary of Chemoprevention Trials Evaluating Alternatives to Tamoxifen

	RUTH	STAR	HOT	IBIS-2	ApreS
Reference (no.)	Mosca et al., 2001 (137)	Vogel et al., 2001 (138)	Decensi et al., 2003 (139)	Cuzick et al., 2001 (140)	Goss et al., 2003 (134)
Accrual goal	10,000	19,000	85,000	10,000	666
Selection	⇑ Risk for heart disease	⇑ Breast cancer risk	⇑ Breast cancer risk	⇑ Breast cancer risk	*BRCA1/2* mutation
Arms	Raloxifene, 60 mg QD vs. placebo	Tamoxifen, 20 mg QD vs. placebo	Tamoxifen, 20 mg QD vs. placebo	Anastrazole, 1 mg QD vs. placebo	Exemestane, 25 mg QD vs. placebo
Duration	5 yr	5 yr	5 yr	5 yr	5 yr

RUTH, Raloxifene for Use in the Heart; STAR, Study of Tamoxifen and Raloxifene; HOT, Hormone Replacement Therapy Opposed by Low-Dose Tamoxifen; IBIS-2, International Breast Intervention Study-2; ApreS, Aromasin Prevention Study.

gression through effects on angiogenesis and apoptosis as well as through effects on intramural aromatase.[143] A large clinical trial is currently evaluating the role of the COX-2 inhibitor celecoxib when used as secondary prevention in conjunction with aromatase inhibitors in women with early-stage breast cancer.[136]

The peroxisome proliferator–activated receptor (PPAR) gamma, whose inactivation occurs during mammary gland carcinogenesis, is a nuclear receptor that is activated by polyunsaturated fatty acids (PUFAs), eicosanoids, and antidiabetic agents. Such activation, which is enhanced by ligands of the retinoic receptor (RAR) and the retinoid X receptor (RXR), suppresses breast carcinogenesis in experimental models and induces differentiation of human liposarcoma cells. Selective PPAR ligands or modulators (SPARMs) are currently being designed to have desired effects on specific genes relevant to breast cancer development. Recent evidence for a synergistic interaction between RAR as well as RXR with PPAR gamma suggests that appropriate selective ligands from these two groups of receptors might be combined in breast cancer chemoprevention studies.[145,146]

Histone deacetylation inhibitors, combined with demethylating agents, are promising as a means of rehabilitating silenced tumor suppressor genes. Inhibitors of activated tyrosine kinases (receptor tyrosine kinase inhibitors) offer a means of inhibiting increased growth factors and growth factor receptor expression and activation.[147]

The statins atorvastatin, fluvastatin, lovastatin, and simvastatin were shown to inhibit proliferation of MCF-7, a human breast cancer cell line, by up to 90%. These data have led to studies to determine whether statins, in addition to their cholesterol-lowering effect, may have clinical significance in chemoprevention of human breast cancer.[148]

The monoterpenes, including limonene and perillyl alcohol, prevent carcinogen-induced and spontaneous rodent mammary tumors during the initiation phase as well as the promotion/progression phase. Limonene, a monocyclic monoterpene that is the major component of the peels of oranges and lemons, has little or no toxicity. Both D-limonene and perillyl alcohol, a more potent analogue of limonene, are in phase I and II prevention trials.[149,150]

The isothiocyanates, thiocyanates, and other sulfur-containing compounds (disulfiram and allyl sulfides) are effective chemopreventive agents in animal models in which they have been utilized as anti-initiators against carcinogen-induced mammary tumors.[151] They inhibit cytochrome P-450 phase I hepatic enzymes or induce phase II detoxification enzymes.[152] Increased consumption of cruciferous vegetables (e.g., cabbage, broccoli, cauliflower, Brussels sprouts), which are rich sources of isothiocyanates, are associated with a reduced incidence of intestinal cancers in humans.[153] Cruciferous vegetables are also rich in indole-3-carbinol, an effective chemopreventive agent in animals.[154] Ingestion of indole-3-carbinol by humans (400 mg/day) produces a significant increase in 2-hydroxyestrone, resulting in decreased production of 16-α-hydroxyestrone.[78] 16-α-Hydroxyestrone is genotoxic to mammary cells, and its production correlates closely with the development of mammary tumors in animals.[155] Women with breast cancer often have a low urinary ratio of 2-hydroxyestrone to 16-α-hydroxyestrone compared with age-matched controls, suggesting that endogenous differences in estrogen metabolism may account for increased

breast cancer risk.[156] Preliminary human trials have demonstrated that indole-3-carbinol is well tolerated and has a sustained estrogen-modifying effect.[157] Therefore, the evidence suggests that indole-3-carbinol, by modulating estrogen metabolism, may be chemopreventive.

Lycopene, a carotenoid present in tomatoes, processed tomato products, and other fruits, is one of the most potent antioxidants among dietary carotenoids. Although some recent studies have suggested that lycopene and other plasma carotenoids may reduce the risk for developing breast cancer, others have not seen an association.[158–160]

Calcium glucarate, which is normally synthesized in human liver cells and is also present in vegetables and fruits, has been shown to inhibit chemically induced mammary tumors in the rat. Oral supplementation of calcium-D-glucarate has been shown to inhibit β-glucuronidase, an enzyme whose elevated expression is associated with an increased risk for breast cancer. The chemopreventive ability of this nontoxic agent may be twofold in that it may act as a regulator of estrogen metabolism and also as a detoxifying agent of carcinogens responsible for breast cancer.[161]

Organic and inorganic selenium inhibits both chemically induced and spontaneous mammary tumors in animal models.[162] Although selenium inhibits the initiation and postinitiation phases of carcinogenesis at both the cellular and molecular levels, its toxicity has been of concern. Recently, however, synthetic organoselenium compounds, such as Se-methylselenocysteine, that have optimal chemopreventive potency and low toxicity in animals have been developed and should allow for the adequate investigation of selenium as a chemopreventive agent in human breast cancer.[163]

Dihydroepiandrosterone (DHEA) is an adrenocortical steroid that prevents carcinogen-induced mammary tumors in animal models. DHEA appears to affect the promotion stage of tumorigenesis, suggesting that this agent may be useful in inhibiting the transition from human ductal carcinoma in situ (DCIS) to invasive carcinoma.[164]

REMOVAL OF THE TARGET ORGAN (PROPHYLACTIC BILATERAL MASTECTOMY)

What is the rationale for prophylactic bilateral mastectomy?

Prophylactic bilateral mastectomy (PBM) is a logical, although extreme, measure for the prevention of breast cancer. Indeed, occult cancer has been detected in up to 5% of prophylactic mastectomy specimens in untargeted populations that included low-risk and high-risk patients.[165] On the other hand, occult cancer has been reported to be found incidentally at autopsy in 20% of young and middle-aged women who died of causes other than breast cancer.[166] Mammary tumors can occur in animals, however, despite prophylactic removal of mammary tissue, and risk reduction is not proportional to the percentage of mammary tissue removed.[167,168] In humans treated with mastectomy for breast cancer, residual mammary tissue is often left behind in the axilla and pectoralis fascia.[169]

What are the results of prophylactic bilateral mastectomy?

Hartmann and colleagues retrospectively evaluated all women with a family history of breast cancer who underwent PBM at the Mayo Clinic over a 33-year period.[170] Of the 1065 women who underwent the procedure, 214 met their criteria for "high-risk" family history and 425 met their criteria for "moderate-risk" family history. High-risk family history was defined as established criteria suggestive of a heritable breast cancer predisposition, whereas moderate risk included those who had a family history in first-degree or more distant relatives but who did not meet the high-risk criteria.[171] The median age at mastectomy was 42 years, and the median length of follow-up was 14 years. Using the Gail model to estimate the expected incidence in the moderate-risk group, there was a 90% reduction in the observed-to-expected incidence of breast cancer (0.9% vs. 8.8%). When comparing the 214 high-risk probands with their 403 sisters who had not undergone a mastectomy, there was a significant reduction in the incidence of breast cancer in the probands compared with their sisters (1.4% vs. 38.7%). Recurrent cancers most often were diagnosed only on the chest wall and occurred after a median of 6 years (range, 2–25 years). PBM also resulted in about a 90% reduction in the risk for death from breast cancer. A subsequent report from this same group retrospectively identified 26 women with an alteration in BRCA1 or BRCA2, 18 of which were known to be deleterious.[172] None of the 26 women who had PBM developed breast cancer after a median of 13.4 years of follow-up (range, 5.8–28.5 years), suggesting a beneficial effect in mutation carriers.

Meijers-Heijboer prospectively evaluated the effectiveness of PBM in 139 healthy women known to have BRCA1 or BRCA2 mutations but no prior history of breast cancer, of whom 76 chose PBM and 63 chose surveillance.[173] After a mean follow-up of about 3 years, there were no cases of breast cancer in the PBM group compared with 8 cases in the surveillance group. The annual incidence of breast cancer in the surveillance group was 2.5% and was consistent with the number of cases expected for this population.

Although these studies seem to indicate a clear protective effect for PBM, some experts have pointed out that it is difficult to accept the notion that prevention of the disease by PBM is not too extreme a procedure as a cure of established disease, which can often be managed with breast-conserving surgery.[174] In addition, most women with established disease are cured, and up to 50% of women with heritable mutations may never develop breast cancer. Furthermore, the PBM is not protective against ovarian cancer, which is less common among mutation carriers than breast cancer but much more lethal. Finally, risk-reducing salpingo-oophorectomy is protective against both ovarian and breast cancer (when performed in premenopausal women) and does not induce the physical and psychosocial consequences of breast loss, nor does it result in the need for additional reconstructive breast surgery. For individuals who are more fearful of a breast cancer diagnosis than the surgery required to prevent it, however, PBM may be an appropriate choice.

Is there a role for prophylactic mastectomy in women with a prior history of breast cancer?

McDonnell and coworkers[175] followed 745 women with a first breast cancer and a family history of breast or ovarian cancer who underwent contralateral prophylactic mastectomy (CPM) at the Mayo Clinic over a 33-year period. There was about a 95% reduction in the risk for contralateral breast cancer, a result similar to that obtained for PBM in high-risk women with no prior breast cancer history.

What is the optimal procedure for patients who undergo prophylactic bilateral mastectomy?

Bilimoria and Morrow[176] have recommended that preventive surgery should be simple mastectomy, which encompasses removal of the entire breast, including the nipple, the areola, and the breast tissue that extends into the axilla. Axillary lymph node dissection is not appropriate in these prophylactic procedures. Simple mastectomy may be followed by immediate reconstruction using implant or myocutaneous flaps. Subcutaneous mastectomy may not be adequate because substantially more glandular tissue remains beneath the nipple–areolar complex, beneath the skin flaps, and in the axilla than after simple mastectomy.

What are the physical and psychological consequences of prophylactic bilateral mastectomy and breast reconstruction?

Prophylactic mastectomy and reconstruction are associated with sensate loss, particularly of the nipple–areolar complex. Another important consideration is the need for additional surgery in those individuals who choose breast reconstruction.[177] In the Mayo Clinic experience, approximately one half of those women who had reconstruction with implants required at least one unanticipated reoperation during a median follow-up of 14 years. Implant-related issues were the most common cause for reoperation.

One report indicated that approximately 60% of women indicated negative impact of the surgery on their sex lives, and 20% of women were not satisfied with the cosmetic result.[178] On the other hand, Frost and colleagues reported that among women who chose PBM at the Mayo Clinic, about 70% were satisfied with the procedure, compared with 30% who were either dissatisfied (19%) or neutral (11%).[179] Importantly, 74% reported a diminished level of emotional concern about developing breast cancer. Most women reported no change/favorable effects in levels of emotional stability (68%/23%), level of stress (58%/28%), self-esteem (69%/13%), sexual relationships (73%/4%), and feelings of femininity (67%/8%). In addition, 48% reported no change in their level of satisfaction with body appearance, and 16% reported favorable effects. These findings indicate that most women who choose PBM are satisfied with their decision, although a substantial minority may be dissatisfied.

Who should be offered prophylactic bilateral mastectomy? What are the alternatives to the procedure? How should a woman be counseled?

There are no absolute indications for prophylactic bilateral mastectomy. Close clinical observation and mammographic surveillance are a reasonable alternative for high-risk patients and offer the advantage of sparing the procedure in a substantial proportion of them. On the other hand, advanced disease may still occur in patients who undergo close surveillance, and even patients with early-stage invasive carcinoma are at risk for cancer-related mortality. Furthermore, routine screening mammography in patients younger than 50 years, the age at which close follow-up begins for the high-risk patient, is not associated with reduced breast cancer mortality.[101] In addition, there is no information regarding the efficacy of clinical and mammographic surveillance in high-risk populations. On the other hand, the finding that the 60% to 90% of premenopausal women with breast cancer have mammographically detectable cancers suggests that this approach is reasonable and likely to be efficacious in this population.[176]

It is well known that most women with a family history of breast cancer substantially overestimate their risk for developing the disease, which in turn results not only in unnecessary anxiety but also in diminished compliance with screening recommendations for some women and unnecessary requests for genetic testing or prophylactic mastectomy by others.[180–182] A limited period of regular counseling and education significantly reduces risk perception and enhances compliance with screening.[183] Other investigators have demonstrated, however, that breast cancer risk continues to be overestimated by most patients despite formal, standardized counseling sessions.[184]

CONCLUSION

Is there any effective strategy for a woman to prevent breast cancer at the present time?

The measures that a woman may wish to consider to prevent breast cancer are dependent on her underlying risks for developing the disease (see Table 6–1; see also Chapter 5). Measures that might be taken and previously discussed in detail in this chapter are summarized in Table 6–4 and have also been reviewed by experts in the field.[185] Early or multiple pregnancies, lactation, regular exercise, ingestion of adequate amounts of fruits and vegetables, limiting alcohol consumption,

Table 6–4 Modifiable Factors in Breast Cancer Prevention

Factors	Effect	Comments
Reproductive or Hormonal		
Term pregnancy before age 30 yr	Up to 30% decrease in risk	Increased risk for up to 15 yr after delivery followed by reduced risk
Multiple pregnancies	Up to 20% decrease in risk	
Lactation	Small but significant decrease in risk	Protection for premenopausal women who initiate lactation before age 29 yr and continue for at least 4 mo
Oral contraceptives, ever use	No increased risk ≥ 10 yr after cessation of use	
Oral contraceptives, current use or in past 10 yr	Slight increased risk for having breast cancer diagnosed	
Hormone replacement therapy, ever use	No risk effect	
Hormone replacement therapy, current use for >15 yr	Increases risk up to 50%	Greatest relative risk is for those with a family history
Contraceptive to suppress ovarian function through use of gonadotropin-releasing hormone agonist	May decrease risk by 50% (10-yr use); by 70% (15-yr use)	Not yet tested in large trials
Lifestyle		
Ingestion of adequate amounts of fruits and vegetables, olive oil, and soy products	Decreased risk	
Alcohol consumption	Increased risk	Proportionate to amount consumed
Exercise	Decreased risk	Proportionate to amount
Obesity	Increased risk	Applies to postmenopausal women
Tamoxifen	Decreases risk about 40%	Applies to contralateral breast cancer in women with prior breast cancer history

avoidance of obesity in postmenopausal women, and perhaps the use of olive oil and soy products may all have a protective effect and should be considered sufficient by women at average risk. Preventive measures that include diet, exercise, and avoidance of alcohol may be especially important during adolescence. For high-risk women, all of the aforementioned measures may also afford some protection, although the risk may be sufficiently high to warrant consideration of a chemoprevention trial or screening by those older than 50 years. Close observation and mammographic surveillance are clearly indicated for this group. For very-high-risk women, such as those who have a *BRCA1* or *BRCA2* gene mutation, participation in a chemoprevention trial, close observation, and prophylactic oophorectomy or bilateral mastectomy are reasonable considerations. Screening average-risk individuals with mammography and selected high-risk individuals with magnetic resonance imaging is always an option, not to prevent the disease but rather to detect it at an earlier time. Chemoprevention is not a substitute for screening, and screening should continue in those who elect chemoprevention. In addition, chemoprevention or prophylactic bilateral mastectomy should always be discussed in the context of screening as a possible alternative.

REFERENCES

1. Ries LAG, Eisner MP, Kasary CL (eds). SEER Cancer Statistics Review, 1973–1999. Bethesda, MD, National Cancer Institute, 2002.
2. King M-C, Marks JH, Mandell JB. Breast and ovarian cancer risks due to inherited mutations in *BRCA1* and *BRCA2*. Science 2003;302:643–646.
3. Colditz GA, Willett WC, Hunter DJ, et al. Family history, age, and risk of breast cancer. JAMA 1993;270:338.
4. Claus EB, Risch N, Thompson WD. Autosomal dominant inheritance of early-onset breast cancer: Implications for risk prediction. Cancer 1994;73:643–651.
5. Bruzzi P, Green SB, Byar DP, et al. Estimating the population attributable risk for multiple factors using case-control data. Am J Epidemiol 1985;122:904–910.
6. Spicer DV, Pike MC. Sex steroids and breast cancer prevention. Monogr Natl Cancer Inst 1994;16:139–147.
7. Trichopoulos D, McMahon B, Cole P. The menopause and breast cancer risk. J Natl Cancer Inst 1972;48:605–613.
8. Lambe M, Hsieh CC, Trichopoulos D, et al. Transient increase in the risk of breast cancer after giving birth. N Engl J Med 1994;331:5–9.
9. Gail MH, Brinton LA, Byar DP, et al. Projecting individualized probabilities of developing breast cancer for white females who are being examined annually. J Natl Cancer Inst 1989;81:1879–1886.
10. Toniolo PG, Levitz M, Zeleniuch-Jacquotte A, et al. A prospective study of endogenous estrogens and breast cancer in postmenopausal women. J Natl Cancer Inst 1995;87:190–197.
11. Malins DC, Holmes EH, Polissar NL, et al. The etiology of breast cancer. Characteristic alterations in hydroxyl radical-induced DNA base lesions during oncogenesis with potential for evaluating incidence risk. Cancer 1993;71:3036–3043.
12. Djuric Z, Heilbrun LK, Simon MS, et al. Levels of 5-hydroxymethyl-2′-deoxyuridine in DNA from blood as a marker of breast cancer. Cancer 1996;77:691–696.
13. Janerich DT, Hoff MB. Evidence for a crossover in breast cancer risk factors. Am J Epidemiol 1982;116:737–742.
14. Russo J, Russo IH, van Zwieten MJ, et al. Classification of neoplastic and non-neoplastic lesions of the rat mammary gland. In Jones TC, Mohr U, Hunt RD (eds). Integument and Mammary Glands of Laboratory Animals, Berlin, Springer-Verlag, 1989, pp 275–304.
15. Russo J, Russo IH. Toward a physiological approach to breast cancer prevention. Cancer Epidemiol Biomarkers Prev 1994;3:353–364.
16. Newcomb PA, Storer BE, Longnecker MP, et al. Lactation and a reduced risk of premenopausal breast cancer. N Engl J Med 1994;330:81–87.
17. Byers T, Graham S, Rzepka T, et al. Lactation and breast cancer. Evidence for a negative association in premenopausal women. Am J Epidemiol 1985;12:664–674.
18. Lee SY, Kim MT, Kim SW, et al. Effect of lifetime lactation on breast cancer risk: A Korean women's cohort study. Int J Cancer 2003;105:390–393.
19. Petrakis NL, Wrensch MR, Ernster VL, et al. Influence of pregnancy and lactation on serum and breast fluid estrogen levels: Implications for breast cancer risk. Int J Cancer 1987;40:587–591.
20. Dao TL, Bock FG, Greiner MJ. Mammary carcinogenesis by 3-methylcholanthrene. II. Inhibitory effect of pregnancy and lactation on tumor induction. J Natl Cancer Inst 1960;25:991–1003.
21. Spicer DV, Urskin G, Parisky YR, et al. Changes in mammographic densities induced by a hormonal contraceptive designed to reduce breast cancer risk. J Natl Cancer Inst 1994;86:431–436.
22. Byrne C, Shairer C, Wolfe J, et al. Mammographic features and breast cancer risk: Effects with time, age, and menopause status. J Natl Cancer Inst 1995;87:1622–1629.
23. Meijer WJ, vanLindert ACM. Prophylactic oophorectomy. Eur J Obstet Gynecol Report Biol 1992;47:59–65.
24. Schairer C, Persson I, Falkeborn M, et al. Breast cancer risk associated with gynecologic surgery and indications for such surgery. Int J Cancer 1997;70:150–154.
25. Kauff ND, Satagopan JY, Robson ME, et al. Risk-reducing salpingo-oophorectomy in women with a *BRCA1* or *BRCA2* mutation. N Engl J Med 2002;346:1609–1615.
26. Thomas RB. Oral contraceptives and breast cancer. Review of the epidemiologic literature. Contraception 1991;43:597–642.
27. Romieu I, Berlin JA, Colditz G. Oral contraceptives and breast cancer. Review and meta-analysis. Cancer 1990;66:2253–2263.
28. White E, Malone KE, Weiss NE, et al. Breast cancer among young U.S. women in relation to oral contraceptive use. J Natl Cancer Inst 1994;86:505–514.
29. Kay CR, Hannanford PC. Breast cancer and the pill: A further report from the Royal College of General Practitioners' Oral Contraception Study. Br J Cancer 1988;58:675–680.
30. Romieu I, Willett WC, Colditz GA, et al. Prospective study of oral contraceptive use and risk of breast cancer in women. J Natl Cancer Inst 1989;81:1313–1321.
31. Vessey MP, McPherson K, Villard-Makintosh L, et al. Oral contraceptives and breast cancer: Latest findings in a large cohort study. Br J Cancer 1989;59:613–617.
32. Pike MC, Henderson BE, Krailo MD, et al. Breast cancer in young women and use of oral contraceptives: Possible modifying effect of formulation and age at use. Lancet 1983;2:926–929.
33. Ferguson D, Anderson T. Morphologic evaluation of cell turnover in relation to the menstrual cycle in the "resting" human breast. Br J Cancer 1981;44:177–181.
34. Althius MD, Brogan DR, Coates RJ, et al. Hormonal content and potency of oral contraceptives and breast cancer risk among young women. Br J Cancer 2003;88:50–57.
35. Collaborative Group on Hormonal Factors in Breast Cancer. Breast cancer and hormonal contraceptives: Collaborative reanalysis of individual data on 53,297 women with breast cancer and 100,239 women without breast cancer from 54 epidemiological studies. Lancet 1996;347:1713–1727.
36. Manson JE, Hsia J, Johnson KC, et al., for the Women's Health Initiative Investigators. Estrogen plus progestin and the risk of coronary heart disease. N Engl J Med. 2003;349:523–534.
37. Chlebowski RT, Hendrix SL, Langer RD, et al., for the WHI Investigators. Influence of estrogen plus progestin on breast cancer and mammography in healthy postmenopausal women: The Women's Health Initiative Randomized Trial. JAMA 2003;289:3243–3253.
38. Bernstein L, Henderson BE, Hanisch R, et al. Physical exercise and reduced risk of breast cancer in young women. J Natl Cancer Inst 1994;86:1403–1408.
39. Dirx M, Voorips L, Goldbohn R, vandenBrandt P. Baseline recreational physical activity, history of sports participation, and postmenopausal breast carcinoma risk in the Netherlands Cohort Study. Cancer 2001;92:1638–1649.
40. Lee IM, Cook NR, Rexrode KM, Buring JE. Lifetime physical activity and risk of breast cancer. Br J Cancer 2001;85:962–965.

41. Moradi T, Adami HO, Ekboom A, et al. Physical activity and risk for breast cancer: A prospective cohort study among Swedish twins. Int J Cancer 2002;100:76–81.

42. Bonen A, Long WY, MacIntyre KP, et al. Effects of exercise on the serum concentrations of FSH, LH, progesterone, and estradiol. Eur J Appl Physiol 1979;42:15–23.

43. Ellison PT, Lager C. Moderate recreational running is associated with lowered salivary progesterone profiles in women. Am J Obstet Gynecol 1986;143:1000–1003.

44. Bernstein L, Ross RK, Lobo RA, et al. The effects of moderate physical activity on menstrual cycle patterns in adolescence: Implications for breast cancer prevention. Br J Cancer 1987;55:681–685.

45. Russell JB, Mitchell D, Musey PI, et al. The relationship of exercise to anovulatory cycles in female athletes: Hormonal and physical characteristics. Obstet Gynecol 1984;63:452–456.

46. Powell KE, Casperson CJ, Koplan JP, et al. Physical activity and chronic diseases. Am J Clin Nutr 1989;49:999–1006.

47. Sternfeld B. Cancer and the protective effect of physical activity: The epidemiologic evidence. Med Sci Sports Med 1992;24:1195–1209.

48. Levi F, LaVecchia C, Negri E. Selected physical activities and the risk of endometrial cancer. Br J Cancer 1993;67:846–851.

49. National Research Council, Committee on Diet and Health, Food and Nutrition Board, Commission of Life Sciences, Diet and Health. Implications for Reducing Chronic Disease Risk. Washington, DC, National Academy Press, 1989.

50. Block G, Patterson B, Subar A. Fruit, vegetables, and cancer prevention: A review of the epidemiological evidence. Nutr Cancer 1992; 18:1–29.

51. Howe GR. Dietary fat and breast cancer risks. Cancer 1994;74:1078–1084.

52. Shimizu H, Ross RK, Bernstein L, et al. Cancer of the prostate and breast among Japanese and white immigrants in Los Angeles County. Br J Cancer 1991;63:963–966.

53. Armstrong B, Doll R. Environmental factors and cancer incidence and mortality in different countries, with special reference to dietary practices. Int J Cancer 1975;15:617–631.

54. Anderson JW, Johnstone BM, Cook-Newell ME. Meta-analysis of the effects of soy protein intake on serum lipids. N Engl J Med 1995; 333:276–282.

55. Etkind PR, Qiu L, Lumb K. Dietary fat: Gene expression and mammary tumorigenesis. Nutr Cancer 1995;24:13–21.

56. Rose DP, Connolly JM, Meschier CL. Effect of dietary fat on human breast cancer growth and lung metastasis in nude mice. J Natl Cancer Inst 1991;83:1491–1495.

57. Welsch MA, Cohen LA, Welsch CW. Inhibition of growth of human breast carcinoma xenografts by energy expenditure via voluntary exercise in athymic mice fed a high-fat diet. Nutr Cancer 1995;23:309–318.

58. Welsch CW. Interrelationship between dietary lipids and calories and experimental mammary gland tumorigenesis. Cancer 1994;74:1055–1062.

59. Cohen LA, Thompson DO, Chio K, et al. Dietary fat and mammary cancer. II. Modulation of serum and lipid tumor composition and tumor prostaglandin by different dietary fats: Association with tumor incidence patterns. J Natl Cancer Inst 1986;77:43–51.

60. Bagga D, Ashley JM, Geffrey SP, et al. Effects of a very low fat, high fiber diet on serum hormones and menstrual function: Implications for breast cancer prevention. Cancer 1995;76:2491–2496.

61. Hunter DJ, Spiegelman D, Adami HO, et al. Cohort studies of fat intake and the risk of breast cancer—a pooled analysis. N Engl J Med 1996;334:356–361.

62. Howe GR, Hirohata T, Hislop TG, et al. Dietary factors and the risk of breast cancer: Combined analysis of 12 case-control studies. J Natl Cancer Inst 1990;82:561–569.

63. Cho E, Spiegelman D, Hunter DJ, et al. Premenopausal fat intake and risk of breast cancer. J Natl Cancer Inst 2003;95:1079–1085.

64. Trichopoulou A, Toupadaki N, Tzonou A, et al. The macronutrient composition of the Greek diet: Estimates derived from six case control studies. Eur J Clin Nutr 1993;47:549–558.

65. Trichopoulou A, Katsouyanni K, Stuver S, et al. Consumption of olive oil and specific food groups in relation to breast cancer risk in Greece. J Natl Cancer Inst 1995;87:110–116.

66. Martin-Morena JM, Willett WC, Gorgojo L, et al. Dietary fat, olive oil intake and breast cancer risk. Int J Cancer 1994;58:774–780.

67. Toniolo P, Riboli E, Protta F, et al. Calorie-providing nutrients and risk of breast cancer. J Natl Cancer Inst 1989;81:278–286.

68. Messian MJ, Pinsky V, Setchall KD. Soy intake and cancer risk: A review of the in vitro and in vivo data. Nutr Cancer 1994;21:113–131.

69. Lee HP, Gourley L, Duffy SE, et al. Dietary effects on breast cancer risk in Singapore. Lancet 1991;337:1197–1200.

70. Yamamota S, Sobue T, Kobayashi M, et al. Japan Public Health Center-based prospective study on cancer cardiovascular diseases group. J Natl Cancer Inst 2003;95:906–913.

71. Adlercreutz H. Phytoestrogens and breast cancer. J Steroid Biochem Mol Biol 2002;83:113–118.

72. Kelsey JL, Berkowitz GS. Breast cancer epidemiology. Cancer Res 1988;48:5615–5623.

73. Wasserman L, Flatt SW, Natarajan L, et al. Correlates of obesity in postmenopausal women with breast cancer: Comparison of genetic, demographic, disease-related, life history and dietary factors. Int J Obes Relat Metab Disord 2004;28:49–56.

74. Senie RT, Rosen PP, Rhodes P, et al. Obesity at diagnosis of breast cancer influences duration of disease-free survival. Ann Intern Med 1992;116:26–32.

75. Calle EE, Rodriquez C, Walker-Thurmond K, Thun MJ. Overweight, obesity, and mortality from cancer in a prospectively studied cohort of U.S. adults. N Engl J Med 2003;348:1625–1638.

76. Willett WC. Dietary fat and breast cancer. Toxicol Sci 1999;52:127–146.

77. Cohen LA, Kendall ME, Zang E, et al. Modulation of N-nitrosomethylurea-induced mammary tumor promotion by dietary fiber and fat. J Natl Cancer Inst 1991;83:496–501.

78. Goldin BR, Adlercreutz H, Gorbach SL, et al. The relationship between estrogen levels and diets of Caucasian American and Oriental immigrant women. Am J Clin Nutr 1986;44:945–953.

79. Goldin BR, Woods MN, Spiegelman DL, et al. The effect of dietary fat and fiber on serum estrogen concentrations in premenopausal women under controlled dietary conditions. Cancer 1994;74:1125–1131.

80. Bradlow HL, Michnovicz JJ, Halper M, et al. Long-term responses of women to indole-3-carbinol or a high fiber diet. Cancer Epidemiol Biomarkers Prev 1994;3:591–595.

81. Willett WC, Hunter DJ, Stampfer MJ, et al. Dietary fat and fiber in relation to risk of breast cancer. JAMA 1992;268:2037–2044.

82. Rohan TE, Howe GR, Friedenreich CM, et al. Dietary fiber, vitamins A, C, and E, and risk of breast cancer: A cohort study. Cancer Causes Control 1993;4:29–37.

83. Graham S, Zielenyy M, Marshall J, et al. Diet in the epidemiology of postmenopausal breast cancer in the New York state cohort. Am J Epidemiol 1992;136:1327–1337.

84. Bala DV, Patel DD, Duff SW, et al. Role of dietary intake and biomarkers in risk of breast cancer: A case control study. Asian Pac J Cancer Prev 2001;2:123–130.

85. Moon RC, McCormick DL, Mehta RG. Inhibition of carcinogenesis by retinoids. Cancer Res 1983;42:2469S–2475S.

86. Boone CW, Kellof GJ, Malone WE. Identification of candidate cancer chemopreventive agents and their evaluation in animal models and human clinical trials: A review. Cancer Res 1990;50:2–9.

87. King DM, McCay PB. Modulation of tumor incidence and possible mechanisms of mammary carcinogenesis by dietary antioxidants. Cancer Res 1983;43(Suppl):2485S–2490S.

88. Hunter DJ, Manson JE, Colditz GA, et al. A prospective study of the intake of vitamins C, E, and A and the risk of breast cancer. N Engl J Med 1993;329:234–240.

89. Michels KB, Holmberg L, Bergkvist L, et al. Dietary antioxidant vitamins, retinol, and breast cancer incidence in a cohort of Swedish women. Int J Cancer 2001;91:563–567.

90. Garland FC, Garland CF, Gordham CF, et al. Geographic variation in breast cancer mortality in the United States: A hypothesis involving exposure to solar irradiation. Prev Med 1990;19:614–622.

91. Jacobson EA, James KA, Newmark HL, et al. Effects of dietary fat, calcium, and vitamin D on growth and mammary tumorigenesis induced by 7,12-dimethylbenz[a]anthracene in female Sprague-Dawley rats. Cancer Res 1989;49:6300–6303.

92. Pirianov G, Colston KW. Interactions of vitamin D analogue CB1093, TNF alpha, and ceramide on breast cancer cell apoptosis. Mol Cell Endocrinol 2001;172:69–78.

93. Baker MR, Peacock M, Nordin BE. The decline in vitamin D status with age. Age Ageing 1980;9:249–252.

94. Schatzkin A, Longnecker MP. Alcohol and breast cancer: Where are we now and where do we go from here? Cancer 1994;74:1101–1110.

95. Rehm J, Room R, Graham K, et al. The relationship of average volume of alcohol consumption and patterns of drinking to burden of disease: An overview. Addiction 2003;98:1209–1228.

96. Reichman ME, Judd JT, Longcope C, et al. Effects of moderate alcohol consumption on plasma and urinary hormone concentrations in premenopausal women. J Natl Cancer Inst 1993;85:722–727.

97. Hildreth NG, Shore RE, Dvoretsky PM. The risk of breast cancer after irradiation of the thymus in infancy. N Engl J Med 1989;321:1281–1284.

98. Foss Abrahamsen J, Andersen A, Hannisdal E, et al. Second malignancies after treatment of Hodgkin's disease: The influence of treatment, follow-up time, and age. J Clin Oncol 1993;11:255–261.

99. Miller AB, Howe GR, Sherman GJ, et al. Mortality from breast cancer after irradiation during fluoroscopic examinations in patients being treated for tuberculosis. N Engl J Med 1989;321:1285–1289.

100. Tokunaga M, Lind LE, Yamamato T, et al. Incidence of female breast cancer among atomic bomb survivors. Hiroshima and Nagasaki. Radiat Res 1987;112:243–272.

101. Fletcher SW, Black W, Harris R, et al. Report of the International Workshop on Screening for Breast Cancer. J Natl Cancer Inst 1993;85:1644–1656.

102. Swift M. Ionizing radiation, breast cancer, and ataxia-telangiectasia. J Natl Cancer Inst 1994;86:1571–1572.

103. Meyn MS. Ataxia-telangiectasia and cellular responses to DNA damage. Cancer Res 1995;55:5991–6001.

104. Swift M, Morrell D, Massey RB, et al. Incidence of cancer in 161 families affected by ataxia-telangiectasia. N Engl J Med 1991;325:1831–1836.

105. Lavin MF, Bennett I, Ramsay J. Identification of a potentially radiosensitive subgroup among patients with breast cancer. J Natl Cancer Inst 1994;86:1627–1634.

106. Loomis DP, Savitz DA, Ananth CV. Breast cancer mortality among female electrical workers in the United States. J Natl Cancer Inst 1994;86:921–925.

107. Matanoski GM, Breysse PN, Elliot EA. Electromagnetic field exposure and male breast cancer. Lancet 1991;337:737.

108. Guenel P, Rasmah P, Anderson JD, et al. Incidence of cancer in persons with occupational exposure to electromagnetic fields in Denmark. Br J Ind Med 1993;50:758–764.

109. Vogero D, Ahebom A, Olin R, et al. Cancer morbidity among workers in the telecommunications industry. Br J Ind Med 1985;42:191–195.

110. Vagero D, Olin R. Incidence of cancer in the electronics industry: Using the new Swedish Cancer Environment Registry as a screening instrument. Br J Ind Med 1983;40:188–192.

111. London SJ, Pogoda JM, Hwang KL, et al. Residential magnetic field exposure and breast cancer risk: A nested case-control study from a multiethnic cohort in Los Angeles County, California. Am J Epidemiol 2003;158:969–980.

112. Schoenfeld ER, O'Leary ES, Henderson K, et al., for the EBCLIS Group. Electromagnetic fields and breast cancer on Long Island: A case-control study. Am J Epidemiol 2003;158:47–58.

113. Riggs BL, Hartmann LC. Selective estrogen-receptor modulators: Mechanisms of action and application to clinical practice. N Engl J Med 2003;348:618–629.

114. Khovidhunkit W, Shoback DM. Clinical effects of raloxifene hydrochloride in women. Ann Intern Med 1999;20:253–278.

115. Early Breast Cancer Trialists' Collaborative Group. Tamoxifen for early stage breast cancer: An overview of the randomized trials. Lancet 1998;351:1451–1467.

116. Cummings SR, Eckert S, Krueger KA, et al. The effect of raloxifene on risk of breast cancer in postmenopausal women: Results from the MORE randomized trial. JAMA 1999;281:2198–2197 [erratum, JAMA 1999;282:2124].

117. Cauley JA, Lucas FL, Kuller LH, et al. Bone mineral density and risk of breast cancer in older women: The study of osteoporotic fractures. JAMA 1996;276:1404–1408.

118. Fisher B, Costantino JP, Wickerham DL, et al. Tamoxifen for prevention of breast cancer: Report of the National Surgical Adjuvant Breast and Bowel Project P-1 study. J Natl Cancer Inst 1998;90:1371–1388.

119. Powles T, Ecles R, Ashley S, et al. Interim analysis of the incidence of breast cancer. I. The Royal Marsden Hospital tamoxifen randomized chemoprevention trial. Lancet 1998;352:98–101.

120. Veronesi U, Maisonneuve P, Costa A, et al. Prevention of breast cancer with tamoxifen: Preliminary findings from the Italian randomized trial among hysterectomised women. Italian Tamoxifen Prevention Study. Lancet 1998;352:93–97.

121. IBIS Investigators. First results from the International Breast Cancer Intervention Study (IBIS-I): A randomized prevention trial. Lancet 2002;360:817–824.

122. Cuzick J, Powles T, Veronesi U, et al. Overview of the main outcomes in breast-cancer prevention trials. Lancet 2003;361:296–300.

123. Chlebowski RT, Col N, Winer EP, et al. American Society of Clinical Oncology technology assessment of pharmacologic interventions for breast cancer risk reduction including tamoxifen, raloxifene, and aromatase inhibitors. J Clin Oncol 2002;20:3328–3343.

124. Levine M, Moutquin JM, Walton R, et al. Chemoprevention of breast cancer: A joint guideline from the Canadian Task Force on Preventive Health Care and the Canadian Breast Cancer Initiative's Steering Committee on Clinical Practice Guidelines for the Care and Treatment of Breast Cancer. CMAJ 2001;164:1681–1690.

125. NCCN Breast Cancer Risk Reduction Guideline. The Complete Library of NCCN Oncology Practice Guidelines. Rockledge, PA, National Comprehensive Cancer Network, 2002. Available at *www.nccn.org.*

126. Gail MH, Brinton LA, Byar DP, et al. Projecting individualized probabilities of developing breast cancer for white females who are being examined annually. J Natl Cancer Inst 1989;81:1879–1886.

127. Costantino JP, Gail MH, Pee D, et al. Validation studies for models projecting the risk of invasive and total breast cancer incidence. J Natl Cancer Inst 1999;91:1541–1548.

128. Gail MH, Costantino JP. Validating and improving models for projecting the absolute risk of breast cancer. J Natl Cancer Inst 2001;93:334–335.

129. Claus EB, Risch N, Thompson WD. Autosomal dominant inheritance of early-onset breast cancer: Implications for risk prediction. Cancer 1994;73:643–651.

130. Day R, Ganz PA, Costantino JP, et al. Health-related quality of life and tamoxifen in breast cancer prevention: A report from the National Surgical Adjuvant Breast and Bowel Project P-1 study. J Clin Oncol 1999;17:2659–2669.

131. Gail MH, Costantino JP, Bryant J, et al. Weighing the risks and benefits of tamoxifen treatment for preventing breast cancer. J Natl Cancer Inst 1999;91:1829–1846.

132. King MC, Wieand S, Hale K, et al. Tamoxifen and breast cancer incidence among women with inherited mutations in BRCA1 or BRCA2 mutations: National Surgical Adjuvant Breast and Bowel Project (P-1) Breast Cancer Prevention Trial. JAMA 2001;286:2251–2256.

133. Narod SA, Brunet JS, Ghadirian P, et al. Tamoxifen and risk of contralateral breast cancer in BRCA1 and BRCA2 mutation carriers: A case-control study. Hereditary Breast Cancer Clinical Study Group. Lancet 2000;356:1876–1881.

134. Goss PE, Ingle JN, Martino S, et al. A randomized trial of letrozole in postmenopausal women after five years of tamoxifen therapy for early stage breast cancer. N Engl J Med 2003;349:1793–1802

135. Baum M, Buzdar AU, Cuzick J, et al. Anastrazole alone or in combination with tamoxifen versus tamoxifen alone for adjuvant treatment of postmenopausal women with early breast cancer: First results of the ATAC randomized trial. Lancet 2002;359:2131–2139 [erratum, Lancet 2002;360:1520].

136. Goss PE. Breast cancer prevention: Clinical trials strategies involving aromatase inhibitors. J Steroid Biochem Mol Biol 2003;86:487–493.

137. Mosca L, Barrett-Connor E, Wenger NK, et al. Design and methods of the Raloxifene Use for the Heart (RUTH) study. Am J Cardiol 2001;88:392–395.

138. Vogel BV. Followup of the breast cancer prevention trial and the future of breast cancer prevention efforts. Clin Cancer Res 2001:4413s–4418s.

139. Decensi A, Galli A, Veronesi U. HRT opposed to low-dose tamoxifen (HOT study): Rationale and design. Recent Results Cancer Res. 2003;163:104–111; discussion, 264–266.

140. Cuzick J. A brief review of the International Breast Cancer Intervention Study (IBIS), the other current breast cancer prevention trials, and proposal for future trial. Ann N Y Acad Sci 2001;949:123–133.

141. Veronesi U, DePalo G, Marubini E, et al. Randomized trial of fenretinide to prevent second breast malignancy in women with early stage breast cancer. J Natl Cancer Inst 1999;91:1847–1856.

142. Eng ET, Williams D, Mandava U, et al. Anti-aromatase chemicals in red wine. Ann N Y Acad Sci 2002;963:239–246.

143. Howe LR, Dannenberg AJ. COX-2 inhibitors for the prevention of breast cancer. J Mammary Gland Biol Neoplasia 2003;8:31–43.

144. Harris RE, Chlebowski RT, Jackson RD, et al. Breast cancer and nonsteroidal antiinflammatory drugs: Prospective results from the Women's Health Initiative. Cancer Res 2003;63:6096–6101.

145. Stoll BA. Linkage between retinoid and fatty acid receptors: Implication for breast cancer prevention. J Cancer Prev 2002;11:319–325.

146. Kzystyniak KL. Current strategies for anticancer chemoprevention and chemoprotection. Acta Pol Pharm 2002;59:473–478.

147. Fabian CJ, Kimler BF. Beyond tamoxifen: New endpoints for breast cancer prevention, new drugs for breast cancer prevention. Ann N Y Acad Sci 2001;952:44–59.

148. Seeger H, Wallwiener D, Mueck AO. Statins can inhibit proliferation of human breast cancer cells in vitro. Exp Clin Endocrinol Diabetes 2003;111:47–48.

149. Crowell PL. Monoterpenes in breast cancer prevention. Breast Cancer Res Treat 1997;46:191–197.

150. Fabian CJ. Breast cancer chemoprevention: Beyond tamoxifen. Breast Cancer Res 2001;3:99–103.

151. El-Bayoumy K. Evaluation of chemopreventive agents against breast cancer and proposed strategies for future clinical interventions. Carcinogenesis 1994;15:2395–2420.

152. Bradlow HL, Michnovicz JJ, Telang NT, et al. Diet, oncogenes, and tumor viruses as modulation of estrogen metabolism in vivo and in vitro. Cancer Detect Prev 1992;16:S35–S42.

153. Graham S, Schotz W, Martino P. Alimentary factors in the epidemiology of gastric cancer. Cancer 1972;30:927–938.

154. Wattenberg LW, Loub WD. Inhibition of polycyclic hydrocarbon-induced neoplasia by naturally-occurring indoles. Cancer Res 1978;38:1410–1413.

155. Telang NT, Suto A, Wong GY, et al. Induction by estrogen metabolite 16-alpha-hydroxyestrone of genotoxic damage and aberrant proliferation in mouse mammary epithelial cells. J Natl Cancer Inst 1992;84:634–638.

156. Kabat G, Chang CJ, Sparano JA, et al. Urinary estrogen metabolites and breast cancer: A case-control study. Cancer Epidemiol Biomarkers Prev 1997;6:505–509.

157. Brignall MS. Prevention and treatment of cancer with indole-3-carbinol. Altern Med Rev 2001;6:580–589.

158. La Vecchia C. Tomatoes, lycopene intake, and digestive tract and female hormone-related neoplasms. Exp Biol Med 2002;227:860–863.

159. Hulton K, VanKappel AL, Winkvist A, et al. Carotenoids, alpha-tocopherols, and retinol in plasma and breast cancer risk in northern Sweden. Cancer Causes Control 2001;12:529–537.

160. Agarwal S, Rao AV. Tomato lycopene and its role in human health and chronic diseases. CMAJ 2000;163:739–744.

161. Heerdt AS, Young CW, Borgen PI. Calcium glucarate as a chemopreventive agent in breast cancer . Isr J Med Sci 1995;31:101–105.

162. Ip C. Prophylaxis of mammary neoplasia by selenium supplementation in the initiation and promotion phase of chemical carcinogenesis. Cancer Res 1981;41:2683–2686.

163. Medina D, Thompson H, Ganther H, Ip C. Se-methylselenocysteine: A new compound for chemoprevention of breast cancer. Nutr Cancer 2001;40:12–17.

164. Kavanaugh C, Green JE. The use of genetically altered mice for breast cancer prevention studies. J Nutr 2003;133:2402S–2409S.

165. Pennisi VR, Capozzi A. Subcutaneous mastectomy data: A final statistical analysis of 1500 patients. Aesthetic Plast Surg 1989;13:15–21.

166. Nielsen M, Thomsen JL, Primdahl S, et al. Breast cancer and atypia among young and middle-aged women: A study of 110 medicolegal autopsies. Br J Cancer 1987;56:814–819.

167. Nelson H, Miller SH, Buck D, et al. Effectiveness of prophylactic mastectomy in the prevention of breast carcinomas in C3H mice. Plast Reconstr Surg 1989;83:662–669.

168. Jackson CF, Palmquist M, Swanson J, et al. The effectiveness of prophylactic subcutaneous mastectomy in Sprague-Dawley rats induced with 7,12-dimethylbenzathracene. Plast Reconstr Surg 1984;73:249–255.

169. Temple WJ, Lindsay RL, Magi E. Technical considerations for prophylactic mastectomy in patients at high risk for breast cancer. Am J Surg 1991;161:413–415.

170. Hartmann L, Schaid DJ, Woods JE, et al. Efficacy of bilateral prophylactic mastectomy in women with a family history of breast cancer. N Engl J Med 1999;340:77–84.

171. Hoskins KF, Stopfer JE, Calzone KA, et al. Assessment and counseling for women with a family history of breast cancer. A guide for clinicians. JAMA 1995;273:577–585.

172. Hartmann LC, Sellers TA, Schaid DJ, et al. Efficacy of bilateral prophylactic mastectomy in BRCA1 and BRCA2 gene mutation carriers. J Natl Cancer Inst. 2001;93:1633–1637.

173. Meijers-Heijboer H, van Geel B, van Putten WLJ, et al. Breast cancer after prophylactic bilateral mastectomy in women with BRCA1 or BRCA21 mutation. N Engl J Med 2001;345:159–164.

174. Eisen A, Weber BL. Prophylactic mastectomy for women with BRCA1 and BRCA2 mutations: Facts and controversy. N Engl J Med 2001;345:207–208.

175. McDonnell SK, Schaid DJ, Myers JL, et al. Efficacy of contralateral prophylactic mastectomy in women with a personal and family history of breast cancer. J Clin Oncol 2001;19:3938–3943.

176. Bilimoria MM, Morrow M. The woman at increased risk for breast cancer: Evaluation and management strategies. CA Cancer J Clin 1995;45:263–278.

177. Zion SM, Slezak JM, Sellers TA, et al. Reoperations after prophylactic mastectomy with or without implant reconstruction. Cancer 2003;98:2152–2160.

178. Stefanek ME, Helzlsouer KJ, Wilcox PM, et al. Predictors of and satisfaction with bilateral prophylactic mastectomy. Prev Med 1995;24:412–419.

179. Frost MH, Schaid DJ, Sellers TA, et al. Long-term satisfaction and psychological and social function following bilateral prophylactic mastectomy. JAMA 2000;284:319–324.

180. Lerman C, Daly M, Sands C, et al. Mammography adherence and psychological distress among women at risk of breast cancer. J Natl Cancer Inst 1993;85:1074–1080.

181. Lerman C, Kash K, Stefanek M. Young women at increased risk for breast cancer: Perceived risk, psychological well-being, and surveillance behavior. Monogr J Natl Cancer Inst 1994;16:171–176.

182. Lerman C, Daly M, Masny A, et al. Attitudes about genetic testing for breast-ovarian cancer susceptibility. J Clin Oncol 1994;12:843–850.

183. Kash KM, Holland JC, Osborne MP, et al. Psychologic counseling strategies for women at high risk of breast cancer. Monogr J Natl Cancer Inst 1995;17:73–79.

184. Lerman C, Lustbader E, Rimer B, et al. Effects of individualized breast cancer risk counselling: A randomized trial. J Natl Cancer Inst 1995;87:286–292.

185. Chlebowski RT. Reducing the risk of breast cancer. N Engl J Med 2000;343:191–198.

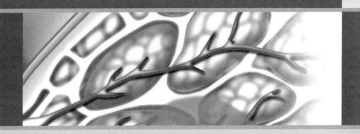

SECTION II

PATHOLOGY

CHAPTER 7

Pathologic Evolution of Preinvasive Breast Cancer: The Atypical Hyperplasias

David L. Page

The precursors of breast cancer are unknown, but there are histologic patterns associated with an increased risk for developing breast cancer. The associations are of differing magnitude for different anatomic lesions and are potentially useful for determining prevention strategies. They also provide current guidelines for clinical management and patient counseling.

How do the atypical hyperplastic lesions differ in clinical significance from ductal carcinoma in situ?

The major thrust of this chapter is to differentiate the atypical hyperplastic lesions from ductal carcinoma in situ (DCIS), which is discussed in detail in Chapter 8. When minimal examples of DCIS are identified and these samples are incompletely removed, the invasive cancer that may develop later is regularly in the same breast at the same site.[1,2] This differs from the later cancers developing after identification of atypical hyperplasia (AH) of the lobular or ductal type, which are largely and evenly distributed within each breast at any site.[3–5] Thus, it has become well established (Table 7–1) that the AHs, including lobular carcinoma in situ (LCIS), are markers of increased risk for cancer development anywhere within either breast over the next 10 to 15 years at least. This is very different from the obviously local progression to malignant behavior of the DCIS lesions, although there is a regional implication for the lesions of atypical lobular hyperplasia (ALH) that is strongly supported by the fact that 70% of the later-developing invasive carcinomas are in the ipsilateral breast, with the biopsy showing ALH. This tendency toward favoring one breast rather than having the even and bilateral distribution found with atypical ductal hyperplasia (ADH) has been recognized since the 1970s, when contralateral biopsies for lobular neoplasia (ALH) and LCIS frequently demonstrated no disease in the contralateral breast. However, there are differences of risk magnitude and site of later cancers, as discussed elsewhere.

What is the magnitude and location of risk for later invasive breast cancer after atypias?

Prediction of later untoward events, specifically the development of invasive breast carcinoma, is the important practical and biologic association of the specifically defined AHs. Although there are some characteristics that are especially relevant to either the *lobular* or *ductal* pattern of AH, the practical consequences of the AHs may be discussed as a cohesive group because in the important age group of 35 to 55 years, the consequences and presentations are similar.[6,7]

A major part of this discussion is the difference between AHs (see Table 7–1) and the conceptual "parent" carcinoma in situ (CIS) lesions.[8–10] Before the 1980s, a woman with benign breast disease was understood to have had a history of a benign breast biopsy. It was accepted as common knowledge that these women had a threefold increased risk for breast cancer.[11] Since the late 1980s, we have widely accepted the fact that most women undergoing breast biopsy for a benign lesion have no increased risk for subsequent breast cancer, and that a subset of these women may be identified as being at some risk of later breast cancer on the basis of histologic patterns of disease[4,5,10,12,13] (see Table 7–1).

Figures 7–1 and 7–2 present data from follow-up studies of women with hyperplastic lesions of various types and the philosophic underpinnings of these and analogous observations. Only three other cohort studies[12,14,15] similar to the one presented in Figure 7–1 have been performed using the same criteria for stratification of hyperplastic lesions. These have been essentially confirmatory, with small differences discussed elsewhere.[6,7,15,16] Other studies using analogous criteria or criteria derived from different pathologists without using criteria-driven terminology are essentially supportive in that the more complex (or "atypical") the hyperplastic lesions, the more elevated the risk.[17,18] However, the cancer risk of the atypical hyperplastic lesions is highest when strict criteria are used for their evaluation. Considering that none of these predictions is absolute, there may actually be little practical difference between a patient with extensive usual-pattern hyperplasia and a patient with a small amount of AH. These risk implications may also vary somewhat with age and are

Table 7–1   Characterization of Breast Histopathology, from Benign through Carcinoma In Situ

Definition	Clinical Implications	Diagnoses
Benign	No increased risk for later invasive cancer compared with similar women (age most important)	Cysts, fibrosis, apocrine change, most fibroadenomas
Benign; similar to above group in practical terms	Slightly increased cancer risk, reliably approaching double that of comparable women	Well-developed patterns of usual hyperplasia; sclerosing adenosis; subsets of fibroadenoma; possibly, many larger and recurring cysts
Benign; elevated cancer concern in some age groups	Moderate magnitude, and generalized (anywhere in breasts) increased risk	Specific patterns of atypia; cytologic and histologic criteria of ADH and ALH/LCIS
CIS, low-grade DCIS	Prolonged, local evolution into invasive carcinoma	Low-grade DCIS, <1 cm
CIS, high-grade DCIS	Shorter and more certain local evolution into invasion, about 50% in 3 yr for larger lesions incompletely removed	High-grade CIS, ductal pattern, regional disease, regularly >1 cm in greatest extent; can be large

ADH, atypical ductal hyperplasia; ALH, atypical lobular hyperplasia; LCIS, lobular carcinoma in situ; CIS, carcinoma in situ; DCIS, ductal carcinoma in situ.

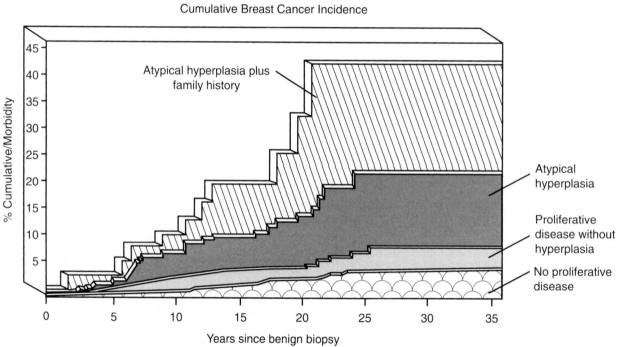

Figure 7–1   This Kaplan-Meier life table presents the experience of women after benign breast biopsy and records the incidence of later development of invasive breast cancer. Patients were excluded when lost to follow-up and if they died of other conditions, which accelerates the apparent incidence after 15 years; thus, the absolute risk indicated by the findings on breast biopsy should properly be cut off at 10 to 15 years. Note that this represents an average experience of women of average age (mid- to late mid-40s) in the initial Nashville series. Thus, a woman of that age with atypical hyperplasia experiences a risk for invasive carcinoma in the next 10 to 15 years of 10%. This risk might be slightly higher for older women, certainly for those into their 50s at the time of biopsy, but other causes of death after that age (certainly in the late 60s) would not increase this incidence. The incidence in women without proliferative disease may be extrapolated from the incidence in the general population, with an error rate of about 10%. In this series from the premammographic era, women developing invasive breast carcinoma had a death rate of only 28% at 10 years after mastectomy.

certainly of less importance in older women, who are more likely to develop cancers of increasingly lower malignant capacity and whose mortality is increasingly likely to result from cardiovascular causes.

The occurrence of fibroadenomas has also been studied, with attempts made to stratify the 1.4 to 1.7 times increased risk found for all fibroadenomas. One large study has found that some elements occurring with fibroadenomas identify

women as being at a slightly increased risk for breast cancer, and about 70% of women with fibroadenomas and without the added risk elements are left without an increased risk (Table 7–2).[19]

Figure 7–1 presents percentages of women developing invasive breast cancer and indicates that the most relevant and practical information is obtained in the first 15 or so years after diagnosis. The information more than 15 years after

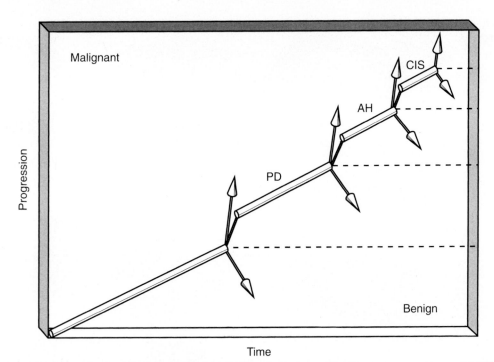

Figure 7–2   This graph indicates levels of likelihood of developing true malignancy over time as measured by anatomic lesions at benign biopsy. The implication is that women who developed proliferative disease (PD) or atypical hyperplasia (AH) are more likely to proceed to the next step, carcinoma in situ (CIS). This is certainly not a guaranteed progression but must be viewed as one that is likely; for that reason, the connections between the different levels are in *dotted lines,* indicating a more tenuous link. The *arrows* pointing up and down indicate that lesions may recede or progress; the *dashed lines* indicate that they may maintain stability over a long period of time. It is believed that as one progresses, certainly to and past the level of atypical hyperplasia, recession of lesions is less likely. However, there is good indication that even low-grade ductal carcinoma in situ may remain stable or regress about 50% of the time.

Table 7–2   Features Associated with Fibroadenoma* That Elevate Breast Cancer Risk

Complex histology: any combination of apocrine change, cysts, sclerosing adenosis, or calcification (epithelium related)
Usual patterns of hyperplasia; moderate and florid in surrounding parenchyma (similar to women without fibroadenoma)
History of breast cancer in first-degree relative (slightly higher than the history of cancer in a relative alone)

*Most of the risk is operative 10 to 15 years after diagnosis.

biopsy is fragmentary and related to a small number of women. It also should be recognized that those women are now on average almost 20 years older than when their risk was evaluated initially. Because this is a cumulative risk statement, women who have developed cancer in the early years are also included in the statement. Basically, the relative risk for these older women (15 to 20 years after biopsy) may change to be more like that of comparable women of the same age at that period of time. Because of this somewhat confusing aspect, we believe that for practical reasons, predictiveness should be truncated at 10 to 15 years.[6,20] The relationship of relative risk (a comparison with similar women in magnitude of risk) to absolute risk (an indication of the specific risk in percentage likelihood applying to the woman being counseled) is presented by Dupont and Plummer.[21] One of the most important aspects of risk assessment is that breast disease and its treatment are constantly changing. Any decision based on what might happen to a woman more than 15 or 16 years in the

future would seem best made at that time, rather than at a time 10 to 20 years earlier that does not integrate the other events that may occur in that time.

Figure 7–2 presents a stochastic model proposing that cancer development takes place through a series of steps whose recognition determines the likelihood or probability of development of carcinoma. The individual lesions cannot be identified as specific precursors. This model must take into consideration the fact that any lesion that is viewed under the microscope and categorized has been removed from the breast. Presumably, then, lesions remaining within the breast or nonanatomically defined factors are the causative or provoking agents for later cancer development. Thus, the DCIS lesions that proved to be local precursors may be so because even the smallest lesions usually have dimensions in the 5- to 10-mm range[1,21] and are more likely to remain after biopsy than after planned wide excision (see Chapter 8).

What is the histologic definition of atypical ductal hyperplasia and its special features?

Atypical ductal hyperplasia (ADH) is most often a solitary lesion on biopsy and confined within a single lobular unit, seldom larger than about 3 mm overall. Figure 7–3 presents a theoretical progression of lesions to invasion through levels of hyperplasia, although in reality very few lesions progress. Some of the particulars of histologic diagnosis were discussed earlier, but Figure 7–4 indicates more precisely the criteria used to arrive at a specifically defined lesion of ADH.[22] Three

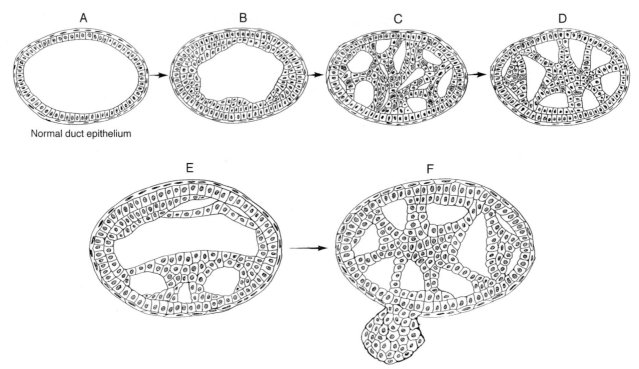

Normal duct epithelium

Figure 7–3   The hypothetical progression of lesions to invasion through levels of hyperplasia is presented. Note that each of these units is a space bounded by a basement membrane. These are usually acini or terminal ducts within the breast, but they could be major ducts as well. *A,* Normally, there is a single luminal layer of cells and a single outer layer of basal or myoepithelial cells. *B,* A slight increase in cell number, three to four cells above the basement membrane, is not associated with a measurable increase in likelihood of breast cancer incidence in the next 10 to 15 years. *C,* The usual hyperplasia, with irregularity in placement of cells and irregularity of intercellular spaces. *D,* More regular arches are present, similar to those seen in low-grade ductal carcinoma in situ (DCIS), with maintenance of normally polarized cells around the outside. *E,* Patterns of atypical ductal hyperplasia or DCIS of very low grade are indicated, with the arches and bars formed by a uniform population of cells. *F,* It is suggested that microinvasion into stroma occurs from the in situ lesions, with the protrusion of cells in the lower portion indicating loss of basement membrane materials and invasion. However, an in situ component is often absent, and invasive lesions can form basement membrane components, a further example of the heterogeneity of these processes.

criteria are important: cytology, histologic pattern, and extent (or size) of lesion.[23] Agreement among pathologists is usually obtained when consistent criteria are used.[24]

Recognizing that these specifically defined, atypical lesions are clinically important indicators of increased risk will also lead to the recognition of anatomic patterns that mimic and may be confused with these lesions. An excellent example is that of "collagenous spherulosis," originally described by Clement and colleagues.[26] Further studies have confirmed that this hyaline element is usually related to basement membrane materials.[27] The importance of collagenous spherulosis lies in the fact that with its sharply defined, round spaces it strongly mimics the histologic pattern of ADH. However, the lack of a uniform population of neoplastic-appearing cells makes its recognition as an AH (identifying moderate risk) inappropriate. Both the cytologic features of an appropriate population of cells and the histologic pattern criteria are necessary for a diagnosis of AH, which is indicative of a moderately increased cancer risk (four to five times that of comparable women; see Table 7–1). The risk implications of ADH are slightly smaller in the studies from the Nurses' Health Study at Harvard. This may relate to the selection of cases during the mammographic era.

The incidence of ADH probably continues to rise for 10 to 20 years after menopause, a major differential feature

from ALH, which tends to decrease in incidence after menopause.[4,6,9]

What is the histologic definition of atypical lobular hyperplasia and its special features?

Special considerations of ALH relate to its regular multicentricity. Although usually complete lobular units are involved, many units may be involved without involvement of intervening ducts. This multicentricity has been thought to be the reason for dispersion of sites of later-developing carcinomas, although the breast with identified ALH is twice as likely to be the site of later invasive cancer.[28]

Of special note is the terminology related to ALH and LCIS. The histologic criteria demand alteration of lobular units as well as a characteristic and uniform cytology. The diagnosis is less difficult than with ADH, but problems with the use of the term LCIS remain. These problems may be considered resolved when one recognizes the slightly different criteria used to describe the same spectrum of change from "fully developed" (LCIS) to "minor deformity of lobular units" (just a few atypical cells without distention). When pathologists agree on criteria, they usually agree on diagnostic assessment.[25] Basically, this is a problem in terminology only

DCIS vs. ADH vs. FHWA
cytology & histology

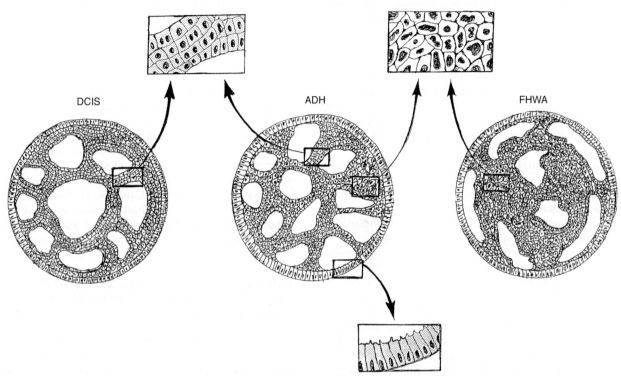

DCIS   ADH   FHWA

Figure 7–4   The specific histologic features in the sequence of ductal pattern lesions. Florid hyperplasia without atypia (FHWA) is shown with irregular spaces between the cells. The *insert* above FHWA shows the irregularity of cell placement and nuclear features. These irregularities may indicate atypia in another organ but within the breast usually indicate the variation of ordinary hyperplasia, unless advanced nuclear atypia, as seen in comedocarcinoma in situ, is present. The anatomically intermediate lesion of atypical ductal hyperplasia (ADH) has specific features of ductal carcinoma in situ (DCIS) in less than completely developed form, usually best measured by the extent of the lesion (see text). Note that the even placement of similar-appearing cells is seen in both low-grade DCIS and ADH but that remaining areas within the same basement membrane–bounded space of normally polarized cells (*insert* below ADH) and also intermixtures of the varied cell population of usual hyperplasia are present. In DCIS, the uniform population of cells is present throughout the space without another cell population (although myoepithelial cells can be present). Usually, at least two spaces are completely involved, and the area of discernible atypia is greater than approximately 3 mm in overall size.

because recently performed studies in fairly large groups of patients[4,29–32] have shown that lesser changes within the lobular units indicate a lesser risk than the more fully developed lesions that may be identified as LCIS.[27,29–33] In this way, use of the term ALH is understood to mean an implication of increased risk only, without an implication of "carcinoma attached with LCIS." Others accept *lobular neoplasia* as a clinically useful term,[31,32,34] although the term ALH for most of these cases is appropriate and clinically useful. The term LCIS, which has historical precedent and wide clinical acceptance, is then reserved for the most fully developed lesions, which probably have a greater associated cancer risk.[9,29,31] Also, dense local disease, approaching 1 cm in size, may have lobular cytology. Fisher and coworkers have presented a group of such patients with excellent follow-up after excision.[29]

In 1996, Bodian and associates[30] stated that all of the changes should be called "lobular neoplasia,"[34] while documenting that lesser examples of this phenomenon, called "ALH" by others, are associated with a significantly lower risk. It would seem immaterial whether one calls these "lobular neoplasia types 1 and 2" rather than "ALH" or whether one

calls the fully developed examples of LCIS by that name or by "lobular neoplasia number 3."

Fisher and coworkers[29] document the cases of LCIS presenting within the National Surgical Adjuvant Breast Project (NSABP). These cases are particularly valuable because they document a subset of LCIS that is quite advanced and that mimicked DCIS in the view of the original pathologist. These cases have a significant risk for later cancer development, which is not as high if the changes are not as advanced.

What are the nonclassic forms of atypical hyperplasia?

In addition to the relatively common and verified lobular and ductal series of AHs, other lesions presenting in the breast may also be considered "atypical" in the sense that they are close in their characteristics to those recognized as CIS. Such lesions include the hypersecretory atypias and the apocrine atypias.[35,36] Basically, the available literature has not proceeded beyond the stage of recognizing these as a potential

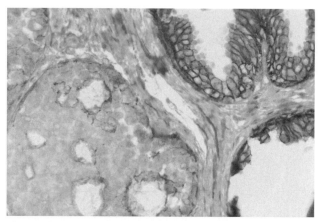

Figure 8–3 E-cadherin immunohistochemistry. Three duct spaces on the right represent columnar alteration with prominent apocrine snouts. Note the uniform cell membrane reaction product with E-cadherin antiserum characteristic of ductal proliferations. On the left, pleomorphic lobular carcinoma in situ shows no such reaction product, except for myoepithelial elements at the duct periphery and surrounding the pseudocribriform spaces, which are invaginations of the ductal wall.

whom had undergone needle-localized excision and had a breast at risk. Only one of these five had a recurrence; this patient had an initial margin smaller than 1 mm that was additional pleomorphic lobular neoplasia. Georgian-Smith and Lawton[21] reported that two of five patients with pleomorphic lobular neoplasia undergoing excision exhibited invasive lobular carcinoma but provided no follow-up data on cases with pleomorphic lobular neoplasia alone after excision. Fisher and colleagues[7] relegated all comparable cases of pleomorphic lobular neoplasia (*ductolobular* carcinoma in situ, in their terminology) to treatment as DCIS in the NSABP B-17 protocol.

Because knowledge of the biology of pleomorphic lobular neoplasia, particularly of the type detected by microcalcification, is presently so limited, treatment will necessarily represent speculative projections based on the significance of more pleomorphic nuclear morphology, higher proliferative index, or p53, but not on outcome studies. Although it would appear reasonable to excise pleomorphic lobular neoplasia in cases in which the mammographic target has only been sampled, re-excision for the presence of the histologic finding alone near or at a margin may be over-reaching.

How does lobular carcinoma in situ differ from atypical lobular hyperplasia?

LCIS differs from ALH only by degree morphologically and biologically; both are risk markers. Current criteria for LCIS established by Page and Anderson[22] require uniform effacement of the ductular architecture and uniform involvement of the entire lobule with significant distention of each terminal ductule. In practice, this generally requires distention of the affected ductule equivalent to the sum of the diameters of six to seven neoplastic cells or more. Lesser degrees of involvement are classified as ALH. Biologically, ALH is associated with a lesser relative risk for breast cancer; women with ALH have about four or five times the risk of the general population, and their risk is also influenced by a first-order

family history (mother, sister, daughter) and menopausal status. The presence of a first-order family history in a premenopausal patient essentially doubles the relative risk for ALH.[23,24] Such a patient experiences a risk similar to that associated with LCIS itself. In patients with ALH who are postmenopausal, in contrast, the relative risk is lower than that associated with proliferative breast disease in a premenopausal patient (relative risk [RR] of 2.6).[24]

From the therapeutic point of view, patients with LCIS and ALH, both of which generically are lobular neoplasia, receive no benefit for local control from attempts at re-excision—the risk remains the same. Lobular neoplasia tends to be diffuse in the ipsilateral breast, in contrast to the segmental distribution of DCIS, and may occur in the contralateral breast in some 30% to 35% of cases. There is no medical rationale for the ipsilateral treatment of lobular neoplasia, and the cumulative risk even at 20 years of follow-up does not warrant the treatment popular 20 years ago, which was bilateral total mastectomy. Well-documented cases of invasive carcinoma occurring after mastectomy for LCIS exist[25] and emphasize the limitations of a surgical approach to a diffuse disease in a nonencapsulated organ system.

What is ductal carcinoma in situ?

DCIS and Paget's disease of the nipple, by contrast with lobular neoplasia, are variably obligate precursors to invasive growth with risk limited to the ipsilateral breast. Unlike LCIS, DCIS and Paget's disease are infrequently bilateral at their discovery, and in follow-up series of treated DCIS, the risk for contralateral disease remains low, comparable to that seen for invasive carcinoma.

In contrast to LCIS, DCIS exhibits an exceedingly heterogeneous appearance in regard to both nuclear morphology or grade and histologic (i.e., architectural) pattern. Moreover, a significant number of DCIS cases exhibit a spectrum of nuclear grades and architectural patterns within a single lesion.[26]

How is ductal carcinoma in situ detected?

DCIS has only recently been clearly separated from invasive carcinoma and had been considered the same disease in actual practice.[27] In the early 1970s, DCIS constituted 2% to 5% of all new breast cancer diagnoses. Mammographic technology increased this rate 7- to 10-fold within a few years of its introduction.[28,29] Before mammography became available, DCIS was generally an extensive or diffuse disease that presented as a clinical mass, nipple discharge, or concurrent Paget's disease. DCIS was frequently associated with occult areas of invasive growth detected at mastectomy (the only available treatment at the time) but was rarely associated with axillary metastases. Mammographically detected DCIS, in contrast, had generally progressed to a far more limited extent, was less frequently associated with invasive growth, and never exhibited axillary metastases. The small size at which DCIS was detected with mammography led to attempts at BCT, and this shift in approach formed the basis for the explosive interest in the disease that followed. These studies have demonstrated that DCIS comprises numerous entities, all with distinctive

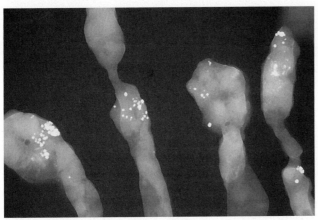

Figure 8–4 Specimen radiograph of 11-gauge cores. Note that most of the microcalcification is spherical.

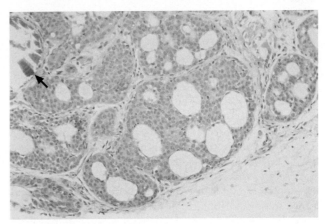

Figure 8–5 Uniform proliferation with pseudocribriform spaces in pleomorphic lobular carcinoma in situ. Note the large psammomatous microcalcification (*arrow*).

biologies and risks for progression. Clearly, DCIS is biologically as well as morphologically very heterogeneous, like invasive breast carcinoma itself. It became clear from studies of BCT that not all DCIS progresses to invasive growth within a given follow-up period; rather, it is possible to provide for local control of this disease without a mastectomy. Moreover, there is a relationship between the morphology of the DCIS and the risk for local recurrence and invasion,[30–34] as well as a relationship between extent of disease and the risk for invasion.[29,35] More recently, the impact of the size and margin status of DCIS on local recurrence rate has become clear.[33,36]

What are the pathologic determinants of clinical outcome for ductal carcinoma in situ with breast conservation?

Three features largely determine clinical outcome for attempts at BCT in DCIS: (1) the *grade* of the DCIS; (2) the *extent* or size in the carcinoma; and (3) the *width* and adequacy of the resection margins.

The grade or subtype of the DCIS is currently based on the nuclear grade and the presence of comedonecrosis. This system has begun to supersede an older, conventional classification based largely on the architectural features of DCIS (e.g., solid, cribriform). The older system provides little prognostic separation for DCIS patients and has been largely abandoned. Nuclear grading for DCIS follows the Bloom Richardson System (see Table 8–1). For purposes of clinical classification, patients with NG III lesions and comedonecrosis of any extent are classified as having high-grade lesions (Fig. 8–4). A small group of NG III DCIS cases in which comedonecrosis is not detected are also included in the high-grade subset. Intermediate-grade lesions are variously defined as NG II with or without necrosis or NG I and II with necrosis[28,30,33]; low-grade DCIS is variously defined as NG I without necrosis or NG I and II without necrosis (Fig. 8–5). Analyses of outcome by grade, whether by the criteria of Lagios and associates[32,37] or Silverstein and colleagues,[30,33] are comparable (Table 8–2).

High-grade DCIS as defined here has been shown to have the highest frequency of local recurrence and invasive

Table 8–2 Van Nuys Prognostic Index Scores in Ductal Carcinoma In Situ*

	Margin Width (mm)		
Extent (mm)	**>10**	**1–9**	**<1**
High grade			
1–15	5	6	7
16–40	6	7	8
>41	7	8	9
Intermediate grade			
1–15	4	5	6
16–40	5	6	7
>41	6	7	8
Low grade			
1–15	3	4	5
16–40	4	5	6
>41	5	6	7

*See text for explanation of scores.

transformation of the three subtypes.[32–34,38] Comparably defined high-grade DCIS[39,40] shows similar high frequencies of local failure.

Outcomes of BCT for high-grade DCIS depend a great deal on the extent of the DCIS in the breast and the adequacy of the resection margins. For example, high-grade DCIS of small size (<15 mm) and with margins of 10 mm or more has an 8% local recurrence rate at 7 years of follow-up without irradiation and a 0% recurrence rate with irradiation. Patients with high-grade DCIS with more extensive disease in the breast or narrower margins are at greater risk for local recurrence, but the risk can be somewhat reduced with successful attempts at re-excision to produce more adequate margins.[33,38]

The Van Nuys Prognostic Index (VNPI) provides a method for weighing these three prognostic features (grade, extent, and width) that is most useful for high-grade DCIS (Table 8–3).

In the VNPI system, scores of 3 and 4 are associated with excellent local recurrence-free survival at 8 years without irradiation. Patients with scores of 5, 6, and 7 have an intermediate local recurrence-free survival and benefit from radiation therapy, but the actual benefit is only 14% over those who do not receive radiation. Patients with scores of 8 and 9 have very poor local recurrence-free survival with BCT and are candidates for mastectomy. For high-grade DCIS, two thirds of the nine prognostic subtypes are amenable to breast conservation (with or without irradiation), and the remaining three may be candidates if their margins were reduced by re-excision (see Table 8–3).

In intermediate-grade DCIS (group II, NG I and II with necrosis), all VNPI scores are compatible with BCT except for a single prognostic subset with the largest extent of disease (>41 mm) and with inadequate margins (Table 8–4).

Among low-grade DCIS (NG I and II without necrosis), all nine subsets are amenable to BCT. One third would expect no benefit from irradiation, and two thirds could achieve a lower score after a successful re-excision with wider margins (Table 8–5).

Conventional pathologic classification of DCIS has been based predominantly on architectural pattern. Papillary, cribriform, micropapillary, and solid growth patterns were recognized as specific types of DCIS. Central coagulative or comedonecrosis within DCIS was often interpreted as a specific type of DCIS with the term *comedo-type DCIS*. A solid growth pattern and central necrosis would define most cases of comedo-type DCIS, although it was the only conventionally defined DCIS for which a specific nuclear morphology (i.e., high grade or NG III) was included as a characteristic if not requisite diagnostic feature. The remainder of conventionally classified DCIS cases were defined on the basis of predominant architectural patterns regardless of nuclear grade (Figs. 8–6, 8–7, 8–8, and 8–9).

Table 8–3 Van Nuys Prognostic Index Scores in High-Grade Ductal Carcinoma in Situ

Extent (mm)	Margin Width (mm)		
	>10	1–9	<1
1–15	5	6	7
16–40	6	7	8
>41	7	8	9

Table 8–4 Van Nuys Prognostic Index Scores in Intermediate-Grade Ductal Carcinoma in Situ

Extent (mm)	Margin Width (mm)		
	>10	1–9	<1
1–15	4	5	6
16–40	5	6	7
>41	6	7	8

Table 8–5 Van Nuys Prognostic Index Scores in Low-Grade Ductal Carcinoma in Situ*

Extent (mm)	Margin Width (mm)		
	>10	1–9	<1
1–15	3	4	5
16–40	4	5	6
>41	5	6	7

*Nuclear grades I and II plus necrosis.

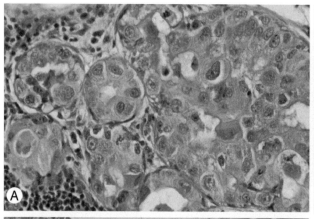
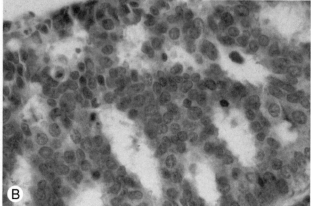
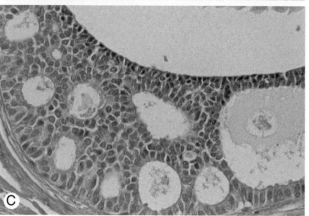

Figure 8–6 Duct carcinoma in situ (DCIS). Examples of different nuclear grades at the same magnification. *A,* DCIS involving a small, minimally distended lobule (cancerization of a lobule). Note the large nuclear size, prominent degree of pleomorphism, and presence of nucleoli and mitotic figures. Nuclei are grade III (NG III, high grade). *B,* Larger duct space demonstrates DCIS with cribriform pattern. Note the smaller nuclear size and absence of nucleoli and mitotic figures. Nuclei are grade II (NG II, intermediate grade). *C,* A large duct space with a rigidly cribriform DCIS composed of small uniform (monomorphous) cells. Note the small nuclear size, diffuse chromatin pattern, and absence of nucleoli and mitotic figures. These nuclei are grade I (NG I, low nuclear grade).

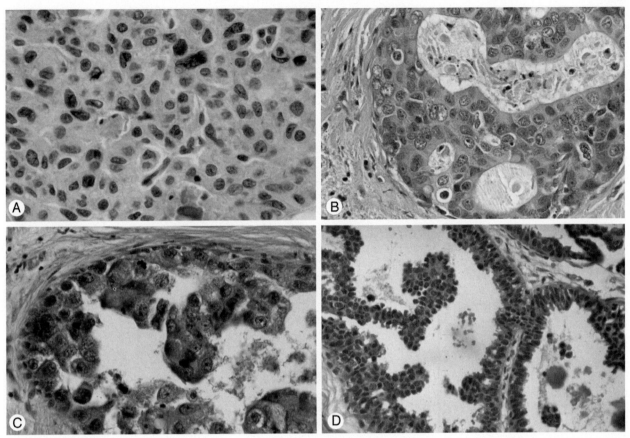

Figure 8–7   *A–D,* Architectural features of ductal carcinoma in situ (DCIS). *A–C,* Three examples of high-nuclear-grade (NG III) DCIS with different architectural patterns. Follow-up studies have shown that such features are not significant as prognostic indicators. *A,* Solid growth pattern; *B,* cribriform growth pattern; *C,* micropapillary growth pattern; *D,* contrasting micropapillary DCIS with low nuclear grade (NG I) at the same magnification.

How does age affect local recurrence rate in ductal carcinoma in situ?

Age at diagnosis is frequently cited as one of the significant, nonpathologic prognostic variables for local control in programs of breast conservation with irradiation for DCIS. Vicini and colleagues[41,42] noted a greater than threefold increase in local failure among patients younger than 45 years (26.1% vs. 8.6%) in their series of DCIS patients. However, the high rate of local failure in these patients was associated with smaller excision volumes. Among patients who underwent re-excision, the actuarial rate of true recurrence–to–marginal miss was significantly greater only in those patients with excision volumes of less than 40 mL. This variable had the highest *P* value (*P* = .005) for ipsilateral breast failure at 10 years in their study.

Silverstein[38] has shown a significant increase in local in-breast failures for DCIS patients younger than 40 years—a relative risk 2.5 times that of women 60 years of age and older. However, if this small subset of patients (7% of the patient database) is stratified by margin width 10 mm or greater or negative re-excision, the added risk of younger age disappears for low- and intermediate-grade DCIS patients and is markedly reduced for younger patients even with high-grade lesions.

These observations suggest that much of the adverse impact of younger age on local recurrence reflects a bias toward breast cosmesis resulting in smaller excision volumes with a greater likelihood of inadequate surgical resection. An extensive intraductal component (EIC) previously had been shown in analogous fashion to affect local control only when the margins of resection were inadequate or the entire extent of the component was not included in the resection.

What is the importance of pathology practice in determining treatment of ductal carcinoma in situ?

All discussions of DCIS must take into consideration the variations in tissue sampling and capabilities of identifying margins that are encountered in pathology practice. These limitations, not obvious in a statistical analysis of a population, come into sharp focus in a second-opinion practice for individual patients. A recent example illustrates this point: A 49-year-old grammar school teacher sought a consultation for a palpable and mammographically evident focus of DCIS. Formal request for the slide materials resulted in receipt of 2 of 4 slides prepared of a biopsy described as 5 × 4 × 3 cm. The 2 slides demonstrated intermediate-grade DCIS extending to the margins and no microinvasion. An inquiry to the reference laboratory obtained the release of the remaining slides and also revealed that sufficient unsampled wet tissue

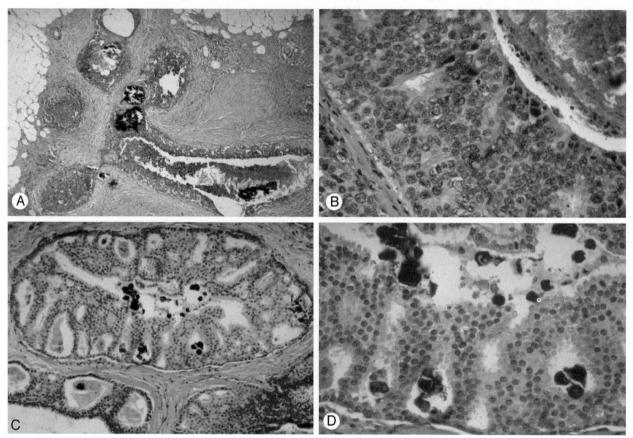

Figure 8–8   Necrosis and microcalcification. *A,* Central zones of necrosis in this high-grade ductal carcinoma in situ (DCIS) have a linear distribution following the anatomy of the extralobular ducts and terminal ductolobular units. Dystrophic microcalcification deposited in the necrotic debris results in a linear and branching mammographic pattern characteristic of DCIS with comedonecrosis. *B,* High-grade DCIS with central comedo-type necrosis (*top right*). Note karyorrhectic fragments with the debris. *C* and *D,* Psammomatous microcalcifications tend to be rounded both mammographically and microscopically. They can be seen as laminated in favorable preparations. They are characteristic of DCIS, exhibiting a papillary and cribriform architecture, and are generally associated with lower-nuclear-grade DCIS. Psammomatous microcalcifications do not require necrotic debris but represent calcification within proteinaceous secretions of the neoplastic epithelium.

remained to require 9 additional blocks. One of the 9 additional slides, 1 of the total of 13 now prepared, contained a T1a invasive carcinoma. Such foci of microinvasion and minimal invasion profoundly affect local recurrence rates in the ipsilateral breast, particularly in situations in which radiation therapy is not offered.

Some would argue that because of current practice standards in pathology, all presumptive DCIS patients would benefit (statistically) from radiation therapy, given that pathology practice is "immutable." This is a costly presumption given the expense, time, and in some cases morbidity that radiation therapy entails. In addition, it is important to remember that radiation therapy can be utilized only once, and its use in a prophylactic setting will obviate its more effective use for a future invasive recurrence. In this specific example, the cost saved by not processing the additional 9 blocks is about $56.70 (at $6.30 total cost per slide for processing). In contrast, the expense, on average, of radiation therapy is $15,000 (80% Medicare reimbursement for whole breast exclusive of node bearing tissues = $7000).

Data on local recurrence-free survival from my prior work[29,32,43] was obtained with thorough pathologic evaluation of the biopsy and the re-excision. This type of examination

mandates that all of the biopsy sample be processed and in sequence, that all margins be inked and evaluated, and that microinvasion or greater areas of invasion be excluded. This requirement is now generally recognized.[35,44,45] Treatment options for DCIS that exclude radiation therapy in programs of BCT will not be successful without the requisite thorough pathologic examination.

Although this discussion focuses on the pathologic aspects of noninvasive carcinoma, some mention must be made of the controversy surrounding radiation therapy for DCIS. Our work on DCIS antedates the first of the more recent publications on radiation therapy for DCIS by 9 years,[46] at which time we had a growing experience with BCT for DCIS without irradiation.[29] Most of the studies on radiation for DCIS have been conducted by single institutions without a comparison arm.

Three published randomized trials of radiation therapy in programs of breast conservation for DCIS have all shown a 50% significant benefit in reducing ipsilateral local recurrences. However, the outcome data from these trials are limited by the now historic, suboptimal pathologic practice employed at the time. Both NSABP B-17 and EORTC 10853[40,47–51] entered patients without prospective mammographic pathologic correlation and with incomplete sampling

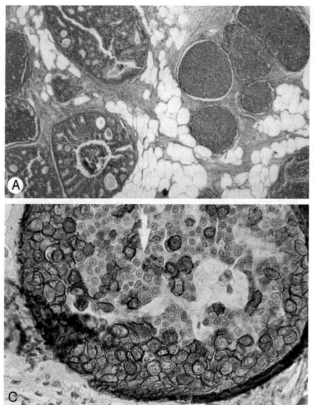
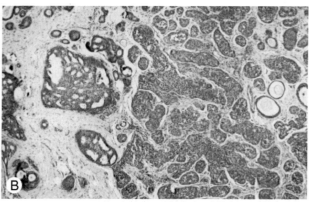

Figure 8–9 Heterogeneity in ductal carcinoma in situ (DCIS). DCIS can be markedly heterogeneous in its morphology and ploidy, in the expression of oncogenes, and in its biology. *A,* Two adjacent lobules (terminal ductolobular unit [TDLU]) demonstrate DCIS of different nuclear grade, architecture, and ploidy. The cribriform-pattern DCIS exhibited NG II, necrosis, and aneuploidy; the solid-pattern DCIS exhibited NG I morphology, absence of necrosis, and diploid DNA status. *B,* Sometimes heterogeneity is expressed *within* a single lobule (TDLU). In this case, the lobule exhibits a solid, discohesive pattern of lobular neoplasia, but the terminal extralobular duct exhibits a cribriform architecture. *C,* Single duct exhibiting DCIS with heterogeneous population of larger *HER-2/neu*–positive and smaller *HER-2/neu*–negative cells.

of the resected tissue and therefore with an inherent inability to define margin status accurately and exclude invasion. Inking of margins was not required in B-17 or the UK/ANZ trial, and margins were defined as positive only when transected in all three trials.[40,48,52–54] The local control rate achieved with radiation therapy in these circumstances was suboptimal. In B-17, a local recurrence rate of 7% at 43 months was reported, with 16% at 12 years in the irradiated arm. In EORTC 10853, the local recurrence rate was 11% at 8 years. The UK/ANZ trial achieved a superior local control rate of 4.8% (vs. 9% EORTC and 10% B-17) at 5 years of follow-up.

Because the age of the patients was comparable in the EORTC 10853 trial and the UK/ANZ trial, this difference probably reflects a well-developed pathologic protocol that requires determination of disease extent and mammographic pathologic correlation, with extensive excision of margins and with inking of margins advised in the UK/ANZ trial. However, 3% of patients had "microinvasion," and breast cancer mortality at 52 months' median follow-up was 2.6%, comparable to the rates in the EORTC and B-17 trials. A similar overall breast cancer mortality rate is seen in the VNPI database only at 12 years, but this largely reflects progressive disease in patients whose previous radiation therapy obscured and delayed discovery of local invasive recurrences.[55]

In summary, all of the published randomized trials are limited by a type of pathology practice that was current at their inception in 1985 and 1986. The quality of mammography, localization procedures, and need for correlation and pathologic techniques today are quite different from those that existed at that time. The conclusions of these trials cannot be projected into contemporary practice, for which they were not designed and for which they are largely noninformative. This is particularly true regarding their inability to define low-risk subsets, for which irradiation provides little if any benefit.

Previous studies of radiation therapy in DCIS had shown that local recurrences increase substantially after 5 years, and in all studies with 5- and 8-year comparisons, the local recurrence rate at least doubled by 8 years.[56,57] These studies had shown that radiation therapy is very effective for local control within the first 5 years, but as noted by Solin and coworkers, the in-breast local recurrence rate is 16% by 86 months (i.e., 7 years) and 19% at 15 years.[31,57] Fisher and colleagues,[50] in a further update of B-17, noted a local recurrence rate of 16% in the irradiated arm at 12 years. Although these local recurrence rates are roughly half of the rate in the nonirradiated arm in B-17 and EORTC 10853, they are very high relative to control rates for invasive breast cancer with radiation therapy. An actuarial analysis of our initial 79 patients,[32] none of whom received irradiation or tamoxifen, demonstrates a 19% local recurrence rate at 15 years of follow-up.[37] Although these patients were carefully selected for size and margin status, this recurrence rate is comparable to that reported by Solin and coworkers[58] and Fisher and colleagues[50] in studies that included irradiation.

The conclusions of Silverstein and associates[33,36,38] provide a marked contrast. These studies were all based on complete tissue processing, evaluation of margins, and a consistent analysis of pathologic subtype. All cases reported were complete with regard to grade size and margin analysis. There was no difference in local recurrence-free survival with or without irradiation in patients with low- and intermediate-grade DCIS at 82 months, and there was only a modest benefit of radiation therapy (14%) in patients whose sum prognostic index score was 5, 6, or 7. Because low- and

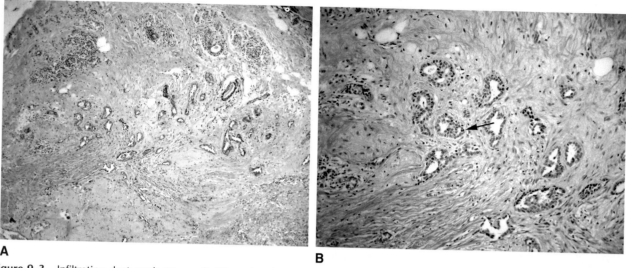

Figure 9–3   Infiltrating duct carcinoma, well differentiated. *A,* Nearly all the tumor is composed of glands invading stroma in a disorganized fashion. Normal terminal ducts and lobules are present in the upper third of the photograph. *B,* Higher power of the infiltrating glands reveals uniform nuclei in terms of size and shape and minimal mitotic activity (*arrow*).

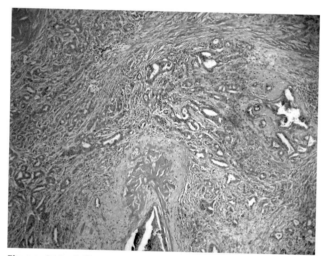

Figure 9–4   Infiltrating duct carcinoma, moderately differentiated. Whereas parts of this invasive tumor are forming glands, other areas are not. Higher power (not shown) would reveal an intermediate degree of nuclear atypia and occasional mitoses.

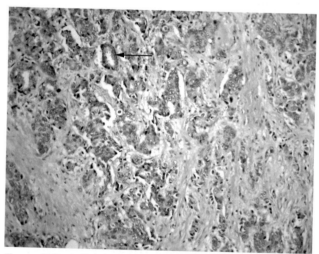

Figure 9–5   Infiltrating duct carcinoma, poorly differentiated. Only a minority of this invasive tumor is gland forming (*arrow*), and there is severe nuclear pleomorphism with frequent mitoses.

What is invasive lobular carcinoma?

Invasive lobular carcinoma is the second most commonly encountered type of invasive carcinoma of the breast and was first described in 1946 by Foote and Stewart,[5] who deemed it the invasive counterpart to lobular carcinoma in situ (LCIS), previously described by the same authors. Modern thinking does not, however, classify LCIS as an obligate precursor lesion to invasion but rather as a risk factor for its development. In fact, most invasive carcinomas that develop in patients with LCIS are ductal in type, and it is not uncommon to encounter an invasive lobular carcinoma accompanied by an intraductal component (DCIS).

In contrast to infiltrating duct carcinoma, most invasive lobular carcinomas either provoke no desmoplastic reaction at all or do so to a far lesser degree. Rather, the cells grow around or in between normal glandular structures of the breast and may even invade adipose tissue without inducing a fibrous reaction. The result is that the radiologic, clinical, and even gross estimation of size of invasive lobular carcinoma may be inaccurate or misleading. Yet, invasive lobular carcinomas typically are as irregular in shape as most invasive duct carcinomas and, in our experience, do not form well-circumscribed lesions. Grossly, the tumor may consist of a firm tan-white area, but it may merge imperceptibly with the surrounding breast tissue. There is also a distinct tendency for invasive lobular carcinoma to be multifocal (i.e., multiple, often tiny, areas of invasion separated from each other by benign tissue or intraductal carcinoma), complicating the assessment of both size and margins (discussed later).

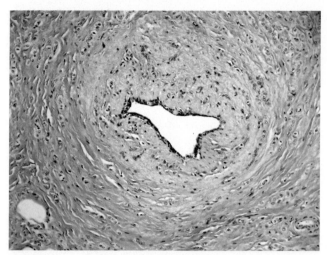

Figure 9–6 Invasive lobular carcinoma, classic form. Tumor cells surround a benign ductal structure, creating a targetoid pattern. The cells invade in a linear fashion (single file) and have relatively uniform nuclei without mitoses.

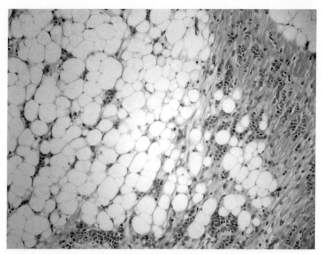

Figure 9–7 Invasive lobular carcinoma, classic form. At the periphery of a mass tumor cells invade adipose tissue (*clear areas*) without provoking a desmoplastic reaction.

What is the classic form of invasive lobular carcinoma?

Invasive lobular carcinoma, in its classic, originally described form, is composed of a uniform population of cells that infiltrate the breast parenchyma in so-called single file, following each other in a linear fashion to surround both benign ductal or lobular structures and those containing in situ carcinoma. This centripetal array is the basis of the designation "targetoid" for this pattern (Fig. 9–6). The cytology, however, truly defines the classic form of invasive lobular carcinoma and consists of relatively small cells with minimal cytoplasm, large but nonpleomorphic nuclei, and few if any mitoses (see Fig. 9–6). Desmoplastic reaction is minimal and sometimes nonexistent, particularly at the periphery of lesions (Fig. 9–7). It is extremely unusual to identify lymphatic invasion in such cases, and lymph node metastases may be difficult to identify without the aid of immunohistochemical stains.

What are the histologic variants of invasive lobular carcinoma?

Several forms of invasive lobular carcinoma have been characterized since the initial description of the classic type. These variants are only rarely seen in isolation because they nearly always coexist with at least some areas of the classic type. As a group, the variants tend to exhibit more aggressive histologic characteristics and a greater tendency for lymph node metastasis. Although the variant classifications are based on either cytologic or growth pattern characteristics, in practice, mixtures of each are frequently encountered. The cytologically based designators are pleomorphic, histiocytoid, and signet-ring cell; the pattern-based classifications are alveolar, solid, and tubulolobular (considered by some authors to be a variant of invasive duct carcinoma). The common thread among all the variants, in our experience, is that they share the same clinical and radiologic characteristics described earlier for the classic invasive lobular carcinoma in general.

Pleomorphic invasive lobular carcinoma was first described by Weidner and Semple[6] and is characterized by larger cells with pleomorphic nuclei and mitotic activity but maintenance of the growth pattern of the classic form (Fig. 9–8). The criteria for such a designation are somewhat arbitrary and overlapping with other designations such as alveolar. Furthermore, the distinction of pleomorphic lobular carcinoma from invasive poorly differentiated duct carcinoma may be difficult or arbitrary, particularly if the classic pattern of invasion is completely lacking. The signet-ring cell variant[7,8] similarly is rarely pure, and it is debatable what percentage of such cells is necessary for the designation; however, the cells contain nuclei that are indented or pushed peripherally by mucinous cytoplasm (Fig. 9–9). The cells of histiocytoid invasive lobular carcinoma[9] are so designated because they have abundant, lightly eosinophilic foamy or granular cytoplasm and resemble histiocytes (Fig. 9–10) to such an extent that the diagnosis may be difficult, necessitating the use of immunohistochemical stains for cytokeratins for confirmation.

Alveolar invasive lobular carcinoma[10] is composed of cells forming small, well-circumscribed nests devoid of a fibrous wall around them (Fig. 9–11). Because the nuclei of these nests are frequently pleomorphic, the designation of this as an entity separate from the pleomorphic type is an unsettled issue. The appellation "solid"[11] is applied when the invasive tumor cells form large sheets without a dominant pattern, except at the periphery, where a single-file pattern of invasion is typically seen (Fig. 9–12).

What is the prognostic significance of classic and variant forms of invasive lobular carcinoma?

As a group, invasive lobular carcinomas are prognostically not different from tumors of ductal type.[12] Because of methodologic differences and variation in inclusion criteria, it is difficult to compare studies; however, some authors have reported slightly better survival rates for invasive lobular carcinoma, at least at 5 and 10 years,[13] whereas survival curves may merge with longer term (>15 year) follow-up.[10,13] Others

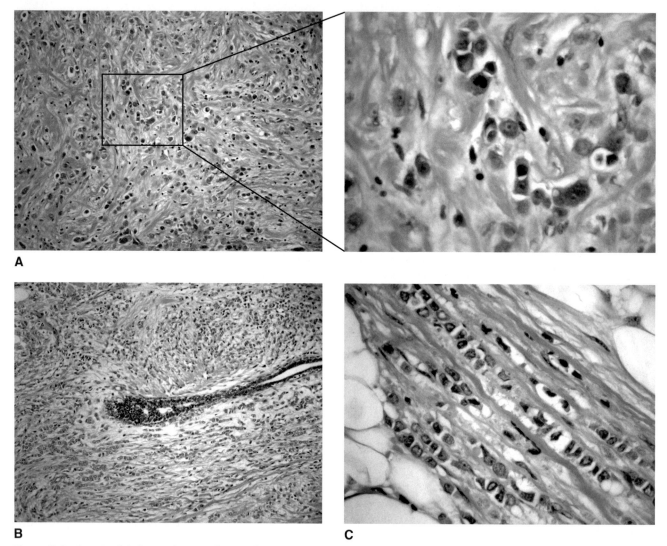

A

B   **C**

Figure 9–8   Invasive lobular carcinoma, pleomorphic type. *A,* The nuclei of these cells are extremely pleomorphic with mitoses (*inset*), but both the targetoid (*B*) and linear (*C*) growth patterns are maintained.

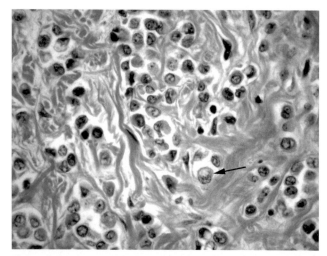

Figure 9–9   Invasive lobular carcinoma, signet-ring cell type. The nuclei of these tumor cells are indented or pushed to the periphery of the cells by abundant eosinophilic cytoplasm or by mucin globules (*arrow*).

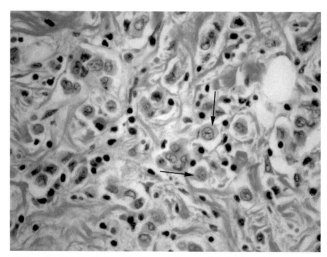

Figure 9–10   Invasive lobular carcinoma, histiocytoid type. These tumor cells contain so much eosinophilic cytoplasm and such low-grade nuclei that they are extremely difficult to distinguish from histiocytes (*arrows*).

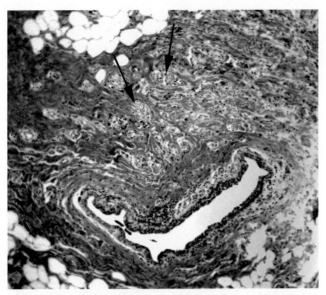

Figure 9–11 Invasive lobular carcinoma, alveolar type. Tumor cells are grouped into nests (*arrows*) of variable size and shape invading around a benign duct.

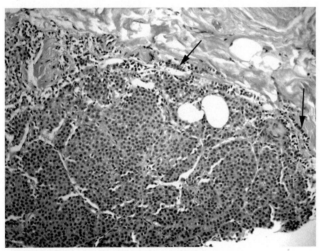

Figure 9–12 Invasive lobular carcinoma, solid type. Tumor cells form a solid sheet that envelops adipose tissue. Linear growth of the tumor is seen peripherally (*arrows*).

report a statistically significant improved 10-year survival for invasive lobular carcinoma (with inclusion of tubulolobular).[14] When considered separately, the classic invasive lobular phenotype conferred a small but significant survival advantage.[14] When allowing for variant lobular forms, the literature becomes difficult to interpret because of overlapping inclusion and classification criteria, differences in treatment protocols, and relatively small numbers of patients. In general, the classic pattern seems to have a relatively better prognosis when compared with the solid and alveolar patterns[10,14,15]; however, in practice, these patterns are rarely pure. It is also possible that the poorer prognosis may actually be due to the pattern variants' frequent admixture with the cytologic variant pleomorphic lobular carcinoma. Weidner and Semple showed a markedly increased recurrence rate and nonstatistically significant decreased survival for pleomorphic lobular carcinoma.[6] In Eusebi and colleagues' small series, 9 of 10 patients with invasive pleomorphic lobular carcinoma either developed recurrence or metastasis very rapidly or died within 42 months.[16] Prognostically, the difference may be due to the higher rate of lymph node positivity for this variant (9 of 10 of Eusebi's patients exhibited positive axillary lymph nodes). The signet-ring cell variant is generally thought to have a relatively poor prognosis,[17] whereas the histiocytoid type may mirror the classic form in outcome.[18] In our experience, pure populations are rare, and the variants do not vary in prognosis, stage for stage; however, the poorer prognosis associated with some variants (i.e., pleomorphic) may be ascribed to their higher rate of lymph node positivity. Thus, pleomorphic lobular carcinoma may represent an innately more aggressive phenotype in that lymph node metastasis may be occurring more frequently in smaller lesions with nuclear atypia and mitoses than in those without. This might explain the lack of prognostic difference between invasive lobular carcinoma as a whole relative to invasive duct carcinoma.

What is invasive tubulolobular carcinoma?

Invasive tubulolobular carcinoma was first described by Fisher and colleagues as part of the early National Surgical Adjuvant Breast Project (NSABP) studies.[19] Although historically it has constituted only a small percentage of invasive carcinoma, our experience is that this is due to its infrequent recognition by pathologists. As its name implies, it is histologically a combination of tubular carcinoma and invasive lobular carcinoma in which well-formed glands or tubules merge directly into a linear single-cell pattern of invasion surrounding normal structures (Fig. 9–13). Both patterns contain identical tumor cells and are contiguous with each other. Calcifications may also be seen in the invasive tumor. Although some authors have classified this lesion as a variant form of invasive duct carcinoma, we believe it is more accurate to consider it a form of invasive lobular carcinoma because it has a propensity for multifocality, has the same clinical and radiographic characteristics as lobular type, and provokes less desmoplastic reaction than a routine invasive duct carcinoma. In our experience, it is not infrequent to encounter cases in which areas separate from an invasive tubulolobular carcinoma are histologically composed purely of tubular carcinoma or invasive lobular carcinoma.

Are mixed duct and lobular invasive tumors possible?

Although most invasive carcinomas are easily classified as ductal or lobular, a significant subset of tumors has growth or cytologic features of both. The different forms may be in separate areas of the same mass or intimately admixed. In either case, the lesion is probably best treated with respect to the dominant type of tumor present. In practice, such cases are frequently designated as invasive carcinoma with mixed ductal and lobular features.

What features distinguish metastatic lobular from metastatic duct carcinoma?

The growth pattern of metastatic breast carcinoma typically recapitulates that of the primary lesion. Thus, the classic

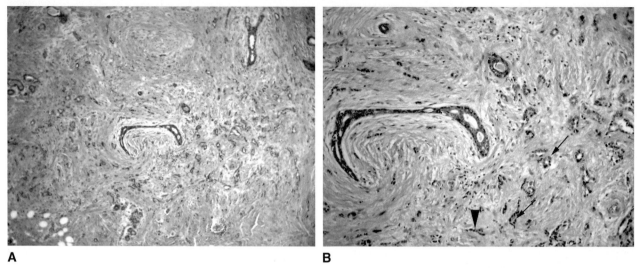

A   **B**

Figure 9–13   Invasive tubulolobular carcinoma. *A,* At low power, this invasive tumor grows in a lobular targetoid fashion (*center*) and is largely composed of small angulated glands with uniform nuclei (tubular component). *B,* The glands (*arrows*) merge almost imperceptibly with the linear growth pattern (*arrowhead*) of classic invasive lobular carcinoma.

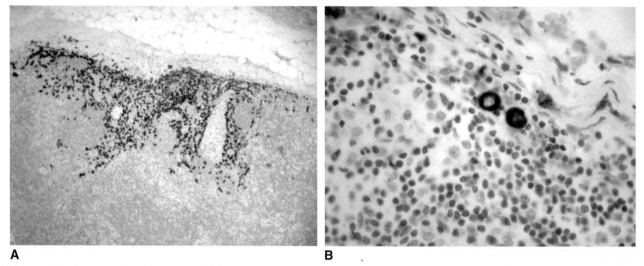

A   **B**

Figure 9–14   Lymph node with metastatic lobular carcinoma. Immunohistochemical stains for cytokeratin reveal tumor cells spreading into the nodal parenchyma from the peripheral sinuses (*A*) and as individual cells (*B*).

single-file pattern of lobular carcinoma is often seen in distant metastases. Deposits of lobular carcinoma in lymph nodes, however, may consist of nests of cells, more diffuse involvement of the sinuses, or scattered individual cells usually found in the peripheral sinuses. Metastatic lobular carcinoma in lymph nodes is often very subtle and may be difficult to distinguish from histiocytes, especially in classic and histiocytoid forms. In such cases, immunohistochemical stains for cytokeratins are extremely helpful and often reveal far more tumor cells than were evident on examination with routine stains (Fig. 9–14). Metastatic duct carcinoma grows in cohesive clusters, occasionally provoking a fibrous reaction (Fig. 9–15).

Several studies have documented a different spread pattern for distant metastasis of lobular carcinoma as opposed to duct carcinoma.[20,21] Ductal carcinomas favor bony sites, followed by lung, liver, and brain. Lobular metastases tend to occur after a longer lag period, sometimes up to 15 to 20 years, and its metastatic sites are far more variable, including peritoneum, retroperitoneum, ovaries, gastrointestinal tract, and meninges, in addition to those sites typical of ductal spread. Patients with metastatic lobular carcinoma may present in unusual ways, such as with gastric outlet or ureteral obstruction. There may be diffuse involvement of pelvic and peritoneal structures, and involvement of the stomach can closely mimic a primary gastric signet-ring cell carcinoma. Immunohistochemical stains are invaluable in the resultant differential diagnosis.

Are patients with invasive lobular carcinoma candidates for breast conservation?

Given the predilection for invasive lobular carcinoma to form multiple separate tumors apart from the main mass, often

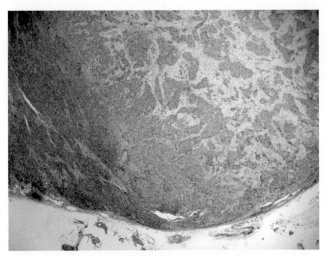

Figure 9–15 Lymph node with metastatic duct carcinoma. A large area of the lymph node parenchyma is replaced by metastatic tumor cells arranged in large cohesive, irregular groups with extensive fibrosis.

clinically and radiographically undetectable because of their small size and lack of desmoplastic reaction, it would be logical to assume that lumpectomy margins in such patients may be falsely negative owing to the presence of tiny areas of invasion retained in the breast. In fact, a lobular phenotype has been used as a rationale for mastectomy as opposed to lumpectomy. Yeatman and associates[22] reported a higher rate of mastectomy in patients with lobular tumors than in those with ductal carcinomas. In more than half of patients in whom breast conservation was unsuccessful because of persistently positive margins, the tumor was lobular.

One therefore would expect that such patients would have an increased local recurrence rate when compared with identically treated patients with invasive duct carcinoma. Recent studies of large numbers of patients, however, have not confirmed this and in fact show no difference in 5-year recurrence rates between such groups of patients treated with lumpectomy and radiation.[23] Schnitt and colleagues[24] showed similar results, with 5-year local recurrence rates of 12% for lobular and 11% for ductal carcinoma. Kurtz and coworkers[25] showed a slightly higher 5-year recurrence rate for lobular (13.5%) than ductal (9%) carcinoma, but the result was not statistically significant. These authors noted, however, that lobular recurrences tended to be multifocal and multicentric. Thus, the available data would appear to indicate that breast conservation with radiation is feasible in patients with invasive lobular carcinoma.

What pathologic factors are of particular significance in breast conservation specimens?

Breast conservation specimens are commonly termed *lumpectomy*, but the synonymous terms *partial mastectomy*, *quadrantectomy*, and *tumorectomy* have also been applied. However labeled, these specimens demand attention to several factors that are less relevant in mastectomies. In most current practices, a diagnosis of invasive breast carcinoma is initially made upon examination of a mammographically or sonographi-

cally directed core biopsy. It is crucial that the pathologist histologically identify the site of this biopsy in the subsequent lumpectomy specimen, regardless of whether there is residual tumor. This ensures that the correct, originally targeted area of the breast has been removed. Occasionally, core biopsies remove the entire invasive tumor, typically when the target lesion consists of mammographic calcifications, and a small or microinvasive carcinoma is found incidental to the imaging findings. Complete removal can be confirmed only by identification and examination of the biopsy site in the lumpectomy specimen. Finding the biopsy site in a mastectomy specimen of such a patient is to be strongly encouraged; however, it is not nearly as important as in breast conservation therapy.

Margins of resection are also of particular importance in the pathologic examination of a lumpectomy specimen and are known to affect the likelihood of local recurrence, although the subsequent impact of local recurrence on disease-free and overall survival is controversial. Several pathologic factors are important in assessing the surgical adequacy of a lumpectomy specimen: status of the margins, closest distance of tumor to a margin, presence or absence of an extensive intraductal component, and lymphatic and blood vessel invasion.

How are breast conservation specimens evaluated by pathologists?

Proper pathologic evaluation of lumpectomy specimens actually begins with their proper handling by the surgeon. Ideally, such specimens should be removed intact, with surgeons resisting the temptation to incise them to have a gross peek at the tumor. At least two margins (or one if a segment of skin is attached) should be designated, usually with sutures. This, along with the specimen's laterality, allows the pathologist to orient any lumpectomy specimen in six planes. The external surface of the specimen is then painted, usually with India ink, and sections are typically taken perpendicular to the inked surfaces or as pieces of tissue shaved from the surfaces. Many color inks are available so that each individual margin (e.g., superior, lateral) can be assigned a color, keeping in mind that the borders between these planes cannot be delineated and are subjective at best. These inks are visible under the microscope and thus histologically represent the surgical margins. Seepage of these inks into folds and crevices presents a significant problem, particularly in fatty breast tissue, and methods are available that fix the ink to the external surface, decreasing its tendency to run. Only after the inks are applied to the intact specimen's surface does the pathologist slice into the specimen and grossly evaluate the internal aspect of the lumpectomy. The macroscopic tumor or biopsy site is identified and measured in three dimensions, and its apparent distance from the margins is noted, particularly with respect to its closest approach to a margin. Often, the latter assessment is made during the surgical procedure so that the surgeon can immediately re-excise that specific margin. Frozen section can be performed and is reasonably accurate in assessing invasive tumor margins, especially in invasive duct carcinoma; however, it is inadequate in ruling out intraductal carcinoma at margins because of a combination of sampling issues and technical difficulties inherent in freezing of fatty tissue. Frozen sections should be discouraged because they can hamper

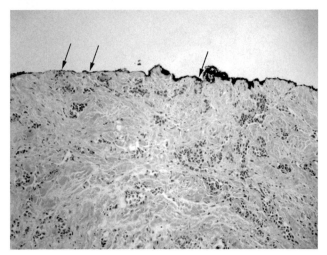

Figure 9–16   Invasive tumor involving a margin. The tumor cells of this invasive lobular carcinoma are present at the inked surface of this tissue (*arrows*), representing a positive margin.

permanent histologic assessment, especially in small mammographically detected lesions; thus, they are usually performed only in the currently unusual circumstance in which the diagnosis of invasive carcinoma has not already been established by prior core biopsy. Sections of the tumor are taken so that its largest grossly measured size as well as its relation to the inked margins may be confirmed microscopically.

The India or multiple-colored inks are visible under the microscope, and thus slides are examined such that if the cells of intraductal or invasive carcinoma touch an inked surface, that margin is considered positive (Fig. 9–16). The closest proximity of tumor to individual margins can also be assessed and reported. The use of cautery also produces specific histologic effects and can be used as an adjunct to ink (or in lieu of ink if the specimen is received in fragments or if ink is unavailable). It should be kept in mind, however, that margin evaluation is by no means precise. Microscopic examination is a two-dimensional representation of a three-dimensional process, and thus deeper sections of tissue in a paraffin block may reveal a positive margin where the original was read as close or even negative. Nowhere is this more apparent than in the situation of intraductal carcinoma or invasive carcinoma with extensive intraductal component (discussed later). The actual protocols and methods of sampling such specimens are beyond the scope of this chapter but are highly variable and dependent on institutional and individual practice.

What is the significance of margins?

The evaluation of margins in carcinoma of the breast builds on the pivotal work of Holland and colleagues,[26] who used a mapping technique to document areas of malignancy separate from a known "index" invasive tumor in mastectomy specimens. These investigators found that the incidence of additional intraductal or invasive carcinoma decreased in direct proportion to the distance of the margin from the index lesion. Furthermore, intraductal carcinoma was found to be a lesion of contiguous spread through the ductolobular tree rather than one of multiple widely separated foci. Thus, such

tumors are generally unicentric even if large, and pathologic assessment of margins should therefore theoretically be predictive of complete excision of the tumor. In practice, however, positive margins do not absolutely predict the presence of residual tumor on re-excision, nor do negative margins necessarily dictate its absence. This can be attributed to several issues of sampling, including those described previously, and the fact that it is impossible to examine histologically every area of the margin even if all of the tissue of a lumpectomy is embedded in paraffin blocks (not the typical situation). In general, however, the more tumor found at or close to the margins and the shorter the distance to the margins, the more likely it is that residual tumor will be found. Put another way, the likelihood of complete excision of a tumor is inversely related to the amount of tumor at the margins and its proximity to them.[27–29]

Numerous studies have addressed the importance of margins in terms of assigning risk for local recurrence, but a few deserve special mention. Although radiation is currently included for most lumpectomy patients, an early test of the importance of margins alone was provided by Lagios and associates,[30] who reported relatively short follow-up time (mean, 24 months) of a group of such patients in whom radiation therapy was not given. The local recurrence rate was 45% in those patients with positive margins versus 9% when the margins were clear. The short interval until recurrence and the corresponding margin status indicate that local recurrence is probably a phenomenon of progression of persistent disease rather than the development of true de novo tumor. The addition of radiation therapy decreases the local recurrence rate, but most studies indicate that it does not substitute for negative margins, with local recurrence rates ranging from 0% to 9% with negative margins, compared with 10% to 21% in patients with positive margins.[29,31,32] Other authors have expanded this idea, showing that risk for local recurrence is directly proportional to the amount of tumor at the margins and its proximity to them.[33,34] For example, Schnitt and colleagues[33] reported 5-year recurrence rates of 0%, 4%, 6%, and 21% for groups of irradiated lumpectomy patients with negative (no tumor within 1 mm), close (tumor within 1 mm), focally positive, or positive margins, respectively. Similar findings have been derived from studies of relatively larger surgical procedures, that is, quadrantectomy versus tumorectomy.[35]

The extreme variations of technique, evaluation criteria, and treatment in such studies makes direct comparison difficult; however, it seems clear from all the accumulated data that (1) the goal of breast-conserving surgery should be to achieve negative margins; (2) the closer a tumor is histologically to the margin, the greater the likelihood that the margin is, in fact, occultly positive; (3) the greater the amount of tumor at or close to the margins, the higher the risk for local recurrence; and (4) more extensive surgery decreases the risk for local recurrence by increasing the likelihood of attaining truly negative surgical margins.

What is meant by "extensive intraductal component" and what is its significance?

Extensive intraductal component (EIC) is a term that was first introduced by Schnitt and colleagues.[36] It applies only to invasive carcinomas and refers to cases in which either (1) at least

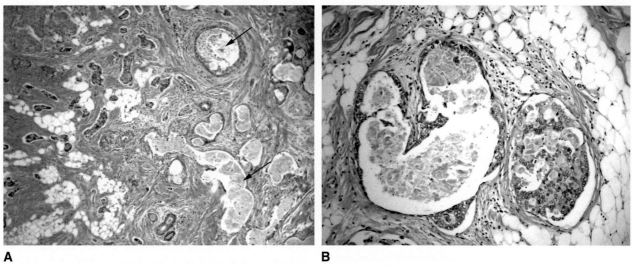

A   **B**

Figure 9–17   Invasive duct carcinoma with extensive intraductal carcinoma (EIC). *A,* The majority of this tumor mass is composed of invasive carcinoma, especially on the left side of the picture; however, more than 25% of the lesion is histologically intraductal carcinoma, the rounded structures containing central necrosis (*arrows*) on the right side. *B,* Areas of intraductal carcinoma are also present in fatty breast tissue outside of the mass. The two together fulfill criteria for the first definition of EIC.

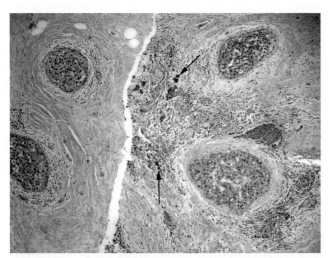

Figure 9–18   Microinvasive duct carcinoma. An area of invasive, poorly differentiated duct carcinoma measuring just below 1 mm is present between the *arrows.* Four duct spaces containing intraductal carcinoma surround it. This fulfills the criteria for the second definition of extensive intraductal carcinoma (EIC).

25% of the mass of invasive tumor is histologically composed of intraductal carcinoma, and the intraductal component is also present in breast tissue clearly outside the tumor mass (Fig. 9–17), or (2) there is microinvasive carcinoma (measuring <1 mm) accompanying intraductal carcinoma (Fig. 9–18). Cases classified as EIC positive were more likely to have residual DCIS in their respective re-excision specimens than cases designated EIC negative.[37] In irradiated patients, regardless of whether margins were actually evaluated, EIC-positive cases had higher local recurrence rates than those deemed to be EIC negative.[36] Furthermore, when margins were categorized as negative, close, focally positive, or positive, the recurrence rate for EIC-negative patients was half that of EIC-positive cases, arguing for the importance of attaining negative margins for local control.[33]

Because, at least theoretically, local recurrence risk should be entirely attributable to the DCIS outside the invasive mass, we additionally categorize tumors as EIC negative but DCIS in surrounding breast tissue for those cases in which the amount of DCIS within the invasive tumor is minimal or below 25%. In our care, such cases have local recurrence rates identical to those designated EIC positive. Other studies have cited no difference or a nonsignificant difference in local recurrence rates between EIC-positive and EIC-negative groups of patients with clear margins and radiation.[38] Thus, achieving negative margins is of paramount importance. Some clinicians have used the designation EIC positive as a justification for mastectomy as opposed to lumpectomy. Whereas the extent and location of the tumor relative to the size of the individual patient's breast may necessitate mastectomy, the appellation EIC positive can be applied to both large and small tumors and should be interpreted to signify that a larger excision will be necessary to achieve negative margins than in an EIC-negative case. EIC positive is not an absolute contraindication to breast conservation.[33,37–39]

What is the significance of lymphatic and vascular invasion?

The terms *lymphatic invasion, vascular invasion,* and *lymphovascular invasion* are commonly invoked by pathologists but are applied somewhat loosely to what nearly always represents lymphatic invasion. Strictly speaking, the term vascular invasion should be reserved for the histologic finding of tumor cells within a vessel containing a muscular wall; the presence of red blood cells in its lumen is helpful but not specific. Defined in this way, true vascular invasion in the breast is identified exceedingly rarely. Lymphatic invasion, conversely, is not infrequent and depends on the identification of intraluminal groups of tumor cells usually conforming to the shape of the endothelial-lined space. The space may or may not contain red blood cells, but usually small arterial or venous

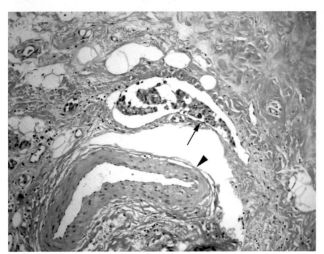

Figure 9–19 Lymphatic invasion. Cohesive clusters of tumor cells are present in a dilated endothelial-lined (*arrow*) space adjacent to a muscular vein (*arrowhead*). The tumor cells conform to the shape of the lymphatic space but appear to float in it.

structures will be immediately adjacent to the lymphatic channel (Fig. 9–19). In practice, lymphatic invasion can be difficult to differentiate from retraction artifacts because of tissue processing (in invasive carcinoma) or from DCIS. Thus, the diagnosis should only be considered in breast tissue outside the invasive carcinoma. There is considerable disagreement in the literature about the reproducibility of this diagnosis even with careful adherence to diagnostic criteria.[40,41] The use of immunohistochemical markers has been attempted but not universally accepted,[42] in part because of the lack, until recently, of antibodies able to differentiate lymphatic channels from other endothelial lined vessels.[43]

All studies have shown a greater than 50% predictive value of lymphatic invasion for the presence of axillary lymph node metastasis.[44,45] Curiously, the amount of lymphatic invasion (extensive areas may be termed *lymphatic permeation*) does not imply the extent of lymph node involvement. The presence of any lymphatic invasion simply correlates with axillary disease in a qualitative, not quantitative, sense. Most studies have indicated a decrease in disease-free survival for patients with lymphatic invasion or lymphatic and vascular invasion as a group, mostly in lymph node–negative patients;[41,42,44–47] however, these were carried out before the current era of identifying microscopic metastases in sentinel lymph nodes, and it is possible that lymphatic invasion may not contribute additional prognostic information in terms of survival. Although there are far fewer data available, it does appear that lymphatic invasion is a risk factor for local recurrence in patients treated with lumpectomy and radiation, especially when the lymphatic invasion is present at or close to a surgical margin.[47] Most studies have shown blood vessel invasion alone to be a negative indicator of disease-free and overall survival.[27,41,48,49]

What is the importance of the size of the invasive tumor and how is it determined?

Size of the invasive tumor is arguably the most important factor determined by the pathologic evaluation of breast carcinoma.[50] A classic study by Rosen and coworkers[51] showed that node-negative patients with invasive tumors greater than 1 cm had a significantly decreased survival compared with those who had tumors smaller than 1 cm. Decisions regarding the use or withholding of systemic therapy are often made on the basis of tumor size regardless of lymph node status. Thus, it is crucial to assess size accurately. Generally, the size of a breast cancer is the measurement of the largest pathologically identifiable area of contiguous invasive carcinoma. Although, in our experience, tumor measurement using modern sonographic equipment is often quite accurate, pathologic size may or may not correspond to the clinical or radiographically determined size. Clinically and radiographically determined sizes should be regarded as estimates because they cannot account for the possible contribution of adjacent benign fibrous tissue or other masses (e.g., fibroadenoma, intraductal papilloma) to their size assessment. In fact, this holds true, although to a lesser degree, even for the examiner of the gross specimen, particularly in cases of invasive lobular carcinoma (discussed earlier). In practice, therefore, the grossly suspicious mass is measured in three dimensions, and at least one section is taken of the largest gross diameter to confirm the largest size microscopically. In the case of multiple invasive tumors, as is frequent in infiltrating lobular carcinoma, the largest microscopic area of contiguous invasive tumor is used for purposes of staging and systemic therapy decisions, while noting the presence of the other invasive areas and their relationship to margins. This situation is created iatrogenically by the use of preoperative chemotherapy when a large invasive tumor is shrunken into multiple tiny dispersed areas of invasion separated by fibrous tissue, often making postchemotherapy pathologic size determination a futile exercise.

The current era of imaging-directed core biopsy followed by sometimes multiple surgical specimens has added a layer of complexity to the evaluation of tumor size. Substantial amounts of invasive tumor may be removed by core biopsy, sometimes leading to the situation in which the largest area of invasive tumor is present in the core biopsy specimens rather than in the lumpectomy. More commonly, however, the bulk of the invasive tumor is present in the lumpectomy and, despite the granulation tissue that forms in the interval between core biopsy and surgery, the microscopic size of tumor in the surgical specimen closely mirrors that measured by imaging,[52] with sonography being especially accurate. It is incorrect to add the size of the invasive tumor seen on core to that seen on excision, and it is similarly misleading to add the size of any residual invasive tumor on re-excision of a positive lumpectomy margin to the original size. Thus, it is important that the same pathologist review the slides of each diagnostic procedure in order to assign the proper size and therefore provide accurate information for staging purposes.

What other additional histologic factors are prognostic?

Numerous other histopathologic characteristics have been evaluated as possible indicators of favorable or unfavorable prognostic factors, among them inflammatory infiltrate, stromal fibrosis, circumscribed versus irregular tumor border, necrosis of invasive tumor, and perineural invasion.[27,41,49] Most of these have not consistently yielded additional

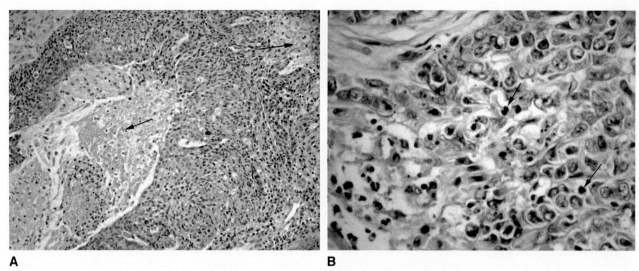

A   **B**

Figure 9–20   Necrosis in invasive duct carcinoma. This infiltrating duct carcinoma is poorly differentiated. *A,* Only minimal gland formation is evident, there is extreme nuclear pleomorphism, and there is extensive necrosis (*arrows*). Such tumors are often well circumscribed (*top left corner*) and exhibit very rapid growth. *B,* This is histologically seen as numerous mitoses (*arrows*) adjacent to areas of necrosis (*lower left corner*).

prognostic information in the literature; however, necrosis of the invasive component may impart additional poor prognosis,[53] probably because it is associated with rapid tumor growth (Fig. 9–20). Perineural invasion does not, by itself, impart a worse prognosis, but it is associated with lymphatic invasion and therefore, by extension, with positive axillary lymph nodes.

What additional prognostic and predictive actors should be tested for in invasive carcinoma?

A vast number of additional immunohistochemical and other markers have been studied over the years with varying success, and it is beyond the scope of this chapter to describe all of them. Currently, testing for estrogen receptor protein, progesterone receptor protein, and HER-2/neu oncoprotein is standard for any newly diagnosed invasive carcinoma.[54] Although other methods are available, all of these parameters are most commonly evaluated by direct immunohistochemistry, allowing the pathologist to visually evaluate the number of tumor cells staining and the intensity of the reaction (Fig. 9–21). Most important, direct immunohistochemistry permits the confirmation that it is truly the invasive tumor contributing to the test result, as opposed to normal tissue or in situ carcinoma. Immunohistochemical testing for HER-2/neu is often inconclusive and may be supplanted by fluorescence in situ hybridization if clinically necessary. Other, less frequently performed tests include flow cytometry and immunohistochemical evaluation for p53 protein and proliferation markers such as Ki-67, but conflicting data can be found in the literature as to the prognostic value of each.[54] Newer tests, including molecular characterization of invasive breast cancer by gene expression assays,[55] appear to hold great promise in separating invasive carcinomas into prognostically relevant groups irrespective of their histologic categorization.

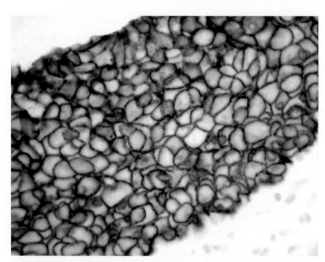

Figure 9–21   Immunohistochemical stain for HER-2/neu oncoprotein. Each individual cell in this carcinoma shows intense cytoplasmic membrane staining, creating a mosaic pattern.

REFERENCES

1. Simpson JF, Page DL. Status of breast cancer prognostication based on histopathologic data. Am J Clin Pathol 1994;102(Suppl 1):53–58.
2. Bloom HJG, Richardson WW. Histological grading and prognosis in breast cancer. A study of 1409 cases of which 359 have been followed for 15 years. Br J Cancer 1957;9:359–377.
3. Frierson HF Jr, Wolber RA, Beran KW, et al. Interobserver reproducibility of the Nottingham modification of the Bloom and Richardson histologic grading scheme for infiltrating ductal carcinoma. Am J Clin Pathol 1995;103:195–198.
4. Sidoni A, Bellezza G, Cavaliere R, et al. Prognostic indexes in breast cancer: Comparison of the Nottingham and Adelaide indexes. Breast 2004;13:23–27.
5. Foote FW Jr, Stewart FW. A histologic classification of carcinoma of the breast. Surgery 1946;19:74–99.
6. Weidner N, Semple JP. Pleomorphic variant of invasive lobular carcinoma of the breast. Hum Pathol 1992;23:1167–1171.

7. Steinbrecher JS, Silverberg SG. Signet-ring cell carcinoma of the breast. The mucinous variant of invasive lobular carcinoma? Cancer 1976;37: 828–840.

8. Merino MJ, Livolsi VA. Signet ring carcinoma of the female breast. A clinicopathologic analysis of 24 cases. Cancer 1981;48:1830–1837.

9. Walford N, Ten Velden J. Histiocytoid breast carcinoma: An apocrine variant of lobular carcinoma. Histopathology 1989;14:515–522.

10. Dixon JM, Anderson TJ, Page DL, et al. Infiltrating lobular carcinoma of the breast. Histopathology 1982;6:149–161.

11. Fechner RE. Histologic variants of infiltrating lobular carcinoma of the breast. Hum Pathol 1975;6:373–378.

12. Mersin H, Yildirim E, Gulben K, Berberoglu U. Is invasive lobular carcinoma different from invasive ductal carcinoma? Eur J Surg Oncol 2003;29:390–395.

13. Dixon JM, Anderson TJ, Page DL, et al. Infiltrating lobular carcinoma of the breast: An evaluation of the incidence and consequence of bilateral disease. Br J Surg 1983;70:513–516.

14. Ellis IO, Galea M, Broughton N, et al. Pathological prognostic factors in breast cancer. II. Histological type. Relationship with survival in a large study with long-term follow-up. Histopathology 1992;20:479–489.

15. DiCostanzo D, Rosen PP, Gareen I, et al. Prognosis in infiltrating lobular carcinoma. An analysis of "classical" and variant tumors. Am J Surg Pathol 1990;14:12–23.

16. Eusebi V, Magalhaes F, Azzopardi JG. Pleomorphic lobular carcinoma of the breast: An aggressive tumor showing apocrine differentiation. Hum Pathol 1992;23:655–662.

17. Frost AR, Terahata S, Yeh I-T, et al. The significance of signet ring cells in infiltrating lobular carcinoma of the breast. Arch Pathol Lab Med 1995;119:64–68.

18. Eusebi V, Foschini MP, Bussolati G, et al. Myoblastomatoid (histiocytoid) carcinoma of the breast. A type of apocrine carcinoma. Am J Surg Pathol 1995;19:553–562.

19. Fisher ER, Gregorio RM, Redmond C, et al. Tubulolobular invasive breast cancer: A variant of lobular invasive cancer. Hum Pathol 1977;8: 679–683.

20. Dixon AR, Ellis IO, Elston CW, et al. A comparison of the clinical metastatic patterns of invasive lobular and ductal carcinoma of the breast. Br J Cancer 1991;63:634–635.

21. Borst MJ, Ingold JA. Metastatic patterns of invasive lobular versus invasive ductal carcinoma of the breast. Surgery 1993;114:637–642.

22. Yeatman TJ, Cantor AB, Smith TJ, et al. Tumor biology of infiltrating lobular carcinoma. Implications for management. Ann Surg 1995;222: 549–561.

23. White JR, Gustafson FS, Wimbish K, et al. Conservative surgery and radiation therapy for infiltrating lobular carcinoma of the breast. The role of preoperative mammograms in guiding treatment. Cancer 1994;74:640–647.

24. Schnitt SJ, Connolly JL, Recht A, et al. Influence of infiltrating lobular histology on local tumor control in breast cancer patients treated with conservative surgery and radiotherapy. Cancer 1989;64:448–454.

25. Kurtz JM, Jacquemier J, Torhorst J, et al. Conservation therapy for breast cancers other than infiltrating duct carcinoma. Cancer 1989;63: 1630–1635.

26. Holland R, Veling SHJ, Mravunac M, et al. Histologic multifocality of Tis, T1-2 breast carcinomas. Implications for clinical trials of breast-conserving surgery. Cancer 1985;56:979–990.

27. Fisher ER, Sass R, Fisher B, et al. Pathologic findings from the National Surgical Adjuvant Breast Project (protocol 6). II. Relation of local breast recurrence to multicentricity. Cancer 1986;57:1717–1724.

28. Frazier TG, Wong RWY, Rose D. Implications of accurate pathologic margins in the treatment of primary breast cancer. Arch Surg 1989;124: 37–38.

29. Smitt MC, Nowels KW, Zdeblick MJ, et al. The importance of the lumpectomy surgical margin status in long-term results of breast conservation. Cancer 1995;76:259–267.

30. Lagios MD, Richards VE, Rose MR, et al. Segmental mastectomy without radiotherapy. Short-term follow-up. Cancer 1983;52:2173–2179.

31. Anscher MS, Jones P, Prosnitz LR, et al. Local failure and margin status in early-stage breast carcinoma treated with conservation surgery and radiation therapy. Ann Surg 1993;218:22–28.

32. Borger J, Kemperman H, Hart A, et al. Risk factors in breast-conserving therapy. J Clin Oncol 1994;12:653–660.

33. Schnitt SJ, Abner A, Gelman R, et al. The relationship between microscopic margins of resection and the risk of local recurrence in patients with breast cancer treated with breast-conserving surgery and radiation therapy. Cancer 1994;74:1746–1751.

34. Goldstein NS, Kestin L, Vicini F. Factors associated with ipsilateral breast failure and distant metastases in patients with invasive breast carcinoma treated with breast-conserving therapy. A clinicopathologic study of 607 neoplasms from 583 patients.

35. Veronesi U, Luini A, Galimberti V, et al. Conservation approaches for the management of stage I/II carcinoma of the breast: Milan Cancer Institute trials. World J Surg 1994;18:70–75.

36. Schnitt SJ, Connolly JL, Silver B, et al. Updated results on the influence of pathologic features on treatment outcome in stage I and II breast cancer patients treated by primary radiation therapy. Radiat Oncol Biol Phys 1985;11(Suppl 1):104–105.

37. Schnitt SJ, Connolly JL, Khettry U, et al. Pathologic findings on re-excision of the primary site in breast cancer patients considered for treatment by primary radiation therapy. Cancer 1987;59:675–681.

38. Fisher ER, Anderson S, Redmond C, et al. Ipsilateral breast tumor recurrence and survival following lumpectomy and irradiation: Pathological findings from NSABP protocol B-06. Semin Surg Oncol 1992;8:161–166.

39. Vicini FA, Eberlein TJ, Connolly JL, et al. The optimal extent of resection for patients with stages I and II breast cancer treated with conservative surgery and radiotherapy. Ann Surg 1991;214:200–205.

40. Gilchrist KW, Gould V, Hirschl S, et al. Interobserver variation in the identification of breast carcinoma in intramammary lymphatics. Hum Pathol 1982;13:170–172.

41. Roses DF, Bell DA, Flotte TJ, et al. Pathologic predictors of recurrence in stage 1 (T1N0M0) breast cancer. Am J Clin Pathol 1982;78:817–820.

42. Lee AKC, DeLellis R, Silverman ML, et al. Prognostic significance of peritumoral lymphatic and blood vessel invasion in node-negative carcinoma of the breast. J Clin Oncol 1990;8:1457–1465.

43. Kahn HJ, Marks A. A new monoclonal antibody, D2-40, for detection of lymphatic invasion in primary tumors. Lab Invest 2002;82:1255–1257.

44. Bettelheim R, Penman HG, Thornton-Jones H, et al. Prognostic significance of peritumoral vascular invasion in breast cancer. Br J Cancer 1984;50:771–777.

45. Pinder SE, Ellis IO, Galea M, et al. Pathological prognostic factors in breast cancer. III. Vascular invasion: Relationship with recurrence and survival in a large study with long-term follow-up. Histopathology 1993;24:41–47.

46. Barbareschi M, Dall Palma P, Bevilacqua P, et al. Invasive node negative breast carcinoma: Multivariate analysis of the prognostic value of peritumoral vessel invasion compared with that of conventional clinicopathologic features. Anticancer Res 1994;14:2229–2236.

47. Celemente CG, Boracchi P, Andreola S, et al. Peritumoral lymphatic invasion in patients with node negative mammary duct carcinoma. Cancer 1992;69:1396–1403.

48. Sampat MB, Sirsat MV, Gangadharan P. Prognostic significance of blood vessel invasion in carcinoma of the breast in women. J Surg Oncol 1977;9:623–632.

49. Dawson PJ, Karrison T, Ferguson T. Histologic features associated with long-term survival in breast cancer. Hum Pathol 1984;17:1015–1021.

50. Michaelson JS, Silverstein M, Wyatt J, et al. Predicting the survival of patients with breast carcinoma using tumor size. Cancer 2002;95: 713–723.

51. Rosen PP, Groshen S, Kinne DW, Norton L. Factors influencing prognosis in node-negative breast carcinoma: Analysis of 767 T1N0M0/T2N0M0 patients with long-term follow-up. J Clin Oncol 1993;11: 2090–2100.

52. Charles M, Edge SB, Winston JS, et al. Effect of stereotactic core needle biopsy of pathologic measurement of tumor size of T1 invasive breast carcinomas presenting as mammographic masses. Cancer 2003;97: 2137–2141.

53. Jimenez RE, Wallis T, Visscher DW. Centrally necrotizing carcinomas of the breast: A distinct histologic subtype with aggressive clinical behavior. Am J Surg Pathol 2001;25:1557–1558.

54. Bast RC, Ravdin P, Hayes DF, et al. 2000 Update of recommendations for the use of tumor markers in breast and colorectal cancer: Clinical practice guidelines of the American Society of Clinical Oncology. J Clin Oncol 2001;18:1865–1878.

55. Sorlie T, Perou CM, Tibshirani R, et al. Gene expression patterns of breast carcinomas distinguish tumor subclasses with clinical implications. Proc Natl Acad Sci U S A 2001;98:10869–10874.

CHAPTER 10

Pathology of Special Forms of Breast Cancer

Shabnam Jaffer

Invasive carcinomas of the breast are ductal (65% to 80%), lobular (5% to 15%), or mixed (6%).[1,2] Most invasive duct carcinomas (IDCs) are of the conventional type (see Chapter 9), also known as *ordinary, classic, usual,* and *not otherwise specified.* A smaller proportion of breast carcinomas (10% to 25%) constitute the *special* or *unusual* variants of infiltrating breast carcinoma owing to distinct cytoarchitecture and pattern of spread.[1] This chapter describes the pertinent clinical, morphologic, and biologic features of these special types of breast carcinomas.

How are the variants of breast cancer defined?

These distinct carcinoma variants are separated from IDC owing to unique features, such as specific cell types (e.g., apocrine), secretion (e.g., mucinous carcinoma), architectural features (e.g., papillary carcinoma), pattern of spread (e.g., micropapillary carcinoma), and biologic behavior (e.g., good prognosis—tubular carcinoma; poor prognosis—metaplastic carcinoma).

What is the implication of a diagnosis of a variant of invasive breast cancer when it coexists with ordinary invasive breast carcinoma?

For prognostic reasons, it is important to qualify whether a variant of IDC is present in pure or mixed form. In contrast to the mixed forms, the pure types are endowed with unique biologic behavior. Second, in most cases, the mixed form is more common than the pure form. Inaccurate distinction of the pure from the mixed forms leads to conflicting data in the literature regarding the behavior of these variants. For the purposes of this chapter, we will discuss only the salient features of the pure and not the mixed variants of IDC.

TUBULAR CARCINOMA

A well-differentiated invasive carcinoma, tubular carcinoma is characterized by the formation of neoplastic tubules that closely resemble breast ductules. It constitutes less than 2% of all breast carcinomas[3-7] and 9% of carcinomas smaller than 1.0 cm.[8] Tubular carcinoma may commonly be admixed with invasive lobular carcinoma, known as tubulolobular carcinoma.

What are the clinical features of tubular carcinoma?

Compared with IDC, tubular carcinoma is more likely to occur in older patients and to be multicentric (10% to 56%), bilateral (38%), and associated with a family history of breast carcinoma (40%).[9,10] Most tubular carcinomas (80% to 87%) are less than 1cm, suggestive of slow growth.[11-13] They are usually not palpable and thus are detected primarily by mammography, presenting as spiculated densities or as trabecular distortion.

Tubular carcinoma is associated with a favorable prognosis owing to a combination of its small size at presentation, well-differentiated histology, and low rate of axillary lymph node metastases (0% to 29%).[3,6,7,12-17] This favorable prognosis is maintained even when axillary lymph nodes are involved. Multifocal tumor with its associated greater tumor volume has a predisposition to lymph node metastases. Cumulative survival rates for tumors of all sizes were 97.3% at 5 years, 87.8% at 10 years, and 77.3% at 20 years, compared with 45.3%, 32.6%, and 19.8%, respectively, for IDC.[3] The rate of recurrence over an interval of 2 to 22 years is reported to be about 3% to 4% and occurs more commonly in patients with axillary lymph node metastases.[5,6,11,12,15,18]

A study comparing tubular carcinoma and tubulolobular carcinoma found a higher incidence of multifocality (20% versus 29%), axillary lymph node metastases (12% versus 43%), and recurrence rate (1% versus 12%) for the latter.[18] However, analyses of these results failed to find any statistical significance.[19] Thus, the prognosis of these tumors is thought to be intermediate between tubular carcinomas and invasive lobular carcinomas. Additional studies are indicated to further delineate the clinical features of these two tumors.

What are the pathologic features of tubular carcinoma?

Grossly and microscopically, tubular carcinomas recapitulate the mammographic appearance of a stellate mass (Fig. 10–1).

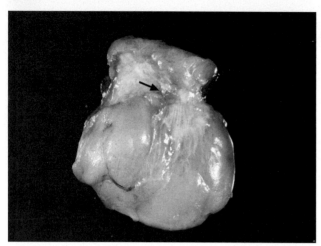

Figure 10–1 Gross appearance of tubular carcinoma showing a spiculated mass.

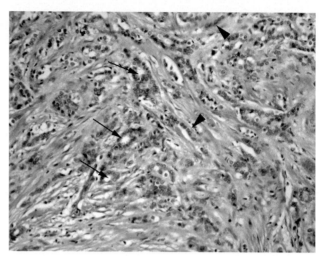

Figure 10–3 Histologic appearance of tubulolobular carcinoma showing features of both tubular carcinoma (*arrows*) and lobular carcinoma (*arrowheads*).

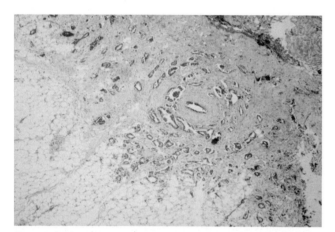

Figure 10–2 Histologic appearance of tubular carcinoma showing neoplastic glands with angulated contours infiltrating fat.

Morphologically, it is composed of a haphazard distribution of small open glands or tubules with irregular shapes and angular contours lined by a single layer of neoplastic columnar or cuboidal ductal cells infiltrating fat (Fig. 10–2). The nuclei are bland, basally oriented, hyperchromatic, and round to oval with inconspicuous nuclei. The cytoplasm is usually amphophilic, rarely clear or eosinophilic. Apocrine-type cytoplasmic tufts or snouts may be present along the luminal border of the cells and are seen in one third of cases. Alternatively, the glands may have open lumina containing basophilic secretions or calcifications. Mitoses are rare to nil.

There is a lack of agreement with regard to the extent of tubular differentiation necessary to make a diagnosis of tubular carcinoma. Criteria range from being strict, requiring 100% tubular differentiation,[3,4] to others ranging from 75% to 90%.[6,12,20,21] Most authors agree with a cutoff at 90%, such that tumors with 50% to 90% tubular differentiation are labeled as mixed type.

The interglandular stroma may be composed of altered collagen that may contain myofibroblasts, myxoid matrix, calcifications, and/or elastin. Elastin may be seen in other IDC and radial scars, raising the differential diagnosis and possible origin from radial scar. In fact, in some cases, tubular carcinoma has been found to arise from or to be associated with radial scars.[20,22] Microscopically, the distinction from radial scar is made by the presence of glands lined by a single cell type, that is, devoid of myoepithelial cells and infiltrating adipose tissue (see Fig. 10–2). Associated low-grade intraductal carcinoma, micropapillary or cribriform types, may be present in 60% to 84% of tubular carcinomas.[5,11,14,16]

As the name indicates, tubulolobular carcinoma is the morphologic sum of tubular carcinoma intimately admixed with invasive lobular carcinoma that is characterized by cords of small, uniform cells arranged in single linear file fashion (Fig. 10–3). It is more likely to be admixed with lobular carcinoma in situ.

Most tubular and tubulolobular carcinomas are estrogen and progesterone hormone receptor positive.[23]

CRIBRIFORM CARCINOMA

As the name suggests, the morphology of this tumor is characterized by a cribriform pattern. It is a form of well-differentiated IDC whose incidence ranges from 0.3% to 4%.[24–26]

What are the clinical features of cribriform carcinoma?

As with IDC, cribriform carcinoma can present as a spiculated mass or calcifications. Multifocal tumors are present in 20% of cases.[25] The rate of axillary lymph node metastases (11%) is lower than in conventional IDC, portending a favorable prognosis.[24,25]

However, studies on cribriform carcinoma are few in number, and the data are not standardized in terms of tumor size or surgical treatment. Nevertheless, postmastectomy disease-free survival approaches almost 100%, with follow-up times ranging from 5 to 21 years.[24–26] The role of conservative surgery is currently unknown but worthy of future study.

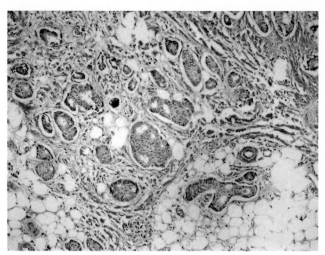

Figure 10–4 Histologic appearance of cribriform carcinoma showing a fenestrated pattern with sharp cookie-cutter spaces in a desmoplastic stroma and associated focal tubular carcinoma.

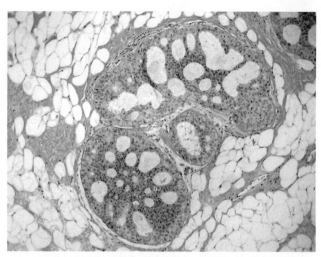

Figure 10–5 Histologic appearance of cribriform intraductal carcinoma showing prominent basement membrane and absence of desmoplastic stroma.

What are the pathologic features of cribriform carcinoma?

A cribriform pattern is characterized by the presence of nests of tumor cells containing sharply outlined cookie-cutter type round to oval arched glandular spaces imparting a fenestrated or sievelike appearance with a desmoplastic stroma (Fig. 10–4). The cells within these nests have low-grade nuclei and rare mitoses. Cribriform carcinoma may also have tubular differentiation (see Fig. 10–4) and still qualify as cribriform carcinoma as long as the tubular differentiation is less than 50%.[24]

A similar pattern is observed in cribriform intraductal carcinoma, distinguished by the presence of basement membrane around the cribriform nests, rare myoepithelial cells, and lack of stromal invasion (Fig. 10–5). Nevertheless, distinction of the in situ form from the invasive component may be difficult, particularly because the invasive form is usually associated with the in situ form. A cribriform growth pattern is also seen in adenoid cystic carcinoma (described later) and is differentiated by the absence of the cylindromatous basement membrane in cribriform carcinoma. All tumors express estrogen hormone receptor, and up to 70% also express progesterone receptor.[25]

MEDULLARY CARCINOMA

The term *medullary carcinoma* was coined by Ewing in 1940[27] to describe a small group (1% to 7% of all IDC)[6,28–33] of well-circumscribed, poorly differentiated tumors, paradoxically associated with good prognosis. It is for this reason that strict morphologic criteria must be met in order to diagnose medullary carcinoma. Alternatively, when most, but not all, diagnostic criteria are met, a diagnosis of atypical medullary carcinoma or IDC with medullary features is made, both of which are associated with a prognosis similar to that of IDC.

What are the clinical features of medullary carcinoma?

Medullary carcinoma affects younger women (range, 45 to 54 years).[28,34–36] It occurs more frequently in native Japanese women[37,38] and black women[39] in the United States. Of all *BRCA1* tumors analyzed, 19% were pure medullary carcinomas,[40,41] a higher rate than that of IDC. Radiologically, the circumscription of these tumors leads them to be mistaken for fibroadenomas.[42] Whereas in the past they were designated as bulky adenocarcinomas, today smaller tumors are detected (<3.0 cm).

The favorable prognosis associated with medullary carcinoma in older series, even with involved axillary lymph nodes (10%), has been confirmed in several newer series with postmastectomy survival rates as follows: 5 years, 78% to 88.5%; 10 years, 64%; and 20 years, 95% (stage I) and 61% (stage II).[31,33,34,43–46] In a few other series, patients have been treated with conservative surgery followed by radiotherapy, also with favorable results.[47,48] Despite a higher reported rate of axillary lymph node metastases in some series (42% to 45%), the prognosis is still better than in IDC.[31,43] Patients with medullary carcinoma typically experience reactive lymphadenopathy that is readily palpable and may lead to clinical upstaging. However, the actual number of involved nodes is usually less than three and limited to the lower axillary group. When metastases occur in medullary carcinoma, they do so within the first 5 years and are usually systemic, associated with poor survival.[27,43]

What are the pathologic features of medullary carcinoma?

Grossly, these tumors differ from IDC by being brown, soft, lobulated, and bulging (Fig. 10–6). Foci of necrosis and cystic degeneration may also be present. Despite strict criteria for the diagnosis of medullary carcinoma, this entity is unfortunately overdiagnosed, as seen in previous series.[49,50] As stressed before, the pathologist should diagnose medullary carcinoma

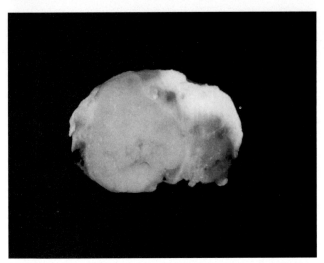

Figure 10–6 Gross appearance of medullary carcinoma showing a well-circumscribed brown soft tumor.

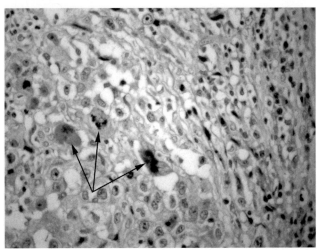

Figure 10–8 High-power histologic appearance of medullary carcinoma showing a syncytial growth pattern, admixed rich lymphoid reaction, high-grade nuclei, and frequent mitoses (*arrows*).

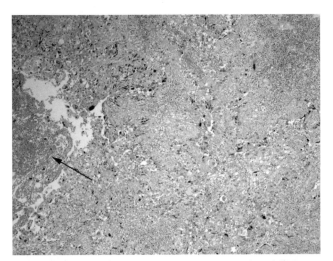

Figure 10–7 Low-power histologic appearance of medullary carcinoma showing a well-circumscribed tumor with central cystic necrosis (*arrow*).

only using strict histologic criteria to preserve its predictive favorable prognosis.

First, the carcinoma must be microscopically circumscribed, characterized by a smooth rounded pushing border (Fig. 10–7). Second, a lymphoplasmacytic reaction must be present both within and at the periphery of the tumor (see Fig. 10–7). Germinal centers may occasionally be present, such that distinguishing a true medullary carcinoma from an intramammary lymph node with metastatic carcinoma may be difficult, particularly on core biopsy. Thus, medullary carcinomas are rich in activated cytotoxic and HLA-DR–positive lymphocytes, both of which may be related to its favorable prognosis.[51,52] In addition, the level of immunoglobulin G (IgG) can be high and may be inversely related to diminished expression of estrogen hormone receptor (<10%).[53,54] Third, a syncytial growth pattern, a prognostically important finding,[55] is present, characterized by broad irregular sheets or islands of cells devoid of any glandular differentiation, such that the borders between the cells are indiscriminant. Finally, the

carcinoma must be poorly differentiated, consisting of cells with high nuclear grade and mitotic activity (Fig. 10–8). This correlates with an increased expression of *p53* and *Ki-67* but low *bcl-2*, consistent with rapid cell turnover and possibly related to a good prognosis. *HER-2/neu* expression is variable but usually negative.

Other microscopic features associated with, but not diagnostic for, medullary carcinoma may be present. The first is the presence of high-grade intraductal carcinoma, usually at the periphery of the tumor, also associated with a lymphoplasmacytic reaction. Second, metaplastic change, particularly of the squamous type, may be found in up to 16% of medullary carcinomas.[33] Finally, necrosis may be present, directly related to size, such that with increasing tumor size, cystic degeneration may occur.

The term *atypical medullary carcinoma* was introduced to classify carcinomas that differ from typical medullary carcinomas by one or more histologic features. One or more of the following may characterize them: invasive growth pattern, diminished lymphoplasmacytic reaction, well-differentiated carcinoma, and low mitotic count. The distinction is crucial so as to make clear the favorable prognosis of medullary carcinoma versus atypical medullary carcinoma, which has a prognosis equivalent to that of IDC.

MUCINOUS CARCINOMA

Initially recognized in 1826,[56] mucinous carcinoma constitutes 2% of all breast carcinomas. Also known as colloid or gelatinous carcinoma, these tumors, as their name implies, are composed of large amounts of extracellular mucus that is visible both grossly and microscopically.

What are the clinical features of mucinous carcinoma?

Mucinous carcinoma affects mostly elderly women (average age, 62 years), with the exception of Japanese women (average

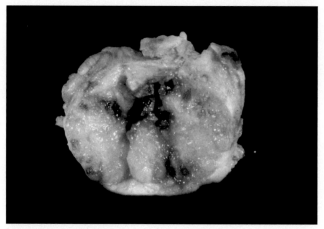

Figure 10–9   Gross appearance of mucinous carcinoma showing a well-circumscribed tumor with a gelatinous or mucoid cut surface.

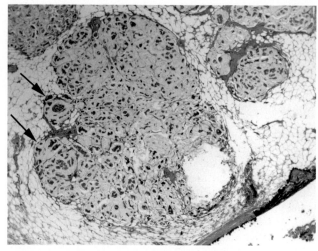

Figure 10–10   Low-power histologic appearance of mucinous carcinoma showing a predominantly well-circumscribed tumor with focal pushing borders (*arrows*).

age, 49 years)[57–59] Clinical presentation is that of a soft to moderately firm lesion, which may rarely be crepitant ("swish sign"). The average time from onset of symptoms to biopsy and diagnosis may be 3 months or less.[60] Delay in seeking treatment, particularly in elderly women, may lead to larger tumor size at presentation.[61] Although most mucinous carcinomas are mammographically occult, some may present as either a circumscribed, lobulated mass lesion, deceptively resembling a benign lesion, or rarely with calcifications.[62–64] Based on serial mammograms, these carcinomas most likely have a slow growth rate. This is further supported by the low incidence of axillary lymph node metastases reported by several series, ranging from 0% to 29%.[60,64,65] Second, the survival rate is also favorable, ranging from 79% to 90% at 10 to 20 years,[59,61,66] with death from disease usually occurring after more than 10 years.[67] Thus, a small node-negative mucinous carcinoma can be appropriately treated without the need for systemic adjuvant therapy.[61,68,69] However, postmastectomy chest wall recurrence has been reported in up to 15% of cases, and systemic recurrences have been described as long as 25 to 30 years after mastectomy.[70–73] Rarely, cerebral metastases have been described that manifest as a mucin embolus, leading to fatal cerebral infarction.[74,75]

What are the pathologic features of mucinous carcinoma?

In contrast to IDC, mucinous carcinomas are usually well-circumscribed, larger (range, 1 to 20 cm; mean, 2.8 cm) tumors, with a soft, currant-jelly gelatinous cut surface (Fig. 10–9). Larger tumors may also have cystic degeneration. Despite their gross circumscription, microscopically most tumors (70%) have pushing borders demonstrated by irregular knobby contours protruding into normal breast tissue[66] (Fig. 10–10). The key microscopic feature is the presence of well-differentiated tumor cells floating in a sea of extracellular mucin separated by fibrous septa (Fig. 10–11). Rarely, the carcinomas are poorly differentiated, probably representing admixed invasive micropapillary carcinoma (described later), the two being difficult to separate. The cells may be arranged

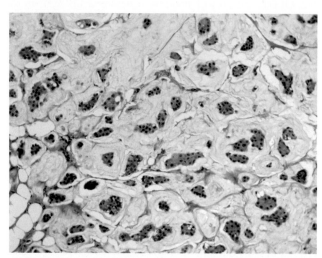

Figure 10–11   High-power histologic appearance of mucinous carcinoma showing well-differentiated tumor cells in a sea of mucin.

in strands, alveolar nests, macropapillae, or cribriform clusters, usually correlating with the intraductal pattern that is present in 20% to 75% of cases. The ratio of cells to mucin may vary from case to case but is usually consistent within a case. The mucin is composed of neutral and acidic mucopolysaccharides[76] and expresses MUC-5 and MUC-2 (gel-forming mucin),[77] the latter being highly specific for mucinous carcinoma. The typical indolent behavior of mucinous carcinoma is probably related to MUC-2, which not only confers tumor suppressor activity but also acts as a containing factor, hindering the spread of cells.[78]

In contrast to mucin-rich tumors, hypercellular tumors with diminished mucin are associated with a worse prognosis.[59,65,71] Occasionally, the entire tumor may consist of mucin and needs to be thoroughly sampled to identify the cells. Thus, the margin of a mucinous carcinoma may be deemed positive based on the presence of mucin with or without admixed cells. Based on ultrastructural studies, the extent of neuroendocrine differentiation ranges from 25% to 50%

but is not prognostically significant.[57,79–81] Most mucinous carcinomas express estrogen (>90%) and progesterone (>50%) hormone receptors and only rarely (<5%) express *HER-2/neu*.[59,65,71]

APOCRINE CARCINOMA

Apocrine carcinomas constitute less than 1% to 4% of all breast carcinomas.[82,83] It is hypothesized that these carcinomas originate from ductal cells with apocrine differentiation because of their normal existence in the breast and their capacity to proliferate into atypical and eventually neoplastic lesions. In fact, this spectrum of lesions may be found adjacent to an invasive apocrine carcinoma.

What are the clinical features of apocrine carcinoma?

The clinical features of apocrine carcinoma are similar to those of IDC and thus will be excluded from discussion, with the exception of one report stating the frequent association of older age and or postmenopausal status with apocrine carcinoma.[84]

What are the pathologic features of apocrine carcinoma?

Although the architectural features of apocrine carcinoma include the usual growth patterns found in IDC, it is the cytologic features that justify its distinction as a unique entity. The cells contain large pleomorphic nuclei with prominent eosinophilic nucleoli (Fig. 10–12). The cytoplasm contains abundant granular eosinophilia that is periodic acid–Schiff (PAS) stain positive after diastase digestion. Alternatively, the cytoplasm may contain fine empty vacuoles, such that the cells may resemble histiocytes. Immunohistochemically, gross cystic disease fluid protein (GCDFP-15) marks more than half of

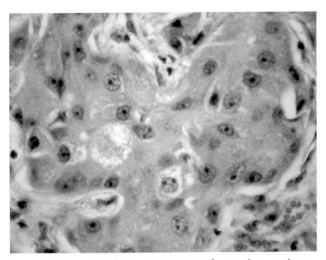

Figure 10–12 Histologic appearance of apocrine carcinoma showing cells containing granular eosinophilic cytoplasm and pleomorphic nuclei with conspicuous nucleoli.

all apocrine carcinomas and is thus considered a putative marker of apocrine differentiation.[83,85] These cytologic and immunohistochemical features are also seen and overlap with the histiocytoid variant of infiltrating lobular carcinoma, making the distinction difficult.[85]

Studies on hormone receptor expression in apocrine carcinomas have been conflicting, with estrogen receptor positivity ranging from 0% to 50% of cases, whereas progesterone receptor expression is usually negative or low.[82,83,86,87] Interestingly, some apocrine carcinomas express androgen receptors,[88] a finding of uncertain significance at present.

MICROPAPILLARY CARCINOMA

First recognized in 1979 and later described in 1993,[89,90] this is the most recently described variant of IDC. It makes up less than 2% of all IDC and is characterized by a distinctive "exfoliative" morphology and lymphotropism.

What are the clinical features of micropapillary carcinoma?

Women with invasive micropapillary carcinoma tend to be older than those with other types of IDC. Patients may present with a palpable mass or radiologic abnormality. Mammographically, a spiculated, irregular, or round, high-density mass with or without calcifications may be present. Sonographically, a homogeneously hypoechoic irregular or microlobulated mass may be present.

The aggressive nature of these carcinomas is reflected in high rates of both lymphatic invasion (>50%)[91,92] and axillary lymph node metastases (72% to 77%),[93] regardless of size or extent of differentiation.[94] Thus, they are best treated with mastectomy and axillary dissection[93–98]; chemotherapy is advocated for tumors larger than 1.0 cm regardless of lymph node status. However, the treatment of smaller tumors is not clear. Despite studies indicating a shorter disease-free and overall survival, when cases are stratified by involved lymph nodes and other prognostic features, multivariate analysis failed to show any difference between invasive micropapillary carcinoma and IDC.[95,96]

What are the pathologic features of micropapillary carcinoma?

The distinctive growth pattern of this carcinoma is characterized by solid morules or nests floating within punched-out spaces with a serrated border in the fibrous stroma (Fig. 10–13). On cross-section, the aggregates of malignant cells have a tubular appearance with minimal to no lumina formation. These artifactual spaces represent shrinkage owing to fixation, as proved by their absence on frozen sections. They deceptively resemble angiolymphatic spaces but lack an endothelial lining. Cytologically, the cells are cuboidal to columnar, containing finely granular or densely eosinophilic cytoplasm and intermediate- to high-grade nuclei. Apocrine and mucinous differentiation may be present. In fact, as mentioned previously, mucinous carcinomas with high-grade

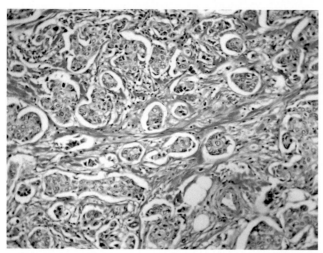

Figure 10–13 Histologic appearance of micropapillary carcinoma showing morules of cells floating in punched-out spaces.

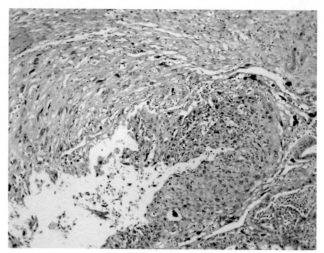

Figure 10–14 Histologic appearance of metaplastic squamous cell carcinoma showing a cystic tumor with spindled (*left*) and dyskeratotic cells with intercellular bridges and keratin pearl formation (*right*).

nuclear features may actually represent admixed invasive micropapillary carcinoma, and the distinction may not always be feasible. A high mitotic rate and calcifications in the form of psammoma bodies may be present. Intraductal carcinoma, micropapillary type, with intermediate- to high-nuclear-grade and associated necrosis may be present.

Ultrastructurally, microvilli have been observed on the peripheral cell surfaces, suggesting that the spaces around the clusters are glandular lumina with an inside-out growth pattern."[97] Furthermore, immunohistochemical staining with epithelial membrane antigen (EMA) demonstrates staining of these peripheral spaces, supporting this hypothesis. It is this reverse polarization that is hypothetically responsible for the lymphotropic behavior.

Invasive micropapillary carcinoma is usually estrogen positive (73% to 90%) and progesterone positive (45% to 70%) but paradoxically may also be *HER-2/neu* positive (36% to 100%).[91,92,94,98]

METAPLASTIC CARCINOMA

Metaplasia is defined as the change from one cell type to another. In metaplastic breast carcinomas, it is the transformation of IDC into a nonglandular component (i.e., mesenchymal differentiation). Composed of a heterogeneous group of neoplasms, metaplastic carcinomas are characterized by an admixture of mammary carcinoma with spindle, squamous, chondroid, or osseous elements. The incidence of these neoplasms ranges from 1% to 5%. Low-grade adenosquamous carcinoma, a distinct variant of metaplastic carcinoma, has unique morphologic and clinical features, described next.

What are the clinical features of metaplastic carcinoma?

These tumors usually present clinically and radiologically as well-circumscribed, firm, palpable masses. They tend to be rapidly growing with a short duration before detection. They are larger than IDC, ranging in size from 1 to 21 cm (mean, 3

to 4 cm), with more than half greater than 5 cm. They may reach massive sizes (>20 cm) with consequent ulceration and displacement of the skin and nipple. Relative to their large size, the frequency of axillary lymph node metastases is low, ranging from 0% to 54%.[99–105] Five-year mortality rates range from 25% to 86%.[99–101,103,105] The higher end of these two incidences is true mostly for tumors with spindle and squamous differentiation.[98] Metastases are composed of ductal or metaplastic elements or both.

After adjusting for nodal status and tumor size, metaplastic carcinoma has a more favorable prognosis than IDC; however, this difference is not statistically significant.[106] In fact, with the exception of extensive spindle cell metaplasia in a squamous cell carcinoma, heterologous metaplasia does not negatively affect prognosis.[107] The above data are derived from treatment by mastectomy and axillary dissection; the roles of lumpectomy, chemotherapy, and radiotherapy are currently unknown.

What are the pathologic features of metaplastic carcinoma?

Grossly, these tumors are large, cystic, and necrotic, with pushing or infiltrative borders. Morphologically, they are usually poorly differentiated IDC that are further subdivided into two arbitrary categories: squamous and heterologous differentiation. Tumors with mixed components also occur.

Squamous Metaplasia
Given the identical histologic features of squamous cell carcinoma from other body sites (i.e., formation of intercellular bridges, dyskeratotic cells, and keratin pearl formation; Fig. 10–14), metastasis must be excluded. The most common manifestation of metaplastic squamous cell carcinoma is focal squamous metaplasia within a typical IDC, described in up to 3.7% of IDC.[108] The IDC can range from poorly to well differentiated, the latter known as *low-grade adenosquamous carcinoma*, described later. When squamous differentiation is

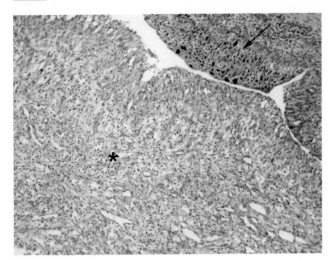

Figure 10–15 High-power histologic appearance of metaplastic squamous cell carcinoma (*arrow*) showing acantholytic areas with a pseudovascular stroma resembling angiosarcoma (*asterisk*).

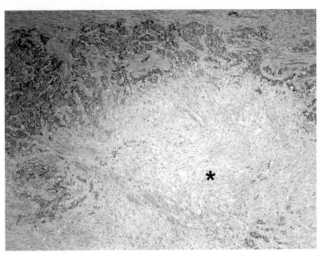

Figure 10–16 Histologic appearance of metaplastic carcinoma with heterologous metaplasia showing an intermediate myxoid stroma (*asterisk*) bridging between the chondroid elements and invasive ductal carcinoma.

predominant or diffuse, a spectrum of histologic patterns can emerge singly or in combination as follows: keratinizing, large cell, spindle cells, and acantholytic.

Tumors may be cystic, lined by bland-appearing cells that become focally spindled as they invade the stroma (see Fig. 10–14). The acantholytic variant of squamous cell carcinoma, associated with aggressive behavior, contains degenerated squamous cells embedded in a rich spindle cell and pseudovascular stroma and can be mistaken for angiosarcoma (Fig. 10–15). The distinction of pure spindle cell variants of squamous cell carcinoma from primary or metastatic sarcoma is difficult, if not impossible. Extensive sampling may be necessary to find areas of squamous differentiation; in situ and/or invasive duct carcinoma usually presents at the periphery. In the absence of any epithelial components, one can resort to immunohistochemistry (discussed later). These tumors are usually negative for hormone receptors.

Low-grade adenosquamous carcinomas, a distinct variant of squamous metaplastic carcinoma, are similar to adenosquamous carcinoma of the skin and are also known as syringomatous squamous tumors.[109] Smaller than other metaplastic carcinomas, they range in size from 0.5 to 3.4 cm. They are composed of varying proportions of three components of IDC: glands, solid nests, and stroma. The solid nests may be cystic or solid, the latter composed of squamous cells or keratin pearl formation. The stroma can also be variable, ranging from fibrotic to having osseous and chondroid metaplasia. Some low-grade adenosquamous carcinomas may be associated with radial sclerosing papillary lesions or sclerosing adenosis. Most of these carcinomas have an excellent prognosis, but some can be locally aggressive because of infiltrative borders.

Heterologous Metaplasia

Carcinomas with heterologous metaplasia are biphasic, composed of an epithelial component and a heterologous component. The latter can range from bland to malignant and more commonly consist of spindle cells, bone, and cartilage; less frequently, they consist of muscle, adipose, and vascular differentiation.[111] When both the epithelial and mesenchymal

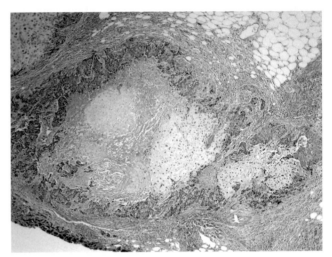

Figure 10–17 Histologic appearance of metaplastic carcinoma, "matrix-producing" type, showing an abrupt transition between the chondroid and ductal carcinoma.

elements are poorly differentiated, it is called *carcinosarcoma*. When the heterologous elements are osseous or chondroid, it is known as *matrix-producing carcinoma*. Although some metaplastic carcinomas have a transitional myxoid or spindle cell component bridging the two components (Fig. 10–16), in both carcinosarcoma and matrix-producing carcinomas, there is a sharp transition between these two elements without an intermediary[110] (Fig. 10–17). Multinucleated osteoclast giant cells may accompany carcinomas with osseous, chondroid, and spindle cell differentiation.

Despite numerous immunohistochemical studies attempting to analyze the relation between the epithelial and mesenchymal components, the results are inconsistent.[112–114] Typically, the epithelial elements express cytokeratin and EMA, and the mesenchymal elements express vimentin and actin, but these results can overlap. For instance, cytokeratin expression may be present in 63% of spindle cell carcinomas,[115] and EMA reactivity has been observed in 31% of heterologous carcinomas.[103] However, the sarcomatous elements in carcinosarcomas and matrix-producing carcinomas is usually negative for cytokeratin. The sarcomatous areas may also stain with 34βE12, suggesting myoepithelial derivation. Estrogen and progesterone hormone receptor expression is usually negative, depending on the grade of the invasive component.

MAMMARY CARCINOMA WITH OSTEOCLAST-LIKE GIANT CELLS

As mentioned earlier, osteoclast giant cells may be admixed with chondroid and osseous elements in metaplastic carcinoma. However, mammary carcinoma with osteoclast-like giant cells is distinguished by the association with only IDC and no heterologous elements. They constitute 0.5% to 1.2% of all IDCs.[116,117] The clinical features of this tumor are similar to IDC and will not be discussed.

What are the pathologic features of mammary carcinoma with osteoclast-like giant cells?

Grossly, these tumors are fleshy, firm, and well circumscribed, with a bulging, dark brown-red cut surface. The IDC component is moderately to poorly differentiated but can occasionally also be lobular. The osteoclast giant cells can be present in the periphery, center, or glandular lumina of the IDC (Fig. 10–18). The stroma may contain extravasated erythrocytes or hemosiderin, suggestive of recent or old hemorrhage. It is unknown what induces the presence of the osteoclast giant cells, but one in vitro study suggested a role played by interleukin-1 (IL-1).[116] Both immunohistochemical and ultrastructural studies definitively show these cells to be of mesenchymal rather than epithelial origin. They are hypothesized to be a specific type of macrophage with osteoclastic functional ability. Interestingly, they have higher progesterone than estrogen hormone receptor expression.[115,117–120]

LIPID-RICH CARCINOMA

As the name suggests, this variant of breast carcinoma is characterized by the predominant presence (>90%) of cells containing abundant cytoplasmic neutral lipids.[121] The incidence ranges from 1% to 6% of all IDCs.[122–124]

What are the clinical features of lipid-rich carcinoma?

Because of a limited number of series in the literature with short follow-up data, clinical data on these cases are also limited. These series indicate that these tumors are larger and more aggressive than IDC, with a higher incidence of axillary lymph node metastases.[123]

What are the pathologic features of lipid-rich carcinoma?

These carcinomas are characterized by cells containing neutral lipids such that they contain clear, foamy to vacuolated cytoplasm as a result of lipid extraction during histologic processing. Morphologically, they are poorly differentiated tumors characterized by large pleomorphic cells arranged in an alveolar pattern with a hobnail appearance.

The differential diagnosis includes other IDCs containing similar-appearing vacuolated cells (Fig. 10–19) and includes apocrine carcinoma, glycogen-rich carcinoma, and secretory carcinoma (described later). Metastatic carcinomas with clear cells, such as renal cell carcinoma, should also be excluded. The presence of lipids can be confirmed by specialized tissue processing that preserves cytoplasmic lipids, electron microscopy, or histochemical analysis (oil red O stain) of fresh-frozen tissue for cytoplasmic lipid. When the latter is done, up to 75% of IDCs are reactive, but only 6% contain lipids in large enough amounts to qualify as lipid-rich carcinoma.[119]

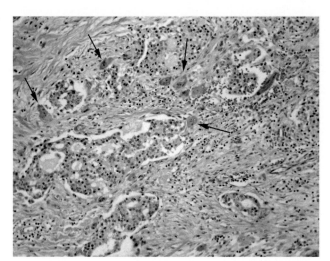

Figure 10–18 Histologic appearance of mammary carcinoma with osteoclast giant cells (*arrows*) showing both components with associated hemorrhage.

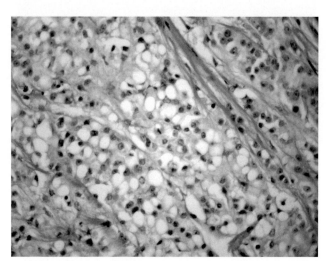

Figure 10–19 Histologic appearance of an invasive duct carcinoma with clear cell features raising the differential diagnosis of lipid-rich, glycogen-rich, and secretory carcinoma.

The carcinomas are usually negative for estrogen and progesterone hormone receptors but may express α-lactalbumin and lactoferrin.

GLYCOGEN-RICH CLEAR CELL CARCINOMA

This is yet another carcinoma that contains cells with predominantly (>90%) clear cytoplasm, but it is composed of glycogen. It constitutes 1% to 3% of all breast carcinomas.[125,126]

What are the clinical features of glycogen-rich clear cell carcinoma?

Based on limited number of series, these tumors appear to be more aggressive than conventional IDCs,[127] with a high rate (30%) of axillary lymph node metastases.[126] This is reflected in a low disease-free and overall survival rate, with up to 30% to 50% of patients reported dying from metastatic disease.[125,128]

What are the pathologic features of glycogen-rich clear cell carcinoma?

This carcinoma is usually composed of architectural features of IDC but rarely may also be of lobular origin. The cells have sharply defined cell borders and polygonal contours. As with lipid-rich clear cell carcinomas, extraction of cytoplasmic substances during processing causes the cytoplasm to acquire a clear vacuolated to granular appearance, raising the same differential diagnoses. However, in up to 58% of cases, these carcinomas may have no significant clear cell change.[125] The cells stain with the diastase-labile PAS stain. About half of these tumors are estrogen hormone receptor positive, but they are never positive for progesterone.[125,128]

SECRETORY CARCINOMA

Secretory carcinoma is a rare neoplasm with an incidence of 0.15% of all breast carcinomas. Because of its original description in children,[129] it was labeled "juvenile" carcinoma. Today, we know this carcinoma to occur over a wide age range (3 to 73 years),[130,131] and it has thus been renamed *secretory carcinoma*. Most patients are younger than 30 years of age.[132]

What are the clinical features of secretory carcinoma?

These tumors portend a good prognosis in children, but they are slightly more aggressive in adults.[133] Specifically, recurrences in children are rare. However, the incidence of axillary lymph node metastases (15% to 27%) is similar in both age groups.[134,135] Recurrences can occur as late as 20 years, thus warranting long-term follow-up.[136] Although most patients are treated by mastectomy, local excision should be attempted in adolescents to maximize preservation of the breast bud.

The role of radiotherapy and chemotherapy is currently unknown.

What are the pathologic features of secretory carcinoma?

Grossly, these carcinomas are usually circumscribed and lobulated owing to the presence of fibrous septa within the tumor. Morphologically it is a compact tumor with solid, papillary, tubular, and microcystic areas (Fig. 10–20). Cytologically, the cells contain small, round, low-grade–appearing nuclei with inconspicuous nucleoli. Secretions can be extracellular or intracellular; the latter can be abundant and variable from small to large, fusing to impart a microcystic appearance (Fig. 10–21). Some of the cells may contain vacuolated, granular, or eosinophilic cytoplasm, making the distinction from apocrine carcinoma difficult. Few to rare mitoses may be present. Low-grade intraductal car-

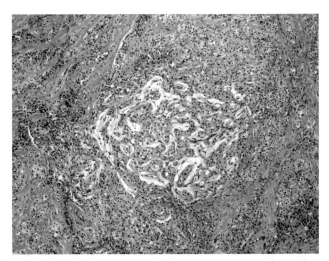

Figure 10–20   Low-power histologic appearance of secretory carcinoma showing peripheral solid and central cystic and papillary areas.

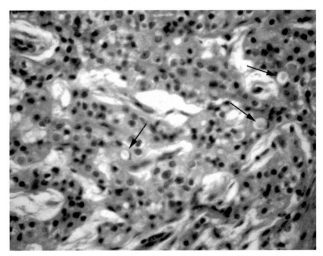

Figure 10–21   High-power histologic appearance of secretory carcinoma showing cells with low-grade cytology associated with intraluminal (*arrows*) and extraluminal eosinophilic secretions.

cinoma may also be present. Histochemically, the secretory material stains with mucin and PAS, consistent with its mucopolysaccharide nature. Immunohistochemically, reaction with α-lactalbumin, S-100, and carcinoembryonic antigen (CEA) is present. Ultrastructurally, the secretions correspond to membrane-bound vacuoles. Most of the carcinomas are nonreactive with estrogen and progesterone hormone receptors.

NEUROENDOCRINE CARCINOMA

These neoplasms encompass a heterogeneous group of neoplasms defined by the presence of one or more of the following: most important, an endocrine growth pattern; argyrophilic granules (positive Grimelius silver stain); expression of neuroendocrine markers (>50%); or ultrastructural finding of neurosecretory granules. They make up 1% to 5% of breast carcinomas. Although many carcinomas (mucinous carcinoma, infiltrating lobular carcinoma) may exhibit some of these features, to qualify as a neuroendocrine carcinoma, these features must be predominant. The cell of origin is hypothesized to be neuroendocrine, located between the basal myoepithelial and luminal epithelial cell.[137–140]

What are the clinical features of neuroendocrine carcinoma?

Neuroendocrine carcinomas tend to occur in elderly women in the sixth to seventh decade of life.[138] Rarely, they may present with systemic ectopic endocrine hormone-related syndromes such as adrenocorticotropic hormone (ACTH), parathyroid hormone (PTH), calcitonin, and epinephrine. Prognostic data on these carcinomas are limited owing to the lack of case-controlled studies.

What are the pathologic features of neuroendocrine carcinoma?

Histologic features typical of endocrine neoplasms as seen in other organs must be present and include cells with uniform, low-nuclear-grade cytology arranged in solid nests, trabeculae, rosettes, and alveolar arrangements (Figs. 10–22 and 10–23). A morphologic spectrum akin to neuroendocrine neoplasms in other organs, ranging from carcinoid tumors to small and large cell carcinomas, may be present. Although small and large cell carcinomas represent poorly differentiated carcinomas, most (85%) endocrine neoplasms in the breast are well to moderately differentiated.

Immunohistochemically, they stain with neuroendocrine markers such as neuron-specific enolase (NSE) (100%), and about half are positive for chromogranin and synaptophysin. Most of these carcinomas express estrogen and progesterone hormone receptors, including half of all small cell carcinomas.[141]

Finally, it is important to be aware that extramammary neuroendocrine metastases can rarely occur in the breast. The presence of intraductal carcinoma and hormone receptor positivity helps confirm the mammary origin of these tumors.

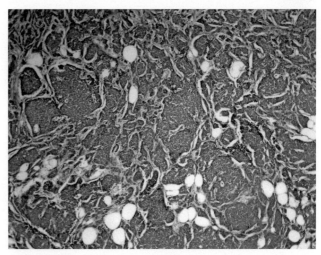

Figure 10–22 Low-power histologic appearance of neuroendocrine carcinoma showing cells arranged in nests, trabeculae, and rosettes.

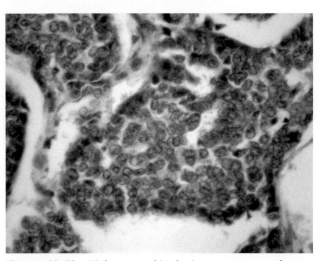

Figure 10–23 High-power histologic appearance of neuroendocrine carcinoma showing uniform cells with low-grade cytology.

ADENOID CYSTIC CARCINOMA

These low-grade tumors predominantly arise in salivary glands and rarely occur in the breast (0.1%).[142]

What are the clinical features of adenoid cystic carcinoma?

Adenoid cystic carcinoma usually forms a palpable discrete firm mass that may present later than conventional IDC (mean, 24 months).[143] About half occur in the subperiareolar region and can be painful, tender, or cystic. By mammography, adenoid cystic carcinoma appears as either a well-defined lobulated mass or an ill-defined lesion.

As in the salivary gland, these tumors are low grade and associated with a good prognosis, mastectomy being curative. Few cases of axillary lymph node metastases are described in

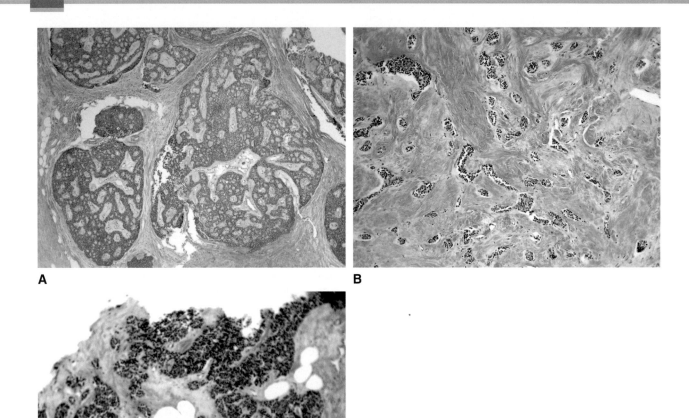

A

B

C

Figure 10–24 Histologic appearance of adenoid cystic carcinoma showing patterns of increasing aggressive potential. *A,* Cribriform. *B,* Tubular. *C,* Solid.

the literature.[144] Distant metastases occur in 10% of cases, usually to the lungs.[145]

What are the pathologic features of adenoid cystic carcinoma?

Despite their circumscribed and nodular gross appearance, histologically, more than half of adenoid cystic ademomas demonstrate an invasive growth pattern. Cystic areas may be present in up to 25% of cases, particularly in larger tumors with cystic degeneration. Morphologically, they are characterized by a variable mixture of proliferating glands and stromal and basement membrane material (type IV collagen), creating much intratumoral heterogeneity. The glandular component may present in a myriad of patterns, including cribriform, tubular, trabecular, solid, basaloid, and scirrhous (Fig. 10–24).

The cribriform pattern is the most characteristic, formed by nests of cells perforated by a sieve or fenestrated pattern. The spaces contain small spherules or cylinders of hyaline material (Fig. 10–25), consistent with basal lamina, which stains immunohistochemically with laminin and collagen IV. The surrounding cells consist of predominantly

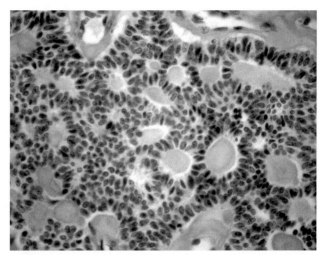

Figure 10–25 High-power histologic appearance of adenoid cystic carcinoma with cribriform pattern with associated basement membrane material.

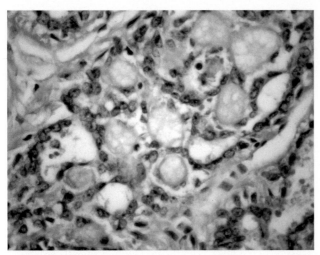

Figure 10–26 Histologic appearance of collagenous spherulosis showing a benign glandular proliferation consisting of spherules of basement membrane material.

myoepithelial cells with basaloid features, followed by cells with more eosinophilic cytoplasm and thirdly by cells with sebaceous elements.

Cribriform carcinoma is differentiated from adenoid cystic carcinoma by the uniformity of its cells and absence of stromal component (see Fig. 10–4). Furthermore, whereas adenoid cystic carcinomas are hormone receptor negative, cribriform carcinomas are positive. Nevertheless, the distinction of cribriform carcinoma from adenoid cystic carcinoma may be challenging on limited core biopsy material. Another entity in the differential diagnosis is collagenous spherulosis (Fig. 10–26), a benign proliferation composed of ductal and myoepithelial cells associated with spherules of basement membrane material.

A grading system using morphologic features such as cytology, mitoses, and architecture is proposed.[146] Architecturally, adenoid cystic carcinoma is divided into a three-tiered system—cribriform, tubular, and solid, in order of increasing aggressive potential. These features are directly associated with large tumor size and increased rate of recurrence. In a minority of cases, an associated in situ carcinoma may be present. In fact, intraductal carcinoma is an important contributing factor for recurrence. Although perineural invasion and resultant pain is a common finding in salivary gland type tumors, it is rare in the breast. It has been suggested that adenoid cystic carcinoma probably develops in a background of and is continuous with microglandular adenosis, a benign proliferative lesion. Atypical microglandular adenosis, a more complex proliferative lesion both cytologically and architecturally, is found to have areas of transition with adenoid cystic carcinoma and is interpreted as adenoid cystic carcinoma in situ by some.[147]

INFLAMMATORY CARCINOMA

Inflammatory carcinoma is not a true variant of IDC, but rather a specific mode of local spread of breast carcinoma. Clinically, it is defined by the distinct appearance of erythema of the skin of the breast. Morphologically, lymphatic

obstruction from an underlying IDC is almost always present. It is a misnomer because it lacks any inflammatory condition clinically or morphologically. It is an advanced form of breast cancer classified as T4d. The frequency of inflammatory carcinoma ranges from 1% to 10% of all IDCs, depending on the diagnostic criteria used and the nature of the institution (community versus tertiary medical center),[148–150] and inflammatory carcinoma occurs more commonly in younger women. A strikingly high incidence of 28% has been reported from Tunisia.[151]

What are the clinical features of inflammatory carcinoma?

On physical examination, the cardinal signs of inflammation characterized by color, tumor, rubor, and dolor are present. The mammary skin is thickened 2 to 8 mm (mean, 4 mm),[152] manifesting with a palpable ridge at the edge of the involved skin, and also has peau d'orange changes. Depending on the stage of the tumor, the breast may contain a central palpable tumor or may be diffusely indurated. The size of the tumor can be large, ranging from 2 to 12 cm (mean, 6 cm).[153] Most patients present with lymphadenopathy, affecting axillary lymph nodes more commonly than supraclavicular. Mammography confirms clinical findings of skin thickening, an underlying mass, stromal coarsening, and increased parenchymal density. Although magnetic resonance imaging (MRI) cannot distinguish between mastitis and inflammatory carcinoma, it shows more than 100% enhancement in the first minute after contrast administration.

Secondary inflammatory carcinoma occurs as a result of metastases in the skin of patients who initially present with axillary lymph node metastases and is clinically similar to primary inflammatory carcinoma. These patients can also present with palpable tumor infiltrates in the chest wall, at the site of prior mastectomy, within or outside of the radiated field. They are more likely to be IDC, particularly of the apocrine type.

The presence of morphologic changes in the absence of clinical findings of inflammatory carcinoma is known as occult inflammatory carcinoma. These patients have a large central or multicentric tumor and are prone to inflammatory recurrences. Although they have a less acute clinical course, survival is similar to that of conventional inflammatory carcinoma. Thus, irrespective of the clinical findings of inflammatory carcinoma, dermal lymphatic involvement portends a poor prognosis,

Before the advent of combined-modality intensive chemotherapy, the prognosis of inflammatory carcinoma was dismal. Although earlier studies indicated that patients with clinical but no morphologic evidence of inflammatory carcinoma did better than those with histologically proven inflammatory carcinoma,[148] additional later studies refuted these findings.[154–156] Today, systemic chemotherapy, particularly preoperative anthracycline-based neoadjuvant chemotherapy followed by radiotherapy, provides better local control and an improved disease-free survival (5-year survival rate of 40% to 50%).[156–158] Radiation and chemotherapy decrease or eliminate the skin erythema, edema, and tumor size. Clinical features associated with a poor prognosis include diffuse erythema, chest wall adhesions, and axillary lymph node metastases.

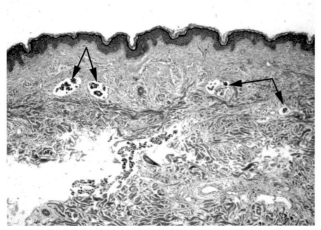

Figure 10–27 Histologic appearance of inflammatory carcinoma showing dermal lymphatics (*arrows*) containing tumor emboli.

What are the pathologic features of inflammatory carcinoma?

There are no specific histologic features of inflammatory carcinoma, and up to half of all skin biopsy samples may be negative.[159,160] In fact, when the characteristic skin findings are clinically present, a skin biopsy may not be required for diagnosis. Histologic changes in skin may be variable and may not necessarily correlate with the clinical findings. The typical histologic finding includes tumor emboli in dermal lymphatics (Fig. 10–27). Other histologic changes in skin include a broad reticular dermal layer due to edema and collagen deposition, and dilated lymphocytes surrounded by a lymphoplasmacytic cell population. A widespread, poorly differentiated IDC with extensive carcinomatosis of lymphatics in the breast and skin is usually present. In secondary inflammatory carcinoma, in addition to tumor emboli in dermal lymphatics, dermal plaques and nodules of IDC are also present. Estrogen hormone receptor positivity ranges from 31% to 47%, whereas progesterone positivity ranges from 30% to 34%.[161–163] *HER-2/neu* amplification has been observed in some tumors.[164]

PHYLLODES TUMOR

First characterized in 1838,[165] this group of fibroepithelial tumors was named *cystosarcoma phyllodes* because of its leaflike and fleshy gross appearance. Although most phyllodes tumors (PTs) are benign, the biologic behavior, that is, the potential for recurrence and metastasis, cannot be reliably predicted. Thus, today, we more appropriately call them phyllodes tumors and histologically subclassify them as benign, low-grade (borderline), or malignant. PTs make up 0.3% to 1% of all breast tumors.

What are the clinical features of phyllodes tumor?

Patients present with a discrete, painless, palpable mass that is firm to hard, ranging in size from 1 to more than 20 cm

(range, 4 to 5 cm).[166–169] Infrequently, PT may present as diffuse enlargement of the breast. The nipple may become flattened from the underlying PT, but skin changes are rare. PTs occur in women over a wide age range (10 to 86 years), with a mean and median of 45 years (at least 15 years later than the mean age for fibroadenomas), and are rare in adolescents.[166–169] An unusual presentation with bloody nipple discharge due to spontaneous infarction has been described in a few adolescents.[170,171] The age-adjusted incidence of PT is 2.1 per 1 million women per year.[172] A threefold to fourfold higher incidence has been observed in foreign-born Latino women from Mexico or the Americas compared with those born in the United States.[173] A younger age of onset (average, 25 to 30 years) has been described in Asian and Latino patients.[174]

There are no specific clinical or radiologic features that can reliably differentiate among the three histologic grades of PT. By mammography, PTs are rounded, lobulated, sharply defined opaque masses, occasionally with indistinct borders. On sonography, a circumscribed heterogeneous mass is present resulting from the presence of cysts and epithelial-lined clefts. Even though size is not a reliable indicator of clinical behavior, a diagnosis of PT is favored if the tumor is larger than 4 cm. History of rapid growth suggests malignant transformation of a benign PT or origin from a previous fibroadenoma. The latter has further been supported by clonal analysis of three fibroadenomas that recurred as PT.[175] Furthermore, in up to 40% of cases, coexistent fibroadenomas may be present histologically.[176]

Based on histologic features, PTs are classified into benign, low-grade/borderline, and high-grade/malignant (described later) tumors. Although these features correlate with the frequency of recurrence, metastases, and mortality, the biologic behavior of PT cannot be reliably predicted, and there is much interseries variability. Benign PT almost never metastasizes and has a low probability (8% to 20%) of local recurrence.[176–178] Low-grade PT has a low probability (<5%) of metastasis and a slightly higher risk (25%) for recurrence. High-grade PT metastasizes in about 22% to 25% of cases and has the highest risk for recurrence (27% to 71%). Time to recurrence was shortest in malignant PT, recurrence almost always happening within a year of diagnosis. In contrast, less than half of all benign PTs recurred within a year, the remainder from 3 to 17 years. Slightly more than half of low-grade malignant PTs recurred within a year, most within 10 years. Morphologically, the recurrences are usually of higher grade (75%),[175] may invade the chest wall, and are fibroepithelial or stromal; the amount of stroma increases with each recurrence.

In addition to histologic classification, factors predictive of recurrence include, most importantly, incomplete excision, invasive tumor border, and secondary peripheral tumor nodules. Higher recurrence rates were reported for low-grade/borderline PT (29% to 46%) and malignant PT (36% to 65%) when treated by lumpectomy,[179] the lower rates reflecting wider local excisions. Although smaller tumors may be treated by lumpectomy and still be cosmetically acceptable, mastectomy is indicated for larger tumors. Axillary dissection is not necessary because of infrequent involvement (10% to 15%).[178]

Although metastases are more common in malignant PT, it may not always be preceded by recurrence. However, in benign and low-grade PT, metastases are rare and are usually preceded by recurrence. They usually spread hematogenously to the lungs, bone, and heart and infrequently to the axillary lymph nodes. If the cancer is unresponsive to chemotherapy and radiotherapy, death from metastatic disease usually occurs in malignant PT (primary or recurrent) within 5 years of diagnosis.[176,180] Whereas the 5-year overall survival rate for all PT is about 90%,[176] for malignant PT it decreases to 65%.[169,181] By histologic grade, death from disease is estimated as follows: benign, 0.3%; low-grade/borderline, 6.6%; and malignant, 20%.

What are the pathologic features of phyllodes tumor?

Grossly, PTs are well-circumscribed, unencapsulated, firm, bulging, singular to multinodular masses, which are amenable to being shelled out surgically. Foci of degeneration, necrosis, and infarction may be present, suggestive of malignancy. An arborizing pattern can be grossly appreciated (Fig. 10–28), owing to the histologic presence of elongated epithelial clefts consisting of ductal and myoepithelial cells (Fig. 10–29). These cells may show hyperplasia or metaplasia (apocrine or squamous).

As members of the family of fibroepithelial tumors, PTs are distinguished from fibroadenomas by the expanded and increased cellularity of the stromal component, particularly along the periductal stroma, the favored site of origin of PT (Fig. 10–30). The distinction of fibroadenoma with cellular stroma from a benign PT is not always straightforward, particularly on limited core needle biopsies. Furthermore, the stroma in PT can be heterogeneous, with hypocellular, hyalinized (Fig. 10–31), and myxoid areas, as in fibroadenomas. These areas may be adjacent to more cellular areas typical of PT, creating diagnostic difficulties on core biopsies.

At a microscopic level, PTs are classified as benign, low-grade malignant/borderline and high-grade/malignant tumors based on the following histologic features: stromal cellularity, cytologic atypia, tumor borders, mitotic rate, and necrosis. Benign PTs (Fig. 10–32) are characterized by a uniform mild to moderate stromal cellular overgrowth, slight to moderate cytologic pleomorphism, well-defined tumor

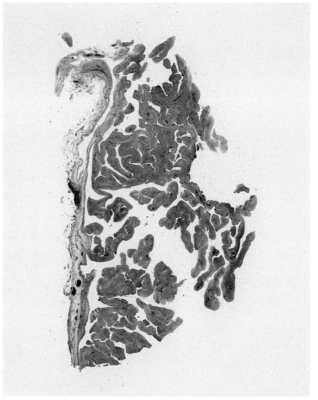

Figure 10–29 Whole-mount section of phyllodes tumor showing arborizing microscopic appearance owing to elongated epithelial clefts.

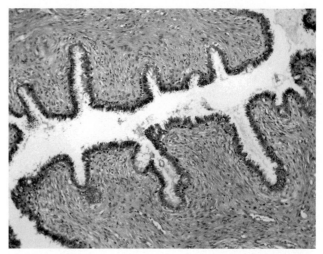

Figure 10–30 Histologic appearance of a phyllodes tumor showing cellular periductal stroma, the favored site of origin of a phyllodes tumor.

borders, and few mitoses (1 or 2 per 10 high-power fields [hpf]). Benign lipomatous (Fig. 10–33), chondroid, and osseous metaplasia may occur in the stroma. Borderline PTs have more aggressive histologic features that include greater stromal cellularity and atypia, microscopically invasive border, and moderate mitotic activity (2 to 5 per 10 hpf) (Fig. 10–34). Metaplastic areas are infrequently present. At the other end of the spectrum, malignant PT is characterized by

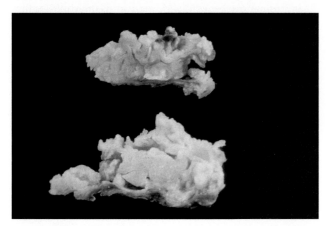

Figure 10–28 Gross appearance of phyllodes tumor showing a fleshy tumor with leaflike growth pattern.

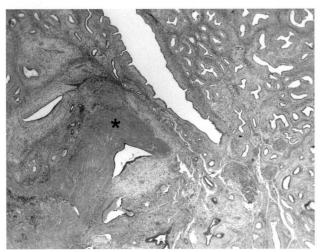

Figure 10–31   A phyllodes tumor with a hyalinized area (*asterisk*), raising questions regarding histogenesis of phyllodes tumor from fibroadenoma.

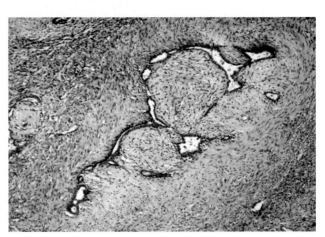

Figure 10–34   Histologic appearance of a borderline phyllodes tumor showing more stromal cellularity, cellular atypia, and mitoses than a benign phyllodes tumor.

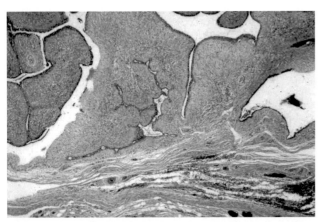

Figure 10–32   Histologic appearance of a benign phyllodes tumor showing low stromal cellularity and minimal cellular atypia.

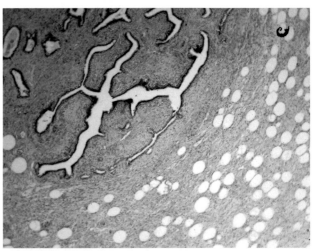

Figure 10–35   Histologic appearance of a malignant phyllodes tumor showing infiltration into adipose tissue.

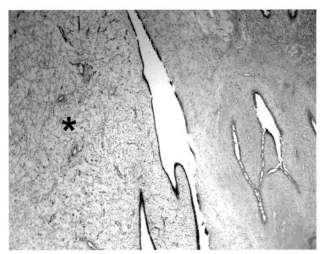

Figure 10–33   Histologic appearance of a benign phyllodes tumor showing a section of phyllodes tumor adjacent to an area of lipomatous metaplasia (*asterisk*).

extensively invasive tumor border (Fig. 10–35) and hypercellular stromal overgrowth, with marked pleomorphism, high mitotic rate (>5 per 10 hpf) (Fig. 10–36), and necrosis. An important diagnostic criterion of malignancy is stromal overgrowth (Fig. 10–37), defined as stromal proliferation to the extent that the epithelial elements are not identifiable in at least one low-power field and may be seen only after extensive sampling.[182,183] In rare cases, the stroma may exhibit heterologous stromal elements, such as angiosarcoma, liposarcoma (Fig. 10–38A), rhabdomyosarcoma, chondrosarcoma, and osteosarcoma (see Fig. 10–38B); the latter two more prone to systemic metastases.[184,185] Proliferative immunohistochemical markers, such as Ki-67 and MIB-1, show a concordance with the classification of PT, such that such markers are lowest in benign PTs and highest in the malignant tumors. Progesterone receptor positivity has been described in the stromal component both biochemically and immunohistochemically.[186]

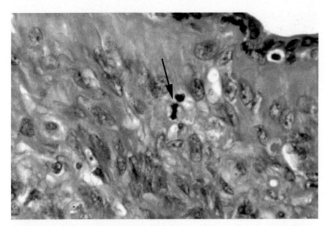

Figure 10–36   Histologic appearance of a malignant phyllodes tumor showing highly pleomorphic cells associated with frequent mitoses (*arrow*).

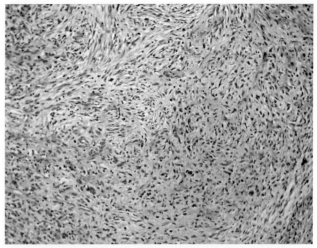

Figure 10–37   Histologic appearance of a malignant phyllodes tumor showing stromal overgrowth such that no epithelial elements are identified in one low-power field.

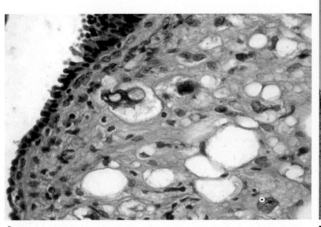

A

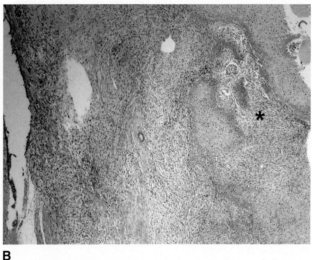

B

Figure 10–38   Histologic appearance of a malignant phyllodes tumor showing malignant heterologous elements. *A*, Liposarcoma showing lipoblasts. *B*, Osteosarcoma (*asterisk*).

SARCOMAS

This heterogeneous group of malignant mesenchymal neoplasms is thought to arise from the interlobular mesenchymal elements that constitute the supporting mammary stroma. Given the rarity of mammary sarcomas, the diagnosis should be made only after excluding metaplastic carcinoma and PT, both of which can have sarcomatoid elements, as discussed previously. Thus, sarcomas should be extensively sampled to detect in situ and invasive carcinoma or PT.

Histogenetically, sarcomas in the breast are identical to those from other body sites and include angiosarcoma, leiomyosarcoma, liposarcoma, osteosarcoma, chondrosarcoma, malignant fibrous histiocytoma, rhabdomyosarcoma, and fibrosarcoma, among others. Given that angiosarcoma is the only sarcoma that has a predilection for the breast, we will discuss only this sarcoma.

What are the clinical features of sarcomas?

Patients usually present with a rapidly enlarging mass. Grading is prognostically important, with 5- and 10-year survival rates as follows: low-grade, 75% and 63%, respectively; intermediate-grade, 55% and 40%, respectively; and high-grade, 29% and 19%, respectively.[187] Whereas low-grade lesions may be treated by local excision, higher grade sarcomas should be treated by mastectomy. As with PTs, axillary dissection is not indicated because sarcomas are blood borne. Death results from metastatic disease, especially to the lungs. The role of radiation and chemotherapy is still investigative.

Postradiation sarcomas can occur in soft tissue or bone after mastectomy and radiation to the chest wall and axilla and include almost always angiosarcoma (discussed later), fibrosarcoma, malignant fibrous histiocytoma, and osteosarcoma.

What are the pathologic features of sarcomas?

Grossly, sarcomas can range in size from 1 to 30 cm (mean, 3 to 4 cm). They are typically fleshy with areas of hemorrhage and necrosis. Despite their gross circumscription, they are usually microscopically infiltrative. Grading of sarcomas is three tiered (low, intermediate, high) based on the extent of cytologic atypia, necrosis, pushing borders, and mitoses. Immunohistochemically, all sarcomas express vimentin, a nonspecific mesenchymal marker. As mentioned previously, cytokeratin can serve as a useful marker to exclude metaplastic carcinoma. To determine further histogenetic differentiation, more specific connective tissue markers can be used.

ANGIOSARCOMA

Angiosarcomas of the chest wall, mammary skin, and parenchyma are rare (0.05%), described almost exclusively after radiation treatment. Although the incidence of primary angiosarcoma has remained constant, the rate of postradiation angiosarcoma (PRA) has risen. On the other hand, the incidence of Stewart-Treves syndrome, characterized by angiosarcoma in the skin and soft tissues of the arm after radical mastectomy, radiation, and lymphedema, has declined as a result of more frequent lumpectomies versus mastectomies.

All postradiation sarcomas in the breast are almost always angiosarcoma. The risk for developing PRA of the skin or breast after breast conservation and radiation ranges from 0.06% to 1.35% from 3 to 12 years (mean, 6 years) and is inversely related to age.[188–192] No relationship has been found between PRA and radiation dose, tumor site, and lymphedema. Morphologically heterogeneous, the grading of these neoplasms is prognostically important.

What are the clinical features of angiosarcoma?

Patients with primary angiosarcoma range in age from 17 to 70 years (mean, 38 years). PRA usually occurs in older women (range, 61 to 78 years) and more frequently affects the skin rather than the breast. Mammary angiosarcomas usually also involve the skin, are multifocal, and are high grade. In PRA, age is inversely linked to tumor grade, with median ages as follows: low grade, 43 years; intermediate grade, 34 years; and high grade, 29 years. Pregnancy-associated PRA is usually high grade and portends a poor prognosis.

Skin changes may be subtle, with areas of blue or purple discoloration. Hemorrhagic discoloration in adjacent breast is indicative of tumor spread away from the primary lesion. Patients with high-grade lesions may present with multiple subcutaneous and dermal tumor nodules. Tumors may be avascular and present as skin thickening or induration. Patients with mammary lesions usually present with a painless mass and rarely with diffuse breast enlargement. By mammography, these neoplasms are noted to be ill-defined lobulated tumors, whereas sonography demonstrates high and low echogenicity, and MRI shows markedly enhancing lesions.

Initially angiosarcoma was regarded as a fatal disease; occasional cases with prolonged survival (up to 18 years) are described today.[193] Stratified by grade, the disease-free and recurrence-free survival rates at 5 years are as follows, respectively: low-grade, 91% and 76%; intermediate-grade, 68% and 70%; and high-grade, 14% and 15%.[192] All patients with high-grade tumors died of recurrent disease within 5 years.[193] Duration of disease-free survival was also directly related to grade as follows: low-grade, 15 years or longer; intermediate-grade, 12 years or longer; and high-grade, 15 months or longer.[192] Metastases occur soon after primary diagnosis, most frequently to bone, lungs, liver, skin, and the contralateral breast. The latter may prove challenging to distinguish from a new primary. However, bilateral primary angiosarcomas are much rarer than metastases, particularly given the cutaneous tropism of these tumors.

As with PT, the recommended treatment is total mastectomy without axillary dissection. The efficacy of radiation and chemotherapy is presently investigative, even though studies, albeit not statistically significant, indicate that recurrences are consistently less frequent after treatment with radiation and chemotherapy.[192–194]

What are the pathologic features of angiosarcoma?

Grossly, the tumors range in size from 1 to 20 cm (average, 5 cm). Smaller tumors (<2 cm) are rare and usually detected by mammography. The cut surface reveals a friable, firm, spongy, hemorrhagic tumor. Whereas well-differentiated tumors may have a rim of vascular engorgement, poorly differentiated tumors are ill-defined, indurated, fibrous lesions.

Morphologically, angiosarcomas consist of an infiltrative tumor composed of vascular channels. There are two similar proposed systems that divide angiosarcomas into three categories that directly correlate with prognosis: low grade (type I), intermediate grade (type II), and high grade (type III).[193,195] Low-grade tumors contain large open anastomosing vascular channels with red blood cells that diffusely dissect the intralobular stroma, causing lobular atrophy. Atypical endothelial cells with prominent hyperchromatic nuclei line the vessels in a flat, single cell fashion (Fig. 10–39). Occasional papillary formation and few to rare mitoses may be present. The differential diagnosis of low-grade angiosarcoma includes atypical vascular lesions that may also occur after radiation and may be difficult to differentiate.

Low-grade components may be the predominant constituent in an intermediate- or high-grade lesion. In fact, intermediate-grade lesions may contain mostly (75%) low-grade elements, with scattered hypercellular areas, the transition between the two being sharp. Thus, limited material from a core biopsy may cause erroneous grading of a tumor. They are best graded on excision specimens and require extensive sampling to identify the minor but prognostically more important higher grade lesion. Intermediate-grade lesions (Fig. 10–40) are distinguished from low-grade lesions by higher cellularity and more frequent mitoses. They are composed of spindle and polygonal cells forming small papillae that bud into the vascular luminal spaces.

High-grade angiosarcomas (Fig. 10–41) have obviously malignant features consisting of interanastomosing vascular channels admixed with solid and spindle cell areas. The vessels show endothelial tufting and solid papillary formations

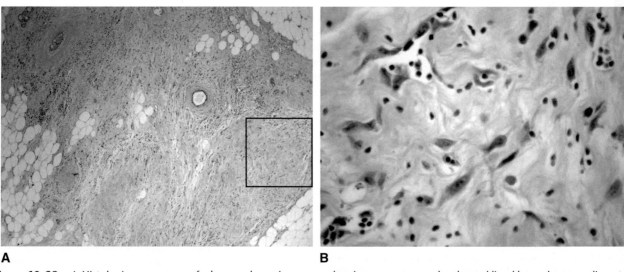

A   **B**

Figure 10–39   *A*, Histologic appearance of a low-grade angiosarcoma showing an open vascular channel lined by and surrounding atypical endothelial cells. *B*, High-power view of marked area in *A*.

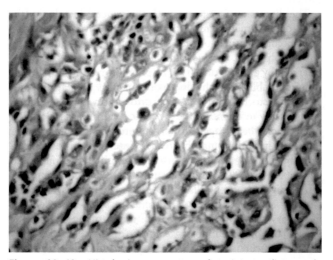

Figure 10–40   Histologic appearance of an intermediate-grade angiosarcoma showing higher cellularity and atypia.

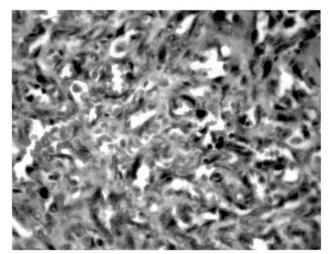

Figure 10–41   Histologic appearance of a high-grade angiosarcoma in skin (*arrow*) showing solid and spindle cell areas and a blood lake (*asterisk*).

composed of malignant endothelial cells (Figs. 10–42 and 10–43), frequent mitoses (>5 per 10 hpf), and necrosis. Grossly and microscopically, areas of hemorrhagic necrosis, also known as "blood lakes" (see Fig. 10–41), are only found in malignant angiosarcomas. In more than half of the high-grade tumors, the solid and spindle cell tumors are predominant without any vascular component, a finding that can be mistaken for a metaplastic spindle cell carcinoma. Immunohistochemically, as mentioned earlier, metaplastic carcinoma stains with cytokeratin but not with endothelial antigens (CD34, factor VIII–related antigen).

MALIGNANT LYMPHOMA

Another rare neoplasm of the breast, malignant lymphoma, occurs either as a primary (<5%) or, more commonly, as a secondary form; the two forms are morphologically indistinguishable. Criteria[196] established to diagnose primary

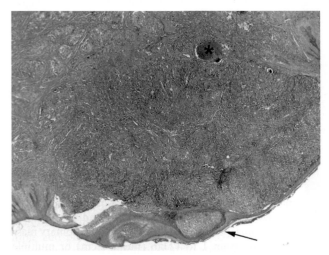

Figure 10–42   High-power histologic appearance of a high-grade angiosarcoma in skin showing malignant spindle cells lining vessels.

15. Sandrucci S, Mussa A. Sentinel lymph node biopsy and axillary staging of T1-T2 N0 breast cancer: Multicenter study. Semin Surg Oncol 1998;15:278–283.
16. Waddington WA, Keshtgar MRS, Taylor I, et al. Radiation safety of the sentinel lymph node technique in breast cancer. Eur J Nucl Med Mol Imaging 2000;27:377–391.
17. Harlow S, Krag DN, Weaver D, et al. Extra-axillary sentinel lymph nodes in breast cancer. Breast Cancer 1999;6:159–165.
18. Veronesi U. The sentinel node and breast cancer. Br J Surg 1999;86:1–2.
19. Johnson N, Soot L, Nelson J, et al. Sentinel node biopsy and internal mammary lymphatic mapping in breast cancer. Am J Surg 2000;179:386–388.
20. Fitzgibbons PL, Page DL, Weaver D, et al. Prognostic factors in breast cancer: College of American Pathologists consensus statement. Arch Pathol Lab Med 2000;124:966–978.
21. Cserni G. Mapping metastases in sentinel lymph nodes of breast cancer. Am J Clin Pathol 2000;113:351–354.
22. Lundell C, Kadir S. Lymph vessels and nodes. In Kadir S (ed). Atlas of Normal and Variant Angiographic Anatomy. Philadelphia, WB Saunders, 1991, pp 495–519.
23. Craeger AJ, Geisinger KR. Intraoperative evaluation of sentinel lymph nodes for breast carcinoma: Current methodologies. Adv Anat Pathol 2002;9:233–243.
24. Turner RR, Ollila DW, Krasne DL, et al. Histopathologic validation of the sentinel lymph nodes hypothesis for breast carcinoma. Ann Surg 1997;226:271–276.
25. Cserni G. Metastases in axillary sentinel lymph nodes in breast cancer as detected by intensive histopathological work up. Clin Pathol 1999;52:922–924.
26. Turner RR, Ollila DW, Stern S, et al. Optimal histopathologic examination of the sentinel lymph node for breast carcinoma staging. Am J Surg Pathol 1999;23:263–267.
27. Noguchi S, Aihara T, Motomura K, et al. Detection of breast cancer micrometastases in axillary lymph nodes by means of reverse transcriptase-polymerase chain reaction: Comparison between MVC1 mRNA and keratin 19 mRNA amplification. Am J Pathol 1996;148:649–656.
28. Yun K, Gunn J, Merine AE, et al. Keratin 19 mRNA is detectable by RT-PCR in lymph nodes of patients without breast cancer. Br J Cancer 1997;76:1112.
29. Bostick PJ, Chatterjee S, Chi DD, et al. Limitations of specific reverse-transcriptase polymerase chain reaction markers in the detection of metastases in the lymph nodes and blood of breast cancer patients. J Clin Oncol 1998;16:2632–2640.
30. Hansen NM, Grube BJ, Te W, et al. Clinical significance of axillary micrometastases in breast cancer: how small is too small? [abstract 91]. Pro Am Soc of Clinical Oncology 2001;20:24a.
31. Greene FL, Page DL, Fleming ID, et al. AJCC Cancer Staging Manual. New York, Springer, 2002.
32. Dowlatshahi K, Fan M, Bloom KJ, et al. Occult metastases in the sentinel lymph nodes of patients with early stage breast carcinoma. A preliminary study. Cancer 1999;86:990–996.
33. Nasser IA, Lee AKI, Bosari S, et al. Occult axillary lymph metastases in node-negative breast carcinoma. Hum Pathol 1993;24:950–957.
34. McGuckin MA, Cummings ML, Walsh MD, et al. Occult axillary node metastases in breast cancer: Their detection and prognostic significance. Br J Cancer 1996;73:88–95.
35. Dowlatshahi K, Fan M, Snider HC, et al. Lymph node micrometastases from breast carcinoma: Reviewing the dilemma. Cancer 1997;80:1188–1197.
36. International (Ludwig) Breast Cancer Study Group. Prognostic importance of occult axillary lymph node micrometastases from breast cancers. Lancet 1990;35:1565–1568.
37. Chen Z-L, Wen D-R, Coulson WF, et al. Occult metastases in the axillary lymph nodes of patients with breast cancer node negative by clinical and histologic examination and conventional histology. Dis Markers 1991;9:239–248.
38. Clare SE, Sener SF, Wilkens W, et al. Prognostic significance of occult lymph node metastases in node-negative breast cancer. Ann Surg Oncol 1997;4:447–451.
39. De Mascarel I, Bonichon F, Coindre JM, et al. Prognostic significance of breast cancer axillary lymph node micrometastases assessed by two spe-

cial techniques: Reevaluation with longer follow-up. Br J Cancer 1992;66:523–527.
40. Hainsworth PJ, Tjandra JJ, Stillwell RG, et al. Detection and significance of occult metastases in node-negative breast cancer. Br F Surg 1993;80:459–463.
41. Friedman S, Bertin F, Mouriesse H, et al. Importance of tumor cells in axillary node sinus margins ("clandestine" metastases) discovered by serial sectioning in operable breast carcinoma. Acta Oncol 1988;27:483–487.
42. Trojan M, de Mascarel I, Bonichon F, et al. Micrometastases to axillary lymph nodes from carcinoma of breast: detection by immunohisto-chemistry and prognostic significance. Br J Cancer 1987;55:303–306.
43. Nasser IA, Lee AKC, Bosari S, et al. Occult axillary lymph node metastases in "node-negative" breast carcinoma. Hum Pathol 1993;24:950–957.
44. Degnim AC, Griffith KA, Sabel MS, et al. Clinicopathologic features of metastasis in nonsentinel lymph nodes in breast carcinoma patients. Cancer 2003;98:2307–2335.
45. Chu KU, Turan RR, Hansen NM, et al. Sentinel node metastasis accurately predicts immunohistochemically detectable nonsentinel node metastasis. Ann Surg Oncol 1999;6:756–761.
46. Weaver DL, Krap ND, Ashikaga T, et al. Pathologic analysis of sentinel and nonsentinel lymph nodes in breast carcinoma: A multicenter study. Cancer 2000;88:1099–1107.
47. Chu KU, Turner RK, Hansen NM, et al. Do all patients with sentinel node metastasis from breast carcinoma need complete axillary dissection? Ann Surg 1999;229:536–541.
48. Reynolds C, Mick R, Donohue JH, et al. Sentinel lymph node biopsy with metastasis: Can axillary dissection be avoided in some patients with breast cancer? J Clin Oncol 1999;17:1720–1726.
49. Turner RR, Chuk U, Oik K, et al. Pathologic features associated with nonsentinel lymph node. Metastases in patients with metastatic breast cancer in a sentinel lymph node. Cancer 2000;89:574–581.
50. Viale G, Maiorano E, Mazzarol G, et al. Histologic detection and clinical implication of micrometastases in axillary sentinel lymph nodes for patients with breast cancer. Cancer 2001;92:1378–1384.
51. Pierce LJ, Oberman HA, Strawderman MH, et al. Microscopic extra-capsular extension in the axilla: Is this an indication for axillary radio-therapy? Int J Radiat Oncol Biol Phys 1995;33:253–259.
52. Leonard C, Corkill M, Tompkin J, et al. Are axillary recurrence and overall survival affected by axillary extranodal tumor extension in breast cancer? Implications for radiation therapy. J Clin Oncol 1995;13:47–53.
53. Fisher BJ, Perera FE, Cooke AL, et al. Extracapsular axillary node extension in patients receiving adjuvant systemic therapy: an indication for radiotherapy? Int J Radiat Oncol Biol Phys 1997;38:551–559.
54. Mignano JE, Zahurak ML, Chakravarthy A, et al. Significance of axillary lymph node extranodal soft tissue extension and indications for post-mastectomy irradiation. Cancer 1999;86:1258–1262.
55. Fisher ER, Gregorio RM, Redmond C, et al. Pathologic findings from the National Surgical Adjuvant Breast Project (Protocol No. 4). III. The significance of extranodal extension of axillary metastases. Am J Clin Pathol 1976;65:439–449.
56. Turner DR, Millis RR. Breast tissue inclusions in axillary lymph nodes. Histopathology 1980;4:631–636.
57. Holdsworth PJ, Hopkinson JM, Leverson SH. Benign axillary epithelial lymph node inclusions: A histological pitfall. Histopathology 1988;13:226–228.
58. Fisher CJ, Hills S, Millis RR. Benign lymph node inclusions mimicking metastatic carcinoma. J Clin Pathol 1994;47:245–247.
59. Ridolfi RL, Rosen PP, Thaler H. Nevus cell aggregates associated with lymph nodes. Estimated frequency and clinical significance. Cancer 1977;39:164–171.
60. McCarthy SW, Palmer AA, Bale PM, et al. Nevus cells in lymph nodes. Pathology 1974;6:351–358.
61. Bautista NC, Cohen S, Anders KH. Benign melanocytic nevus cells in axillary lymph nodes: A prospective incidence and immunohistochem-ical study with literature review. Am J Clin Pathol 1994;1:102–108.
62. Lamovec J. Blue nevus of the lymph node capsule: report of a new case with review of the literature. Am J Clin Pathol 1984;81:367–372.
63. Douglas-Jones AG. Benign lymph node inclusions mimicking metasta-tic carcinoma. J Clin Pathol 1994;47:868–869.

CHAPTER 12

Molecular Pathology Assays for Breast Cancer

W. Fraser Symmans and Giorgio Inghirami

Breast cancer is a biologically, pathologically, and clinically complex disease in which a patient's chance of survival remains uncertain despite intensive efforts to assess prognosis. Markers that are molecular targets for assay are numerous and complex. Different assays, different types of samples, small clinical studies, inconsistent conclusions, and complex associations between markers can prevent independent statistical significance. As a result of the explosion in knowledge concerning the molecular pathology of breast cancer, there is urgency to address clinical issues with these assays. However, before a new assay can be clinically useful, it must be compared with existing assays and markers and proved to be reproducible in different laboratories. There is a major shift in the way molecular pathologic assays are viewed: a shift from prognostic assessment to prediction of therapeutic response. In the past, these assays were used to supplement the prognostic information that was already obtained from tumor stage and grade. Two of those prognostic markers, estrogen receptor (ER) and HER-2/neu, began to be used to select patients for specific treatments when targeted molecular therapies were developed to block the ER and HER-2/neu cellular pathways. We provide a detailed discussion of the molecular pathologic assays to detect ER and HER-2/neu in breast cancer.

There are a growing number of other potential uses for molecular pathologic assays in the selection of treatments and prediction of likely response. A number of novel molecular therapies are either currently or soon to be in clinical trials, and the medical and pharmaceutical communities are actively pursuing the development of new assays to determine which patients are likely to benefit from specific molecular therapies. Furthermore, molecular pathologic assays are being studied for prediction of response to different cytotoxic chemotherapy agents. Increasing choice of effective treatments for breast cancer (itself a heterogeneous disease) enhances the need for laboratory tests that will help oncologists to select the best treatment regimen for each patient.

The biology of cancer cells involves disruptions of normal cell biology,[1,2] and several excellent review articles address these cellular changes and their clinical implications in breast cancer.[3-13] This chapter discusses the molecular pathologic assays that presently have relevance to the biologic and clinical understanding and management of breast cancer. We start with an overview of different clinical reasons for using molecular assays, then discuss performance of the different assays, the critical pathologic steps in breast cancer, specific markers and their relationships to biologic and pathologic systems within breast cancer cells and the host response, and specific issues relating to molecular pathologic assays for breast cancer.

What is most important in evaluating a molecular pathologic assay?

An ideal breast cancer marker would provide prognostic information and therapeutic information, represent a critical step in tumor biology, and be a target for therapeutic intervention. In addition, the assay should be accurate, reliable and reproducible, time and cost efficient, and applicable to routine clinical samples. At this time, although no single marker fulfills all these criteria, certain markers are clinically useful, and others are promising.

What are the reasons for performing molecular assays?

Molecular assays have the potential to be used to identify women who are at increased risk for developing breast cancer or who have an early stage of breast cancer. Furthermore, assays may provide additional information about the prognosis and therapeutic possibilities for a woman with breast cancer, and they may have the potential to detect recurrent or metastatic disease.

Genetic Screening

Abnormalities of tumor suppressor genes (p53, BRCA1, and BRCA2) have been identified in women whose families have a higher frequency of breast cancer.[14,15] These women represent a minority of breast cancer cases in the population, but they are targets for genetic screening. The genetics and epidemiology are fully discussed in Section I of this text.

Early Detection

Molecular pathologic assays do not at this time play a role in the early detection of breast cancer. Strategies to develop an assay of blood to detect breast cancer (analogous to prostate-specific antigen screening for prostate cancer) have not yet

proved
target h
is ubiqu
specific
diagnos
than fo
formed
tissues,
exclude

Cyto
develop
strateg
used to
analyse
suited
tion. R
ferent
occur
analys
investi
molec
of int
those
risk fo
be sep
hybric
whole
(mRN

Th
syster
for w
pretre
than
faster
cann
the t
lavag
Gene
samp
proce
nipp
lar a
Epitl
vary
prot
teins
duct
loca
glob
shec

**Ado
Pri**
Mos
or i
the
The
in I
in t
the
tha

concentrations, incubation periods, buffers and washers) are established. Optimal conditions are essential if clinical decisions or prospective research studies are to rely on the assay.[42] This immunologic technique can also be used to detect cancer cell proteins within the blood. Proteins within cells can also be quantitated using image analysis to measure the concentration of colored chromogen. Alternatively, proteins can be accurately quantitated using biochemical assays—for example, dextran charcoal ligand binding assays for ER and progesterone receptor (PR). Such biochemical assays may have the advantage of greater accuracy. However, biochemical assays often require considerable amounts of tissue, which are not available when small lesions are being studied. Biochemical assays also do not distinguish normal cells from cancer cells; hence, accurate tissue sampling is also essential.

In Situ Hybridization

In situ hybridization uses synthesized DNA probes to recognize specific DNA or RNA sequences within the cell. Probes can be designed to specifically identify sequences that represent molecular markers of breast cancer oncogenes.[43] Increased expression of the RNA sequence generally represents overexpression of the oncogene, and increased presence of the DNA sequence represents amplification of the oncogene. The specific DNA probe is labeled (radioactively or chemically), and the labeled probe can then be seen microscopically.

The main application of in situ hybridization in breast cancer diagnosis is to determine the number of copies of c-erbB-2 gene that codes for HER-2/neu growth factor receptor protein (Fig. 12–4). The most common FISH assay is a commercially available kit that provides fluorescent-labeled probes that detect c-erbB-2 and a centromeric sequence of chromosome 17 (cep17) and are visualized with different light filters. Therefore, the FISH assay for c-erbB-2 is reported as the average number of copies of c-erbB-2 per cancer cell nucleus (≥5 copies defined as amplification) or the ratio of the average numbers of gene copies of c-erbB-2 compared with the

average number of copies of chromosome 17 (>2 defined as amplification). There are subtle implications for each method because the absolute number of copies of c-erbB-2 gene may determine the protein expression level of HER-2/neu in the breast cancer, whereas the ratio of c-erbB-2 to cep17 may correct for aneuploidy of chromosome 17 and select tumors with amplification of c-erbB-2 gene on each copy of chromosome 17.[44] A CISH test is newly available for detection of c-erbB-2 gene using a chromogen that is stable and visible with light microscopy.[45,46] The hybridization signal is slightly less distinct than with fluorescence, and it is not possible to compare c-erbB-2 copy number with a cep17 probe using CISH, but the method does not require a fluorescence microscope for interpretation. Cytologic samples provide FISH signals of excellent quality because the entire nucleus is present on the slide, so that all cep17 and c-erbB-2 signals are represented in every cell.[47]

Polymerase Chain Reaction

Specific hybridization assays can be performed on purified DNA and RNA from digested tumor samples. For direct hybridization, whole (entire) DNA is digested using selected enzymes that cleave DNA at known restriction sites, and the digested DNA is then hybridized to a selected DNA probe (currently synthesized as a specific sequence of bases) to detect the corresponding target sequence of DNA. The development of PCR has been a significant advance because it uses specific primers at each end of a selected DNA sequence to amplify that DNA sequence using a thermodynamic enzyme (taq polymerase). This allows small amounts of the target DNA to be amplified and detected, has diminished the number of tumor cells required to perform DNA studies, and has accelerated the progress of DNA and RNA studies. Cellular mRNA can be reverse transcribed into cDNA and then amplified using PCR (RT-PCR), and the product can be sequenced (automated) or detected by hybridization to a specific cDNA or oligonucleotide probe. Amplification and hybridization techniques are routinely used in the study of clinical research samples.

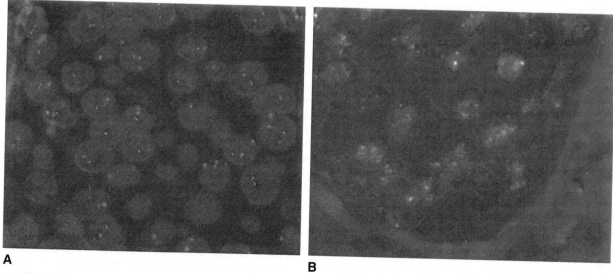

A   B

Figure 12–4 Fluorescence in situ hybridization assay for c-erbB-2 gene copy number relative to chromosome 17 centromere (Cep17) copy number on fine-needle aspiration slides of breast cancer. A, Tumor without amplification. B, Tumor with amplification.

Molecular Cytogenetics

Newer techniques in cytogenetics are increasingly applied to breast cancer. FISH and nonfluorescent chromogenic in situ hybridization (CISH) are assays that are in use as clinical tests for *HER-2/neu.* FISH uses fluorescent-labeled DNA probes to specific regions of individual chromosomes[48] and can detect loss of regions of chromosomes (potential sites of tumor suppressor genes) as well as aneusomy of chromosome numbers and regions of increased copy number (potential sites of oncogenes). A related technique, called *comparative genomic hybridization* (CGH), uses whole-chromosome hybridization in which labeled normal chromosomes are hybridized to labeled metaphase cancer cell chromosomes. The distribution and intensity of the two labels (represented as two different colors) along the fusion chromosomes are measured using computerized image analysis.[49] Regions of the fusion chromosome where the cancer cell DNA is deleted will have the color of the normal chromosome label, whereas regions of fusion chromosome where the cancer cell DNA is amplified will have the color of the cancer cell chromosome label. CGH is currently a research assay.

Technical Considerations

The presence and quantity of any marker must also be assessed in benign and preneoplastic breast conditions as well as other disease states. This is particularly important for assays to detect residual or metastatic cancer. These different assays employ sensitive techniques requiring multiple sequential steps, and the results can therefore vary depending on the status of the marker within the cancer sample (e.g., degradation, clinical fixation, nature of the target marker), the reagents used (e.g., antigen retrieval methods, antibodies, probes, primers, buffers), and the conditions of reaction for each step (e.g., incubation period, concentration, temperature, washes). These variables can limit the clinical interpretation for a sample from a laboratory at a given time. Nevertheless, some markers have been shown to be prognostically relevant in breast cancer. Others may prove to be valuable in the future.

What is the clinical potential for gene expression microarrays in breast cancer?

Gene expression microarrays are high-density arrays of specific cDNA or oligonucleotide sequences that are printed onto a medium such as silicone or glass. Purified RNA from a breast cancer sample is reverse-transcribed to cDNA before colorimetric labeling and hybridization to the array. In the popular Affymetrix GeneChip platform (Affymetrix, Inc., Santa Clara, CA), the cDNA is then transcribed into cRNA before colorimetric labeling of the cRNA and hybridization to the array. The colored hybridization product is then detected and quantified using image analysis, and the numeric data are represented by computer software for viewing of the array with high expression of a gene shown as a red spot at the site of that probe and low expression of a gene shown as a green spot at the site of that probe. The numeric results are used for analysis, and those data are mathematically normalized to known controls. The relative expression levels of tens of thousands of known genes can be simultaneously evaluated from a single sample. This high-throughput technology can even be applied

to a single needle biopsy sample of breast cancer.[50,51] To date, the results from this technology using clinical breast cancer samples have been promising. Unsupervised analysis of the overall gene expression profiles of different breast cancer samples have consistently demonstrated that ER activity is the principal determinant of overall gene expression in 50% to 60% of breast cancers and that the activity of *HER-2/neu* gene expression is an important secondary determinant of overall transcription.[51–53] We already know from decades of clinical and laboratory studies that ER and *HER-2/neu* are critically important molecules in breast cancer, which supports the interpretation that information derived from microarray experiments is probably meaningful. ER and *HER-2/neu* are the most intensively studied molecules in breast cancer, and preliminary results indicate that the relative expression of these two genes from microarray experiments correlates well with the results of well-validated immunohistochemistry (IHC) and FISH assays performed on corresponding tumor sections.[51]

Gene expression data from transcriptional profiling of breast cancers can be used for different purposes, including molecular pathologic classification, selection of specific molecular therapies, prognostic analysis, and prediction of likely benefit from different available treatments.[52–55] There is potential for this technology to address currently unmet medical needs in clinical oncology, such as prediction of response to different cytotoxic chemotherapy regimens and selection of molecular therapies.[56] Transcriptional profiling might even be adopted as an all-in-one testing modality for multiple prognostic and molecular markers and so realize its technologic potential for high-throughput analysis. Most known genes are represented in transcriptional profiles and can potentially be interpreted for clinical purposes. This presents a challenge because specific information gained from transcriptional profiles should first be defined and compared with existing pathologic assays, and then validated in clinical trials.[57] Only then can the information be used with confidence to decide patient care. There is already detailed knowledge about the coding base-pair sequence for many genes and the fidelity of DNA hybridization, and these support genomic microarrays as a testing platform. Available data are limited, but overall transcriptional profiles of human invasive breast cancers appear to be maintained in individual breast cancers during progression and after chemotherapy, indicating that the profile of transcriptional expression is generally quite stable.[52,58] Relative stability of the gene expression profile in breast cancers also supports transcriptional profiling as an attractive platform for the development of molecular pathologic tests for routine diagnostics and patient care decisions.

What are the general biologic concepts in breast cancer progression?

Important biologic steps include the development of breast cancer cells from the epithelial lining of the ductal lobular system (neoplasia), independently accelerated cell growth and proliferation, then the invasion of these neoplastic cells through their surrounding basement membrane. Once invasive, the tumor cells can invade lymphatic and blood vessels and thereby spread to other sites in the body (metastasis)

(Fig. 12–5A). Metastatic cells can form clusters in association with blood components and are therefore able to withstand the physical stresses of the bloodstream (see Fig. 12–5B). These cells must adhere to the endothelial cells at the metastatic site, pass between these cells, and invade through the basement membrane of the blood vessels. Once at the metastatic site, they repeat the biologic steps of adhesion, invasion, and angiogenesis in order to produce a viable colony of metastatic carcinoma cells. It is unlikely that a single cancer cell has all the biologic abilities required to invade, spread, metastasize and continue to grow. Therefore, it is probably communities of tumor cells that collectively produce all the steps required for cancer dissemination.

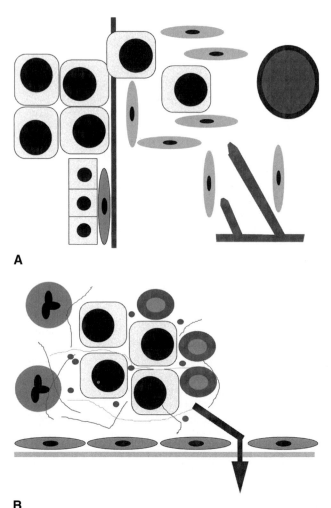

A

B

Figure 12–5   *A,* Neoplastic transformation and invasion: normal breast epithelial cells fixed to a myoepithelial cell layer and basement membrane (*lower left*) develop in situ neoplastic transformation (*upper left*) and then become invasive through the basement membrane and interstitium with associated desmoplastic stroma (*center*) and angiogenesis (*lower right*). Once invasive, the cancer cells are capable of dissemination by vascular routes (*upper right*). *B,* To survive circulatory forces, cancer cells form microemboli binding to red and white blood cells, platelets, and fibrin. The attached white blood cells also augment intercellular adhesion to the vascular endothelium. Once adherent, the cancer cells must invade through the vascular basement membrane and interstitium before establishing a new tumor growth.

Which types of markers are important in breast cancer cells?

Markers in breast cancer cells can be grouped into different cellular systems (see Fig. 12–1), which will be discussed in greater detail next. These include the following:

1. *Cell growth and proliferation,* including growth factors, growth factor receptors, signal transduction proteins, DNA transcription proteins, control of the cell cycle, indicators of cell proliferation, and nuclear hormone receptors
2. *Cell death,* such as through apoptosis and necrosis
3. *Invasive and metastatic potential,* including cell adhesion molecules, stromal digestive enzymes, and the metastasis suppressor gene
4. *Other markers of chromosome and DNA content within cancer cells* (ploidy and cytogenetics), which can be used to study breast cancer cell populations

How are growth signals transmitted to the nucleus in breast cancer cells?

Cell Surface Receptors

There are many signaling pathways within cancer cells, but in breast cancer, the two most important growth factor receptors presently identified are *HER-2/neu* (*c-erbB-2*) and epidermal growth factor receptor (EGFR). Both receptors are of the membrane-bound tyrosine kinase receptor family and act by similar mechanisms (Fig. 12–6). Briefly, two adjacent receptors dimerize when the growth factor (ligand) binds. The ligand for *HER-2/neu* has been a subject of intensive recent research (see Chapter 3). Binding of the ligand to the extracellular domain of the paired receptors stimulates the tyrosine residues within the cytoplasmic component of the receptor molecules, which in turn activates a phosphorylation cascade involving the SH2 (src homology 2) proteins, transferring the growth signal onto the *ras* signal transduction pathway.

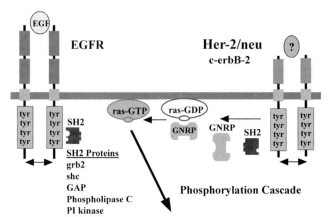

Figure 12–6   Comparison of *HER-2/neu* and epidermal growth factor receptor (EGFR; membrane-bound tyrosine [tyr] kinase receptor dimers), and demonstration of the ensuing phosphorylation cascade involving SH2 molecules and the ras pathway to relay the growth signal toward the nucleus. GAP, GTPase-activating protein; GNRP, guanine-nucleotide-releasing protein; GTP, guanosine triphosphate; PI kinase, phosphotidylinositol 3-kinase; SH2, src homology 2.

HER-2/neu

The oncogenic abnormality of *HER-2/neu* in breast cancer is principally amplification of the gene and overexpression of the protein. The role of the ligand of *HER-2/neu* is not certain at this time. The effect of *HER-2/neu* overexpression is to enhance growth signals within the breast cancer cell. The *HER-2/neu* gene is located on chromosome 17 (17q21), and DNA probes, as well as monoclonal antibodies, for the protein are available for use with clinical specimens.[59] *HER-2/neu* protein is overexpressed in about 20% to 30% of invasive breast carcinomas[60-62] (Fig. 12–7). Of interest, *HER-2/neu* is overexpressed in 10% to 20% of cases of noncomedo ductal carcinoma in situ (DCIS) but is overexpressed in most (60% to 80%) cases of higher-grade comedo DCIS.[62-64] Some studies have shown a prognostic predictive value for *HER-2/neu*—more strongly in node-positive cancers and less clearly in node-negative cancers.[61,65-67] There are also data to suggest that *HER-2/neu* overexpression may predict response to adjuvant chemotherapy (discussed later).

Assays for *HER-2/neu* have become standard in clinical samples of invasive breast cancer to select patients who are eligible to receive trastuzumab (Herceptin) therapy. The importance of critical interpretation has been highlighted with IHC for *HER-2/neu*. IHC staining with antibodies to *HER-2/neu* is commonly seen in the cytoplasm of tumor and normal cells, but only circumferential cell membrane localization should be interpreted as true positive staining. Membrane staining is then assessed using a semiquantitative score (1+ to 3+) depending on intensity, and 2+ and 3+ staining is considered to be positive. The preanalytic fixation and antigen retrieval methods for *HER-2/neu* IHC are less problematic than for ER IHC (discussed later), but there is consistent discrepancy in the interpretation between central review and community pathologists that mostly affects scoring of 1+ and 2+ staining.[68] Normal breast epithelial cells do not express enough *HER-2/neu* on the cell membrane for IHC detection; therefore, interpretation of tumor staining should always be compared with normal breast epithelium as a negative control.

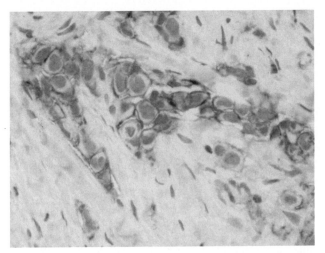

Figure 12–7 Immunohistochemical stain showing a circumferential membranous staining pattern for *HER-2/neu* that is of moderate intensity (2+) and restricted to the invasive breast cancer cells in a paraffin tissue section (×400). There was no amplification of the *HER-2/neu* gene copy number with the fluorescence in situ hybridization assay (*c-erbB-2*: cep17 = 1.29).

The IHC scoring system is semiquantitative and inevitably subjective; thus, there is known variability in the interpretation of negative versus 1+ staining, and for 1+ versus 2+ staining.[69-72] Generally, 3+ staining is accepted as true overexpression for clinical purposes, and more than 90% have gene amplification. Although 2+ staining is defined as positive and 1+ staining is defined as negative by IHC, many laboratories perform FISH assay to assess *c-erbB-2* gene copy number in those cases because only 10% to 15% of 2+ tumors have gene amplification and less than 5% of 1+ tumors have gene amplification.[72-74] If normal epithelial staining is present, some authors suggest subtracting the intensity score of the normal cells from the intensity score of the carcinoma cells to prevent false-positive results.[75]

Epidermal Growth Factor Receptor

Epidermal growth factor receptor has been shown by immunocytochemistry to be overexpressed in about 35% of invasive breast carcinomas and has equivocal prognostic significance.[76-78] There is an inverse correlation with estrogen receptor expression.[76] To date, treatment with targeted therapies to inhibit EGFR signaling has had limited success in breast cancer, and IHC expression of EGFR does not accurately predict therapeutic response.[79] However, a recent study in lung cancer demonstrated that tumors responsive to gefitinib (Iressa) treatment have deletion or mutation of the DNA sequence for the tyrosine kinase domain of EGFR.[80] If that proves to be the case in breast cancer, a better approach might be performing an assay to identify that genetic change rather than performing IHC for EGFR. Both epidermal growth factor (EGF) and transforming growth factor-α (TGF-α) stimulate EGFR.[81] Other growth factor receptor molecules that can be amplified in breast cancer cells (but in fewer tumors) include insulin-like growth factor receptor,[82] *int-2* oncogene product,[83,84] *pS2*, and TGF-β receptor (which has an inhibitory effect on breast cancer cell growth).[85,86]

Signal Transduction

Signal transduction proteins represent important biologic pathways of growth and survival signals in breast cancer cells. The main growth factor receptors in breast cancer (*HER-2/neu*, EGFR, and insulin-like growth factor receptor [IGFR]) signal through transduction networks from the cell membrane to the nucleus. The ras protein (p21) is an important membrane-bound signal transduction protein that recruits receptors and signaling molecules to coordinate a phosphorylation signal cascade (see Fig. 12–6). It is a guanosine triphosphate (GTP)-binding protein that is active when bound to GTP and inactive when bound to guanosine diphosphate (GDP). The ras protein contains a GTPase enzyme component that cleaves a phosphate group from the bound GTP and deactivates the ras protein. Mutations of the *ras* gene are one of the more important and common oncogene abnormalities in human cancer. These are usually point mutations that disrupt the GTPase enzymatic function of the *ras*, so that the protein cannot deactivate itself and is permanently turned on. Mutations of *ras* are uncommon in breast cancer,[87] but little is known about expression of nonmutated *ras* in this disease. This is partly because of a lack of specific antibodies to the different members of the ras protein family. Preliminary immunocytochemistry studies have indicated that ras protein (p21) is overexpressed in a significant proportion (20% to

60%) of invasive human breast cancers.[88–91] Signal transduction from *ras* is mediated through raf and then bifurcates along a mitogen-activated protein (MAP) kinase pathway to stimulate growth and proliferation or along a PI3 kinase/AKT (protein kinase B) pathway to promote cell survival.[92–94] *PTEN* (at 10q23) is a tumor suppressor gene that encodes a proapoptotic inhibitor of the PI3K/AKT pathway, and loss of *PTEN* function occurs from loss of heterozygosity (>40%), mutation (2% to 20%), or methylation in sporadic breast cancer, or from germline mutation in breast cancer that is associated with Cowden's syndrome.[94] It is passed on by the ras protein through a cascade of other enzyme transduction proteins (raf, MAP kinase-kinase, MAP kinase). MAP kinase is a common end point for other signal transduction pathways within cells.

Transcription Factors

MAP kinase phosphorylates nuclear proteins, including important DNA-binding proteins that control DNA transcription and cell proliferation. Two important examples of these proteins are fos and jun, which are the DNA-binding transcription factors involved in the proliferative response to growth factors and estrogen. These two proteins bind another transcription factor (AP-1), leading to direct DNA binding. Another important transcription factor in breast cancer is *myc* oncogene product, which has direct DNA binding in association with another protein called max. This myc-max pair binds to DNA in the regions known as E boxes, thereby activating promoters for genes (leading to transcription and replication of DNA). The control of myc activation is believed to be related to a third protein called mad, which replaces myc, binds to max at the E-box domains within DNA, and becomes inhibitory for promoters for the genes which had been activated by myc. Antibodies are available to detect these activating transcription factors (fos, jun, myc), and detection of these proteins is increased in a small proportion (<20%) of invasive human breast cancers.[90] Although these proteins provide an essential function in cells, increased levels have not been shown to be of independent prognostic significance in women with breast cancer.

Breast cancer cell proliferation— which assays are informative?

In clinical samples of breast cancer, the DNA histogram obtained by flow cytometry (sometimes by image analysis) provides a mathematical determination of the proportion of the cell population that is synthesizing DNA (in S phase) and the proportion of cells in G_2-M phase (Fig. 12–8). Clinical studies have indicated that S phase has prognostic value and correlates with histologic grade in breast cancer.[95–102] Two markers associated with DNA proliferation are the antigen recognized by Ki-67 and proliferating cell nuclear antigen (PCNA). Ki-67 recognizes a large, nonhistone nuclear protein,[103,104] and PCNA is a protein associated with a DNA polymerase enzyme.[101] Both are expressed in proliferating cells[102,105] and can be identified in nuclei in late G_1, S, or G_2-M phases of the cell cycle.[106] The immunocytochemical assay for PCNA gives less reliable results than that for Ki-67. A newer antibody (MIB-1) recognizes the same antigen as the Ki-67 antibody, can be reliably employed on paraffin tissue,[107–110]

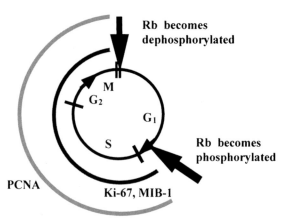

Figure 12–8   Diagram of the cell cycle showing when phosphorylation and dephosphorylation of retinoblastoma (Rb) protein occur, and the general phases when proliferation markers (Ki-67, MIB-1, and PCNA) are believed to be positive by immunocytochemical assay.

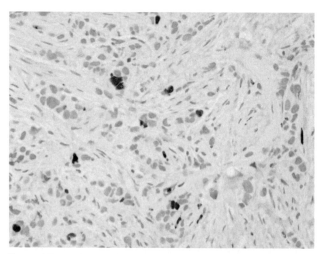

Figure 12–9   Immunohistochemical stain showing expression of the antigen detected by Ki-67 (MIB-1) in the nuclei of breast cancer cells in a paraffin tissue section (×200). The percentage of positive (*dark-colored*) cancer nuclei was calculated and expressed as a proliferation index of 5% to 10% (low).

and is the antibody of choice for immunocytochemical assays of formalin-fixed breast cancer specimens[111] (Fig. 12–9). There is generally an excellent correlation between expression of these proliferation markers and cell cycle analysis by flow cytometry,[105,112,113] with mitotic figure counts,[110] and with histologic grade.[110,113,114] Some studies do not show close correlation of proliferation markers with S phase, but still show prognostic relevance.[115] The immunocytochemical assays detect a greater population of cycling cells than S-phase alone. Numeric values for percentage cells in S phase or percentage cells expressing these other markers of proliferation are variable, and exact clinical cutoff points are not reliable. However, ranges of values that give relative prognostic information can be assigned. Generally, 10% to 15% and 25% to 35% are the ranges for the cutoffs among low, intermediate, and high proliferation indices in breast cancers.

How is the cell cycle controlled in breast cancer?

Breast epithelial cell proliferation is striking in some benign conditions (fibroadenomas) and even protective conditions of the breast (pregnancy). Increased proliferation is therefore not sufficient alone to explain the abnormal proliferation of breast cancer cells.[116] There are two major checkpoints in the cell cycle, in late G_1 phase and in late G_2-M phase (see Fig. 12–8). The major controls of the cell cycle are pairs of cyclins and bound cyclin-dependent kinases (CDKs; cyclin-CDK pairs).[117,118] The levels of these complexes determine cellular progression through the cell cycle by their interactions with other important transcription factors, such as retinoblastoma (Rb) protein.

Cyclin D and its complex with CDK (CDK-4 or -6) controls the checkpoint near the end of G_1 phase for cells to enter DNA synthesis (S phase) and become committed to replicate. When a cell passes through the late G_1 checkpoint, Rb becomes phosphorylated and remains so during the proliferation phases of the cell cycle. At the end of G_2-M phase, the Rb protein becomes dephosphorylated, and the cell exits the replicative phase (see Fig. 12–8). Cyclin D–CDK-4 complexes control Rb protein phosphorylation and therefore help to control the late G_1 checkpoint of the cell cycle (Fig. 12–10). During the resting phases of the cell cycle, the Rb protein binds to the E2F transcription factor, thereby preventing the transcription and proliferation effects of E2F binding to DNA. As cyclin D–CDK-4 levels increase at the end G_1 phase, they form complexes and bind to Rb protein. The Rb protein then releases E2F, which binds to DNA and activates transcription of target genes involved in cell proliferation and DNA replication (see Fig. 12–10), and the cell thereby enters the DNA synthesis phase. The Rb protein is an essential component of the cell cycle; however, abnormalities of this gene and protein are very rare in breast cancer.

Amplification of the cyclin D gene (located on chromosome 11q13) has been identified in about 20% of invasive breast carcinomas, and overexpression of the protein by

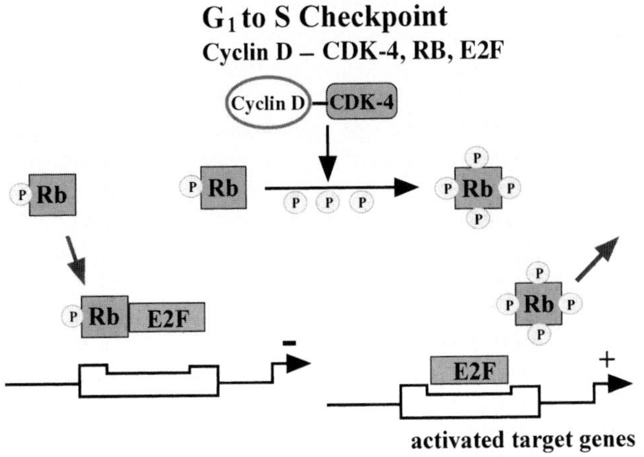

Figure 12–10 Diagram illustrating the role of cyclin D–CDK-4 complexes in phosphorylation of retinoblastoma (Rb) protein in a checkpoint between G_1 and S phase of the cell cycle. The E2F transcription factor is released to activate replication-associated gene transcription.

immunocytochemistry has been identified in about 80%.[6,83] Few studies, however, and only limited sample numbers are available at present. There are specific inhibitors of the activity of cyclin D–CDK-4 complexes in late G_1 phase. These serve to prevent the phosphorylation of Rb protein and thereby prevent cells from entering S phase from G_1 phase. These inhibitors include *p16, p21,* and *p14.* One of these (*p21*) is induced by the *p53* tumor suppressor gene (discussed next). There are molecular inhibitors for all the cyclin-CDK pairs involving the cell cycle. An inhibitor of all of these cyclin-CDK pairs, *p21* probably has global inhibitory effects of the cell cycle progression.

An inhibitor of cyclin E–CDK-2 in late G_1 phase of the cell cycle (after cyclin D–CDK-4), *p27* was cloned from estrogen-treated MCF7 breast cancer cells and is frequently expressed and infrequently mutated (point mutation) in breast cancers.[119,120] Recent clinical studies, using an immunocytochemical assay, suggest that elevated levels of cyclin E expression and decreased levels of *p27* expression have independent prognostic significance in breast cancer, including node-negative breast cancer in premenopausal women.[121,122] Expression of *p27* was reduced in high-grade, but not low-grade, DCIS and was reduced in 20% of low-grade, 67% of moderate-grade, and 97% of high-grade invasive ductal carcinomas.[122] Identification of a low-molecular-weight isoform of cyclin E has been described as a molecular marker of poor prognosis.[123] However, those assays require fresh tumor sample collection and more sophisticated laboratory techniques than standard IHC on a paraffin tissue section. The cyclin E isoform assay is currently performed in a single research laboratory, still needs independent validation, and hence is not currently used for routine clinical practice. These assays may well have a future role in the clinical laboratory. In summary, there are several levels of cell cycle control at specific checkpoints that use different tumor suppressor genes, cyclins, and their inhibitors.

Which tumor suppressor genes are important markers in breast cancer?

p53

The most important tumor suppressor gene in human cancer, *p53* is believed to play a significant role in breast cancer.[124,125] The gene is located on chromosome 17 (17p21), and its protein product is a DNA-binding transcription factor for growth inhibitory factors that regulate the cell cycle and prevent entry into S phase.[126–130] Expression of normal (wild-type) *p53* is increased in stressed cells, such as those exposed to ionizing radiation or chemotherapy.[130,131] Wild-type *p53* is also able to induce apoptosis (active cell death) in damaged or stressed cells,[132,133] activates genes involved in DNA repair,[125] and promotes differentiation and senescence of cells.[129] The overall effects are to prevent damaged cells from cycling, differentiate them into nonproliferative terminal stages, or kill severely damaged cells. Wild-type p53 protein binds DNA as a tetramer,[134] enhances transcription of several genes (including *p21, GADD45,* and *mdm-2*), and also represses transcription of other genes (*fos, jun, myc*).[129,135–137] Expression of *p53* is induced in late G_1 through the S phase of the cell cycle.[127,131] It delays cells in G_1 phase so that DNA damage can be corrected

p53 and the Cell Cycle

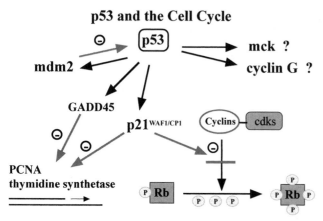

Figure 12–11   Diagram of the inhibitory influence of p53 protein on DNA synthesis (*bottom left*) and the G_1- to S-phase checkpoints of the cell cycle (*bottom right*) by inducing inhibitory molecules (p21 and GADD45).

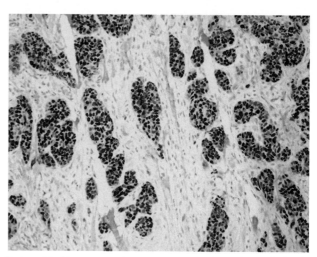

Figure 12–12   Immunohistochemical stain showing expression of p53 in the nuclei of breast cancer cells in a paraffin tissue section (×100). The proportion of positive (*dark-colored*) cancer nuclei is calculated and reported as more than 90% (high).

before replication.[129,130] The p53 protein is expressed in the nucleus; however, wild-type p53 is rapidly cleared, and therefore the protein is usually not detectable by immunocytochemical assays.[124,129] Mutation of the *p53* gene (the most common abnormality) leads to a dysfunctional p53 protein, which can be detected by immunocytochemistry as increased amounts of p53 protein due to the delayed clearance of the abnormal protein.[124,129] The genes induced by p53 binding to DNA include *p21 (WAF-1/CP1), GADD45, bax,* and *mdm-2*[129] (Fig. 12–11). The p21 protein product inhibits cyclin D–CDK-4 binding of Rb protein (the late G_1 cell cycle checkpoint) and also inhibits DNA replication enzymes such as PCNA and thymidine synthetase.[126,138] The ras, MAP kinase signal transduction pathway has also been shown to induce *p21* expression in a *p53*-independent manner.[139] *GADD45* also inhibits these DNA replication enzymes. The mdm-2 protein binds to and inhibits p53 protein in a negative feedback effect.[140] This protein has not yet been shown in breast cancer but is a significant abnormality in some sarcomas.[141]

The role of wild-type *p53* in apoptosis is more definitive in breast cancer cells than in hemopoietic and lymphoid cells.[142] This may partly explain why hematologic malignancies respond to chemotherapy and ionizing radiation more reliably than most solid malignancies.[142] Activation of wild-type *p53* stimulates transcription of proapoptotic molecules, such as bax, PIG3, PUMA, Noxa, and *p53*AIP1, and there is also evidence that wild-type *p53* can directly enter mitochondria and stimulate apoptosis.[125] Mutant *p53* may be involved in cellular resistance to necrosis in the center of expanding tumors. One study has suggested that clones of *p53* mutant cancer cells may be able to survive in this anoxic environment.[143] Whether this mechanism is due to an influence of *p53* on necrosis or apoptosis has not been completely determined.

Detection of *p53* by immunocytochemistry (Fig. 12–12) implies dysfunctional (mutated or bound) p53 protein. This can be detected in about 40% of invasive breast carcinomas[42,144–146] and in 20% to 40% of DCIS (particularly higher-grade comedo DCIS).[63,144,145,147] Overexpression of p53 is believed to have prognostic significance, particularly in node-positive and higher-grade breast cancer.[148] Overall, the literature contains mixed results concerning the prognostic

value of *p53* overexpression in node-negative patients.[67,149] Overexpression of *p53* is associated with increased cell proliferation (S phase, Ki-67, PCNA, MIB-1), histologic grade, and lack of hormone receptor expression.[42,144,146,148,150–153] Some data suggest an association between *p53* expression and *HER-2/neu* overexpression,[144] perhaps only in high-grade carcinomas,[148] although other data indicate no correlation.[42,146] Loss of the stabilizing effect of wild-type *p53* is associated with greater genomic instability in breast cancers,[154] which could lead to the development of new, biologically aggressive clones within the tumor.

BRCA1 *and* BRCA2

BRCA1 is a tumor suppressor gene on chromosome 17 (17q) that is sometimes mutated in hereditary breast cancer.[15,155] Women with *BRCA1* mutations often have cancers with aneuploidy, high histologic grade, and an increased frequency of medullary features,[156–158] but their long-term survival may not be different.[157,159] *BRCA1* encodes a 220-kD protein that has nuclear localization and inhibits the cell cycle through G_1-S, S, and G_2-M phases.[160] *BRCA1* regulates expression of genes during cellular stress and repairs double-stranded DNA damage.[159] The *BRCA1* gene can be screened for mutations; this technique is presently employed in genetic screening programs for heritable breast cancer (see Chapter 20). *BRCA1* expression is increased during lactation and late pregnancy (times at which a woman is relatively protected from breast cancer)[161,162] and can be induced by estrogen (and possibly tamoxifen).[163,164] Germline mutation of *BRCA2*, a tumor suppressor gene located on chromosome 13 (13q), accounts for a similar proportion of hereditary breast cancer families as *BRCA1*.[165] The gene product of *BRCA2* is critical for the repair of double-stranded DNA breaks.[166] Unlike *p53*, somatic mutation of *BRCA2* (or *BRCA1*) in solid tumors is extremely rare.[166] Decreased expression of *BRCA1* or *BRCA2* does occur in sporadic breast cancer, and this is thought to be due to somatic deletion of one copy of the gene.[166] Hypermethylation of the promoter sequence for the remaining copy of *BRCA1* is occasionally identified, and this completely silences the expression of *BRCA1*, but this is not the case for *BRCA2*.[166] However, EMSY is a novel protein that was recently shown to bind *BRCA2* after its induction following irradiation.[167] The normal function for EMSY is to inactivate *BRCA2* after DNA repair, but the authors identified amplification of the gene for EMSY (11q13.5) in 13% of breast cancers, and this was associated with node positivity and worse survival.[167] In 60% of these tumors, EMSY was coamplified with cyclin D1 (also at 11q13), suggesting a possible double oncogenic lesion in those cases.[167]

What assays are used to evaluate hormone receptors in breast cancer?

Hormone receptor expression may indicate a better prognosis in premenopausal woman (PR slightly stronger than ER), although the main reason for routinely performing these assays is the predictive value of response to hormonal therapy. ER and PR levels are often similar within a breast cancer. PRs are closely related to ER activity. There are several forms with different tissue expression and activity. The PR level is widely considered to be an indicator of the integrity of the ER pathway. Immunocytochemical,[168] immunoenzymatic,[169] and biochemical (ligand binding)[170] assays are available for ER and PR

(Table 12–1). Fresh or frozen cancer tissue is required for immunoenzymatic and biochemical analyses. Many carcinomas are small and require fixation and complete histologic evaluation of the entire tumor. In these cases, hormone receptors can be studied using immunocytochemistry. There is excellent correlation between biochemical and immunocytochemical techniques.[171–173] Biochemical assays can be limited by sampling of normal (instead of malignant) cells, by endogenous hormone bound to and blocking recognition of receptors (in premenopausal women),[174] and by truncated or mutated receptor protein, which does not bind hormone but is still transcriptionally active.[175] In recent years, antibodies have been developed to reliably detect ER and PR in formalin-fixed paraffin-embedded tissue.[176,177] These antibodies are readily used on routine histologic materials (Fig. 12–13) and have largely replaced biochemical assays as the standard assay.[174,176,178,179]

The reagents to be used for clinical ER testing using IHC now require approval by the U.S. Food and Drug Administration (FDA) because the results of the ER IHC test are the main determinant of whether a patient with breast cancer is eligible for hormonal therapy.[180,181] This recent measure by the FDA acknowledges the change in how ER status is used in patient care. Although it is important to maintain the quality and reliability of reagents used to perform IHC for ER,

Table 12–1   Summary of Assays Used to Measure Estrogen and Progesterone Receptors in Clinical Breast Cancer Specimens

		Hormone Receptor Assays			
Assay	*Tissue*	*Paraffin?*	*Amount*	*Measure*	*Positive*
Biochemical	GT	No	1 mg	Quantitation of ligand binding	>10–15 fmol/mg
Immunoenzymatic	GT	No	1 μg	Immunologic quantitation of receptor in cytosol	>10–15 fmol/mg
Immunocytochemical	FroT, FixT, TI, FNA	Yes	1 slide ea	Positive nuclei (%) (image analysis)	>10%

Paraffin?, can assay be used on formalin-fixed paraffin-embedded tissue sections?; Amount, recommended minimum amount of pure tumor; Positive, values representing positive receptors status; GT, ground tissue piece (fresh or frozen); FixT, fixed tissue section (5 μm usually); FroT, frozen tissue section; TI, tissue imprint onto glass slide; FNA, fine-needle aspirate; ea, each assay.

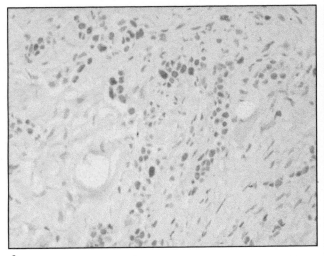 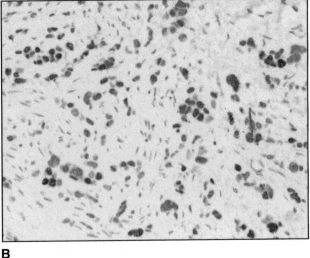

A   B

Figure 12–13   Immunohistochemical stain for estrogen receptor (ER) in the nuclei of breast cancer cells in paraffin tissue sections from a core biopsy (×200). One tissue core (*A*) demonstrates weak, equivocal nuclear staining (low expression), but the other tissue core (*B*) from the same paraffin block demonstrates stronger staining in the nuclei of most cancer cells. This case demonstrates the differences that can occur in the ER immunohistochemistry assay from tissue fixation and antigen-retrieval methods, even in a single tissue block.

and standardization of reagents is enforceable by the FDA, this measure does not resolve two main problems with the IHC assay for ER.[180,181] Stringent evaluation of the IHC test for ER has shown that the antigen-retrieval protocol is the most important variable of staining result.[182–184] Generally, fixed tissue sections are immersed in a buffered solution and cooked in a microwave oven at high temperature setting for 30 minutes.[182] Insufficient antigen retrieval can produce false-negative IHC results. Excessive antigen retrieval can lead to nonspecific background staining or loss of the antigen epitope. Antigen-retrieval methods also depend on the type and duration of tissue fixation and histochemical processing; thus, many laboratories optimize their own retrieval methods using control tissues.[182] A standardized antigen-retrieval protocol is not an FDA requirement, and tissue fixation and processing methods are also not standardized.[181] A recent study indicated that the duration of microwave cooking was the most important determinant of staining quality.[182] Obviously, the quality and extent of antigen retrieval determines staining intensity in paraffin-embedded tissues, and this significantly influences the interpretation of staining results.

Most pathologists report the percentage of positively stained cancer nuclei and use a 10% threshold for definite positive status, ignoring the overall intensity of staining.[182] Limited staining of less than 10% of the cancer nuclei can occur and is considered to be low expression that is equivocal. The H score was devised to combine the product of nuclear staining intensity (0 to 4) and the percent tumor area with each intensity score, to give a total of 0 to 400. The H score is time-consuming to perform and has not been widely adopted.[182] A semiquantitative interpretation of ER IHC (combines percent positivity and intensity) has been proved in clinical studies to predict response to tamoxifen more accurately than ligand-binding assays,[185,186] but this method is still not widely used.[182] Systems that include the intensity and frequency of nuclear staining demonstrate higher response rates in metastatic breast cancer related to level of ER expression (responses in 25% negative, 46% intermediate, and 66% high expressors).[186] Computerized image analysis systems also seek to quantify intensity and distribution of staining but require additional cost and time to perform.

The gain from IHC has been greater confidence that ER expression is being assessed in the cancer cells and applicability of IHC to archival and routine diagnostic materials that can be performed in any laboratory (see Fig. 12–13). However, during this time, the quality of information provided by these different assays has not improved much, whereas the clinical utilization of ER information has radically changed from ER status as one of the prognostic markers to ER status as the main determinant to choose endocrine treatment.

ER in the nucleus is composed of three main components: a central DNA-binding domain, flanked by AF-1 and AF-2 domains. Estrogen (ligand) binds into a central site in the AF-2 domain, and a hydrophobic cleft forms, attracting coactivator proteins to bind. Coactivator proteins also bind the AF-1 domain. Coactivation is greatly enhanced by the changed conformation when estrogen is bound and enables the DNA-binding domain to bind to specific estrogen response elements in the promoter regions of certain genes, directly influencing their transcription. Nuclear ER is present in every breast epithelial cell but is detectable using IHC only when the level of expression is increased. This is the concept behind use of IHC for ER as the assay to select patients for endocrine therapy.[187] Binding of the receptor hormone complexes to DNA induces promoters for a variety of genes, which are then transcribed. Those genes define the ER-related transcriptional profile and encode a variety of growth, proliferative, and secretory proteins that define the biology of ER-positive breast cancer.[52,53,188,189]

ER has recently been described in the cell membrane and is bound to caveolin within cell membrane rafts.[190,191] Transactivation of other receptors present in these rafts (EGFR, IGFR, HER-2/neu) leads to signaling to multiple kinase cascades, such as MAPK (ERK) and PI3K/AKT, that influence cell proliferation and transcription of genes.[190,192–194] This occurs in tumors that are positive for ER and EGFR or HER-2/neu.[194,195] There is also activation of bcl-2 and bcl-XL (phosphorylated by JNK) to promote survival.[196] This membrane signaling by ER probably contributes to tamoxifen resistance because it bypasses the antagonistic action of tamoxifen in the nucleus.[190] However, because aromatase inhibitors markedly reduce estrogen levels in the tissues, the combination of aromatase inhibitors with agents that inhibit signal transduction molecules (tyrosine kinases, farnesyl transferase, cyclin-dependent kinases) has been proposed.[190,197]

Are markers of breast cancer cell death available and informative?

The relevance of this question pertains to the ability of cancer cells to survive in conditions that would normally lead to cell death, to continued proliferation with severe DNA abnormalities that would normally be fatal, and to the effectiveness of chemotherapy and radiation therapy against cancer cells. Breast cancer cells can die by two different mechanisms. One mechanism is necrosis, due, for example, to inadequate blood supply to a region of tumor; the other mechanism is apoptosis (active individual cell death). Necrosis is documented histologically, without need for molecular assays.

Apoptosis is an active, multistep process by which cells release proteases and DNAses to digest themselves. This process is seen in normal cells as a response to endocrine effects; damage (radiation, toxins, drugs, viral infection); cytokines (tumor necrosis factor, TGF-β); and disruption of cells from their extracellular matrix or neighboring cells, from electrolyte disturbances, or from disrupted linkage between growth and proliferative signals.[198] It is proposed that the common mechanism for inducing apoptosis is disruption of the link between proliferative drive within the cell nucleus and the required growth signal from receptors and transduction pathways.[198] For example, cells that overexpress c-myc (transcription factor) are very susceptible to apoptosis.[199] The specific DNAse enzymatic destruction of DNA in apoptosis leads to fragmented DNA.[198,200] In situ detection of DNA fragments allows detection of apoptotic cells and determination of apoptotic indices within tissue sections of tumors.[201]

A normal protein (bcl-2) is expressed in the cytoplasm of cells and prevents them from undergoing apoptosis.[202] The bcl-2 protein binds to another protein (bax), negating the apoptosis-promoting activity of bax.[203] Antibodies are available for the immunocytochemical detection of bcl-2, and this has been studied in breast cancer, showing favorable prognosis in women whose cancer strongly expresses bcl-2.[204,205] There is a functional relationship between ER activity and bcl-2,[205,206] as well as between wild-type p53 activity and bcl-2.[207] Survivin is an upstream inhibitor of mitochondrial apoptosis that has increased nuclear expression in up to 60% of breast cancers and is associated with improved survival.[208,209] Activation of estrogen receptor increases the expression of both bcl-2 and survivin.[210] Preliminary data suggest that reduced bcl-2 expression may indicate response to chemotherapy.[211] Transcription factors (myc and E2F) and tumor suppressor genes (p53 and PTEN) have a role in the control of apoptosis.[199] Therefore, the systems of cell growth, proliferation, and death are related.

How does chromosomal telomere integrity affect breast cancer?

Mortality of normal cell lineages occurs in normal aging because the telomeric ends of chromosomes are shortened with successive divisions until eventually the lineage is exhausted. Activation of telomerase is common in breast cancer but not normal breast tissue.[212] This enzyme maintains the ends of chromosomes, effectively producing immortality of the cancer cell lineage. A PCR-based telomere repeat amplification protocol (TRAP assay) was developed to identify a specifically repeating nucleotide sequence that is synthesized on the ends of the telomeres by telomerase.[213,214] Newer assays are easier to perform; they use RT-PCR or IHC to recognize the active enzyme domain and use human telomerase reverse transcriptase (hTERT) or in situ hybridization to recognize an internal RNA component (hTR).[215,216] These assays have demonstrated that increased telomerase expression is associated with more proliferative breast cancers and poorer disease-free survival.[215,216]

Which markers assess breast cancer invasion and metastasis?

An invasive breast cancer has the ability to spread by metastasis to other organs, and it is this systemic disease that is the most important determinant of patient survival. Normal breast cells are strongly bound to their neighboring cells and to the underlying basement membrane by adhesion proteins. To invade, breast cancer cells must be able to dissociate from their neighbors, pass through the basement membrane and the extracellular matrix, and bind to new structures in order to pull themselves through the tissues (see Fig. 12–5A). The fact that pathologists detect stromal desmoplastic response in invasive breast cancer indicates that the invasive component of the tumor and the host stromal response are intimately associated (see Fig. 12–2). These same processes are required when the cells invade through tissue and through blood vessel walls, travel in the bloodstream, attach to distant endothelial sites, invade outside vessels, and establish tumor growths at distant sites (metastasis) (see Fig. 12–5B).

Cell Adhesion

Cell adhesion molecules join adjacent cells and the extracellular matrix and link the cell membrane to the underlying protein cytoskeleton. In breast cells, these cell adhesion proteins

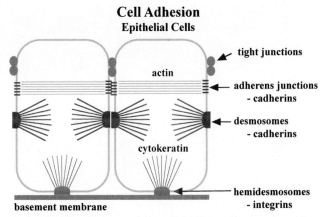

Cell Adhesion
Epithelial Cells

Figure 12–14   Diagram of the main cellular adhesions in epithelial cells. Cadherins are involved in intercellular adhesion, whereas integrins generally mediate adhesion of the cell to basement membrane. Cytoskeletal filaments (actins, cytokeratins) attach to the adhesion units.

include cadherins and integrins (Fig. 12–14), which are families of different proteins. Reduced expression of E-cadherin has been shown in invasive breast cancer, correlating with higher histologic grade.[217–219] The different pattern of invasive growth seen in lobular carcinoma is largely explained by loss of expression of E-cadherin (Fig. 12–15). E-cadherin gene encodes an adhesion molecule that is critical for intercellular attachment of epithelial cells. In lobular carcinomas, there is no expression of E-cadherin protein at the cell membrane, owing to loss of a gene allele (loss of heterozygosity [LOH]), mutation (encoding a protein that is secreted and not able to form intercellular attachments), or silencing of gene expression due to hypermethylation of the promoter site.[220–223] Therefore, E-cadherin is not expressed at the cell membrane, and the carcinoma cells have minimal intercellular attachment. Loss of E-cadherin expression also occurs in lobular carcinoma in situ (LCIS), explains the characteristic discohesive appearance of the epithelial cells in that lesion, and is related to subsequent development of invasive lobular carcinoma.[224] A recent publication compared the overall gene expression profiles between ductal and lobular types of invasive cancer and identified differential gene expression in very few genes.[225] The most significant difference was reduced expression of E-cadherin in lobular carcinomas.[225] Expression of osteopontin, survivin, and cathepsin B genes was also significantly decreased in invasive lobular cancer.[225] Although complete loss of expression of E-cadherin is usual in invasive lobular carcinoma, reduced expression of E-cadherin does occur in some invasive ductal carcinomas and is related to a more infiltrative growth pattern[226] (see Fig. 12–15). In this context, it is possible to consider lobular carcinoma of the breast as a variant of invasive carcinoma (rather than a specific histologic type), in which lost expression of a single gene product (E-cadherin) influences intercellular attachment and imparts a characteristic pattern of infiltrative growth.

Integrins are heterodimer pairs of different α and β chains (many combinations exist), which form attachments to the extracellular matrix and to adjacent cells and also act as growth-signaling peptides through their interactions with other cytoplasmic proteins beneath the cell membrane.[227] In normal breast, these molecules are preferentially expressed in

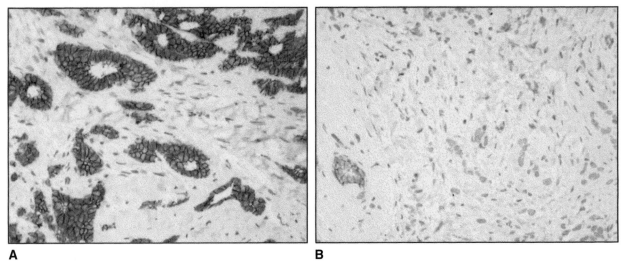

Figure 12–15   Immunocytochemical stain demonstrates a membranous staining pattern of E-cadherin in invasive ductal carcinoma cells (*A*) that is lost in poorly differentiated invasive carcinoma with a single-cell invasive pattern (*B*). Note that epithelial cells of a normal duct (*B, lower left*) stain for E-cadherin (×200).

myoepithelial cells and the base of epithelial cells.[228,229] In invasive cancers, there is loss of polarity and reduced overall expression of integrins in the malignant cells.[228,229] Reduced expression of β_1 and β_4 chains has been shown in DCIS.[230] The hyaluronic acid receptor (CD44) has also been indicated as a marker of tumor differentiation in breast cancer.[231]

Enzymes

Proteolytic degradation of the extracellular matrix occurs by three main enzyme families. These are cathepsins, plasminogen activators, and matrix metalloproteinases (stromelysins, type IV collagenases, and interstitial type I collagenases). These enzymes can be secreted by breast cancer cells or by desmoplastic host stromal cells; all have been identified in invasive breast cancers and have been related to the likelihood of metastasis. These enzymes are usually secreted in an inactive proenzyme state and then activated in the extracellular space. Specific molecular inhibitors can inhibit their activity. In addition, growth factor and hormone effects permit transcriptional control of the genes for these enzymes, with transcription factors binding to specific gene control sites and subsequent inhibition or promotion of gene transcription.

Cathepsin D is a lysosomal proteolytic enzyme that also has growth factor properties and can be secreted by breast cancer or stromal cells.[232] The prognostic significance of cathepsin D expression has been evaluated in numerous studies using different assays. Studies using Western blot assays (cytosol protein levels) have shown increased enzyme levels to be associated with more aggressive outcome,[233] although immunocytochemical assays have not detected significant independent prognostic value for cathepsin D.[234] Therefore, the prognostic significance of cathepsin D levels remains controversial. Cathepsin D levels are closely associated with ER activity in breast cells[235]; therefore, in breast cancer cells, they may be related to the integrity of the ER system.[236]

Urokinase plasminogen activator (uPA) binds to a cell membrane receptor; activates plasminogen, matrix metalloproteinases, and collagenase IV; and can digest fibronectin.[234] Immunoassays of cytosol extracts have indicated that high uPA levels correlate with poor prognosis in breast cancer.[234] This effect may be more marked when there are low levels of the inhibitor of uPA (PAI-2).[237] The cell membrane receptor for uPA has been identified on breast cancer cells as well as macrophages in the desmoplastic stroma.[238,239] Recently, ELISAs for the cytosolic ratio of uPA to inhibitor of plasminogen activator inhibitor type 1 (PAI-1), and for tissue inhibitor of metalloproteinase type 1 (TIMP-1), have been reported to achieve independent prognostic significance.[240–243]

The matrix metalloproteinases are a family of enzymes that include interstitial (type I) collagenases, type IV collagenases, stromelysins, and membrane-type metalloproteinases.[234,244–246] As a group of enzymes, they can digest almost any protein in the extracellular matrix. Type IV collagen is the main component of basement membranes and is presumed to be a major barrier to invasion; however, there are inconsistent (and limited) data concerning the utility of immunocytochemical assays for type IV collagenases as prognostic markers in breast cancer.[247,248]

Other Markers of Invasion and Metastasis

A metastasis suppressor gene (*nm-23*) has been described.[249] Loss of this suppressor gene product has been associated with more frequent metastatic disease[250]; however, there are also conflicting prognostic data.[251]

How is the host desmoplastic stromal response related to breast cancer markers?

The invasiveness of breast cancer cells is histologically related to the desmoplastic stromal response. The major components of the stromal response are the activity of stromal fibroblasts and histiocytes and the induction of angiogenesis to create a new capillary network to supply the tumor.

Stromal cells can influence tumor growth through paracrine simulation or inhibition of cancer cells through cytokines and growth factors. These stromal cells can also secrete enzymes to degrade the extracellular matrix. These are normal functions for these cells in wound healing, and it is believed that cancer cells may use these natural processes to their own advantage in the process of invasion. Tenascin is an extracellular matrix glycoprotein expressed in embryogenesis (mediating epithelial–mesenchymal interactions) as well as in some malignancies. Cancer and stromal cell expression of tenascin has been reported as an adverse prognostic marker in breast cancer.[252]

Angiogenesis is a critical component of tumor growth. Tumor cells and the associated host cells can induce angiogenesis through cytokines such as fibroblast growth factor-β. This again is a normal activity in wound healing but is uncontrolled in breast cancer. There is increased requirement for blood supply in rapidly growing and invasive tumors, leading to angiogenesis. Immunocytochemical assays for endothelial cell antigens (factor VIII, CD34) will demonstrate these capillaries, and vessel density within the tumor can be counted. Vessel density correlates with invasiveness, metastasis, and clinical behavior in breast cancers,[253–256] but not all results have supported vessel density as a prognostic marker.[257,258] Breast cancer cells produce and secrete vascular endothelial growth factor (VEGF) to stimulate angiogenesis by activating VEGF receptors on endothelium. VEGF expression is probably higher in HER-2/neu–positive breast cancers.[259] High levels of cytosolic VEGF in tumor extracts (measured by ELISA) are associated with significantly shorter disease-free survival.[260–262]

The immune response to breast cancer cells involves cytotoxic T lymphocytes (cell-mediated immunity), which can kill cancer cells by releasing toxic granules (perforin) or by binding Fas antigen and inducing apoptosis.[263] However, this probably has a negligible influence on the growth, invasiveness, and clinical outcome of invasive breast cancers. Tumor-associated lymphocytes are infrequently a significant histologic component of these tumors.

How heterogeneous are cells within breast cancer?

Most studies of molecular pathologic assays involve single samples from breast cancers. There is some evidence that breast cancers can be quite heterogeneous. Evaluation of DNA content (ploidy) shows heterogeneity in 30% to 50% of breast cancers if samples are studied from four or more areas of each cancer.[264–266] Analysis of all lymph node metastases and multiple primary tumor samples in heterogeneous tumors (by DNA ploidy) showed that DNA clones are stable during metastasis.[267,268] These clones are identifiable as a significant population (≥25%) in the primary tumor, but different nodal metastases contain different DNA clones.[267] These findings indicate established heterogeneity of DNA ploidy clones within the primary tumor and the different metastases and show that different clones from the tumor can metastasize (retaining their DNA indices) and establish a majority in each metastasis.[267] However, neither diploid nor aneuploid clones appeared to have a metastatic advantage.[267] Cytogenetic analysis showed loss of specific chromosomal regions in only some of the tumor cells in 15% to 45% of breast cancer samples,[269] indicating clonal heterogeneity within the tumor. Cytogenetic clones within the lymph node metastases were always present within the primary tumor,[269] consistent with the DNA ploidy studies discussed earlier.[267]

Single samples of primary tumor and nodal metastases have approximately similar proliferative indices, although there is considerable variance.[270] There is marked heterogeneity of proliferative activity if multiple samples are studied by any of the assays for proliferative activity.[267,271,272] In one study of 101 patients followed for 5 years, only the means of the proliferation indices (three to eight samples measured) were of prognostic significance, whereas the highest values and the degrees of heterogeneity (coefficients of variance) were not significant.[271]

Little is known about heterogeneity of HER-2/neu or p53 expression. Generally, if the primary tumor overexpresses HER-2/neu, its nodal metastases will mostly overexpress this oncoprotein.[267,273] Cancer cells frequently develop genetic damage because of inherent genetic instability. Breast cancer cells with abnormal p53 have been shown to have greater genomic instability.[154] This is associated with more frequent oncogene activation, such as HER-2/neu expression.[154] Many genetic alterations are fatal or are not advantageous to the tumor cells; however, as dominant subclones develop, they overtake the tumor population.[274–276] This is a mechanism of cancer progression, and clonal heterogeneity should be considered as part of the evolving biology of breast cancer.

It is important to appreciate that there is no single definition of clonality in breast cancer; therefore, the concept of multiclonality depends on which molecular assay is being studied. For example, some breast cancers have been shown to be clonal by some molecular techniques (X-chromosome inactivation pattern and restriction fragment length polymorphisms of other chromosomes), whereas DNA indices of the same breast cancers were heterogeneous.[277] A different group used similar techniques and found monoclonality of the X chromosome in predominantly intraductal carcinoma compared with heterogeneity in atypical ductal hyperplasias and papillomas.[278] This may be evidence that breast neoplasia begins as a monoclonal cell population but that heterogeneous subclones emerge as the disease progresses. The degree of heterogeneity within a single tumor would therefore depend on the state of tumor progression and the relative biologic aggressiveness of the different subclones that emerge.

Should molecular pathologic assays achieve independent prognostic significance?

The molecular pathologic pathways within breast cancer cells are complicated, and there is considerable overlap between different biochemical pathways and systems. Examples we have discussed include p53 and its role in the cell cycle, gene transcription, and cell death; ER activation and its influence on PRs, growth factors, signal transduction, and proteolytic enzymes; the interactions between cancer cells and host stromal cells; and the overlap between different cell surface receptor systems, signal transduction pathways, and DNA transcription factors. It is understandable, therefore, that an individual molecular pathologic assay is unlikely to serve as a single independent prognostic determinant in such a complex biologic system. These assays do, however, study critical cancer cell functions that relate directly to growth survival, invasion, and metastasis. It is hoped that further refinement of these biologic pathways in cancer cells, and a more critical interpretation of the results of expanding clinical studies using these assays, may focus attention on molecular systems within cancer cells rather than placing the emphasis on the prognostic significance of an individual molecule.

Can molecular pathologic assays predict response to therapy?

The difficulties in determining the prognostic significance of molecular markers from clinical outcome studies (outlined earlier) also apply to studies on the effects of therapy. However, the role of breast markers in predicting therapeutic responses will be an important area for future prospective clinical studies. Studies have found that certain markers do provide indications of potential therapy responses; some (ER and PR) have established clinical utility, whereas most require further research before any clinical value can be ascribed.

Antiestrogens

About 50% to 60% of newly diagnosed breast cancer patients are eligible for endocrine therapy on the basis of a positive IHC result (ER staining of ≥10% cancer cell nuclei).[187] The current IHC test for ER has a high negative predictive value because patients with ER-negative breast cancer are highly unlikely to benefit from endocrine therapy.[187] However, the positive predictive value of response for patients with ER-positive breast cancer is weaker (50%), depending on whether the tumor is positive for ER and PR (50% to 70% respond) or ER only (30% respond).[187] The hormone receptor assays (estrogen and progesterone) provide reliable and valuable information concerning response to antiestrogen therapy. Expression of pS2 in ER-positive cancers implies a good response to antiestrogens.[279] This probably reflects the integrity of the ER pathway because pS2 is an estrogen-induced gene. There are also data to suggest that patients with ER-positive cancer may not respond as well to antiestrogen therapy if the cancer cells overexpress HER-2/neu.[280] A breast cancer cell line transfected with mutant p53 did not develop antiestrogen resistance,[281] but clinical studies are not available.

Trastuzumab (Herceptin)

Monoclonal antibodies to HER-2/neu are available for clinical use and were used in the initial clinical trials of trastuzumab therapy[282] (clones 4D5 and CB11), but these may not be optimally sensitive. The FDA-approved HercepTest (DAKO) uses a polyclonal antibody cocktail that enhances the sensitivity of HER-2/neu detection but may compromise its specificity. Indeed, the HercepTest yielded a positive score in nearly 60% of breast carcinomas (expected frequency of 25% to 30%) and in 54% of samples from a group of 59 cases in which there had been no prior IHC staining using a monoclonal antibody (CB11).[283] This was attributed to poor specificity of the polyclonal antibody used in the HercepTest.[283] However, the HercepTest yielded a positive score in 58% of samples from a group of 48 cases in which there had been no prior IHC staining using the concentrate for the polyclonal HercepTest antibody (DAKO) and in which FISH had also shown no HER-2/neu gene amplification.[74] It was claimed that the scoring system of the HercepTest is prone to overestimation of IHC staining intensity because the normal epithelium is also positive in some cases.[74] This depends on the antibody selected and the laboratory methods. In our study of HercepTest, the

normal breast epithelium was always negative.[284] Response rates from trastuzumab are lower for 2+ IHC staining tumors compared with 3+ staining tumors. In many laboratories, IHC is used as a primary screen, with FISH testing of all 2+ cases or primary FISH-based testing.[285] In a study of single-agent trastuzumab in 111 patients, the response rates for 3+ IHC staining was 35%, versus 0% for 2+ IHC staining, and the response rate was 34% for FISH amplified, compared with 7% for nonamplified, breast cancer.[285] In another study of breast cancer treated with trastuzumab and paclitaxel, patients with HER-2/neu–overexpressing tumors had overall response rates from 67% to 81%, versus 41% to 46% in patients with normal expression of HER-2/neu.[286] FISH-based testing is more expensive and not as widely available as IHC, but some have suggested that FISH is actually more cost-effective if trastuzumab therapy is restricted to those with HER-2/neu amplification.[287]

Radiation Therapy

Radiation is most effective in proliferating cells; therefore, cell cycle–related proteins are likely molecular targets for predictive assays. Abnormalities of p53 have been suggested to increase cellular resistance to radiotherapy,[288] but reliable clinical data relating to breast cancer are not yet available.

Chemotherapy

High S-phase fraction has been shown to predict for improved response to chemotherapy.[289–291] Other data suggest that HER-2/neu overexpression may adversely predict outcome to CMF (cyclophosphamide, methotrexate, 5-fluorouracil) chemotherapy[292–294]; however, contradictory findings were published for doxorubicin-based therapy.[295] Cultured human breast cancer cells with HER-2/neu overexpression have recently been shown to develop resistance to paclitaxel (Taxol) chemotherapy.[296] Recent data suggest that patients whose tumors express p53 (immunocytochemistry of paraffin-embedded tissue) may have a poorer response to CMF chemotherapy; the study sample was small, however, and results were not statistically significant.[297] Matched-pair analysis of tissues before and after CMF chemotherapy showed altered p53 expression in 40% of cases, suggesting clonal selection after therapy.[298] There is strong evidence that apoptosis (and the role of bcl-2 and bax) is important in the response of hematologic malignancies to chemotherapy and radiotherapy,[299] but the influence of this cellular process in breast cancer is not fully understood.[142] Early data indicate a possible role for bcl-2 assays in predicting response to therapy.[204,205,300] Immunocytochemical assays may be performed to detect drug resistance proteins, most importantly P glycoprotein (MDR-1). This is a multidrug resistance protein that, if present, actively pumps drug molecules out of cancer cells and is associated with resistance to chemotherapy.[291]

There is considerable potential for high-throughput technologies, such as gene expression arrays, to identify responsive and resistant molecular profiles to predict likely response to chemotherapy regimens. To achieve this, the molecular profiles must be obtained and validated in the context of clinical trials that have meaningful outcomes. An example of this is complete pathologic response (pCR) from neoadjuvant chemotherapy that has an associated excellent long-term survival.[301,302] Using gene expression microarrays from needle biopsies in a training set of 24 newly diagnosed breast cancers, a 74-gene-expression profile was developed to distinguish the tumors that subsequently achieved pCR from those that had residual invasive carcinoma after 6 months of preoperative chemotherapy with paclitaxel, then 5-fluorouracil, doxorubicin, and cyclophosphamide.[303] The same methods were then used to evaluate a validation set of 18 new patients who received the same medical and surgical management. The 74-gene profile from the pretreatment needle biopsy sample predicted there would be pCR for three patients, and all three achieved pCR.[303] There were three additional pCRs in the other 15 patients for whom the 74-gene-expression profile did not predict complete response.[303] These pilot data are promising but far from mature. The training set was limited (24 patients) and probably did not encounter the diversity of gene expression profiles that are associated with complete response, and hence some complete responses in the validation set were not correctly predicted.[303] It is hoped that expansion of this and other clinical studies will lead to new predictive assays for response to chemotherapy.

What are the effects of chemotherapy and radiotherapy on breast cancer markers?

There are few data to address this question, and the results are not consistent. Some evidence suggests that proliferative activity is reduced, whereas HER-2/neu and p53 expression is increased.[304] It has also been shown that proliferative activity decreases following chemotherapy if the cancer had a high level of proliferation originally, that this phenomenon is dependent on the chemotherapeutic regimen, and that p53 expression is decreased.[305] The data from these studies may only reflect the more advanced stage of tumors that are treated with chemotherapy before surgery and may not be relevant to earlier stages of disease.

What are surrogate end-point biomarkers?

The concept of surrogate end points for breast cancer broadly encompasses any marker that predicts for future outcome. The more specific context in which this term is used here involves molecular pathologic markers as predictors of risk for future breast cancer or for response to chemoprevention strategies. The purpose is to speed up clinical trials by studying earlier, intermediate changes without having to wait years for prospective clinical follow-up before results are known. These biomarkers can be sought in samples from FNA, nipple fluid aspiration, or tissue from previous breast biopsies. Identification of aneuploidy and abnormal expression of several markers (ER, EGFR, HER-2/neu, p53) has been reported in fine-needle aspirates of "normal" breast in women at higher risk for developing breast cancer (family history or previous atypical or neoplastic breast biopsy) than women at lower risk.[306] These data are very early, however. Chemoprevention biomarkers should be related to the mechanism of action of the therapeutic agent to be tested (e.g., PR expression in an antiestrogen trial) and should be identifiable in precancerous breast tissue.[307] At this time, there are no clinically accepted surrogate end-point biomarkers, although potential targets include cell proliferation markers, HER-2/neu, p53, hormone receptors, and cytogenetic imbalances.[307–309] Heterogeneity of biomarkers in breast cancer is an important issue to be addressed before this approach will be clinically meaningful.

Should molecular pathologic assays be performed on in situ breast cancer?

Presently, the most important information concerning DCIS is the histologic absence of invasion and the cytologic-histologic grade. Sometimes, the histopathologic appearance is indefinite. In such cases, immunohistochemical stains that recognize myoepithelial cells are used to determine whether a myoepithelial cell layer surrounds the groups of cancer cells. These assays detect antigens associated with myofilament organization (e.g., smooth muscle actin and calponin) or nuclear p63 expression.[310–312] Absence of myoepithelium indicates invasion (see Fig. 12–6). The interpretation of these stains for myoepithelium in such cases is often challenging because there are increased numbers of myofibroblastic cells in the reactive stroma of invasive or in situ carcinoma (and these share expression of many of the same markers), and preexisting myoepithelial cells in a duct or lobule distended by in situ carcinoma can become attenuated and difficult to identify. Furthermore, these studies are often performed on small needle biopsy samples with known limitations of incomplete sampling and artifacts of tissue compression and disruption. Nonetheless, the implications of determining the presence or absence of invasion for patient management justify the use of these stains in biopsy samples to address this important diagnostic issue.[312]

Conceptually, in situ carcinoma is a preinvasive, localized phase of breast carcinoma and thus is managed by surgical or radiotherapy management; it does not require systemic therapy. There has been a recent shift in this paradigm since adjuvant hormonal therapy with tamoxifen has been shown to prevent (or delay) the onset of subsequent invasive breast cancer in women with previous DCIS.[313] Tamoxifen is currently being offered to women with DCIS.[314] Therefore, many laboratories have begun to test DCIS routinely for ER and PR (see Fig. 12–5), although there is not yet a published paper to confirm that the benefit is restricted to hormone receptor–positive DCIS. It is expected that most LCIS and low-grade DCIS should be positive for ER (see Fig. 12–5), whereas the ER status of intermediate- and high-grade DCIS is unpredictable from histopathologic appearance alone.[315] High-grade DCIS has interesting biologic and molecular characteristics. This lesion tends to be locally extensive within the ductal system and may involve single-cell (pagetoid) intraductal spread. Typically, the lesion is histopathologically associated with necrosis, apoptosis, and evidence of cellular proliferation. There is usually a high proliferation index (Ki-67 expression), and most high-grade DCIS cases have abnormal p53 or overexpression of HER-2/neu.[62,316] The frequency of p53 and HER-2/neu abnormalities in high-grade DCIS (50% to 70%) is much higher than in invasive cancer (20% to 30%).[62,317,318] In concurrent high-grade DCIS and invasive cancer, the status of HER-2/neu is usually the same.[317] High-grade DCIS with abnormal p53 expression and high proliferation may be more likely to develop local recurrence.[319] This suggests that some high-grade DCIS lesions are locally aggressive but are delayed in their progression to invasive disease, despite frequent abnormalities of p53 and HER-2/neu.[317] At

87. Rochlitz CF, Scott GK, Dodson JM, et al. Incidence of activating ras oncogene mutations associated with primary and metastatic human breast cancer. Cancer Res 1989;49(2):357–360.

88. Gulbis B, Galand P. Immunodetection of the p21-ras products in human normal and preneoplastic tissues and solid tumors: a review. Hum Pathol 1993;24(12):1271–1285.

89. Spandidos DA, Karaiossifidi H, Malliri A, et al. Expression of ras Rb1 and p53 proteins in human breast cancer. Anticancer Res 1992;12(1):81–89.

90. Bland KI, Konstadoulakis MM, Vezeridis MP, Wanebo HJ. Oncogene protein co-expression. Value of Ha-ras, c-myc, c-fos, and p53 as prognostic discriminants for breast carcinoma. Ann Surg 1995;221(6):706–718; discussion, 18–20.

91. Going JJ, Anderson TJ, Wyllie AH. Ras p21 in breast tissue: Associations with pathology and cellular localisation. Br J Cancer 1992;65(1):45–50.

92. Craven RJ, Lightfoot H, Cance WG. A decade of tyrosine kinases: From gene discovery to therapeutics. Surg Oncol 2003;12(1):39–49.

93. Navolanic PM, Steelman LS, McCubrey JA. EGFR family signaling and its association with breast cancer development and resistance to chemotherapy [review]. Int J Oncol 2003;22(2):237–252.

94. Mills GB, Kohn E, Lu Y, et al. Linking molecular diagnostics to molecular therapeutics: Targeting the PI3K pathway in breast cancer. Semin Oncol 2003;30(5 Suppl 16):93–104.

95. Frierson HF Jr. Ploidy analysis and S-phase fraction determination by flow cytometry of invasive adenocarcinomas of the breast. Am J Surg Pathol 1991;15(4):358–367.

96. Merkel DE, Winchester DJ, Goldschmidt RA, et al. DNA flow cytometry and pathologic grading as prognostic guides in axillary lymph node-negative breast cancer. Cancer 1993;72(6):1926–1932.

97. Stal O, Dufmats M, Hatschek T, et al. S-phase fraction is a prognostic factor in stage I breast carcinoma. J Clin Oncol 1993;11(9):1717–1722.

98. Clark GM, Mathieu MC, Owens MA, et al. Prognostic significance of S-phase fraction in good-risk, node-negative breast cancer patients. J Clin Oncol 1992;10(3):428–432.

99. Balslev I, Christensen IJ, Rasmussen BB, et al. Flow cytometric DNA ploidy defines patients with poor prognosis in node-negative breast cancer. Int J Cancer 1994;56(1):16–25.

100. Hedley DW, Rugg CA, Gelber RD. Association of DNA index and S-phase fraction with prognosis of nodes positive early breast cancer. Cancer Res 1987;47(17):4729–4735.

101. Bravo R, Frank R, Blundell PA, Macdonald-Bravo H. Cyclin/PCNA is the auxiliary protein of DNA polymerase-delta. Nature 1987;326(6112):515–517.

102. Garcia RL, Coltrera MD, Gown AM. Analysis of proliferative grade using anti-PCNA/cyclin monoclonal antibodies in fixed, embedded tissues. Comparison with flow cytometric analysis. Am J Pathol 1989;134(4):733–739.

103. Gerdes J, Li L, Schlueter C, et al. Immunobiochemical and molecular biologic characterization of the cell proliferation-associated nuclear antigen that is defined by monoclonal antibody Ki-67. Am J Pathol 1991;138(4):867–873.

104. Schluter C, Duchrow M, Wohlenberg C, et al. The cell proliferation-associated antigen of antibody Ki-67: a very large, ubiquitous nuclear protein with numerous repeated elements, representing a new kind of cell cycle-maintaining proteins. J Cell Biol 1993;123(3):513–522.

105. van Dierendonck JH, Wijsman JH, Keijzer R, et al. Cell-cycle-related staining patterns of anti-proliferating cell nuclear antigen monoclonal antibodies. Comparison with BrdUrd labeling and Ki-67 staining. Am J Pathol 1991;138(5):1165–1172.

106. Leonardi E, Girlando S, Serio G, et al. PCNA and Ki67 expression in breast carcinoma: Correlations with clinical and biological variables. J Clin Pathol 1992;45(5):416–419.

107. Cattoretti G, Becker MH, Key G, et al. Monoclonal antibodies against recombinant parts of the Ki-67 antigen (MIB 1 and MIB 3) detect proliferating cells in microwave-processed formalin-fixed paraffin sections. J Pathol 1992;168(4):357–363.

108. McCormick D, Chong H, Hobbs C, et al. Detection of the Ki-67 antigen in fixed and wax-embedded sections with the monoclonal antibody MIB1. Histopathology 1993;22(4):355–360.

109. Barbareschi M, Girlando S, Mauri FM, et al. Quantitative growth fraction evaluation with MIB1 and Ki67 antibodies in breast carcinomas. Am J Clin Pathol 1994;102(2):171–175.

110. Weidner N, Moore DH 2nd, Vartanian R. Correlation of Ki-67 antigen expression with mitotic figure index and tumor grade in breast carcinomas using the novel "paraffin"-reactive MIB1 antibody. Hum Pathol 1994;25(4):337–342.

111. Keshgegian AA, Cnaan A. Proliferation markers in breast carcinoma. Mitotic figure count, S-phase fraction, proliferating cell nuclear antigen, Ki-67 and MIB-1. Am J Clin Pathol 1995;104(1):42–49.

112. Dawson AE, Norton JA, Weinberg DS. Comparative assessment of proliferation and DNA content in breast carcinoma by image analysis and flow cytometry. Am J Pathol 1990;136(5):1115–1124.

113. Isola JJ, Helin HJ, Helle MJ, Kallioniemi OP. Evaluation of cell proliferation in breast carcinoma. Comparison of Ki-67 immunohistochemical study, DNA flow cytometric analysis, and mitotic count. Cancer 1990;65(5):1180–1184.

114. Gasparini G, Dal Fior S, Pozza F, Bevilacqua P. Correlation of growth fraction by Ki-67 immunohistochemistry with histologic factors and hormone receptors in operable breast carcinoma. Breast Cancer Res Treat 1989;14(3):329–336.

115. Brown RW, Allred CD, Clark GM, et al. Prognostic value of Ki-67 compared to S-phase fraction in axillary node-negative breast cancer. Clin Cancer Res 1996;2(3):585–592.

116. Farber E. Cell proliferation as a major risk factor for cancer: A concept of doubtful validity. Cancer Res 1995;55(17):3759–3762.

117. Pines J. Cyclins, CDKs and cancer. Semin Cancer Biol 1995;6(2):63–72.

118. Bates S, Peters G. Cyclin D1 as a cellular proto-oncogene. Semin Cancer Biol 1995;6(2):73–82.

119. Rasmussen UB, Wolf C, Mattei MG, et al. Identification of a new interferon-alpha-inducible gene (p27) on human chromosome 14q32 and its expression in breast carcinoma. Cancer Res 1993;53(17):4096–4101.

120. Spirin KS, Simpson JF, Takeuchi S, et al. p27/Kip1 mutation found in breast cancer. Cancer Res 1996;56(10):2400–2404.

121. Porter PL, Malone KE, Heagerty PJ, et al. Expression of cell-cycle regulators p27Kip1 and cyclin E, alone and in combination, correlate with survival in young breast cancer patients. Nat Med 1997;3(2):222–225.

122. Catzavelos C, Bhattacharya N, Ung YC, et al. Decreased levels of the cell-cycle inhibitor p27Kip1 protein: Prognostic implications in primary breast cancer. Nat Med 1997;3(2):227–230.

123. Keyomarsi K, Tucker SL, Buchholz TA, et al. Cyclin E and survival in patients with breast cancer. N Engl J Med 2002;347(20):1566–1575.

124. Vogelstein B, Kinzler KW. p53 Function and dysfunction. Cell 1992;70(4):523–526.

125. Gasco M, Shami S, Crook T. The p53 pathway in breast cancer. Breast Cancer Res 2002;4(2):70–76.

126. Morris GF, Bischoff JR, Mathews MB. Transcriptional activation of the human proliferating-cell nuclear antigen promoter by p53. Proc Natl Acad Sci U S A 1996;93(2):895–899.

127. Lin D, Shields MT, Ullrich SJ, et al. Growth arrest induced by wild-type p53 protein blocks cells prior to or near the restriction point in late G1 phase. Proc Natl Acad Sci U S A 1992;89(19):9210–9214.

128. Yin Y, Tainsky MA, Bischoff FZ, et al. Wild-type p53 restores cell cycle control and inhibits gene amplification in cells with mutant p53 alleles. Cell 1992;70(4):937–948.

129. Harris CC, Hollstein M. Clinical implications of the p53 tumor-suppressor gene. N Engl J Med 1993;329(18):1318–1327.

130. Kuerbitz SJ, Plunkett BS, Walsh WV, Kastan MB. Wild-type p53 is a cell cycle checkpoint determinant following irradiation. Proc Natl Acad Sci U S A 1992;89(16):7491–7495.

131. Kastan MB, Zhan Q, el-Deiry WS, et al. A mammalian cell cycle checkpoint pathway utilizing p53 and GADD45 is defective in ataxia-telangiectasia. Cell 1992;71(4):587–597.

132. Shaw P, Bovey R, Tardy S, et al. Induction of apoptosis by wild-type p53 in a human colon tumor-derived cell line. Proc Natl Acad Sci U S A 1992;89(10):4495–4499.

133. Lane DP. Cancer. A death in the life of p53. Nature 1993;362(6423):786–787.

134. Friedman PN, Chen X, Bargonetti J, Prives C. The p53 protein is an unusually shaped tetramer that binds directly to DNA. Proc Natl Acad Sci U S A 1993;90(8):3319–3323.

135. Seto E, Usheva A, Zambetti GP, et al. Wild-type p53 binds to the TATA-binding protein and represses transcription. Proc Natl Acad Sci U S A 1992;89(24):12028–12032.

136. Ragimov N, Krauskopf A, Navot N, et al. Wild-type but not mutant p53 can repress transcription initiation in vitro by interfering with the binding of basal transcription factors to the TATA motif. Oncogene 1993;8(5):1183–1193.

137. Kley N, Chung RY, Fay S, et al. Repression of the basal c-fos promoter by wild-type p53. Nucleic Acids Res 1992;20(15):4083–4087.

138. Waga S, Hannon GJ, Beach D, Stillman B. The p21 inhibitor of cyclin-dependent kinases controls DNA replication by interaction with PCNA. Nature 1994;369(6481):574–578.

139. Liu Y, Martindale JL, Gorospe M, Holbrook NJ. Regulation of p21WAF1/CIP1 expression through mitogen-activated protein kinase signaling pathway. Cancer Res 1996;56(1):31–35.

140. Oliner JD, Pietenpol JA, Thiagalingam S, et al. Oncoprotein MDM2 conceals the activation domain of tumour suppressor p53. Nature 1993;362(6423):857–860.

141. Oliner JD, Kinzler KW, Meltzer PS, et al. Amplification of a gene encoding a p53-associated protein in human sarcomas. Nature 1992;358(6381):80–83.

142. Kastan MB, Canman CE, Leonard CJ. P53, cell cycle control and apoptosis: Implications for cancer. Cancer Metastasis Rev 1995;14(1):3–15.

143. Graeber TG, Osmanian C, Jacks T, et al. Hypoxia-mediated selection of cells with diminished apoptotic potential in solid tumours. Nature 1996;379(6560):88–91.

144. Poller DN, Hutchings CE, Galea M, et al. p53 Protein expression in human breast carcinoma: Relationship to expression of epidermal growth factor receptor, c-erbB-2 protein overexpression, and oestrogen receptor. Br J Cancer 1992;66(3):583–588.

145. Davidoff AM, Kerns BJ, Iglehart JD, Marks JR. Maintenance of p53 alterations throughout breast cancer progression. Cancer Res 1991;51(10):2605–2610.

146. Haerslev T, Jacobsen GK. An immunohistochemical study of p53 with correlations to histopathological parameters, c-erbB-2, proliferating cell nuclear antigen, and prognosis. Hum Pathol 1995;26(3):295–301.

147. O'Malley FP, Vnencak-Jones CL, Dupont WD, et al. p53 Mutations are confined to the comedo type ductal carcinoma in situ of the breast. Immunohistochemical and sequencing data. Lab Invest 1994;71(1):67–72.

148. Martinazzi M, Crivelli F, Zampatti C, Martinazzi S. Relationship between p53 expression and other prognostic factors in human breast carcinoma. An immunohistochemical study. Am J Clin Pathol 1993;100(3):213–217.

149. Barbareschi M. Prognostic value of the immunohistochemical expression of p53 in breast carcinomas: A review of the literature involving over 9000 patients. Appl Immunohistochem 1996;4:106–116.

150. Allred DC, Clark GM, Elledge R, et al. Association of p53 protein expression with tumor cell proliferation rate and clinical outcome in node-negative breast cancer. J Natl Cancer Inst 1993;85(3):200–206.

151. Stenmark-Askmalm M, Stal O, Sullivan S, et al. Cellular accumulation of p53 protein: An independent prognostic factor in stage II breast cancer. Eur J Cancer 1994;30A(2):175–180.

152. Stenmark-Askmalm M, Stal O, Olsen K, Nordenskjold B. p53 As a prognostic factor in stage I breast cancer. South-East Sweden Breast Cancer Group. Br J Cancer 1995;72(3):715–719.

153. Domagala W, Markiewski M, Harezga B, et al. Prognostic significance of tumor cell proliferation rate as determined by the MIB-1 antibody in breast carcinoma: its relationship with vimentin and p53 protein. Clin Cancer Res 1996;2(1):147–154.

154. Eyfjord JE, Thorlacius S, Steinarsdottir M, et al. p53 Abnormalities and genomic instability in primary human breast carcinomas. Cancer Res 1995;55(3):646–651.

155. Futreal PA, Swensen J, Shattuck-Eidens D, et al. A strong candidate for the breast and ovarian cancer susceptibility gene BRCA1. Science 1994;266(5182):66–71.

156. Eisinger F, Stoppa-Lyonnet D, Longy M, et al. Germ line mutation at BRCA1 affects the histoprognostic grade in hereditary breast cancer. Cancer Res 1996;56(3):471–474.

157. Marcus JN, Watson P, Page DL, et al. Hereditary breast cancer: Pathobiology, prognosis, and BRCA1 and BRCA2 gene linkage. Cancer 1996;77(4):697–709.

158. Breast Cancer Linkage Consortium. Pathology of familial breast cancer: Differences between breast cancers in carriers of BRCA1 or BRCA2 mutations and sporadic cases. Lancet 1997;349(9064):1505–1510.

159. Kennedy RD, Quinn JE, Johnston PG, Harkin DP. BRCA1: Mechanisms of inactivation and implications for management of patients. Lancet 2002;360(9338):1007–1014.

160. Chen Y, Farmer AA, Chen CF, et al. BRCA1 is a 220-kDa nuclear phosphoprotein that is expressed and phosphorylated in a cell cycle-dependent manner. Cancer Res 1996;56(14):3168–3172.

161. Lane TF, Deng C, Elson A, et al. Expression of Brca1 is associated with terminal differentiation of ectodermally and mesodermally derived tissues in mice. Genes Dev 1995;9(21):2712–2722.

162. Marquis ST, Rajan JV, Wynshaw-Boris A, et al. The developmental pattern of Brca1 expression implies a role in differentiation of the breast and other tissues. Nat Genet 1995;11(1):17–26.

163. Jensen RA, Thompson ME, Jetton TL, et al. BRCA1 is secreted and exhibits properties of a granin. Nat Genet 1996;12(3):303–308.

164. Gudas JM, Nguyen H, Li T, Cowan KH. Hormone-dependent regulation of BRCA1 in human breast cancer cells. Cancer Res 1995;55(20):4561–4565.

165. Wooster R, Neuhausen SL, Mangion J, et al. Localization of a breast cancer susceptibility gene, BRCA2, to chromosome 13q12–13. Science 1994;265(5181):2088–2090.

166. King MC. A novel BRCA2-binding protein and breast and ovarian tumorigenesis. N Engl J Med 2004;350(12):1252–1253.

167. Hughes-Davies L, Huntsman D, Ruas M, et al. EMSY links the BRCA2 pathway to sporadic breast and ovarian cancer. Cell 2003;115(5):523–535.

168. Pertschuk LP, Eisenberg KB, Carter AC, Feldman JG. Immunohistologic localization of estrogen receptors in breast cancer with monoclonal antibodies. Correlation with biochemistry and clinical endocrine response. Cancer 1985;55(7):1513–1518.

169. Klijanienko J, Laine-Bidron C, Vielh P, Magdelenat H. Immunoenzymatic (EIA) assays of estrogen and progesterone receptors in fine-needle and surgical samples in breast cancer patients. Am J Clin Pathol 1995;104(3):289–293.

170. Kiang DT, Frenning DH, Goldman AI, et al. Estrogen receptors and responses to chemotherapy and hormonal therapy in advanced breast cancer. N Engl J Med 1978;299(24):1330–1334.

171. Katz RL, Patel S, Sneige N, et al. Comparison of immunocytochemical and biochemical assays for estrogen receptor in fine needle aspirates and histologic sections from breast carcinomas. Breast Cancer Res Treat 1990;15(3):191–203.

172. Bacus S, Flowers JL, Press MF, et al. The evaluation of estrogen receptor in primary breast carcinoma by computer-assisted image analysis. Am J Clin Pathol 1988;90(3):233–239.

173. Alberts SR, Ingle JN, Roche PR, et al. Comparison of estrogen receptor determinations by a biochemical ligand-binding assay and immunohistochemical staining with monoclonal antibody ER1D5 in females with lymph node positive breast carcinoma entered on two prospective clinical trials. Cancer 1996;78(4):764–772.

174. Battifora H, Mehta P, Ahn C, Esteban J. Estrogen receptor immunocytochemical assay in paraffin-embedded tissue: A better gold standard? Appl Immunohistochem 1993;1:39–45.

175. Fuqua SA, Chamness GC, McGuire WL. Estrogen receptor mutations in breast cancer. J Cell Biochem 1993;51(2):135–139.

176. Goulding H, Pinder S, Cannon P, et al. A new immunohistochemical antibody for the assessment of estrogen receptor status on routine formalin-fixed tissue samples. Hum Pathol 1995;26(3):291–294.

177. De Rosa CM, Ozzello L, Greene GL, Habif DV. Immunostaining of estrogen receptor in paraffin sections of breast carcinomas using monoclonal antibody D75P3 gamma: Effects of fixation. Am J Surg Pathol 1987;11(12):943–950.

178. Pertschuk LP, Feldman JG, Kim YD, et al. Estrogen receptor immunocytochemistry in paraffin embedded tissues with ER1D5 predicts breast cancer endocrine response more accurately than H222Sp gamma in frozen sections or cytosol-based ligand-binding assays. Cancer 1996;77(12):2514–2519.

179. Taylor CR. Paraffin section immunocytochemistry for estrogen receptor: The time has come. Cancer 1996;77(12):2419–2422.

180. Medical devices; classification/reclassification of immunohistochemistry reagents and kits—FDA. Final rule. Federal Register 1998;63:30132–30142.

181. Taylor CW. FDA issues final rule for classification and reclassification of immunochemistry reagents and kits. Am J Clin Pathol 1999;111(4):443–444.

182. Rhodes A, Jasani B, Barnes DM, et al. Reliability of immunohistochemical demonstration of oestrogen receptors in routine practice: Interlaboratory variance in the sensitivity of detection and evaluation of scoring systems. J Clin Pathol 2000;53:125–130.

183. Rüdiger T, Höfler H, Kreipe H, et al. Quality assurance in immunohistochemistry: Results of an interlaboratory trial involving 172 pathologists. Am J Surg Pathol 2002;26(7):873–882.

184. Rhodes A. Quality assurance in immunohistochemistry. Am J Surg Pathol 2003;27(9):1284–1285.

185. Harvey JM, Clark GM, Osborne CK, Allred DC. Estrogen receptor status by immunohistochemistry is superior to the ligand-binding assay for predicting response to adjuvant endocrine therapy in breast cancer. J Clin Oncol 1999;17(5):1474–1481.

186. Elledge RM, Green S, Pugh R, et al. Estrogen receptor (ER) and progesterone receptor (PgR), by ligand-binding assay compared with ER, PgR and pS2, by immuno-histochemistry in predicting response to tamoxifen in metastatic breast cancer: A Southwest Oncology Group study. Int J Cancer 2000;89(2):111–117.

187. Buzdar A. Endocrine therapy in the treatment of metastatic breast cancer. Semin Oncol 2001;28:291–304.

188. Brown M. Estrogen receptor molecular biology. Hematol Oncol Clin North Am 1994;8(1):101–112.

189. Gruvberger S, Ringner M, Chen Y, et al. Estrogen receptor status in breast cancer is associated with remarkably distinct gene expression patterns. Cancer Res 2001;61:5979–5984.

190. Johnston SRD, Head J, Pancholi S, et al. Integration of signal transduction inhibitors with endocrine therapy: An approach to overcoming hormone resistance in breast cancer. Clin Cancer Res 2003;9:524S–32S.

191. Schlegel A, Wang C, Katzenellenbogen BS, et al. Caveolin-1 potentiates estrogen receptor alpha (ERalpha) signaling: Caveolin-1 drives ligand-independent nuclear translocation and activation of ERalpha. J Biol Chem 1999;274(47):33551–33556.

192. Atanaskova N, Keshamouni VG, Krueger JS, et al. MAP kinase/estrogen receptor cross-talk enhances estrogen-mediated signaling and tumor growth but does not confer tamoxifen resistance. Oncogene 2002;21(25):4000–4008.

193. Razandi M, Pedram A, Park ST, Levin ER. Proximal events in signaling by plasma membrane estrogen receptors. J Biol Chem 2003;278(4):2701–2712.

194. Ellis MJ, Coop A, Singh B, et al. Letrozole inhibits tumor proliferation more effectively than tamoxifen independent of HER1/2 expression status. Cancer Res 2003;63:6523–6531.

195. Ellis MJ, Coop A, Singh B, et al. Letrozole is more effective neoadjuvant endocrine therapy than tamoxifen for ErbB-1- and/or ErbB-2-positive, estrogen receptor-positive primary breast cancer: Evidence from a phase III randomized trial. J Clin Oncol 2001;19(18):3808–3816.

196. Razandi M, Pedram A, Levin ER. Plasma membrane estrogen receptors signal to antiapoptosis in breast cancer. Mol Endocrinol 2000;14(9):1434–1447.

197. Gee JMW, Harper ME, Hutcheson IR, et al. The antiepidermal growth factor receptor agent gefitinib (ZD1839/Iressa) improves antihormone response and prevents development of resistance in breast cancer in vitro. Endocrinology 2003;144(11):5105–5117.

198. Bellamy CO, Malcomson RD, Harrison DJ, Wyllie AH. Cell death in health and disease: The biology and regulation of apoptosis. Semin Cancer Biol 1995;6(1):3–16.

199. Canman CE, Kastan MB. Induction of apoptosis by tumor suppressor genes and oncogenes. Semin Cancer Biol 1995;6(1):17–25.

200. Eastman A. Survival factors, intracellular signal transduction, and the activation of endonucleases in apoptosis. Semin Cancer Biol 1995;6(1):45–52.

201. Gavrieli Y, Sherman Y, Ben-Sasson SA. Identification of programmed cell death in situ via specific labeling of nuclear DNA fragmentation. J Cell Biol 1992;119(3):493–501.

202. Hockenbery D, Nunez G, Milliman C, et al. Bcl-2 is an inner mitochondrial membrane protein that blocks programmed cell death. Nature 1990;348(6299):334–336.

203. Oltvai ZN, Milliman CL, Korsmeyer SJ. Bcl-2 heterodimerizes in vivo with a conserved homolog, Bax, that accelerates programmed cell death. Cell 1993;74(4):609–619.

204. Joensuu H, Pylkkanen L, Toikkanen S. Bcl-2 protein expression and long-term survival in breast cancer. Am J Pathol 1994;145(5):1191–1198.

205. Gasparini G, Barbareschi M, Doglioni C, et al. Expression of bcl-2 protein predicts efficacy of adjuvant treatments in operable node-positive breast cancer. Clin Cancer Res 1995;1(2):189–198.

206. Wang TT, Phang JM. Effects of estrogen on apoptotic pathways in human breast cancer cell line MCF-7. Cancer Res 1995;55(12):2487–2489.

207. Miyashita T, Krajewski S, Krajewska M, et al. Tumor suppressor p53 is a regulator of bcl–2 and bax gene expression in vitro and in vivo. Oncogene 1994;9(6):1799–1805.

208. Blanc-Brude OP, Mesri M, Wall NR, et al. Therapeutic targeting of the survivin pathway in cancer: Initiation of mitochondrial apoptosis and suppression of tumor-associated angiogenesis. Clin Cancer Res 2003;9(7):2683–2692.

209. Kennedy SM, O'Driscoll L, Purcell R, et al. Prognostic importance of survivin in breast cancer. Br J Cancer 2003;88(7):1077–1083.

210. Frasor J, Danes JM, Komm B, et al. Profiling of estrogen up- and down-regulated gene expression in human breast cancer cells: insights into gene networks and pathways underlying estrogenic control of proliferation and cell phenotype. Endocrinology 2003;144(10):4562–4574.

211. Buchholz TA, Davis DW, McConkey DJ, et al. Chemotherapy-induced apoptosis and Bcl-2 levels correlate with breast cancer response to chemotherapy. Cancer J 2003;9(1):33–41.

212. Herbert BS, Wright WE, Shay JW. Telomerase and breast cancer. Breast Cancer Res 2001;3(3):146–149.

213. Aldous WK, Grabill NR. A fluorescent method for detection of telomerase activity. Diagn Mol Pathol 1997;6(2):102–110.

214. Carey LA, Kim NW, Goodman S, et al. Telomerase activity and prognosis in primary breast cancers. J Clin Oncol 1999;17(10):3075–3081.

215. Bieche I, Nogues C, Paradis V, et al. Quantitation of hTERT gene expression in sporadic breast tumors with a real-time reverse transcription-polymerase chain reaction assay. Clin Cancer Res 2000;6(2):452–459.

216. Poremba C, Heine B, Diallo R, et al. Telomerase as a prognostic marker in breast cancer: High-throughput tissue microarray analysis of hTERT and hTR. J Pathol 2002;198(2):181–189.

217. Moll R, Mitze M, Frixen UH, Birchmeier W. Differential loss of E-cadherin expression in infiltrating ductal and lobular breast carcinomas. Am J Pathol 1993;143(6):1731–1742.

218. Glukhova M, Koteliansky V, Sastre X, Thiery JP. Adhesion systems in normal breast and in invasive breast carcinoma. Am J Pathol 1995;146(3):706–716.

219. Palacios J, Benito N, Pizarro A, et al. Anomalous expression of P-cadherin in breast carcinoma. Correlation with E-cadherin expression and pathological features. Am J Pathol 1995;146(3):605–612.

220. Kanai Y, Oda T, Tsuda H, et al. Point mutation of the E-cadherin gene in invasive lobular carcinoma of the breast. Jpn J Cancer Res 1994;85(10):1035–1039.

221. Berx G, Cleton-Jansen AM, Strumane K, et al. E-cadherin is inactivated in a majority of invasive human lobular breast cancers by truncation mutations throughout its extracellular domain. Oncogene 1996;13(9):1919–1925.

222. Droufakou S, Deshmane V, Roylance R, et al. Multiple ways of silencing E-cadherin gene expression in lobular carcinoma of the breast. Int J Cancer 2001;92(3):404–408.

223. Sarrio D, Moreno-Bueno G, Hardisson D, et al. Epigenetic and genetic alterations of APC and CDH1 genes in lobular breast cancer: relationships with abnormal E-cadherin and catenin expression and microsatellite instability. Int J Cancer 2003;106(2):208–215.

224. Reis-Filho JS, Cancela Paredes J, Milanezi F, Schmitt FC. Clinicopathologic implications of E-cadherin reactivity in patients with lobular carcinoma in situ of the breast. Cancer 2002;94(7):2114–2115; author reply, 5–6.

225. Korkola JE, DeVries S, Fridlyand J, et al. Differentiation of lobular versus ductal breast carcinomas by expression microarray analysis. Cancer Res 2003;63(21):7167–7175.

226. Goldstein NS. Does the level of E-cadherin expression correlate with the primary breast carcinoma infiltration pattern and type of systemic metastases? Am J Clin Pathol 2002;118(3):425–434.

227. Clark EA, Brugge JS. Integrins and signal transduction pathways: the road taken. Science 1995;268(5208):233–239.

228. Pignatelli M, Cardillo MR, Hanby A, Stamp GW. Integrins and their accessory adhesion molecules in mammary carcinomas: loss of polarization in poorly differentiated tumors. Hum Pathol 1992;23(10):1159–1166.

229. Koukoulis GK, Virtanen I, Korhonen M, et al. Immunohistochemical localization of integrins in the normal, hyperplastic, and neoplastic breast. Correlations with their functions as receptors and cell adhesion molecules. Am J Pathol 1991;139(4):787–799.

230. Hanby AM, Gillett CE, Pignatelli M, Stamp GW. Beta 1 and beta 4 integrin expression in methacarn and formalin-fixed material from in situ ductal carcinoma of the breast. J Pathol 1993;171(4):257–262.

231. Friedrichs K, Franke F, Lisboa BW, et al. CD44 isoforms correlate with cellular differentiation but not with prognosis in human breast cancer. Cancer Res 1995;55(22):5424–5433.

232. Vignon F, Capony F, Chambon M, et al. Autocrine growth stimulation of the MCF 7 breast cancer cells by the estrogen-regulated 52 K protein. Endocrinology 1986;118(4):1537–1545.

233. Tandon AK, Clark GM, Chamness GC, et al. Cathepsin D and prognosis in breast cancer. N Engl J Med 1990;322(5):297–302.

234. Duffy MJ. Proteases as prognostic markers in cancer. Clin Cancer Res 1996;2(4):613–618.

235. Rochefort H, Capony F, Garcia M. Cathepsin D in breast cancer: from molecular and cellular biology to clinical applications. Cancer Cells 1990;2(12):383–388.

236. Henry JA, McCarthy AL, Angus B, et al. Prognostic significance of the estrogen-regulated protein, cathepsin D, in breast cancer. An immunohistochemical study. Cancer 1990;65(2):265–271.

237. Foekens JA, Buessecker F, Peters HA, et al. Plasminogen activator inhibitor-2: Prognostic relevance in 1012 patients with primary breast cancer. Cancer Res 1995;55(7):1423–1427.

238. Grondahl-Hansen J, Peters HA, van Putten WL, et al. Prognostic significance of the receptor for urokinase plasminogen activator in breast cancer. Clin Cancer Res 1995;1(10):1079–1087.

239. Pyke C, Graem N, Ralfkiaer E, et al. Receptor for urokinase is present in tumor-associated macrophages in ductal breast carcinoma. Cancer Res 1993;53(8):1911–1915.

240. Look MP, van Putten WL, Duffy MJ, et al. Pooled analysis of prognostic impact of urokinase-type plasminogen activator and its inhibitor PAI-1 in 8377 breast cancer patients. J Natl Cancer Inst 2002;94(2):116–128.

241. Harbeck N, Dettmar P, Thomssen C, et al. Risk-group discrimination in node-negative breast cancer using invasion and proliferation markers: 6-Year median follow-up. Br J Cancer 1999;80(3–4):419–426.

242. Harbeck N, Kates RE, Look MP, et al. Enhanced benefit from adjuvant chemotherapy in breast cancer patients classified high-risk according to urokinase-type plasminogen activator (uPA) and plasminogen activator inhibitor type 1 (n = 3424). Cancer Res 2002;62(16):4617–4622.

243. Schrohl AS, Holten-Andersen MN, Peters HA, et al. Tumor tissue levels of tissue inhibitor of metalloproteinase-1 as a prognostic marker in primary breast cancer. Clin Cancer Res 2004;10(7):2289–2298.

244. Aznavoorian S, Murphy AN, Stetler-Stevenson WG, Liotta LA. Molecular aspects of tumor cell invasion and metastasis. Cancer 1993;71(4):1368–1383.

245. Sato H, Takino T, Okada Y, et al. A matrix metalloproteinase expressed on the surface of invasive tumour cells. Nature 1994;370(6484):61–65.

246. Puente XS, Pendas AM, Llano E, et al. Molecular cloning of a novel membrane-type matrix metalloproteinase from a human breast carcinoma. Cancer Res 1996;56(5):944–949.

247. Daidone MG, Silvestrini R, D'Errico A, et al. Laminin receptors, collagenase IV and prognosis in node-negative breast cancers. Int J Cancer 1991;48(4):529–532.

248. Visscher DW, Hoyhtya M, Ottosen SK, et al. Enhanced expression of tissue inhibitor of metalloproteinase-2 (TIMP-2) in the stroma of breast carcinomas correlates with tumor recurrence. Int J Cancer 1994;59(3):339–344.

249. Leone A, Flatow U, King CR, et al. Reduced tumor incidence, metastatic potential, and cytokine responsiveness of nm23-transfected melanoma cells. Cell 1991;65(1):25–35.

250. Steeg PS, de la Rosa A, Flatow U, et al. Nm23 and breast cancer metastasis. Breast Cancer Res Treat 1993;25(2):175–187.

251. Sawan A, Lascu I, Veron M, et al. NDP-K/nm23 expression in human breast cancer in relation to relapse, survival, and other prognostic factors: an immunohistochemical study. J Pathol 1994;172(1):27–34.

252. Ishihara A, Yoshida T, Tamaki H, Sakakura T. Tenascin expression in cancer cells and stroma of human breast cancer and its prognostic significance. Clin Cancer Res 1995;1(9):1035–1041.

253. Horak ER, Leek R, Klenk N, et al. Angiogenesis, assessed by platelet/endothelial cell adhesion molecule antibodies, as indicator of node metastases and survival in breast cancer. Lancet 1992;340(8828):1120–1124.

254. Weidner N, Folkman J, Pozza F, et al. Tumor angiogenesis: A new significant and independent prognostic indicator in early-stage breast carcinoma. J Natl Cancer Inst 1992;84(24):1875–1887.

255. Bosari S, Lee AK, DeLellis RA, et al. Microvessel quantitation and prognosis in invasive breast carcinoma. Hum Pathol 1992;23(7):755–761.

256. Fox SB, Leek RD, Weekes MP, et al. Quantitation and prognostic value of breast cancer angiogenesis: Comparison of microvessel density, Chalkley count, and computer image analysis. J Pathol 1995;177(3):275–283.

257. Costello P, McCann A, Carney DN, Dervan PA. Prognostic significance of microvessel density in lymph node negative breast carcinoma. Hum Pathol 1995;26(11):1181–1184.

258. Goulding H, Abdul Rashid NF, Robertson JF, et al. Assessment of angiogenesis in breast carcinoma: An important factor in prognosis? Hum Pathol 1995;26(11):1196–1200.

259. Linderholm B, Andersson J, Lindh B, et al. Overexpression of c-erbB-2 is related to a higher expression of vascular endothelial growth factor (VEGF) and constitutes an independent prognostic factor in primary node-positive breast cancer after adjuvant systemic treatment. Eur J Cancer 2004;40(1):33–42.

260. Gasparini G, Toi M, Gion M, et al. Prognostic significance of vascular endothelial growth factor protein in node-negative breast carcinoma. J Natl Cancer Inst 1997;89(2):139–147.

261. Nakamura Y, Yasuoka H, Tsujimoto M, et al. Prognostic significance of vascular endothelial growth factor D in breast carcinoma with long-term follow-up. Clin Cancer Res 2003;9(2):716–721.

262. Linderholm BK, Lindh B, Beckman L, et al. Prognostic correlation of basic fibroblast growth factor and vascular endothelial growth factor in 1307 primary breast cancers. Clin Breast Cancer 2003;4(5):340–347.

263. Graubert TA, Ley TJ. How do lymphocytes kill tumor cells? Clin Cancer Res 1996;2(5):785–789.

264. Beerman H, Smit VT, Kluin PM, et al. Flow cytometric analysis of DNA stemline heterogeneity in primary and metastatic breast cancer. Cytometry 1991;12(2):147–154.

265. Fuhr JE, Frye A, Kattine AA, Van Meter S. Flow cytometric determination of breast tumor heterogeneity. Cancer 1991;67(5):1401–1405.

266. Ottesen GL, Christensen IJ, Larsen JK, et al. DNA aneuploidy in early breast cancer. Br J Cancer 1995;72(4):832–839.

267. Symmans WF, Liu J, Knowles DM, Inghirami G. Breast cancer heterogeneity: Evaluation of clonality in primary and metastatic lesions. Hum Pathol 1995;26(2):210–216.

268. Bonsing BA, Beerman H, Kuipers-Dijkshoorn N, et al. High levels of DNA index heterogeneity in advanced breast carcinomas. Evidence for DNA ploidy differences between lymphatic and hematogenous metastases. Cancer 1993;71(2):382–391.

269. Chen LC, Kurisu W, Ljung BM, et al. Heterogeneity for allelic loss in human breast cancer. J Natl Cancer Inst 1992;84(7):506–510.

270. Daidone MG, Silvestrini R, Valentinis B, et al. Proliferative activity of primary breast cancer and of synchronous lymph node metastases evaluated by (3H)-thymidine labelling index. Cell Tissue Kinet 1990;23(5):401–408.

271. Paradiso A, Mangia A, Barletta A, et al. Heterogeneity of intratumour proliferative activity in primary breast cancer: Biological and clinical aspects. Eur J Cancer 1995;31A(6):911–916.

272. Meyer JS, Wittliff JL. Regional heterogeneity in breast carcinoma: thymidine labelling index, steroid hormone receptors, DNA ploidy. Int J Cancer 1991;47(2):213–220.

273. Nesland JM, Ottestad L, Borresen AL, et al. The c-erbB-2 protein in primary and metastatic breast carcinomas. Ultrastruct Pathol 1991;15(3):281–289.

274. Theodorescu D, Cornil I, Sheehan C, et al. Dominance of metastatically competent cells in primary murine breast neoplasms is necessary for distant metastatic spread. Int J Cancer 1991;47(1):118–123.

275. Itaya T, Judde JG, Hunt B, Frost P. Genotypic and phenotypic evidence of clonal interactions in murine tumor cells. J Natl Cancer Inst 1989;81(9):664–668.

276. Kerbel RS. Growth dominance of the metastatic cancer cell: cellular and molecular aspects. Adv Cancer Res 1990;55:87–132.

277. Bonsing BA, Devilee P, Cleton-Jansen AM, et al. Evidence for limited molecular genetic heterogeneity as defined by allelotyping and clonal analysis in nine metastatic breast carcinomas. Cancer Res 1993;53(16):3804–3811.

278. Noguchi S, Motomura K, Inaji H, et al. Clonal analysis of predominantly intraductal carcinoma and precancerous lesions of the breast by means of polymerase chain reaction. Cancer Res 1994;54(7): 1849–1853.

279. Foekens JA, Rio MC, Seguin P, et al. Prediction of relapse and survival in breast cancer patients by pS2 protein status. Cancer Res 1990; 50(13):3832–3837.

280. Wright C, Nicholson S, Angus B, et al. Relationship between c-erbB-2 protein product expression and response to endocrine therapy in advanced breast cancer. Br J Cancer 1992;65(1):118–121.

281. Elledge RM, Lock-Lim S, Allred DC, et al. p53 Mutation and tamoxifen resistance in breast cancer. Clin Cancer Res 1995;1(10):1203–1208.

282. Allred DC, Swanson PE. Testing for erbB-2 by immunohistochemistry in breast cancer. Am J Clin Pathol 2000;113:171–175.

283. Roche PC, Ingle JN. Increased HER2 with U.S. Food and Drug Administration-approved antibody. J Clin Oncol 1999;17:434.

284. Hoang MP, Sahin A, Ordoñez NG, Sneige N. HER-2/neu gene amplification compared with HER-2/neu protein overexpression and interobserver reproducibility in invasive breast carcinoma. Am J Clin Pathol 2000;113:852–859.

285. Vogel CL, Cobleigh MA, Tripathy D, et al. Efficacy and safety of trastuzumab as a single agent in first-line treatment of HER2-overexpressing metastatic breast cancer. J Clin Oncol 2002;20(3):719–726.

286. Seidman AD, Fornier MN, Esteva FJ, et al. Weekly trastuzumab and paclitaxel therapy for metastatic breast cancer with analysis of efficacy by HER2 immunophenotype and gene amplification. J Clin Oncol 2001;19(10):2587–2595.

287. Fornier MN, Risio M, Van Poznak C. HER-2 testing and correlation with efficacy in trastuzumab therapy. Oncology 2003;16:1340–1358.

288. Lee JM, Bernstein A. p53 Mutations increase resistance to ionizing radiation. Proc Natl Acad Sci U S A 1993;90(12):5742–5746.

289. Gamel JW, Meyer JS, Province MA. Proliferative rate by S-phase measurement may affect cure of breast carcinoma. Cancer 1995;76(6): 1009–1018.

290. Hietanen P, Blomqvist C, Wasenius VM, et al. Do DNA ploidy and S-phase fraction in primary tumour predict the response to chemotherapy in metastatic breast cancer? Br J Cancer 1995;71(5):1029–1032.

291. Chevillard S, Pouillart P, Beldjord C, et al. Sequential assessment of multidrug resistance phenotype and measurement of S-phase fraction as predictive markers of breast cancer response to neoadjuvant chemotherapy. Cancer 1996;77(2):292–300.

292. Gusterson BA, Gelber RD, Goldhirsch A, et al. Prognostic importance of c-erbB-2 expression in breast cancer. International (Ludwig) Breast Cancer Study Group. J Clin Oncol 1992;10(7):1049–1056.

293. Lippman M, Weisenthal L, Paik S. erb-2 Positive specimens from previously untreated breast cancer patients have in-vitro drug resistance profiles which resemble profiles of specimens obtained from patients who have previously failed combination chemotherapy. Proc Am Soc Clin Oncol 1990;9:88–92.

294. Allred DC, Clark GM, Tandon AK, et al. HER-2/neu in node-negative breast cancer: Prognostic significance of overexpression influenced by the presence of in situ carcinoma. J Clin Oncol 1992;10(4):599–605.

295. Muss HB, Thor AD, Berry DA, et al. c-erbB-2 Expression and response to adjuvant therapy in women with node-positive early breast cancer. N Engl J Med 1994;330(18):1260–1266.

296. Yu D, Liu B, Tan M, Li J, et al. Overexpression of c-erbB-2/neu in breast cancer cells confers increased resistance to Taxol via mdr-1-independent mechanisms. Oncogene 1996;13(6):1359–1365.

297. Elledge RM, Gray R, Mansour E, et al. Accumulation of p53 protein as a possible predictor of response to adjuvant combination chemotherapy with cyclophosphamide, methotrexate, fluorouracil, and prednisone for breast cancer. J Natl Cancer Inst 1995;87(16):1254–1256.

298. Moll UM, Ostermeyer AG, Ahomadegbe JC, et al. p53 Mediated tumor cell response to chemotherapeutic DNA damage: A preliminary study in matched pairs of breast cancer biopsies. Hum Pathol 1995;26(12): 1293–1301.

299. McDonnell TJ, Meyn RE, Robertson LE. Implications of apoptotic cell death regulation in cancer therapy. Semin Cancer Biol 1995;6(1): 53–60.

300. Krajewski S, Blomqvist C, Franssila K, et al. Reduced expression of proapoptotic gene BAX is associated with poor response rates to combination chemotherapy and shorter survival in women with metastatic breast adenocarcinoma. Cancer Res 1995;55(19):4471–4478.

301. Bonadonna G, Valagussa P, Brambilla C, et al. Primary chemotherapy in operable breast cancer: Eight year experience at the Milan Cancer Institute. J Clin Oncol 1998;16:93–100.

302. Kuerer HM, Newman LA, Smith TL, et al. Clinical course of breast cancer patients with complete pathologic primary tumor and axillary lymph node response to doxorubicin-based neoadjuvant chemotherapy. J Clin Oncol 1999;17:460–469.

303. Ayers M, Symmans WF, Stec J, et al. Gene expression profiles predict complete pathologic response to neoadjuvant paclitaxel and fluorouracil, doxorubicin, and cyclophosphamide chemotherapy in breast cancer. J Clin Oncol 2004;22:2284–2293.

304. Rasbridge SA, Gillett CE, Seymour AM, et al. The effects of chemotherapy on morphology, cellular proliferation, apoptosis and oncoprotein expression in primary breast carcinoma. Br J Cancer 1994;70(2):335–341.

305. Daidone MG, Silvestrini R, Luisi A, et al. Changes in biological markers after primary chemotherapy for breast cancers. Int J Cancer 1995;61(3):301–305.

306. Fabian CJ, Zalles C, Kamel S, et al. Biomarker and cytologic abnormalities in women at high and low risk for breast cancer. J Cell Biochem Suppl 1993;17G:153–160.

307. Dhingra K, Vogel V, Sneige N, et al. Strategies for the application of biomarkers for risk assessment and efficacy in breast cancer chemoprevention trials. J Cell Biochem Suppl 1993;17G:37–43.

308. Hilsenbeck SG, Clark GM. Surrogate endpoints in chemoprevention of breast cancer: Guidelines for evaluation of new biomarkers. J Cell Biochem Suppl 1993;17G:205–211.

309. Dressler LG. DNA flow cytometry measurements as surrogate endpoints in chemoprevention trials: Clinical, biological, and quality control considerations. J Cell Biochem Suppl 1993;17G:212–218.

310. Mukai K, Schollmeyer JV, Rosai J. Immunohistochemical localization of actin: Applications in surgical pathology. Am J Surg Pathol 1981;5(1):91–97.

311. Ribeiro-Silva A, Zamzelli Ramalho LN, Garcia SB, Zucoloto S. Is p63 reliable in detecting microinvasion in ductal carcinoma in situ of the breast? Pathol Oncol Res 2003;9(1):20–23.

312. Damiani S, Ludvikova M, Tomasic G, et al. Myoepithelial cells and basal lamina in poorly differentiated in situ duct carcinoma of the breast. An immunocytochemical study. Virchows Arch 1999;434(3): 227–234.

313. Fisher B, Dignam J, Wolmark N, et al. Tamoxifen in treatment of intraductal breast cancer: National Surgical Adjuvant Breast and Bowel Project B-24 randomised controlled trial. Lancet 1999;353(9169): 1993–2000.

314. Yen TW, Hunt KK, Mirza NQ, et al. Physician recommendations regarding tamoxifen and patient utilization of tamoxifen after surgery for ductal carcinoma in situ. Cancer 2004;100(5):942–949.

315. Baqai T, Shousha S. Oestrogen receptor negativity as a marker for high-grade ductal carcinoma in situ of the breast. Histopathology 2003;42(5):440–447.

316. Bose S, Lesser ML, Norton L, Rosen PP. Immunophenotype of intraductal carcinoma. Arch Pathol Lab Med 1996;120(1):81–85.

317. Latta EK, Tjan S, Parkes RK, O'Malley FP. The role of HER2/neu overexpression/amplification in the progression of ductal carcinoma in situ to invasive carcinoma of the breast. Mod Pathol 2002;15(12): 1318–1325.

318. Eriksson ET, Schimmelpenning H, Aspenblad U, et al. Immunohistochemical expression of the mutant p53 protein and nuclear DNA content during the transition from benign to malignant breast disease. Hum Pathol 1994;25(11):1228–1233.

319. Ringberg A, Anagnostaki L, Anderson H, et al. Cell biological factors in ductal carcinoma in situ (DCIS) of the breast: Relationship to ipsilateral local recurrence and histopathological characteristics. Eur J Cancer 2001;37(12):1514–1522.

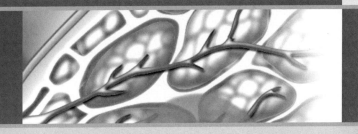

SECTION III

DIAGNOSIS

CHAPTER 13

Surveillance Strategy for Detection of Breast Cancer

Stephen A. Feig

Breast cancer screening, the periodic examination of women to detect previously unrecognized disease, has usually been performed by mammography, physical examination (PE), and breast self-examination (BSE), alone or in combination. By definition, a breast cancer screening test is performed only on women with no clinical abnormality to suggest breast cancer, although they may be at increased risk because of factors such as age, family history, or nulliparity. Requirements for a screening test differ from those for a diagnostic test and include adequate sensitivity to detect early disease, acceptable specificity to minimize false-positive examinations, low risk, and acceptable cost and cost-to-benefit ratio. Because the ultimate goal of screening is reduction in deaths from breast cancer, demonstration of a statistically significant reduction in breast cancer mortality in a randomized clinical trial (RCT) is considered the gold standard of success. Thus far, this result has been documented for mammography but not for PE or BSE alone.

BENEFIT FROM EARLY DETECTION

How effective are clinical examination, mammography, and other imaging tests?

Mammography, PE, and BSE are complementary: each should be capable of detecting cancers that are missed by one or both of the other modalities. However, smaller tumors with higher survival rates are more likely to be detected by mammography than PE or BSE.[1,2]

The Breast Cancer Detection Demonstration Project (BCDDP) screened 280,000 women throughout the United States with both mammography and PE from 1973 to 1981.[1] In this program, which was sponsored by the American Cancer Society (ACS) and National Cancer Institute (NCI), 39% of cancers were found by mammography alone, 7% by PE alone, and 51% by both mammography and PE. Detection at PE was lowest among earlier-stage lesions. BCDDP results indicated that mammography was the most sensitive means of early detection but that screening will be most effective when both modalities are used. Today, major improvements in mammography allow detection of even earlier lesions than was possible during the BCDDP era.[3] However, the relative efficacy of any detection method depends on the quality of the examination being performed.

Both ultrasound and magnetic resonance imaging (MRI) may detect some cancers missed by mammography and are currently under investigation to determine whether they might be effective as supplementary screening tests, especially in women at high risk and in those with dense breasts.[2] However, many questions regarding detection rates, false-positive biopsy results, costs, examination, and interpretation time need to be answered before ultrasound or MRI can be recommended for routine screening.

Digital mammography appears to have comparable sensitivity and specificity to conventional mammography. A large multicenter screening study of digital mammography is currently in progress to obtain a more precise comparison.[2]

Other modalities, such as thermography, which measures variation in breast temperature; light scanning (transillumination), which records transmission of light through the breast; and radionuclide scans, such as ^{99m}Tc sestamibi, should not be used for screening because they are much less effective than mammography in detecting very small lesions.

Why is decreased mortality a better measure of benefit than improved survival?

The 20-year survival rate for breast cancers detected at the BCDDP was 81%, substantially higher than the 20-year survival rate of 53% for breast cancers in the largely nonscreened U.S. population.[4] Although these results are impressive, there are several reasons why "improved" survival rates among women who volunteer to be screened do not necessarily establish benefit from screening. These include selection bias, lead-time bias, length bias, and interval cancers.[5]

Selection bias refers to the possibility that women who volunteer for screening differ from those who do not volunteer in ways that may affect their respective survival rates. Lead-time bias implies that screening may advance the date of detection but not alter the date of death from breast cancer. Length bias postulates that cancers detected at screening contain a disproportionate number of less aggressive lesions. Even if undetected, such cancers might never result in death. Finally, higher survival rates among screen-detected cancers may be negated by lower survival rates among faster-growing interval cancers that are undetected by mammography and surface clinically between screenings.

Considering these potential biases, benefit from screening cannot be proved by observation of improved survival rates. Rather, such proof requires prospective comparison of breast cancer death rates among study group women offered screening and control group women not offered screening in an RCT.

What are the results from randomized clinical trials?

Protocols and results for seven randomized trials of breast cancer screening by mammography alone or in combination with physical examination are shown in Table 13–1.[6–12] Among seven randomized screening trials, six have shown evidence of benefit. Breast cancer mortality reduction was statistically significant in each of three trials (Health Insurance Plan of Greater New York [HIP], Swedish Two-County, and Edinburgh) and in combined results from the Stockholm, Malmö, Östergötland, and Gothenburg, Sweden, trials, and marginally significant in the Gothenburg trial. Only one trial, the National Breast Screening Study of Canada (NBSS-2), failed to show any benefit for mammography. In that trial, women receiving annual mammography and physical examinations were compared with those being screened by physical examination alone.[10] Possible explanations for the NBSS-2 results include poor technical quality of mammography and a faulty protocol that allowed preferential allocation of women with advanced breast cancer into the study group.[13]

Why has screening of women aged 40 to 49 years been controversial?

Initial reports from the HIP trial found a difference in breast cancer death rates between study and control groups for women aged 50 years and older at entry that was apparent by year 4. Such a difference for women aged 40 to 49 years did not emerge until 7 to 8 years of follow-up. By 18 years of follow-up, the reduction in breast cancer deaths among study women aged 40 to 49 years at entry was 23%, the same as for those aged 50 to 64 years at entry. Yet even then, benefit for younger women was not statistically significant according to Shapiro and colleagues.[6] This lack of statistical significance was a consequence of the relatively smaller number of younger women enrolled and their lower breast cancer incidence. Despite these explanations, the HIP trial results led to controversy regarding screening women in their 40s.[5]

The fact that the data for women aged 50 to 59 years and for those aged 60 years and older at entry when analyzed separately also lacked statistical significance was largely ignored. Moreover, Chu and associates subsequently found a statistically significant mortality reduction of 24% for women aged 40 to 49 years at entry into the HIP trial.[14]

There were two reasons why some observers were still not convinced. First, the delay in benefit for younger women in the HIP trial was also seen in all subsequent RCTs. Second, statistically significant benefit for younger women was not seen in any other individual trial until 1997.

The controversy intensified in 1992 with publication of the 7-year follow-up report from the NBSS-1 trial that found no evidence of benefit from screening women aged 40 to 49 years.[15] There are several explanations for these disappointing

Table 13–1   Randomized Trials: Results for All Ages Combined

Trial (Dates)	Age at Entry (yr)	No. of Mammography Views	Mammography Frequency (mo)	Rounds (No.)	CBE	Follow-up (yr)	RR (95% CI)	Mortality Reduction (%)
HIP (1963–1969)	40–64	2	12	4	Annual	18	0.77 (0.61–0.97)	23*
Malmö (1976–1986)	45–69	1–2	18–24	5	None	12	0.81 (0.62–1.07)	19
Two-county: Kopparberg, Östergötland (1979–1988)	40–74	1	23–33	4	None	20	0.68 (0.59–0.80)	32*
Edinburgh (1979–1988)	45–64	1–2	24	4	Annual	14	0.71 (0.53–0.95)	29*
NBSS-2 (1980–1987)	50–59	2+ CBE versus CBE	12	5	Annual	13	1.02 (0.78–1.33)	−2
Stockholm (1981–1985)	40–64	1	28	2	None	8	0.80 (0.53–1.22)	20
Gothenburg (1982–1988)	40–59	2	18	4	None	14	0.77 (0.60–1.00)	23

*Statistically significant. Mortality reduction = 1 − RR.
CBE, clinical breast examination; CI, confidence interval; HIP, Health Insurance Plan of Greater New York; NBSS, Canadian National Breast Screening Study; RR, relative risk for death from breast cancer in study group/control group.
Data from references 6 to 12.

results. First, the technical quality of mammography was poor. During most of the trial, more than 50% of the mammograms were poor or completely unacceptable, even as assessed by the standards of the day.[13] Second, the randomization process through which women were assigned into study and control groups was flawed and may have allowed preferential allocation of women with breast masses into the study group. As a likely consequence, an excess of late-stage breast cancers was found in the study group compared with the control group.[13]

Is there now proof of benefit for screening women aged 40 to 49 years?

Beginning in 1993, several successive meta-analyses of combined data for multiple RCTs were performed to accrue a greater number of women-years of follow-up than possible from any one RCT alone. Although the earliest meta-analyses suggested little if any benefit, subsequent meta-analyses published in 1995 and 1996 based on longer-term follow-up showed a statistically significant mortality reduction of 24% for women aged 40 to 49 years at entry into the seven population-based RCTs[16–18] (Table 13–2). The most recent meta-analysis, published in 1997, found statistically significant mortality reductions among women invited to screening in their 40s: 18% for all eight RCTs (NBSS-1 included) and 29% for the five Swedish RCTs (see Table 13–2).[18] Thus, with increasing length of follow-up, successive meta-analyses have shown progressively greater and statistically significant mortality reductions from screening for women in their 40s.

Table 13–2 Most Recent Meta-analyses of Randomized Clinical Trials Showing Statistically Significant Mortality Reduction for Women Aged 40 to 49 Years

Trials	Follow-up (yr)	Mortality Reduction (%)
All eight trials*	10.5–18.0	18
Seven trials†	7.0–18.0	24
Five Swedish trials	11.4–15.2	29

*All eight trials: Health Insurance Plan of Greater New York (HIP), five Swedish trials (Two-County, Stockholm, Malmö, Gothenburg), Edinburgh, National Breast Screening Study of Canada (NBSS-1).
†Seven trials: all trials except NBSS-1.
Data from references 16 to 18.

Moreover, meta-analyses are no longer necessary because two other RCTs besides the HIP study[14] have now shown statistically significant mortality reductions for younger women: 45% for women who began screening at ages 39 to 49 years in the Gothenburg, Sweden, trial and 36% for women who began screening at ages 45 to 49 years in the Malmö, Sweden, trial[19,20] (Table 13–3).

Should women aged 75 years and older be screened?

The question of mammographic screening for elderly women is clinically relevant because there are almost 10 million women aged 75 years and older in the United States. The life expectancy for an average woman at age 75 is 12 years[21] and is even longer for those in good general health. Reduction in breast cancer mortality among women aged 50 years and older becomes apparent within 4 years from entry into randomized trials.[22] Therefore, older women have a long enough life expectancy to benefit from screening long before they might die from other causes. Strictly speaking, benefit from screening women aged 75 years and older has not been proved because this age group was not included in any RCT. Nevertheless, there is no biologic reason why early detection should not be effective for these women. Survival rates according to stage of disease are almost as high in older as in younger women. The detection sensitivity of mammography is higher in elderly women owing to their generally more fatty breast composition. Therefore, screening mammography should be performed on women aged 75 years and older if their general health and life expectancy are good.[2]

Why do randomized trials underestimate the benefit from screening?

There are several reasons why results from all RCTs have underestimated the benefit to an individual woman undergoing screening with modern mammography. These include (1) mammographic image quality below today's standards, (2) use of only one mammographic view per breast, (3) noncompliance of some study group women, (4) contamination of the control group, (5) excessively long screening intervals, and (6) inadequate number of screening rounds.

Table 13–3 Most Recent Follow-up of Randomized Clinical Trials Showing Statistically Significant Breast Cancer Mortality Reduction for Women Aged 40 to 49 Years

Trial (Dates)	Age at Entry (yr)	No. of Mammography Views	Mammography Frequency (mo)	Clinical Breast Examination	Follow-up (yr)	Mortality Decrease (%)
HIP (1963–1969)	40–49	2	12	Annual	18.0	24
Malmö, Sweden (1976–1990)	45–49	1–2	18–24	None	12.7	36
Gothenburg, Sweden (1982–1988)	39–49	2	18	None	12.0	45

HIP, Health Insurance Plan of Greater New York.
Data from references 14, 19, 20.

First, there have been many technical improvements in mammographic technique since the early 1980s when nearly all trials were conducted. Better image quality facilitates detection of early breast cancer.[3] Second, women in the RCTs were mostly screened with one view per breast. A two-views-per-breast examination, today's standard, has been shown to detect more cancers than are found using a mediolateral oblique (MLO) view alone.[23]

Two other reasons why RCTs underestimate the benefit from screening are that not all study group women accept the invitation to be screened (noncompliance), whereas some control group women obtain screening outside the trial (contamination). Yet, to avoid selection bias, an RCT must compare the breast cancer death rate among all study group women, both screened and unscreened, with that among all control group women, including those who are screened on their own initiative. Thus, both "noncompliance" of some study women and "contamination" of control group women reduce the calculated benefit from RCTs.

Fifth, randomized trials have also underestimated the potential benefit because screening intervals have been generally much longer than the annual intervals now recommended.[2] Numerous studies indicate that greater benefit should result from annual screening, especially for women in their 40s, in whom breast cancer growth rates are faster.[24-26] Based on a tumor growth rate model, Michelson calculated that annual screening would result in a 51% reduction in the rate of distant metastatic disease, compared with a 22% reduction at a screening interval of 2 years.[27]

Several investigators have used mathematical models of actual RCT data to calculate the benefit to an average woman who is screened every year and where results are not affected by noncompliance and contamination.[17,23,26] For example, based on an observed 45% reduction in breast cancer mortality among women aged 39 to 49 years offered screening every 18 months at the Gothenburg trial, Feig calculated that the mortality reduction could have been as high as 65% with annual screening at the observed 80% compliance rate and as high as 75% at a 100% compliance rate.[26]

Finally, the fact that no randomized trial had more than four or five screening rounds represents a sixth reason why such trials may underestimate the potential benefits from screening. Such relatively short trials limit the mortality reduction with estimates that can be made using standard methods of measurement. Screening needs to be performed not only frequently but also over much longer time periods in order to reach a steady state, when the greatest mortality reduction will be apparent. Using a new method of moving averages, Miettinen and colleagues calculated a 55% reduction in breast cancer deaths for women aged 55 to 69 years at entry into the Malmö Screening Trial.[28] This value was much higher than the 26% mortality reduction reported by Andersson and Nystrom, who had included data from before year 8, when benefit had not yet peaked, and from after year 11, when benefit was being diluted.[28]

What are the current screening mammography guidelines?

Less than 5% of all breast cancers occur before age 40 years and less than 0.3% before age 30 years, compared with 19%

for women aged 40 to 49 years. Therefore, screening mammography is not advised for most women until age 40 years. Screening in their 30s may be considered only for those very few women who are in an extremely high-risk group for developing breast cancer at an early age.[2]

The time between screenings can affect the benefits. Mounting evidence indicates that breast cancer in younger women has a shorter lead time than cancer in older women.[23,25,29] Lead time is the average time between actual detection at screening and clinical finding in the absence of screening. Accordingly, many major medical organizations now recommend that women aged 40 to 49 years be screened annually[2,25,30] (Table 13-4). This recommendation replaces the previous recommendation that women in this age group receive screening mammography every 1 to 2 years and is justified by the more rapid growth of breast tumors among younger women. Some individuals have suggested that the interval between screenings can be lengthened as a woman ages. Nevertheless, it is likely that even in older women, some faster-growing cancerous tumors will become clinically apparent between biennial screenings, reducing the screening benefit. Women and their physicians should be aware that the major reason for accepting a longer screening interval at any age is a presumed reduction in screening cost, but some consequent reduction in screening benefit will occur. Screening guidelines of major medical organizations and advocacy groups are also shown in Table 13-4.

How valid is the most recent screening controversy?

Based on results from randomized trials conducted over the past quarter of a century and involving more than 500,000 women, there has been consensus in the medical community in favor of screening mammography. In the face of such near-unanimous agreement, two recent articles by Gøtzsche and

Table 13-4 Current Screening Mammography Guidelines

Group (Date)	Screening Frequency 40–49 yr	Screening Frequency ≥50 yr
Government and Foundations		
American Cancer Society (2003)	1	1
National Cancer Institute (2002)	1–2	1–2
U.S. Preventive Services Task Force (2002)	1–2	1–2
Medical Specialty Societies		
American Academy of Family Physicians (2001)	No	1–2*
American College of Obstetricians and Gynecologists (2000)	1–2	1
American College of Preventive Medicine (1996)	No	1–2
American College of Radiology (1998)	1	1
Society of Breast Imaging (2000)	1	1
Advocacy Groups		
National Alliance of Breast Cancer Organizations (2002)	1	1
Susan B. Komen Foundation (2002)	1	1

*American Academy of Family Physicians does not recommend screening after age 70 years.

Olsen made the seemingly incredible claim that none of the trials provided any convincing evidence that screening prevents breast cancer deaths.[31,32] The Gøtzsche and Olsen papers received enormous publicity because of the sensational nature of their claim, which questioned the widely held belief in the efficacy of early detection. The arguments and counter-arguments are complex and have been summarized in detail elsewhere.[33,34] Fortunately, all of the conclusions reached by Gøtzsche and Olsen have been subsequently refuted in the peer review literature.

For example, Gøtzsche and Olsen suggested that the reductions in breast cancer death rates were due to age differences between study and control groups rather than the screening process itself. Gøtzsche and Olsen were unaware that when screening trials use cluster randomization rather than individual randomization, such relatively small age differences are not only expected but also acceptable.[34] In fact, after adjustment for age, mortality rates were only minimally different: 31% versus 30% for women aged 40 to 70 years, in the Swedish Two-County Trial, and 45% instead of 46% for women aged 39 to 49 years in the Gothenburg, Sweden, trial.[34,35] Thus, there was no way that these small differences in age could have altered the overall conclusion that screening results in a substantial reduction in deaths from breast cancer.

Gøtzsche and Olsen also jumped on the fact that no statistically significant decrease in death rates from all causes combined had yet been shown in any of the Swedish trials. This observation was interpreted by Gøtzsche and Olsen to mean that any benefit from reduction in breast cancer deaths would be countered by increased deaths from other causes. This incorrect conclusion disregarded the fact that breast cancer accounts for only about 5% of total mortality. Thus, even the largest individual trial would be unlikely to demonstrate any statistically significant decrease in all-cause mortality. On this issue too, Gøtzsche and Olsen were proven wrong. Subsequent to publication of the second Gøtzsche and Olsen paper, Nystrom and coworkers were in fact able to find a 2% decrease in all-cause mortality among study group women in five Swedish trials combined.[36] Additionally, Tabár and colleagues observed a significant 19% reduction in deaths from all causes among breast cancer cases in the group invited to screening in the Two-County trial.[37] Thus, the Gøtzsche and Olsen conjecture regarding all-cause mortality was incorrect.

Although the reports by Gøtzsche and Olsen received considerable publicity in the U.S. media, no medical organization or government has changed its screening policy on the basis of their conclusions. Indeed, after review of the Gøtzsche and Olsen papers, 10 leading medical organizations, including the American Academy of Family Physicians, American Cancer Society, American College of Obstetricians and Gynecologists, American College of Physicians–American Society of Internal Medicine, American College of Preventive Medicine, American Medical Association, Cancer Research Foundation of America, National Medical Association, Oncology Nursing Society, and the Society of Gynecologic Oncologists, reaffirmed their support of screening in a full-page public service announcement in the *New York Times* on January 31, 2002. Also, the National Cancer Institute and the U.S. Preventive Services Task Force concluded that despite the Gøtzsche and Olsen contentions, the results from randomized screening trials were still valid. Elsewhere, the Swedish National Board of Health and Welfare, the Danish National Board of Health,

the Health Council of the Netherlands, the European Institute of Oncology, and the World Health Organization dismissed the Gøtzsche and Olsen arguments and concluded that the evidence for benefit was convincing.[33,34]

Have breast cancer death rates been reduced by service screening in Scandinavia?

After the success of the Swedish randomized trials, organized service screening mammography became routine in nearly all Swedish counties by the 1990s. Unlike randomized trials, which are primarily conducted as clinical research studies, service screening is mainly performed as a public health initiative. Nevertheless, results from service screening projects have provided strong confirmation that screening mammography is effective in reducing breast cancer mortality.[38]

A recent study by Tabár and colleagues measured the effect of mammography in a population in whom service screening is offered to all women aged 40 years and older.[39] The authors compared breast cancer death rates in two Swedish counties over three periods of time: 1968 to 1977, when virtually no women were screened; 1978 to 1987, when half the population was offered screening in the RCT; and 1988 to 1996 after completion of the trial, when screening was offered to all women and 85% of the population was being screened.

When compared with breast cancer death rates among women aged 40 to 69 years in the prescreening era, breast cancer death rates in 1988 to 1996 were reduced 63% for screened women and 50% for the entire population (85% screened plus 15% nonscreened) (Table 13–5). During this time, reduction in death rates from breast cancer for screened women were similar to those for women screened during the trial, that is, 63% versus 57%. However, during the RCT trial period (1978 to 1987), only half of the population was offered screening. For that era, breast cancer death rate reduction in the entire population was only 21%.

It seems probable that screening, rather than advances in treatment, was responsible for nearly all the benefit. The relative risk for breast cancer death among nonscreened women age 40 to 69 years was similar (1.0, 1.7, and 1.19, respectively) during the three consecutive periods. Moreover, the breast cancer death rate for women aged 20 to 39 years, virtually none of whom were screened, showed no significant

Table 13–5 Reduction in Population Death Rates from Breast Cancer, Women Diagnosed Between Ages 40 and 69 Years in Two Swedish Counties*

Screening Status	1978–1987 Randomized Trial	1988–1996 Service Screening
Screened	57%	63%
Invited to screening	43%	48%
Screened plus nonscreened	21%	50%

*Time of diagnosis either 1978–1987 or 1988–1996, compared with death rates from cancers diagnosed during 1969–1977 before screening began. All results were statistically significant at 95% confidence interval.
Data from Tabär L, Vitak B, Chen H-H, et al. Beyond randomized controlled trials: Organized mammographic screening substantially reduces breast carcinoma mortality. Cancer 2001;91:1724–1731.

difference (1.0, 1.10, and 0.81, respectively) during these three consecutive periods.

Possibly, women who agree to be screened have selection bias factors that apart from the screening process improved their survival rates. Even assuming the maximum effect of selection bias, screening was shown to reduce breast cancer deaths by at least 50%.

A study by Duffy and associates assessed the effect of service screening in seven Swedish counties.[40] Among women aged 40 to 69 years, breast cancer mortality was reduced 44% for screened women and 39% for women offered screening compared with the prescreening era. Based on breast cancer mortality trends, it was estimated that only 12% of the mortality reduction was due to improved therapy and patient management apart from the screening process.

Results from these and other service screening studies in Sweden and Finland indicate that the reductions in breast cancer mortality found in the randomized trials can be obtained and exceeded in non–research-organized service screening settings.[38] These programs effectively refute the claim by Gøtzsche and Olsen that the benefits seen in the randomized screening trials were not real because of supposed flaws in randomization and ascertainment of cause of death.[33]

ADVERSE CONSEQUENCES AND COSTS OF SCREENING

The ability of screening mammography to substantially reduce breast cancer deaths is now well established and should no longer be subject to debate. Comparison of screening benefits with costs and adverse consequences, however, may reveal legitimate concerns. Such comparisons are discussed in the remainder of this chapter and can help determine when screening should begin and how often it should be performed. We must also seek ways to reduce these risks without reducing cancer detection rates.

Breast compression: can discomfort be avoided?

The benefits from breast compression include the ability to obtain better images at a lower radiation dose. Improvement in breast compression devices and techniques over the past 30 years have allowed higher cancer detection rates and more comfortable examinations.[3] When properly performed, mammography usually is not painful.[41] Following some simple recommendations can minimize discomfort. First, vigorous compression is not necessary; rather, the breast should be compressed only until the skin is taut. Compression should be applied gradually and gently. The patient should let the technologist know of any excessive discomfort so that no further compression will be applied. Patients who experience tenderness just before their menstrual periods may want to schedule mammography at some other time. In such cases, a mild analgesic before mammography may be helpful. It is important to minimize any discomfort from mammography so that women will not be reluctant to undergo periodic screening.

How often should screening patients be recalled for additional imaging?

When screening mammograms are "batch interpreted," the patient leaves the imaging center immediately after her standard two-views-per-breast screening mammogram is performed and checked for image quality by the technologist. The images are then placed on a rotating film viewer and interpreted in batches by a radiologist at some later time. Patients receive their results by mail. If mammographic findings indicate that supplementary views or sonography are needed, the patient is telephoned and asked to return another day.

Because batch reading is much more efficient and cost-effective than on-line interpretation, it is the only practical way to perform screening mammography at the current low reimbursement levels and high demand for screening. In contradistinction, on-line interpretation is necessary for diagnostic mammography because of the high percentage of abnormal studies and the need to tailor each examination to the patient's clinical problem.

Recall rates refer to the percentage of patients asked to return for additional imaging workup after batch interpretation of screening mammography. Batch interpretation can be performed successfully only if recall rates are maintained within acceptable limits. Recall rates that are too high cause patient inconvenience and anxiety as well as increasing the cost and reducing the efficiency of the screening process. If recall rates are too low, some subtle cancers may be missed, and some benign lesions may be subjected to biopsy unnecessarily because supplementary views and sonography were not performed.

On the basis of published reports of recall rates for well-conducted screening programs, the American College of Radiology recommends that recall rates be maintained at 10% or less.[42] The upper limit should probably be 7% or less for women who have had a recent previous mammogram. Hunt and colleagues found that recall rates for such women could be 30% lower than those for women having their initial mammogram.[43]

What are acceptable rates for false-positive biopsy results?

Excessive biopsies lead to anxiety and discomfort for the patient and also increase the cost of screening mammography. Positive predictive value (PPV) refers to the percentage of biopsies in which malignancy is found. The American College of Radiology recommends that the positive predictive value when biopsy is recommended (PPV_2) should be 25% to 40%.[42] PPV results will be affected by patient age, risk factors, and presence of clinical signs and symptoms. Results from several centers have found that the PPV_3 (number of cancers detected per number of biopsies performed) for screening women aged 40 to 49, 50 to 59, 60 to 69, and 70+ years are about 22%, 35%, 45%, and 50%, respectively.[44,45] Although the PPV is lower for women in the 40- to 49-year-old group, it is still acceptable. Complete imaging workup, including supplementary mammographic views and sonography; follow-up rather than biopsy for lesions that appear probably benign;

and second opinions for problematic cases can all reduce false-positive biopsy rates.

Is screen-detected ductal carcinoma in situ a real cancer?

Coincident with the increasing use of mammography has been a marked increase in the incidence of ductal carcinoma in situ (DCIS). Before the era of mammographic screening, DCIS represented less than 5% of all malignancies of the breast.[46] DCIS now accounts for 20% to 40% of all nonpalpable cancers detected at screening.[46] With appropriate treatment, the survival rate for patients with DCIS should be 99.5%.[46] DCIS may be considered a frequent but nonobligate precursor of fatal breast cancer. In other words, all cases of invasive ductal carcinoma are believed to develop from DCIS, but not all cases of DCIS may progress to invasive ductal carcinoma.

Justification for the use of DCIS as an index of benefit from screening depends on how often and how rapidly DCIS evolves into invasive ductal carcinoma. As of yet, no direct method exists for determining the natural progression of DCIS. If patients with DCIS were never to undergo biopsy and the DCIS were left to develop into invasive ductal carcinoma, there would be no way to establish that the initial lesion was DCIS. If DCIS is completely excised, then its natural history has been stopped, and there is no proof that it would have evolved into invasive ductal carcinoma.

Several follow-up studies of DCIS treated with biopsy alone also shed light on the invasive potential of DCIS. The lesions in these studies were categorized as benign at initial histologic review, so wide excision was not performed. In one study, researchers found development of invasive ductal carcinoma at the biopsy site in 53% of cases within 9.7 years.[46] Another study showed development of invasive ductal carcinoma in 28% of cases by 10 years and 36% of cases within 24 years.[46] Recurrence rates for DCIS in series such as these have suggested to some observers that DCIS is unlikely to progress to invasive disease.

There are two reasons why these studies should lead to just the opposite conclusion. First, these studies underestimate the invasive potential of DCIS because they involved only cases of low-grade DCIS, that is, all histologic subtypes of DCIS except for comedocarcinoma, the most aggressive subtype. Comedocarcinoma typically accounts for 32% to 50% of all cases of DCIS detected at mammographic screening.[46] Second, these studies included some cases in which the DCIS lesion was completely removed and other cases in which some DCIS remained in the breast when biopsy margins were not sufficiently wide. Invasive ductal carcinoma would be expected only in this latter subgroup.

Are detection rates too low and false-positive biopsy rates too high to justify screening women aged 40 to 49 years?

Women aged 40 to 49 years have a lower incidence of breast cancer, a faster rate of breast cancer growth, and a tendency to have denser, more fibroglandular breast tissue, for which mammography is less sensitive. As a consequence, screening detection rates for women in their 40s are somewhat lower than those for women in succeeding decades. Biopsy PPV is also lower for women in their 40s. However, both detection rates and PPVs for women aged 40 to 49 years are well within acceptable limits.

Some investigators have used inappropriate methods of comparison to suggest that detection rates are too low and false-positive rates too high to support screening women aged 40 to 49 years. Methods such as pooling data for women aged 40 to 49 years with data from younger women, pooling data for women aged 50 to 59 years with data from older women, and the exclusive use of data from the initial (prevalence) screening result in an inaccurate portrayal of screening outcomes for women in their 40s. Such improper assessment led Kerlikowske and colleagues to make the misleading statement that screening women younger than 50 years old will detect only 20% as many cancers per 1000 women screened, will require 4 times as many diagnostic procedures per cancer detected, and will cause 2.5 times as many false-positive biopsy results for each cancer detected, compared with screening older women.[47]

Proper assessment of the accuracy of screening mammography for women aged 40 to 49 years requires comparing data from that age group only with data for women aged 50 to 59 years. The use of data from initial (prevalence) screening alone may be misleading. The use of data from subsequent (incidence) screening alone is preferred, but combined data from prevalence and incidence screenings may also be used. Such an assessment will indicate that screening of women aged 40 to 49 years will detect at least 63% to 80% as many cancers, require 1.7 times as many diagnostic imaging procedures, and result in 1.3 to 1.4 times as many false-positive biopsy results for cancers detected[48] (Table 13–6).

What is the radiation risk from screening mammography?

Misperceptions regarding radiation risk from mammography persist even though no woman has ever been shown to have developed breast cancer as a result of mammography, not even from multiple examinations over many years' time at doses much higher than the current dose of 0.40 rad (0.004 Gy) for a two-view-per-breast examination. Such concern is based on the observation that some groups of women, such as Japanese atomic bomb survivors and North American women given radiation therapy for benign breast conditions such as postpartum mastitis or monitored with multiple chest fluoroscopies during treatment for tuberculosis before 1940, were found to be at increased risk for breast cancer.[49] Among these women, excess risk was observed for doses from 100 to more than 1000 rad (1 to 10 Gy).

The hypothetical risk for mammography is based on a linear extrapolation from these high-dose studies. If there is any risk from mammography, it is extremely low and is lowest for those who are exposed at ages older than 35 years. The current mean breast dose of 0.4 rad (0.004 Gy) from mammography is markedly less than the mean glandular dose of 3.2 rad (0.032 Gy) from the mammography film systems that were used at most facilities until 1973.[49]

Screening benefits can be compared with radiation risks. On the basis of results from screening trials, we know that

Table 13–6   Relative Benefits and Risks of Screening According to Age Groups Being Compared

	Age Groups Being Compared (yr)	
	30–49 vs. 50–69*	40–49 vs. 50–59†
Detection rates	20%	63%–80%
Diagnostic procedures per cancer detected	4×	1.7×
False-positive biopsy results per cancer detected	2.5×	1.3–1.4×

*Prevalent screen data.
†Prevalent and incident screen data.
Data from Feig SA. Age-related accuracy of screening mammography: How should it be measured? Radiology 2000;214:633–640.

Table 13–7   Detection Benefits and Radiation Risks from Annual Screening Mammography of 1,000,000 Women Aged 40 to 74 Years

Parameter	No. of Women
Lives saved	18,900
Possible deaths caused	21.6
Benefit-to-risk ratio	875 : 1
Net benefit in lives	18,878

Data from Feig SA. Risk, benefit and controversies in mammographic screening. In Haus AG, Yaffe MJ (eds). Physical Aspects of Breast Imaging: Current and Future Considerations. 1999 Syllabus, Categorical Courses in Radiology Physics. Oak Brook, IL, Radiological Society of North America, 1999, pp 99–108.

Table 13–8   Median Cost Per Life-Year Saved for Annual Mammographic Screening of Women Aged 40 to 79 Years and Other Selected Types of Lifesaving Interventions

Intervention	Median Cost per Year of Life Saved ($)
Colorectal screening	3000
Cholesterol screening	6000
Cervical cancer screening	12,000
Antihypertensive drugs	15,000
Osteoporosis screening	18,000
Mammography screening	18,800
Coronary artery bypass surgery	26,000
Automobile seat belts and air bags	32,000
Hormone replacement therapy	42,000
Renal dialysis	46,000
Heart transplantation	54,000
Cholesterol treatment	154,000

Data on nonmammographic interventions from Tengs TO, Adams M, Pliskin J, et al. Five hundred life-saving interventions and their cost-effectiveness. Risk Anal 1995;15:369–390; data on cost-effectiveness estimate for screening mammography from Rosenquist CJ, Lindfors KK. Screening mammography beginning at age 40 years: A reappraisal of cost-effectiveness. Cancer 1998;82:2235–2240.

annual screening can reduce deaths from breast cancer detected among women aged 40 to 49 years by at least 35% and deaths from breast cancer detected among women at 50 and older by at least 46%.[50] Possible deaths from radiation exposure from mammography can be estimated using a linear relative risk extrapolation of risk found among populations that received extremely high doses. Calculations based on these assumptions indicate that 18,900 deaths from breast cancer can be averted when 1,000,000 women are screened annually from age 40 years until age 74 years, and that at most 21.6 excess deaths might be caused by radiation (Table 13–7). Thus, even if there is a risk from multiple mammographic examinations at a dose of 0.4 rad (0.004 Gy) each, the benefit from annual screening for women aged 40 years onward exceeds that theoretical risk by at least 875 : 1.[50]

Is screening mammography cost-effective?

The cost-effectiveness of screening mammography can be calculated based on the mortality reduction observed in the Swedish screening trials and current costs of screening in the United States. A recent study estimated that annual screening mammography beginning at age 40 years and continuing until age 79 years would cost $18,800 per year of life expectancy saved.[51] This estimate for the cost-effectiveness of screening mammography is in the same general range of other commonly accepted interventions such as screening for cervical cancer and osteoporosis[52] (Table 13–8). The cost per year of life gained from annual screening mammography is higher than that for screening for colorectal cancer but is much lower than that for the use of seat belts and air bags in automobiles.

Although the cost per year of life gained for screening mammography is less than that for renal dialysis or heart transplantation, these interventions are needed for only a tiny fraction of the population. Because screening mammography is advised for all women aged 40 years and older, its total program cost must also be considered. In the United States, 62.6 million women are 40 to 89 years of age. If every one of these women obtained an annual screening mammogram at a cost of $90, the total cost would come to $5.6 billion per year. The total annual cost for all U.S. health care expenditures, however, is even more staggering: $1.3 trillion for the year 2000. Thus, even if every woman 40 to 89 years of age obtained an annual mammogram, the total cost would be only 0.43% of the national expenditure on health care. At present, 59% of all U.S. women aged 40 to 89 years report having had a screening mammogram in the past year. At this compliance rate, screening mammography at a cost of $90 would account for 0.25% of all U.S. health care expenditures.[53]

This year, 192,200 women in the United States will develop breast cancer, and 40,200 women will die from previously diagnosed breast cancer. It is often stated that when women living to age 85 years are included, 1 of every 8 U.S. women will eventually develop breast cancer during her lifetime. Because of screening mammography and early treatment, most women who develop breast cancer today will not die from their disease. Breast cancer, although the most common cancer among women and the second-most common cause of cancer death among women, accounts for only 3.9% of all causes of death among women in the United States.[53] Nevertheless, allocation of 0.4% of all national health expenditures (or about 0.8% of all national health expenditures for women) to substantially reduce the death rate from a disease that accounts for 3.9% of all deaths among women would seem to be a reasonable policy.

Moreover, early detection will also reduce other health care expenditures, including treatment of advanced primary cancers, diagnosis and treatment of distant metastases or recurrent disease, loss of work productivity, short-term disability, long-term disability, and terminal care costs.

REFERENCES

1. Seidman H, Gelb SK, Stilverberg E, et al. Survival experience in the breast cancer detection demonstration project. CA Cancer J Clin 1987;37:258–290.
2. Smith RA, Saslow D, Sawyer KA, et al. American Cancer Society guidelines for breast cancer screening: Update 2003. CA Cancer J Clin 2003;53:141–169.
3. Feig SA. Screening mammography: Effect of image quality on clinical outcome. AJR Am J Roentgenol 2002;178:805–807.
4. Smart CR, Byrne C, Smith RA, et al. Twenty-year follow-up of the breast cancers diagnosed during the Breast Cancer Detection Demonstration Project. CA Cancer J Clin 1997;47:134–149.
5. Feig SA. Methods to identify benefit from mammographic screening. Radiology 1996;201:309–316.
6. Shapiro S, Venet W, Strax P, et al. Periodic Screening for Breast Cancer: The Health Insurance Plan Project and Its Sequelae, 1963–1986. Baltimore, Johns Hopkins University Press, 1988.
7. Andersson I, Aspegren K, Janzon L, et al. Mammographic screening and mortality from breast cancer: The Malmö Mammographic Screening Trial. BMJ 1998;297:943–948
8. Tabar L, Vitak B, Chen H-H, et al. The Swedish Two-County trial twenty years later. Radiol Clin North Am 2000;38:625–652.
9. Alexander FE, Anderson TJ, Brown HK, et al. 14 Years of follow-up from Edinburgh randomized trial of breast cancer screening. Lancet 1999;353:1903–1908.
10. Miller AB, To T, Baines CJ, Wall C. Canadian National Breast Screening Study—2: 13–Year results of a randomized trial in women aged 50–59 years. J Natl Cancer Inst 2000;92:1490–1499.
11. Frisell J, Lidbrink E, Hellstrom L, Rutqvist LE. Follow-up after 11 years: Update of mortality results in the Stockholm mammographic screening trial. Breast Cancer Res Treat 1997;45:263–270.
12. Bjurstam N, Bjorneld L, Warwick J, et al. The Gothenburg Breast Screening Trial. Cancer 2001;97:2387–2396.
13. Kopans DB, Feig SA. The Canadian National Breast Screening Study: A critical review. AJR Am J Roentgenol 1993;161:755–760.
14. Chu KC, Smart CR, Tarone RE. Analysis of breast cancer mortality and stage distribution by age for the Health Insurance Plan clinical trial. J Natl Cancer Inst 1998;80:1125–1132.
15. Miller AB, Baines CJ, To T, et al. Canadian National Breast Screening Study. I. Breast cancer detection and death rates among women aged 40–49 years. CMAJ 1992;147:1477–1488.
16. Smart CR, Hendrick RE, Rutledge JH III, et al. Benefit of mammography screening in women ages 40–49 years: Current evidence from randomized controlled trials. Cancer 1995;75:1619–1626 [erratum appears in Cancer 1995;75:2788].
17. Falun Meeting Committee and Collaborators. Falun meeting on breast cancer screening with mammography in women aged 40–49 years: Report of the organizing committee and collaborators. Int J Cancer 1996;68:693–699.
18. Hendrick RE, Smith RA, Rutledge JH III, et al. Benefit of screening mammography in women aged 40–49: A new meta-analysis of randomized controlled trials. Monogr Natl Cancer Inst 1997;33:87–92.
19. Andersson I, Janzon L. Reduced breast cancer mortality in women under 50: Updated results from the Malmö Mammographic Screening Program. Monogr Natl Cancer Inst 1997;22:63–68.
20. Bjurstam N, Bjorneld L, Duffy SW. The Gothenburg Breast Screening Trial: First results on mortality, incidence, and mode of detection for women ages 39–49 years at randomization. Cancer 1997;20:2091–2099.
21. U.S. Bureau of the Census: Statistical Abstract of the United States, 204th ed. Washington DC, U.S. Government Printing Office, 2004.
22. Feig SA. Mammographic screening of elderly women. JAMA 1996;276: 446.
23. Feig SA. Estimation of currently attainable benefit from mammographic screening of women aged 40–49 years. Cancer 1995;75:2412–2419.
24. Feig SA. Determination of mammographic screening intervals with surrogate measures for women aged 40–49 years. Radiology 1994;193: 311–314.
25. Feig SA, D'Orsi CJ, Hendrick RE, et al. American College of Radiology Guidelines for Breast Cancer Screening. AJR Am J Roentgenol 1998;171:29–33.
26. Feig SA. Increased benefit from shorter screening mammography intervals for women ages 40–49 years. Cancer 1997;80:2035–2039.
27. Michaelson JS, Halpern E. Kopans DB. Breast cancer computer simulation method for estimation of optimal intervals for screening. Radiology 1999;212:551–560.
28. Miettinen OS, Henschke CI, Pasmantier MW, et al. Mammographic screening: No reliable supporting evidence? Lancet 2002;359:404–406.
29. Duffy SW, Day NE, Tabar L, et al. Markov models of breast tumor progression: Some age-specific results. Monogr Natl Cancer Inst 1997;22: 93–98.
30. Council on Scientific Affairs. Mammography screening for asymptomatic women: Report No. 16. Chicago, American Medical Association, 1999.
31. Gøtzsche PC, Olsen O. Is screening for breast cancer with mammography justifiable? Lancet 2000;355:129–134.
32. Olsen O, Gøtzsche PC. Cochrane review on screening for breast cancer with mammography. Lancet 2001;358:1340–1342.
33. Feig SA. How reliable is the evidence for screening mammography? Recent Results Cancer Res 2003;163:129–139.
34. Duffy SW. Interpretation of the breast screening trials: A commentary on the recent paper by Gøtzsche and Olsen. Breast 2001;10:209–212.
35. Bjurstam N, Bjorneld L, Dufy SW, Prevost TC. The Gothenburg Breast Screening Trial (authors' reply). Cancer 1998;83:188–190.
36. Nystrom L, Andersson, I, Bjurstam N, et al. Long-term effects of mammography screening: Updated overview of the Swedish randomized trials. Lancet 2002;359:909–919.
37. Tabar L, Duffy SW, Warwick J, et al. All cause mortality among breast cancer patients in a screening trial: Support for breast cancer mortality as an endpoint. J Med Screening 2002;9:159–162.
38. Feig SA. Effect of service screening mammography on population mortality from breast carcinoma. Cancer 2002;95:451–457.
39. Tabar L, Vitak B, Chen H-H, et al. Beyond randomized controlled trials: Organized mammographic screening substantially reduces breast carcinoma mortality. Cancer 2001;91:1724–1731.
40. Duffy SW, Tabar L, Chen H-H, et al. The impact of organized mammography service screening on breast cancer mortality in seven Swedish counties: A collaborative evaluation. Cancer 2002;95:458–469.
41. Stomper PC, Kopans DB, Sadowsky NL, et al. Is mammography painful? A multicenter patient study. Arch Intern Med 1988;148: 521–524.
42. D'Orsi CJ, Bassett LW, Berg W, et al. Breast Imaging Reporting and Data System: Mammography, 4th ed. Reston, VA, American College of Radiology, 2003, p 234.
43. Hunt KA, Rosen EL, Sickles EA. Outcome analysis for women undergoing annual versus biennial screening mammography: A review of 24,211 examinations. AJR Am J Roentgenol 1999;173:285–289.
44. Kopans DB, Moore RH, McCarthy KA, et al. Positive predictive value of breast biopsy performed as a result of mammography: There is no abrupt change at age 50 years. Radiology 1996;200:357–360.

45. Sickles EA. Auditing your practice. In Kopans DB, Mendelson EB (eds). Syllabus: A Categorical Course in Breast Imaging. Oak Brook, IL, Radiological Society of North America, 1995, pp 81–91.

46. Feig SA. Ductal carcinoma in situ: Implications for screening mammography. Radiol Clin North Am 2000;38:653–668.

47. Kerlikowske K, Grady D, Barclay J, et al. Positive predictive value of screening mammography by age and family history of breast cancer. JAMA 1993;270:2444–2450.

48. Feig SA. Age-related accuracy of screening mammography: How should it be measured? Radiology 2000;214:633–640.

49. Feig SA, Hendrick RE. Radiation risk from screening mammography of women aged 40–49 years. Monogr Natl Cancer Inst 1997;22:119–124.

50. Feig SA. Risk, benefit and controversies in mammographic screening. In: Haus AG, Yaffe MJ (eds). Physical Aspects of Breast Imaging: Current and Future Considerations. 1999 Syllabus, Categorical Courses in Radiology Physics. Oak Brook, IL, Radiological Society of North America, 1999, pp 99–108.

51. Rosenquist CJ, Lindfors KK. Screening mammography beginning at age 40 years: A reappraisal of cost-effectiveness. Cancer 1998;82:2235–2240.

52. Tengs TO, Adams M, Pliskin J, et al. Five hundred life-saving interventions and their cost-effectiveness. Risk Anal 1995;15:369–390.

53. Feig SA. Projected benefits and national health care costs from screening mammography. Semin Breast Dis 2001;4:62–67.

CHAPTER 14

Clinical Assessment of Breast Cancer and Benign Breast Disease

Matthew N. Harris

Breast cancer ranks highest among women's health concerns, and the incidence rates are highest in industrialized nations such as the United States, Australia, and countries in Western Europe.[1,2] The incidence of breast cancer increased in many countries during the 20th century, largely reflecting global changes in reproductive patterns and regional increases in mammography.[3] In spite of this, many women have rarely if ever had a mammogram or physical examination of their breasts. Breast cancer is a progressive disease, and small tumors are more likely to be at an early stage, have a better prognosis, and are more successfully treated.[4]

ASSESSMENT OF BREAST CANCER

What are the reasons for patient delay in seeking medical attention for breast problems?

Delay in seeking medical attention falls into three general categories: (1) economic, (2) ignorance, and (3) psychological. First, the costs of medical attention are significant for the poor, those with inadequate insurance coverage, and those with other financial obligations.[5] Second, many older women were not taught to recognize the significance of a breast mass or other presenting symptoms. There is a notion that as long as pain is not present, there is no problem. Third, an in-depth study of the psychological reasons for patient delay in diagnosis by Gold[6] identified six psychological causes: (1) fear of cancer, mutilation, or a change in the relationship with the husband; (2) shyness or false modesty regarding examination of the breast; (3) negativism—some women raised in a hostile environment may become introverted and delay attention until the process is advanced; (4) depression causing the woman to ignore her health; (5) compulsion toward another goal so that all other aspects of life are ignored; (6) lack of breast tactility. In Gold's study, 47% of women never experienced emotional sensations associated with their breasts and tended to ignore them and therefore were not likely to discover an abnormality.

The fact that a patient consults a physician concerning breast disease may suggest knowledge about the importance of early detection, but it may also reflect a situation of "desperation" after a long period of procrastination, doubt, and misunderstanding.

What are the essential components of the clinical history?

The physician must bear in mind that the patient may be very anxious and that much can be done to allay apprehension. It is advantageous to have a second person present to participate and lend moral support. The patient may not hear or understand the discussion both before and after the physical examination. Although the patient or her partner often requests to take notes, it should be discouraged during the initial interview and can be reserved for the postexamination discussion.

In many instances, an anxious patient will volunteer information quickly and without pause. The patient should be asked to listen to the questions and answer them individually. If at the end of the interview all of the details of the history have not been covered, additional information can be added.

The physician must be discreet at all times during the interview, and patients must be informed of their Protected Health Information (PHI).[7] Certain questions may embarrass the patient in front of her partner or significant other, and these questions can be reserved for the more private setting of the examining room. This is particularly important when dealing with younger women who have been accompanied to the interview by a parent. One cannot predict the relationship between patient and parent; if this relationship is open and is made known to the physician, a full discussion can be carried out without hesitation. Records of previous examinations and consultations, prior biopsy results, mammograms, and other pertinent data should be available at the time of the initial examination.

When a physician is asked to provide a second opinion, it is preferable that the physician review the history with the patient without the prior discussion or conclusion revealed, so that an unprejudiced decision can be made. At the end of the consultation, the previous opinion can be critically reviewed, and the patient will have confidence that she has received a truly independent opinion.

The interview is opened with a personal greeting, and the patient who has not been referred by a physician is asked the source of the referral. Not uncommonly, this is another patient, and a sense of rapport rapidly develops between patient and physician.

The chief complaint is often a "lump in the breast." The history regarding a "lump" should include the date of onset or the date of detection, whether it is tender, and whether the patient conducts self-examinations and at what frequency. A careful history may help differentiate between the acute onset of a cyst of the breast and a mass of a more chronic nature, more likely a solid tumor, whether benign or malignant. Skin retraction, often a sign of a neoplasm, may be extremely subtle, but certainly the patient should be asked if she has noted any such changes.

If the complaints are nonspecific, the patient is questioned about whether she has a mass, any nipple discharge, and a history of injury to her breasts. The patient is asked whether she has had previous breast surgery and what the findings were. Tenderness and pain in the breast are the second most common complaints, and these may or may not be associated with a mass or what is perceived as a mass by the patient or her referring physician. The duration of symptoms should be recorded, as should whether the patient has sought other opinions in the past for a similar or the same problem.

Menstrual history is important and should include the age at menarche, the regularity of the menstrual cycle, and the date of the most recent menstrual period. The time of the menstrual cycle may be reflected in breast changes and may influence the findings on physical examination. Menstrual history should include the date of onset of menopause. Frequently, this is a protracted period of time, and the patient notes "irregularity" consistent with early menopausal changes. In addition, she may describe symptoms of menopause such as "hot flushes," dyspareunia, and irritability.

Both age at menarche and age at menopause are related to a woman's chance of developing breast cancer. Early menarche and late menopause lead to an increased total lifetime number of menstrual cycles and a corresponding 30% to 50% increase in breast cancer risk.[8] Conversely, late menarche and early menopause lead to reduction in breast cancer risk of a similar magnitude. Oophorectomy before a woman reaches menopause lowers her risk for breast cancer by about two thirds. Pregnancy at a young age, especially before 20 years of age, markedly reduces the incidence of subsequent breast cancer. Nulliparity and age older than 30 years at first live birth are associated with nearly a doubling of the risk for subsequent breast cancer. Pregnancies not ending in the birth of a viable fetus do not reduce the risk for breast cancer. A nursing history should be obtained as well, although it may have little impact on breast cancer risk.

Nipple discharge, although relatively common and usually benign in origin, is often frightening. Evaluation of the patient with nipple discharge should begin with a thorough history. It is important to differentiate spontaneous from induced discharge, single duct from multiple duct discharge, and unilateral from bilateral discharge. The character of the discharge should be categorized as potentially related to a neoplasm (serous, serosanguineous, bloody, or watery) or probably benign (various shades of green, gray, or brown).

What are the relevant issues related to the patient's history of hormonal therapy?

The patient is questioned on the use of hormones, both parenterally and by suppository, and the use of oral contraceptives. The type of hormone and the reason it is being taken are important.

The Women's Health Initiative, in a large multi-institutional study, enrolled more than 16,000 postmenopausal women aged 50 to 79 years to prospectively assess the risks and benefits of hormone replacement therapy using the most commonly prescribed form of estrogen plus progestin or estrogen alone.[9] In July 2002, the National Institutes of Health suddenly halted the estrogen plus progestin arm of the study because interim analysis of the data indicated that the risks of continued hormone replacement therapy outweighed the benefits. In addition to the expected increase in the risk for stroke, women in the study arm also showed an unexpected increase in the risk for coronary disease. Of relevance here as well, this large randomized prospective study demonstrated a 26% increase in the risk for breast cancer over a 5-year period. The study indicates that an increased risk for breast cancer is only in current or recent users of hormone replacement therapy. Of known users who stopped hormone replacement therapy more than 5 years previously, the risk was no greater than in someone who had never used it.

Olsson and associates,[10] in a study from Sweden, reported that longer use of hormone replacement therapy containing progestins significantly elevates breast cancer risks, whereas hormonal therapy containing estradiol does not.

In a randomized trial conducted by Chlebowski and associates on the influence of estrogen plus progestin on breast cancer and mammography in healthy postmenopausal women, 16,608 postmenopausal women aged 50 to 79 years with an intact uterus were randomly assigned to receive conjugated equine estrogens plus medroxyprogesterone acetate or placebo.[11] Significantly, relatively short-term combined estrogen plus progestin use increased the incident breast cancers, which were diagnosed at a more advanced stage, compared with placebo use, and also substantially increased the percentage of women with abnormal mammograms. The results suggest that estrogen plus progestin may stimulate breast cancer growth and hinder breast cancer diagnosis.

Additional data presented by Li and associates on the relationship between long durations and different regimens of hormone therapy and the risk for breast cancer concluded that the use of combined estrogen and progestin hormone replacement is associated with an increased risk for breast cancer, particularly invasive lobular carcinomas, whether the progestin component was taken in a sequential or a continuous manner.[12] Of interest is the fact that women using unopposed estrogen replacement therapy even for 25 years or longer have no appreciable increase in the risk for breast cancer, although the associated odds and ratios were not inconsistent with a possible small effect. The increase in risk is greater in those using combination hormone replacement therapy for longer durations (uses for 5 to 14.9 years), and those who used combination hormone replacement therapy for more than 15 years had a 1.5-fold increased risk for invasive ductal carcinoma and a 3.7-fold increase in the risk for invasive lobular carcinoma.

Postmenopausal women have a greater risk than men of developing Alzheimer's disease. The use of estrogen plus progestin and the incidence of dementia and mild cognitive impairment in 4532 postmenopausal women was evaluated as part of the Women's Health Initiative memory study in a randomized controlled trial by Schumaker and associates.[13] In this well-controlled study, it was concluded that estrogen plus progestin therapy increased the risk for probable dementia in women aged 65 years or older. In addition, estrogen plus progestin therapy did not prevent mild cognitive impairment in these women. The data support the conclusion that the risks of estrogen plus progestin outweigh the benefits.

In another study from the Women's Health Initiative, a randomized trial was conducted by Wassertheil-Smoller and associates concerning the effect of estrogen plus progestin on stroke in postmenopausal women.[14] This study, involving 16,608 women aged 50 to 79 years, with an average follow-up of 5.6 years, concluded that estrogen plus progestin increased the risk for ischemic stroke in generally healthy postmenopausal women. Excess risk for all strokes attributed to estrogen plus progestin appeared to be present in all subgroups of women examined.

Rapp and associates,[15] as part of the Women's Health Initiative memory study, conducted a randomized controlled trial of the effect of estrogen plus progestin on global cognitive function in postmenopausal women. They, too, found that although most women receiving estrogen plus progestin did not experience a clinically relevant adverse effect on cognition compared with placebo, a small increased risk for clinically meaningful cognitive decline occurred in the estrogen plus progestin group.

Clinically, hormone replacement therapy may cause swelling and tenderness of the breasts as well as increased density on mammography. Benign breast problems such as cysts are uncommon after menopause in the absence of exogenous hormones. Signs and symptoms include breast pain, a change in the size and shape of the breast, nipple discharge, and changes in the appearance of the skin.

What questions related to family history are relevant?

A family history of breast cancer is of great importance because heredity is a major risk factor.[16–18] About 7% of breast cancers and 10% of ovarian cancers are thought to be associated with an autosomal dominant pattern of inheritance. Two high-penetrance breast cancer susceptibility genes, BRCA1 and BRCA2, have been identified as accounting for most (about 85%) hereditary breast cancers. Mutations in these two genes are also responsible for most hereditary ovarian cancers, with 70% attributed to BRCA1 and 20% to BRCA2.[19–24] Genetic testing may be an important risk-assessment tool for patients whose family histories include multiple or early-onset breast or ovarian cancers. The BRCA mutations are also associated with an increased risk for prostate, pancreatic, and male breast cancer, although the risk for these is still small compared with breast and ovarian cancer. Hereditary risk for breast or ovarian cancer should be considered when there is early-onset breast cancer (usually before age 50 years) or

ovarian cancer, especially in more than one family member. Therefore, any woman diagnosed with breast cancer before age 50 years or with ovarian cancer at any age should be asked about first-, second-, and third-degree relatives on either side of the family with either of these diagnoses. In addition, the threshold for genetic testing should be lower in individuals who are members of ethnic groups in which BRCA mutations are known to be more prevalent, such as those of Ashkenazi Jewish descent. The patient's ethnicity may also influence her decision to have BRCA testing. For the near future, precisely estimating an individual woman's absolute risk for breast cancer must mainly rest on reproductive, family, and clinical history as well as genetic testing as detailed in Chapters 2 and 20.

The American Society of Clinical Oncology (ASCO) recommends that cancer predisposition testing be done to search for mutations of the BRCA1 and BRCA2 genes when (1) the patient has a strong family history of cancer or very early onset of disease, (2) the tests can be adequately interpreted, and (3) the results will influence the medical management of the patient or family member.[25] Genetic testing for breast and ovarian cancer susceptibility should be performed only with the individual's fully informed consent. Pretest and post-test counseling are important components of genetic testing, and genetic testing should be preceded by appropriate pretest and post-test follow-up care. Counseling should include a discussion of the risk to relatives as well as the availability and success of risk-reducing options such as surveillance, prophylactic mastectomy, prophylactic bilateral salpingo-oophorectomy, or risk-reducing drug therapy.

The recommended surveillance for patients with hereditary breast-ovarian cancer mutations includes breast self-examination (BSE) starting at age 18 years, semiannual breast examinations by a physician starting at age 20 years, annual mammography starting at age 25 years, and transvaginal ultrasound, Doppler color-flow imaging, and CA-125 testing annually after age 30 years.

What are the risks with a past history of treatment for Hodgkin's disease?

Prior treatment for Hodgkin's disease is a known risk factor for a second malignancy. A study by Ng and Mauch from the Brigham and Women's Hospital and Dana-Farber Cancer Institute in Boston indicated that survivors of Hodgkin's disease have a 4.6-fold increased risk for developing a second malignancy compared with the general population.[26] The effect of age and Hodgkin's disease diagnosis on subsequent cancer risk was most pronounced for breast cancer, and the relative risk for breast cancer was significantly increased in women diagnosed with Hodgkin's disease when younger than 30 years. The increased risk for breast cancer was of borderline significance in women diagnosed between 30 and 35 years of age. After age 35 years, the risk was not significantly increased. The risk for a second malignancy was significantly associated with extent of treatment exposure, including the radiation field size and the addition of chemotherapy to radiation therapy. The risk appeared to be the highest among patients who relapsed after combined-modality therapy and those who received further salvage therapy.

Travis and associates[27] conducted a matched case-control study of breast cancer within a cohort of 3817 female 1-year survivors of Hodgkin's disease diagnosed at 30 years of age or younger. There was a greater risk for the development of breast cancer in patients who received moderately high doses of radiation to the breast than in those who received lower doses and no alkylating agents. Risk increased to eightfold with high doses of radiation. Increased risks persisted for 25 years or more following radiotherapy. Treatment with alkylating agents alone resulted in a decreased risk for breast cancer compared with treatment with combined alkylating agents and radiotherapy, which resulted in a 1.4-fold increased risk. Those who received radiation to the ovaries had a lower risk, suggesting that hormonal stimulation is important for the development of radiation-induced breast cancer.

What is the relevance of a past history of breast surgery?

If there is a past history of surgical procedures on the breast, the reports should be obtained.[28,29] "Atypical" breast disease, including lobular neoplasia, noted on a previous biopsy, is important for final decision making.[30-34] Mammograms with full reports should be available for review. The remainder of the history should be devoted to obtaining information elicited at all thorough examinations, including previous surgery, medical problems, and medications, particularly those medications that may affect hemostasis at surgery, such as aspirin, anti-inflammatory drugs, vitamins, and some herbal remedies.

What is the role of breast self-examination?

The main thrust in the treatment of breast cancer has been toward earlier diagnosis. The patient's role in diagnosis may include performing periodic BSE.

Beginning in their 20s, women should be told of the benefits and limitations of BSE. The importance of prompt reporting of any new breast symptoms to a health professional should be emphasized. Women who choose to do BSE should receive instruction and have their technique reviewed on the occasion of their periodic health examination. It is acceptable for women to choose not to do BSE or to do BSE irregularly.

An additional role of BSE is to increase awareness of normal breast composition so that changes can be detected. Even regular BSE performers commonly detected their breast cancer incidentally, suggesting that there was a component of increased body awareness in addition to the self-performed physical examination.

Recent data have indicated that the rate of biopsy for benign disease is higher in women who regularly perform BSE as compared with women who do not regularly perform BSE.[35] The U.S. Preventive Services Task Force concluded that the evidence is insufficient to recommend for or against teaching or performing routine BSE.[36] However, incidental self-detection of breast cancer still accounts for a significant percentage of cases.

Up to 50% of patients presenting with breast complaints have no evidence of a breast abnormality. If the health professional is unable to appreciate any breast abnormality, it is prudent to have the patient return for reexamination within a relatively short period of time, or a referral can be made to an appropriate facility with experience in breast examination. Skinner and associates,[37] in a multivariate analysis, noted that treatment for breast cancer by a surgical oncologist resulted in a 33% reduction in the risk for death at 5 years.

What is the recommendation for clinical breast examination?

In addition to BSE, it is recommended that average-risk, asymptomatic women in their 20s and 30s have clinical breast examination (CBE) performed at least every 3 years. Asymptomatic women aged 40 years and older should have CBE annually. Women at average risk should begin annual mammography at age 40 years, and older women in reasonable good health should continue to be screened with annual mammography as well. Women at increased risk for breast cancer, as determined by a qualified health professional, may require earlier initiation of screening and shorter screening intervals.

How is the patient instructed in breast self-examination?

At the New York University (NYU) Medical Center and the NYU Cancer Institute, "shower cards" describing BSE have been made available to patients (Fig. 14–1).

BSE is performed monthly, and the patient looks for lumps, thickening, discharge, or any changes in the breast. If the patient is menstruating, the best time to perform self-examination is a week after the start of the period. It is important that pregnant and lactating women continue to perform monthly self-examinations. If the menopause has been passed, an easy date to remember is chosen, such as the first day of the month.

The patient is instructed to stand in front of a mirror. With arms at the sides and then raised above the head, she should look carefully for changes in the size, shape, and contour of each breast (Fig. 14–2). Specifically, she should observe for puckering, dimpling, or changes in the skin texture. Each nipple should be *gently* squeezed and any discharge recorded (Fig. 14–3). BSE can also be performed lying down. A pillow is placed under the right shoulder, and the right hand is placed behind the head. The right breast is examined with the left hand (Fig. 14–4). With the fingers flat, the breast is gently pressed in a circular motion, starting at the outside top edge and spiraling toward the nipple (Fig. 14–5A and B). The underarms and the area below the breast should be included (Fig. 14–6). This is then repeated for the left breast. In the shower, the right arm is raised, and the left hand is used to examine the right breast (Fig. 14–7). With the fingers flat and using a circular motion, every part of the breast is palpated, including the underarm, gently feeling for a lump or thickening. This is repeated for the left breast.

It is important to remind the patient that the purpose of regular BSEs is not to diagnose breast cancer but rather to detect any changes in the breast. If a lump or thickening is felt or a discharge or change in breast size or shape is noted, a health professional should be contacted as soon as possible. Most lumps are not indicative of cancer, and BSEs are free and take only a few minutes each month.

Breast Self-Examination

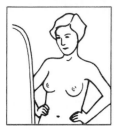

In Front of a Mirror

With arms at your sides, look carefully for changes in the size, shape and contour of each breast. Look for puckering, dimpling or changes in the skin texture. Gently squeeze each nipple and look for discharge. Repeat with your arms raised above your head.

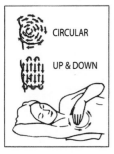

CIRCULAR

UP & DOWN

Lying Down

Place a pillow under your right shoulder, and your right hand behind your head. Examine your right breast with your left hand. With fingers flat, gently press using an up and down pattern or a circular motion, starting at the outside top edge and spiraling toward the nipple. Include your underarm and the area above and below your breast. Repeat for your left breast.

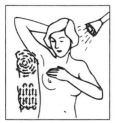

In The Shower

Raise your right arm and use your left hand to examine your right breast. With fingers flat (using the up and down or circular pattern as you used lying down) touch every part of the breast, including the underarm, gently feeling for a lump or thickening. Repeat for your left breast.

Donated by the Landsberg Zale Surgical Oncology Research Fund

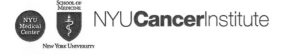

What You Should Know

Breast cancer is a progressive disease, and small tumors are more likely to be successfully treated. The purpose of breast self-examination (BSE) is to encourage you to be aware of how your breasts look and feel in order to recognize any changes and promptly report them to a health-care professional. Although there is some disagreement about the value of BSE, the self-detection of breast cancer still accounts for a significant percentage of cases found at an early stage.

REGULAR MONTHLY SELF-EXAMS ARE FREE AND TAKE ONLY A FEW MINUTES.

What You Can Do

As part of monthly BSE, you should look and feel for lumps, thickening, nipple discharge, or any changes in the shape or size of your breasts. Most lumps are not cancer.

If you are menstruating, the best time to perform a self-exam is a week after the start of your period. It is important for pregnant and nursing women to continue to perform monthly breast self-exams. Your obstetrician-gynecologist should review any modifications needed for you to perform the exam. If you are past menopause, choose an easy date to remember, such as the first day of each month.

Clinical Breast Exams and Mammography

For women in their 20s and 30s at average risk of breast cancer who do not have symptoms, it is recommended that clinical breast examinations (CBE) be performed at least every three years by a health-care professional. Asymptomatic women age 40 and over should have CBE annually. Women at average risk should begin having a mammogram each year starting at age 40, and older women in reasonably good health should continue to have regular mammograms. Women at increased risk of developing breast cancer, as determined by a qualified health-care professional, may need screening earlier and more frequently.

Donated by the Landsberg Zale Surgical Oncology Research Fund

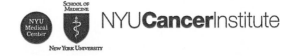

Figure 14–1 "Shower card" describing breast self-examination.   (Courtesy of Landsberg Zale Research Fund in Surgical Oncology.)

What are the components of the physician's breast examination?

The patient should be escorted into a well-lighted examining room with an available x-ray view box. She is asked to undress at least to the waist and should be given a gown or similar appropriate covering so that she can feel comfortable if there is a short delay until the time of the physical examination. Although the patient has given a complete history and has informed the physician of the area of concern, it is suggested that the patient not show the physician the specific area until the physical examination is completed. In this way, the findings can be corroborated without prejudice. If, of course, the physician does not ascertain the area, the patient should be questioned directly about where she feels there is a problem.

The examination begins with the head and neck and the skin, including the skin of the upper extremities and the back.

It is not uncommon to find disorders of the thyroid, cervical lymph nodes, and the skin, some even suggestive of carcinoma or melanoma (Figs. 14–8 and 14–9). The size of the breasts should be noted, and difference in size recorded (Fig. 14–10). Many women have breasts that are not identical in size, and small size discrepancies are rarely a sign of malignancy. The patient should be questioned about whether she was aware of a difference in size, if present, as a recent change in size may indicate a pathologic process. One specific abnormality related to chest wall asymmetry is Poland's syndrome, which consists of hand and digital abnormalities in association with absence or hypoplasia of the pectoralis major muscle, asymmetry of the chest wall, and hypomastia on the involved side.

The patient is asked to raise her arms, and the breasts are examined for evidence of skin retraction, dimpling, or a mass that protrudes from the breast (Figs. 14–11, 14–12, and 14–13). Although retraction is often a sign of malignancy, benign lesions of the breast such as fat necrosis can also cause retraction. Other benign causes include previous surgical biopsy and superficial thrombophlebitis of the breast (Mondor's disease) (Fig. 14–14).

Edema of the skin of the breast (peau d'orange) may be present as a result of obstruction of dermal lymphatics by tumor cells. However, it may also be caused by extensive metastatic axillary lymph node involvement, by primary disease of the axillary nodes, or subsequent to axillary lymph node dissection with or without radiation therapy. Erythema of the breasts may have an infectious cause, as with cellulitis or abscess, but a diagnosis of inflammatory carcinoma should be considered as well (Figs. 14–15 and 14–16).

It is extremely important to inspect the inframammary regions because this component of the examination is often overlooked by patient and physician alike (Fig. 14–17). Lesions in this area are often neglected and diagnosed at an advanced stage because they are not perceived on casual examination by the physician on palpation or by the patient unless she looks in the mirror when doing BSE. Skin lesions of

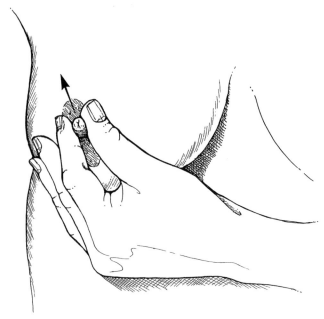

Figure 14–3   Breast self-examination. Each nipple is *gently* squeezed.

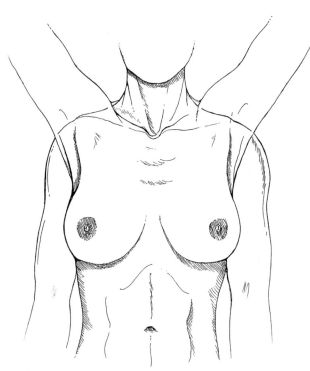

Figure 14–2   Breast self-examination. The patient stands in front of a mirror with arms at the sides and then raised above the head.

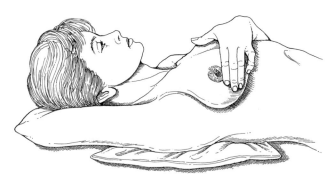

Figure 14–4   Breast self-examination. The patient lies down with a pillow under the shoulder. Each breast is examined with the opposite hand.

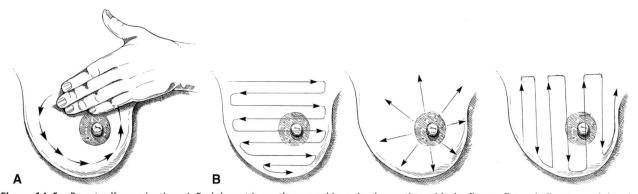

Figure 14–5   Breast self-examination. *A,* Each breast is gently pressed in a circular motion with the fingers flat, spiraling toward the nipple. *B,* Alternative methods of examination.

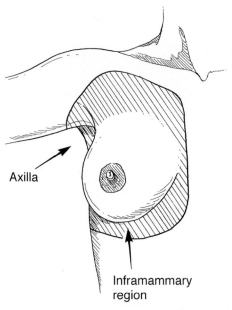

Axilla

Inframammary
region

Figure 14–6 Breast self-examination. The axilla (armpit) and the inframammary region (area below the breast) are included in the examination.

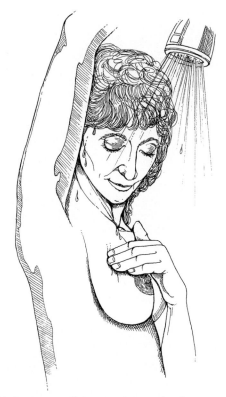

Figure 14–7 Breast self-examination. In the shower, each breast is examined with the opposite hand.

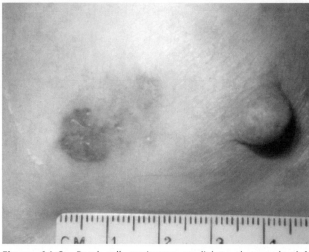

Figure 14–8 Basal cell carcinoma medial to the areola, left breast.

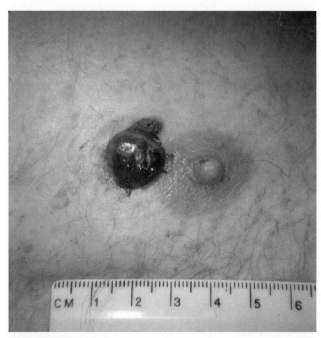

Figure 14–9 Malignant melanoma adjacent to the areola of a male breast.

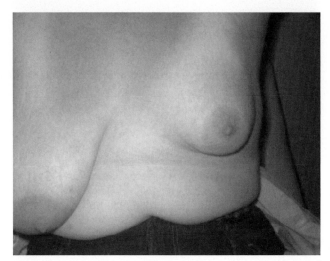

Figure 14–10 Difference in breast size secondary to congenital hypoplasia of the left breast.

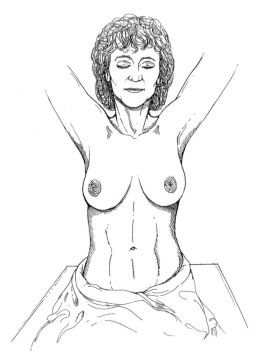

Figure 14–11   Breast examination by the physician. The patient's arms are raised, and skin retraction, dimpling, or a mass can be observed.

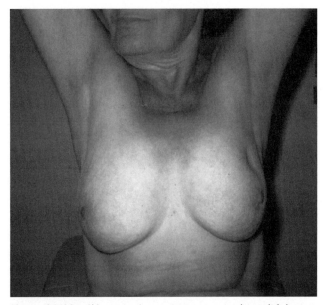

Figure 14–12   Skin retraction, upper outer quadrant, left breast.

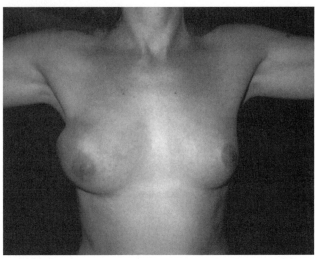

Figure 14–13   Obvious tumor mass in the right breast on inspection.

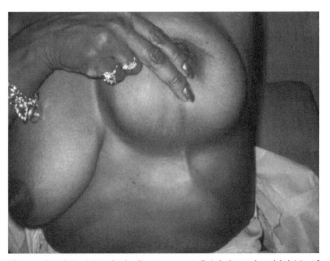

Figure 14–14   Mondor's disease: superficial thrombophlebitis of the breast.

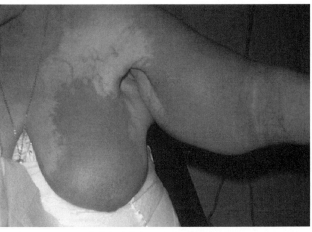

Figure 14–15   Cellulitis, left breast and upper arm.

the breast should be noted and the area of the nipple-areolar complex carefully examined for evidence of crusting, eczematoid changes, and other epithelial changes (Fig. 14–18). If dimpling, skin retraction, nipple inversion, or a mass is observed on inspection, attention should be directed to those areas by palpation with the patient in the sitting position and again in the supine position.

Inspection is completed with the patient contracting her pectoral muscles by pressing her hands against her hips (Fig.

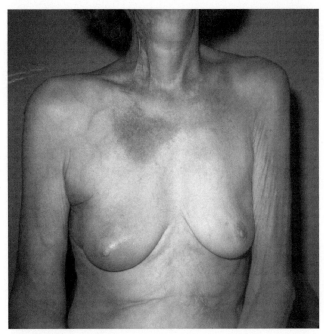

Figure 14–16   Inflammatory carcinoma of the right breast. There is erythema and edema of the skin.

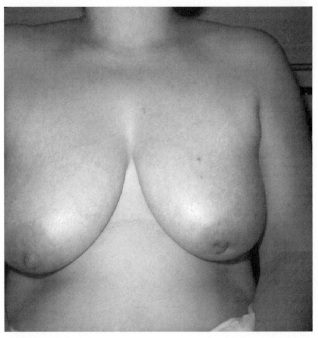

Figure 14–18   Nipple retraction, left breast, secondary to subareolar carcinoma.

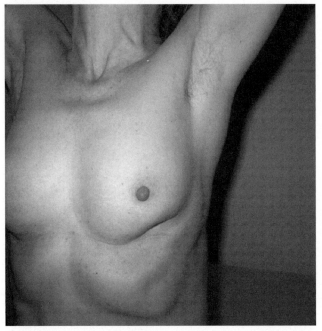

Figure 14–17   Skin retraction, left inframammary region, readily apparent with the arms raised.

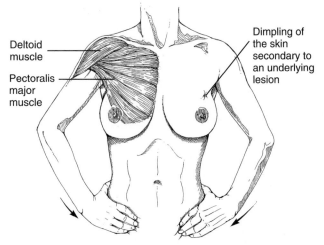

Deltoid muscle

Pectoralis major muscle

Dimpling of the skin secondary to an underlying lesion

Figure 14–19   Breast examination by the physician. The patient contracts the pectoral muscles by pressing against the hips, highlighting any areas of retraction.

14–19). This maneuver, which puts tension on the suspensory ligaments, often highlights areas of skin retraction not readily apparent with the arms relaxed.

The breast examination is continued by palpation with the patient in the sitting position. The breasts are examined simultaneously with attention to any differences in contour or a palpable thickening or mass (Fig. 14–20).

Palpation of breast tissue between fingers or squeezing the breast may result in a false perception of a mass; this is a common error of inexperienced examiners and women attempt-

ing self-examination (Fig. 14–21). Comparing the breasts is often helpful in determining whether a questionable area requires further evaluation.

The relative sparsity of breast tissue in the subareolar region often gives the impression of a periareolar "shelf" or "ridge," particularly in larger breasts. This should not be mistaken for a mass and is usually bilateral.

The axillae should be thoroughly examined with the patient in the sitting position, with the arms relaxed and with the patient supported by the physician's nonexamining hand. The axillary tissue should be firmly palpated under the pectoralis muscle, with pressure exerted and the axillary tissue pressed against the chest wall (Fig. 14–22A and B). The examining hand is then gently rolled over any palpable mass. This examination may be somewhat uncomfortable for the patient but

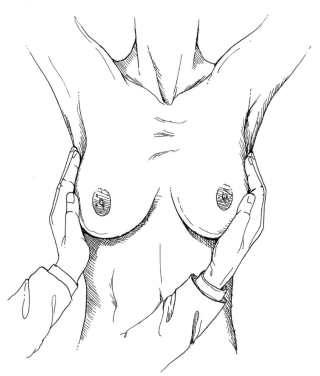

Figure 14–20   Breast examination by the physician. The breasts are palpated simultaneously for changes in contour, thickening, or a mass.

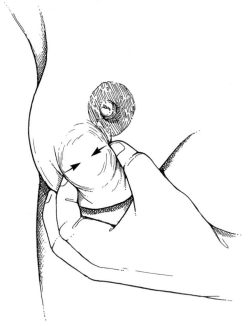

Figure 14–21   Breast examination by the physician. Palpation of breast tissue between the fingers or "squeezing" may result in the *false* perception of a mass.

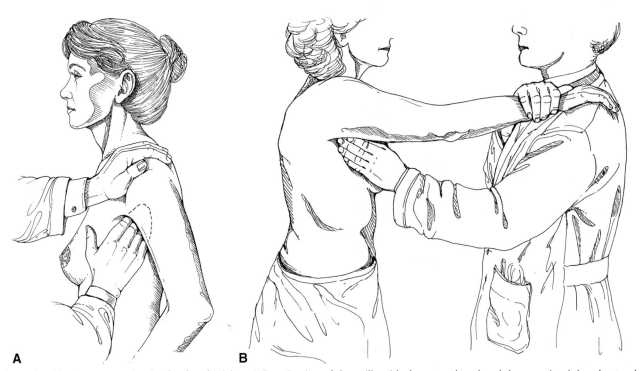

A   B

Figure 14–22   Breast examination by the physician. *A,* Examination of the axilla with the arm relaxed and the examiner's hand extending high into the axilla. *B,* Alternative technique for examination of the axilla.

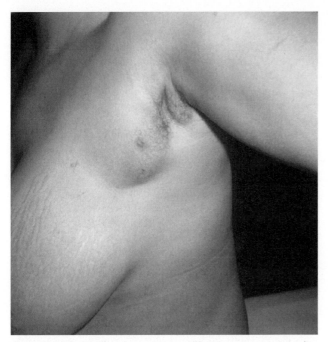

Figure 14–23   Axillary breast tissue with supernumerary nipple.

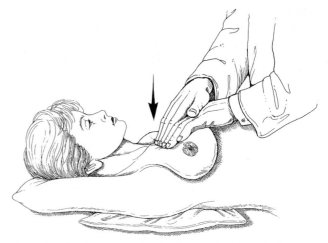

Figure 14–25   Breast examination by the physician. The breast is palpated with the tufts of the fingertips applying gentle pressure.

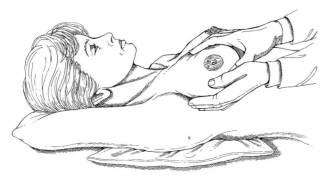

Figure 14–24   Breast examination by the physician. The patient is supine and the breasts are palpated for changes in contour, thickening, or a mass.

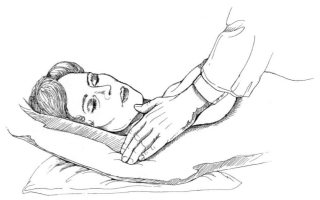

Figure 14–26   Breast examination by the physician. The axillae are palpated with the patient supine.

need not be a prolonged process. The skin of the axillae should be observed. A patient may believe she has a breast mass when the problem is really one of the skin, such as an epidermoid inclusion cyst, a cyst of the sweat gland apparatus, or hidradenitis suppurativa. Axillary breast tissue can be appreciated as well and should be carefully evaluated (Fig. 14–23). In obese patients, the axillae, and sometimes the supraclavicular areas, may contain a soft to rubbery fat pad that can be mistaken for adenopathy. Lymph nodes may be palpable or present within them.

The patient is then asked to assume the supine position, and the breast examination is carried out as described in the discussion of BSE (Figs. 14–24 and 14–25). Note is made of any mass in the breast, tenderness, nipple discharge, or skin retraction. The axillae are again palpated in this position (Fig. 14–26).

It may be difficult to determine whether a palpable mass is solid or cystic. The history may be of some help in that cystic lesions are more likely to be of sudden onset and tender. If a mass feels like a cyst, aspiration is attempted to obtain fluid.

If the mass is no longer palpable after aspiration, one of the criteria for a benign cyst of the breast has been met. If, however, the fluid appears to be bloody or if the mass does not disappear completely on palpation after aspiration, further investigation is warranted. If the lesion is not a cyst but solid, further diagnostic procedures are mandatory with fine-needle aspiration biopsy, image-directed biopsy, or excision. If there is some doubt about whether a palpable mass is cystic or solid, breast ultrasonography with attention to the area in question is helpful. The radiologist or surgeon may then proceed with cyst aspiration under ultrasound guidance or with other appropriate biopsies. Of course, if a mammogram or an ultrasonogram is available at the time of the examination and an obvious cyst is both palpable and seen on the imaging studies, a cyst aspiration should be performed.

In patients who have had an augmentation mammoplasty, the prosthesis may be palpable, most often as a globular smooth mass underlying the breast. On occasion, the valve of the prosthesis can be felt and may be mistaken for a significant breast lesion. These valves have a characteristic discoid outline on palpation. If there is any question concerning the findings on palpation, confirmation can usually be obtained by history and ultrasound imaging, if necessary.

Any palpable finding not matched in a mirror-image location in the opposite breast is a reason for concern, including ill-defined asymmetrical thickenings. It is impossible to rule out breast cancer on clinical grounds alone. Failure to be impressed with physical examination findings was cited as the most common reason for a delay in the diagnosis of breast cancer and the second most frequent cause of legal action against physicians, and the most expensive.[38]

It is appropriate, and often helpful, to review mammographic findings on the x-ray view box with the patient so that she has a clear perception of what microcalcifications or a solid or cystic lesion looks like and the extent of the process. With the use of image-guided biopsies and the availability of a well-trained cytologist, the patient can be given at least a preliminary diagnosis within a short period of time. This will help allay apprehension and will allow the patient and the physician to discuss further treatment if indicated. With the increased use of image-guided biopsies, most patients will have definitive surgery with a fairly accurate preliminary diagnosis.

What is the role of screening in the clinical assessment?

The American Cancer Society estimates that in 2005, 212,930 women will be diagnosed with invasive breast cancer and an additional 58,490 with in situ breast cancer. It estimates that 1690 men will be diagnosed with breast cancer, and 40,410 women and 460 men will die of the disease.[39] It is widely acknowledged that when breast cancer is diagnosed and treated at an early stage, the chances for long-term survival are better; and furthermore, smaller lesions are more amenable to breast-conserving surgery.

Ghafoor and associates,[40] in a recent report from the American Cancer Society, described the trends in incidence, mortality, and survival rates of female breast cancer in the United States by race and ethnicity. Breast cancer incidence has increased among women of all races combined and among white women since the early 1980s. The increasing incidence in white women predominantly involves small (<2 cm) and localized-stage tumors, although a small increase in the incidence of regional-stage tumors and those larger than 5 cm occurred since the early 1990s. The incidence among African American women stabilized during the 1990s for all breast cancers and for localized tumors. African American women are more likely than white women to be diagnosed with large tumors and distant-stage disease. Other racial and ethnic groups have a lower incidence than white or African American women. However, the proportion of disease diagnosed at advanced stage and with larger tumor size in all minorities is greater than in white persons. Death rates decreased by 2.5% per year among white women since 1990 and by 1% per year among African American women since 1991. A disparity in mortality rates increased progressively between 1980 and 2000, so that by 2000, the age-standardized death rate was 32% higher in African Americans than in white women. The authors point out that 63% and 29% of breast cancers, respectively, are diagnosed at local- and regional-stage disease, for which the 5-year relative survival rates are 97% and 79%, respectively.

O'Malley and associates,[41] using data from the Surveillance, Epidemiology and End Results program (SEER), noted that after adjustment for multiple factors, African Americans continued to have slightly but significantly poorer survival after breast carcinoma compared with whites, whereas the survival of Hispanics and Asians did not differ from that of whites.

Naik and associates[42] studied the epidemiologic and pathologic characteristics of indigent breast cancer patients in a public city hospital in comparison to national standards. The medical records of 188 patients were retrospectively reviewed. The authors concluded that indigent patients among all ethnic and racial backgrounds present with more advanced disease when compared with national statistics reported by the SEER program.

Two components of delay have been identified: (1) delay by a woman in seeking care for breast cancer symptoms, and (2) delay by the patient, provider, and system during the evaluation, diagnosis, and initiation of treatment of breast cancer. A study by Bedell and associates[43] addressed the problem of delay in diagnosis and treatment of breast cancer. They noted that nearly half of the diagnostic interval delay in the public hospital results from systemic factors such as general scheduling delays or time spent waiting for appointments and diagnostic procedures to be scheduled and completed, waiting for reports and results, and waiting for retrieval of lost or missing records. Missed diagnosis was the most common reason for provider delays in the diagnostic interval. Missed diagnoses occurred when cancer symptoms were ignored, treatment for presumed infection was instituted, a mass was present and biopsy was not performed, or a suspect finding was not followed up. Complaints of a breast mass must be aggressively pursued, and dominant masses should undergo biopsy. A normal mammogram does not rule out the need for a biopsy. Education of women to follow routine screening recommendations, to recognize breast cancer symptoms early, and to recognize benefits of early detection is important. Minority and uninsured women are at particular risk. Language, culture, and financial barriers in this population may necessitate more outreach and support.

The Gothenburg Breast Screening Trial[44] reported a randomized controlled trial of mammographic screening for breast carcinoma with 21,650 women in the screened group and 29,961 women in a control group. The screening interval was 18 months. Age-specific analyses yielded greater mortality rate reduction for the groups of women aged 39 to 44 years, 45 to 49 years, and 55 to 59 years, but there was no mortality rate reduction in the group of women aged 50 to 54 years. The authors observed a 20% to 30% reduction in breast carcinoma mortality with mammographic screening. The results also suggested that a reduction in mortality in women younger than 50 years of age might also be achieved with a short screening interval.

A Swedish trial conducted by Tabar and associates[45] reported a 30% reduction in mortality associated with the invitation to screening of women aged 40 to 74 years, with the reduction being 34% for women aged 50 to 74 years and 13% for women aged 40 to 49. These authors suggest that much, although not all, of the smaller effect of screening on mortality in women aged 40 to 49 years was due to faster progression of a substantial proportion of tumors in this age group and the rapid increase in incidence during this decade of life. It was estimated that a 19% reduction in mortality would result from an annual screening regimen.

What is the radiation risk from mammography?

The possibility of radiation risk from mammography has been a subject of debate, specifically in the screening of women between the ages of 40 and 49 years. In 1975, Dr. John Bailar, Editor of the *Journal of the National Cancer Institute*, called public attention to the potential radiation risk of screening mammography. Although conceding that for women older than 50 or 60 years, "the radiation risk may be small in relation to the expected benefit," he concluded that the routine use of mammography in screening asymptomatic women "may eventually take as many lives as it saves"[46] Since that time, concerns have lessened as randomized trials have proved the benefit of screening in women between the ages of 40 and 49 years. In addition, with improvements in technology, there has been a sevenfold national reduction in mean glandular dose to the breast from 1974 to 1992, and there are numerous studies indicating that the risk from radiation is negligible compared with the benefit from screening.

Feig[47] summarized the assessment of radiation risk from screening mammography. The female Japanese survivors of the Hiroshima and Nagasaki atomic bombings represent the largest of all available populations of women who received high doses of radiation and from which estimates of the risk for radiation-induced breast cancer can be derived. The longest follow-up of the Japanese women to date was reported by Tokunaga and associates in 1994.[48] Excess relative risk for breast cancer in exposed women compared with nonexposed women was found with doses of 250 to 500 mGy among Japanese atomic bomb survivors, but there was no evidence of excessive risk below 250 mGy. After the hypothetical risk for developing a fatal breast cancer from mammography is calculated from the relative risk estimate that Tokunaga and associates derived from the follow-up of Japanese atomic bomb survivors, it may then be compared with the number of fatal cancers prevented by mammographic screening as observed in randomized screening trials. Mettler and associates[49] have made it clear that the risk is negligible compared with the proven benefit from screening.

In a meta-analysis of seven randomized trials by Smart and associates, a significant reduction in mortality from breast cancer resulted from screening frequencies that ranged from 12 to 33 months, when combined with adequate follow-up.[50] Feig[47] concluded that over a period of 20 years, studies comparing benefits and risks of mammographic screening have reduced the level of concern regarding radiation exposure of asymptomatic women, and the benefit-to-risk ratios from actual screening may be even more favorable than those calculated in the Mettler study.

What special considerations apply to the clinical evaluation of young women?

Breast cancer in women younger than 40 years requires special consideration. These women are often more aware of the necessity for examination and mammography than their older counterparts. In view of this, particularly with the increasing use of mammography in women between the ages of 30 and 40 years, it appears that the incidence of breast cancer in young women is rising. However, the nature of the lesion discovered in many instances may be quite different from that seen in older women. The findings range from minute intraductal neoplasms, manifested by a tiny cluster of microcalcifications on mammography, to invasive lobular carcinoma, which is difficult to detect on mammography in dense breasts and is often discovered on physical examination at a more advanced stage.

Among the 211,300 new cases of breast cancer diagnosed in 2003, about 6% were in women younger than 40 years. The absolute number of breast cancer cases nearly doubled in young women from 1970 to 1990, but the incidence of disease has changed very little because of the marked increase in the young population as a whole.

Examination of young women's breasts is more difficult, and the examiner usually has a low index of suspicion, which may lead to delay in diagnosis. Young women's breasts are often nodular, may be disparate in size, and may change with menstrual cycle. If cyclic changes are suspected, the patient can be reexamined after a short interval, usually 10 to 12 days after onset of the menstrual period. The importance of a short-term physical reexamination cannot be overemphasized. However, in very young women, the most common tumor is a fibroadenoma, and the patient can be reassured that these are common and benign and can be safely excised.

What are the most common breast lesions in younger women?

Fibroadenomas and fibronodular breast tissue are the most common masses in women younger than 25 years, as discussed later in this chapter. It is uncommon for women in this age group to have either a breast cyst or breast cancer. Fibroadenomas are perhaps the easiest to diagnose clinically because the mass is smooth and mobile. In contrast, as women approach the fourth decade of life, breast cysts become common. One of the major responsibilities of the clinician is to establish that a palpable abnormality is a cyst and not a solid mass. This can be done with either needle aspiration or ultrasound, although needle aspiration is preferred because it provides simultaneous therapeutic drainage if a cyst is present. Palpable cysts should be drained for several reasons: (1) to establish the diagnosis of the cyst as benign, (2) to provide an expeditious diagnosis, (3) to provide relief of pain in a woman who has a cyst under tension, and (4) to provide an optimal breast examination interpretation free of interfering masses.[51]

What are the potential problems in the clinical evaluation of younger women?

Approaching the fourth decade, when breast cysts become more common, the incidence of breast cancer also rises. During these years, breast examination may become difficult and the cause of any palpable breast mass equally difficult to predict with any certainty. The use of estrogen replacement therapy additionally confounds the issue.

A review of the litigation literature found that more than two thirds of women who sued physicians over delay in the

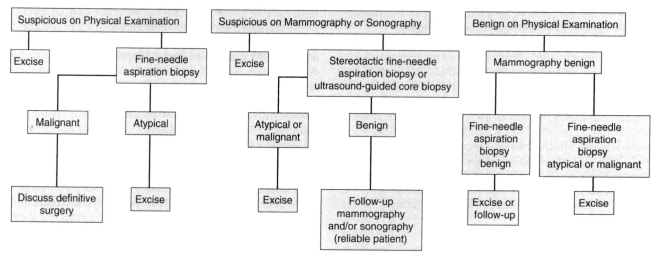

Figure 14–30   Management of solid breast masses.

The accuracy of fine-needle biopsy has been established. The false-positive rate for the procedure is low, averaging about 0.17%.[86] The advantage of the procedure is that it can rapidly establish a preliminary diagnosis of malignancy or possible malignancy, offering the patient the opportunity to discuss treatment options within a very short time. Some surgeons use the results of fine-needle aspiration biopsy for definitive diagnosis. In many instances, however, it may be more prudent to confirm the impression gained from aspiration biopsy with a core biopsy, mammotome biopsy, or an open biopsy with frozen section, especially if there is any question clinically.

The false-negative rate of fine-needle aspiration biopsy has been found to be between 0.4% and 35%. The most common reason for a false-negative result is inadequate sampling, which may be due to lack of communication between surgeon and cytopathologist or due to an inexperienced cytopathologist. Other reasons for false-negative results include tumors 1.0 cm or smaller, which may have been missed by the aspirating needle. The use of stereotactic fine-needle aspiration biopsy as well as ultrasound-guided aspiration biopsy enhances the ability to detect lesions and reduces the false-negative rate.

Aspiration of fibrotic tumors may result in a false-negative result, as may aspiration of tumors with necrosis or edema. The surgeon must be particularly aware of the possibility of a well-differentiated neoplasm (i.e., tubular carcinoma) as well as infiltrating lobular carcinoma, in situ ductal and lobular carcinoma, colloid carcinoma, and papillary carcinoma. In these instances, aspiration biopsies often are read as showing "atypia," and open biopsy is necessary.

At present there is no proven, feasible, reliable, and noninvasive method of identifying high-risk women who have occult atypical hyperplasia. Random, periareolar bilateral breast fine-needle aspirations in women at elevated risks for developing breast cancer on the basis of a family history or an elevated 10-year Gail risk score have been shown to detect breast epithelial cell atypia in 21%. In the series by Fabian and associates, an additional 49% of high-risk women were found to have epithelial hyperplasia without atypia.[87] Bilateral breast fine-needle aspiration is a promising method for detecting cellular atypia in high-risk women. However, there is a large possibility of sampling error inherent in this procedure, and the extent of atypia cannot be determined reliably. In addition, if atypical cells are detected in nipple aspirate fluid, it is generally not possible to localize the duct or segment that yielded the atypical cells because fluid from several ducts can pool on the nipple during the aspiration procedure.

Does ductal lavage complement clinical assessment?

Ductal lavage (DL) is a procedure that has been developed to enhance the tolerability, efficiency, and reproducibility of collecting breast duct epithelial cells for cytologic analysis as part of breast cancer risk evaluation. Appropriate candidates for DL include women who are at elevated risk for development of breast cancer and for whom a finding of atypical breast epithelial cells on cytology would alter their clinical management.[88] Regardless of whether a woman is at elevated risk for development of breast cancer, DL has no proven clinical utility in the evaluation of an abnormal breast examination, mammogram, or other breast imaging study.

Brogi and associates[89] performed DL in the affected breast of 26 women undergoing mastectomy for carcinoma and in the clinically normal breast of 4 additional women undergoing risk-reducing mastectomy. Four (14%) of 29 DL samples showed marked atypia, 10 (34%) showed mild atypia, and 15 (52%) were benign. No DL sample was clearly malignant. Two DL samples from breasts with extensive lobular carcinoma in situ showed mild atypia. The study confirmed that sampling of mammary epithelium by DL is not useful in the diagnostic screening and identification of carcinoma.

DL is not a breast cancer early-detection tool, and any abnormal imaging or physical exam finding requires standard evaluation and consideration for biopsy. Likewise, DL should not be used as a screening test in high-risk women who have dense breasts on mammograms or who otherwise wish or require another breast screening evaluation, because there are no data indicating that DL is useful in detecting occult breast cancer. High-risk women who have a history of estrogen receptor– or progesterone receptor–positive breast cancer, ductal carcinoma in situ or biopsy-proven atypical ductal hyperplasia, atypical lobular hyperplasia, or lobular carcinoma in situ are generally not suitable candidates for DL because a finding of atypical cells in duct fluid does not further elevate risk. Women who are already taking tamoxifen or who have finished 5 years of treatment for invasive breast cancer, ductal carcinoma in situ, atypical ductal hyperplasia, atypical lobular hyperplasia, or lobular carcinoma in situ; women who have a family history of breast cancer; or women with an elevated Gail risk are not appropriate candidates for DL because there are no data to guide treatment recommendations in this setting. There is no proven role for DL in serially monitoring breast cytology in high-risk women who are taking or have taken tamoxifen.

Is there a role for galactography in the evaluation of nipple discharge?

Galactography, a specialized radiologic procedure involving contrast injection of the ductal system, may allow for more accurate localization of lesions and thus a more conservative surgical excision. However, accurate differentiation of benign from malignant lesions is not possible with this technique. The procedure is useful for distally or peripherally located lesions that otherwise might be missed by standard major duct excision. A negative galactographic, mammographic, or cytologic result should not deter surgical excision if neoplasm is suspected.

How does breast endoscopy complement clinical assessment?

The presence of a single-duct spontaneous bloody nipple discharge is an indication for surgical biopsy. The most common lesion identified is an intraductal papilloma in the immediate retroareolar region. Because duct excision often requires resection of the entire ductal system, intraoperative mammary duct endoscopy has been used for direct visualization of intraductal abnormalities during surgical resection. This may be particularly useful in young patients in whom complete duct excision may not be warranted and may lead to subsequent inability to nurse. Smith[90] described a minimally invasive method of excising nipple ducts using cannulation in order to preserve nipple function in women of childbearing age.

Submillimeter endoscopes are now available. Dooley,[91–93] who described operative breast endoscopy for bloody nipple discharge in 27 patients, found a lesion accounting for the bleeding in 26 of them. Cancers were identified in 2 patients, and in these patients, a more proximal papilloma was noted in the same ductal system. The author concluded that the high incidence of multiple lesion identification suggests that the classic blind resection of a limited distance of duct in the retroareolar space may significantly underestimate the extent of proliferative disease.

Dietz and associates[94] reviewed their experience with 119 patients with pathologic nipple discharge undergoing ductoscopy-directed duct excision. In this study, a preoperative ductogram was obtained in 70 patients and was positive in 53 (76%). In the same group, ductoscopy was positive in 63 (90%). They found 5 carcinomas, 84 papillomas, and 16 instances of hyperplasia. Hyperplasia and carcinoma were significant predictors of unsuccessful cannulation. In 22 patients, ductoscopy visualized multiple lesions or abnormalities beyond 4 cm. Their conclusions are similar to those of Dooley in noting that lesions deep within the ductal system can be identified and removed and that these would likely have been missed by blind duct excision.

BENIGN BREAST DISEASE

Benign breast disease is far more frequent in clinical practice than is cancer of the breast. Many patients with symptomatic breast conditions will assume that they harbor a malignancy because of the publicity that surrounds cancer of the breast. The problems facing the clinician are to ensure an accurate diagnosis and to reassure the patient that the condition is benign.

How is fibrocystic disease characterized?

The various entities that are classified under the term *fibrocystic disease* include cystic disease, fibrous disease, and sclerosing adenosis. Fibrocystic disease represents a spectrum of clinical entities, from an epithelium-lined cyst at one end to sclerosing adenosis at the other. Histopathologic changes seen in fibrocystic disease consist of hyperplasia of duct epithelium, duct papillomatosis, blunt duct adenosis, apocrine metaplasia, and adenosis. The usual patient with true cystic disease is in her 30s or 40s. Breast discomfort or frank pain frequently accompanies cystic changes and tends to be increased at the time of menstruation.

Benign breast abnormalities consisting of nodularity on physical examination lead to biopsy by age 50 years in just under 20% of women in North America.[95] Benign breast disease that on pathologic examination is nonproliferative, including cysts, ductal ectasia, mild hyperplasia, and simple fibroadenoma, does not increase breast cancer risk.

Fewer than 5% of women without proliferative changes on biopsy develop breast cancer over the subsequent 25 years, but nearly 40% of women with a family history of breast cancer and atypical hyperplasia subsequently develop breast cancer.[96] Biopsy before the age of 50 to 55 years is associated with a fivefold to sixfold increase in the risk for breast cancer, whereas biopsy at older ages is associated with only half this risk.

Proliferative benign breast disease, however, including lobular and ductal hyperplasia, sclerosing adenosis, intraductal papilloma, and lobular or ductal hyperplasia with atypia and radial scar, does elevate breast cancer risk. Proliferative disease with atypia has been shown to increase the relative risk for developing invasive breast cancer by fourfold to fivefold.[97] Most atypical ductal and lobular hyperplasia lesions are diagnosed as incidental findings on breast biopsy, and about 10% to 12% of these lesions are detectable as mammographic or palpable abnormalities.

About 60,000 breast biopsies per year in the United States are found to contain atypical hyperplasia. Considerable epidemiologic evidence supports atypical hyperplasia as a significant risk marker and one that is associated with a 0.8% to 1% risk per year of developing invasive breast cancer. In addition, two large prospective studies have provided insights into the

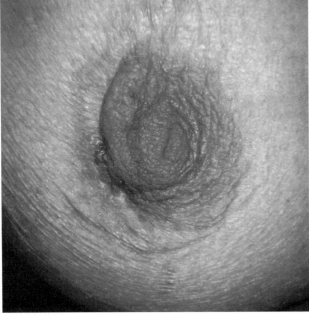

Figure 14–34 Periareolar fistula secondary to subareolar abscess.

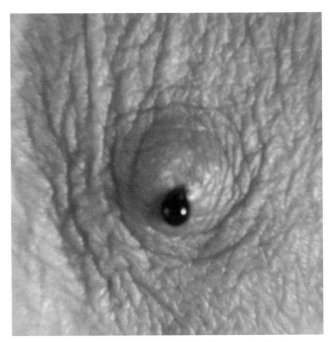

Figure 14–35 Bloody nipple discharge from a single duct secondary to intraductal papilloma.

mimics carcinoma), an excisional biopsy is required. Enlarged lymph nodes can sometimes occur with this condition. Careful examination of the remainder of the breast and mammography are important adjuncts in the management of these patents because a coexisting carcinoma may be present. Another indication for surgery with this entity is a persistent fistula in the periareolar region (Fig. 14–34). Excision of the fistula sometimes requires removal of the entire ductal system as well as partial excision of the nipple.

What are the causes of nipple discharge?

The most common causes of nipple discharge identified from surgical specimens are solitary papillomas and papillomatosis, which are benign conditions (Fig. 14–35). A second common cause of nipple discharge is duct ectasia, a benign condition associated with the loss of elastin within the duct walls and a chronic plasma cell inflammatory infiltrate. Fibrocystic disease may lead to a spontaneous nipple discharge. The discharge may come from several ducts, with fluid of varied coloration, often green (Fig. 14–36). The least frequently observed cause of nipple discharge is carcinoma. Because carcinoma is occasionally associated with bloody nipple discharge, it is imperative that a biopsy of involved ducts be performed. Intraductal papillomas are more common in premenopausal women; the older the patient, the more likely that a bloody discharge is due to carcinoma.

Intraductal papilloma may also produce a clear, yellowish discharge. Mammography should be performed in patients who are to undergo surgery for spontaneous nipple discharge. Nevertheless, a biopsy is required. To ensure that the involved duct or ducts are included in the specimen, careful palpation of the periareolar region with pressure applied toward the nipple, one quadrant at a time, should be performed before surgery. This will help localize the most likely source of bleeding.

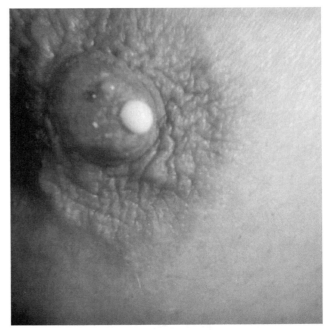

Figure 14–36 Multiple-duct, multicolored discharge secondary to fibrocystic disease and duct ectasia.

When there is a spontaneous bloody discharge by history but the physician is unable to elicit this in the office, the nipple may be coated with collodion and the patient asked to return in a week. The collodion is then stripped from the nipple or dissolved with acetone, and if the duct has become engorged with blood, the source can be easily demonstrated with mild pressure.

At times, it is difficult to determine the color of the discharge as it exits from the nipple. It is best to visualize the discharge against a white background, such as a white surgical

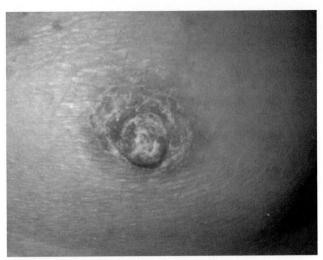

Figure 14–37 Eczema of the nipple, indistinguishable from Paget's disease. The diagnosis was made by biopsy.

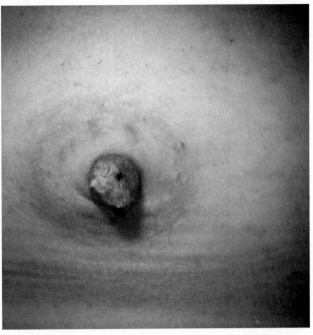

Figure 14–39 Papillomatosis of the nipple. The diagnosis was made by biopsy.

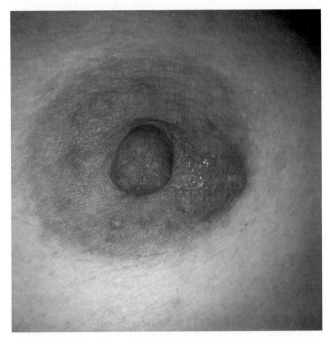

Figure 14–38 Psoriasis of the areola.

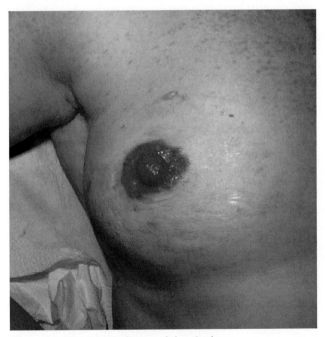

Figure 14–40 Paget's disease of the nipple.

sponge. A discharge that appears bloody at a quick glance may actually be dark green. It should also be emphasized that the nipple discharge should be *spontaneous* to be considered pathologic. Persistent squeezing may produce a discharge in many *normal* patients.

Changes in the epithelium of the nipple and areola, often associated with itching or nipple discharge, warrant nipple biopsy (Figs. 14–37 and 14–38). A wedge of the nipple–areolar complex can be obtained under local anesthesia and the edges reapproximated with minimal deformity.

An occasional patient may present with extensive papillomatosis of the nipple, a benign condition often clinically indistinguishable from Paget's disease (Figs. 14–39 and 14–40). An appropriate biopsy will establish the diagnosis.

A spontaneous nipple discharge may not be pathologic in all instances. A serous or milky discharge can occur in patients using oral contraceptives.[102,103] This discharge is usually bilateral and may be accompanied by a limited increase in breast size. As already mentioned, a bloody nipple discharge may occur in the last trimester of pregnancy and should resolve after delivery.

Persistent nonpuerperal bilateral milky discharge may be caused by a pituitary adenoma, particularly when associated with amenorrhea, infertility, and visual field loss. Further diagnostic evaluation should include determination of prolactin levels; if they are persistently elevated, the patient should undergo imaging studies (computed tomography scans, MRI) of the sella turcica region and visual field testing. Other endocrine causes of galactorrhea are drugs (antihypertensives, phenothiazines, and tranquilizers) and transient hyperprolactinemia secondary to nipple stimulation and chest trauma, including thoracotomy.

The clinical features suggesting a benign or a malignant neoplasm as the origin of nipple discharge include the following: spontaneous discharge; unilateral localization; confinement to one duct associated with a mass; bloody, serous, serosanguineous, or watery discharge; old age; and male gender. The results of cytologic evaluation of the discharge may be inconclusive or misleading, and the utility of this procedure is questionable.

As discussed previously in this chapter, ductoscopy, galactography, and possibly DL may be used to diagnose lesions causing nipple discharge.

How are benign papillary lesions of the breast characterized clinically?

Solitary intraductal papillomas are tumors of the major lactiferous ducts, most frequently observed in women 30 to 50 years of age. The clinical presentation in most patients is a bloody nipple discharge, as discussed previously. A palpable mass close to the areola may be present, but most of these lesions range in size from 0.3 to 0.5 cm. Bilaterality is uncommon. Solitary intraductal papilloma does not represent a major risk for subsequent cancer development. However, surgical excision and analysis is necessary to differentiate this lesion from intraductal papillary carcinoma.

Gutman and associates[104] questioned the hypothesis concerning the benign nature of solitary breast papillomas. In a retrospective analysis of 95 papillary lesions, they noted that 10% of solitary papillomas were associated with breast carcinoma, and an additional 9% presented with invasive or noninvasive carcinoma within the papillomas. The risk for associated malignancy was not significantly different between solitary ductal papilloma and multiple papillomas.

Multiple peripheral papillomas occur less frequently than solitary papillomas and are often bilateral. Although they may present as a mass, or much less often with nipple discharge, with the current increased use of ultrasonography, small peripheral papillomas are being discovered and the diagnosis confirmed by ultrasound-guided biopsy. Studies have indicated that there is an increased risk for cancer associated with multiple peripheral intraductal papillomas, and complete excision with careful follow-up of both breasts is recommended.[105]

How is fat necrosis characterized clinically?

A large portion of the breast is composed of fat, particularly in the older patient, in whom it replaces glandular tissue. An area of fat necrosis may follow trauma or may result from erosion of stagnant lactiferous ducts with extrusion of the contents into the surrounding fat. Initially, an inflammatory reaction will develop as macrophages envelop degenerated lipids. A healing phase then occurs, with proliferation of connective tissue clinically resulting in a firm lesion that can mimic cancer.

The incidence of prior trauma is probably quite high, but many patients may not remember a minor traumatic incident. Evidence of ecchymosis may be present on physical examination, but often this has resolved before the patient is seen.

Surgical trauma secondary to biopsy and reduction mammoplasty can also lead to fat necrosis, as can the injection of foreign materials such as paraffin, silicone, and narcotics into the breast. More important today is the fact that conservative treatment of breast carcinoma with lumpectomy and radiation therapy may also result in fat necrosis. Autologous fat injection using the liposuction technique to fill in irregular contours and small soft tissue defects in the breast may lead to fat necrosis secondary to the poor blood supply in the injected fat. A more common occurrence of fat necrosis may be seen in patients who, after total mastectomy with or without axillary dissection, choose reconstruction with a TRAM flap. These patients may present with a firm, nontender mass at the periphery of the transplanted flap. The findings mimic recurrent carcinoma. However, the temporal relationship of this occurrence to the flap procedure militates against a recurrence. If there is any doubt, aspiration biopsy is indicated.

The classic mammographic findings associated with fat necrosis include dystrophic calcifications and lipid cysts that may or may not be calcified. Patients who present soon after trauma with physical sequelae such as ecchymoses and painful masses in the breast can be safely observed. Breast masses may initially increase in size and later become smaller as the acute inflammatory process resolves. If patients present later with painless masses and histories of trauma that cannot be substantiated, a diagnosis of fat necrosis must be established by biopsy.

How are fibroadenomas characterized clinically?

Fibroadenoma is the most commonly appearing tumor in the female breast between puberty and 30 years of age. It usually presents as a palpable mass and may be present on a mammogram as a nodular density. The mass is classically well defined, rubbery in texture, and mobile. Mammographically, it may be seen as a well-circumscribed nodule that may or may not contain coarse calcifications. Although they present most frequently in younger patients, the exact prevalence of fibroadenomas is unknown. Once thought to be benign neoplasms, fibroadenomas are now believed to represent a hyperplastic process that involves the terminal ductulolobular unit and its surrounding connective tissue. A study by Dupont and associates[106] noted a small but definite increased risk for breast cancer development (relative risks of 1.3 to 1.9). Unlike other benign breast lesions, such as atypical hyperplasia, in which the breast cancer risk decreases over time, the risk associated with fibroadenomas appears to be persistent. However, this has little impact on clinical management. Infrequently, carcinoma may occur in association with a fibroadenoma. The most frequent finding is lobular carcinoma in situ, but intraductal, infiltrating ductal, and infiltrating lobular carcinoma have also been observed. The prognosis of carcinoma limited to a fibroadenoma is excellent.

In older lesions and in postmenopausal patients, the stroma may become hyalinized, calcified, or even ossified. Fibroadenomas may undergo partial, subtotal, or total

Fibroadenoma

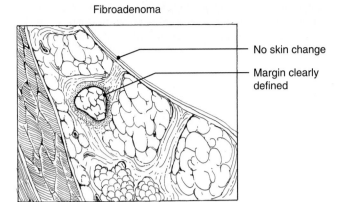

No skin change

Margin clearly
defined

Malignant Lesion

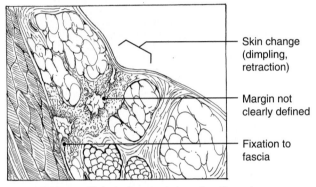

Skin change
(dimpling,
retraction)

Margin not
clearly defined

Fixation to
fascia

Figure 14–41   Clinical characteristics of a fibroadenoma compared with those of a malignant lesion.

infarction, with pregnancy and lactation the most common predisposing factors.

Fibroadenomas may occur in any part of the breast and are frequently multiple (Fig. 14–41). Subsequent fibroadenomas (after initial excision) are common as well. In the younger age group, in which a malignant diagnosis is extremely remote, reassurance of the patient and her family is most important. Reexamination after a short time in the middle of the patient's menstrual cycle has been useful because occasionally a prominent mammary lobule may be mistaken for a fibroadenoma and may regress. Because these lesions may increase in size, particularly under the influence of oral contraceptives, other hormonal stimulants, or pregnancy, excision seems most prudent to establish a diagnosis with certainty and eliminate the presence of a dominant mass. Recently, with the availability of accurate cytologic evaluation, many physicians are recommending stereotactic or ultrasound-guided core biopsies of suspected small and nonpalpable fibroadenomas, particularly to differentiate them from phyllodes tumors.[107,108] If the diagnosis is confirmed, the patient may be observed with follow-up physical examination and follow-up imaging procedures.

How are adenomas of the breast characterized clinically?

Adenomas of the breast are well-circumscribed tumors composed of benign epithelial elements with sparse, inconspicuous stroma. This differentiates these lesions from fibroadenomas. The so-called tubular adenoma usually occurs in young women as well-defined, freely movable nodules that resemble fibroadenomas. Clinically, they present in a similar fashion as the fibroadenoma and the differentiation is only noted on pathologic examination.

Lactating adenomas occur as one or more freely movable masses during pregnancy or in the postpartum period. These lesions are well circumscribed, lobulated, and usually softer than the tubular adenoma. They may represent nodular foci of hyperplasia in the lactating breast. Diagnosis can be established by aspiration biopsy.

How are adenomas of the nipple characterized clinically?

Adenomas of the nipple have been described by a variety of names, including florid papillomatosis of the nipple ducts, subareolar duct papillomatosis, papillary adenoma of the nipple, and erosive adenomatosis of the nipple. They may appear as solid, gray-tan, poorly demarcated tumors in the nipple and subareolar region or as no gross lesion in evidence at all. In advanced lesions, glandular epithelium extends onto the surface of the nipple, a phenomenon that results in the clinically evident reddish, glandular appearance, making it somewhat difficult to distinguish from Paget's disease of the nipple. In most instances, the lesion is entirely benign; however, biopsy and subsequent total excision are necessary to distinguish the lesion from carcinoma. Reports of recurrence most likely represent instances in which the initial resection failed to remove the lesion completely.

How is juvenile papillomatosis characterized clinically?

Rosen and associates[109] described a clinical pathologic entity known as juvenile papillomatosis in 1980. These patients, usually younger than 30 years, most often present with a discrete mass, mistaken clinically for a fibroadenoma. Pathologic findings included duct papillomatosis, apocrine and nonapocrine cysts, papillary apocrine hyperplasia, sclerosing adenosis, and duct stasis. Cytologic atypia (74%) and necrosis (17%) were not uncommon.

Several studies have indicated that juvenile papillomatosis may represent a marker for families at risk for coincidental or subsequent breast cancer.[110,111] The frequency of a positive family history exceeds 50%, and affected family members are most likely to be their mothers or maternal aunts. From 10% to 15% of patients with juvenile papillomatosis also have breast carcinoma, and these women are usually in the upper quartile of the age distribution for the lesion. With few exceptions, the carcinoma is within, and appears to arise from, the juvenile papillomatosis. A review of 41 patients with at least 10 years of follow-up after the diagnosis of juvenile papillomatosis (median, 14 years) found that 10% of patients subsequently developed breast carcinoma after an interval of 5 to 15 years. The carcinomas were intraductal; one with microinvasion.[112] Presently, the frequency of carcinoma in juvenile papillomatosis patients does not warrant considering this to be a precancerous lesion.

How is Mondor's disease of the breast characterized clinically?

Mondor's disease of the breast is an uncommon condition first reported in 1869 by Fagge[113] and later discussed in detail in 1939 by Mondor[114] as superficial thrombophlebitis of the lateral thoracic or superior thoracoepigastric veins (see Fig. 14–14). It usually presents as a tender subcutaneous cord in the breast sometimes associated with dimpling of the overlying skin but without systemic signs of infection. Its causes include benign conditions such as trauma, infections, breast surgery, excessive physical strain, and rheumatoid arthritis. Associated carcinoma has been reported in 5% to 12.7% of cases.[115] Mammography should be performed to rule out an underlying malignancy. It has also been found following breast conservation surgery and radiation therapy. The process is usually self-limited and resolves spontaneously in 2 to 10 weeks. Local application of heat and nonsteroidal anti-inflammatory agents can give some relief of symptoms.

How are granular cell tumors of the breast characterized clinically?

Granular cell tumors, uncommonly found in the breast, may simulate carcinoma on clinical, mammographic and pathologic examination.[116] These tumors typically appear between puberty and menopause and most often occur in the upper inner quadrant of the breast, in contrast with carcinoma, which occurs most frequently in the upper outer quadrant. Patients present with a palpable mass, and retraction or fixation to the underlying muscle or chest wall is not uncommon. In addition, they resemble scirrhous carcinoma on mammography.

Granular cell tumors are almost invariably benign and are treated by wide local excision. They are most likely of neurogenic rather than myogenic origin.[117]

How is warfarin-induced breast necrosis characterized clinically?

Flood and associates[118] in 1943 first described a patient with an unusual type of localized hemorrhagic necrosis of skin and subcutaneous tissue of the breast caused by therapy with oral anticoagulation, warfarin. Subsequently, several other cases have been reported. Heparin does not appear to be a predisposing agent. Warfarin-induced breast necrosis is self-limited and fails to respond to a variety of treatments, including steroids, vasodilators, vitamin K, dextran, hypothermia, and symptomatic nerve blocks. Wide excision or simple mastectomy, which may require skin graft for flap closure, is the only effective treatment.

CONCLUSION

Clinical assessment, with attention to a thorough history and physical examination and the use of the adjunctive procedures described in this chapter, will hopefully lead to earlier diagnoses and an improved outlook for women and men with breast cancer. The ultimate goal is prevention, but until that time, early detection is the key to prolonged survival and possible cure.

REFERENCES

1. Smith R, Saslow D. Breast cancer. In Wingood GM, DiClemente RJ (eds). Handbook of Women's Sexual and Reproductive Health. New York, Kluwer Academics/Plenum Publishers, 2002, pp 345–356.
2. Chu K, Tarone R, Kessler L, et al. Recent trends in US breast cancer incidence, survival, and mortality rates. J Natl Cancer Inst 1996;88: 1571–1579.
3. Garfinkel L, Boring CC, Heath CW Jr. Changing trends. An overview of breast cancer incidence and mortality. Cancer 1994;74:222–227.
4. Tabar L, Duffy SW, Vitak B, et al. The natural history of breast carcinoma: What have we learned from screening? Cancer 1999;86: 449–462.
5. Rosato FE, Rosenberg AL. Examination techniques: Role of the physician and patient in evaluating breast diseases. In Bland KI, Copeland EM II (eds.). The Breast. Comprehensive Management of Benign and Malignant Disease. Philadelphia, WB Saunders, 1991.
6. Gold MA. Causes of patients' delay in diseases of the breast. Cancer 1964;17:564–567.
7. Department of Health and Human Services. Federal Register 2002; 76:53182–53273.
8. Vogel VG. Management of the high risk patient. In Jatoi I, Singletary SE, eds. Breast cancer: New concepts in management. Surg Clin North Am 2003;83:733–751.
9. Nelson HD, Humphrey LL, Nygren P, et al. Postmenopausal hormone replacement therapy: Scientific review. JAMA 2002;288:872–881.
10. Olsson HL, Ingvar C, Bladstrom A. Hormone replacement therapy containing progestins and given continuously increases breast carcinoma risk in Sweden. Cancer 2003;97:1387–1392.
11. Chlebowski RT, Hendrix SL, Langer RD, et al. Influence of estrogen plus progestin on breast cancer and mammography in healthy postmenopausal women. The women's health initiative randomized trial. JAMA 2003;289:3243–3252.
12. Li CI, Malone KI, Porter PL, et al. Relationship between long durations and different regimens of hormone therapy and risk of breast cancer. JAMA 2003;289:3254–3263.
13. Shumaker SA, Legault C, Rapp SR, et al. Estrogen plus progestin and the incidence of dementia and mild cognitive impairment in postmenopausal women. The Women's Health Initiative Memory Study: A randomized controlled trial. JAMA 2003;289:2651–2662.
14. Wassertheil-Smoller S, Hendrix SL, Limacher M, et al. Effect of estrogen plus progestin on stroke in postmenopausal women. The Women's Health Initiative: A randomized trial. JAMA 2003;289:2673–2684.
15. Rapp SR, Espeland MA, Shumaker SA, et al. Effect of estrogen plus progestin on global cognitive function in postmenopausal women. The Women's Health Initiative study: A randomized controlled trial. JAMA 2003;289:2663–2672.
16. Israeli D, Tartter PI, Brower ST, et al. The significance of family history for patients with carcinoma of the breast. J Am Coll Surg 1994;179: 29–32.
17. Colditz GA, Willett WC, Hunter DJ, et al. Family history, age, and risk of breast cancer. Prospective data from the nurses' health study. JAMA 1993;270:338–343.
18. Singletary SE. Rating the risk factors for breast cancer. Ann Surg 2003;237:474–482.
19. Langston AA, Malone KE, Thompson JD, et al. BRCA-1 mutations in a population-based sample of young women with breast cancer. N Engl J Med 1996;334:137–142.
20. Fitzgerald MG, MacDonald DJ, Kramer M, et al. Germ-line BRCA-1 mutations in Jewish and non-Jewish women with early-onset breast cancer. N Engl J Med 1996;334:143–149.
21. Offit K. A new marker in the management of patients with breast cancer? Cancer 1996;77:599–601.
22. Claus EB, Schildkraut JM, Thompson WD, et al. The genetic attributable risk of breast and ovarian cancer. Cancer 1996;77:2318–2324.

23. Easton DF, Ford D, Bishop DT, et al. Breast and ovarian cancer incidence in BRCA-1 mutation carriers. Am J Hum Genet 1995;56:265–271.

24. Weitzel JN, McCaffrey SM, Nedelcu R, et al. Effect of genetic cancer risk assessment on surgical decisions at breast cancer diagnosis. Arch Surg 2003;138:1323–1328.

25. American Medical Association. Identifying and managing hereditary risk for breast and ovarian cancer. August 2002.

26. Ng AK, Mauch PM. Second malignancy after Hodgkin's disease. Am J Oncol Rev 2003;2:190–200.

27. Travis LB, Hill DA, Dores GM, et al. Breast cancer following radiotherapy and chemotherapy among young women with Hodgkin's disease. JAMA 2003;290:465–475.

28. Ahmed S, Tartter PI, Jothy S, et al. The prognostic significance of previous benign breast disease for women with carcinoma of the breast. J Am Coll Surg 1996;183:101–104.

29. Connolly JL, Schnitt SJ. Benign breast disease. Resolved and unresolved issues. Cancer 1993;71:1187–1189.

30. Dupont WD, Park FF, Hartmann WH, et al. Breast cancer risk associated with proliferative breast disease and atypical hyperplasia. Cancer 1993;71:1258–1265.

31. Bodian CA, Perzin KH, Lattes R, et al. Prognostic significance of benign proliferative breast disease. Cancer 1993;71:3896–3907.

32. Rosen, PP. Proliferative breast "disease." An unresolved diagnostic dilemma. Cancer 1993;71:3798–3807.

33. Simpson JF, Page DL. The role of pathology in premalignancy and as a guide for treatment and prognosis in breast cancer. Semin Oncol 1996;23:428–435.

34. Bodian CA, Perzin KH, Lattes R. Lobular neoplasia. Long-term risk of breast cancer and relation to other factors. Cancer 1996;78:1024–1034.

35. Smith RA, Saslow D, Sawyer KA, et al. American Cancer Society guidelines for breast cancer screening: Update 2003. CA Cancer J Clin 2003;53:141–169.

36. U.S. Preventive Services Task Force. Screening for breast cancer: Recommendations and rationale. Ann Intern Med 2002;137:344–346.

37. Skinner DA, Helsper JT, Deapen D, et al. Breast cancer: Do specialists make a difference? Ann Surg Oncol 2003;197:334–338.

38. Brenner JR. Medicolegal aspects of breast cancer evaluation and treatment. In Harris JR, Lippman ME, Morrow M, et al. (eds). Diseases of the Breast. Philadelphia, Lippincott-Raven, 1996.

39. Jemal A, Murray T, Ward E, et al. Cancer statistics, 2005. CA Cancer J Clin 2005;55:10–30.

40. Ghafoor A, Jemal A, Ward E, et al. Trends in breast cancer by race and ethnicity. CA Cancer J Clin 2003;53:342–355.

41. O'Malley CD, Lee GM, Glaser SL, et al. Socioeconomic status and breast carcinoma survival in four racial/ethnic groups. Cancer 2003;97:1303–1311.

42. Naik AM, Joseph K, Harris M, et al. Indigent breast cancer patients among all racial and ethnic groups present with more advanced disease compared with nationally reported data. Am J Surg 2003;186:400–403.

43. Bedell MB, Wood ME, Lezotte DC, et al. Delay in diagnosis and treatment of breast cancer: Implication for education. J Cancer Educ 1995;10:223–228.

44. Bjurstam N, Bjorneld L, Warwick J, et al. The Gothenburg Breast Screening Trial. Cancer 2003;97:2387–2396.

45. Tabar L, Fagerberg G, Chen HH, et al. Efficacy of breast cancer screening by age. New results from the Swedish two-county trial. Cancer 1995;75:2501–2507.

46. Bailar JC. Mammography: A contrary view. Ann Intern Med 1976;84:77–84.

47. Feig SA. Assessment of radiation risk from screening mammography. Cancer 1996;77:818–822.

48. Tokunaga M, Land CE, Tokuoka S, et al. Incidence of female breast cancer among atomic bomb survivors, 1950–1985. Radiat Res 1994;38:209–223.

49. Mettler FA, Upton AC, Kelsey CA, et al. Benefits versus risks from mammography: A critical reassessment. Cancer 1996;77:903–909.

50. Smart CR, Hendrich RE, Rutlege JH III, et al. Benefit of mammography screening in women ages 40 to 49 years. Cancer 1995;75:1619–1626.

51. Osuch JR. Abnormalities on physical examination. In Harris JR, Lippman ME, Morrow M, et al (eds). Diseases of the Breast. Philadelphia, Lippincott-Raven, 1996.

52. Lannin DR, Harris RP, Swanson FH, et al. Difficulties in diagnosis of carcinoma of the breast in patients less than fifty years of age. Surg Gynecol Obstet 1993;177:457–462.

53. Winchester DP. Breast cancer in young women. In Lopez MJ (ed). Special Problems in Breast Cancer Therapy. Surg Clin North Am 1996;76:279–287.

54. Velentgas P, Daling JR. Risk factors for breast cancer in younger women. Monogr Natl Cancer Inst 1994;16:15–22.

55. Wallack MK, Wolf JA, Bedwinek J, et al. Gestational carcinoma of the female breast. Curr Probl Cancer 1983;7:1–58.

56. DiFrongo AL, O'Connell TX. Breast cancer in pregnancy and lactation. In Lopez MJ (ed). Special Problems in Breast Cancer Therapy. Surg Clin North Am 1996;76:267–278.

57. Siegelman-Danieli N, Tamir A, Zohar H, et al. Breast cancer in women with recent exposure to fertility medications is associated with poor prognostic features. Ann Surg Oncol 2003;10:1031–1038.

58. Bunker ML, Peters MV. Breast cancer associated with pregnancy or lactation. Am J Obstet Gynecol 1963;85:312–321.

59. Petrek JA, Dutcoff R, Rogatko A. Prognosis of pregnancy-associated breast cancer. Cancer 1991;67:869–872.

60. Costanza M. Issues in breast cancer screening in older women. Cancer 1994;74:2009–2015.

61. Law TM, Hesketh PJ, Parker ICA, et al. Breast cancer in elderly women. In Lopez MJ (ed). Special Problems in Breast Cancer Therapy. Surg Clin North Am 1996;76:289–308.

62. Davis S, Karrer F, Moor B, et al. Characteristics of breast cancer in women over 80 years of age. Am J Surg 1985;15:655–658.

63. Swanson R, Sawicker J, Wood W. Treatment of carcinoma of the breast in the older geriatric patient. Surg Gynecol Obstet 1991;173:465–469.

64. Singletary SE, Shallenberger R, Guinee VF. Breast cancer in the elderly. Ann Surg 1993;218:667–671.

65. Donegan WL, Redlich PN. Breast cancer in men. In Lopez MJ (ed). Special Problems in Breast Cancer Therapy. Surg Clin North Am 1996;76:343–363.

66. Campagnaro EL, Woodside KJ, Xiao S-Y, et al. Cystosarcoma phyllodes (phyllodes tumor) of the male breast. Surgery 2003;133:689–691.

67. Soler NG, Khadori R. Fibrous disease of the breast, thyroiditis, and cheiroarthropathy in type I diabetes mellitus. Lancet 1984;1:193–195.

68. Gump FE, McDermott J. Fibrous disease of the breast in juvenile diabetes. N Y State J Med 1990;90:356–357.

69. Byrd BF Jr, Hartmann WH, Graham LS, et al. Mastopathy in insulin-dependent diabetics. Ann Surg 1987;205:529–532.

70. Logan WW, Hoffman NY. Diabetic fibrous breast disease. Radiology 1989;172:667–670.

71. Frassica DA, Bajaj GK, Tsangaris TN. Treatment of complications after breast-conservation therapy. Oncology 2003;17:1118–1141.

72. Holmich LR, Friis S, Fruzek JP, et al. Incidence of silicone breast implant rupture. Arch Surg 2003;138:801–806.

73. Staren ED, Klepac S, Smith AP, et al. The dilemma of delayed cellulitis after breast conservation therapy. Arch Surg 1996;131:651–654.

74. Stewart FW, Treves N. Lymphangiosarcoma in postmastectomy lymphedema. Cancer 1948;1:64–81.

75. Petrek JA. Post-treatment sarcomas. In Harris JR, Hellman SH, Henderson IC, et al. (eds). Breast Diseases. Philadelphia, JB Lippincott, 1991.

76. Howard J. Using mammography for cancer control: An unrealized potential. Cancer 1987;37:33–48.

77. Layfield LJ, Chrischilles EA, Cohen MB, et al. The palpable breast nodule: A cost-effectiveness analysis of alternate diagnostic approaches. Cancer 1993;72:1642–1651.

78. Stavros AT, Thickman D, Rapp CL, et al. Solid breast nodules: Use of sonography to distinguish between benign and malignant lesions. Radiology 1995;196:123–134.

79. Vetto JT, Pommier RF, Schmidt WA, et al. Diagnosis of palpable breast lesions in younger women by the modified triple test is accurate and cost-effective. Arch Surg 1996;131:967–974.

80. Louie L, Velez N, Earnest CST, Staren ED. Management of nonpalpable ultrasound-indeterminate breast lesions. Surgery 2003;134:667–674.

81. Chen S-C, Yang H-R, Hwang T-L, et al. Intraoperative ultrasonographically guided excisional biopsy or vacuum-assisted core needle biopsy for nonpalpable breast lesions. Ann Surg 2003;238:738–742.

82. Bodrosian I, Mick R, Orel SG, et al. Changes in the surgical management of patients with breast carcinoma based on preoperative magnetic resonance imaging. Cancer 2003;98:468–473.

83. Quan ML, Scalafani L, Heerdt AS, et al. Magnetic resonance imaging detects unsuspected disease in patients with invasive lobular cancer. Ann Surg Oncol 2003;10:1048–1053.

84. Liberman L, Morris EA, Benton CL, et al. Probably benign lesions at breast magnetic resonance imaging. Preliminary experience in high-risk women. Cancer 2003;98:377–388.

85. Vazquez MF, Mitnick JS, Pressman P, et al. Stereotactic aspiration biopsy of nonpalpable nodules of the breast. J Am Coll Surg 1994;178:17–23.

86. Layfield LJ, Glasgow BJ, Cramer H. Fine-needle aspiration in the management of breast masses. Pathol Annu 1989;24:23–62.

87. Fabian CJ, Kimler BF, Zalles CM, et al. Short-term breast cancer prediction of random periareolar fine-needle aspiration cytology and the Gail risk model. J Natl Cancer Inst 2000;92:1217–1227.

88. O'Shaughnessy JA. Ductal lavage: Clinical utility and future promise. In Jatoi I, Singletary SE (eds). Breast Cancer: New Concepts in Management. Surg Clin North Am 2003;753–769.

89. Brogi E, Robson M, Panageas KS, et al. Ductal lavage in patients undergoing mastectomy for mammary carcinoma. Cancer 2003;98:2170–2176.

90. Smith JS. Minimally invasive approach preserves function in nipple discharge. Contemp Surg 2003;59:518–522.

91. Dooley WC. Routine operative breast endoscopy during lumpectomy. Ann Surg Oncol 2003;10:38–42.

92. Dooley WC. Routine operative breast endoscopy for bloody nipple discharge. Ann Surg Oncol 2002;9:920–923.

93. Dooley WC. Ductal lavage, nipple aspiration and ductoscopy for breast cancer diagnosis. Curr Oncol Rep 2003;5:63–65.

94. Dietz JR, Crowe JP, Grundfest S, et al. Directed duct excision by using mammary ductoscopy in patients with pathologic nipple discharge. Surgery 2002;132:582–587.

95. Vogel VG. High-risk populations as targets for breast cancer prevention trials. Prev Med 1991;20:86–100.

96. Gail MH, Brinton LA, Byar DP, et al. Projecting individualized probabilities of developing breast cancer for white females who are being examined annually. J Natl Cancer Inst 1989;81:1879–1886.

97. Dupont WD, Page DL. Risk factors for breast cancer in women with proliferative breast disease. N Engl J Med 1985;312:146–151.

98. Wrensch MR, Petrakis NJ, King EB, et al. Breast cancer incidence in women with abnormal cytology in nipple aspiration of breast fluid. Am J Epidemiol 1992;135:130–134.

99. Wrensch MR, Petrakis NJ, King EB, et al. Cancer risk in women with abnormal cytology in nipple aspirates of breast fluid. J Natl Cancer Inst 2001;93:1791–1798.

100. Minton JP, Fosking MK, Wilsher DJ, et al. Response of fibrocystic disease to caffeine withdrawal and correlation of cyclic nucleotides with breast disease. Am J Obstet Gynecol 1979;135:157–158.

101. Minton JP, Abon-Issa H, Reiches N, et al. Clinical and biochemical studies on methyl-xanthine-related fibrocystic breast disease. Surgery 1981;90:299–304.

102. Winchester DP. Nipple discharge. In Harris JR, Lippman ME, Morrow M, et al. (eds). Diseases of the Breast. Philadelphia, Lippincott-Raven, 1996.

103. Haagensen CD. Abnormalities of breast growth, secretion, and lactation, of physiologic origin. In Diseases of the Breast. Philadelphia, WB Saunders, 1971.

104. Gutman H, Schlachter J, Wasserberg N, et al. Are solitary breast papillomas entirely benign? Arch Surg 2003;138:1330–1333.

105. Carter D. Intraductal papillary tumors of the breast. Cancer 1977;39:1689–1692.

106. Dupont WD, Page DL, Parl FF, et al. Long-term risk of breast cancer in women with fibroadenoma. N Engl J Med 1994;331:10–15.

107. Komenaka IK, El-Tamer M, Pile-Spellman E, et al. Core needle biopsy is a diagnostic tool to differentiate phyllodes tumor from fibroadenoma. Arch Surg 2003;138:987–990.

108. Sperber F, Blank A, Metser V, et al. Diagnosis and treatment of breast fibro-adenomas by ultrasound-guided vacuum-assisted biopsy. Arch Surg 2003;138:796–800.

109. Rosen PP, Cantrell B, Mullen DL, et al. Juvenile papillomatosis (Swiss cheese disease) of the breast. Am J Surg Pathol 1980;4:3–12.

110. Bazzocchi F, Santini D, Martinelli G, et al. Juvenile papillomatosis (epitheliosis) of the breast. Am J Clin Pathol 1986;86:745–748.

111. Rosen PP, Holmes G, Lasser ML, et al. Juvenile papillomatosis and breast carcinoma. Cancer 1985;55:1345–1352.

112. Rosen PP, Kimmel M. Juvenile papillomatosis of the breast: A follow-up study of 41 patients having biopsies before 1979. Am J Clin Pathol 1990;98:599–603.

113. Fagge CH. Remarks on certain cutaneous affections. Guy's Hospital Report 1869–70;15:302.

114. Mondor H. Tronculite sous-cutanee subaigte de la paroi thoracique antero-laterale. Mem Acad Chir Paris 1939;65:1271–1278.

115. Catania S, Zurrida S, Veronesi P, et al. Mondor's disease and breast cancer. Cancer 1992;69:2267–2270.

116. Turnbull AD, Huvos AG, Ashikari R, et al. Granular-cell myoblastoma of the breast. N Y State J Med 1971;71:436–438.

117. Ingram DL, Mossler JA, Snowhite J, et al. Granular cell tumors of the breast. Steroid receptor analysis and localization of carcinoembryonic antigen, myoglobin and S100 protein. Arch Path Lab Med 1984;108:897–901.

118. Flood E, Redish M, Rociek S, et al. Thrombophlebitis migrans disseminata: Report of a case in which gangrene of a breast occurred. N Y State J Med 1943;43:1121–1124.

CHAPTER 15

Mammographic Diagnosis of Breast Cancer

Julie Mitnick

Mammography has become accepted as the single most effective technique to detect breast cancer before it becomes palpable and to aid in decreasing mortality from this cancer.[1] Improvements in mammography have been responsible for the current high proportion of breast cancers that are detected as ductal carcinoma in situ (DCIS)—that is, tumors less than 1 cm in diameter and without axillary lymph node metastases.[2] The benefits of mammographic screening were first defined by the early study of Shapiro and his colleagues, who participated in the Health Insurance Plan of Greater New York (HIP).[3] They demonstrated that women older than 50 years who had screening mammography had cancers that were significantly smaller and had an improved survival compared with women who did not have screening mammography. The efficacy of mammography for the detection of breast cancer in younger women was first shown in the Breast Cancer Detection Demonstration Project (BCDDP), in which 35% of cancers in women younger than 50 years were detected only by mammography.[4] Subsequently, other studies have become available to demonstrate the benefit of screening women younger than 50 years.[5] A controversial report by Olsen and Gøtzsche received a great deal of attention in the media.[6,7] These authors cited technical flaws in early studies of screening mammography and concluded that there is no reduction in mortality from mammography. However, other experts after considerable analysis found the critique itself biased and continue to support the benefits of screening mammography.[8,9]

When did mammography enter into standard diagnostic practice?

The first reproducible technique for radiographic imaging of the breast was described by Egan in 1960.[10] His report of 53 cases of clinically occult malignancies detected by mammography in 2000 consecutive patients suggested that mammography might be used for breast cancer screening in asymptomatic women.[11] The prototype x-ray units "dedicated" to mammography were produced in France in 1965. A molybdenum target and a built-in compression device provided more detailed images with better contrast and lower radiation dose.[12] The initial high-definition intensifying screen was developed for use in mammography in 1970.[13]

Xeroradiography became the predominant method for mammography after its introduction in 1971. The Xerox image was preferred because microcalcification visibility was amplified by an edge enhancement effect and xeromammograms could be viewed in ambient light without a view box. Further improvement in the film-screen combination led to better contrast and visibility of calcifications with decreased scattered radiation. When radiation exposure by the film-screen technique was decreased and the detail of the images obtained by the film-screen combination was improved, this technique came to be preferred over xeromammography.[14] In 1989, the Xerox corporation discontinued production of its xeromammography units because of declining interest. Since then, attention has been focused on obtaining optimal imaging with the film-screen combination, and more recently with digital full-field mammography.

What are the two types of mammography?

There are two types of mammography, screening and diagnostic. Screening mammography aims to detect breast cancer in an asymptomatic individual. Screening examinations use two standard mammographic views. Processing of the films may take place later, at a separate site, termed "batch" processing. Diagnostic mammography is considered to be a problem-solving type of study. The patient may be symptomatic; for example, she may feel a lump in her breast, or her physician may have a concern based on the clinical examination. This study often includes additional views such as magnification views or spot films. The diagnostic evaluation determines whether a mammographic finding is suspicious for cancer. According to Kopans, the distinction between the two types of mammography is that screening detects breast abnormalities that may represent cancer, whereas diagnostic evaluation attempts to determine, with the greatest possible specificity, which of the abnormalities is actually cancer.[15] A second type of diagnostic mammogram is one performed on a woman who has had an abnormal screening mammogram and for whom further evaluation has been requested.

What are the current recommendations for mammography?

Current recommendations for performing mammography by age for asymptomatic women with average risk according to the American Cancer Society are presented below.[16] These guidelines were issued in 1997 and confirmed in 2003:

- Screening should begin by age 40 years
- Screening should be performed every year after age 40 years
- Yearly clinical breast examination should begin at age 40 years; it should be performed every 3 years during ages 20 to 39 years

These guidelines are not accepted as optimal by everyone, and the interval for appropriate screening in women younger than 50 years is controversial. The U.S. Preventive Services Task Force recommended as of 2002 that women 40 years and older receive a mammogram every 1 to 2 years with or without a clinical breast examination.[17] This represents a change over the previous guidelines by including women in their 40s for routine screening. The American Cancer Society guidelines do not have an upper age limit for screening. As long as a woman is in good health, screening is suggested.

Using current high-quality technique, mammography is now considered by many to be as effective in detecting cancer in the 40- to 49-year age group as in the over-50 age group.[5] Technical improvements in mammography, such as full-field digital mammography, have made the evaluation of younger women with denser breasts less problematic than in the past. The composition of the individual's breast tissue (e.g., the relative amount of fat and glandular components) may be more important than the specific age. Women may have breasts that are quite dense even though they are older than 50 years of age, and some women younger than 50 years can easily be assessed by mammography because their breasts are not dense. Aggressive screening of women 40 to 49 years of age to detect occult cancers has been urged, and technical problems and poor study design have been cited as responsible for the failure of the Canadian National Breast Screening Study to demonstrate a decrease in mortality in the under-50 age group.[18] Liberman and associates suggest that the benefits of screening may apply to even younger women.[19] They reviewed the results of screening mammography and breast biopsy results in women 30 to 39 years old screened through the Memorial Hospital BE SMART! Program and found that the rate of cancer detection was comparable to that for women 40 to 49 years of age.

It has been suggested that certain high-risk individuals be screened yearly below age 40 years. These include women with a personal history of breast cancer, high-risk conditions such as lobular carcinoma in situ, atypical duct hyperplasia, or *BRCA1*- or *BRCA2*-positive genetic testing. Also included are women who have had chest irradiation for lymphoma or who have a strong family history of premenopausal breast cancer.

What is the radiation dosage of mammography?

The average radiation dose at the present time of two-view mammography at an American College of Radiology–approved facility is 0.25 cGy.[20] At this dose range, the benefit has been estimated to exceed the risk by a factor of about 100 in women older than 50 years and by a factor of more than 25 in women younger than 50 years.[17] According to Feig, the benefit to women younger than 50 years may be even greater.[20] A more detailed discussion of the benefits of screening mammography is provided by Feig in Chapter 13.

What is full-field digital mammography?

Because the sensitivity of mammography has been demonstrated to reveal only about 75% of breast cancers, there has been an emphasis on developing newer technologies for screening. The prototype for digital mammography occurred in 1996 and was approved by the U.S. Food and Drug Administration (FDA) in 2000. The fluorescent film and screen used with standard mammography is replaced with a digital detector. This detector records the x-rays as electrical signals that are then converted to digital information. Digital detectors have greater latitude and contrast resolution. The digital mammograms can be interpreted from a computer workstation rather than film. At some sites film is still printed because of greater ease in performing comparison with prior film-screen examinations. However, Pisano and associates found that there was no significant difference in the diagnostic accuracy and speed of interpretations with soft-copy and printed-film displays.[21] Digital mammography is particularly valuable for imaging women with dense breasts, for the evaluation of subtle microcalcifications, and for the timely performance of needle localization procedures. The use of digital mammography has been shown to decrease the radiation exposure of needle localizations by as much as 50%.[22] The clinical performance of digital mammography is to some extent dependent on the physician's familiarity with the technique. Published reports, to date, do not demonstrate a significant difference in cancer detection between prototype digital and film-screen mammography in initial studies. Digital mammography has been found to result in fewer recalls for screening.[23] Further benefit may be demonstrated in the future with technologic advances of digital mammography.

What are the standard mammographic views?

High-quality mammography depends on proper technique and skillful performance of positioning as well as accurate interpretation of the films. There has been a renewed emphasis on the importance of technical aspects of mammography with the implementation of the Mammography Quality Standards Act in 1992, which requires that specific standards be met for a facility to receive accreditation. For a mammogram to be of optimal quality, adequate compression must be applied to the breast to separate overlapping structures, decrease the amount of radiation required to produce the image, and obtain sharp images[24] (Fig. 15–1). The standard mammogram consists of the mediolateral oblique (MLO) and the craniocaudal (CC) views, both of which are included in a two-view screening mammogram and a diagnostic mammogram. The MLO is considered the most important view because it includes most of the breast when performed correctly[24] (Fig. 15–2). The pectoral muscle is in an oblique position, extending down to at least the level of the nipple.

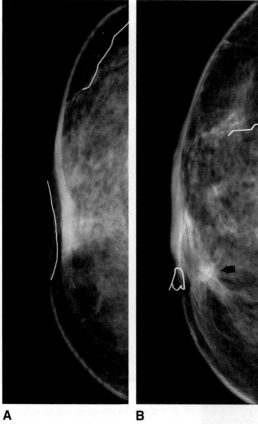

A   **B**

Figure 15–1   Importance of adequate compression during the mammogram. *A,* Implant-displaced craniocaudal view with inadequate compression. *B,* Adequate compression of the implant-displaced view has a 0.3-cm infiltrating carcinoma (*arrow*). Scar markers are at the sites of previous benign biopsies.

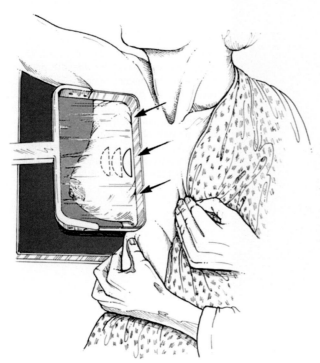

Figure 15–2   Correct patient positioning for the mediolateral oblique view. Note inclusion of the axillary tail and inframammary fold.

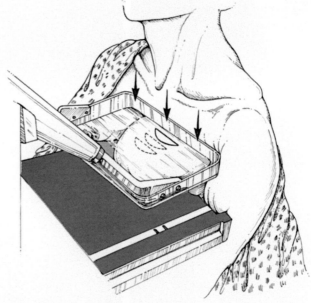

Figure 15–3   Schematic representation of the compressed breast for the craniocaudal view. This view can optimally visualize the medial aspect of the breast.

The axilla is at the superior aspect of the image, and the inframammary fold should be present at the lower. The CC view optimally visualizes the medial aspect of the breast, and in many mammograms it shows the pectoral muscle at the posterior aspect of the film (Figs. 15–3 to 15–5). According to Eklund and Cardenosa, in the exaggerated CC view (XCC), the lateral aspect of the breast can be pulled in as a final maneuver by the technologist when performing this film, thus reducing the need for an extra view.[24] The XCC view is helpful if there is a prominent tail of the breast.

In some cases, additional views are necessary to evaluate a physical or a mammographic finding that is not completely defined by the routine views. Most frequently required additional views include spot compression and magnification views (Figs. 15–6 to 15–10). With spot compression, intense compression is applied to a specific area of the breast, improving the detail of the region. Magnification views can be obtained with or without spot compression and are used to assess microcalcifications and to determine the details of a specific area of the breast such as the border characteristics of a mass (see Fig. 15–4). The 90-degree lateral view is helpful to remove overlapping breast tissue that is seen on the MLO view. In combination with the MLO view, it is possible to determine whether a lesion is medial or lateral in position when it is not seen on the CC view.

Other views may also be needed when performing a diagnostic mammogram. These include angled views, in which the breast is rolled to remove adjacent or overlying tissue; the cleavage view, which images the most medial portion of both breasts on the same film; and the Cleopatra view, to visualize the lateral aspect of the breast in an angled position. A tangential view has the tube angled to bring a specific region of the breast close to the skin surface. It is frequently used to differentiate whether calcifications are within the skin or the breast tissue. "Lumpograms" are performed by pulling on a palpated abnormality, thereby removing adjacent breast and

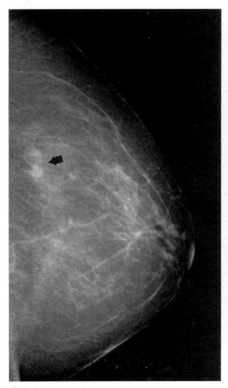

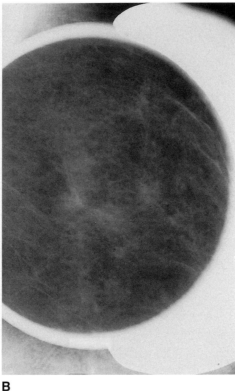

A   **B**

Figure 15–10 *A,* Subtle, low-density irregular mass *(arrow)* at the outer right breast. *B,* The spot film has a persistent mass. An ultrasound-guided core biopsy revealed a 0.4-cm infiltrating lobular carcinoma.

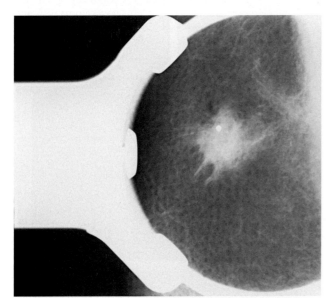

Figure 15–11 A "lumpogram" of a desmoid tumor. The mammographic findings simulate the findings of an infiltrating cancer.

compressing that region with a spot film, to obtain better detail (Fig. 15–11).

What is the mammographic appearance of breast cancer?

The mammographic appearance of breast cancer is varied, and its detection depends on the interpretive skills of the radiologist. In many instances, there is overlap between benign

Table 15–1   Mammographic Appearance of Proven Cancers of the Breast (n = 1314)

Mammographic Finding	Number (%)
Clustered microcalcifications	589 (45%)
Spiculated mass	355 (27%)
Round, oval, lobular, or irregular mass	249 (19%)
Architectural distortion	87 (7%)
Focal asymmetric density	34 (2%)

and malignant entities, and mammography alone may not be specific enough to differentiate them. Even the most suspicious appearance for cancer, a spiculated mass, can have benign histology, such as surgical scarring, fat necrosis, or radial scar. Further evaluation of a finding that the radiologist determines is suspicious for cancer may require additional films, sonography, or percutaneous or surgical biopsy.

The Breast Imaging Reporting and Data System (BI-RADS) lexicon has been developed to obtain uniformity in the description of findings on the mammogram.[25] This descriptive system enhances understanding of the likelihood that a particular mammographic finding is a cancer. We retrospectively reviewed the mammographic appearance of our proven cancers, both palpable and nonpalpable, according to the American College of Radiology (ACR) terminology (Table 15–1). These are cases for which a malignant diagnosis was confirmed by histopathology. Clustered microcalcifications were the most common indicator of cancer in this series. The term *focal asymmetrical density,* according to the ACR lexicon, is used to describe a density with a similar shape on two views but lacking the borders of a discrete mass. Asymmetrical breast tissue is judged relative to other areas in the breast and includes a greater volume of breast tissue, greater density, or more prominent ducts. There is no focal mass present, and it usually represents a normal variation. It may be deemed significant when there is an associated palpable mass. Other less common findings are skin thickening, nipple retraction, trabecular thickening, and axillary adenopathy.

According to federal regulations, every mammogram must have, in its impression, an overall assessment of the likelihood of a finding's being cancer. This promotes understanding among the radiologist, clinician, and patient of the relative risk for cancer's being present. The overall assessment categories for the BI-RADS coding is as follows:

- Category 0: Incomplete: needs additional imaging evaluation, or comparison with prior studies
- Category 1: Negative
- Category 2: Benign finding
- Category 3: Probably benign; short term follow-up suggested
- Category 4: Suspicious for malignancy
- Category 5: Highly suspicious for malignancy
- Category 6: Proven breast cancer

According to Liberman and associates,[19] the findings that are most likely to have a positive predictive value for being cancer (BI-RADS category 4 or 5) are spiculated masses or linear or branching calcifications.

Why obtain mammography for patients with palpable masses?

Suspicious palpable masses detected by clinical examination should be evaluated by mammography to determine the extent of the cancer within the breast and to identify other occult sites of cancer within the same and the opposite breast. Identification of other sites of cancer will likely affect the surgical treatment (e.g., whether conservation is possible). Most palpable findings detected by clinical examination prove to be benign following surgery, and mammography helps to identify the nonmalignant palpable mass and thereby avoid surgery. When a benign mass such as a cyst is suspected, mammography should be performed before aspiration or core biopsy. A breast sonogram may also be of help to further evaluate the nature of the mass. The dominant mass that is palpated and aspirated may be a cyst, but an occult cancer adjacent to it may be detected on the mammogram (Fig. 15–12). If a cancer is palpated, imaging of the same and contralateral breasts may detect other clinically occult sites of cancer.

How frequently are breast cancers missed by mammography?

Mammography cannot detect all breast cancers. For women with dense breasts, such as young women and those with a fibrocystic condition, it may be difficult to visualize a cancer. With problem-solving additional views or technique tailored to the individual, however, information may often be obtained even in young symptomatic women with dense breasts.

The sensitivity of mammography is in the range of 68% to 92%.[26] The problem of missed breast cancers has been attributed to several causes: technical faults, observer errors, and the intrinsic limitations of mammography itself. Technical factors include proper positioning and adequate compression (see Fig. 15–7). Observer errors have been analyzed by Bird and associates, who reviewed 320 cancers, 77 (24%) of which they

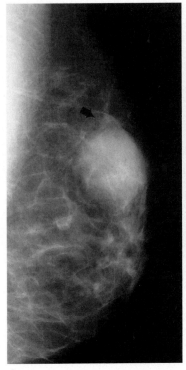
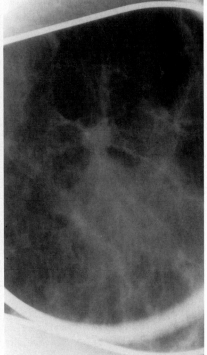

Figure 15–12 *A,* Small carcinoma is partially obscured by a large cyst. Architectural distortion is present at the superior aspect of the 3-cm oval mass. *B,* The mass was aspirated and was a cyst. A spot film of the distorted area showed a tiny invasive duct carcinoma.

A   B

missed mammographically.[27] They found that diagnostic errors were more likely to occur for developing densities and that missed cancers were most often small, irregular densities in the retroareolar or retroglandular portions of the breast. Missed cancers were unlikely to demonstrate microcalcifications and were more likely to occur in women with dense breasts. Forty (52%) of their missed cancers could be identified in retrospect, on earlier mammograms. Fourteen (18%) of the cases that were missed, according to the authors, were incorrectly interpreted as benign. Dense breasts, diffuse nodularity, and breast implants may cause difficulty in detecting a cancer by mammography.

The use of double reading for mammographic interpretation has been demonstrated to detect 15% more cancers than interpretations by a single radiologist.[28]

An alternative to double reading is the use of computer programs to help in detecting an abnormality on the mammogram. Reports have shown that computer-aided detection (CAD) algorithms are able to detect breast abnormalities on screening mammograms and reduce the number of false-negative findings. In a prospective study of 12,860 patients who had screening mammography with CAD, there was a 19.5% increase in the number of cancers found.[29] In a different study, the CAD system was found to have no effect on radiologist performance, despite high sensitivity, probably owing to the many false-positive markings.[30] Zheng and coworkers reported that the sensitivity for the detection of clustered microcalcifications is high at 96% but that sensitivity for mass is only 66.7% to 70.8%.[31] The authors also noted that the abnormalities in their study were visible on both views and that they were not particularly subtle. Further improvements must be achieved in the detection of masses for CAD systems to be sufficiently reliable for general use, and for the possibility of achieving the increased sensitivity of a second reader. These authors also cautioned that the use of CAD may be problematic from a medicolegal viewpoint if an area marked on an earlier mammogram later develops into a cancer.[31] CAD has not been found beneficial for the detection of architectural distortion on the mammogram, an often subtle and important presentation of breast cancer.[32] It has been reported that the reproducibility of the CAD systems is currently insufficient for clinical routines.[33]

What are the medicolegal ramifications of mammography?

Publicity regarding the success of mammography has been accompanied by unrealistic claims for the reliability of this technique to detect breast cancer. The rise in lawsuits charging delay in diagnosing breast cancer may be partially due to a misunderstanding that all breast cancers can be detected by mammography. Summarized data from the Physicians Insurance Association of America (PIAA), based on the pooled results of selected insurance companies with lawsuits instituted for a claim of a missed diagnosis of breast cancer, were issued in 1990 and again in 1995.[34,35] These two reports found that most claimants were younger than 50 years, frequently found their own breast mass, and often were incorrectly diagnosed as having a fibrocystic condition. Our own review of lawsuits in New York State and other reports confirmed these findings[36–38] (Table 15–2). The PIAA reports

Table 15–2 Complaint of Plaintiff in Legal Actions (n = 37)*

Complaint Category	Complaint	No. (%)
1	Plaintiff felt a lump; physician failed to obtain a biopsy specimen or refer to a specialist	22 (60)
2	Plaintiff felt a lump; physician failed to order mammography	6 (16)
3	Physician failed to examine properly and palpate breasts, and detect a palpable lump	2 (5)
4	Physician failed to read mammogram properly	3 (8)
5	Physician failed to warn that pregnancy can reactivate breast cancer	1 (3)
6	Physician ignored suspicious findings on mammogram and recommendation of biopsy	1 (3)
7	Physician failed to properly treat already diagnosed breast cancer	2 (5)

*Several of these actions involved more than one category of complaint. Modified from Mitnick JS, Vazquez MF, Plesser KP, et al. Breast cancer malpractice litigation in New York State. Radiology 1993;189:673–676.

showed that in 1990, gynecologists were the physician specialty most frequently sued. In 1995, radiologists were more often cited, probably owing to the increased number of screening mammograms being performed. Both the failure to perform mammograms and an over-reliance on this technique when it is negative have led to lawsuits in which a delay in diagnosis was purported.

Ikeda and associates have reported that there is a subset of nonspecific mammographic findings that do not warrant recall but that were the subtle findings where cancer later developed.[39] They believe that a failure to act on these nonspecific findings does not constitute an interpretation below the standard of care. In their study, the most common nonspecific finding on prior mammograms that they believed should not be considered an error was a density seen on only one view. They found that these densities are indistinguishable from randomly distributed islands of breast tissue that are common in fibrocystic disease. They have noted that in the setting of a malpractice allegation, the mere presence of a finding on a prior mammogram does not indicate liability. Mammograms should be viewed in the temporal sequence in which they were obtained, and a retrospective analysis of a nonspecific finding at the site of cancer development is not malpractice. They noted that just because "something is visible where cancer develops subsequently does not mean that a defendant radiologist was negligent in choosing not to recommend recall for additional imaging."

Because of the highly litigious nature of mammography, fewer radiology residents are choosing to practice breast imaging. In a survey of radiology residents, causes of disinterest in interpreting mammograms included fear of lawsuits, low pay, and mental stress.[40] There is currently a nationwide shortage of radiologists willing to read mammograms.

Berlin has reported that the current system of malpractice awards is such that even if a panel of highly educated experts agree that no negligence has occurred, if a woman has a witness who will testify that a breast cancer was missed on an earlier mammogram, she is likely to be successful in the lawsuit.[41]

What are interval breast cancers?

Interval breast cancers are cancers diagnosed during the 12 months after a normal screening mammogram and clinical examination (Figs. 15–13 to 15–15). They have traditionally been thought to be more aggressive forms of breast cancer, with a poor prognosis for survival. DeGroote and colleagues reported 21 patients with interval breast cancers, with 24% having stage II and 25% having stage III disease at the time of diagnosis.[42] In contrast, Koivunen and associates did not find their interval cancers to be more aggressive.[43] They evaluated 24 patients with interval breast cancers and found that 54% had stage II disease and none had more advanced disease. Their patients with interval breast cancers were characterized by increased density of the breasts and greater difficulty in diagnosis by mammography. Physical examination was also less reliable in their patients because they had diffuse nodularity or fibrocystic conditions. Their conclusion was that interval breast cancers are not a subset of biologically more aggressive cancers but are cancers that are more difficult to diagnose by mammography and clinical examination. A series by Burrell and associates of 90 interval cancers had 51 (57%) true positive, 20 (22%) false negative, 7 (8%) mammographically occult, and 12 (13%) unclassified.[44] The false-negative cases were most often found to be areas of architectural distortion at mammography. There was no significant difference in the patterns of breast parenchyma for these categories of interval cancer. Their interval cancers were larger and more likely to have lymph node metastases and to have a poorer prognosis than screening-detected cancers.

What is the radiologist's role in the surgical excision of a clinically occult lesion?

Clinically occult mammographic abnormalities that require excision, such as suspicious microcalcifications or architectural distortion, should be preoperatively localized by the radiologist to achieve a successful surgical biopsy. Outpatient needle localization breast biopsies (NLBBs) for nonpalpable abnormalities have become a standard surgical practice similar to that used for the removal of palpable abnormalities. A report from the New England Medical Center in Boston found that when local anesthesia for NLBB is used, the chance of missed lesions is less than 2%, and complication rates are comparable to those for biopsy of palpable lesions.[45] This failure rate using NLBB was slightly lower than that found from 17 series in the literature that the authors reviewed, which was 2.8%. Reported complications related to the needle localizing device and cited as causes for missing the lesions included transection or breakage of the localizing device, retraction of the wire into the breast, entrapment of the wire below the pectoralis fascia, and poor positioning of the localizing wire. We have found these complications to be extremely rare, with the most common rare complication being a minor vasovagal reaction. A similar experience was reported by Helvie and associates, who evaluated complications of patients undergoing needle localization and aspiration procedures: of 172 patients

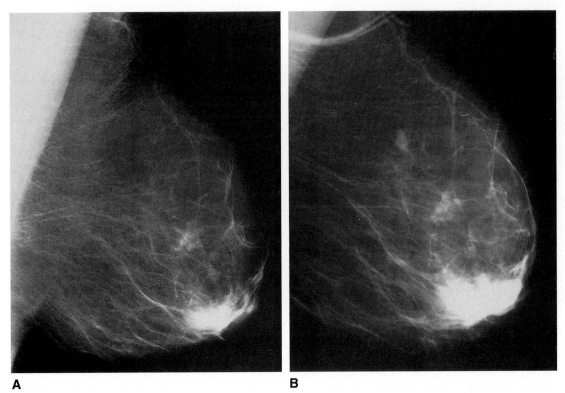

A   **B**

Figure 15–13   Interval breast cancer. *A,* Mediolateral oblique view of the right breast is unremarkable. *B,* One year later, a 1.2-cm lobular carcinoma developed in the superior breast.

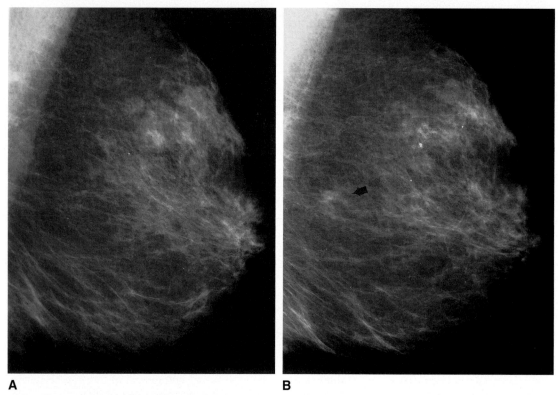

A   B

Figure 15–14   Interval breast cancer. *A,* The mediolateral oblique view of a screening mammogram was normal. *B,* One year later, there is a subtle asymmetrical density (*arrow*) that was poorly differentiated duct carcinoma.

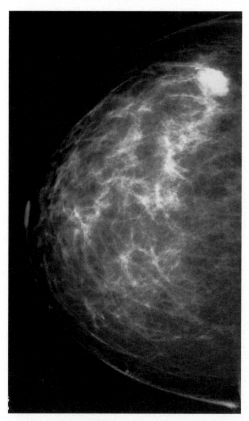

Figure 15–15   Craniocaudal view of the right breast was negative (not shown). One year later, there has been development of an interval high-grade invasive duct carcinoma. The mass was circumscribed with irregular borders, findings that were highly suggestive of the malignant diagnosis.

who underwent needle localization, 13 (8%) had vasovagal reactions.[46]

Several needle localizer systems are widely used. The three most popular systems are the Kopans, Homer, and Hawkins needle localizer systems. The Kopans system (Cook, Bloomington, IN) allows for a moderate amount of traction on the wire during surgery. The disadvantage is that the wire cannot be repositioned (Figs. 15–16 and 15–17). The Homer system (North American Instrument, Glens Falls, NY) is easy to use and has a retractable wire. When the J-shaped memory wire is delivered, the needle may be left in place and used as a nontransectable guide for the surgeon. The disadvantage is that the needle and wire are relatively easy to pull out with moderate traction. The Hawkins I system (National-Standard Medical Products, Gainesville, FL) has a tip that is withdrawn into an outer cannula once the barb is deployed. The barb exits from the cannula at an acute angle, allowing for moderate traction at surgery. It is reported to have greater anchoring strength than the Kopans system.[47]

The approach for the needle localization procedure should be carefully planned. Generally, the shortest distance from the skin to the lesion is used. Some surgeons prefer a needle entry close to the areolar margin. Once the suspicious area is localized within the fenestrated grid, an intradermal injection of local anesthetic can be given at the site of approach of the localizer needle. Using the tube light as a guide, the needle is inserted to the proper coordinate location indicated on the scout film. As the needle is inserted into the breast, a change in texture may occasionally be noted as the needle reaches the suspicious lesion. The needle should be advanced just beyond that point. It is better to "overshoot" the lesion than to be short of it. Next, the compression device is released while

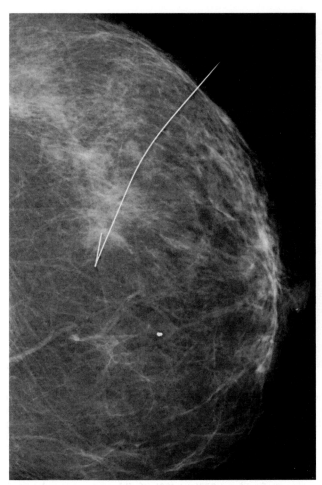

Figure 15–16 Kopans wire in place for the preoperative localization of invasive lobular carcinoma. The wire extends through a subtle area of distortion of the breast architecture.

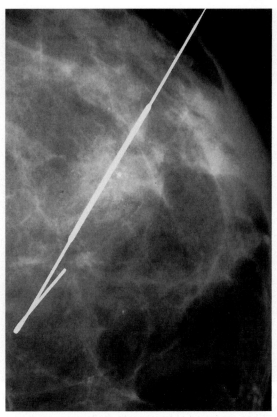

Figure 15–17 Kopans wire has microcalcifications at the thick segment of the wire. The microcalcifications were excised, and the histology was solid and cribriform ductal carcinoma in situ.

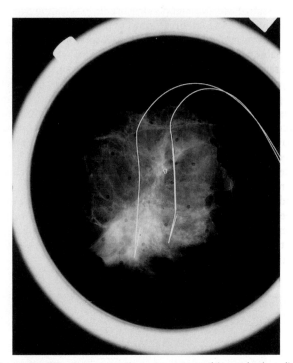

Figure 15–18 A stereotactic mammotome biopsy had malignant microcalcifications. The Micromark clip and residual microcalcifications were bracketed with preoperative localization wires seen in the specimen radiograph. Bracketing of malignant microcalcifications may aid the surgeon to achieve clear margins.

the needle is protected from contacting the edges of the coordinated grid window. Final films are obtained with the wire in place, and the site to be excised is marked on both films. These films accompany the patient to the operating room as a guide for the surgeon. Needle localizations can also be performed using ultrasound guidance. Mammographic films are obtained after placement of the wire to confirm the correct wire placement. Bracketing wires may be used for preoperative needle localization to delineate the boundaries of a mammographic lesion, such as a broad region of suspicious microcalcifications, to help encompass the entire lesion (Fig. 15–18). In a report by Liberman and colleagues, bracketing wires were most often used for large calcified lesions that were highly suggestive of malignancy (e.g., BI-RADS category 5 lesions).[48] These authors emphasize that the complete removal of the calcifications does not ensure clear histologic margins at resection. The advantage of ultrasound localization is that there is no radiation exposure except for the final films demonstrating wire position. Also, because the patient is supine, there are fewer vasovagal reactions, and the time to perform the localization is lessened. With the increasing use of sonography to evaluate the breast, more needle localizations are being performed with this technique. We routinely use sonography to localize most nonpalpable entities, except for microcalcifications.

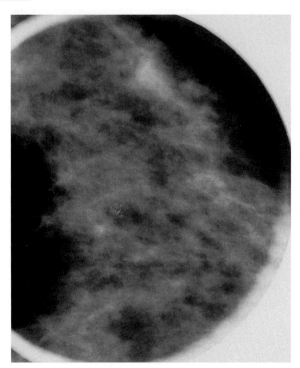

Figure 15–24   Comedocarcinoma. A screening mammogram has a new cluster of microcalcifications. There is a linear calcification in the center of the cluster. A faint separate site of microcalcifications was also ductal carcinoma in situ (DCIS) in this patient with multifocal DCIS.

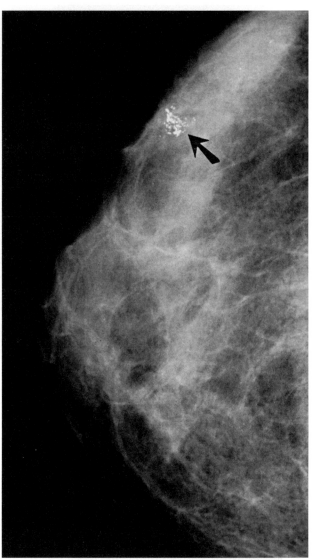

Figure 15–25   A cluster of calcifications on a screening mammogram in a young woman with a positive family history of breast cancer (*arrow*). On initial inspection the calcifications appear coarse, but numerous fine microcalcifications were also within the cluster. Although not typical of ductal carcinoma in situ, coarse calcifications may also occur with this entity.

reported a case of DCIS that appeared as a branching tubular opacity with peripheral coarse calcifications. With this appearance, DCIS may be difficult to distinguish from vascular calcifications.[56] In a review by Stomper and coworkers of 100 cases of DCIS, an indistinct round or oval mass was present in 18%, an irregular or poorly defined mass in 64%, a spiculated mass in 14%, and architectural distortion in 4%.[57] These soft tissue findings were attributed to direct involvement by tumor into an expanded lobule and to periductal fibrosis or elastosis. In an early report, we described 13 small, round, or oval masses that were well circumscribed and had microcalcifications that proved to be DCIS.[58]

Liberman and associates have reported that calcifications highly suggestive of malignancy account for about 10% of nonpalpable lesions referred for biopsy.[59] These calcifications include linear or branching clustered microcalcifications. Based on their experience, they recommend sterotactic biopsy of the calcifications using an 11-gauge vacuum-assisted automated device because there is a greater likelihood that a single operation for definitive treatment may be performed. They found that only 16.2% of women with breast cancer who had a diagnostic surgical biopsy had a single operation for treatment. This compared with 71.4% of women who had a stereotactic biopsy. They report that the significantly greater chance of having a single operation after stereotactic biopsy allows for better treatment planning by anticipating the need for wide excision or mastectomy.

What is the role of specimen radiographs?

Careful correlation between intraoperative specimen radiography and preoperative mammography is important to verify complete excision of the mammographic lesion. Because successful breast conservation therapy is believed to be dependent on the demonstration of complete removal of the lesion, preoperative magnification views may be obtained for assessment of other sites of involvement by DCIS manifested as microcalcifications. Some of the microcalcifications may be extremely faint and not visualized by conventional radiographs (see Fig. 15–27). Morrow reviewed a study by Holland and concluded that there is underestimation of DCIS by as much as 20 mm if magnification views are not performed.[60] These films may be useful to diagnose multicentric

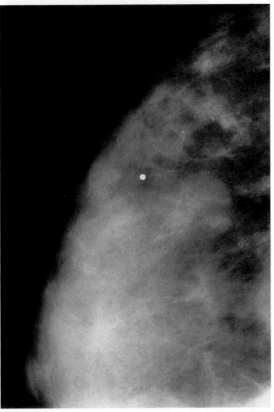

Figure 15–26 Multiple clusters of punctate microcalcifications were micropapillary ductal carcinoma in situ in a 33-year-old patient. There is also a palpable, partially obscured mass that was infiltrating duct carcinoma.

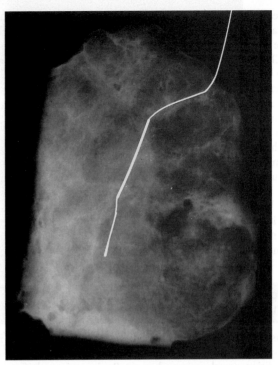

Figure 15–27 This specimen radiograph has heterogeneous clustered microcalcifications at the thickened segment of a wire used for preoperative needle localization. There was a barely perceptible new cluster of microcalcifications on the mammogram. A 0.3-cm focus of comedo-type DCIS was excised.

Figure 15–28 Recurrent carcinoma. *A,* A 37-year-old woman had a prior excision of microcalcifications that were ductal carcinoma in situ (DCIS). A routine mammogram performed 3 years later has pleomorphic microcalcifications that were recurrent DCIS. At times, it may be difficult to differentiate recurrence from fat necrosis in the lumpectomy site. *B,* Heterogeneous microcalcifications and architectural distortion were recurrent cancer. Multiple foci of invasive ductal and cribriform DCIS were found at excision. The DCIS extended beyond the edges of the infiltrating cancer.

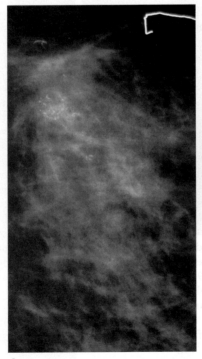

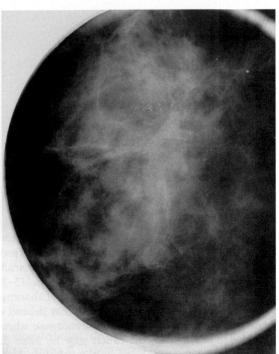

A   B

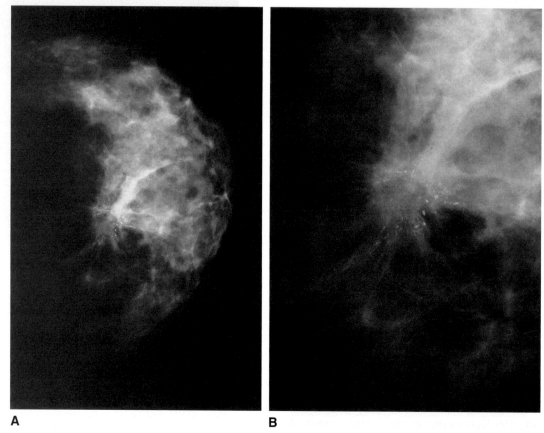

Figure 15–33 *A,* A spiculated mass has linear microcalcifications extending along ducts. *B,* The microcalcifications indicate the associated ductal carcinoma in situ.

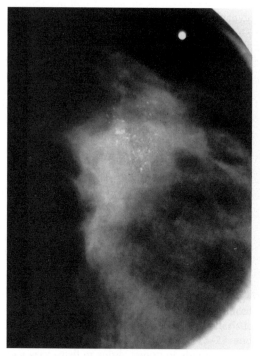

Figure 15–34 A spot film of a palpable irregular mass that was infiltrating poorly differentiated duct carcinoma also had ductal carcinoma in situ as indicated by microcalcifications.

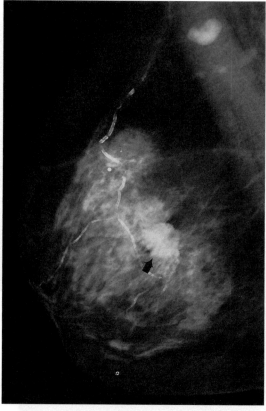

Figure 15–35 Infiltrating duct carcinoma. A high-density mass (*arrow*) with irregular borders in the central left breast. There is a dense axillary lymph node that was positive for metastatic disease.

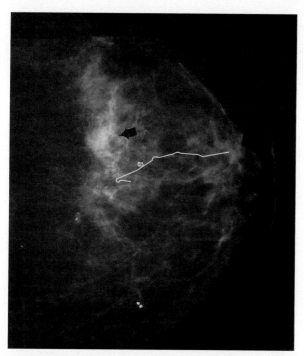

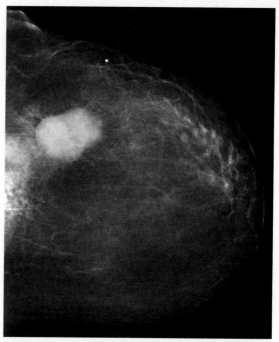

Figure 15–36 A round mass (*arrow*) with partially obscured borders developed adjacent to a prior benign biopsy. The border characteristics made this mass suspicious, and the needle biopsy showed infiltrating duct carcinoma.

Figure 15–37 A 75-year-old woman had a rapidly growing mass with irregular borders that was found to be poorly differentiated infiltrating duct carcinoma with metaplasia.

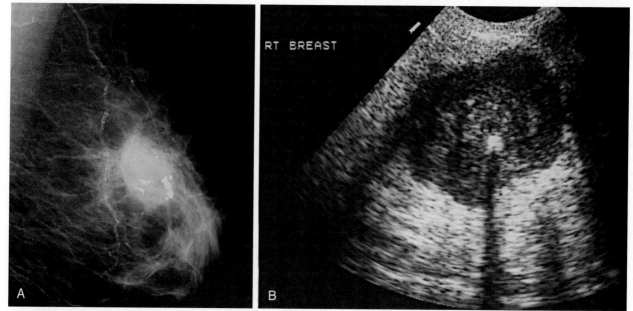

Figure 15–38 *A,* Well-circumscribed carcinoma. A lobular mass in the outer half of the right breast on the craniocaudal view has distinct borders. Although medullary, colloid, and intracystic carcinomas are known to present as well-circumscribed masses, the most common well-circumscribed carcinoma is infiltrating ductal, not otherwise specified, which this proved to be. *B,* Corresponding sonogram shows the hypoechoic lobulated mass.

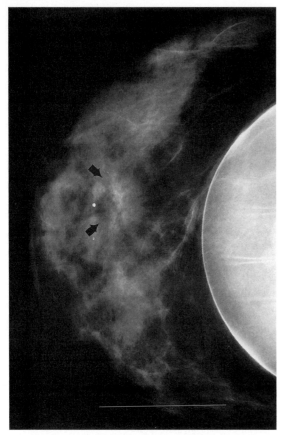

Figure 15–39   A subtle region of architectural distortion corresponded to palpable thickening in this patient with a silicone breast implant. It proved to be a well-differentiated infiltrating duct carcinoma, visualized on this implant-displaced view. *Arrows* outline an area of architectural distortion that proved to be an invasive duct carcinoma.

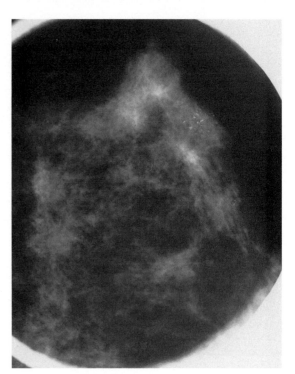

Figure 15–40   Multifocal carcinoma. A spot magnification view has multiple masses and sites of architectural distortion, all of which were invasive ductal cancer. Ductal carcinoma in situ was also present at the site of microcalcifications.

mammography and by palpation. Five patterns of mammographic presentation of ILC were described by Mendelson, with the most frequent being a focal region of asymmetrical density[58] (Figs. 15–44 and 15–45). The spread of this cancer in the classic single-file configuration was proposed as being responsible for its subtle appearance as a poorly delimited mass. Sickles refers to the mammographic findings of ILC as "atypical," often preventing early diagnosis of this cancer.[59] Our experience, based on a retrospective review of 102 cases of proven ILC, had a spiculated mass as the most common appearance, similar to the findings of Helvie.[60,61] Negative mammography has traditionally been described as occurring more frequently with ILC than IDC. Microcalcifications have also been found less frequently with ILC than with IDC in most series. There is a high incidence of bilaterality and multifocality with ILC, and of metastatic spread with unusual sites of deposits, including the gastrointestinal tract, ovary, uterus, and peritoneum.[62] Various studies have found the prognosis to be either better, the same as, or worse than that of IDC.[62]

How is tubular carcinoma characterized radiographically?

Tubular carcinoma, a variant of infiltrating ductal carcinoma, is being detected with increasing frequency and at a smaller

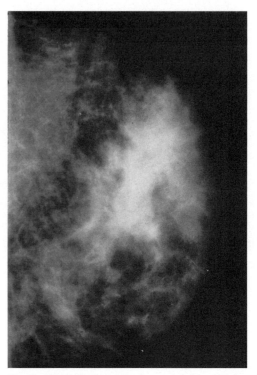

Figure 15–41   Virtually the entire breast has been replaced with high-grade infiltrating duct carcinoma that is extending from the superior to inferior right breast.

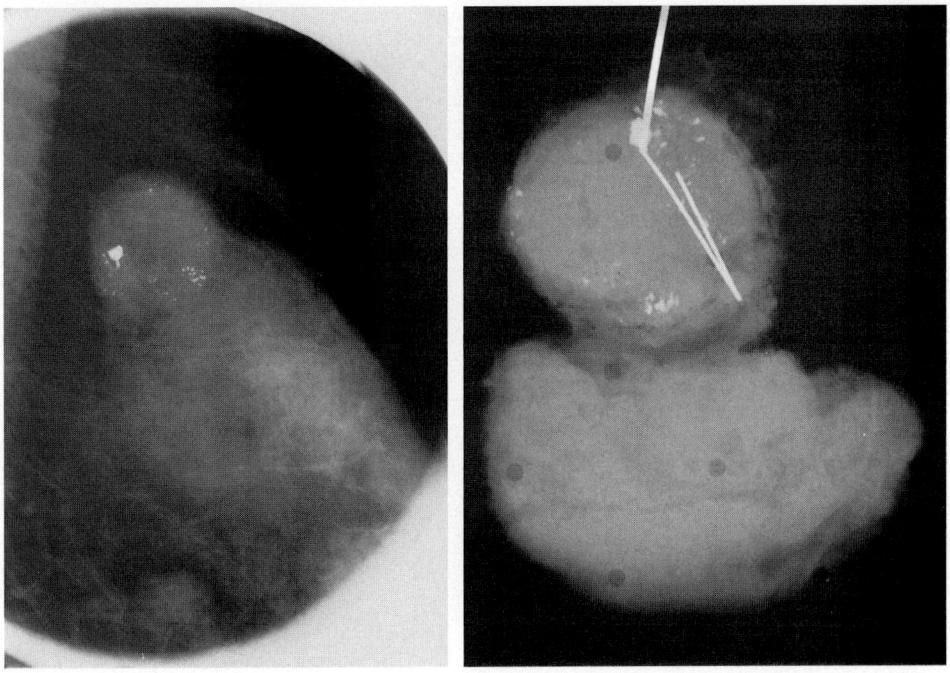

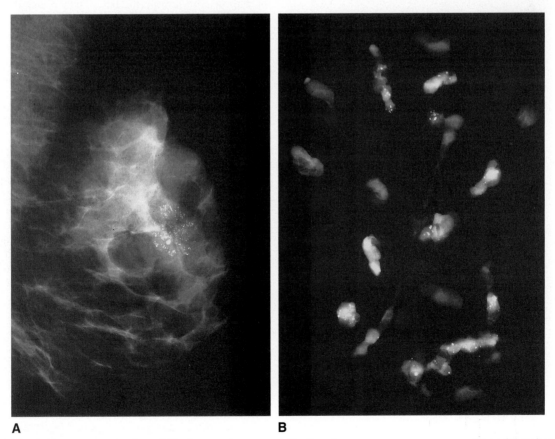

Figure 15–42 *A,* Round mass in the outer right breast has heterogeneous, mainly peripherally located microcalcifications and coarse calcifications. Although the preoperative impression was that of a fibroadenoma, because of the atypical appearance of the calcifications, the lesion was excised. *B,* The specimen radiograph has the fibroadenoma and the localizing wire.

A   **B**

A   **B**

Figure 15–43 *A,* Heterogeneous microcalcifications and coarse calcifications in a young woman were suspicious for malignancy. The patient underwent a stereotactic mammotome biopsy, and a benign fibroadenoma was diagnosed. *B,* The specimens have abundant calcium.

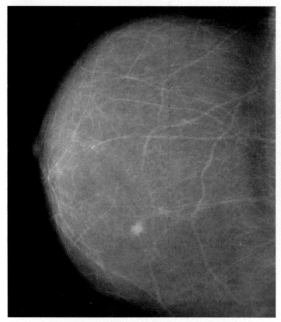

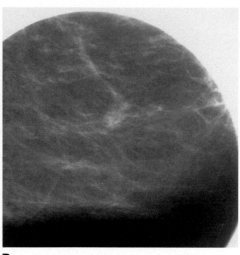

Figure 15–44 *A* and *B*, A tiny mass with irregular borders in the right breast at the 6-o'clock axis was a 0.5-cm invasive lobular carcinoma. Despite its small size and moderate density, the cancer was detectable because of the surrounding fatty tissue.

A

B

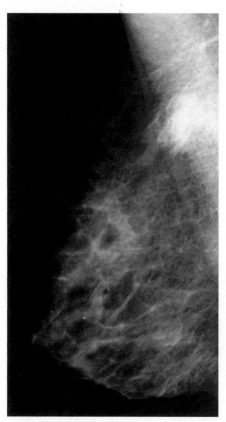

Figure 15–45 An asymmetrical density in the upper outer left breast was infiltrating lobular carcinoma. This represented an interval change on the mammogram.

average size as a result of screening mammography. Winchester and associates recently reported the median tumor diameter to be 1 cm[64] (Fig. 15–46). They suggest that the larger tubular cancers may have a more aggressive course and are evolving into typical IDC. Tubular carcinomas are usually found when they are nonpalpable, in women younger than those with nonspecific IDC. The pathologic use of the term *tubular carcinoma* requires that at least 75% of the lesion be composed of tubular elements. Some pathologists suggest that tubular carcinomas arise from papillary or cribriform intraductal carcinoma, whereas others suggest that they evolve from radial scars.[65,66] Regarded as a well-differentiated cancer with a favorable prognosis, it has also been reported to be associated with an increased incidence of multicentricity and contralateral cancers. A 32% rate of incidental DCIS within this tumor following excision has been reported.[64] Although there is controversy regarding the proper treatment for this cancer, 20% of Winchester's patients had axillary nodal metastases.[64] These cancers most frequently appeared as spiculated masses at mammography in the series by Liebman and coworkers.[67] They suggest that the spiculated appearance of tubular carcinoma is characteristic and that because of its smallness, it can be differentiated by mammography from other cancers. However, Elson and associates found a variety of mammographic presentations for this type of cancer, including a mass, mass with calcifications, architectural distortion, and asymmetrical density.[68]

How is mucinous carcinoma characterized radiographically?

Mucinous (colloid) carcinoma of the breast, accounting for 1% to 7% of breast cancers, has received relatively little attention in the radiologic literature. It is a well-differentiated, distinct type of invasive adenocarcinoma characterized by the extracellular mucin that embeds the tumor cells. It is usually detected in older patients with an average age of 65 years. Although it was traditionally thought to have a favorable prognosis and a lower incidence of metastases than less differentiated infiltrating ductal carcinoma NOS, one series noted metastatic disease in about 30% of patients.[69] The classic

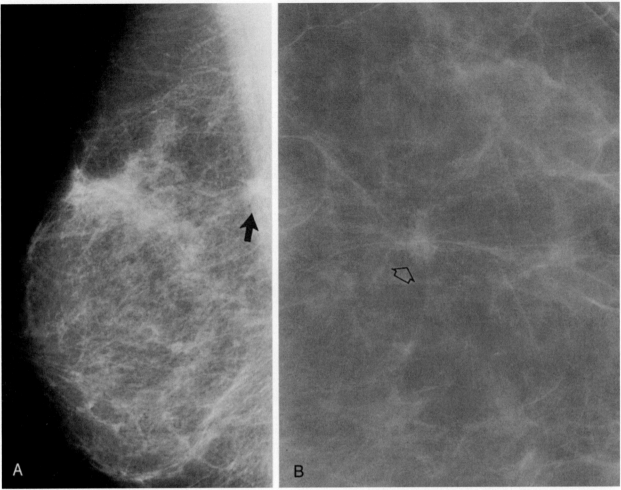

Figure 15–46 Tubular carcinoma. *A,* The mediolateral oblique view shows a 5-mm spiculated mass overlying the pectoral muscle (*arrow*). These slow-growing, well-differentiated neoplasms often present as tiny spiculated lesions. *B,* Spot magnification views may be necessary to delineate the spiculated nature of these lesions (*arrow*).

mammographic features of pure mucinous carcinoma have been described by Conant and associates as a mass with either indistinct or microlobulated margins rarely having calcifications[70] (Figs. 15–47 and 15–48). We have found several mucinous carcinomas that had coarse calcifications simulating those in fibroadenomas. Wilson and associates evaluated 20 patients with mucinous carcinoma and found that a more sharply circumscribed and distinct border was found for the pure mucinous carcinomas and that irregular margins were found with tumors of mixed mucinous and NOS type.[71] The irregularity of contour is thought to result from fibrosis associated with the nonmucinous component of the tumor. Mixed-type mucinous tumors tend to be larger at the time of diagnosis and to have a less favorable prognosis than the pure type.

How is medullary carcinoma characterized radiographically?

Medullary carcinoma of the breast, an uncommon subtype of infiltrating ductal carcinoma, is associated with an improved survival rate and younger age compared with survival and age of women with infiltrating ductal carcinoma NOS. The specific pathologic characteristics associated with this tumor include a predominantly syncytial growth pattern, microscopic completely circumscribed margins, mononuclear stromal infiltrate, and anaplastic cytologic details.[65] A report by Rubens and associates of 30 cases of breast cancer originally diagnosed as medullary carcinoma at Massachusetts General Hospital stated that only 9 (30%) were in fact typical medullary carcinomas.[72] Using strict histologic criteria for medullary carcinoma, the remaining cases were reclassified as atypical medullary carcinomas in 7 (23%) and infiltrating ductal carcinoma NOS in 14 (47%). It has been suggested that the too frequent diagnosis of this type of cancer may lead to a false impression of a more favorable outcome and undertreatment.[72] The typical appearance of medullary carcinoma at mammography is an oval or round circumscribed mass, with varying degrees of lobulation without calcifications (Figs. 15–49 and 15–50). At ultrasound, there is a well-defined hypoechoic mass with an inhomogeneous texture and enhanced through transmission. Central necrosis may be seen in large mucinous cancers.[73] According to Kopans, despite the so-called typical imaging characteristics of medullary carcinoma, there are no criteria to reliably distinguish medullary carcinomas from infiltrating ductal carcinomas NOS.[74] Liberman and coworkers found that mammography could not

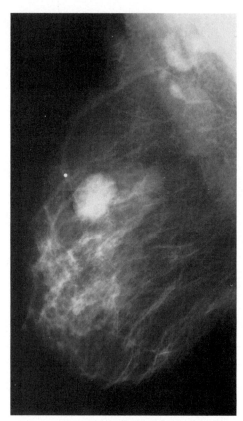

Figure 15–47 A 63-year-old woman had a palpable mass that was colloid carcinoma. It is sharply circumscribed, as is typical of this type of cancer. Colloid carcinoma may also appear as low-density masses when there is abundant mucin within the tumor.

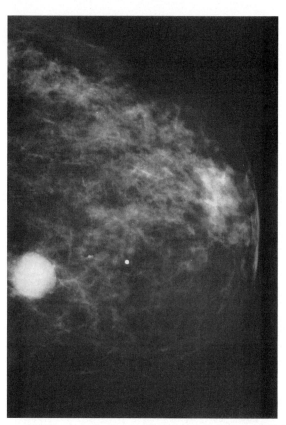

Figure 15–48 A well-circumscribed mass in the medial left breast was colloid carcinoma. The sonogram (not shown) showed a corresponding hypoechoic mass with microlobulated borders. The diagnosis was made by a needle biopsy under ultrasound guidance.

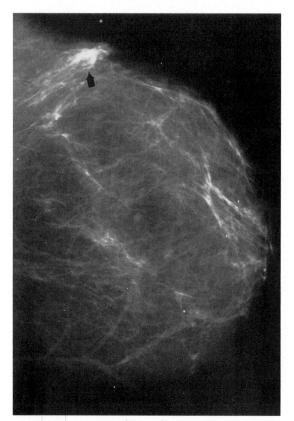

Figure 15–49 A craniocaudal view of a medullary carcinoma (*arrow*) has ill-defined and lobulated borders. Medullary carcinomas may also have sharply circumscribed borders.

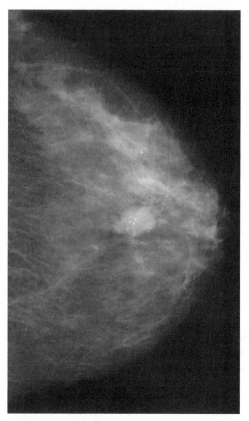

Figure 15–50 Medullary carcinoma may have associated coarse calcifications, as in this mass in the center of the left breast.

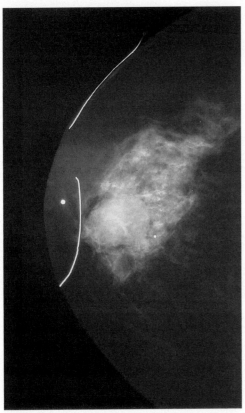

Figure 15–51   Papillary carcinoma. This 65-year-old woman who had previous benign biopsies found a mass in the subareolar region of the left breast. The location and age of the patient were suggestive of this diagnosis.

distinguish medullary carcinoma from atypical medullary carcinoma (e.g., cancers that had most, but not all, the requisite histopathologic criteria).[75] Most cancers diagnosed as medullary carcinomas by mammography ultimately prove to be infiltrating ductal carcinoma NOS after excision, with the usual survival prognosis.

How is papillary carcinoma characterized radiographically?

Papillary carcinomas are rare, comprising only 1% to 2% of breast cancers.[76] With their indolent growth, excellent prognosis, and low incidence of metastases, recognition of the presence of this cancer relies on mammography when there is no palpable mass or nipple discharge.[76–78] The mammographic appearance has been described by Soo and associates, who differentiate the in situ papillary cancer into an intraductal type and an intracystic type.[76] The in situ papillary cancer can extend within a ductal system, the intraductal type, or may be within a cystic structure, the intracystic type. Intraductal papillary carcinomas are most often detected as clustered microcalcifications, and the intracystic type is usually seen as a well-circumscribed mass or multiple adjacent masses, usually in the retroareolar region (Figs. 15–51 and 15–52). Sonography of the intracystic papillary cancer can show both cystic and solid components in the mass.[79] It may appear as a cystic mass with or without septations. Solid

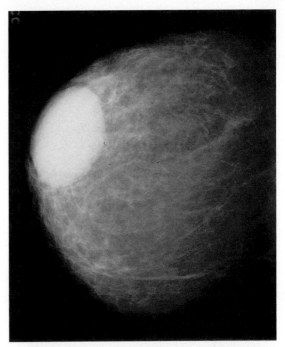

Figure 15–52   A large subareolar mass was an intracystic papillary carcinoma. It is indistinguishable from a benign papilloma by mammography. A giant fibroadenoma and a phyllodes tumor may also have an identical appearance.

papillary masses may project into the cyst. Invasive papillary carcinomas may have either mammographic pattern but more often occur as intracystic lesions.[76] A focus of irregularity in a round mass may suggest invasion. Intracystic fluid is thought to result from secretory activity by the neoplastic epithelial cells and from intracystic hemorrhage.[80] Cytology of the aspirated fluid has been reported as being negative for malignant cells and cannot be relied on for diagnosis.[80] The differential diagnosis of the intracystic type of cancer includes benign lesions, such as fibroadenomas and papillomas, and circumscribed malignant lesions, such as medullary carcinoma, colloid carcinoma, and metastatic lesions to the breast. When there are multiple peripheral masses that are solid on ultrasound, it may be impossible to distinguish papillary carcinoma from multiple papillomas, which is considered to be a precursor to this type of cancer.[81]

A nipple discharge may be caused by a solitary papilloma or by cancer. A ductogram may be used to identify the site of origin of the discharge. This may facilitate a more minimal volume excision of the responsible intraductal lesion. A solitary filling defect is most commonly associated with an intraductal papilloma, whereas multiple filling defects are more likely to be malignant.

How is malignant phyllodes tumor characterized radiographically?

Malignant phyllodes tumor (cystosarcoma phyllodes) is a relatively rare tumor that is distinguished from benign phyllodes tumor by the high mitotic count, cellular atypia, stromal overgrowth, and infiltrating margins. Local recurrences and hematogenous metastases occur in 20% to 25% of cases.[82]

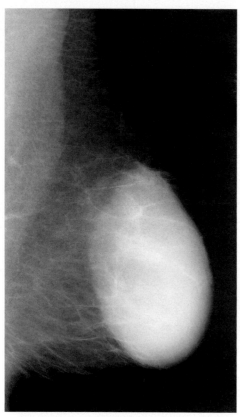

Figure 15–53   Phyllodes tumor. This large oval mass has almost entirely replaced the normal breast tissue and produced asymmetrical enlargement of the right breast.

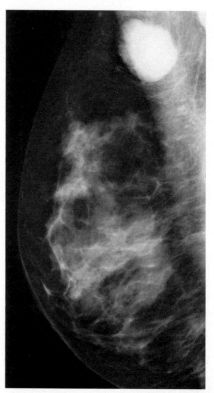

Figure 15–54   This patient had a rapidly enlarging mass in the axillary region. It proved to be a benign phyllodes tumor. It has circumscribed borders and increased density.

Mammographically, these tumors often appear identical to fibroadenomas, with sharply circumscribed margins of a round, ovoid, or lobulated mass (Figs. 15–53 and 15–54). A report by Liberman and associates of 51 phyllodes tumors showed nonspiculated soft tissue masses in 49, with only 4 having calcifications.[83] They found that benign and malignant phyllodes tumors could not be distinguished by either mammography or ultrasound, which demonstrated hypoechoic masses. The sonographic features have been described as showing a lobulated, smoothly marginated mass with a heterogeneous echo pattern. At times, cystic spaces within the mass can be identified. Fine-needle aspiration may also be unreliable to distinguish benign from malignant phyllodes tumors. The history of rapid growth of a circumscribed mass found on interval mammography may be helpful when considering this diagnosis before excision or core biopsy. Magnetic resonance imaging (MRI) has been investigated as a modality to distinguish benign and malignant phyllodes tumors, but overlapping enhancement patterns have made this technique unreliable.[84] Treatment of phyllodes tumor is complete excision with wide margins. Mastectomy may be performed for recurrent phyllodes tumor.[85]

How are extramammary metastases to the breast characterized radiographically?

Breast metastases from extramammary primary sites are uncommon, but the incidence varies depending on whether lymphoma and leukemia are included in the series (Fig. 15–55). The classic mammographic appearance of a cancer metastatic to the breast is a sharply delineated solid round mass that can be superficial in location and mobile by clinical examination.[86] At times, multiple round masses that may be confused with benign masses such as fibroadenomas may be detected. Calcifications within the metastatic lesions are unusual, but there are case reports of calcifications in the metastases of ovarian and medullary thyroid cancer.[87,88] The most common origin of extramammary metastases are melanoma, lung, sarcomas, ovary, and, less often, gastrointestinal and genitourinary tract primaries (Figs. 15–56 to 15–58). In males, carcinoma of the prostate may metastasize to the breast and the nipple. When metastatic cancer cells involve the lymphatics and blood vessels diffusely, skin thickening may be observed at mammography and, if extensive, may even simulate an inflammatory carcinoma. When lymphoma involves the breast, enlarged dense axillary lymph nodes may be visualized at mammography (Fig. 15–59). On occasion, these nodes may be distinguished from those secondary to metastatic breast cancer; in the latter case, they may be spiculated. The spiculated appearance correlates with extranodal extension of tumor into perinodal fat.[89]

How is inflammatory carcinoma characterized radiographically?

Inflammatory carcinoma of the breast, accounting for only 1% of all breast cancers, is defined by its clinical presentation with a specific inflamed appearance. The involved breast has

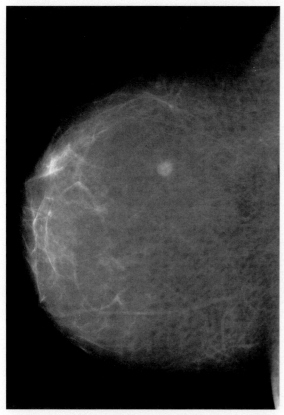

Figure 15–55 A woman with a known diagnosis of melanoma presented for a screening mammogram and was found to have a circumscribed mass that was a metastasis. This mass has slightly indistinct borders. Other lesions that may metastasize to the breast include lung, lymphoma, ovarian, and renal cell carcinoma.

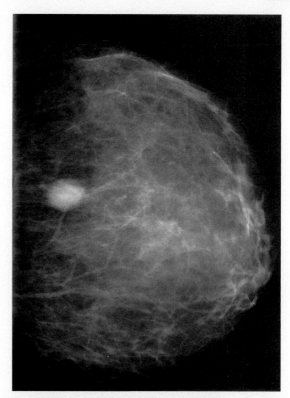

Figure 15–56 A solitary mass of increased density was found on a routine screening mammogram. The diagnosis of metastatic lymphoma was made by needle biopsy in this patient, who had a history of previously treated lymphoma.

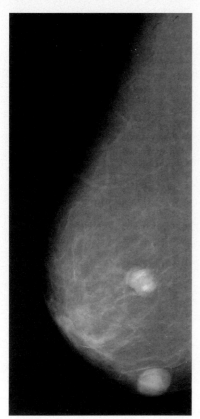

Figure 15–57 Metastatic bladder cancer was responsible for these circumscribed round masses.

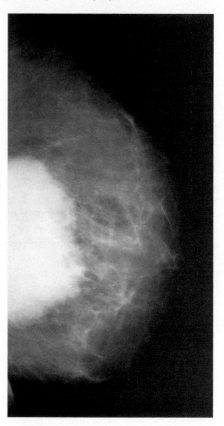

Figure 15–58 Metastatic renal cell carcinoma. A large lobulated mass with irregular borders in the center of the breast is an unusual appearance for a metastatic lesion. Metastatic lesions are more commonly sharply demarcated lesions.

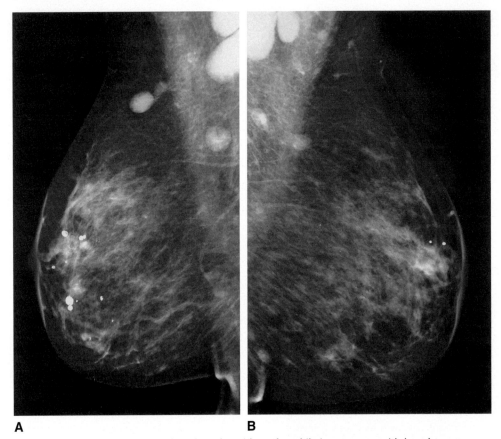

A   B

Figure 15–59   *A* and *B*, Bilateral enlarged axillary lymph nodes without fatty hila in a woman with lymphoma.

erythema and edema of the skin, often with a peau d'orange appearance. Inflammatory carcinoma is most often the result of a poorly differentiated ductal carcinoma with vascular dilation and lymphatic reaction and blockage owing to tumor emboli. Mammography may not demonstrate the underlying primary cancer, but it typically shows diffuse trabecular thickening or increased density secondary to the obstructed lymphatic drainage (Figs. 15–60 and 15–61). There is skin thickening, which may be difficult to appreciate without digital mammography. Enlarged axillary lymph nodes may be seen; these can shrink following chemotherapy. Other causes of edema of the breast may give an identical pattern. Loprinzi and associates found that patients who have undergone partial mastectomy, breast biopsy, or axillary lymph node biopsy may present with a clinical syndrome that may mimic inflammatory carcinoma.[90] Surgical biopsy was required to rule out inflammatory carcinoma in several of their patients with this syndrome. In these patients, the clinical syndrome resembling inflammatory carcinoma is due to interruption of lymphatic vessels and associated lymphostasis. A retrospective review of 43 women with inflammatory carcinoma found the most frequent mammographic finding to be skin thickening, present in 92% of patients.[91] Diffuse increased density was present in 81%, trabecular thickening was seen in 62%, axillary adenopathy was present in 58%, and malignant-appearing microcalcifications were seen in 23%. A mass was present in only 15% of the patients. An earlier report had a higher incidence of masses in their series.[92]

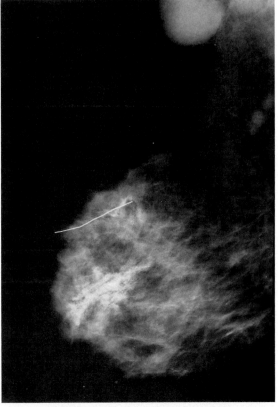

Figure 15–60   Inflammatory carcinoma of the breast. The left mediolateral oblique view shows diffuse trabecular thickening and enlarged axillary lymph nodes.

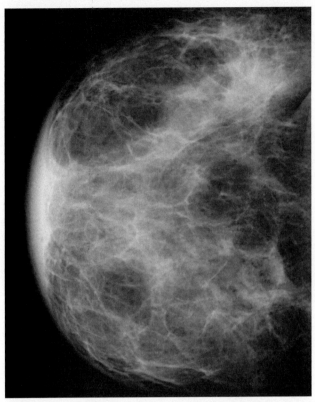

Figure 15–61 Inflammatory carcinoma. Note the skin and tra-becular thickening that is most prominent in the anterior aspect of the breast seen on this craniocaudal view. The differential diagnosis for this appearance includes inflammatory mastitis, postradiation change, edema, and metastatic disease.

What are the radiographic characteristics of unusual tumors of the breast?

Unusual tumors of the breast do not generally have a distinct appearance and are diagnosed by histology after core biopsy or excision. *Adenoid cystic carcinoma* of the breast has histology similar to that found in salivary glands. Buchbinder and Baker reported a case of a slow-growing, well-defined, mammographically benign-appearing mass that proved to be an adenoid cystic carcinoma.[93] About 125 cases have been reported. The prognosis of this tumor is favorable, with a 3% mortality rate and metastases in 6%.[93] Other tumors of the breast with histology related to the salivary glands have included benign tumors such as *pleomorphic adenoma* and *myoepithelioma*, malignancies, and *mucoepidermoid carcinoma* of the breast. *Apocrine carcinoma* is characterized histologically by granular eosinophilic cells and by masses at mammography that may be of low density. *Granular cell tumors*, with histologic features of neural differentiation, are generally considered benign, but rare malignant granular cell tumors have been reported.[94] Both the benign and malignant granular cell tumors may have mammographic and clinical features that mimic a scirrhous carcinoma of the breast. *Fibromatosis*, or *desmoid tumor* of the breast, is a rare benign tumor in young patients characterized by proliferation of spindle cells that invade the involved breast tissue locally (see Fig. 15–11). This lesion does not metastasize but has been reported to invade the chest wall. Complete excision with wide

margins is required because it tends to recur; in one series, the recurrence rate was 23%.[95] These tumors can appear identical to scirrhous carcinomas at mammography and by physical examination.

Sarcomas of the breast often have a history of a rapidly increasing breast mass, which may be mobile by clinical examination. At mammography, they may have smooth margins and may be identical in appearance to giant fibroadenomas or phyllodes tumors, with increased density with respect to the surrounding breast tissue (see Fig. 15–54). *Osteogenic sarcomas* of the breast mass have osseous trabeculae within the mass and in the metastatic lesions. *Angiosarcomas* of the breast are smoothly marginated or lobulated masses, rapidly enlarging in size. They may occur as a complication of radiation treatment. A metaplastic carcinoma of the breast is a high-density mass that may be microlobulated and may have solid and cystic components on sonography. Variations of metaplastic carcinoma include matrix-producing carcinoma, spindle cell carcinoma, squamous cell carcinoma, and carcinosarcoma. These cancers are extremely rare and have been published as case reports.[96,97]

How is male breast cancer characterized radiographically?

Male breast cancer is an unusual occurrence, accounting for only 0.5% of all breast cancers and for less than 1% of all cancers in men.[98] A painless, hard subareolar mass is the most common presentation, with a median duration of symptoms before diagnosis of 6 to 18 months. The mammogram demonstrates a noncalcified mass in most instances (Fig. 15–62). The mass is usually spiculated but can also appear well circumscribed. In a review of 23 cases of proven male breast cancer at Memorial Hospital, Dershaw and associates found a noncalcified mass in 17 (74%) and a mass with microcalcifications in 2 (9%).[99] Three of their male breast cancers had negative mammography; in one, the cancer was reported to be obscured by gynecomastia. Only one of the cases in their series presented with microcalcifications without an associated mass, and these were punctate. Eighty-two percent of their cancers were subareolar in location. Because benign tumors of the breast are rare in males, the differential diagnosis is usually gynecomastia, in which there is a characteristic proliferation of the ducts in the subareolar region.[100] Either fine-needle aspiration biopsy or core needle biopsy can be performed to differentiate cancer from gynecomastia, and biopsy is useful if there is a question of gynecomastia obscuring cancer. Most cases of male breast cancer are infiltrating ductal carcinomas; noninvasive cancer is rare. Because screening mammography is not performed for men, patients with DCIS have their disease detected when they are already symptomatic, with the usual mode of presentation being a mass or nipple discharge. Other histologic subtypes of breast cancer occur in men less commonly than in women. Owing to the rarity of lobules in men, infiltrating lobular carcinoma and lobular carcinoma in situ are noted only as case reports in the literature.[101] The prognosis of breast cancer is less favorable for men than for women.[102] It has been recommended that men whose physical examinations show a mass, ulceration, or inflammatory changes should have aspiration or surgical biopsy.[100]

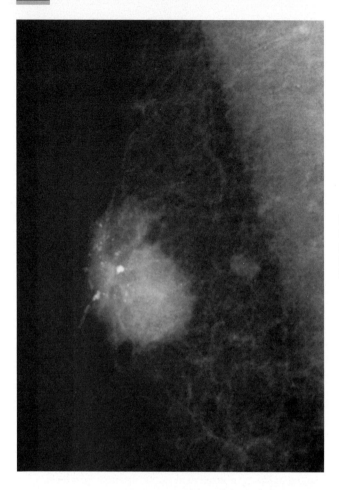

Figure 15–62 Male breast cancer. This 70-year-old man had a nontender palpable subareolar mass with associated nipple inversion. A large ill-defined subareolar mass has associated pleomorphic microcalcifications on the oblique view. There is an intramammary lymph node that was positive for metastatic disease.

What are the radiographic benign simulators of infiltrating ductal carcinoma?

There are specific entities that may simulate the spiculated mass that occurs with infiltrating ductal carcinoma. These include surgical scar, radial scar, desmoid tumor, and stromal fibrosis. Surgical scars can be identified by the history of a previous biopsy and by demonstrating stability or decreasing mass when compared with previous mammograms. They are usually not problematic to diagnose by mammography, particularly if there is changing appearance on different views.

A radial scar, or radial sclerosing lesion, has a fibroelastic core surrounded by a spiculated arrangement of ductal structures. Although it is considered entirely benign by some pathologists, others focus on its premalignant potential, possibly as a precursor to tubular carcinoma of the breast.[66,103] Mammographic criteria used to identify radial scar and to distinguish it from carcinoma include the presence of elongated radiating spicules with a central lucency and the absence of a palpable mass[104–106] (Figs. 15–63 to 15–66). The presence of microcalcifications associated with a spiculated lesion has been described as being more frequent with both radial scar and cancer.[106,107] The mammographic criteria to diagnose radial scars are not completely reliable. We retrospectively reviewed 255 spiculated lesions that were excised

and found that translucent centers could be identified in cancer, and that a radial scar could have a central density (see Fig. 15–63). Whenever a spiculated density that is suspected of being a radial scar is identified, it should be excised because it can be a low-grade cancer, and histologic evaluation is required to differentiate a radial scar from carcinoma.[107]

Desmoid tumors, composed of spindle cells, are unusual and invade the breast locally (see Fig. 15–11). They have a high rate of recurrence if not completely excised, but they do not metastasize. Although the involved breast tissue is generally clearly identifiable by mammography and by physical examination, at surgery it may be difficult to differentiate involved from uninvolved tissue, resulting in re-excision for wider margins.[95]

Fat necrosis secondary to scarring may appear as a spiculated mass with or without calcifications (Fig. 15–67). Focal fibrosis of the breast (FFB) is an entity that has hypocellular fibrous tissue that may appear on mammography as a mass, architectural distortion, or asymmetrical density. Revelon and colleagues found that in their series of 44 patients with FFB, 37 were present on mammography; two lesions with architectural distortion were reported as highly suggestive of malignancy and were surgically excised.[108]

A minor indicator of breast cancer, prominent veins, may also occur when there is superior vena cava obstruction. This may be seen with advanced lung cancer (Fig. 15–68).

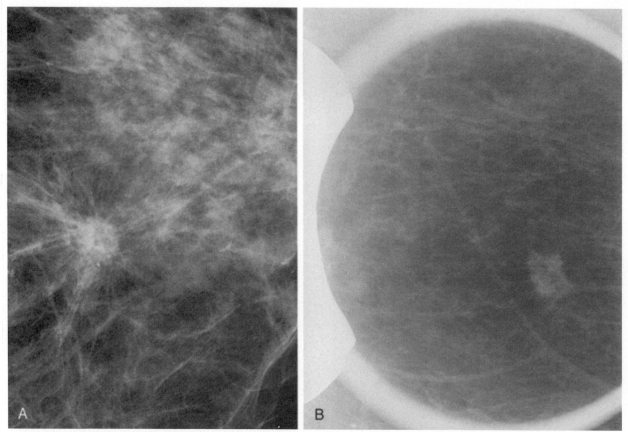

Figure 15–63   *A,* Radial scar. This benign entity has the long, fine spicules radiating from the center of the lesion with a lucent center and associated microcalcifications. The central lucency is due to entrapped fat. A radial scar may have an appearance identical to cancer, and the diagnosis must be confirmed by histology. *B,* This spot magnification film of a tiny spiculated mass with a central lucency may be confused with a radial scar. It proved to be an infiltrating duct carcinoma.

Figure 15–64   This radial scar with its characteristic long spicules involves almost the entire breast.

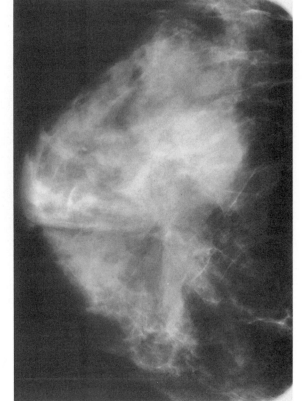

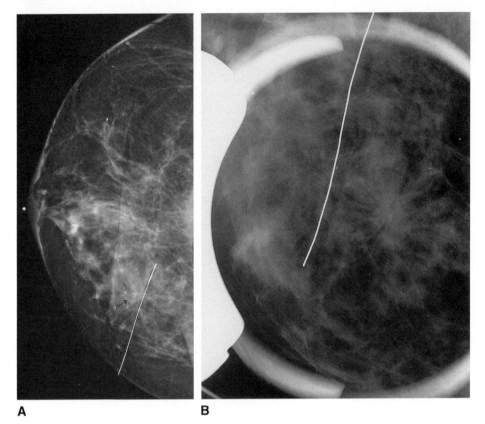

A   **B**

Figure 15–65 *A,* Tiny spiculated lesion (*arrow*) developed posterior to a lumpectomy scar for infiltrating lobular carcinoma. The core biopsy performed under ultrasound guidance had atypia. It was excised after needle localization. The lesion proved to be a radial scar. *B,* The spot magnification view of the spiculated mass shows that its mammographic features are identical to those of an infiltrating cancer. There is a skin marker at the lumpectomy site, where the patient previously had an infiltrating duct cancer removed.

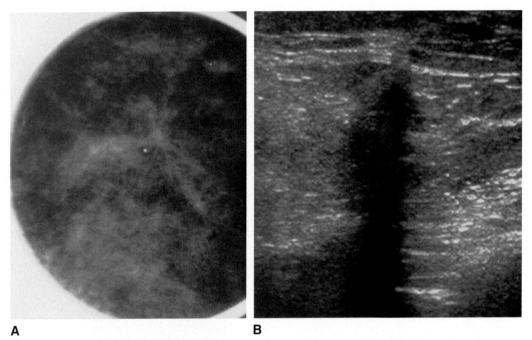

A   **B**

Figure 15–66 *A,* Spot film has a subtle spiculated mass with a dense nidus that proved to be a radial scar. The central density is unusual for this lesion and, when present, makes differentiation from cancer more difficult. *B,* The sonogram of the radial scar has a hypoechoic mass with shadowing.

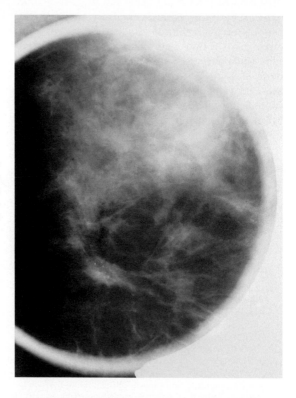

Figure 15–67 Fat necrosis may simulate cancer. This woman had a tubular carcinoma excised and 8 years later developed a spiculated mass with calcifications. The mainly peripheral location of the coarse calcifications and the lucency in the center of the mass are mammographic features that are suggestive of the diagnosis of fat necrosis. Because of the overlapping features with cancer, biopsy was performed to confirm the diagnosis.

Figure 15–68 Superior vena cava obstruction may cause dilation of veins in the breast, as in this patient with advanced lung cancer. Note the enlargement of the vein at the medial aspect of the left breast. There is obstruction of the drainage of the tributaries of the veins of the breast. Dilated veins can also be one of the minor mammographic findings that may indicate the presence of breast cancer.

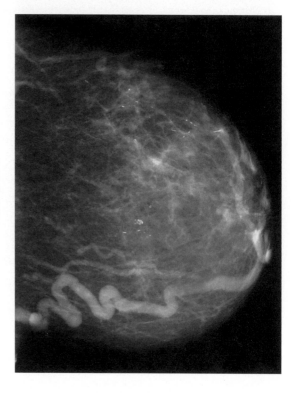

CONCLUSION

While efforts to diagnose breast cancer by techniques other than mammography are being investigated, mammography remains the most effective modality to detect this cancer before it becomes clinically evident. As a result of mammography, in many cases an early diagnosis of breast cancer is possible, when the lesions are small and axillary lymph nodes are more likely to be negative for metastatic disease. It can be expected that further improvements in mammography will continue to increase the yield of lesions that are detected before they become invasive.

REFERENCES

1. Tabar L. Control of breast cancer through screening mammography. Radiology 1990;174:655–656.
2. Cady B, Stone MD, Schuler JG, et al. The new era in breast cancer. Arch Surg 1996;131:301–308.
3. Shapiro S, Venet W, Strax P, et al. Periodic Screening for Breast Cancer: The Health Insurance Plan Project and Its Sequelae, 1963–1986. Baltimore, Johns Hopkins University Press, 1988.
4. Baker LH. Breast cancer detection demonstration project: Five-year summary report. CA Cancer J Clin 1982;32:258–290.
5. Kopans DB, Moore RH, McCarthy KA, et al. Positive predictive value of breast biopsy performed as a result of mammography: There is no abrupt change at 50 years. Radiology 1996;200:357–360.
6. Olsen O, Gøtzsche PC. Screening for breast cancer with mammography (Cochrane Review). Cochrane Database Syst Rev 2001;4:CD001877.
7. Olsen O, Gøtzsche PC. Cochrane review on screening for breast cancer with mammography. Lancet 2001;358:1340–1342.
8. Tabar L, Smith RA, Duffy SW. Update on effects of screening mammography. Lancet 2002;360:337;339–340.
9. Nystrom L, Andersson I, Bjurstam N, et al. Long-term effects of mammography screening: Updates overview of the Swedish randomized trials. Lancet 2002;359:909–919.
10. Egan R. Experience with mammography in a tumor institution: Evaluation of 1,000 studies. AJR Am J Roentgenol 1960;75:894–900.
11. Egan R. Fifty-three cases of carcinoma of the breast, occult until mammography. AJR Am J Roentgenol 1962;88:1095–1101.
12. Gold RH. The evolution of mammography. Radiol Clin North Am 1992;30:1–19.
13. Price JL, Butler PD. The reduction of radiation and exposure time in mammography. Br J Radiol 1970;43:251–255.
14. Basset LW, Gold RH, Kimme-Smith C. History of technical development of mammography. In Haus AG, Yaffe MJ (eds). Syllabus: A Categorical Course in Physics, Technical Aspects Breast Imaging. Oak Brook, IL, Radiological Society of North America, 1992, pp 9–20.
15. Kopans DB. Imaging analysis of breast lesions. In Harris JR, Lippman ME, Morrow M, et al. (eds). Disease of the Breast. Philadelphia, Lippincott-Raven, 1996, pp 71–84.
16. Smith RA, Cokkinides V, Eyre HJ. American Cancer Society guidelines for the early detection of cancer, 2003. CA Cancer J Clin 2003;53: 27–43.
17. Mettler FA, Upton AC, Kelsey CA, et al. Benefits versus risks from mammography. Cancer 1996;77:903–909.
18. Kopans DB, Feig SA. The Canadian National Breast Screening Study: A critical review. AJR Am J Roentgenol 1993;161:755–760.
19. Liberman L, Dershaw DD, Deutch BM, et al. Screening mammography: Value in women 35–39 years old. AJR Am J Roentgenol 1993;161: 53–56.
20. Feig SA. Mammographic screening in women aged 40–49 years: Benefit, risk and cost considerations. Cancer 1995;76:2097–2105.
21. Pisano ED, Cole EB, Kistner EO, et al. Interpretation of digital mammograms: Comparison of speed and accuracy of soft-copy versus printed-film display. Radiology 2002;223:483–488.
22. Dershaw DD, Fleischman RC, Liberman L, et al. Use of digital mammography in needle localization procedures. AJR Am J Roentgenol 1993;161:559–562.
23. Lewin JM, D'Orsi CJ, Henrick, RE, et al. Clinical comparison of full-field digital mammography and screen-film mammography for detection of breast cancer. AJR 2002;179:671–677.
24. Eklund GW, Cardenosa G. The art of mammographic positioning. Radiol Clin North Am 1992;30:21–53.
25. American College of Radiology (ACR). Breast Imaging Reporting and Data Systems (BI-RADS), 2nd ed. Reston, VA, American College of Radiology, 1995.
26. Yankaskas BC, Schell MJ, Bird RE, Desrochers DA. Reassessment of breast cancers missed during routine screening mammography. A community based study. AJR Am J Roentgenol 2001;3:535–549.
27. Bird RE, Wallace TW, Yankaskas BC. Analysis of cancers missed at screening mammography. Radiology 1992;184:613–617.
28. Thurfjell EL, Lernevall KA, Taube AS. Benefit of independent double reading in a population-based mammography screening program. Radiology 1994;191:241–244.
29. Freer TW, Ulissey MJ. Screening mammography with computer-aided detection: Prospective study of 12,860 patients in a community based breast center. Radiology 2001;220:781–786.
30. Brem RF, Schoonjans JM. Radiologist detection of microcalcifications with and without computer-aided detection: a comparative study. Clin Radiol 2001;56:150–154.
31. Zheng B, Hardesty LA, Poller WR, et al. Mammography with computer-aided detection: Reproducibility assessment—initial experience. Radiology 2003;228:58–62.
32. Baker JA, Rosen EL, Lo JY, et al. Computer aided detection (CAD) in screening mammography: Sensitivity of commercial CAD systems for detecting architectural distortion. AJR Am J Roentgenol 2003;181: 1083–1088.
33. Malich A, Zahari T, Bohm T, et al. Reproducibility: An important factor determining the quality of computer-aided detection (CAD) systems. Eur J Radiol 2000;36(3):170–174.
34. Data Sharing Reports, Breast Cancer Study. Washington, DC, Physician Insurers Association of America, 1990.
35. Data Sharing Reports, Breast Cancer Study. Washington, DC, Physician Insurers Association of America, 1995.
36. Mitnick JS, Vazquez MF, Plesser KP, et al. Breast cancer malpractice litigation in New York state. Radiology 1993;189:673–676.
37. Mitnick JS, Vazquez MF, Kronovet SZ, et al. Malpractice litigation involving patients with carcinoma of the breast. J Am Coll Surg 1995; 181:315–321.
38. Brenner RJ. Screening mammography: Medical legal considerations. Cancer 1990;66(Suppl):1348–1350.
39. Ikeda DM, Birdwell RL, O'Shaughnessy KO, et al: Analysis of 172 subtle findings on prior normal mammograms in women with breast cancer detected at follow-up screening. Radiology 2003;226:494–503.
40. Basset LW, Monsees BS, Smith RA, et al. Survey of radiology residents: Breast imaging training and attitudes. Radiology 2003;227:862–869.
41. Berlin L. Missed mammographic abnormalities, malpractice, and expert witnesses: Does majority rule in the courtroom? [letter]. Radiology 2003;229:288–289.
42. DeGroote R, Rush BF Jr, Milazzo J, et al. Interval breast cancer: A more aggressive subset of breast neoplasias. Surgery 1983;94:543–547.
43. Koivunen D, Zhang X, Blackwell C, et al. Interval breast cancers are not biologically distinct—just more difficult to diagnose. Am J Surg 1994;169:538–542.
44. Burrell HC, Sibbering M, Wilson ARM, et al. Screening interval breast cancers: Mammographic features and prognostic factors. Radiology 1996;199:811–817.
45. Kaelin CM, Smith TJ, Jomer MJ, et al. Safety, accuracy and diagnostic yield of needle localization biopsy of the breast performed using local anesthesia. J Am Coll Surg 1994;179:267–272.
46. Helvie MA, Ikeda DM, Adler DD. Localization and needle aspiration of breast lesions: Complications in 370 cases. AJR Am J Roentgenol 1991;157:711–714.
47. Czarnecki DJ, Berridge DL, Splittgerber GF, et al. Comparison of the anchoring strengths of the Kopans and Hawkins II needle-wire systems. Radiology 1992;183:573–574.
48. Liberman L, Kaplan J, VanZee KJ, et al. Bracketing wires for preoperative breast needle localization. AJR Am J Roentgenol 2001;177: 565–572.
49. Kopans DB, Gallagher WJ, Swann CA, et al. Does preoperative needle localization lead to an increase in local breast cancer recurrence? Radiology 1988;167:667–668.

50. Youngston BJ, Cranor M, Rosen PP. Epithelial displacement in surgical breast specimens following needling procedures. Am J Surg Pathol 1994;18:896–903.
51. Frykberg ER, Masood S, Copeland EM, et al. Ductal carcinoma in situ of the breast. Surg Gynecol Obstet 1993;177:424–440.
52. Lagios MD. Duct carcinoma in situ, pathology and treatment. Surg Clin North Am 1990;70:853–870.
53. Evans AJ, Pinder S, Ellis IO, et al. Screening-detected and symptomatic ductal carcinoma in situ: Mammographic features with pathologic correlation. Radiology 1994;191:237–240.
54. Kinkel K, Giles R, Feger C, et al. Focal areas of increased opacity in ductal carcinoma in situ of the comedo type: Mammographic-pathologic correlation. Radiology 1994;192:443–446.
55. Ikeda DM, Andersson I. Ductal carcinoma in situ: Atypical mammographic appearance. Radiology 1989;172:661–666.
56. Harris AT. Case 41: Ductal carcinoma in situ. Radiology 2001;221:770–773.
57. Stomper PC, Connolly JL, Meyer JE, et al. Clinically occult ductal carcinoma in situ detected with mammography: Analysis of 100 cases with radiologic-pathologic correlation. Radiology 1989;172:235–241.
58. Mitnick JS, Roses DF, Harris MN, et al. Circumscribed intraductal carcinoma of the breast. Radiology 1989;170:423–425.
59. Liberman L, Gougoutas CA, Zakowski MF, et al. Calcifications highly suggestive of malignancy. AJR Am J Roentgenol 2001;177:165–172.
60. Morrow M. The natural history of ductal carcinoma is situ. Cancer 1995;76:1113–1115.
61. DiPiro PJ, Meyer JE, Shaffer K, et al. Usefulness of the routine magnification view after breast conservation therapy for carcinoma. Radiology 1996;198:341–343.
62. Kopans DB. Science, not snake oil [letter]. Radiology 1996;200:283.
63. Stomper PC, Connolly JL. Mammographic features predicting an extensive intraductal component in early-stage infiltrating ductal carcinoma. AJR Am J Roentgenol 1992;158:269–272.
64. Winchester DJ, Sahin AA, Tucker SL, Singletary SE. Tubular carcinoma of the breast-predicting axillary nodal metastases and recurrence. Ann Surg 1996;223:342–347.
65. Rosen PP. Invasive mammary carcinoma. In Harris JR, Lippman ME, Morrow M, et al (eds). Diseases of the Breast. Philadelphia, Lippincott-Raven, 1984, pp 393–444.
66. Linell F, Ljungberg O. Atlas of Breast Pathology. Philadelphia, Lippincott, 1984, pp 120–154.
67. Liebman JA, Lewis M, Kruse B. Tubular carcinoma of the breast: Mammographic appearance. AJR Am J Roentgenol 1993;160:263–265.
68. Elson BC, Helvie MA, Frank TS, et al. Tubular carcinoma of the breast: Mode of presentation, mammographic appearance, and frequency of nodal metastases. AJR Am J Roentgenol 1993;161:1173–1176.
69. Cardenosas G, Doudna C, Eklund GW. Mucinous (colloid) breast cancer: Clinical and mammographic findings in 10 patients. AJR Am J Roentgenol 1994;162:1077–1079.
70. Conant EF, Dillon RL, Palazzo J, et al. Imaging findings in mucin-containing carcinomas of the breast: Correlation with pathologic features. AJR Am J Roentgenol 1994;163:821–824.
71. Wilson TE, Helvie MA, Oberman HA, et al. Pure and mixed mucinous carcinoma of the breast: Pathologic basis for differences in mammographic appearance. AJR Am J Roentgenol 1995;165:285–289.
72. Rubens JR, Lewandrowski KB, Kopans DB, et al. Medullary carcinoma of the breast: Overdiagnosis of a prognostically favorable neoplasm. Arch Surg 1990;125:601–604.
73. Meyer JE, Amin E, Lindfors KK, et al. Medullary carcinoma of the breast: Mammographic and US appearance. Radiology 1989;170:79–82.
74. Kopans DB, Rubens J. Medullary carcinoma of the breast [letter]. Radiology 1989;171:876.
75. Liberman L, LaTrenta LR, Billur S, et al. Overdiagnosis of medullary carcinoma: A mammographic-pathologic correlative study. Radiology 1996;201(2):443–445.
76. Soo MS, Williford ME, Walsh R, et al. Papillary carcinoma of the breast: imaging findings. AJR Am J Roentgenol 1995;164:321–326.
77. Schneider JA. Invasive papillary breast carcinoma: Mammographic and sonographic appearance. Radiology 1989;171:377–379.
78. Mitnick JS, Vazquez MF, Harris MN, et al. Invasive papillary carcinoma of the breast: Mammographic appearance. Radiology 1990;177:803–806.
79. Dogan BE, Whitman GJ, Middleon LP, Phelps M. Intracystic papillary carcinoma of the breast. AJR Am J Roentgenol 2003;181:186.
80. Kyriazis AP, Kyriazis AA. Intracystic papillary carcinoma of the female breast with secretory activity: The significance of aspiration cytology as diagnostic procedure. Diagn Cytopathol 1995;13:322–324.
81. Cardenosa G, Eklund GW. Benign papillary neoplasms of the breast: Mammographic findings. Radiology 1991;181:751–755.
82. Petrek JA. Phyllodes tumors. In Harris JR, Lippman ME, Morrow M, et al. (eds). Diseases of the Breast. Philadelphia, Lippincott-Raven, 1996, pp 863–869.
83. Liberman L, Bonaccio E, Hamele-Bena D, et al. Benign and malignant phyllodes tumor: Mammographic and sonographic findings. Radiology 1996;198:121–124.
84. Farria DM, Gorczyca DP, Barsky SH, et al. Benign phyllodes tumor of the breast: MR imaging features. AJR Am J Roentgenol 1996;167:187–189.
85. Lifshitz OH, Whitman GJ, Sahin AA, Yang WT. Phyllodes tumor of the breast. AJR Am J Roentgenol 2003;180:332.
86. Chaignaud B, Hall TJ, Powers C, et al. Diagnosis and natural history of extramammary tumors metastatic to the breast. J Am Coll Surg 1994;179:49–53.
87. Soo MS, Williford ME, Elenberger CD. Medullary thyroid carcinoma metastatic to the breast: Mammographic appearance. AJR Am J Roentgenol 1995;161:65–66.
88. McCrea ES, Johnston C, Haney PJ. Metastases to the breast. AJR Am J Roentgenol 1983;141:685–690.
89. Dershaw DD, Selland DG, Tan LK, et al. Spiculated axillary adenopathy. Radiology 1996;201:439–442.
90. Loprinzi CL, Okuno SH, Pisansky TM, et al. Postsurgical changes of the breast that mimic inflammatory breast carcinoma. Mayo Clin Proc 1996;71:522–555.
91. Kushwaha AC, Whitman GJ, Stelling CB, et al. Primary inflammatory carcinoma of the breast. AJR Am J Roentgenol 2000;174:535–538.
92. Dershaw DD, Moore MP, Liberman L, Deutch BM. Inflammatory breast: Mammographic findings. Radiology 1994;190:831–834.
93. Buchbinder SS, Baker SR. Adenoid cystic carcinoma, another cause of slow-growing breast malignancy. Breast Dis 1989;2:117–120.
94. Regalado J, Sitter S, Mies C. Granular cell tumor of the male breast: A report of three cases and review of the literature. Breast Dis 1996;9:235–242.
95. Gump FE, Sternschein MJ, Wolff M. Fibromatosis of the breast. Surg Gynecol Obstet 1981;153:57–60.
96. Günhan-Belgin IG, Memi A, Ustün EE, et al. Metaplastic carcinoma of the breast: Clinical, mammographic, and sonographic findings with histopathologic correlation. AJR Am J Roentgenol 2002;178:1421–1425.
97. Brenner RJ, Turner RR, Schiller V, et al. Metaplastic carcinoma of the breast: Report of three cases. Cancer 1998;82:1082–1087.
98. Jaiyesimi IA, Buzdar AU, Sahin AA, et al. Carcinoma of the male breast. Ann Intern Med 1992;117:771–777.
99. Dershaw DD, Borgen PI, Deutch BM, et al. Mammographic findings in men with breast cancer. AJR Am J Roentgenol 1993;160:267–270.
100. Munn S. When should men undergo mammography? AJR Am J Roentgenol 2002;178:1419–1420.
101. Camus MG, Joshi MG, Mackarem G, et al. Ductal carcinoma in situ of the male breast. Cancer 1994;74:1289–1293.
102. Joshi MG, Lee AKC, Loda M, et al. Male breast carcinoma: An evaluation of prognostic factors contributing to a poorer outcome. Cancer 1995;77:490–497.
103. Fisher ER, Palekar AS, Kotwal N, et al. A nonencapsulated sclerosing lesion of the breast. Am J Clin Pathol 1979;71:240–246.
104. Ciatto S, Morrone D, Catarzi S, et al. Radial scars of the breast: Review of 38 consecutive mammographic diagnoses. Radiology 1993;187:757–760.
105. Frouge C, Tristant H, Guinebretiere JM, et al. Mammographic lesions suggestive of radial scars: Microscopic findings in 40 cases. Radiology 1995;195:623–625.
106. Orel SG, Evers K, et al. Radial scar with microcalcifications: Radiologic-pathologic correlation. Radiology 1992;183:479–482.
107. Mitnick JS, Vazquez MF, Harris MN, et al. Differentiation of radial scar from scirrhous carcinoma of the breast: Mammographic-pathologic correlation. Radiology 1989;173:697–700.
108. Revelon G, Sherman ME, Gatewood OM, Brem RF. Focal fibrosis of the breast: Imaging characteristics and histopathologic correlation. Radiology 2000;216:255–259.

CHAPTER 16

Sonographic Diagnosis of Breast Cancer

Barbara Baskin, Orna Hadar, Stacey Tashman, Stacey Vitiello, and Stefanie Zalasin

Since the early 1990s, breast ultrasound has assumed an important role in the detection and diagnosis of breast cancer. Without using ionizing radiation, it readily provides information regarding the nature of a lesion, often differentiating cystic from solid immediately. It is used to perform preoperative needle localizations and to guide core biopsies expediently and with minimal discomfort to the patient. It has become popular among both patients and physicians as a reliable adjunct to mammography.

ULTRASONOGRAPHY

When should a patient be referred for a breast ultrasound?

A patient older than 30 years with a palpable area of concern should undergo diagnostic mammography followed by a breast sonogram (Figs. 16–1 to 16–9). It is important to note that 3% to 4% of women with breast cancer presenting with a palpable lump will have negative combined mammogram and sonogram results.[1,2] A suspicious clinical impression should not be overruled by negative test results.

Breast sonography is recommended as the initial imaging technique for palpable abnormalities in women younger than 30 years and in lactating and pregnant women.[3]

Breast ultrasound is also indicated to further characterize mammographic masses and for additional evaluation of patients with questionable mammographic findings (Figs. 16–10 to 16–12). Breast sonography can also be used to guide interventional procedures such as fine-needle aspiration, core biopsy, or preoperative wire localization.

Magnetic resonance imaging (MRI) is currently more sensitive and accurate than ultrasound for evaluating silicone implants for possible rupture. When MRI cannot be performed, ultrasound is a less accurate alternative.[4]

Screening ultrasound in patients with known breast cancer is advocated by some investigators. This is a result of studies revealing additional cancer foci in the ipsilateral or contralateral breast in about 14% of screened women with an index

focus of cancer previously diagnosed.[5,6] However, this is not currently considered to be the standard of care.

Although some centers perform whole-breast screening sonograms, especially in patients with mammographically dense breasts, the American College of Radiology and the American Institute of Ultrasound in Medicine consider ultrasound as a screening study for occult masses to be an area for research at the current time.[3]

How should a surgeon respond to a patient who asks to be referred for a screening breast sonogram?

Clinical breast examination and mammography are considered the accepted standard of care as screening tests for breast cancer. However, they are far from ideal. The overall sensitivity of mammographic screening has been estimated at 85%.[7] This sensitivity decreases significantly in women with dense fibroglandular tissue on their mammogram. In fact, a series of 11,130 women screened in a private practice setting revealed a mammographic sensitivity for breast cancer at 98% for fatty breasts, with only 48% sensitivity in the most dense breasts.[8] Even if all women were to comply with annual mammographic screening, the estimated mortality reduction would be only about 50%.[9] These results exacerbate understandable anxiety among many clinicians in the United States, where delay in the diagnosis of breast cancer is a frequent reason for medical malpractice litigation.

Dense breast tissue is common, especially in younger women. About 62% of women in their 30s, 56% of women in their 40s, 37% of women in their 50s, and 27% of women in their 60s have at least 50% parenchymal density on mammography.[10] To better serve these women for whom mammography may be suboptimal, a second-level screening test for breast cancer is sought. Many educated, medically savvy patients are currently requesting screening breast sonograms, before the standard of care has included this examination in the accepted arsenal of screening tools for breast cancer.

To date, there is no randomized blinded controlled trial to evaluate the contribution of ultrasound to breast cancer screening using mortality as an end point. However,

Text continued on p. 252

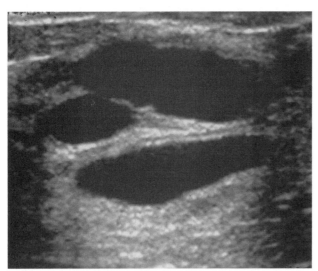

Figure 16–1   A 45-year-old woman with a palpable mass in the left upper outer quadrant. Sonography reveals a cluster of simple cysts corresponding to the palpable finding.

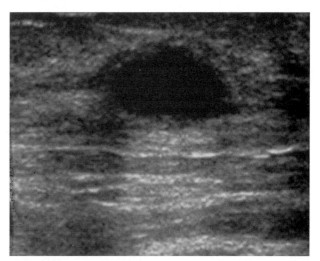

Figure 16–2   A 45-year-old woman with a palpable, tender mass in the left breast at the 12-o'clock axis, which appears as a 1.1-cm hypoechoic mass sonographically, likely representing a complex cyst. Ultrasound-guided aspiration is performed. The lesion aspirates to resolution, confirming its benign cystic nature.

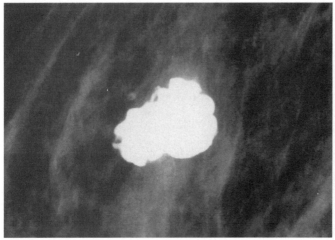

A

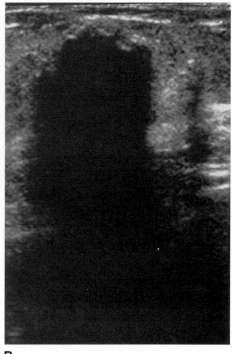

B

Figure 16–3   *A,* A 67-year-old woman with a palpable mass in the right breast at the 6-o'clock axis. Mammographically, this corresponds to a densely calcified mass, consistent with a benign calcified fibroadenoma. *B,* Sonography reveals a hypoechoic mass with intense posterior acoustic shadowing due to the dense calcification.

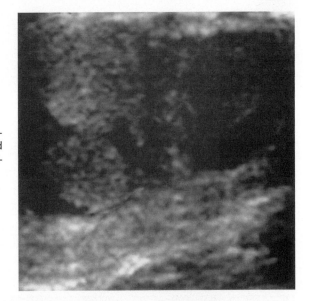

Figure 16–4 A 39-year-old woman with a palpable mass in the right 3-o'clock subareolar location. Sonography reveals a large mixed cystic and solid mass. Ultrasound-guided core biopsy results in a diagnosis of a papilloma, for which surgical excision is recommended.

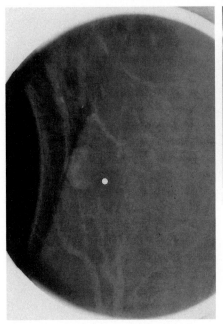

A

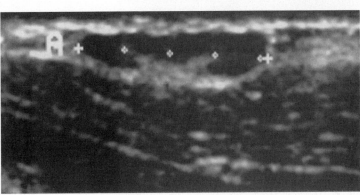

B

Figure 16–5 *A,* A 38-year-old woman with a palpable right axillary mass, marked with a radiopaque "BB" on the mammogram. *B,* Sonography is performed, demonstrating a benign lymph node with a hypoechoic cortex and echogenic hilus, corresponding to the palpable finding.

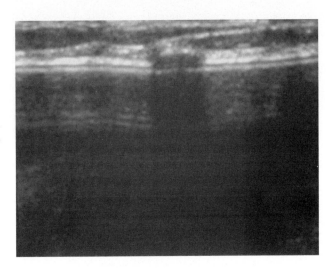

Figure 16–6 A 55-year-old woman with saline implants and a palpable nodule. Sonographically, the palpable finding corresponds to a normal valve on the implant.

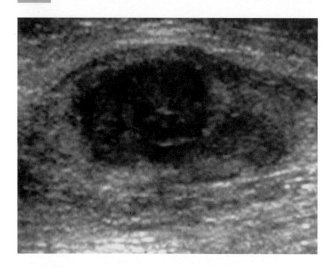

Figure 16–7 An 82-year-old woman taking warfarin sodium (Coumadin) who has a palpable mass in the right axilla. Sonography reveals a mixed hypoechoic and hyperechoic 3-cm mass in the pectoralis muscle, consistent with an intramuscular hematoma. Follow-up to resolution is recommended.

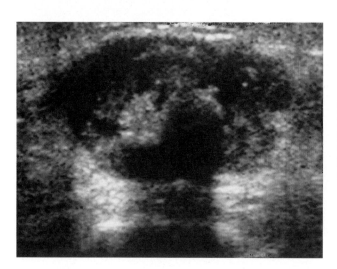

Figure 16–8 A 57-year-old woman with a history of anal cancer treated 10 years ago with radiation therapy. She presents with a palpable mass in the right lateral breast. Sonography is performed, demonstrating a mixed-echogenicity 2.4-cm mass. Ultrasound-guided core biopsy yields a diagnosis of metastatic squamous cell carcinoma, consistent with anal cancer.

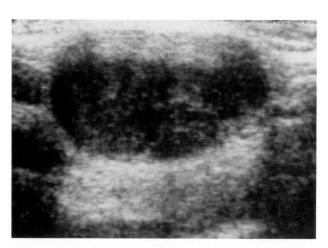

Figure 16–9 A 39-year-old woman with a history of treated melanoma in the left upper arm 3 years ago, presenting with a palpable left axillary mass. This corresponds sonographically to a 2.7-cm solid mass in the left axilla, with a diagnosis of metastatic melanoma in a lymph node on ultrasound-guided core biopsy.

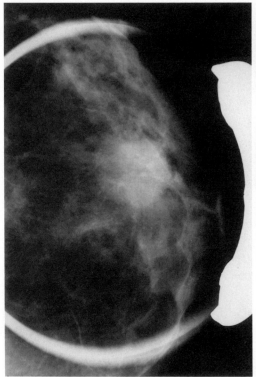

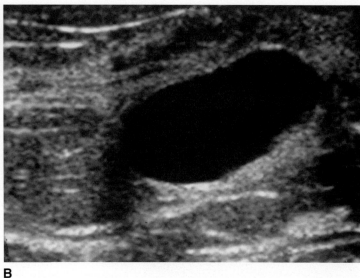

A

B

Figure 16–10   *A,* A 63-year-old woman with a 2-cm partially obscured mass in the right subareolar region on screening mammography. *B,* Sonography demonstrates a benign simple cyst corresponding in size and location to the mammographic finding.

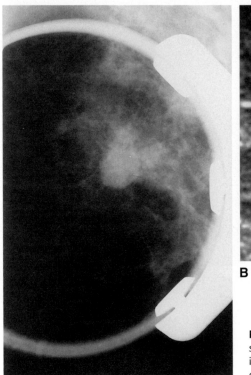

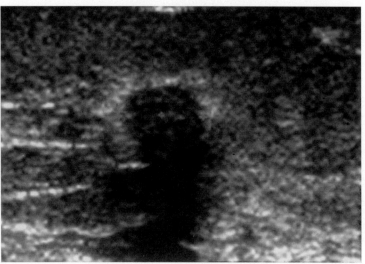

A

B

Figure 16–11   *A,* A 65-year-old woman with a 7-mm spiculated mass in the right subareolar region on screening mammography. *B,* Sonography reveals a 9 × 7 mm irregular mass, corresponding to the mammographic finding. Ultrasound-guided core biopsy yields a diagnosis of invasive ductal carcinoma.

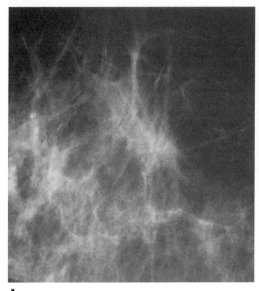

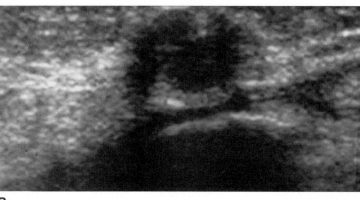

A

B

Figure 16–12 *A,* A 47-year-old woman with a 1-cm mass with indistinct margins in the left lower inner quadrant on her baseline mammogram. *B,* Corresponding to the mammographic mass, in the left breast at the 8:30 axis, there is a 1-cm hypoechoic solid mass, which on ultrasound-guided core biopsy results in a diagnosis of invasive ductal carcinoma.

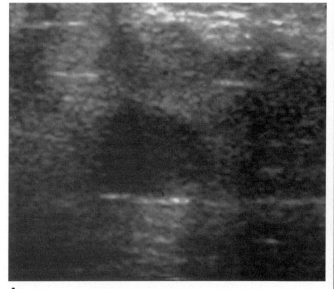

A

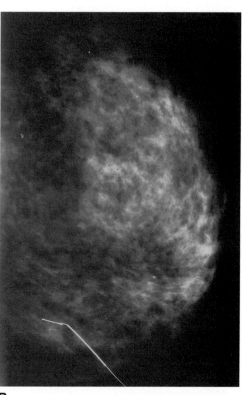

Figure 16–13 *A,* Screening sonography performed on a 67-year-old woman with mammographically dense breasts reveals a 1.1-cm irregular mixed-echogenicity mass. This is diagnosed as an invasive ductal carcinoma on ultrasound-guided core biopsy. *B,* Presurgical wire localization is performed with sonographic guidance. A mammographic view with the localizing wire in place demonstrates the mammographically occult nature of this mass.

B

in several single-center studies, the utility of screening sonography in women with dense breasts for finding mammographically occult, nonpalpable breast cancers has been demonstrated[8,11–15] (Figs. 16–13 to 16–16). Each of these studies has resulted in cancer detection rates of 0.3% to 0.4% for screening sonography alone, which is similar to that of screening mammography.[16–18] In addition, the cancers found in these studies with sonography alone are similar in size and stage to those detected only with mammography. Therefore, it is likely that finding these early cancers at ultrasound before they present mammographically or clinically would result in

improved survival to the women in whom they are found. Among other factors, patient survival is directly related to tumor size at diagnosis.[19]

When discussing screening sonography with a patient, a few key points should be contemplated.[20] First, women with nondense breasts should not be referred for a breast sonogram because the likelihood of discovering a mammographically occult cancer is extremely low. Second, the accuracy of a breast sonogram is highly dependent on the skill of the person performing the study. Most series describe results with radiologist-performed scans, although one study reports

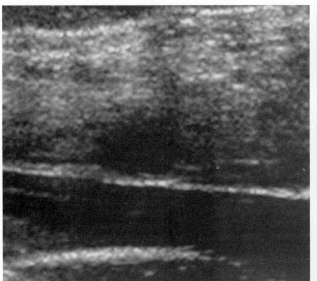

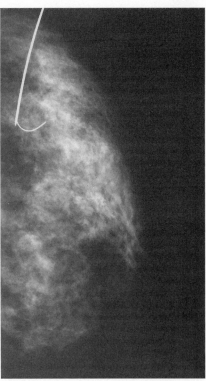

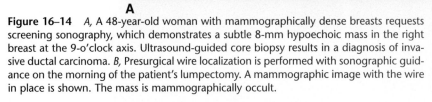

Figure 16–14   *A,* A 48-year-old woman with mammographically dense breasts requests screening sonography, which demonstrates a subtle 8-mm hypoechoic mass in the right breast at the 9-o'clock axis. Ultrasound-guided core biopsy results in a diagnosis of invasive ductal carcinoma. *B,* Presurgical wire localization is performed with sonographic guidance on the morning of the patient's lumpectomy. A mammographic image with the wire in place is shown. The mass is mammographically occult.

B

success with technologists trained specifically in breast screening.[14] Breast ultrasound for the most part is a real-time examination, more akin to physical examination than to other static imaging modalities. The patient should also be aware that in the published series, there was a 2% to 6% risk for an unnecessary aspiration or biopsy as a result of screening sonography[8,11–15] (Figs. 16–17 to 16–19). However, the minimally invasive nature and near-negligible morbidity from an ultrasound-guided aspiration or core biopsy should be taken into account. The likelihood of the excised lesions' being malignant ranged from 5% to 16%,[8,11–15] lower than the expected yield from lesions excised because of an abnormality on screening mammography. The patient needs to be informed that even if both screening mammography and sonography are performed, there is still at least a 2% to 4% risk that a cancer, if present, will not be found.[2,8] Finally, the patient should know that third-party payers currently do not reimburse facilities for screening sonography, and the patient will be expected to accept financial responsibility for the examination.

A large-scale study to assess the efficacy of screening breast sonography is now in its earliest stages. If successful, this may lead to a broader study with death as an end point.[20] Until this is realized, the individual patient and clinician must weigh the potential risks and benefits of screening sonography.

What is the recommended technique for performing breast ultrasound?

Breast ultrasound should be performed with a high-resolution linear array transducer of at least 7.5-MHz frequency. Focal zone settings should be optimized for limited lag time, and gain settings adjusted so that breast fat appears gray. The patient should be positioned so that the area of the breast being evaluated is of minimal thickness. For example, the supine oblique position with the patient's arm above the head is used to study the outer quadrants of the breast. A lesion should be viewed in two perpendicular projections; one view is insufficient. At least one set of images of a finding should be obtained without calipers. The maximum dimensions of a mass should be recorded in at least two dimensions. Labeling should include right or left breast; quadrant or clock face location with distance from the nipple, or location shown on a diagram of the breast; and the orientation of the transducer (i.e., radial or antiradial, longitudinal or transverse). Occasionally, for evaluation of superficial lesions, a standoff pad may be helpful (Figs. 16–20 and 16–21).

The patient's mammogram should be correlated with the sonogram at the time of the examination. Comparison to prior sonograms is necessary if lesion follow-up is to be performed. If indicated, physical examination should also be directly correlated with the sonographic findings.[3,21]

What is the sonographic appearance of breast cancer?

Traditionally, breast sonography has been used to distinguish solid from cystic lesions. Studies have been performed to further characterize solid masses as having either malignant or benign features.[22–24] It is commonly accepted that certain sonographic features are considered suspicious for malignancy and others of benignity. The landmark study by Stavros and colleagues[22] classified masses based on several sonographic characteristics. Characteristics supporting a malignant

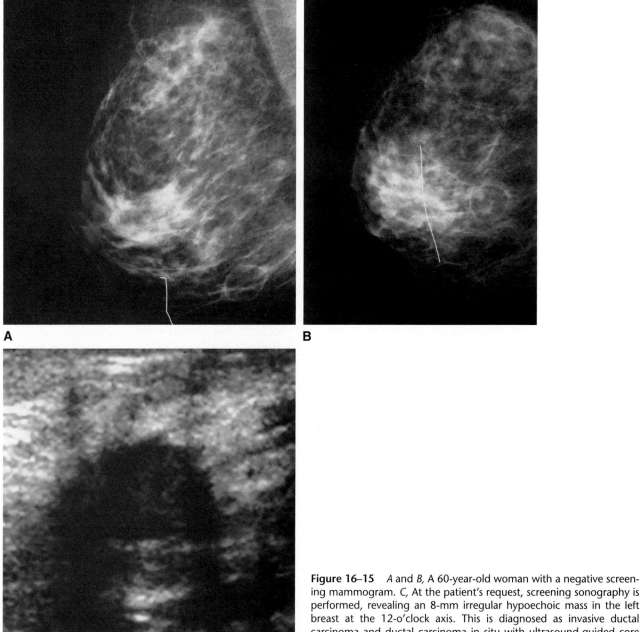

Figure 16–15   *A* and *B,* A 60-year-old woman with a negative screening mammogram. *C,* At the patient's request, screening sonography is performed, revealing an 8-mm irregular hypoechoic mass in the left breast at the 12-o'clock axis. This is diagnosed as invasive ductal carcinoma and ductal carcinoma in situ with ultrasound-guided core biopsy.

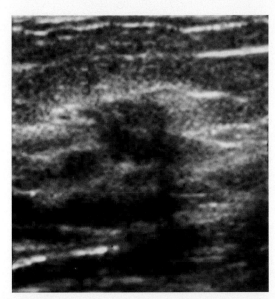

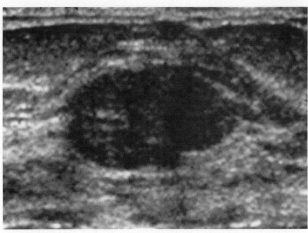

Figure 16–16 Screening sonography demonstrates a 1-cm ill-defined hypoechoic mass in the left breast at the 11:30 axis. Ultrasound-guided core biopsy yields a result of infiltrating tubular carcinoma.

Figure 16–17 A 38-year-old woman has a negative screening mammogram, revealing heterogeneously dense breasts. Screening sonography demonstrates a 1.7-cm circumscribed hypoechoic mass, which is diagnosed as a fibroadenoma on ultrasound-guided core biopsy.

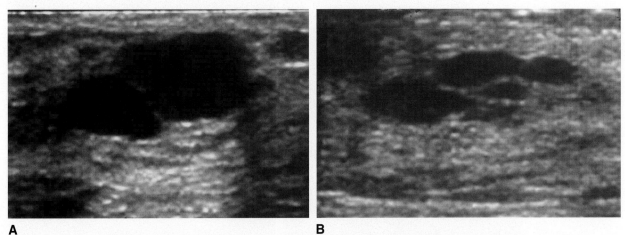

A   **B**

Figure 16–18 *A,* A 31-year-old woman referred for a palpable mass in the right breast at the 12-o'clock axis. Diagnostic mammogram is negative. Sonographically, there is a septated cyst, which corresponds to the palpable finding. This is aspirated to resolution with ultrasound guidance. *B,* Screening sonography of the remainder of the breasts reveals a lobular, septated, hypoechoic mass in the right breast at the 6-o'clock axis. Ultrasound-guided core biopsy is performed, yielding a diagnosis of pseudoangiomatous stromal hyperplasia.

appearance on sonography are spiculation; taller-than-wide (antiparallel) growth; angular margins; marked hypoechogenicity; shadowing; presence of calcifications; duct extension; branching pattern; and microlobulations.[22]

Spiculation (Figs. 16–22 and 16–23) appears as alternating hyperechoic and hypoechoic lines extending out from a mass.[22] As a result of the resolution of sonography, spiculation may appear as an echogenic halo, thicker along the lateral portions of the mass (where the spiculations extend out perpendicular to the sonographic beam) in a hypoechoic fatty background.[25]

Antiparallel growth (see Figs. 16–22 and 16–23) is defined as occurring when any portion of the mass is larger in the anteroposterior dimension than in either the sagittal or transverse plane.

Angular margins (see Fig. 16–23) occur in the bases of Cooper's ligaments.[25]

Hypoechogenicity (see Figs. 16–22 and 16–23) of a mass is defined in relation to the surrounding breast fat. The fibroglandular tissue is echogenic, and all other imaged tissue would appear hypoechoic to the fibroglandular tissue.

Shadowing (see Figs. 16–22 and 16–23) is a result of decreased through transmission of the sound waves as they pass through the mass and its surrounding desmoplastic response.[22]

Calcifications (Fig. 16–24) are not usually seen sonographically; rather, they are visualized on mammography. When calcifications are seen sonographically, they are usually associated with a mass. They may appear as bright punctate echoes that give the impression of being larger than their true size

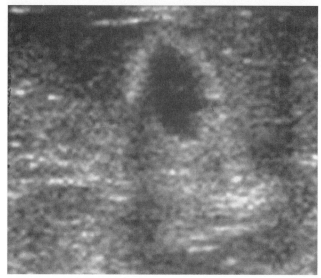

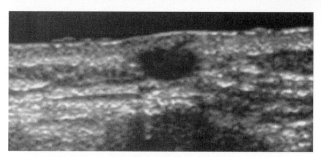

Figure 16–20 A 61-year-old woman with a palpable mass in the left lower inner quadrant. Sonography is performed with a stand-off pad owing to the superficial location of the lesion. Corresponding to the palpable finding, there is an 8-mm hypoechoic mass within the skin, demonstrating a skin tract, consistent with a benign epidermoid inclusion cyst.

Figure 16–19 A 62-year-old woman with a negative mammogram, revealing dense breasts. Screening sonography demonstrates a 7 × 5 mm irregular hypoechoic mass, taller than wide. This is diagnosed as an organizing hematoma fat necrosis on ultrasound-guided core biopsy.

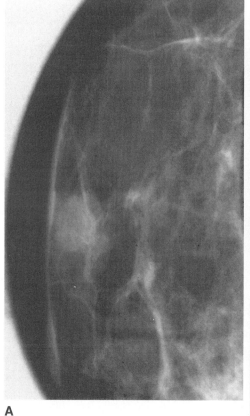

A

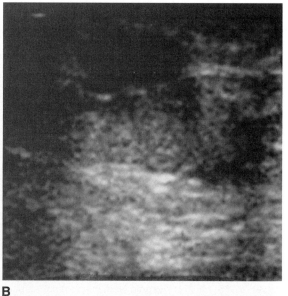

B

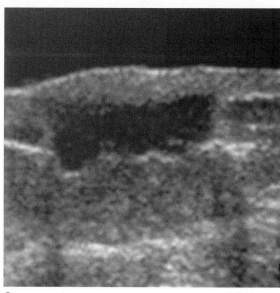

C

Figure 16–21 *A,* Spot compression view from a diagnostic mammogram in a 71-year-old woman with a palpable mass in the right retroareolar region. There is a partially obscured mass in the right medial subareolar location. *B,* Sonography performed without a standoff pad results in a suboptimal image. *C,* Sonography performed with a standoff pad demonstrates a superficial, lobulated, 1.2-cm hypoechoic mass corresponding to the palpable abnormality. Pathology from ultrasound-guided core biopsy reports poorly differentiated ductal carcinoma.

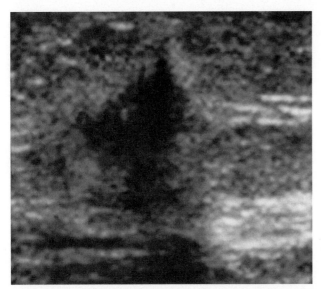

Figure 16–22 This moderately differentiated infiltrating ductal carcinoma is hypoechoic and spiculated and has angular margins.

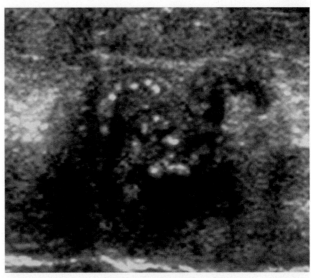

Figure 16–24 Calcifications are present within this heterogeneous poorly differentiated infiltrating ductal cancer.

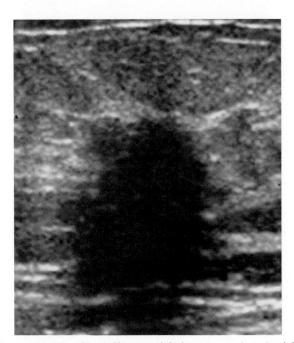

Figure 16–23 This infiltrating lobular cancer is microlobulated, hypoechoic, and spiculated. Growth is in an antiparallel orientation.

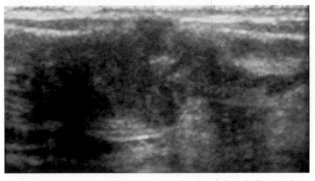

Figure 16–25 This 2.5-cm irregular angulated hypoechoic infiltrating well-differentiated ductal cancer demonstrates duct extension.

but do not create posterior acoustic sound attenuation.[26] The hypoechogenicity of the mass provides more contrast for detection of the calcifications.[4] When the microcalcifications are seen associated with a mass on ultrasound, there is a higher incidence of invasive cancer.[22]

Duct extension can be observed extending from the mass toward the nipple, whereas branching is defined as extending from the mass away from the nipple[22] (Fig. 16–25).

Microlobulated margins measure 1 to 2 mm each, and the risk for malignancy increases with the number of microlobulations[22] (Fig. 16–26).

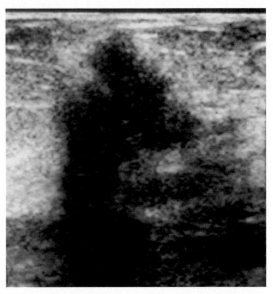

Figure 16–26 This infiltrating lobular carcinoma demonstrates multiple macrolobulations and microlobulations as well as posterior acoustic shadowing.

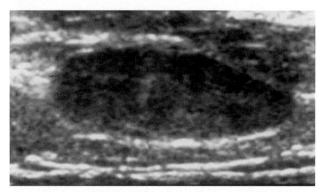

Figure 16–27 This oval hypoechoic, wider than tall, solid, well-circumscribed mass has a pseudocapsule. The stability of morphology and size support a benign etiology.

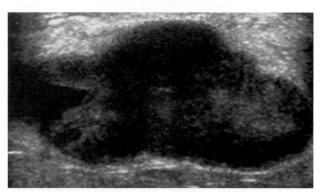

Figure 16–28 This invasive papillary carcinoma is macrolobulated and well circumscribed, with posterior acoustic enhancement. The inferior aspect is heterogeneous.

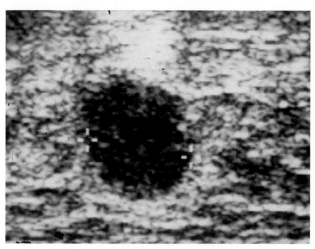

Figure 16–29 A medullary cancer appears as a circumscribed, round mass with homogeneous echoes and posterior acoustic enhancement.

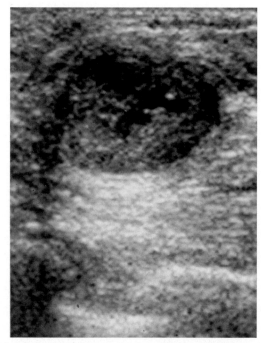

Figure 16–30 A colloid cancer presents as a well-circumscribed complex solid and cystic mass with posterior acoustic enhancement.

If a single malignant feature is present, the sonographic abnormality cannot be called benign, and biopsy must be performed. In the absence of suspicious findings, benign findings must be identified.[25] Benign features include intense hyperechogenicity, an ellipsoid shape, two or three gentle lobulations (at most), and a thin echogenic pseudocapsule[22] (Fig. 16–27).

One study found that a thin echogenic capsule was a feature most predictive of benignity[23]; however, other studies indicate that this characteristic has high interobserver variability and is therefore less useful.[24] Irregular shape, margins, shadowing, echogenic halo, and antiparallel growth are the best predictors of malignancy.[4,23,24]

Despite best attempts to construct clearcut guidelines, malignancies sometimes appear benign. High-grade cancers may appear circumscribed rather than spiculated and can have enhanced through transmission[25] (Fig. 16–28). Cellular cancers that do not generate a desmoplastic response (i.e., medullary carcinomas) would not generate shadowing. Necrotic cancers can have enhanced through transmission but typically possess other suspicious features that would lead to biopsy.

Which cancers have benign characteristics?

Three subtypes of ductal carcinoma, composing 10% of all primary breast cancers,[27] typically appear as well-circumscribed masses that mimic the sonographic appearance of benign entities. These infiltrating carcinomas, which have relatively good prognoses, are medullary, colloid, and papillary carcinoma.

Medullary carcinoma, composing 5% of cancers,[28] is seen as rounded or lobulated, well-circumscribed, almost anechoic masses with enhanced through transmission, similar in appearance to debris-filled cysts[27,29] (Fig. 16–29).

Colloid carcinoma makes up only 1% to 2% of cancers. It contains few malignant cells suspended in abundant mucinous material.[28] It appears as a rounded or oval, well-circumscribed mass with low-level echoes. The through transmission of sound is variable, ranging from posterior acoustic enhancement to posterior shadowing[27] (Fig. 16–30).

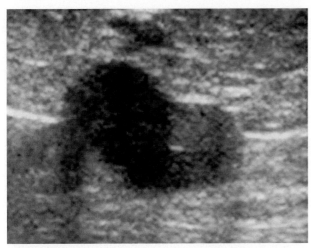

Figure 16–31   A papillary solid cancer with invasive duct carcinoma appears as a sharply circumscribed oval mass.

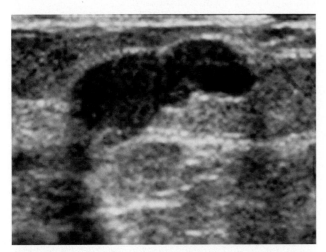

Figure 16–32   A papillary ductal carcinoma in situ with invasion appears as a well-circumscribed, heterogeneously hypoechoic, macrolobulated mass with posterior acoustic enhancement.

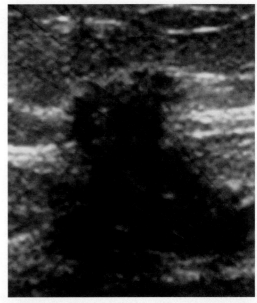

Figure 16–33   Infiltrating lobular cancer appears as an ill-defined, heterogeneous mass with microspiculations and posterior shadowing.

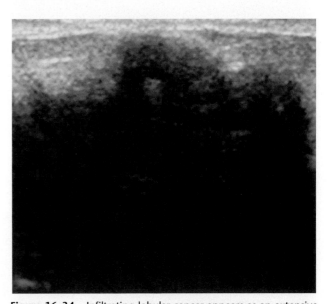

Figure 16–34   Infiltrating lobular cancer appears as an extensive area of intense acoustic shadowing. This patient presented with an extremely firm, immobile right breast. Mammography revealed only bilaterally dense breasts with scattered calcifications.

Papillary carcinoma is a rare malignancy[28] that appears as a well-circumscribed mass with enhanced through transmission. It commonly presents as a complex cystic mass, as solid tissue projecting into a cyst or duct, or as a solid well-circumscribed mass[27] (Figs. 16–31 and 16–32). Papillary cancer may be entirely intraductal or have areas of invasion. It can appear identical to benign papillomas (see Fig. 16–4). Because malignancy and atypia can be focal in this lesion, a papilloma diagnosed with core needle biopsy may require surgical excision.[30,31]

What is the sonographic appearance of infiltrating lobular carcinoma?

Infiltrating lobular carcinoma constitutes 7% to 10% of all breast cancers.[32] It often produces subtle or no mammographic findings. With high-frequency transducers,

sonography has been reported to have a sensitivity of 87.7%[32] and can often confirm the presence of a lesion when mammography shows subtle architectural distortion.[32] The most common appearance of infiltrating lobular carcinoma is a heterogeneous, hypoechoic mass with angular or poorly defined margins and posterior acoustic shadowing (Fig. 16–33). Not uncommonly, focal shadowing without a discrete mass (Fig. 16–34) or a lobulated well-circumscribed mass is seen on ultrasound.[32]

What is the sonographic appearance of inflammatory breast cancer?

Inflammatory breast carcinoma, which presents clinically, has characteristic sonographic features (Fig. 16–35). In a study by Gunhan-Bilgen and associates,[33] 96% of 142 inflammatory breast cancers demonstrated sonographic features of skin thickening, 68% demonstrated dilated lymphatic and vascular channels, and 80% demonstrated a solid mass.

Can benign lesions have a suspicious sonographic appearance?

Several benign lesions mimic the sonographic appearance of cancer. Radial scars, also known as *radial sclerosing lesions*, can be indistinguishable from carcinoma. A radial scar may

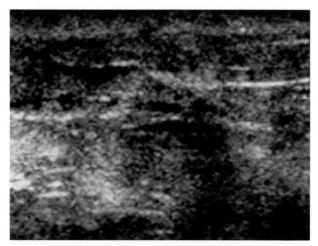

Figure 16–35 Skin thickening and dilated vascular or lymphatic channels are demonstrated within this inflammatory cancer.

appear as an irregular, hypoechoic mass with ill-defined borders and posterior acoustic shadowing (Fig. 16–36). Because the lesion is often more conspicuous on sonography, ultrasound can confirm subtle or equivocal mammographic findings of distortion and be used to direct percutaneous core needle biopsy. Histologically the radial scar is a central fibroelastic core surrounded by cystic proliferative changes. Excisional biopsy is recommended for complete examination of the lesion and to remove any ductal carcinoma in situ (DCIS), atypia, or small cancers with which they are infrequently associated.[34-36]

Diabetic mastopathy is a rare diagnosis of unknown etiology that is made in the setting of long-standing insulin-dependent diabetes mellitus in premenopausal women. It is associated with palpable, hard, irregular, nontender mobile breast masses. Sonographically, it is seen as regions of intense acoustic shadowing (Fig. 16–37), mimicking the sonographic appearance of carcinoma (see Fig. 16–34). The diagnosis can be made on core needle biopsy with histology demonstrating stromal fibrosis, periductal and perivascular lymphocytic opacities, and epithelioid fibroblasts.[37]

Fat necrosis can also be indistinguishable from breast cancer. It often presents as a palpable mass with a history of surgical or noniatrogenic trauma. The process of fat necrosis results from saponification of fat by tissue and blood lipases, resulting in a sterile inflammatory process. It is extremely varied in its sonographic appearance, ranging from that of a benign-appearing, well-circumscribed, anechoic oil cyst (Fig. 16–38), to a complex cystic mass, to that of a malignant-appearing, irregularly marginated, hypoechoic shadowing mass with architectural distortion (Fig. 16–39). The complex cystic lesions may evolve in sonographic appearance over time, becoming either more cystic or more solid. It has been reported that fat necrosis can decrease in sonographic size over time.[38]

Gynecomastia is a benign condition that causes a tender subareolar lump or enlargement of the male breast. It is important to differentiate this process from male breast

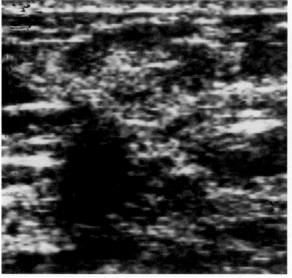
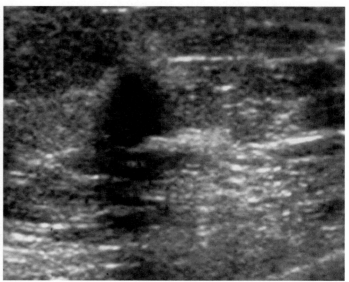

A   **B**

Figure 16–36 A radial scar (*A*) appears identical to a small tubulolobular cancer (*B*). They are spiculated, antiparallel, hypoechoic masses with posterior acoustic shadowing.

cancer. There is an overlap in the appearance of the benign and malignant diseases on both mammography and sonography. The combined use of these modalities may improve the accuracy of the diagnosis. Typically, gynecomastia on ultrasound will be seen as subareolar hypoechoic or hyper-

echoic fibroglandular tissue[4,39,40] (Fig. 16–40). Malignancy in the male breast appears similar to that in the female breast.

Abscesses can also be sonographically indistinguishable from breast cancer. They occur most frequently in the

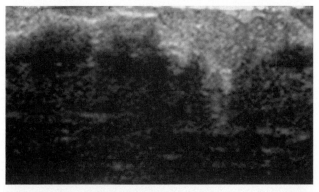

Figure 16–37   Diabetic mastopathy appears as a large, focal, irregularly marginated area of shadowing.

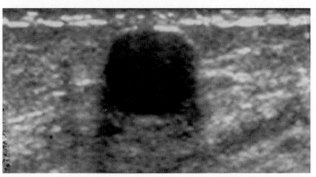

Figure 16–38   An oil cyst appears as a thin-walled anechoic mass at a site of a surgical scar.

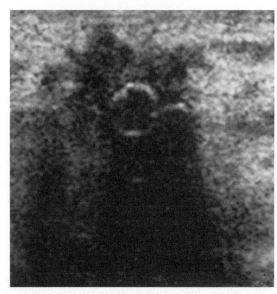

Figure 16–39   The central bright echogenic ring is pathognomonic of a calcified oil cyst typically seen within fat necrosis. This lesion presented as a clinically suspicious, firm, palpable lump. Ultrasound demonstrates, in addition to the ring, an ill-defined, spiculated, hypoechoic mass with posterior acoustic shadowing, identical to cancer. The suspicious mass represented an interval change from a previous sonogram. Biopsy confirmed the lesion to be fat necrosis.

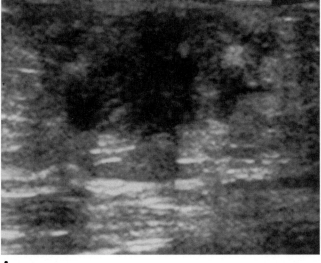

A

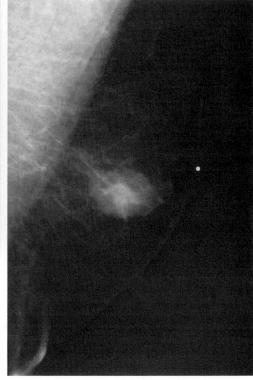

B

Figure 16–40   This case of gynecomastia presented as a palpable, tender mass in a 59-year-old man. It appears as a 3-cm irregularly marginated, heterogeneously hypoechoic, subareolar mass (A). A more typical appearance of gynecomastia was seen on mammography (B), but because of the sonographic discordance, surgical excision was performed.

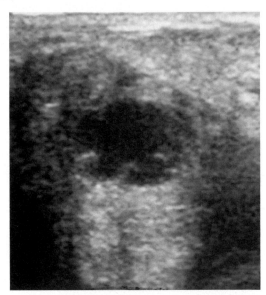

Figure 16–41 An abscess is seen in an 18-year-old woman who presents with a tender inflamed palpable mass. It is seen as a complex cystic mass with thick walls, a few septations, low-level echoes, and posterior acoustic enhancement.

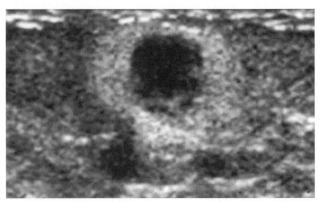

Figure 16–42 This palpable finding demonstrates a hypoechoic round mass with an echogenic halo. This is a hematoma that resolved to sonographic completion.

retroareolar region. Those that are cultured yield multiple organisms, including anaerobes.[41] They may also occur away from the nipple in women with underlying predisposing abnormalities such as diabetes, immunosuppressive conditions, severe skin excoriation, or surgical wounds. The abscess appearance varies from oval lesions with well-circumscribed margins, low-level internal echoes, and posterior acoustic enhancement, to complex cystic masses with thick, irregular walls, internal septa, and debris (Fig. 16–41). Although the diagnosis may be clinically suspected from a painful, warm, erythematous breast mass, fine-needle aspiration biopsy may be necessary to rule out an inflammatory cancer. Needle aspiration also allows for evacuation and culture of the abscess contents. Following treatment, sonography should document resolution of the mass. A treated, unresolved mass may necessitate biopsy.[30]

What is the role of ultrasound in the evaluation of implants?

Because of the high incidence of nonspecific findings in both intact and ruptured implants, the role of sonography is limited. Equivocal or positive findings on sonography merit further evaluation with MRI, which has been shown to be accurate in the diagnosis of implant rupture.[4,42,43] Sonography can, however, provide valuable information regarding the integrity of an implant. The presence of an anechoic interior and a clearly defined contour can reliably predict an intact implant with a negative predictive value for rupture of 91%.[42,44]

The "snowstorm sign," an intensely echogenic focus with echogenic posterior artifactual echoes extending from it, is associated with extracapsular rupture.[45] This is associated with free silicone extending into the surrounding tissue. Although this is 100% diagnostic of rupture, it is a relatively insensitive sign seen in only 23% of ruptured implants.[42,45]

A finding highly suggestive of intracapsular rupture is a "stepladder" arrangement of echogenic lines. This is indicative of the collapsed implant envelope floating within the silicone that is being contained by the fibrous capsule. Generalized increased echogenicity within the implant and coarse echogenic aggregates in the implant have also been found to be indicative of rupture. Linear echoes, however, are not indicative of rupture; they are often seen in intact implants and are related to folds of the intact implant capsule.[42–44]

What is the sonographic appearance of the postoperative breast?

Breast sonography can identify postsurgical alterations. These can include fluid collections, skin thickening, fat necrosis, and scar tissue. These postoperative changes are accentuated and prolonged by radiation therapy. The recurrence of tumor can also be identified at the site of a previous lumpectomy.

Postsurgical fluid collections usually represent seromas or hematomas. A mass at the biopsy or lumpectomy site in the first year after surgery likely reflects a fluid collection.[46] Most fluid collections resolve within the first year, and after 18 months almost 100% of collections have resolved.[46] Fluid collections as a result of benign biopsies typically resolve earlier than those secondary to lumpectomy. The sonographic appearance is commonly that of a complex cystic mass at the biopsy or lumpectomy site. Septations, loculations, or a thickened wall may be evident in a hematoma or seroma (Figs. 16–42 to 16–46).

Edema and skin thickening occur after lumpectomy and radiation therapy, appearing sonographically as increased skin thickness and hypoechogenicity in the areas of edema. In 70% of the cases, these changes have resolved by 2 to 3 years after treatment. In 20% to 30%, however, these changes persist.[46] These changes are more prominent in the periareolar and inferior portions of the breast.[47]

As previously discussed, fat necrosis can occur after surgery. The sonographic appearance is varied. It can appear as an irregular hypoechoic mass with variable shadowing. Mammographically, fat necrosis may appear as a spiculated mass. When the mammographic appearance is that of an oil cyst, the sonographic appearance is usually an anechoic,

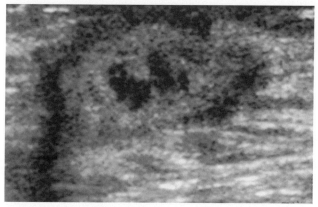

Figure 16–43 This hematoma at a prior biopsy site is a circumscribed, predominantly isoechoic oval mass with heterogeneous hypoechoic areas within it.

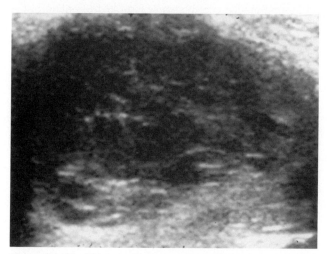

Figure 16–44 This complex cystic mass with septations, loculations, and posterior acoustic enhancement at the lumpectomy site is a hematoma.

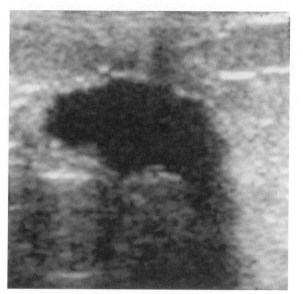

Figure 16–45 A circumscribed hypoechoic oval mass with posterior acoustic shadowing at the lumpectomy site is a postoperative seroma.

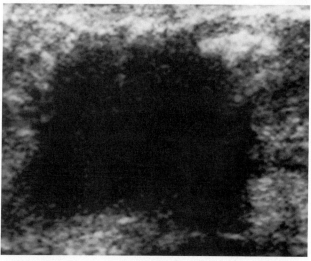

Figure 16–46 An irregular, hypoechoic mass at the biopsy site was aspirated and represents a postoperative seroma.

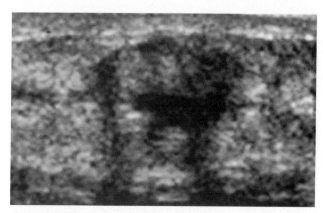

Figure 16–47 A complex mass with variable shadowing at the lumpectomy site represents fat necrosis.

round, well-defined mass with or without posterior acoustic enhancement or shadowing (see Fig. 16–38). It can also appear as a complex cystic mass with internal echoes or soft tissue component (Fig. 16–47). The appearance of fat necrosis should remain stable or decrease in size over time. Biopsy may be needed for a definitive diagnosis, however.

The distinction between postoperative scar and tumor recurrence can often be difficult clinically, mammographically, and sonographically. Both scar and carcinoma can appear spiculated. The history, physical examination, and observation over time are important tools to use for differentiation. Scar tissue contracts and decreases in size and conspicuity over time as it matures. This can occur in the first 1 to 2 years.[46] If a sonographically stable mass changes in appearance, such as increasing in size or nodularity, recurrence should be suspected. The sonographic appearance of a scar is that of a linear hypoechoic area with posterior acoustic shadowing. Scar tissue can have irregular margins. Scar tissue is usually seen deep to the cutaneous scar extending to the skin surface (Fig. 16–48).

Sixty-five percent of recurrences occur within a few centimeters of the site of excision.[46] The sonographic appearance is that of an irregular hypoechoic mass with posterior acoustic shadowing. Difficulty in distinguishing scar tissue from recurrence can be lessened if sonograms are evaluated in sequence (Fig. 16–49). If there is a new or enlarging nodular mass near the known scar, carcinoma should be suspected. Biopsy may be necessary to distinguish between the two.

ULTRASOUND-GUIDED PERCUTANEOUS BIOPSY

What is ultrasound-guided percutaneous biopsy?

With the institution of routine annual mammographic screening at age 40 years, there has been an increase in the number of nonpalpable mammographic abnormalities

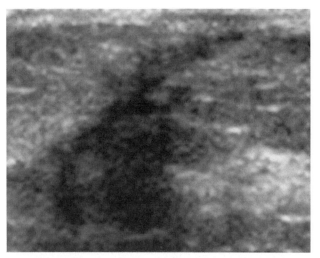

Figure 16–48 A linear hypoechoic band of tissue extending to the skin represents scar tissue.

requiring further diagnostic imaging. As stated earlier in this chapter, ultrasound has become one of the most important diagnostic imaging modalities for lesion characterization. Many of these lesions will be characterized as indeterminate or suspicious, thus requiring biopsy. In the past, it had been customary to obtain histologic confirmation of these nonpalpable lesions using preoperative needle localization followed by surgical excision. Currently, ultrasound provides one means for accurate image-guided percutaneous biopsy[48] as well as preoperative needle localization of nonpalpable lesions. Ultrasound-guided percutaneous biopsies include ultrasound-guided core biopsy, vacuum-assisted biopsy, and fine-needle aspiration.

What are the indications for ultrasound-guided core biopsy?

Ultrasound-guided core biopsy is indicated to obtain histologic diagnoses of indeterminate or suspicious solid masses seen sonographically. These percutaneous core biopsies are performed to obtain tissue diagnosis so that definitive treatment options can be determined. For example, a suspicious mass, detected on a routine mammographic screening examination and sonographically apparent, may undergo percutaneous biopsy under ultrasound guidance. With the confirmation of malignant histology combined with imaging and clinical findings, along with patient preference, the surgical treatment option of lumpectomy with sentinel lymph node biopsy may be selected prior to surgery. Another example is a patient with multiple suspicious or indeterminate masses in the same breast quadrant (multifocal distribution) or in two or more quadrants (multicentric distribution). Masses in varying locations in the breast can undergo percutaneous biopsy under ultrasound guidance to facilitate the planning of the surgical treatment option of mastectomy.[49] In both examples, ultrasound-guided core biopsy allows the patient to undergo one surgery in what traditionally was a two-stage procedure. Additionally, indeterminate sonographically apparent masses may undergo percutaneous biopsy. If

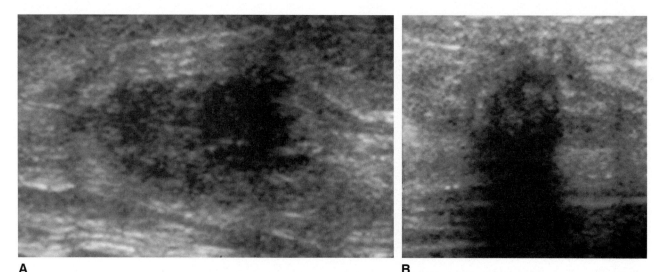

A   **B**

Figure 16–49 An irregular, spiculated, predominantly hypoechoic mass at the lumpectomy site represents recurrence (*A*). An irregular hypoechoic mass with posterior acoustic shadowing at the lumpectomy site represents scar tissue (*B*).

this yields benign histology, these patients do not require surgical excision.

Masses sonographically characterized as probably benign are normally managed with short-term sonographic follow-up.[22] Ultrasound-guided core biopsy can be performed, however, if the patient will be unavailable for follow-up, has planned breast surgery, is pregnant, or is anxious. Ultrasound-guided core biopsy may be performed for probably benign lesions in patients with carcinoma in the ipsilateral breast before breast-conserving surgery.[50]

Finally, ultrasound-guided core biopsy may be performed to obtain tissue diagnosis following insufficient cytology from a prior fine-needle aspiration.

What are the contraindications for ultrasound-guided core biopsy?

Contraindications for ultrasound-guided core biopsy include coagulopathy or anticoagulation therapy in patients who are unable to discontinue it. Other less common contraindications are allergy to local anesthetics and inability to cooperate with the procedure.

How accurate is ultrasound-guided core biopsy?

Excellent accuracy of ultrasound-guided core biopsy has been reported. Parker and coworkers reported 100% agreement in results from 14-gauge automated core needle biopsies of 40 lesions that underwent surgical excision.[48] Another 132 lesions were followed for 12 to 36 months with no cancers found. These authors concluded that ultrasound-guided core biopsy has an accuracy approaching surgical excision and thus provides an alternative to surgical biopsy. Parker and colleagues also reported a low false-negative rate for ultrasound-guided core biopsies of small masses (<1.5 cm) using 11-gauge vacuum-assisted technique.[51] This false-negative rate is attributed to the fact that this technique results in removal of the image-evident lesion 90% of the time. However, the overall accuracy of any image-guided percutaneous biopsy requires that the histopathologic findings be correlated with the imaging findings to establish concordance or discordance. For example, if a lesion exhibited suspicious sonographic characteristics and a core biopsy yielded benign histology, the radiologist would deem this discordant. At this point, surgical excision of the entire lesion would be warranted to confirm histology. On the other hand, if a lesion exhibited primarily benign sonographic morphology and yielded benign histology after ultrasound-guided core biopsy, the radiologist would deem these findings concordant. In this scenario, sonographic follow-up would be recommended for continued surveillance and identification of potential false-negative findings.[52]

What are the advantages of ultrasound-guided core biopsy?

The advantages of ultrasound-guided core biopsy over other image-guided core biopsy techniques include accessibility of ultrasound equipment, patient comfort (because these procedures are performed in the supine and supine oblique positions), and absence of ionizing radiation. Technical advantages include easy accessibility of all areas of the breast, including lesions in proximity to the chest wall and axilla, and the ability to perform these biopsies in real time.[53] Compared with surgical biopsy, ultrasound-guided core biopsies are faster and less invasive, with minimal scarring to the breast.

Ultrasound-guided core biopsies decrease the number of surgical procedures performed on patients. Liberman and associates reported that patients who had not undergone percutaneous biopsies of nonpalpable cancers required significantly more subsequent surgeries than those who had.[54] White and colleagues reported that patients with a preoperative diagnosis of breast cancer from image-guided percutaneous biopsy had fewer positive margins at lumpectomy because preoperative diagnosis facilitated wider margins at initial surgery, resulting in a decreased number of surgical procedures performed in these patients.[55]

Ultrasound-guided core biopsy provides a financial benefit as well. Liberman and coworkers reported a 56% decrease in the cost of diagnosis when percutaneous biopsy is used instead of surgical biopsy.[56]

What are the disadvantages of ultrasound-guided core biopsy?

Because ultrasound-guided core needle biopsy provides a sampling of lesions, the disadvantage of histologic underestimates exists. A sonographically guided core needle biopsy of a mass yielding DCIS may at the time of surgery reveal invasive components of the tumor not detected in the core needle biopsy. Meyer and associates reported that, of lesions yielding atypical ductal hyperplasia at 14-gauge automated core biopsy, 56% yield carcinoma at surgery. Of the 11-gauge vacuum-assisted biopsies of atypical ductal hyperplasia, 11% yield carcinoma at surgery.[57] These data, although not solely based on ultrasound-guided percutaneous biopsy, support the need for surgical excision of lesions yielding the histology of atypical ductal hyperplasia.

Another disadvantage of ultrasound-guided core biopsy is the need for rebiopsy based on histologic findings or sonographic-pathologic discordance. Liberman and colleagues reported a 10% rebiopsy rate when using 14-gauge automated core needles for percutaneous biopsy.[56] As previously discussed, the histologic diagnosis of atypical ductal hyperplasia warrants rebiopsy based on possible histologic underestimation. Another entity that requires rebiopsy is the phyllodes tumor. Although most of these tumors are benign, a small percentage of malignant forms may be missed owing to sampling error on ultrasound-guided percutaneous biopsy.[58]

Other lesions for which rebiopsy is often suggested, although somewhat controversial, include papillary lesions,[31] radial sclerosing lesions,[59] atypical lobular hyperplasia,[59] and lobular carcinoma in situ.[59,60]

What is the patient preparation for ultrasound-guided core biopsy?

The patient is asked to discontinue aspirin, nonsteroidal anti-inflammatory agents, and any other medications that may promote bleeding for the appropriate duration of time before the biopsy. If the patient is taking warfarin sodium (Coumadin), this should be discontinued for at least 4 days, followed by a serum coagulation profile. A pertinent history of adverse drug reactions and allergies is taken. Written and verbal consent is then obtained.

What equipment is necessary for an ultrasound-guided core biopsy?

The necessary equipment includes a tissue acquisition device such as an automated core needle or vacuum-assisted biopsy device. Automated core needle devices use 14-, 16-, or 18-gauge needles. Vacuum-assisted devices use larger-gauge acquisitions. An ultrasound machine using high-frequency transducers ranging from 7 to 15 MHz is essential.

What is the technique used in ultrasound-guided core biopsy?

The patient is positioned on the ultrasound table with the ipsilateral arm raised over her head, at the appropriate obliquity to obtain adequate visualization, and with optimal accessibility of the target lesion.

The area is prepared and draped in a sterile fashion. Superficial and deep local anesthetic is administered under real-time sonographic guidance in the region of the target lesion. Depending on the tissue acquisition device and gauge of needle chosen, a small skin incision made with a scalpel may be necessary. The needle is then inserted under ultrasound guidance, with the needle position in relation to the lesion confirmed in real time. Multiple samples are obtained at varying needle positions to acquire adequate sampling. Hard-copy images are then obtained documenting accurate needle position through the lesion at each pass (Fig. 16–50).

Ultrasound-guided vacuum-assisted breast biopsy is performed by inserting the device through a small skin incision. Under ultrasound guidance, the probe chamber is advanced posterior to the target lesion. The collection chamber of the probe is then opened toward the lesion, away from the chest wall. Using vacuum assistance, tissue is obtained. If there is no remaining sonographic evidence of the lesion, a localizing metallic clip is placed.

Following all procedures, the areas are cleansed and compressed manually to adequate hemostasis. A sterile dressing is applied. At the completion of the procedure, the patient is given postbiopsy instructions.

What is ultrasound-guided fine-needle aspiration and what are its indications?

Ultrasound-guided fine needle aspiration is a technique used to obtain cells for cytologic evaluation.

The primary indication for ultrasound-guided fine-needle aspiration currently in breast image-guided interventions is for cytologic evaluation of complex cysts. These are defined as cysts that do not meet sonographic criteria for simple benign

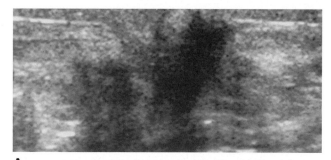

A

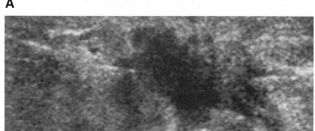

B

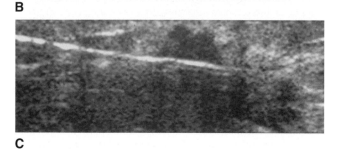

C

Figure 16–50 A, Sonographic image demonstrating a spiculated, irregular highly suspicious mass warranting biopsy. B, The core needle is advanced under ultrasound guidance proximal to the mass in the prefire position. C, Image depicting the core needle through the center of the mass in the postfire position. Histology revealed poorly differentiated infiltrating duct carcinoma.

cysts. Other indications include aspiration of simple cysts for symptomatic relief or to determine mammographic-sonographic correlation for indeterminate masses found on mammography.[61]

With the widespread acceptance, ease, and accuracy of ultrasound-guided core biopsy for tissue diagnosis of solid masses, the practice of ultrasound-guided needle aspiration biopsy for solid masses has somewhat declined. It is often used for patients with coagulopathies or patients who are unable to discontinue anticoagulation when confirmation of benignity or malignancy is needed.

What are the advantages and disadvantages of ultrasound-guided fine-needle aspiration biopsies?

The technical advantages are similar to those for ultrasound-guided core biopsy.

A major disadvantage of fine-needle aspiration is the poor sensitivity and specificity of the procedure compared with other available procedures. Pisano and associates reported the sensitivity of fine-needle aspiration biopsy to range from 85% to 88%, with a specificity ranging from 55.6% to 90.5%.[62] For example, ultrasound-guided fine-needle aspiration of a sonographically suspicious mass may yield malignant cytology, thus confirming a carcinoma. However, ultrasound-guided core biopsy of the same lesion may yield the histology of an infiltrating ductal carcinoma. This specific diagnosis gives the surgeon the vital information of "invasion." The surgeon may then plan to sample axillary lymph nodes at the time of surgery. Pisano and associates also reported that although fine-needle aspiration biopsy was more accurate under ultrasound than stereotaxis, the overall accuracy of the procedure ranged from 62.2% to 89.2%, far lower than the reported accuracy of ultrasound-guided core biopsy.[62]

Other disadvantages include insufficient sampling, often leading to rebiopsy. Pisano and associates reported insufficient sampling of up to 35.4%, requiring additional histopathologic sampling. This, of course, leads to decreased cost-effectiveness of ultrasound-guided fine-needle aspiration biopsy because the patient requires additional procedures.[62] Having an on-site cytopathologist to evaluate immediately for insufficient sampling at the time of biopsy often decreases this possibility.

What equipment is necessary for ultrasound-guided fine-needle aspiration and biopsy?

Needles of various gauges, ranging from 18 to 25 gauge, and standard syringes may be used, depending on the lesion and the desired result. In the diagnosis and drainage of a small breast abscess, an 18-gauge needle may be used. To obtain cytology of a mass, a smaller-gauge needle would likely be employed. An ultrasound machine with a high-frequency transducer (7 to 14 MHz) is needed.

What is the technique for ultrasound-guided fine-needle aspiration and biopsy?

As in ultrasound-guided core needle biopsy, the patient is positioned with the ipsilateral arm over the head and in an obliquity that allows the target lesion to be accessed safely and easily. The patient is prepared and draped in a sterile fashion. Local anesthesia is optional, although recommended.

The needle is advanced to the lesion under real-time sonographic guidance. For cyst or fluid collection aspiration, the needle tip position within the center of the fluid collection is confirmed sonographically. The radiologist draws back on the plunger, creating negative pressure within the needle and syringe. This allows evacuation of the fluid. The fluid may be sent for cytologic analysis, Gram stain, or culture, depending on the sonographic appearance of the lesion, the appearance of the fluid, and the clinical scenario (Fig. 16–51).

To obtain cytology of solid masses, cellular material is obtained by advancing and withdrawing the needle rapidly at different sites in the mass under ultrasound guidance. The samples obtained are then smeared on glass slides and analyzed by a cytopathologist.[61]

When and why do we use ultrasound-guided needle localization?

Preoperative needle localization can be performed under ultrasound guidance. It may be performed for lesions best visualized or only visualized sonographically. If the lesions can be seen both mammographically and sonographically, the radiologist may choose localization under ultrasound guidance because it often is faster, with decreased patient discomfort and lack of ionizing radiation. Ultrasound-guided needle localization may also be performed for lesions that are located

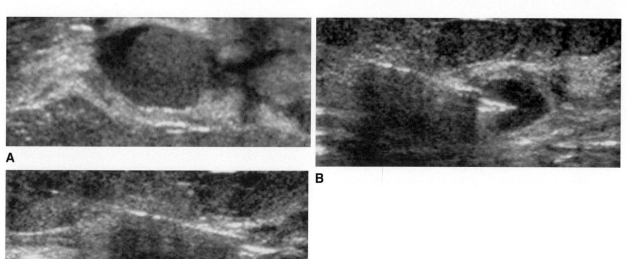

Figure 16–51 *A,* Sonographic image showing a cyst with internal debris (complex cyst), warranting cytologic analysis. *B,* The fine needle is advanced under ultrasound guidance to the center of the cyst. *C,* Image depicting evacuation of the cyst contents and complete sonographic resolution of the lesion. This yielded benign cytology.

in regions of the breast that are difficult to access with the alphanumeric grid necessary for mammographically guided needle localization. These regions include proximity to the chest wall and axillary regions.[63]

What is the technique for ultrasound-guided needle localization?

Patient preparation and positioning are identical to those of ultrasound-guided core biopsy. Again, informed consent is obtained.

After positioning the patient, the target lesion is localized under ultrasound guidance. The overlying skin is prepared and draped in a sterile fashion. Local anesthesia is administered.

Then, using real-time ultrasonography, the localizing wire-needle device is advanced through the center of the lesion, maintaining a position parallel to the chest wall, preferably advancing the needle tip about 1 cm distal to the lesion. Once accurate positioning of the needle and needle tip is confirmed sonographically, the needle is removed, leaving the localizing wire in place. The accurate position of the wire is again confirmed sonographically. A measurement is obtained from the skin surface to the center of the lesion and wire. This depth measurement is conveyed to the surgeon in the dictated procedural report. A mark is placed on the overlying skin in ink, demarcating the position of the center of the lesion.[63]

Whether the lesion is mammographically apparent or not, mammographic images of the breast with the wire in place are obtained and sent with the patient to the surgical suite.

Accurate excision of mammographically apparent lesions after preoperative needle localization is confirmed at the time of excision using specimen radiography. For lesions that are only sonographically apparent, specimen sonography may be performed to confirm lesion removal.[64]

REFERENCES

1. Beyer T, Moonka R. Normal mammography and ultrasonography in the setting of palpable breast cancer. Am J Surg 2003;185:416–419.
2. Moy L, Slanetz P, Moore R, et al. Specificity of mammography and US in the evaluation of a palpable abnormality: Retrospective review. Radiology 2002;225:176–181.
3. American Institute of Ultrasound in Medicine. AIUM Standard for the Performance of Breast Ultrasound Examination. Laurel, MD, American Institute of Ultrasound in Medicine, 2002.
4. Mehta T. Current uses of ultrasound in the evaluation of the breast. Radiol Clin North Am 2003;41:841–856.
5. Berg W, Gilbreath P. Multicentric and multifocal cancer: Whole-breast US in preoperative evaluation. Radiology 2000;214:59–66.
6. Moon W, Noh D, Im J. Multifocal, multicentric and contralateral breast cancers: Bilateral whole-breast US in the preoperative evaluation of patients. Radiology 2002;224:569–576.
7. Bird RE. Increasing the sensitivity of screening mammography. Appl Radiol 1993;Feb:72–73.
8. Kolb TM, Lichy J, Newhouse JH. Comparison of the performance of screening mammography, physical examination, and breast US and evaluation of factors that influence them: An analysis of 27,825 patient evaluations. Radiology 2002;225:165–175.
9. Feig S. Estimation of currently attainable benefit from mammographic screening of women aged 40–49 years. Cancer 1995;75:2412–2419.
10. Stomper PC, D'Souza DJ, DiNitto PA, Arredondo MA. Analysis of parenchymal density on mammograms in 1353 women 25–79 years old. AJR Am J Roentgenol 1996;167:1261–1265.
11. Gordon PB, Goldenberg SL. Malignant breast masses detected only by ultrasound: A retrospective review. Cancer 1995;76:626–630.
12. Kolb TM, Lichy J, Newhouse JH. Occult cancer in women with dense breasts: Detection with screening US—diagnostic yield and tumor characteristics. Radiology 1998;207:191–199.
13. Buchberger W, Niehoff A, Obrist P, et al. Clinically and mammographically occult breast lesions: Detection and classification with high-resolution sonography. Semin Ultrasound CT MR 2000;21:325–336.
14. Kaplan SS. Clinical utility of bilateral whole-breast US in the evaluation of women with dense breast tissue. Radiology 2001;221:641–649.
15. Crystal P, Strano SD, Shcharynski S, Koretz M. Using sonography to screen women with mammographically dense breasts. AJR Am J Roentgenol 2003;181:177–182.
16. Kan L, Olivotto IA, Warren-Burhenne LJ, et al. Standardized abnormal interpretation and cancer detection rates to assess reading volume and reader performance in a breast screening program. Radiology 2000;215:563–567.
17. Thurfjell EL, Lindgren JAA. Breast cancer survival rates with mammographic screening: Similar favorable survival rates for women younger and those older than 50 years. Radiology 1996;201:421–426.
18. Vizcaino I, Salas D, Vilar J, et al. Breast cancer screening: First round in the population-based program in Valencia, Spain. Radiology 1998;206:253–260.
19. Michaelson JS, Silverstein M, Wyatt J, et al. Predicting the survival of patients with breast carcinoma using tumor size. Cancer 2002;95:713–723.
20. Berg W. Rationale for a trial of screening breast ultrasound: American College of Radiology Imaging Network (ACRIN) 6666. AJR Am J Roentgenol 2003;180:1225–1228.
21. American College of Radiology. American College of Radiology Standards. Reston, VA, American College of Radiology, 2002.
22. Stavros TA, Thickman D, Rapp CL, et al. Solid breast nodules: Use of sonography to distinguish between benign and malignant lesions. Radiology 1995;196:123–134.
23. Skaane P, Engedal K. Analysis of sonographic features in the differentiation of fibroadenoma and invasive ductal carcinoma. AJR Am J Roentgenol 1998;170:109–114.
24. Rahbar G, Sie AC, Hansen GC, et al. Benign versus malignant solid breast masses: US differentiation. Radiology 1999;213:889–894.
25. Stavros TA. Sonographic evaluation of solid breast nodules. In Syllabus: Advancements in Breast Imaging. Lenox Hill Hospital, New York, NY, September 2003, pp 1–23.
26. Kasumi F. Can microcalcifications located within breast carcinomas be detected by ultrasound imaging? Ultrasound Med Biol 1998;14(Suppl 1):175–182.
27. McSweeny MB, Murphy CH. Whole-breast sonography. Radiol Clin North Am 1985;23:1157–167.
28. Rosen PP. The pathology of invasive breast carcinoma. In Harris JR, Hellman S, Henderson IC, et al (eds). Breast Diseases, 2nd ed. Philadelphia, JB Lippincott, 1991, pp 245–296.
29. Meyer JE, Amin E, Lindfors KK, et al. Medullary carcinoma of the breast. Radiology 1989;170:79–82.
30. Berg WA, Campassi CI, Ioffe OB. Cystic lesions of the breast: sonographic-pathologic correlation. Radiology 2003;227:183–191.
31. Liberman L, Bracero N, Vuolo MA, et al. Percutaneous large-core biopsy of papillary breast lesions. AJR Am J Roentgenol 1999;172:331–337.
32. Butler RS, Venta LA, Wiley EL, et al. Sonographic evaluation of infiltrating lobular carcinoma. AJR Am J Roentgenol 1999;172:325–330.
33. Gunhan-Bilgen I, Ustun EE, Memis A. Inflammatory breast carcinoma: Mammographic, ultrasonographic, clinical and pathologic findings in 132 cases. Radiology 2002;223:829–838.
34. Sheppard DG, Whitman GJ, Huynh PT, et al. Tubular carcinoma of the breast: Mammographic and sonographic features. AJR Am J Roentgenol 2000;174:253–257.
35. Cohen MA, Sferlazza SJ. Role of sonography in the evaluation of radial scars of the breast. AJR Am J Roentgenol 2000;174:1075–1078.
36. Finlay ME, Liston JE, Lunt LG, et al. Assessment of the role of ultrasound in the differentiation of radial scars and stellate carcinomas of the breast. Clin Radiol 1994;49:52–54.
37. Venta LA, Gabriel H, Adler YT, et al. Reply to letter: Focal fibrosis of the breast in diabetes. AJR Am J Roentgenol 2000;174:870–871.
38. Soo MSS, Kornguth PJ, Hertzberg BS. Fat necrosis in the breast: Sonographic features. Radiology 1998; 206:261–269.

39. Jackson VP, Gilmor RL. Male breast carcinoma and gynecomastia: Comparison of mammography with sonography. Radiology 1983;149:2533–2536.
40. Wigley KD, Thomas JL, Bernardino ME, Rosenbaum JL. Sonography of gynecomastia. AJR Am J Roentgenol 1981;136:5927–5930.
41. Schnitt SJ, Connolly JL. Benign breast disorders. In Harris JR, Hellman S, Henderson IC, et al (eds). Breast Diseases, 2nd ed. Philadelphia, JB Lippincott, 1991, pp 15–50.
42. Venta LA, Salomon CG, Flisak ME, et al. Sonographic signs of breast implant rupture. AJR Am J Roentgenol 1996;166:1413–1419.
43. Palmon LU, Foshager MC, Parantainen H, et al. Rupture or intact: What can linear echoes within silicone breast implants tell us? AJR Am J Roentgenol 1997;168:1595–1598.
44. DeBruhl ND, Gorczyca DP, Ahn CY, et al. Silicone breast implants: US evaluation. Radiology 1993;189:95–98.
45. Harris KM, Ganott MA, Shestak KC, et al. Silicone implant rupture: Detection with US. Radiology 1993;187:761–768.
46. Syllabus for the Mount Sinai 2002 Update. Breast Imaging: New York, 10/2002. Evaluation of the Post-operative Breast. New York, Ellen B. Mendelson, 2002, p 17.
47. Cardenosa G. Breast imaging companion. Philadelphia, Lippincott-Raven, 1997.
48. Parker SH, Jobe WE, Dennis MA, et al. Ultrasound guided automated large core breast biopsy. Radiology 1993;187:507–511.
49. Liberman L, Dershaw DD, Rosen PP, et al. Core needle biopsy of synchronous, bilateral breast lesions: Impact on treatment. AJR Am J Roentgenol 1996;166:1429–1432.
50. Liberman L. Percutaneous imaging-guided core breast biopsy. State of the art at the millennium. AJR Am J Roentgenol 2000;174:1191–1199.
51. Parker SH, Klaus AJ, McWey PJ, et al. Sonographically guided directional vacuum-assisted breast biopsy using a hand-held device. AJR Am J Roentgenol 2001;177:405–408.
52. Kopans DB. Caution on core. Radiology 1994;193:325–325.
53. Harvey JA, Moran RE. US-guided core needle biopsy of the breast: technique and pitfalls. Radiographics 1998;18:867–877.
54. Liberman L, LaTrenta LR, Dershaw DD, et al. Impact of core biopsy on surgical management of impalpable cancer. AJR Am J Roentgenol 1997;168:2459–2499.
55. White RR, Halperin T, Olson JA, et al. Impact of core needle breast biopsy on surgical management of mammographic abnormalities. Ann Surg 2001;233:6769–6777.
56. Liberman L, Feng TL, Dershaw DD, et al. Ultrasound guided core biopsy: Use and cost effectiveness. Radiology 1998;208:3717–3723.
57. Meyer JE, Smith DN, Lester SC, et al. Large core needle biopsy of non-palpable breast lesions. JAMA 1999;281:1638–1641.
58. Kopans D. Breast Imaging. Philadelphia, Lippincott-Raven, 1997, p 291.
59. Reynolds H. Core needle biopsy of challenging benign breast conditions. AJR Am J Roentgenol 2000;174:1245–1250.
60. Liberman L, Sama M, Susnik B, et al. Lobular carcinoma in situ at percutaneous breast biopsy: Surgical biopsy findings. AJR Am J Roentgenol 1999;173:291–296.
61. Fornage D, Coan JD, David CL. Ultrasound guided needle biopsy of the breast and other interventional procedures. Radiol Clin North Am 1992;30:167–185.
62. Pisano ED, Fajardo LL, Caudry DL, et al. Fine-needle aspiration biopsy of non-palpable breast lesions in a multicenter clinical trial: Results from the radiologic diagnostic oncology group V. Radiology 2001;219:785–792.
63. Liberman L, Tashman S. Interventional procedures in breast imaging: Needle localization and image guided core biopsy. In Sostman HD (ed). Taveras & Ferucci's Radiology: Diagnosis, Imaging, Intervention. Philadelphia, Lippincott, 2003.
64. Frenna TH, Meyer JE, Sonnenfeld MR. US of breast biopsy specimens. Radiology 1994;190:573–573.

CHAPTER 17

Needle Biopsy Diagnosis of Breast Cancer

Madeline F. Vazquez

Needle biopsy is a less invasive alternative to surgical biopsy of breast abnormalities. Fine-needle aspiration biopsy (FNAB) is ideal for the triage of a palpable mass and, in experienced hands, may provide a definitive diagnosis. Because of the high insufficiency and false-negative rates for FNAB, however, core needle biopsy (CNB) has become the preferred needle biopsy method for sampling breast lesions, especially under mammographic guidance. Recently, improvements in ultrasound and transducer technology have led to the increased use of ultrasound for the evaluation of dense breast parenchyma; consequently, there has been a resurgence in the number of FNABs of the breast performed under ultrasound guidance, especially of cystic lesions. This chapter answers some practical questions about the performance and interpretation of needle biopsy of the breast. Additionally, the management of malignant and nonmalignant breast lesions diagnosed by needle biopsy is addressed.

FINE-NEEDLE ASPIRATION BIOPSY

What is the diagnostic accuracy of fine-needle aspiration biopsy of the breast for palpable breast masses?

FNAB is an inexpensive and reliable method to triage breast masses, with few complications. In a summary of 18 reported studies from expert laboratories, Grant and colleagues calculated a sensitivity of 92.5%, a specificity of 99.8%, and an accuracy of 96.5% for FNAB of the breast.[1] Zarbo and associates analyzed the results of FNAB procedures in 294 institutions by 988 pathologists and found comparable results: a sensitivity of 97% and a specificity of 97%.[2] Of significance, the mean frequency of unsatisfactory aspirates obtained by nonpathologists was more than double the unsatisfactory aspirates obtained by pathologists (18% vs. 7.2%). In a series of 13 studies with 500 or more cases by Kline and coworkers, the false-negative rate ranged from 2% to 11%.[3] Layfield reported a false-negative rate in the range of 3% to 5% and a false-positive rate of 0.1% to 0.5% for FNAB in experienced hands.[4]

The literature indicates a marked improvement in diagnostic accuracy when the FNAB results are correlated with the clinical and imaging characteristics of the breast mass.[5,6] Proponents of the triple-test method of breast mass evaluation, which includes physical examination, mammogram, and FNAB, recommend excision of all nodules with discordant test results and conservative management of all lesions with concordant negative tests.[5,6] The triple-test method, whereby the results of clinical examination, mammography, and FNAB are combined for diagnosis, increases the accuracy of FNAB to almost 100%.[7] One study showed that FNAB was the most reliable diagnostic component of the triple-test method.[6] Unfortunately, there persists a high insufficiency rate with FNAB. The insufficiency rate can be minimized by increasing the sample size or by performing immediate microscopic assessment of specimen adequacy. In most breast care centers, however, a cytopathologist is not available for on-site evaluation of the specimen while the procedure is being performed.

What is the comparable accuracy of fine-needle aspiration biopsy and core needle biopsy for palpable masses?

One study comparing FNAB of palpable lumps, performed by experienced aspirators and interpreted by experienced cytopathologists, with CNB showed a specificity of 100% for both procedures.[8] Interestingly, the sensitivity for detection of cancer was higher with FNAB than with CNB (99% vs. 92%; $P < .004$). In contrast, the diagnostic accuracy of CNB for the detection of breast cancer under mammographic guidance (stereotactic core needle biopsy [SCNB]) and ultrasound guidance is higher than the diagnostic accuracy of FNAB and stereotactic fine-needle aspiration biopsy (SFNAB).[9] With CNB, experienced operators can obtain sufficient breast tissue for histology in nearly all cases; therefore, there are rarely nondiagnostic samples. Another advantage of CNB is that the pathologist can distinguish invasive ductal breast cancer from ductal carcinoma in situ (DCIS), and invasive lobular cancer from lobular carcinoma in situ (LCIS).[9,10] This distinction cannot be made by aspiration biopsy cytology. Also, specific benign diagnoses can be made more frequently by CNB than by FNAB (Figs. 17–1 and 17–2).

FNAB is an invaluable technique for the detection of breast cancer in nonsuspicious lesions. In one review, FNAB allowed the detection of three unsuspected cancers in 222 screened

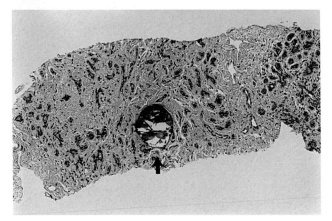

Figure 17–1 Core needle biopsy of microcalcifications (*arrow*) associated with sclerosing adenosis.

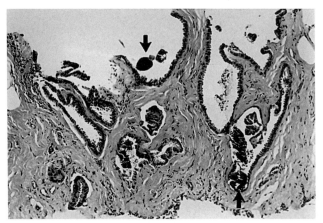

Figure 17–2 Fourteen-gauge core needle biopsy of microcalcifications (*arrows*) associated with microcysts in mild columnar cell hyperplasia (without atypia). Note the columnar cells with apocrine snouts lining the cysts.

patients and of eight unsuspected cancers in 2248 consecutive symptomatic women with palpable masses and normal mammograms.[10] It is also the most cost-effective procedure for the initial evaluation of clinically benign breast lumps.[7] The procedure is performed on an ambulatory basis and requires minimal patient preparation, and the cost of the tools needed for the procedure (a disposable syringe, a needle, a few glass slides, and a few reagents) is minimal.[11] Additionally, the processing in the laboratory is inexpensive, when compared with tissue biopsy by core needle or surgical excision. A study by Layfield and colleagues examined the cost-effectiveness of substituting FNAB for open biopsy in patients with benign clinical and mammographic findings.[7] The outcomes assessed included stage-specific life expectancy, 10-year survival, and total cost. In this study, 92.8% of the patients had benign cytologic results, 4.9% had indeterminate results, and 2.3% had malignant FNAB findings. The authors calculated a savings of more than $700 for the diagnosis of a palpable breast lump at the cost of 0.1% decrease in 10-year overall survival when the following protocol is used: (1) excisional biopsy of all suspicious lesions, (2) mammographic and clinical follow-up of all benign FNAB findings, and (3) one-stage operative management of breast masses with malignant FNAB findings.

What is the proper aspiration technique for palpable lesions?

To perform FNAB properly on a palpable mass requires a needle (usually 25 gauge, $1/2$ inch, with a clear hub) and a syringe (usually 10 mL) attached to the Cameco Syringe Pistol (Precision Dynamics, San Fernando, CA). The skin over the lesion is swabbed with an alcohol pad (local anesthesia is not required). The mass is immobilized between the index and middle fingers of the nondominant hand. Breast cancer is generally firm and fixed by palpation. Benign neoplasms, such as fibroadenomas, are firm and mobile, and cysts are generally mobile and doughy when large but can be quite firm when tiny. The needle is inserted into the target lesion, and the piston of the syringe is retracted to create suction. The needle should be moved back and forth inside the mass using rapid, short excursions. The piston is released before the needle is withdrawn from the mass to prevent the entry of cells and tissue fragments into the barrel of the syringe, where they may be irretrievable. The needle is removed from the syringe, the piston is retracted, the needle is once again attached to the syringe, and the material is expelled onto a glass slide. A modified technique for FNAB described by Kim and coworkers eliminates needle manipulation and reduces the risk for needle-stick injury.[12] In this technique, the FNAB is initiated with 1 to 1.5 mL of air in the syringe; after aspiration, the residual air is used to expel the material from the needle. It is also possible to obtain good specimens by fine-needle sampling without aspiration.[13] In a series of 635 benign and malignant breast lesions sampled with only a needle, a cellular yield comparable to the classic technique was obtained, with an insufficiency rate of 5.5%. This technique reduces the amount of blood and allows for a better perception of tumor consistency, necessary for small lesions.[13]

Fluid should be extracted from cysts until they completely collapse. If there is a residual mass, another aspiration should be performed. For solid lesions, the aim is to keep the cellular sample in the needle; thus, if blood or cellular material is seen in the needle hub, the aspiration should be discontinued. The ideal number of aspirations will depend on the size and nature of the lesion. Sneige and colleagues have stated that the reliability of aspiration cytology depends on a uniform approach to breast sampling and reporting.[14] They standardize the number of aspirations per lesion to three or four.

How are breast samples obtained by fine-needle aspiration biopsy prepared?

All aspirates are prepared as direct smears and stained with both the Diff-Quik method (Baxter Healthcare Corp., Miami, FL) and Papanicolaou method. Adequate specimens are defined as aspirates that contain at least four to six well-preserved cell groups. To prepare an ideal smear, a drop of cellular material should be expressed onto a glass slide, near the label. The slide should be held stationary and firmly in the nondominant hand (Fig. 17–3). A second slide is placed at an angle (of about 45 degrees), with its long edge resting on the specimen slide. It is rotated (dropped slowly without pressure) onto the specimen and spread to the opposite end, again

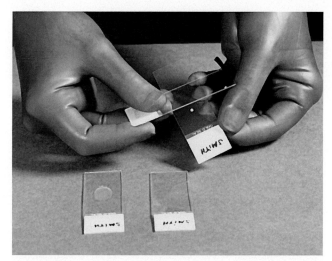

Figure 17–3 Smearing technique. The slide with the specimen is held stationary in the nondominant hand. A second slide is placed with its long edge resting on the specimen slide. It is rotated without pressure onto the specimen and spread to the opposite end, again without additional pressure. The "dab" (*arrow*) technique allows one to make several smears from an overly cellular fine-needle aspiration biopsy.

without additional pressure. In this manner, the smear is oval in shape, thick at the leading edge, and feathered at the tail. This type of smear is the ideal for cytologic analysis of FNAB specimens. The thick portion of the smear is excellent for pattern recognition, and the thin portion allows evaluation of cellular detail. Air-dried smears can be examined immediately using the Diff-Quik method, and slides are placed in 95% alcohol for the Papanicolaou or hematoxylin and eosin stains (which provide better nuclear definition). A rapid Papanicolaou technique using air-dried smears combines some of the advantages of the air-dried smears and Papanicolaou staining.[15]

The "dab" technique is used to make several smears from an overly cellular FNAB sample. In this method of multiple slide preparation, the specimen is lightly touched ("dabbed") and then smeared on multiple slides (see Fig. 17–3). Ancillary stains for organisms, mucin, hormone receptors, and other immunohistochemical stains and image analysis can be done on the additional smears. Material from FNABs can be submitted in culture medium for microbiology, in sterile collection fluid for flow cytometry, in formalin for a cell block, and in glutaraldehyde for electron microscopy.

The Cytospin method of specimen preparation involves flushing the aspirate into 10 mL of special fluid for transport to the laboratory, where cells are sprayed onto one or more special glass slides by centrifugation. It may be convenient in an outpatient setting, in which one physician obtains the specimen and another interprets it. The Cytospin method of processing material aspirated from breasts is equal in sensitivity and specificity to skillful preparation of direct smears[16]; however, it is more expensive and time-consuming. The aspirated material from either a solid mass or a cyst can also be expelled directly in Cytolyt solution (Cytyc Corp., Marlborough, MA) for a Papanicolaou-stained monolayered cell preparation (ThinPrep, Cyte Corp., Marlborough, MA).

Should cyst contents obtained by fine-needle aspiration biopsy be evaluated microscopically?

Benign cysts yield fluid and should collapse when aspirated. Simple cysts have a thin lining and yield fluid with a few foam cells. Complex cysts can have a papillary lining and tend to yield turbid fluid that is more cellular and contains mostly apocrine (metaplastic) cells. Clear or milky fluid is often acellular and may be discarded.

Routine cytologic examination of all breast cyst fluids is not recommended as a cost-effective procedure. Ciatto and colleagues reviewed the cytologic results of 6782 consecutive breast cyst fluids and found only five (0.1%) clinically and mammographically inapparent intracystic papillomas.[17] All of the intracystic papillomas yielded bloody fluid, yet the cytologic diagnoses for these five lesions were not reliable: two papillomas were correctly identified, two were not recognized, and one was falsely diagnosed as malignant. The authors nonetheless concluded that cytologic evaluation of cyst fluids should be done when blood-stained fluid is obtained. The indiscriminate evaluation of all other fluids in their series did not affect the rate of detection of intracystic lesions and is not recommended.

Few cysts contain cancer; 0.5% to 1.0% was reported in one series.[18] The FNAB of a malignant cyst generally yields bloody fluid and may leave a residual mass. There is a high false-negative rate in these cases owing to sparse cellularity and nuclear degeneration of the cells that are present within the bloody fluid. However, an aspiration of the residual mass can increase the accuracy of detecting intracystic cancers. These aspirates may be very bloody. If a clot forms, it can be submitted in 10% formalin for preparation of a cell block.

Apocrine cells represent metaplasia of lobular epithelium and can be abundant in some cysts. They can be found in papillary aggregates, in large monolayered sheets, and also dispersed singly. The cytoplasm of the apocrine cell is usually abundant and finely granular and can show squamous features. The nuclei are central and round and can vary in size. They have smooth nuclear membranes, finely granular chromatin, and a single prominent nucleolus. Occasionally, there is prominent nuclear variability (in size and shape), especially with squamous metaplasia (Fig. 17–4). The cellular atypia is most pronounced when there is inflammation of the cyst. With inflammation, there may be a residual mass following aspiration owing to a thick capsule. This mimics cancer, but inflamed cysts are usually not bloody, and intracystic or cystic cancers are usually not inflamed.

Can fine-needle aspiration biopsy confirm a benign impression of fibrocystic change?

Aspiration biopsy of the breast can confirm a benign clinical or radiographic diagnosis. All specimens that are not clearly benign or clearly malignant are followed clinically, undergo surgical biopsy, or undergo repeat needle biopsy. The main challenge, therefore, with FNAB is the detection of breast cancer with a high sensitivity while reducing the number of benign lesions requiring surgical biopsy.[19] To evaluate the accuracy of benign diagnoses by FNAB, Zemba-Palko and

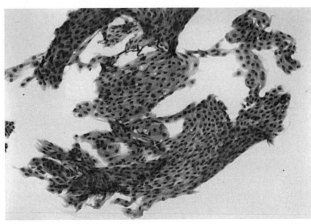

Figure 17–4 Squamous metaplasia in the capsule of a cyst on fine-needle aspiration biopsy. Intact tissue fragments were obtained with a 25-gauge needle by aspirating the cyst capsule following evacuation of its contents. Note the nuclear variability and the spindle-shaped cytoplasm of the cells.

Table 17–1 Smear Characteristics of Benign vs. Malignant Breast Fine-Needle Aspiration Biopsy (FNAB)

	Benign Pattern	Malignant Pattern
Bare myoepithelial nuclei	Present	Usually absent
Cellularity	Low to high*	Usually high
Cohesion	Strong	Poor
Epithelial cell arrangement	Even and flat Few single cells	Marked molding Many single cells
Nuclear size	<2 RBCs	>2 RBCs
Nuclear membranes	Smooth	Irregular
Chromatin	Fine and even	Coarse and irregular
Nucleoli	Inconspicuous	Mostly conspicuous
Intracytoplasmic lumina	Absent	Often present
Apocrine cells	Usually present	Absent
Background	Usually clean	Often necrotic

RBCs, red blood cells.
*The cellularity of a benign FNAB is relative to the degree of epithelial hyperplasia.

associates conducted a 20-year retrospective study of 1518 cytologically benign aspirates from palpable solid breast lesions.[20] Each FNAB was followed by surgical excision within 2 years. The aspirates were taken by clinicians, chiefly surgeons. There were 99 false-negative specimens (99 of 1518; 6.5%) for a sensitivity of 93%. There were 52 specimens available for review. Ten cases had no change in diagnosis, 16 were reclassified as unsatisfactory (fewer than three to six well-preserved epithelial cell groups), and 26 as atypical (cellular dyshesion, nuclear enlargement, or irregularity).

In fibrocystic change, there is a mixture of cysts, fibrosis, and epithelial proliferation. Areas of proliferation are highly cellular, areas of fibrosis are rubbery and yield few cells, and cysts yield fluid.[21] Small regular ductal cells are seen in monolayered sheets with apocrine cells and bare stromal and myoepithelial nuclei. There may be thin proteinaceous fluid coating the slide. The nuclei of the benign ductal cells are generally 1.5 to 2 times the diameter of red blood cells as compared with malignant nuclei, which tend to be larger. Benign epithelial nuclei have smooth nuclear membranes, fine and even chromatin, and inconspicuous nucleoli (Table 17–1). The hallmark of a benign FNAB is the presence of bipolar myoepithelial or stromal nuclei. Although their presence does not exclude malignancy, it warrants caution in making the diagnosis. Myoepithelial nuclei are oval, the chromatin is evenly distributed, the nuclear membrane is smooth, and the nuclei are devoid of nucleoli.

In fibrocystic change, as in cysts, intact apocrine cells may be dispersed singly and must be differentiated from cancer. Important clues to their benign origin are the uniformity of the nuclei and cytoplasm and the low nuclear-to-cytoplasmic ratio. These cells usually are admixed with fluid, foam cells, and benign cell clusters. Many benign diseases of the breast are similar cytologically, but even if a specific benign diagnosis beyond fibrocystic change cannot be rendered by FNAB, the amount of epithelial proliferation and presence of epithelial atypia can be evaluated.[22–24] This distinction is significant because several studies have indicated an increased risk for subsequent breast cancer associated with increasing levels of hyperplasia and atypia.[25,26] Dupont and Page have reported a

1.5 to 2 times increased risk for cancer associated with proliferative breast disease without atypia and a 5 times increased risk with proliferative breast disease with atypia.[25] Bodian and coworkers reported a modest increase in risk, of 2.1, 2.3, and 3.0, for proliferative changes with no atypia, mild atypia, and moderate to severe atypia, respectively.[26] Rosen has suggested caution in making precise risk estimates owing to a lack of reproducibility of the criteria for borderline proliferative breast lesions.[27]

Nonproliferative fibrocystic change is not associated with any increase in risk for developing breast cancer over subsequent years. The aspirates of nonproliferative lesions usually are scanty and hypocellular, containing a few bare bipolar nuclei, pieces of fibroadipose and fibrous tissue, dispersed fat, and rare small round or oval sheets of small regular ductal cells. If microscopic cysts are present, foam and apocrine cells may also be seen.

Proliferative fibrocystic change, which is associated with a mild increased risk for subsequent breast cancer, includes lesions such as sclerosing adenosis, some fibroadenomas, and radial sclerosing lesions. The aspirates generally are more cellular than with nonproliferative change, and the epithelial sheets may be small and round or large and branched, depending on the lesion (Fig. 17–5). The sheets of cells appear regular with sharply defined margins. The shedding of single, intact epithelial cells or small clusters of two to four cells is not commonly observed. Nuclear crowding and pleomorphism are mild but are more commonly present than in the nonproliferative lesion. Numerous bare myoepithelial nuclei are dispersed in the background.

In proliferative fibrocystic change with atypia, the epithelial hyperplasia is accompanied by a loss of nuclear polarity and regularity. There is a mixture of normal and abnormal cells within a group of cells, and the atypical cells are pleomorphic, hyperchromatic, disorganized, and crowded (Fig. 17–6). Proliferative fibrocystic change with atypia is associated with

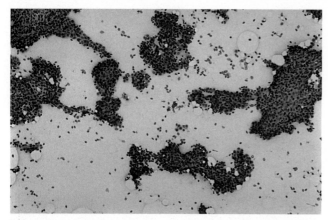

Figure 17–5 Proliferative fibrocystic change on fine-needle aspiration biopsy. There are numerous groups of epithelial cells. They are seen in cohesive clusters and branched fronds. Also note the numerous benign oval myoepithelial nuclei in the background. These features suggest that the lesion is a fibroadenoma. However, the identical cytologic features are observed in proliferative fibrocystic change.

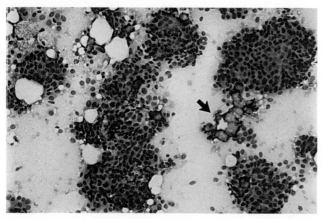

Figure 17–6 Proliferative fibrocystic change with atypia on fine-needle aspiration biopsy. The epithelial groups in these cellular aspirates show nuclear pleomorphism, cellular disorganization, and crowding. Fragments of calcium are also seen in the smear (*arrow*). This case proved to be atypical ductal hyperplasia and focal ductal carcinoma in situ of the solid subtype on histology.

a definite risk for developing subsequent breast cancer and includes such lesions as atypical lobular and ductal hyperplasia. Many lesions diagnosed by FNAB as proliferative fibrocystic change with atypia prove to be DCIS on histology.

In summary, therefore, FNAB does allow an accurate assessment of the degree of proliferation in fibrocystic change, although frequently, specific benign diagnoses cannot be made. When a specific benign pathologic diagnosis is necessary to account for a mammographic or ultrasound finding, a core biopsy or excisional biopsy may be preferable. If a diagnosis of atypia is made by FNAB, excision of the lesion is necessary. In older women, a mass or region of microcalcifications with a high degree of proliferation by FNAB should be excised, even in the absence of cytologic atypia, given the high incidence of carcinoma found on histology when these lesions undergo surgical biopsy.[20,21]

Does a diagnosis of atypia by fine-needle aspiration biopsy accurately reflect a diagnosis of atypical hyperplasia by histology?

A diagnosis of atypia by FNAB correlates poorly with the presence of a prognostically significant proliferation of ductal epithelium on subsequent histology.[28] Instead, atypia by FNAB represents cytologic uncertainty rather than a specific diagnosis of atypical hyperplasia. Some epithelial cells may show some nuclear enlargement or irregularity, or there may be cell dispersal. In some series that analyzed atypical cytologic diagnoses, more than 50% of atypical cases proved malignant by histology.[29,30] In a series by Mulford and Dawson, 134 of 3798 cases, or 3.5%, were diagnosed as atypical.[31] Of these, 72 proved benign (54%), and 62 were malignant (46%). The most common benign diagnoses were fibroadenoma and fibrocystic change, accounting for 46% of the benign cases classified as atypical cytologically. The features responsible for a designation of atypia in benign cases were increased cellularity, single epithelial cells, and reactive nuclear atypia: finely granular, uniform chromatin, and small prominent nucleoli.[4] In general, the diagnosis of atypia suspicious of carcinoma by cytology corresponds to cases with malignant cytologic features but without sufficient cells to evaluate, and to cases of low-grade carcinoma admixed with benign ductal elements.[14]

In a review of 2197 FNAB cases, Al-Kaisi found 39 cases (2%) that represented a "gray zone" of breast cytology where the cytologic features of benign or premalignant breast lesions overlap with those of malignant lesions.[32] Fibroadenomas accounted for 17 of the cases (44%). These tended to be cellular fibroadenomas with some cellular dyshesion, manifested by isolated epithelial cells with intact cytoplasm. Other breast lesions in the gray zone include papillary neoplasms, apocrine carcinoma, and intraductal and atypical hyperplasia.[32] For SFNAB of nonpalpable lesions, there is a higher proportion of atypical or inconclusive diagnoses than for FNAB of palpable lesions.[19] This is related to an increased proportion of DCIS lesions as well as smaller sample size and increased number of bloody smears for SFNAB as compared with FNAB of palpable lesions. Because a diagnosis of atypia by FNAB does not accurately reflect a diagnosis of atypical hyperplasia by histology, a diagnosis of atypia by FNAB should be followed by surgical biopsy.

Can a specific benign diagnosis ever be made by fine-needle aspiration biopsy?

Many benign breast lesions yield cytologic features that allow their subclassification when sampled sufficiently by FNAB. Maygarden and colleagues analyzed the cytology and histology of 265 benign breast masses to determine the ability of FNAB to accurately subclassify benign breast lesions.[33] A nonspecific descriptive diagnosis was given in 135 cases (51%). A specific benign diagnosis was made in 130 cases (49%). Overall, the specific diagnosis was correct in 80% of cases. The distinction between proliferative and nonproliferative fibrocystic change was not highly reliable.[33] Lesions that could be specifically diagnosed with a high reliability included fibroadenoma, papillary lesions, inflammatory lesions, fat necrosis, gynecomastia, and lactational change.

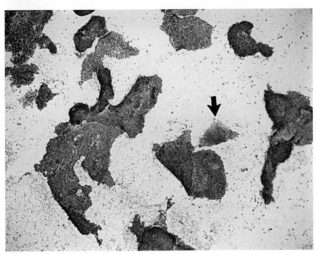

Figure 17–7 Fibroadenoma on fine-needle aspiration biopsy. This highly proliferative fibroadenoma shows folded monolayered sheets of cohesive epithelial cells, bare oval nuclei, and stroma (*arrow*).

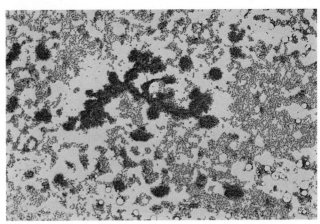

Figure 17–8 Papilloma on fine-needle aspiration biopsy. This low-power magnification of a papilloma shows marked cellularity and dyshesion. The presence of the three-dimensional papillary cluster warrants caution in making a diagnosis of carcinoma. The excised specimen proved to be a highly proliferative papilloma.

Fibroadenoma

The FNABs of fibroadenomas are quite variable. In middle-aged and elderly patients, degenerate (fibrotic) fibroadenomas may have little cellularity and resemble nonproliferative fibrocystic change. In general, typical fibroadenomas are highly cellular and show numerous epithelial cells, bare myoepithelial nuclei, and stromal fragments (Fig. 17–7). Epithelial cells are present in monolayered sheets and branched fronds. Bare oval nuclei are present in abundance and represent myoepithelial and stromal cells.[21] Stromal fragments appear as dense fibromyxoid material with spindle-shaped cells. There may be marked myxoid degeneration of the stroma, and this mimics mucin of colloid carcinoma cytologically. However, there are many bare bipolar nuclei within the strands of myxoid stroma in fibroadenoma, and these are absent in colloid carcinoma. Also, neoplastic epithelial cells are not observed in fibroadenomas. Giant cells, foam cells, and apocrine cells may be seen in fibroadenomas. Some fibroadenomas have high cellularity, nuclear atypia, mitotic figures, and many intact single cells, features mimicking adenocarcinoma.[28,31,34] In one series, intact single atypical cells were seen in 27% of benign fibroadenomas.[34] Generally, the atypical features in fibroadenoma do not dominate the smear and are accompanied by clearcut microscopic markers of benign disease.

A fibroadenoma must be distinguished from a phyllodes tumor. High stromal cellularity, mitotic figures, and single, intact mesenchymal cells that have plump nuclei and a long and wavy cytoplasm favor a diagnosis of phyllodes tumor. Also, phyllodes tumor may show squamous metaplasia, which is rarely seen in fibroadenoma.[35] Phyllodes tumor with atypia must be differentiated from a stromal sarcoma, which lacks the glandular component.

Papillary Lesions

Papillary lesions include florid papillomatosis, papillomas, and papillary adenocarcinoma; it is difficult or impossible to differentiate these lesions cytologically. Three-dimensional papillary clusters with fibrovascular or collagenous cores are the hallmark of papillary neoplasms. Both marked cellularity

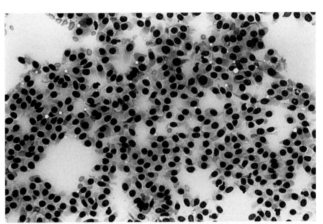

Figure 17–9 Papilloma on fine-needle aspiration biopsy. This high-power magnification of the papilloma in Figure 17–8 shows cellular features that mimic breast cancer. The cells are monotonous and singly dispersed. They show stratification, are tall and columnar with square tops, and have elongated nuclei. In this case, a false-positive diagnosis of adenocarcinoma, papillary type, low nuclear grade was made by stereotactic fine-needle aspiration biopsy. Owing to the small size of the lesion (4 mm) and the good prognosis associated with the presumed carcinoma's subtype and nuclear grade, a lumpectomy without axillary dissection was performed.

and cellular dissociation can be seen in papillomas (Fig. 17–8), and only marked cellular atypia favors malignancy.[36] Mostly, however, papillary adenocarcinomas are composed of monotonous, bland cells. The malignant cells show stratification, are tall and columnar with square tops, and have enlarged, elongated nuclei (Fig. 17–9). When a papilloma is suspected and the FNAB shows marked cellular dissociation and no definitive papillary structures, a CNB can aid in making a more specific diagnosis and ensure that adenocarcinoma is not falsely diagnosed (Fig. 17–10). More commonly, a variation in cell types is actually an important clue to a benign diagnosis in papillomas.[36,37] Regardless of the cytologic features, a cytologic diagnosis of a papillary lesion requires confirmation by open biopsy, and even then the diagnosis may

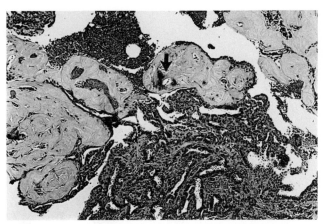

Figure 17–10 Papilloma on core needle biopsy. The papilloma is easily diagnosed by core needle biopsy (14-gauge). Small nests of epithelial cells are seen in collagenized stroma with a myofibroblastic proliferation. Calcifications were seen in the sclerotic portion of the papilloma (*arrow*) and on the mammogram.

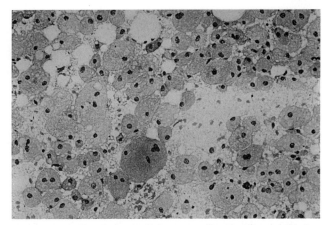

Figure 17–11 Fat necrosis on fine-needle aspiration biopsy. Abundant lipophages are seen, many of which are multinucleated.

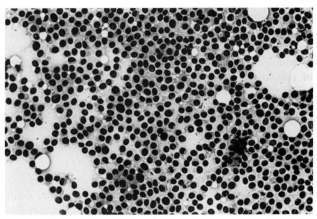

Figure 17–12 Adenocarcinoma, grade II (on fine-needle aspiration biopsy), showing a homogeneous population of noncohesive epithelial cells with enlarged and hyperchromatic nuclei. Note the absence of bare myoepithelial nuclei.

be controversial. Resection of all these papillary lesions is recommended.

Inflammation

When purulent-appearing material is obtained by FNAB, it should be cultured. This occurs in acute mastitis during lactation and in a subareolar abscess that is due to keratin plugging, squamous metaplasia, and rupture of a lactiferous duct or sinus. Subareolar abscess can mimic cancer clinically by its firmness and can be seen in association with nipple invasion and peau d'orange in nearby skin. The aspirate contains inflammatory cells, cellular debris, and a giant cell reaction to keratin. Superficial squamous cells are abundant.

Fat Necrosis

Needle biopsy of the breast is useful in differentiating cancer from postsurgical or trauma-induced fat necrosis. Fat necrosis is firm and fixed when palpable, gritty by needle sensation, and spiculated with calcifications when seen on the mammogram. Therefore, fat necrosis mimics breast cancer clinically, mammographically, and by needle sensation. The smears show multinucleated giant cell lipophages and siderophages (Fig. 17–11). Blood pigment is sometimes present. Fat necrosis can be associated with breast cancer; hence, its presence does not exclude malignancy completely. Multinucleated giant cells are also seen in suture granuloma and, in patients with implants, in silicone granuloma.

Gynecomastia

Gynecomastia presents as a firm, rubbery, subareolar mass that is resistant to the needle excursions during needle biopsy. The FNAB can be quite painful. The cellularity is variable but often scanty. There can be conspicuous cytologic atypia in gynecomastia, including increased cellularity, pleomorphism, and decreased cohesion. Mitotic figures are also frequently seen. The clue to the benign diagnosis is the bare myoepithelial nuclei.

Lactational Change

The aspirates of the lactating breast yield milky fluid with an abundance of acinar cells, are very cellular, and mimic

adenocarcinoma. The cells have enlarged, hyperchromatic nuclei, with prominent nucleoli and dense chromatin. Because the cytoplasm is fragile, dispersed bare nuclei are numerous in the background of vacuolated proteinaceous fluid (milk). These nuclear features may suggest cancer, but when breast cancer is seen in the lactating breast, it usually shows frank malignant features.[38]

Can a definitive diagnosis of breast cancer be made by fine-needle aspiration biopsy?

By FNAB, the diagnosis of breast cancer can be suspected almost immediately by its gritty sensation. A bloody aspirate or a pasty cream-colored or pink aspirate with granules strongly suggests cancer. The diagnosis can be confirmed immediately by examination of a Diff-Quik smear. The smear shows a homogeneous population of atypical epithelial cells in poorly cohesive groups. Most mammary carcinomas have abundant single intact cells with enlarged nuclei but lack bare bipolar nuclei (Fig. 17–12) and can be rapidly and confidently identified by an experienced cytopathologist.

In essence, patients with an equivocal diagnosis by FNAB may benefit from CNB.[42,43] FNAB is less reliable than CNB in the diagnosis of malignancy when there is an invasive lobular carcinoma. In one series by Sadler and colleagues, the FNAB failed to demonstrate malignant cells in 27 of 56 cases (48%) of invasive lobular carcinoma.[43] Ten additional cases of invasive lobular carcinoma were diagnosed by CNB when the FNAB was not diagnostic. Fibrosis and calcifications secondary to surgery or radiation can best be diagnosed by CNB because the aspirates tend to be low in cellularity. But, in general, FNAB is the most efficient, cost-effective, reliable procedure for the diagnosis of palpable breast carcinoma. Ballo and Sneige compared the sensitivity and specificity of CNB and FNAB cytology in detecting breast carcinoma in 124 patients who presented to the University of Texas M. D. Anderson Cancer Center for evaluation of a palpable breast mass.[8] The patients underwent an average of three needle passes and concurrently had a CNB using the 18-gauge Bard Monopty device (C. R. Bard, Inc., Covington, GA). All of the patients had histologic confirmation of their neoplasms. The specificity was 100% for both FNAB and CNB. However, the sensitivity was higher for FNAB than for CNB (97.5% vs. 90%; $P < .004$) and was not dependent on tumor type, size, or differentiation. The addition of CNB to a negative FNAB failed to increase the sensitivity in the detection of breast cancer.

In summary, FNAB is more cost-effective and requires less time and effort than CNB in the diagnosis of palpable lesions. The FNAB procedure allows for greater tactile sensitivity and ease of immobilization. Additionally, FNAB allows for multidirectional passes through the mass. These factors reduce the probability of sampling errors with FNAB compared with CNB for palpable breast masses. When there is discordance with the cytology and imaging findings, a CNB can contribute to a more definitive diagnosis.

What is the optimal number of core biopsy specimens?

Stereotactic and ultrasound-guided percutaneous large core biopsy are now commonly used for the initial histologic diagnosis of nonpalpable breast lesions. A CNB is a sampling procedure; hence, the main concern in the diagnosis of most breast lesions is establishing that the histologic findings on CNB provide an accurate assessment of the mammographically or ultrasound detected target lesion. The first-generation CNB instruments used an automated spring-loaded biopsy gun with a large-core cutting needle (usually 14 gauge) for the procurement of tissue from a target lesion. Second-generation vacuum-assisted CNB devices, such as the Mammotome (Biopsys Medical Instruments, Inc., San Juan Capistrano, CA), use larger-caliber needles (usually 11 gauge) and allow for multiple contiguous specimens to be obtained with a single needle insertion. These vacuum-assisted CNB devices have become a practical alternative to open surgical biopsy for the evaluation of mammographic microcalcifications. They allow for procurement of larger tissue samples, higher retrieval of microcalcifications, sampling of smaller clusters of microcalcifications, and consequently, a reduction in the need for rebiopsy.

If a cytopathologist is not available to determine specimen adequacy of an SFNAB or a touch preparation of a core

biopsy, it is accepted by most radiologists that a minimum of 5 core biopsies be performed for nodules and spiculated densities and that a minimum of 10 core biopsies be performed in cases of microcalcifications.[44] In one series of 145 stereotactic core biopsies using 14-gauge needles, diagnostic material was obtained with one, two, three, four, five, and six core specimens in 102 (70%), 117 (81%), 129 (89%), 132 (91%), 137 (94%), and 140 (97%) of the 145 lesions, respectively.[45] A diagnostic yield of 99% was obtained with five specimens for masses and 87% for calcifications. Obtaining six specimens increased the diagnostic yield to 92% for calcifications but did not improve the yield on masses.[45]

Cancers that elude definitive diagnosis are more often associated with microcalcifications than present as masses. When microcalcifications are the target of stereotactic needle biopsy, increased sampling and specimen radiography documentation are necessary.[46] Automated Tru-Cut biopsy devices are inefficient at sampling small foci of microcalcifications. In one center, a minimum of 12 cores are obtained for microcalcifications.[47] The procedure can take up to 1 hour. A definitive surgical excision may be preferable in cases of high suspicion for malignancy, but the issue remains unresolved at this time.[48]

The Mammotome was developed in 1994 by a radiologist, Fred Burbank, and a medical device engineer, Mark Ritchart, to address the drawbacks of the automated core biopsy devices. These drawbacks included the need for pinpoint accuracy in targeting the lesion and the need for multiple insertions to obtain the requisite number of cores: 5 for masses and 10 for microcalcifications. The Mammotome is a specialized breast biopsy instrument with a probe at its distal end with a piercing tip to penetrate breast tissue. Proximal to the piercing tip of the probe is an aperture into which tissue is drawn by means of a vacuum into a sampling chamber. Tissue in the sampling chamber is cut away from the breast by a coaxial cutter and pulled back into a standard pathology tissue cassette located in a specimen retrieval chamber[49] (Fig. 17–20). The Mammotome can routinely excise an entire cluster of microcalcifications, measuring up to 5×5 mm, in less than 10 minutes.[47,50] The procedure is referred to as stereotactic "mammotomy." With the use of the Mammotome, a breast lesion can be excised quickly and completely because it remains in the breast while the vacuum helps to pull tissue through the probe. The time necessitated for the performance of the CNB procedure is half that needed with the automated CNB devices because of the ability to obtain contiguous sampling of the lesion with one insertion. Another advantage of

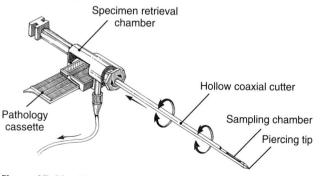

Figure 17–20 Mammotome probe.

the Mammotome vacuum is that there is less accumulation of blood at the biopsy site, and less ecchymosis.[9,51]

Most radiologists now use the Mammotome exclusively for the performance of SCNB. The likelihood of completely removing microcalcifications is higher with the Mammotome when compared with the automated biopsy gun. Liberman and coauthors reported calcification retrieval in 95% of cases with the 11-gauge Mammotome.[52] In one study, the likelihood of completely removing the mammographic lesion with the 14-gauge automated biopsy gun and the 14-gauge and 11-gauge Mammotome was reviewed.[53] Calcified lesions were completely removed in 7%, 26%, and 69% of cases with the 14-gauge automated biopsy gun and the 14-gauge and 11-gauge Mammotome, respectively.[53] Another advantage is that the minimum diameter of microcalcification clusters that can be sampled is 3 mm with the automated gun versus 5 mm with the Mammotome.[54] Consequently, the number of excisions performed following Mammotome biopsy is lower (9% versus 14.9%), the rate of sample insufficiency is lower (1.7% versus 4.4%), and the discrepancy rate between the mammographic findings and CNB diagnosis is lower (0.8% versus 3.4%) than with the automated biopsy gun.[55] Of note, Jackman and associates found that the underestimation of DCIS on SCNB was 1.9 times more frequent with masses than with microcalcifications, 1.8 times more frequent with automated CNB devices than with vacuum-assisted devices, and 1.5 times more frequent with 10 or fewer specimens than with more than 10 specimens per lesion.[56]

A tiny titanium clip for delivery through the Mammotome has been developed to permanently mark the biopsy site.[47] The clip can be deployed to mark the area should re-excision following wire localization be necessary. The contiguous sampling by the Mammotome creates a small air-filled cavity. The clip marks the cavity wall. In one series, 111 cases of CNB with clip deployment were reviewed.[57] The authors showed that 31 (28%) clips were more than 1 cm from the target on at least one postbiopsy image. Postbiopsy mammography in two orthogonal views is therefore necessary to document clip position relative to the biopsy cavity. The radiologist must be aware of the possibility of clip migration.[58] In one rare case, repeat postbiopsy mammograms showed displacement of targeted microcalcifications adjacent to the misplaced clip.[59]

What type of stereotactic needle biopsy equipment is available?

There are two major types of stereotactic breast biopsy apparatuses: upright units that are added to existing mammography machines, and dedicated prone stereotactic biopsy devices. There are two major advantages of the upright, add-on units: low cost and flexibility of use. When the unit is not being used for needle guidance, the mammography unit can be used for screening. The disadvantages of the add-on units are that patient motion is common, there are more episodes of vagal reactions than with the prone unit, and there is limited working space for the physician performing the procedure. All of these factors adversely affect the accuracy of needle guidance and lengthen the time of the procedure. The dedicated prone units (Mammotest, Fischer Imaging, Denver, CO; and Lorad StereoGuide, Hologic Corp., Bedford, MA) (Fig. 17–21) minimize patient movement and vagal reactions and have

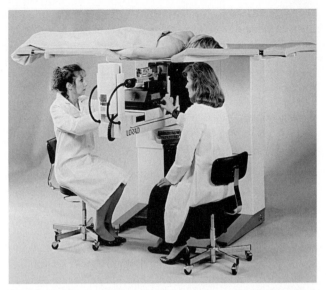

Figure 17–21   Lorad StereoGuide. This stereotactic system minimizes patient movement and vagal reactions and provides ample working space for the operator. (Courtesy of Hologic Corp., Bedford, MA.)

ample working space under the table. The disadvantages of the prone needle guidance systems are the expense and size of the unit. Additionally, the prone units do not allow for versatile use; their sole purpose is to guide needles.[49] It is recommended that another standard mammography unit or breast ultrasound unit (or both) be placed in the same room so that the room does not stand idle when stereotactic needling procedures are not being performed.[9]

How are the stereotactic images obtained and processed?

Stereotactic images can be obtained with conventional film-screen technique or with the digital technique. Direct digital imaging charge-coupled device (CCD) technology is available on both of the prone units and on many of the add-on stereotactic units. The film–screen technique is less costly, and there is no restriction of the field of view. However, there is poor contrast resolution, higher radiation dose, and lengthy film processing time when compared with the digital technique. Digital imaging allows for almost instantaneous image acquisition and display (about 5 seconds). Additionally, there is more contrast resolution, and the operator can postprocess the image by adjusting the image contrast, brightness, and magnification. The digital video display can be reversed to black on white instead of white on black, which can be especially useful in identifying microcalcifications. Edge enhancement algorithms can be applied to evaluate the margins of a nodule.[51]

Parker and coworkers reported a multicenter experience totaling 4744 stereotactic breast core biopsies, using 14-gauge needles. Tissue diagnosis by stereotactic breast core biopsy was found to be accurate and reproducible at 20 sites.[44] The complication rate was 0.2% and included three hematomas and three infections. The breast cancer miss rate was 1.3%. In comparison, surgical biopsy following needle localization may not be successful. Failure rate of 5% was reported even when the technique was performed by those experienced with the procedure.[60]

SCNB is not associated with lasting postbiopsy changes on follow-up mammography.[61,62] Complications include patient motion, vasovagal reactions (up to 7% using upright localization units), bleeding, and, rarely, pneumothorax.[62,63] Needle track seeding of malignant cells occurs in less than 0.01% of cases.[64] The surgical excision can be directed to excise the needle track if there is concern.[65]

How is a stereotactic needle biopsy performed?

Stereotactic localization uses parallax shift principles, apparent movement of the breast lesion, to calculate the position of the lesion in the breast. The three-dimensional coordinates of the mass are calculated from two radiographs taken at an angle of ±15 degrees from a central beam.[66] The needle is inserted into the calculated position and can be positioned within 1 to 2 mm of the target lesion (Fig. 17–22). A second pair of radiographs is obtained to confirm the position of the needle. In SFNAB, 25-gauge spinal needles are generally used. As with palpable lesions, the sensation of the mass provides a clue that the mass has been hit. Multiple specimens from different sites of the target lesion are obtained to minimize inadequate samples.

Variation in the size of the core needle used for SCNB with an automated gun ranges from 14 to 20 gauge, but the best results are obtained using an automated gun with a long throw (2.2 to 2.5 cm) and a 14-gauge needle with a 1.5- to 1.9-cm sample notch.[61] Local anesthesia is used and a small 4- to 5-mm nick is made with an 11-blade scalpel. The small incision is unnecessary with 18- or 20-gauge core needles. The biopsy needle is then manually advanced so that the needle tip alignment is at the front edge of the lesion to be sampled. The proper alignment of the needle with respect to the lesion is confirmed by a set of prefire stereoscopic images. The automated gun is fired, and the proper postfire position of the needle tip is documented by another set of images (Fig. 17–23). The breast is manually compressed to achieve hemostasis, and a Steri-Strip or simple bandage is used to close the skin incision. SFNAB may be preferable to SCNB in women with small breasts because the long throw of the automated gun may hit the backplate of the apparatus, although with experience, this can be avoided by using a side approach to the target.[47] Digital stereotactic imaging provides almost instantaneous image reconstruction with better contrast resolution than film-screen imaging and has eliminated the need for prefire and postfire stereoscopic images; therefore, the patient is subjected to fewer exposures. Additionally, recent software improvements allow for targeting of the lesion orthogonal to the plane of compression. Stereotactic needle biopsy, coupled with stereotactic localization for laser ablation, thermal ablation, or cryotherapy, has been tested on small breast cancers,[67] and excision of the entire breast mass under stereotactic guidance has also been evaluated.[68]

When is an ultrasound-detected lesion diagnosed by needle biopsy?

Many breast surgeons and radiologists are now evaluating nonpalpable breast masses by ultrasound. Up to 90% of mammographically detected nonpalpable breast masses can be identified by ultrasound.[69] Ultrasound-guided biopsy is faster and less expensive than stereotactic biopsy, with no compromise in accuracy.[69,70] Ultrasound offers many other advantages, including no radiation exposure, shorter route to the target, real-time image of the needling procedure, and ability to sample the lesion multidirectionally.[71,72] High-frequency (7.5- to 13-mHz) linear array transducers with a large sole are optimal for use in ultrasound of the breast.[73]

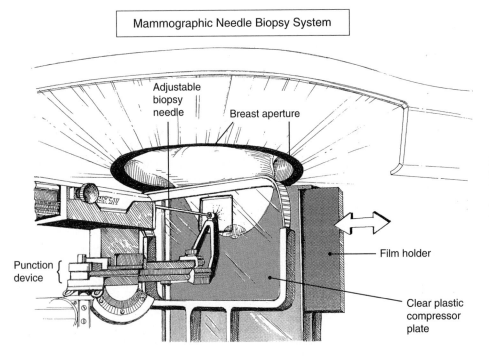

Figure 17–22 Mammographic localization. The needle is inserted into the calculated position, and stereoscopic images are taken to confirm the position of the needle.

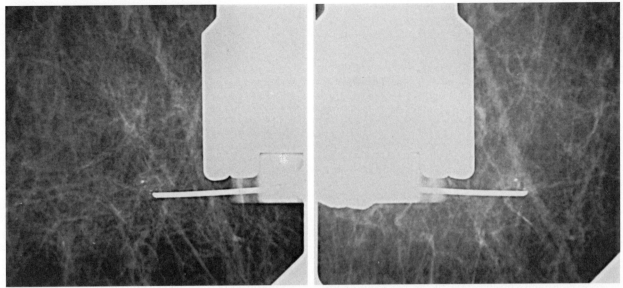

Figure 17–23   Postfire stereotactic images. The needle tip is documented in its proper position with respect to the lesion of concern.

When a complex cyst or an indeterminate lesion is identified by ultrasound, ultrasound-guided needle aspiration can be performed. If the lesion is a cyst, it is managed based on the appearance of the fluid and the degree of cyst resolution; clear colorless fluid can be discarded, but bloody fluid must be analyzed. If the lesion is solid, FNAB or CNB under ultrasound guidance can be done in the same setting. In 1999, a new handheld version of the Mammotome was developed for use under ultrasound guidance.[51] In one series of 71 ultrasound-guided breast biopsies, the device proved to be accurate with a slightly higher risk for bleeding owing to lack of compression of the breast when compared with CNB performed with stereotactic guidance.[74] However, the relative value of sonographically guided Mammotome biopsy compared with stereotactically guided Mammotome biopsy for solid masses remains to be determined.

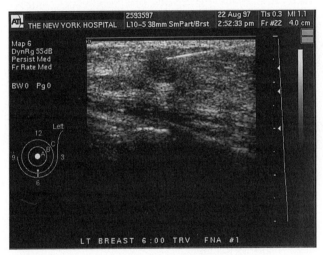

Figure 17–24   Ultrasound-guided core needle biopsy.

How is the ultrasound needle biopsy performed?

The ultrasound-guided breast biopsy is performed with the patient in the supine position. The skin is cleansed, and sterile acoustic gel is placed on the breast. For core biopsy, the needle pathway is anesthetized. The needle is introduced in a direction longitudinal to the long axis of the transducer, which allows for continuous visualization of the hyperechoic (whiter) needle. This orientation is easier to maintain with the aid of biopsy guide attachments for the transducer.[73] Cysts can be evacuated by placing the needle into the center of the mass and then aspirating the fluid. When a core biopsy is performed for solid lesions, the needle is aligned at the edge of the mass, and the automated gun is fired under real-time visualization (Fig. 17–24).

A breast and biopsy device-stabilizing apparatus has been developed for performing three-dimensional ultrasound-guided needle procedures with the patient in the upright position (Sonopsy, NeoVision Corp., Seattle, WA). Four advantages of this method over conventional ultrasound

needle techniques are as follows: (1) there is good immobilization of the lesion with breast compression, (2) there is better visualization of the lesion by three-dimensional ultrasound imaging, (3) there is optimal chest wall access and elimination of the risk for pneumothorax, and (4) it is easy to correlate the ultrasound and radiographic images. All of these factors increase the speed and accuracy of performing the ultrasound-guided needle biopsy procedure.

Should a mammogram be performed following a core biopsy procedure?

Hann and coworkers performed mammograms in 86 cases immediately after stereotactic core biopsy using 14-gauge needles to determine whether mammography should be done routinely to diagnose hematoma, confirm sampling of microcalcifications, and establish a new baseline for future mammograms.[75] The authors found that 57 of 58 hematomas were clinically occult. Postprocedural mammograms showed a decrease in a number of calcifications in 26 of 54 cases (48%), as compared with specimen radiographs, which showed calcium in 50 of 54 cases (93%). Three masses and one cluster of microcalcifications disappeared after biopsy. Hematomas obscured residual microcalcifications at the biopsy site in three cases. The authors concluded that mammography was not necessary immediately after core biopsy for the diagnosis of hematoma and is inferior to specimen radiography for verifying sampling of microcalcifications. The frequent finding of hematoma makes mammograms after core biopsy suboptimal for the establishment of a new baseline.

What are the practical considerations in the reporting of the pathologic diagnosis on core needle biopsy?

The most important consideration in the reporting of the pathologic diagnosis on CNB is to address the specific pathology of the target lesion. For example, for SCNB performed for microcalcifications, the specific diagnosis for the targeted focus of microcalcifications should be noted as the primary finding along with documentation as to whether the microcalcifications on histology correspond to those in the CNB specimen radiograph. Ideally, a SCNB performed for microcalcifications should be submitted in two parts; the first part should include the tissue cores containing mammographic microcalcifications, and the second part (which may constitute most of the specimen volume) should include the additional tissue. A maximum of five intact cores should be submitted in each cassette. Therefore, although a small focus of clustered microcalcifications may be seen in a microscopic fibroadenoma in 1 or 2 of more than 20 tissue cores, the primary diagnosis should be denoted as "fibroadenoma with clustered microcalcifications; *corresponding to those in the CNB specimen radiograph,*" and any additional findings should be delineated separately with attention to the presence of any high-risk lesions.

In cases of fibrocystic change, microcysts and foci of papillary apocrine hyperplasia may be associated with crystals of calcium of oxalate. These may be difficult to identify without polarization. Commonly, sclerosing adenosis (see Fig. 17–1) and columnar cell hyperplasia (CCH) (see Fig. 17–2) may present as suspicious clustered microcalcifications, occasionally of the ossifying type. When multiple sites of microcalcifications are present in one breast, sampling of one can reliably predict the pathology of another.[48]

A diagnosis of atypical ductal hyperplasia (ADH) is rendered when there is hyperplasia and cytologic atypia as well as structural rigidity of the ductal epithelium, but the proliferation is not limited to a monotonous population of cells with distinct cell borders as in DCIS (Fig. 17–25). In most instances in which DCIS is found on CNB, it can be subtyped by its architectural pattern (solid, cribriform, micropapillary, papillary), presence or absence of necrosis, and nuclear grade. The presence of an extensive intraductal component and of microinvasion should be noted to ensure that adequate margins are taken at the time of excisional biopsy. A suspicion of microinvasion can be confirmed or refuted by immunohistochemical staining for basement membrane (collagen IV and

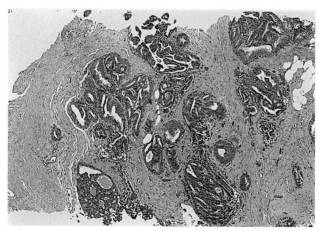

Figure 17–25 Core needle biopsy of atypical ductal hyperplasia (ADH). There is hyperplasia and cytologic atypia of the epithelium as well as structural rigidity of the ducts, but the proliferation is not limited to a monotonous population of cells with distinct cell borders (as in ductal carcinoma in situ [DCIS]). The surgically excised specimen showed DCIS and ADH.

laminin) and myoepithelial cells (smooth muscle actin, CD10, and heavy-chain myosin).[76]

The reporting of the pathology of invasive breast cancer on CNB should include any prognostically relevant findings. A CNB does not permit reliable measurement of tumor size, although a microscopic carcinoma completely incorporated within a tissue core can be very accurately measured by ocular micrometry. Most other prognostic features pertinent to a T1N0 breast carcinoma can be determined on CNB.[77] Grading of the ductal carcinoma by Scarf-Bloom-Richardson scoring (which includes evaluation of gland formation, nuclear grade, and mitotic index) can be done on CNB material. Certain histologic subtypes of invasive carcinoma with favorable outcomes can be identified on CNB, including adenoid cystic carcinoma, which is composed of nests of basaloid cells with a cylindromatous pattern, tubular carcinoma with greater than 75% well-formed glands (see Fig. 17–19), colloid carcinoma characterized by an abundance of extracellular mucin and lack of desmoplastic response, and medullary carcinoma, which is characterized by high-grade nuclear morphology and a syncytial growth pattern accompanied by an infiltrate of lymphocytes and plasma cells.

Invasive lobular carcinoma of the classic variant shows small neoplastic cells infiltrating dense fibrous tissue as linear aggregates, sometimes with prominence of signet-ring cells (see Fig. 17–17). Other variants (alveolar, solid, histiocytoid, or pleomorphic) may need to be confirmed with immunostaining for E-cadherin, a transmembrane glycoprotein involved in the formation of the intercellular junctional complex.[76] E-cadherin immunostaining is typically absent or markedly diminished in mammary carcinoma of the lobular phenotype, as opposed to the intense cytoplasmic membrane staining seen in normal, hyperplastic, and neoplastic ductal epithelial cells. An E-cadherin stain can be useful in distinguishing solid DCIS from LCIS as well. In addition to E-cadherin for diagnostic subtyping of invasive carcinoma, immunohistochemical stains can be performed on CNB specimens for prognostic markers, including estrogen and progesterone receptors and *HER-2/neu.* Feulgen-stained sections of the CNB can be used for determination of ploidy and S-phase fraction with image cytometry. In general, these stains are performed on CNB specimens when the targeted lesion is a small invasive carcinoma that has been completely excised by the needle procedure or when preoperative chemotherapy is to be given.

Evaluation of the CNB for peritumoral lymphatic invasion (PLI) should be done. The lymphatic space should have endothelial cells because artifacts of fixation can cause separation of epithelial cells from the duct wall, mimicking PLI. In CNB material, intraobserver reproducibility for PLI is low.[77]

What is the significance of a diagnosis of atypical ductal hyperplasia by core needle biopsy?

The finding of ADH at SCNB is an indication for surgical biopsy because of the prevalence of carcinoma in the lesions. In one series, ADH was found in 25 of 264 lesions (9%), including 21 of 105 sites of calcification (20%), and 4 of 159 masses (3%).[78] Surgical biopsy was recommended in all 25 instances and was performed in 21. The histopathology of these 21 cases was benign without atypia in 4 (19%), ADH in 6 (29%), and ductal carcinoma in 11 (52%), including 8 cases of DCIS and 3 invasive ductal carcinomas.

Histologic findings of core biopsy and surgical biopsy specimens were concordant in 5 and discordant in 11 cases of ADH diagnosed by core biopsy in a series by Jackman and colleagues.[79] The authors concluded that a diagnosis of ADH by core biopsy is inaccurate and that excisional biopsy is necessary. Also, an unequivocal diagnosis of ADH on a CNB does not preclude the presence of DCIS in the immediate vicinity of the target lesion. It is notable that studies that compare CNB with automated and vacuum-assisted devices show a marked reduction in the underestimation rate for ADH using the 11-gauge Mammotome. In a comprehensive review of the literature, Reynolds and coauthors noted that the underdiagnosis rate for ADH was 41% with the use of the automated biopsy gun, as compared with 15% with the 11-gauge Mammotome.[80] In another review, several subsets of patients with a diagnosis of ADH on CNB with a high likelihood of DCIS in subsequent surgical excisions were identified.[81] These included patients in whom the CNB was diagnosed as ADH bordering on DCIS and patients with a diagnosis of ADH with papillary features, with a 63% and 36% likelihood of DCIS in subsequent surgical biopsies, respectively. The number of atypical foci in CNB and the mammographic span of the microcalcifications, greater than four foci and greater than 2 cm, also correlated with an increased likelihood of DCIS on excision.[81]

What is the accuracy of predicting invasion by stereotactic core biopsy?

Stereotactic core biopsy of breast carcinoma can accurately predict invasion, although absence of invasion is not definitive when only DCIS is found. Liberman and associates correlated the histopathologic findings of stereotactic core biopsy and surgery of 63 breast carcinomas and found concordance in 58 (92%), yielding invasive carcinoma in 46 cases and DCIS in 12 cases.[82] The results were discordant in five cases (8%), including three cases in which the stereotactic core biopsy showed DCIS and surgery showed invasive ductal carcinoma. There was one false-positive case by CNB in which the core biopsies revealed intraductal carcinoma cells displaced in fibroadipose tissue by the needle procedure. The CNB was falsely diagnosed as invasive ductal adenocarcinoma. This case illustrates a potential interpretive pitfall. There is no evidence that the displaced cells are biologically relevant.

There is a high rate of underdiagnosis of invasion by CNB. In a series reported by Jackman and colleagues, there were 8 of 43 (19%) instances in which DCIS diagnosed by CNB proved to be invasive carcinoma by surgical excision.[79] Also, in a multi-institutional study, Parker and associates reported that 33% of the lesions that were diagnosed as low-grade DCIS or ADH and 11% of those diagnosed as high-grade DCIS were underdiagnosed cases of invasive carcinoma.[44] Lee and associates found that SCNB with the 11-gauge Mammotome was as reliable as open surgical excision for diagnosing DCIS without invasion.[83] Nonetheless, in the latter series, DCIS without invasion was diagnosed by CNB in 59 patients, and on excision, 17 (29%) had invasive disease. Despite the high incidence of underdiagnosis by CNB, when a diagnosis of invasive breast cancer is made, CNB is highly reliable and allows for a decision regarding axillary lymph node sampling at the time of mastectomy or segmental excision. The presence of an extensive intraductal component (EIC) on CNB should be reported because in one retrospective review of DCIS in breast CNB with invasive cancer, the authors showed that the presence of an EIC correlated significantly with close or positive margins on subsequent excision.[84]

Is there displacement of carcinomatous epithelium in surgical breast specimens following stereotactic core biopsy?

The attribution of carcinomatous displacement in surgical breast specimens solely by core biopsy is complicated by the fact that these specimens are subjected to other needle procedures. These include local anesthetic injection, needle localization, suture placement, and FNAB. Youngson and coworkers found displaced carcinomatous fragments outside the main tumor mass in 12 of 43 (28%) consecutive cases of breast carcinoma that were initially diagnosed by stereotactic core biopsy using 14-gauge needles.[85] In 18 of these surgical breast specimens, the only needle procedure other than core biopsy was local anesthetic injection by 25-gauge needle. Displaced cancer fragments were seen in 7 of these 18 cases (39%). The authors suggested that the core biopsy was the more likely cause of tumor fragment displacement because they previously documented only one case in which a 25-gauge needle was associated with epithelial displacement.[86] The displaced epithelial fragments may mimic stromal invasion and represent a potential source of misdiagnosis (Fig. 17–26). The biologic and clinical significance of epithelial displacement has not yet been ascertained. As noted previously, there is one reported case of repeat postbiopsy mammograms that showed displacement of targeted microcalcifications adjacent to the misplaced clip.[59]

specimens come from benign lesions.[106] Fewer passes may be needed to support a benign diagnosis in premenopausal women than in postmenopausal women, in whom epithelial atrophy accounts for few diagnostic cells. Zemba-Palko and coauthors undertook a 20-year retrospective review of 52 false-negative diagnoses among 1518 benign breast aspirates followed by surgery.[20] The authors found that among false-negative specimens aspirated from postmenopausal women, 20 or more epithelial cell groups per slide were seen. These findings suggest that among postmenopausal women, high cellularity alone may warrant an excisional biopsy. If the clinical-mammographic-cytologic diagnostic triplet is negative, the false-negative rate can be reduced from an average of 10% to less than 1%.[106] More specific diagnoses can be rendered with a core biopsy.[48,50,61,65,70]

In experienced hands, the false-positive rate of fine-needle biopsy is less than 1%, comparable to intraoperative frozen section.[107] The false-positive rate can be reduced to less than 0.2% with judicious use of the triple-test method.[106] To minimize false-positive diagnoses, DeMay suggested that an unequivocal diagnosis of breast cancer should not be made in these instances: (1) in a poorly cellular aspirate; (2) in the absence of single, intact cells; (3) in the presence of bare bipolar nuclei; and (4) in the absence or paucity of atypia.[21] Most false-positive diagnoses are due to interpretive errors. Many benign breast diseases mimic the patterns of cellularity and atypia of breast cancer. For example, cellular fibroadenoma, proliferative fibrocystic change with atypia, lactational change, and phyllodes tumor are of high cellularity and have conspicuous atypia. There can also be significant cellular atypia following radiation or in fat necrosis, and in the male, gynecomastia. In general, however, these smears are of low cellularity.

By FNAB, papillomas can show a monotonous population of dyshesive, columnar cells that occasionally, in the absence of myoepithelial nuclei, mimic cancer.[108] Therefore, cancer should not be definitively diagnosed in a neoplasm with a papillary pattern unless there is marked cytologic atypia. Even then, excisional biopsy must be done to confirm a diagnosis of papillary carcinoma.

Needle biopsy of a radial scar with adenosis can lead to a false-positive diagnosis. The gritty sensation of the mass, its suspicious spiculated appearance mammographically, and the aspirate are suggestive of tubular carcinoma. The FNAB may show small, angular, and tubular clusters like tubular carcinoma, although it tends to be less cellular, with more bare nuclei.[109] Sclerosing and microglandular adenosis, fibroadenomas, and lactational changes show microacinar structures that may be overinterpreted as carcinoma.

Overdiagnosis and underdiagnosis of cancer may occasionally be due to smearing and drying artifacts in FNAB specimens, and this is even more common in cases in which there is overlap of the cytologic features of benign and malignant lesions (i.e., the gray zone of breast cytology).[32] Therefore, proper preparation of FNAB smears is imperative for accurate diagnoses to be made. When proper smearing techniques cannot be ensured, because of inexperience or a bloody sample, the Cytospin[16] or ThinPrep methods of processing of the FNAB material should be employed.

Difficulty in SCNB interpretation occurs because of fragmentation, hemorrhage, and artifactual distortion of the tissue.[110] These problems can lead to false-positive diagnoses in some benign pseudoinvasive lesions such as florid sclerosing adenosis and radial scar. Distortion of ducts with DCIS may lead to a false impression of invasive cancer. A false-negative SCNB is most commonly due to sampling error. CNB is an invaluable method of determining invasion of a breast cancer preoperatively, although CNB can nonetheless underdiagnose invasive disease.

Histologically, there is significant interobserver variability in the diagnosis of proliferative breast lesions (including epithelial hyperplasia, atypical hyperplasia, and noncomedo DCIS) using standardized criteria.[111–113] SCNB is further limited in the diagnosis of these borderline epithelial lesions by its small sample size as well as by the distortion of the core tissue secondary to the procedure.[110] However, a study by Collins and colleagues showed that there is a high level of diagnostic agreement (90% confidence interval) among pathologists in interpretation of CNB, comparable to that seen for open surgical biopsy.[114]

SUMMARY

No single test can diagnose all breast cancers.[115] The accuracy of diagnosing breast cancer is 90% to 99% by FNAB, 85% to 90% by mammography, and 70% to 90% by physical examination.[116] The diagnostic accuracy of physical examination, mammography, and FNAB together approaches 100% for palpable lesions,[101] as does needle biopsy under stereotactic guidance[117] and under ultrasound guidance for nonpalpable breast masses.[70]

Ideally, needle biopsy procedures will be performed in specialized centers by physicians experienced in the multidisciplinary approach to ambulatory breast care. Symptomatic patients with palpable masses (referred or self-referred) should be treated systematically. A clinical assessment of the breast lesion and of the likelihood that the patient will return for follow-up should be made. If, in the opinion of the clinician, the patient is unlikely to return for follow-up, a mammogram or ultrasound, or both, should be performed and an excisional biopsy scheduled at the initial visit. If, in the opinion of the clinician, the patient is likely to return for follow-up, a mammogram or ultrasound, or both, should be performed, followed by needle aspiration or core needle biopsy. If the lesion is cystic, the procedure will be therapeutic. Malignant, suspicious, and atypical lesions should be excised surgically. If the radiologic, clinical, and cytologic impressions are benign and concordant, a follow-up visit should be scheduled. Discordant results will also require surgical excision.

For the diagnosis of nonpalpable breast lesions that are likely to be benign, ultrasound-guided or stereotactic-guided breast needle biopsies may be performed. Ideally, an aspiration biopsy can be done first, and core needle biopsy can then be performed on all lesions not shown to be cysts. Breast parenchyma with microcalcifications is best sampled stereotactically using the Mammotome core biopsy device. It should be emphasized that a negative needle breast biopsy cannot definitely exclude cancer. It is therefore imperative to follow all palpable and nonpalpable breast masses that are not surgically excised. If a malignant, atypical, or equivocal diagnosis is rendered by CNB, an excisional biopsy is required. Using these clinical measures, breast cancer is rarely missed, whereas the number of open biopsies can be reduced by half.

REFERENCES

1. Grant CS, Goellner JR, Welch JS, et al. Fine-needle aspiration of the breast. Mayo Clin Proc 1986;61:377–381.

2. Zarbo RJ, Howanitz PJ, Bachner P. Interinstitutional comparison of performance in breast fine-needle aspiration cytology. A Q-probe quality indicator study. Arch Pathol Lab Med 1991;115:743–750.

3. Kline TS. Survey of aspiration biopsy cytology of the breast. Diagn Cytopathol 1991;7:98–104.

4. Layfield L. Recommendations, subcommittee V. In NCI Breast Fine Needle Aspiration Conference: Preconference Recommendation. Bethesda, MD, September 9–10, 1996.

5. Hermansen C, Poulsen H, Jensen J, et al. Diagnostic reliability of combined physical examination, mammography, and fine-needle puncture ("triple-test") in breast tumors. A prospective study. Cancer 1987;60:1866–1871.

6. Vetto J, Pommier R, Schmidt W, et al. Use of the "triple test" for palpable breast lesions yields diagnostic accuracy and cost savings. Am J Surg 1995;169:519–522.

7. Layfield LJ, Chrischilles EA, Cohen MB, et al. The palpable breast nodule: A cost-effectiveness analysis of alternative diagnostic approaches. Cancer 1993;72:1642–1651.

8. Ballo MS, Sneige N. Can core needle biopsy replace fine-needle aspiration cytology in the diagnosis of palpable breast carcinoma? A comparative study of 124 women. Cancer 1996;78:773–777.

9. Parker SH, Stavros AT, Dennis MA. Needle biopsy techniques. Radiol Clin North Am 1995;33:1171–1186.

10. Logan-Young WW, Hoffman NY, Janus JA. Fine-needle aspiration cytology in the detection of breast cancer in non-suspicious lesions. Radiology 1992;184:49–53.

11. Koss LG. The palpable breast nodule: A cost-effectiveness analysis of alternative diagnostic approaches. The role of the needle aspiration biopsy. Cancer 1993;72:1499–1502.

12. Kim E, Acosta E, Hilborne L, et al. Modified technique for fine needle aspiration biopsy that eliminates needle manipulation. Acta Cytol 1996;40:174–176.

13. Zajdela A, Zillhardt P, Voillemot N. Cytological diagnosis by fine needle sampling without aspiration. Cancer 1987;59:1201–1205.

14. Sneige N, Staerkel GA, Caraway NP, et al. A plea for uniform terminology and reporting of breast fine needle aspirates. The M. D. Anderson Cancer Center Proposal. Acta Cytol 1994;38:971–972.

15. Yang GCH. Ultrafast Papanicolaou stain is not limited to rapid assessments: Application to permanent fine-needle aspiration smears. Diagn Cytopathol 1995;13:160–162.

16. Howat AJ, Stringfellow HF, Briggs WA, et al. Fine needle aspiration cytology of the breast. A review of 1868 cases using the cytospin method. Acta Cytol 1994;38:939–944.

17. Ciatto S, Cariaggi P, Bulgaresi P. The value of routine cytologic examination of breast cyst fluids. Acta Cytol 1989;33:894–898.

18. Devitt JE, To T, Miller AB. Risk of breast cancer in women with breast cysts. Can Med Assoc J 1992;147:45–49.

19. Sterrett G, Oliver D, Frayne J, et al. Stereotactic fine needle aspiration biopsy (SFNB) of breast: Preliminary results in Perth with the TRC Mammotest machine. Cytological aspects. Pathology 1991;23:302–310.

20. Zemba-Palko V, Klenn PJ, Saminathan T, et al. Benign breast aspirates. Two decades of experience. Arch Pathol Lab Med 1996;120:1056–1060.

21. DeMay RM. Breast. In DeMay RM (ed). Aspiration Cytology, vol 2. The Art and Science of Cytopathology. Chicago, ASCP Press, 1996, pp 847–937.

22. Thomas PA, Cangiarella J, Raab S, et al. Fine needle aspiration biopsy of proliferative breast disease. Mod Pathol 1995;8:130–136.

23. Masood S. Pathological interpretation of fine needle aspiration cytology. In Fajardo LL, Willison KM, Pizzutiello RK (eds). A Comprehensive Approach to Stereotactic Breast Biopsy. Cambridge, MA, Blackwell, 1996, pp 225–239.

24. Malberger E, Yerushalmi R, Tamir A, Keren R. Diagnosis of fibroadenoma in breast fine needle aspirates devoid of typical stroma. Acta Cytol 1997;41:1483–1488.

25. Dupont WD, Page DL. Risk factors for breast cancer in women with proliferative breast disease. N Engl J Med 1985;312:146–151.

26. Bodian CA, Perzin KH, Lattes R, et al. Prognostic significance of benign proliferative breast disease. Cancer 1993;71:3896–3907.

27. Rosen PP. Proliferative breast "disease." Cancer 1993;71:3798–3807.

28. Stanley MW, Henry-Stanley MJ, Zera R. Atypia in breast fine-needle aspiration smears correlates poorly with the presence of a prognostically significant proliferative lesion of ductal epithelium. Hum Pathol 1993;24:630–635.

29. Mitnick JS, Vazquez MF, Roses DF, et al. Stereotaxic localization for fine-needle aspiration breast biopsy: Initial experience with 300 patients. Arch Surg 1991;126:1137–1140.

30. Mitnick JS, Vazquez MF, Feiner HD, et al. Mammographically detected breast lesions: Clinical importance of cytologic atypia in stereotaxic fine-needle aspiration biopsy samples. Radiology 1996;198:319–322.

31. Mulford DK, Dawson AE. Atypia in fine needle aspiration cytology of nonpalpable and palpable mammographically detected breast lesions. Acta Cytol 1994;38:1–17.

32. Al-Kaisi N. The spectrum of the "gray zone" in breast cytology: A review of 186 cases of atypical and suspicious cytology. Acta Cytol 1994;38:898–908.

33. Maygarden SJ, Novotny DB, Johnson DE, et al. Subclassification of benign breast disease by fine needle aspiration cytology. Comparison of cytologic and histologic findings in 265 palpable breast masses. Acta Cytol 1994;38:115–129.

34. Stanley MW, Tani EM, Skoog L. Fine-needle aspiration of fibroadenomas of the breast with atypia: A spectrum including cases that cytologically mimic carcinoma. Diagn Cytopathol 1990;6:375–382.

35. Stanley MW, Tani EM, Rutqvist LE, et al. Cystosarcoma phyllodes of the breast: A cytologic and clinicopathologic study of 23 cases. Diagn Cytopathol 1989;5:29–34.

36. Jeffrey PB, Ljung BM. Benign and malignant papillary lesions of the breast. A cytomorphologic study. Am J Clin Pathol 1994;101:500–507.

37. Dei Tos AP, Giustina DD, Bittesini L. Aspiration biopsy cytology of malignant papillary breast neoplasms. Diagn Cytopathol 1992;8:580–584.

38. Bottles K, Taylor RN. Diagnosis of breast masses in pregnant and lactating women by aspiration cytology. Obstet Gynecol 1985;66:76–78.

39. Ciatto S, Bulgaresi P. Multiple sampling to reduce inadequacy rates in stereotaxic aspiration cytology of the breast. Acta Cytol 1991;35:482.

40. Peterse JL, Thunnissen FBJM, van Heerde P. Fine needle aspiration cytology of radiation-induced changes in nonneoplastic breast lesions: Possible pitfalls in cytodiagnosis. Acta Cytol 1989;33:176–180.

41. Deis Tos AP, Giustina DD, Martin VD, et al. Aspiration biopsy cytology of tubular carcinoma of the breast. Diagn Cytopathol 1994;11:146–150.

42. Carty NJ, Ravichandran D, Carter C, et al. Randomized comparison of fine-needle aspiration cytology and Biopty-cut needle biopsy after unsatisfactory initial cytology of discrete breast lesions. Br J Surg 1994;81:1313–1314.

43. Sadler GP, McGee S, Dallimore NS, et al. Role of fine-needle aspiration cytology biopsy in the diagnosis of lobular carcinoma of the breast. Br J Surg 1994;81:1315–1317.

44. Parker SH, Burbank F, Jackman R, et al. Percutaneous large core breast biopsy: A multi-institutional study. Radiology 1994;193:359–364.

45. Liberman L, Dershaw DD, Rosen PP, et al. Stereotaxic 14-gauge breast biopsy: How many core biopsy specimens are needed? Radiology 1994;192:793–795.

46. Liberman LL, Evans WP, Dershaw DD, et al. Radiography of microcalcifications in stereotaxic mammary core biopsy specimens. Radiology 1994;190:223–222.

47. Burbank F. Stereotactic breast biopsy: Its history, its present and its future. Am Surg 1996;62:128–150.

48. Berg WA, Arnoldus CL, Teferra E, Bhargavan M. Biopsy of amorphous breast calcifications: Pathologic outcome and yield at stereotactic biopsy. Radiology 2001;3:13–32.

49. Parker SH, Dennis MA, Stavros AT. Critical pathways in percutaneous breast intervention. Radiographics 1995;15:946–950.

50. Parker SH. Percutaneous large core breast biopsy. Cancer 1994;74:256–262.

51. Parker SH. The evolution of minimally invasive breast biopsy: From FNA to percutaneous incisional and excisional biopsy. Radiology 2001;3:13–32.

52. Liberman L, Smolkin JH, Dertshaw DD, et al. Calcification retrieval at stereotactic, 11-gauge, directional, vacuum-assisted breast biopsy. Radiology 1998;208:251–260.

53. Jackman RJ, Marzoni FA, Nowels KW. Percutaneous removal of benign mammographic lesions: Comparison of automated large-core and directional vacuum-assisted stereotactic biopsy techniques. AJR Am J Roentgenol 1998;171:1325–1330.

54. Meyer JE, Smith DN, Lester SC, et al. Large-core needle biopsy of nonpalpable breast lesions. JAMA 1999;281:1638–1641.

55. Philpotts LE, Shaheen NA, Carter D, et al. Comparison of rebiopsy rates after stereotactic core needle biopsy of the breast with 11-gauge vacuum suction probe versus 14-gauge needle and automated gun. AJR Am J Roentgenol 1999;172:683–687.

56. Jackman RJ, Burbank F, Parker SH. Stereotactic breast biopsy of nonpalpable lesions: Determinants of ductal carcinoma in situ underestimation rates. Radiology 2001;218(2):497.

57. Rosen EL, Vo TT. Metallic clip deployment during stereotactic breast biopsy: Retrospective analysis. Radiology 2001;218(2):510.

58. Philpotts LE, Lee CH. Clip migration after 11-gauge vacuum-assisted stereotactic biopsy: Case report. Radiology 2002;222(3):794.

59. Lee SG, Piccoli CW, Hughes JS. Displacement of microcalcifications during stereotactic 11-gauge directional vacuum-assisted biopsy with marking clip placement: Case report. Radiology 2001;219(2):495.

60. Homer MJ, Smith TJ, Safaii H. Prebiopsy needle localization: Methods, problems, and expected results. Radiol Clin North Am 1992;30:139–145.

61. Schmidt RA. Stereotactic breast biopsy. CA Cancer J Clin 1994;44:172–191.

62. Helvie MA, Ikeda MD, Adler DD. Localization and needle aspiration of breast lesions: Complications in 370 cases. AJR Am J Roentgenol 1991;157:711–714.

63. Kaufman Z, Shpitz B, Shapiro M, et al. Pneumothorax: A complication of fine needle aspiration of breast tumors. Acta Cytol 1994;38:737–738.

64. Harter LP, Curtis JS, Ponto G, et al. Malignant seeding of the needle track during stereotaxic core needle breast biopsy. Radiology 1992;185:713–714.

65. Sullivan DC. Needle core biopsy of mammographic lesions. AJR Am J Roentgenol 1994;162:601–608.

66. Willison KM. Fundamentals of stereotactic breast biopsy. In Fajardo LL, Willison KM, Pizzutiello RK (eds). A Comprehensive Approach to Stereotactic Breast Biopsy. Cambridge, MA, Blackwell Scientific, 1996, pp 13–72.

67. Robinson DS, Parel JM, Denham DB, et al. Stereotactic uses beyond core biopsy: Model development for minimally invasive treatment of breast cancer through interstitial laser hyperthermia. Am Surg 1996;62:117–118.

68. Lieberman L. Advanced breast biopsy instrumentation (ABBI): Analysis of published experience. AJR Am J Roentgenol 1999;172:1413–1416.

69. Staren ED. Surgical office-based ultrasound of the breast. Am Surg 1995;61:619–627.

70. Parker SH, Jobe WE, Dennis MA, et al. US guided automated large-core breast biopsy. Radiology 1993;187:507–511.

71. Ciatto S, Catarzi S, Morrone D, et al. Fine-needle aspiration cytology of nonpalpable breast lesions. US versus stereotaxic guidance. Radiology 1993;188:195–198.

72. Staren ED, Fine R. Breast ultrasound for surgeons. Am Surg 1996;62:108–112.

73. Staren ED. Physics and principles of breast ultrasound. Am Surg 1996;62:103–107.

74. Simon JR, Kalbhen CL, Cooper RA. Accuracy and complication rates of ultrasonographic (US)-guided vacuum-assisted core breast biopsy: Initial result. Radiology 2000;215–694–697.

75. Hann LE, Liberman L, Dershaw DD, et al. Mammography immediately after stereotaxic breast biopsy: Is it necessary? AJR Am J Roentgenol 1995;165:59–62.

76. Hoda SA, Rosen PP. Practical considerations in the pathologic diagnosis of needle core biopsies of the breast. Am J Clin Pathol 2002;118:101–108.

77. Lagios MD. Prognostic features of breast carcinoma from stereotactic biopsy material. Radiology 1997;1:101–130.

78. Liberman L, Cohen MA, Dershaw DD, et al. Atypical ductal hyperplasia diagnosed at stereotaxic core biopsy of breast lesions: An indication for surgical biopsy. AJR Am J Roentgenol 1995;164:1111–1113.

79. Jackman RJ, Nowels KW, Shepard MJ, et al. Stereotactic large-core needle biopsy of 450 nonpalpable breast lesions with surgical correlation in lesions with cancer and atypical hyperplasia. Radiology 1994;193:91–95.

80. Reynolds HE, Poon CM, Goulet RJ, et al. Biopsy of breast microcalcifications using an 11-gauge directional vacuum-assisted device. AJR Am J Roentgenol 1998;171:611–613.

81. Bonnett M, Wallis T, Rossmann M. Histopathologic analysis of atypical lesions in image-guided core breast biopsies. Mod Pathol 2003;16(2):154–160.

82. Liberman L, Dershaw DD, Rosen PP, et al. Stereotaxic core biopsy of breast carcinoma: Accuracy at predicting invasion. Radiology 1995;194:379–381.

83. Lee CH, Carter D, Philpotts LE. Ductal carcinoma in situ diagnosed with stereotactic core needle biopsy: Can invasion be predicted? Radiology 2000;217:466–470.

84. Jimenez RE, Bongers S, Bouwman D. Clinicopathologic significance of ductal carcinoma in situ in breast core needle biopsies with invasive cancer. Am J Surg Pathol 2000;24(1):123–128.

85. Youngson BJ, Lieberman L, Rosen PP. Displacement of carcinomatous epithelium in surgical breast specimens following stereotaxic core biopsy. Am J Clin Pathol 1995;103:598–602.

86. Youngson BJ, Cranor M, Rosen PP. Epithelial displacement in surgical breast specimens following needling procedures. Am J Surg Pathol 1994;18:896–903.

87. Rubin E, Dempsey PJ, Pile NS, et al. Needle localization biopsy of the breast: Impact of a selective core needle biopsy program on yield. Radiology 1995;195:627–631.

88. Kaufman CS, Delbecq R, Jacobson L. Excising the reexcision: Stereotactic core-needle biopsy decreases need for reexcision of breast cancer. World J Surg 1998;22:1023–1028.

89. Liberman L, Fahs MC, Dershaw DD, et al. Impact of stereotaxic core breast biopsy on cost of diagnosis. Radiology 1995;195:633–637.

90. Doyle AJ, Murray KA, Nelson EW, et al. Selective use of image-guided large-core needle biopsy of the breast: Accuracy and cost-effectiveness. AJR Am J Roentgenol 1995;165:281–284.

91. Jacobs TW, Connolly JL, Schnitt SJ. Nonmalignant lesions in breast core needle biopsies: To excise or not to excise? Am J Surg Pathol 2002;26(9):1095–1110.

92. Liberman L, Sama M, Susnik B. Lobular carcinoma in situ at percutaneous breast biopsy: Surgical biopsy findings. AJR Am J Roentgenol 1999;173:291–299.

93. Burak WE, Owens KE, Tighe MB, et al. Vacuum-assisted stereotactic breast biopsy: Histologic underestimation of malignant lesions. Arch Surg 2000;135:700–703.

94. Shin SJ, Rosen PP. Excisional biopsy should be performed if lobular carcinoma in situ is seen on needle core biopsy. Arch Pathol Lab Med 2002;126:697–701.

95. Reynolds HE. Core needle biopsy of challenging benign breast conditions: A comprehensive literature review. AJR Am J Roentgenol 2000;174:1245–1250.

96. Liberman L, Bracero N, Vuolo MA. Percutaneous large-core biopsy of papillary breast lesions. AJR Am J Roentgenol 1999;172:331–337.

97. Philpotts LE, Shaheen NA, Jain KS. Uncommon high-risk lesions of the breast diagnosed at stereotactic core-needle biopsy: Clinical importance. Radiology 2000;216:831–837.

98. Mercado CL, Hamele-Bana D, Singer C. Papillary lesions of the breast: Evaluation with stereotactic directional vacuum-assisted biopsy. Radiology 2001;221(3):650.

99. Cawson JN, Malara F, Kavanagh A. Fourteen-gauge needle core biopsy of mammographically evident radial scars. Cancer 2003;97:341–351.

100. Brenner RJ, Bassett LW, Fajardo LL. Stereotactic core-needle breast biopsy: A multi-institutional prospective trial. Radiology 2001;218(3):866.

101. Fraser JL, Raza S, Chorny K, Connolly JL, Schnitt SJ. Columnar alteration with prominent apical snouts and secretions. A spectrum of changes frequently present in breast biopsies performed for microcalcifications. Am J Surg Pathol 1998;22:1521–1527.

102. Rosen PP. Columnar cell hyperplasia is associated with lobular carcinoma in situ and tubular carcinoma [letter to the editor]. Am J Surg Pathol 1999;23:1561.

103. Brogi E. Tan LK. Findings at excision biopsy performed after identification of columnar cell change of ductal epithelium in breast core biopsy [abstract]. Mod Pathol 2002;15:29–30.

104. Frable WJ. Fine needle aspiration biopsy. Hum Pathol 1993;14:9–28.
105. Pennes DR, Naylor B, Rebner M. Fine needle aspiration biopsy of the breast: Influence of the number of passes and the sample size on the diagnostic yield. Acta Cytol 1990;34:673–676.
106. Layfield LJ, Glasgow BJ, Cramer H. Fine-needle aspiration in the management of breast masses. Pathol Annu 1989;24:23–62.
107. De Rosa G, Boschi R, Boscaino A, et al. Intraoperative cytology in breast cancer diagnosis: Comparison between cytologic and frozen section techniques. Diagn Cytopathol 1993;9:623–631.
108. Vazquez MF, Mitnick JS, Pressman PI, et al. Stereotactic aspiration biopsy of nonpalpable nodules of the breast. J Am Coll Surg 1994;178:17–23.
109. de la Torre M, Lindholm K, Lindgren A. Fine needle aspiration cytology of tubular breast carcinoma and radial scar. Acta Cytol 1994;38:884–890.
110. Dawson AE. Pathological interpretation of core biopsy. In Fajardo LL, Willison KM, Pizzutiello RK (eds). A Comprehensive Approach to Stereotactic Breast Biopsy. Cambridge, MA, Blackwell Scientific, 1996, pp 211–223.
111. Rosai J. Borderline epithelial lesions of the breast. Am J Surg Pathol 1991;15:599–603.
112. Schnitt SJ, Connolly JL, Tavassoli FA, et al. Interobserver reproducibility in the diagnosis of ductal proliferative breast lesions using standardized criteria. Am J Surg Pathol 1992;16:1133–1143.
113. Bodian CA, Perzin KH, Lattes R, et al. Reproducibility and validity of pathologic classifications of benign breast disease and implications for clinical applications. Cancer 1993;71:3908–3913.
114. Collins LC, Connolly JL, Page DL. Diagnostic agreement in the evaluation of image-guided breast core needle biopsies. Am J Surg Pathol 2004;28:126–131.
115. Negri S, Bonetti F, Capitanio A, et al. Preoperative diagnostic accuracy of fine-needle aspiration in the management of breast lesions: Comparison of specificity and sensitivity with clinical examination, mammography, echography, and thermography in 249 patients. Diagn Cytopathol 1994;11:4–8.
116. Painter RW, Clark WE, Deckers PJ. Negative findings on fine-needle aspiration biopsy of solid breast masses: Patient management. Am J Surg 1988;155:387–390.
117. Rostein S, Nilsson B, Svane G, et al. Clinical examination, mammographic findings and cytological diagnosis in patients with breast disorders. Acta Oncol 1992;31:393–397.

CHAPTER 18

Advanced Technology and Diagnostic Strategy for Breast Cancer

Elisa Rush Port and Elizabeth A. Morris

MAGNETIC RESONANCE IMAGING

What is the role of magnetic resonance imaging in breast cancer screening?

Breast cancer screening with modalities other than mammography is not condoned by any professional organizations or societies at this time. There are, however, emerging data that screening with magnetic resonance imaging (MRI) may benefit some high-risk patients.[1–6] Most of these studies are composed of small groups of patients; nevertheless, MRI screening has been shown to demonstrate a 2% to 4% detection rate of cancers that are not seen on mammography. Most patients with MRI-detected cancers have small cancers, less than 2 cm, and negative axillary nodes (Fig. 18–1). Use of surrogate end points for survival, such as tumor size and nodal status, demonstrates that early cancers can be detected with MRI. It is uncertain, however, whether the detection of small cancers in a high-risk population will positively affect patient mortality because no randomized study has been performed to date. In general, when MRI screening is performed in high-risk populations, 20% to 30% of patients will require biopsy based on MRI findings, and 15% to 65% of patients who undergo biopsy will be found to have breast cancer.

Patient populations that are considered at high risk in the MRI screening trials have differed as well (Table 18–1). Some trials have performed screening on patients with high suspicion for harboring or proven *BRCA1* and *BRCA2* mutations. Other trials have examined patients with a broader range of risk factors, including those with a history of a previous breast cancer, a previous biopsy demonstrating lobular carcinoma in situ or atypical ductal hyperplasia, or a strong family history. Additional studies have used risk-assessment models, such as the Gail model, to determine high risk and have set entry criteria at varying levels. Despite these variations in patient selection for MRI screening, there is a surprising consistency of the data from multiple sites in different countries with different imaging techniques.

What is not consistent in these trials is the ability of MRI to detect ductal carcinoma in situ (DCIS); this may have to do with imaging protocols, patient populations, and radiologic interpretation. Because DCIS is the earliest form of breast carcinoma, a screening test that detects this process is critical (Fig. 18–2). The detection of invasive carcinomas after cells have had access to the breast lymphatics and blood vessels may be too late to positively affect patient survival. Detection of DCIS on mammography has been shown to decrease mortality from breast cancer. It is assumed that DCIS detection by MRI will have a similar impact on mortality. The histologic grade and type of DCIS detected by MRI do not appear to differ from those for DCIS detected mammographically; therefore, it is entirely possible that the MRI-detected DCIS is just as important as that detected mammographically. In addition, the detection of DCIS is one of the advantages that MRI holds over ultrasound as an adjunct screening modality. Whereas ultrasound does not usually detect mammographic occult DCIS unless it presents as a mass, MRI is able to detect ductal enhancement or "clumped enhancement," and the DCIS lesion does not need to manifest as a mass (Fig. 18–3).

Because of the significant rate of false positivity associated with MRI screening, patient selection should be judicious and individualized. A variety of factors should be incorporated in decision making, including risk assessment, breast density on mammography, patient age and menopausal status, and patient overall health.

The role of MRI screening in patients at increased risk for breast cancer remains to be fully defined, and MRI is typically not used for screening in the general population but may be a useful adjunct to further evaluate abnormalities identified on mammography and sonography.

What are the criteria for diagnosing a suspicious lesion?

MRI of the breast uses intravenous contrast to identify areas of increased blood flow; areas on MRI that are suspicious for malignancy will show increased contrast uptake. Although this increased blood flow is often due to increased angiogenesis, other factors are also probably at play because areas of DCIS that have not incited angiogenesis also display increased

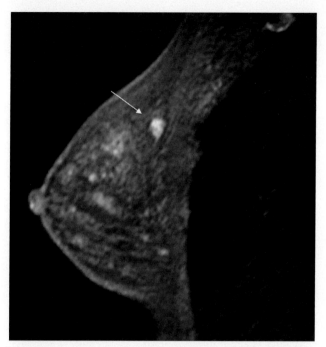

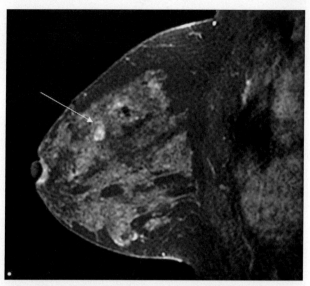

Figure 18–1 This 51-year-old woman underwent right mastectomy 4 years ago for multifocal mixed invasive ductal and lobular carcinoma. Screening MRI was performed of the left breast. Fat-suppressed sagittal three-dimensional fast spoiled gradient-echo pulse sequence image (this and all subsequent images) following contrast administration demonstrates a 5-mm irregular heterogeneously enhancing mass (*arrow*) in the posterior breast. This finding was not seen on mammography or a directed ultrasound examination following MRI. MRI-guided needle localization yielded 5-mm invasive ductal carcinoma with negative sentinel node.

Figure 18–2 A 29-year-old woman with strong family history and prior benign biopsy yielding lobular carcinoma in situ (LCIS). Mammography demonstrated an extremely dense breast with no suspicious findings. Screening MRI examination following contrast injection demonstrates an irregular enhancing mass (*arrow*). Directed ultrasound to this region was negative, and the patient underwent MRI-guided needle localization yielding low-grade cribriform ductal carcinoma in situ (DCIS) and abundant LCIS.

Table 18–1 Summary of Magnetic Resonance Imaging Screening Studies Performed to Date

Studies	Institute	n	Mean Age (yr)	Risk*	No. of Biopsies (%)	PPV (%)	No. of Cancers Detected by MRI Only (%)	No. of DCIS Cases (%)
Kuhl et al. (2000)[1]	U Bonn	192	39	Gene carriers	14 (7%)	9/14 (64)	6/192 (3)	1/6 (17)
Tilanus-Linthorst et al. (2000)[5]	Erasmus MC Rotterdam	109	43	High risk	9 (8%)	3/9 (33)	3/109 (3)	0/3 (0)
Warner et al. (2001)[3]	U Toronto	196	43	High risk	23 (12%)	6/23 (26)	4/196 (2)	0/4 (0)
Stoujesdijk et al. (2001)[4]	Nijmegen	179	NS	High risk	30 (17%)	13/30 (43)	8/170 (4)	2/8 (25)
Lo et al. (2001)[2]	U Penn	157	43	High risk	28 (18%)	5/28 (18)	5/157 (3)	NS
Robson (2003)[42]	MSKCC	54 (129 rounds)	44	Gene carriers	15 (12%)	3/15 (20)	3/129 (2)	NS
Kriege (2003)[43]	Erasmus MC Rotterdam	1869 (3280 rounds)	40	High risk	NS	NS	39/3280 (1)	5/39 (13)
Kuhl (2003)[44]	U Bonn	359 (583 rounds)	39	Gene carriers	63 (11%)	21/63 (34)	21/583 (4)	NS
Morris et al. (2003)[6]	MSKCC	367	50	High risk	64 (17%)	14/59 (24)	14/367 (4)	8/14 (57)
Leach (2002)[45]	UK	1236	<50	High risk	NS	NS	15/1236 (1)	NS
Podo (2002)[46]	Italy	105	46	Gene carriers	8 (8%)	7/8 (88)	7/105 (7)	3/7 (43)

*Risk factor for entrance into the screening study.
DCIS, ductal carcinoma in situ; MSKCC, Memorial Sloan-Kettering Cancer Center; NS, not studied; PPV, positive predictive value.

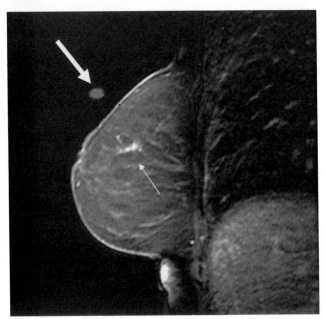

Figure 18–3   A 66-year-old woman with *BRCA1* gene underwent MRI that demonstrated clumped enhancement (*thin arrow*) adjacent to a previous lumpectomy site that is marked with a vitamin E capsule (*thick arrow*). Mammography demonstrated several calcifications that were initially not interpreted as suspicious. Because of the MRI findings, the calcifications were resected under stereotactic guidance, yielding high-grade micropapillary DCIS compatible with recurrent carcinoma. The patient subsequently underwent mastectomy.

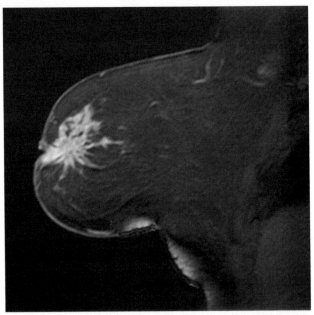

Figure 18–4   A 44-year-old woman with known invasive lobular carcinoma. Note spiculation of mass.

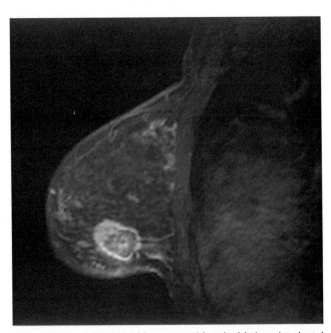

Figure 18–5   A 28-year-old woman with palpable invasive ductal carcinoma demonstrating peripheral rim enhancement, a suspicious sign for malignancy.

contrast uptake.[7–10] In addition, increased uptake alone is not the sole criterion for malignancy because both benign and malignant processes will exhibit increased contrast uptake. Thus, any lesion or condition that results in increased blood flow, such as hormonal stimulation, will generate increased uptake.[11]

An international group of experts in breast MRI has developed a lexicon for interpretation to assist the radiologist in identifying features that may differentiate suspicious-appearing from benign-appearing lesions.[12–14] These guidelines have been published by the American College of Radiology. The lexicon describes both morphologic and kinetic features of lesions. The morphology describes how the lesion "looks," and kinetic analysis evaluates how the contrast is taken up and washed out by the lesion. In general, if the lesion morphology is suspicious, the lesion should undergo biopsy regardless of the kinetic information. The kinetic information is useful if a lesion is not clearly suspicious morphologically. In these cases, the addition of the kinetic information can prompt biopsy rather than close-interval follow-up. Therefore, both the morphology and the kinetics of a particular lesion can be used to facilitate decision making and provide complementary information about a lesion.

Morphologic features that are considered suspicious are spiculated margins (Fig. 18–4) and rim enhancement (Figs. 18–5 and 18–6). Clumped linear enhancement (Fig. 18–7) is suspicious for DCIS, particularly if in a segmental distribution, but can also be seen with benign histology. However, because the descriptor is suspicious, biopsy needs to be performed. Interestingly, kinetic analysis appears not to be reliable in DCIS.

Irregular masses with heterogeneous internal enhancement can also be suspicious and warrant biopsy; however, the positive biopsy rate for these lesions is lower than that for masses without rim enhancement (Figs. 18–8 and 18–9). Well-circumscribed masses with nonenhancing internal septations are considered benign and characteristic of fibroadenoma (Fig. 18–10).

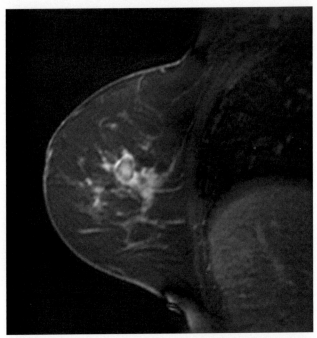

Figure 18–6 A 39-year-old woman with a palpable lump. MRI demonstrated central enhancement, a sign suspicious for malignancy. Pathology yielded invasive ductal carcinoma.

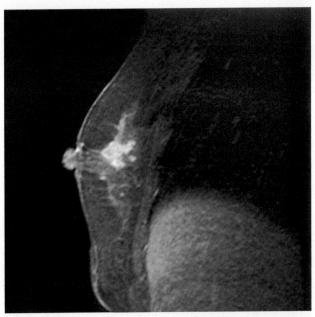

Figure 18–8 A 55-year-old woman with biopsy-proven invasive ductal carcinoma underwent preoperative MRI for extent of disease evaluation. MRI demonstrated an irregular heterogeneously enhancing mass.

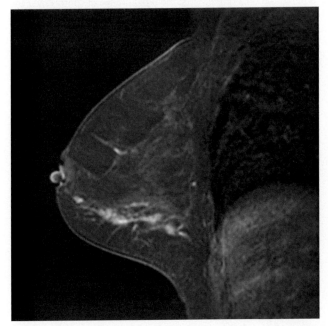

Figure 18–7 A 67-year-old woman treated 2 years ago in the contralateral breast for invasive lobular carcinoma underwent screening breast MRI examination, which demonstrated segmental clumped enhancement along the 6-o'clock axis. Subsequent mammogram and ultrasound were negative. MRI-guided needle localization was performed, yielding high-grade extensive ductal carcinoma in situ, solid and cribriform types.

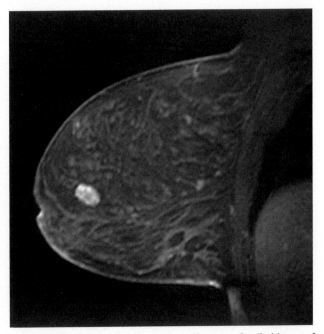

Figure 18–9 A 35-year-old woman with strong family history of breast cancer and a new palpable finding. MRI demonstrated an irregular mass with heterogeneous internal enhancement. Pathology yielded fibroadenoma.

Kinetic features that are suspicious for malignancy are rapid uptake and washout (Fig. 18–11). Because rapid uptake occurs in the first 2 minutes, imaging of the breast should be performed in less than 2 minutes. Washout of the contrast material occurs owing to arteriovenous shunting, which is characteristic of malignant lesions. The problem is that most kinetic MRI features are not highly specific; benign lesions may have some MRI features typically associated with malignancy, and vice versa (Fig. 18–12).

Because overlap exists, it must be expected that there will be false-positive results if biopsies are performed on all lesions

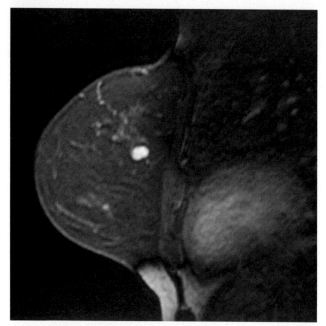

Figure 18–10   A 48-year-old woman with palpable finding. MRI demonstrated a lobulated mass with homogeneous enhancement and nonenhancing internal septations. Subsequent ultrasound demonstrated the mass, and ultrasound core biopsy was performed, yielding fibroadenoma.

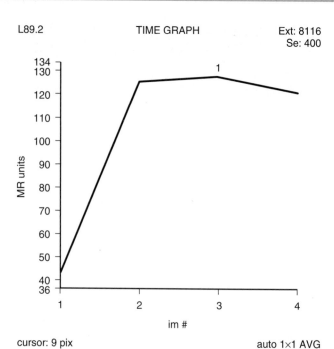

Figure 18–11   A 37-year-old woman with mass suspicious for breast carcinoma underwent MRI evaluation for extent of disease. MRI demonstrated a mass that has washout kinetics. Several images were obtained at time points following contrast injections and plotted on a graph. Note the rapid uptake of contrast and the rapid washout, suspicious for malignancy.

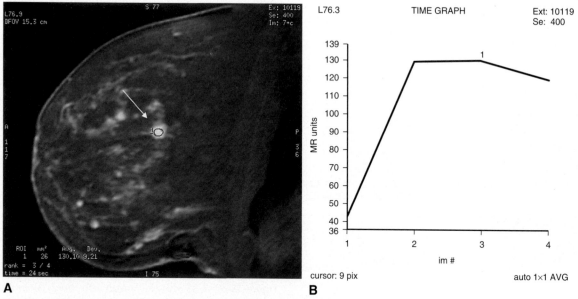

A   B

Figure 18–12   A 42-year-old woman with known right breast carcinoma presented for staging MRI examinations. *A,* In the contralateral left breast, a suspicious enhancing lesion was identified (*arrow*). Region of interest is manually placed over the enhancement. *B,* Curve is generated at three time points following contrast injection. Note the malignant features of the curve. Biopsy was performed that yielded radial scar, concordant with the imaging features. This demonstrates that although morphology and kinetic analysis are important in deciding which lesions are suspicious, there will be false-positive findings.

that demonstrate some suspicious characteristics on MRI. In many reported studies, the positive predictive value (PPV) of MRI biopsy is about 40%. Therefore, most findings prove to be benign. It should be noted that this value of 40% is found in a high-risk population of women—not a general population. Therefore, if MRI were performed on the general population, it would be likely to result in a much lower and unacceptable PPV, one of the many reasons why MRI is not recommended for patients who are not at increased risk for breast cancer.

What is the procedure for biopsy of a suspicious lesion?

If a lesion is identified on MRI and is considered suspicious, a directed ultrasound over the area is often performed. The lesion's location may seem different when viewed with MRI than with ultrasound because MRI is performed with the patient in the prone position and ultrasound with the patient in the supine position. Thus, ultrasound should evaluate the suspected area widely. If ultrasound shows an abnormality corresponding to the MRI finding, ultrasound-guided biopsy can be performed easily. If no ultrasound correlate is found, the patient may need to undergo MRI-guided core biopsy or MRI-guided localization with surgical excision. The position of the lesion in the breast often dictates how biopsy will be performed. Deep, posterior, or subareolar lesions are not optimal candidates for MRI core biopsy, and thus localization with surgical excision is usually necessary.

If an abnormality for which biopsy is recommended is seen only on MRI (and not with ultrasound or mammography), the patient will be required to undergo a second MRI for localization at the time of biopsy. In addition, because currently there is no MRI equivalent of a "specimen radiograph," which is often obtained at the time of needle localization of mammographic findings to verify retrieval of the abnormality in question, a third, "postexcision" MRI may be indicated after surgery to verify that the abnormality has, in fact, been excised. When indicated, this is commonly performed as soon as possible following surgery. From a practical standpoint, the thorough evaluation and ultimate biopsy of an MRI lesion may become quite laborious and stressful, and the patient must fully understand the potential outcomes of having an MRI for breast cancer screening before one is obtained.

What is the role of magnetic resonance imaging in the evaluation of a patient with known breast cancer to evaluate the extent of disease?

MRI has been demonstrated in numerous studies to be the preferred method for detecting disease extent in the breast before surgery.[15–22] MRI can detect additional unsuspected carcinoma in up to 33% of patients. This is particularly true in young patients, patients with dense breasts (Fig. 18–13), and patients with breasts that are difficult to examine. In specific cancer histologies such as invasive lobular carcinoma and invasive ductal carcinomas with an extensive intraductal component, MRI has been shown to provide additional information regarding extent of disease. For example, in one study from our institution, selected patients with newly diagnosed invasive lobular carcinoma, a tumor that is notoriously mammographically occult, underwent MRI screening to determine whether additional unsuspected disease could be detected. The findings demonstrated that 11 of 51 (22%) patients had an additional focus of cancer on the ipsilateral side, and 5 of 53 (9%) had a contralateral cancer not seen on mammography.[23] Interestingly, the MRI data appear to mimic known pathologic data, which have documented that most patients with suspected unifocal disease on clinical examination are found to have residual disease (usually multifocal and less

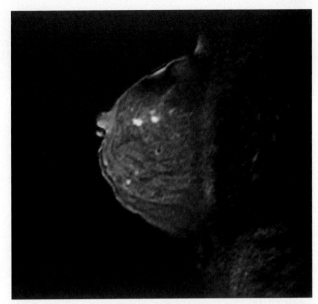

Figure 18–13   A 50-year-old woman with prior history of lobular carcinoma in situ underwent screening bilateral breast MRI. Mammography was negative, demonstrating dense breast tissue. MRI demonstrated two adjacent irregular masses in the superior breast that proved to represent several foci of invasive ductal carcinoma, pure tubular type, ranging in size from 0.2 to 0.7 cm.

likely multicentric). For this and other reasons, postoperative radiation is a mainstay of treatment.[24–26]

Because local failure rates of breast-conservation therapy from the pre-MRI era are much lower than the incidence of detection of additional disease seen on MRI, it is unclear whether the detection and excision of residual disease detected by MRI will actually affect recurrence rates (Fig. 18–14A and B). There may be considerable surgical overtreatment when MRI is used in the staging of breast cancer because these additional areas of carcinoma are now detected and are surgically excised, whereas, previously undetected, they would have been left in the breast and treated with radiation (Fig. 18–15A and B). The use of MRI for determining extent of disease may lead to an increase in the mastectomy rate in some areas of the country because the standard of care is surgical removal of all known or detected disease (Fig. 18–16).

Breast MRI can offer important information in the immediate postoperative period in patients with positive margins following an initial attempt at breast conservation.[27] It is particularly helpful in patients with carcinomas that were difficult to diagnose mammographically or tumors without abundant associated calcifications. The postoperative mammogram is excellent for diagnosing residual calcifications but fares poorly when trying to assess residual mass or residual uncalcified DCIS. In these settings, MRI is able to give information regarding the presence of bulky residual disease at the margin of resection or the presence of additional disease elsewhere in the breast, which may preclude an additional attempt at conservation.

The edges of a postoperative seroma cavity will enhance on MRI because of the presence of granulation tissue that begins to form once the breast parenchyma is cut. The thin rim of enhancement that occurs around the cavity happens

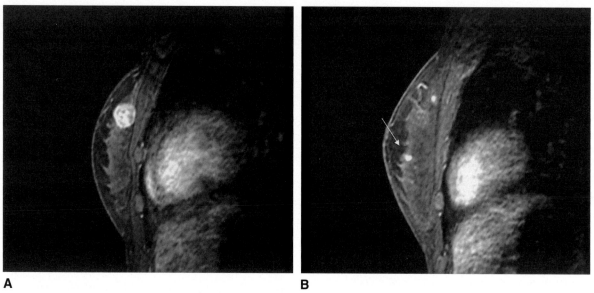

Figure 18–14   A 33-year-old woman presented with a palpable mass. *A,* Staging MRI examination demonstrated a palpable mass that is irregular and heterogeneous enhancement, compatible with invasive ductal carcinoma. *B,* Elsewhere in the breast in a separate quadrant, there was suspicious enhancement that represented a separate focus of invasive ductal carcinoma measuring less than 4 mm (*arrow*). The patient was treated with mastectomy, whereas without the MRI results she would have undergone conservation therapy and postoperative radiation therapy.

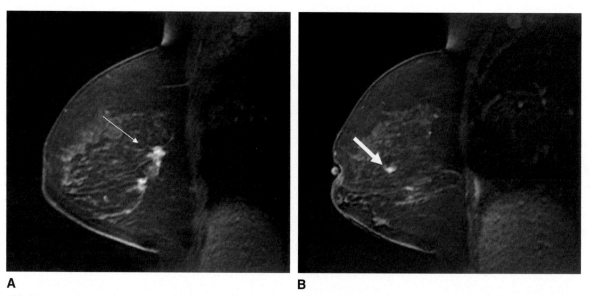

Figure 18–15   A 61-year-old woman with core biopsy–proven right breast invasive lobular cancer. *A,* Mammography demonstrated a spiculated mass in the 10-o'clock axis of the breast confirmed on MRI examination (*thin arrow*). *B,* Elsewhere in the breast on MRI examination in a separate quadrant is a small focus of enhancement (*thick arrow*) that represents multicentric carcinoma. This patient underwent mastectomy, and tumor was located throughout the lower outer quadrant.

uniformly in the postoperative state and is distinguishable from nodular or mass enhancement at the margin of resection, which represents significant and extensive residual disease (Fig. 18–17). The role of MRI, however, is not to assess for microscopic residual disease in those patients known to have positive margins and for whom additional surgery is planned.

What is the accuracy of magnetic resonance imaging?

To understand the sensitivity and specificity of MRI, one must appreciate what he or she is looking at on the MRI. All MRI examinations of the breast parenchyma use intravenous

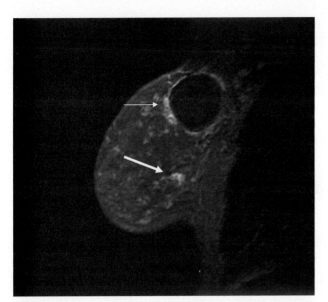

Figure 18–16 A 48-year-old woman with extremely dense breasts underwent excision of calcifications, yielding ductal carcinoma in situ (DCIS) with positive margins. Postexcision mammogram failed to disclose any residual calcifications. MRI was performed 1 week after excision and demonstrated the seroma cavity with thin rim enhancement compatible with postoperative granulation tissue. MRI also demonstrated clumped enhancement surrounding the cavity (*thin arrow*) compatible with residual DCIS. In the lower aspect of the breast, additional clumped enhancement (*thick arrow*) was identified compatible with multicentric DCIS. Following confirmation of this impression, patient received mastectomy.

contrast agent (gadolinium chelate) to assess the inherent vascularity of lesions.[28] Therefore, we can accurately identify invasive carcinomas that have recruited blood vessels and that have greater microvessel density, leaky capillaries, and arteriovenous shunts. For this reason, the sensitivity for invasive carcinomas on MRI is extremely high. Invasive lobular carcinoma, which has a unique growth pattern as well as a less reliable production of vascular endothelial growth factor (VEGF), may rarely be undetectable on MRI. Well-differentiated or slowly growing tumors may not have as robust a vascular supply and therefore may not take up the contrast agent as avidly.

Benign lesions can also have increased vessel density but usually do not have the leaky capillaries or arteriovenous shunting seen with malignant lesions; thus, contrast does not usually "wash out" of benign lesions, as is usually seen in malignancy. Even benign breast parenchyma can enhance, particularly at certain phases of the menstrual cycle, because estrogen has been shown to increase capillary leakiness (Fig. 18–18). Thus, the optimal time for obtaining an MRI in a menstruating woman is during the most quiescent phase of the menstrual cycle, between days 7 and 14 after the last menstrual period (Fig. 18–19).

Enhancement alone is not the only criterion for suspicion; other features of benign and malignant lesions can help discriminate them. A model based on the American College of Radiology Breast Imaging Reporting and Data System (BI-RADS) lexicon is available for MRI. In numerous studies, the positive biopsy rate for MRI is no worse than and is usually even better than the positive biopsy rate for mammography. In general, positive biopsy rates range from 25% to 65%. The accepted positive biopsy rate for mammography is in the range of 25% to 35%.[29–31]

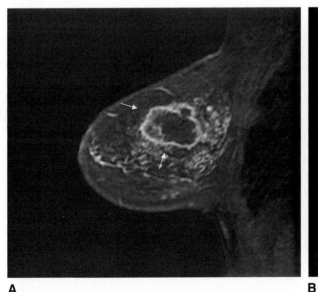
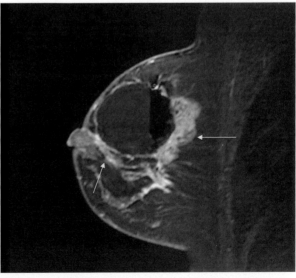

A   B

Figure 18–17 Rim enhancement from recent surgery is typically distinguishable from significant amount of residual disease. *A,* A 50-year-old woman with large palpable breast mass status post surgery with positive margins. MRI demonstrated thin enhancement around the postoperative cavity (*arrows*). *B,* A 42-year-old woman underwent an excisional biopsy yielding invasive lobular carcinoma extending to the margins, and MRI was performed to assess residual disease. A large postoperative seroma cavity with an air-fluid level is seen, compatible with the postoperative state. In addition, residual mass is noted along the posterior margin of the biopsy cavity and extends inferiorly toward the nipple (*arrows*). Mastectomy confirmed the presence of extensive residual invasive lobular carcinoma.

The sensitivity of DCIS detection on MRI has been controversial in the past. When using low-resolution techniques, DCIS detection was low. However, with improvements in the hardware and software used to perform MRI, the resolution has improved over time, and it has become abundantly clear that MRI is able to detect DCIS. The sensitivity of detection is again variable when multiple series are examined. However, it has been demonstrated that with high-resolution techniques, sensitivity can approach 85%. MRI does not replace mammography because some lesions, particularly DCIS, are calcified and are not detected on MRI.[32]

What is the clinical approach to magnetic resonance imaging findings?

Given the multiple and emerging applications of MRI technology, clinical decision making that incorporates MRI findings can be complex (Fig. 18–20).

Patients often indicate that undergoing different screenings for high-risk breast cancer at different intervals (i.e., mammogram every year, staggered with sonography or MRI at alternate 6-month periods) provides an added sense of security and reassurance that they are getting "checked" in some way at least every 6 months. At Memorial Sloan-Kettering Cancer Center, however, our experience has been that different imaging modalities complement each other and that information is most useful when tests are performed synchronously. Thus, if high-risk screening with MRI is performed, we most often recommend that it be done within about 1 month of the yearly mammogram. This way, if a new finding is identified on the MRI, it can be compared with the recent mammogram; the physician would most likely want to obtain a new mammogram if it had been done 6 months earlier.

Findings identified on MRI can vary from minimal and scattered areas of nonspecific enhancement to a highly suspicious mass, and follow-up of MRI findings can thus range from performing a follow-up examination to a recommendation for biopsy. Because MRI contrast enhancement is related to breast tissue blood flow, MRI can vary with the menstrual cycle in premenopausal women. When obtaining a breast MRI, timing the examination with the most quiescent phase of the menstrual cycle, 7 to 14 days after the last period, can reduce the risk for false-positive findings related to hormonal stimulation.

When a suspicious lesion is seen on MRI but a recent mammogram shows no findings, often a targeted sonogram is

Figure 18–18   A 50-year-old woman with strong family history underwent screening MRI examination. Patchy enhancement in the superior breast was noted and thought to represent benign hormonal enhancement, which was confirmed at follow-up MRI examination.

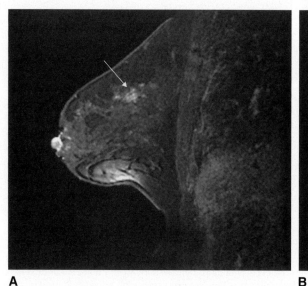

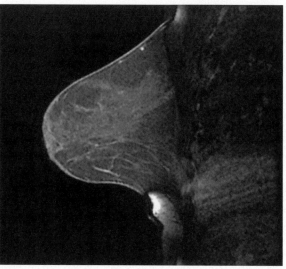

A   **B**

Figure 18–19   A 43-year-old woman with a history of stage II breast cancer underwent screening MRI examination. *A,* Patchy enhancement was noted in the superior breast (*arrow*). *B,* This disappeared on the subsequent follow-up examination, probably owing to hormonal changes.

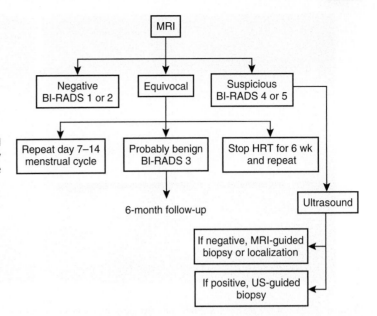

Figure 18–20 Algorithm for clinical decision making based on MRI results. BI-RADS, American College of Radiology Breast Imaging Reporting and Data System; HRT, hormone replacement therapy.

obtained. In our experience, sonography will visualize 24% of abnormalities first identified by screening MRI. If the lesion is visualized by sonography, the patient can undergo the more expeditious procedure of either sonogram-guided core biopsy or surgical excision with ultrasound-guided localization. If the sonogram fails to demonstrate the MRI abnormality, biopsy is typically still pursued and is performed using MRI as a guide. Both MRI-guided core biopsy and MRI localization with surgical excision are feasible options for MRI abnormalities. If multiple abnormalities or one widespread area is identified, often surgical excision with localization is recommended because surgery provides a better opportunity for more extensive sampling.

In our study of MRI screening in 367 women at high risk for developing breast cancer, 59 (15%) underwent biopsy for a suspicious lesion. Of these 59 patients, 50 (85%) had MRI-guided localization, whereas 9 (15%) had sonographically guided biopsies. A total of 14 of the 59 women (24%) who underwent biopsy were found to have cancer. The likelihood of finding cancer when a sonographic correlate was identified (2 of 9 patients; 22%) did not differ significantly from when the lesion was seen only on MRI (12 of 59 patients; 24%).[6]

Performing MRI-guided needle localization requires the patient to undergo another MRI on the day of surgery so that the lesion can be visualized and localized. One or more wires made of titanium, and thus magnetically inert, are inserted by the radiologist into the area or areas in question. A standard mammogram is obtained so that the surgeon can estimate the path and depth of the wire within the breast. Surgical excision is performed in the standard fashion, targeting the area marked by the wire. Because MRI abnormalities are identified by blood flow, once surgical excision is performed and blood flow is severed, the lesion within the removed specimen can no longer be identified. Thus, there is no method for performing a specimen radiograph using MRI. Rather, if a question exists regarding adequate sampling, a postexcision MRI can be performed on the operated breast to verify removal of the area in question.

When MRI is performed for contralateral screening in a patient with a known diagnosis of cancer (Figs. 18–21 and 18–22), identified contralateral abnormalities can undergo biopsy at the time of surgery for the known cancer, using the same localizing techniques. Alternatively, patients can undergo either ultrasound- or MRI-guided core biopsy preoperatively if amenable.

Often, MRI is performed to evaluate the extent of disease or multicentricity in a breast with a known cancer. Importantly, as with other imaging modalities, the decision to perform a mastectomy should not be based on MRI findings alone because false-positive findings are common.

POSITRON EMISSION TOMOGRAPHY

What is the role of positron emission tomography scanning in the detection of breast cancer?

Positron emission tomography (PET) is one of the most promising imaging modalities. In October 2002, the Center for Medicare and Medicaid Services approved expanded coverage for the use of PET scanning in patients with breast cancer; however, appropriate applications relating to breast cancer have yet to be fully defined. PET scanning is most commonly performed using ^{18}F-fluorodeoxyglucose (FDG), a radiolabeled glucose analogue, and is based on the finding that cells with high metabolic rates, such as tumor cells, consume more glucose. Thus, ^{18}F-FDG uptake is more avid than in normal tissue.[33] In addition, FDG is metabolized differently from glucose, getting trapped in cells after it is consumed. Therefore, tumor cells preferentially usurp FDG, which is then trapped within the cell, thereby facilitating imaging of tumor foci with nuclear medicine imaging techniques. The ability of PET scanning to identify primary breast cancer lesions has been extensively studied and documented.[34,35] Although PET scanning can clearly differentiate breast tumors from normal tissue with high levels of specificity, its ability to detect smaller lesions is limited. In one study investigating breast

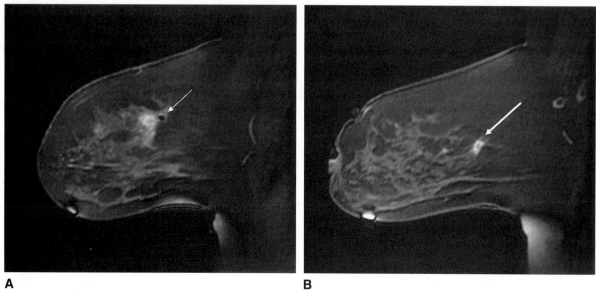

A   **B**

Figure 18–21   A 53-year-old woman with history of lobular carcinoma in situ had new calcifications in the right breast that were excised, yielding ductal carcinoma in situ. MRI was performed for ipsilateral staging and contralateral screening. *A,* Residual clumped enhancement was noted surrounding the clip (seen as signal void) that was placed following right breast stereotactic biopsy for calcifications (*thin arrow*). *B,* Contralateral screening demonstrated a spiculated mass (*thick arrow*) in the left breast that proved to represent an invasive ductal carcinoma, not detected on mammography.

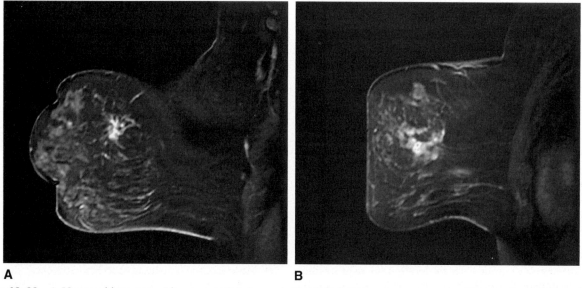

A   **B**

Figure 18–22   A 52-year-old woman with new spiculated mass in the right breast on mammography. Ultrasound-guided core biopsy yielded invasive lobular carcinoma. MRI was performed for ipsilateral staging and contralateral screening. *A,* In the right breast, a unifocal spiculated mass compatible with the known diagnosis of invasive lobular carcinoma was seen. *B,* In the left breast, clumped enhancement in the central breast was proved to represent extensive ductal carcinoma in situ.

imaging with PET, sensitivity for primary tumor detection was 92% for T2 lesions but only 68% for T1 lesions.[36] Given that mammography and MRI can consistently identify lesions that are microscopic, PET scanning pales in terms of its limit of resolution based on size criteria, and thus PET technology, as it exists currently, is not useful as a screening modality for the detection of primary breast cancer lesions. In addition to the possibility of not detecting breast tumors that are small, there is evidence that some histologic types of breast cancer, such as invasive lobular cancers, may be less FDG avid, making them more likely to go undetected by PET scanning.[36,37]

For these reasons, PET scanning is not a standard modality for breast cancer screening.

What is the role of positron emission tomography scanning in the evaluation of a patient with breast cancer?

PET scanning is being investigated as a modality to determine extent of disease in patients with known breast cancer or those suspected of harboring a recurrence. Studies have analyzed

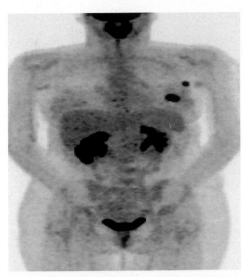

Figure 18–23 Fluorodeoxyglucose positron emission tomography (FDG-PET) scan demonstrating uptake by breast cancer and ipsilateral axillary nodes representing metastatic disease.

the accuracy of PET scanning in demonstrating the presence of lymph node metastases with the goal of obviating removal of negative nodes and the associated morbidity (Fig. 18–23). Although PET scanning has shown high specificity for lymph node metastases, the detection of lymph node metastases with PET seems to be a function of size and amount of tumor burden in lymph nodes, as is seen with primary lesions. Thus, micrometastatic disease in lymph nodes is not detectable by PET imaging. Sentinel lymph node biopsy, in which even isolated tumor cells can be detected pathologically in lymph nodes, is a new standard of care in breast cancer surgery. Because PET scanning currently has no ability to detect such microscopic amounts of disease, the role of PET scanning in staging the axilla is quite limited.[38,39]

PET scanning has been demonstrated to effectively image internal mammary nodal disease in breast cancer as well as other tumor types. PET provides increased specificity over computed tomography (CT) scanning for imaging nodal disease because CT relies only on size estimates to define suspicious nodes, with less than 1 cm being the generally accepted cutoff point for normal size. PET can provide more specific metabolic information that can distinguish benign from malignant adenopathy with a high degree of reliability. However, the assessment of internal mammary nodes is typically not part of standard treatment because previous work has demonstrated that extended radical mastectomy, which incorporates dissection of the internal mammary node chain, does not confer survival benefit over standard modified radical mastectomy. Yet, the detection of metastatic disease in internal mammary nodes could affect adjuvant treatment decisions by resulting in the addition of either chemotherapy or widened radiation fields, particularly if axillary lymph nodes are negative and a patient would not have received adjuvant treatment otherwise. To date, the role of PET scanning to investigate internal mammary node status should be considered exploratory.

There is no standard practice or set of recommendations for evaluating extent of systemic disease in patients with breast cancer. Practice patterns can vary widely, with physicians having different thresholds for obtaining different imaging studies. The yield of discovering foci of metastatic disease is quite low in patients with small primary tumors and clinically negative nodes who are asymptomatic (<1%). However, the yield will be higher in any patient with new symptoms possibly related to the development of metastatic disease, palpable adenopathy, or larger tumors (20% to 30%). In such patients, imaging tests, including PET scanning, may be helpful in determining whether identifiable metastatic disease is present. Definitive findings of metastatic spread could substantially affect the decision to perform surgery and other factors related to patient management.

Because the most likely sites of development of systemic disease include bone, brain, lung, and liver, an extent of disease evaluation may include a CT scan of the chest, abdomen, and pelvis and a bone scan. PET scanning has been shown to be useful in identifying abnormalities in bone as well as viscera and may be complementary to standard imaging modalities.[40] PET may also be more useful in specific clinical scenarios such as when recurrence is suspected. Scar tissue and radiation changes can be difficult to image, and the information that PET scanning provides regarding the presence of hypermetabolic foci may raise or lower the suspicion for the presence of disease. As with other imaging modalities, it should be noted that a variety of different scenarios can lead to either false-positive or false-negative results on PET. The presence of infection or autoimmune disease can cause increased FDG uptake and thus lead to false-positive results. Conversely, PET can miss small foci of disease and cannot be relied on to consistently pick up areas with minimal disease. Thus, as with all imaging modalities, definitive treatment decisions should not be based on PET scan results alone.

What are novel tracers?

The use of fluorodeoxyglucose in detecting tumor is based on the premise that glucose uptake by neoplastic lesions is greater than in surrounding normal tissue. Although the detection of tumor deposits makes PET useful for many reasons, the metabolic property that makes tumors glucose avid is nonspecific relative to tumor type. As a result, much current work is being devoted to identifying novel tracers that are receptor specific and thus have applications for specific tumor types. The development of such technology holds promise for detection, assessment of response to systemic therapy, and even treatment because a radiolabeled ligand that is tumor specific could be developed not only to identify and visualize tumor but also to destroy it.

Some studies have demonstrated the ability of radiolabeled estrogen molecules to image estrogen receptor–positive tumors, and serial scanning after tamoxifen treatment may be useful in assessing response to treatment.[41] At this time the use of tumor-specific ligands in combination with PET scanning is investigational only, but it holds promise for future applications.

What is fusion imaging?

Fusion imaging technology is based on the concept that combining and superimposing two different imaging modalities with different strengths provides better information. Currently, PET/CT is performed at our institution. Although PET provides important biologic and metabolic information, often lesions seen on PET cannot be localized to the specific organ or site of involvement. Superimposing CT images allows foci of uptake on PET to be localized to the site of interest. Currently a biopsy cannot be performed based on PET images alone, but a suspicious site seen on PET and localized with CT can then undergo percutaneous needle biopsy.

Other types of fusion imaging, combining MRI with PET, for example, hold promise for potential future applications but are not used as part of the current standard of care.

REFERENCES

1. Kuhl CK, Schmutzler RK, Leutner CC, et al. Breast MR imaging screening in 192 women proved or suspected to be carriers of a breast cancer susceptibility gene: Preliminary results. Radiology 2000;215:267–279.
2. Lo LD, Rosen MA, Schnall MD, et al. Pilot study of breast MR screening of a high-risk cohort. Radiology 2001;221(P):432.
3. Warner E, Plewes DB, Shumak RS, et al. Comparison of breast magnetic resonance imaging, mammography, and ultrasound for surveillance of women at high risk for hereditary breast cancer. J Clin Oncol 2001;19:3524–3531.
4. Stoutjesdijk MJ, Boetes C, Jager GJ, et al. Magnetic resonance imaging and mammography in women with a hereditary risk of breast cancer. J Natl Cancer Inst 2001;93:1095–1102.
5. Tilanus-Linthorst MMA, Obdeijn IMM, Bartels KCM, et al. First experiences in screening women at high risk for breast cancer with MR imaging. Breast Cancer Res Treat 2000;63:53–60.
6. Morris EA, Liberman L, Ballon DJ, et al. MRI of occult breast carcinoma in a high-risk population. AJR Am J Roentgenol 2003;181: 619–626.
7. Ikeda DM, Birdwell RL, Daniel BL. Potential role of magnetic resonance imaging and other modalities in ductal carcinoma in situ detection. Semin Breast Dis 2000;3(1):50–60.
8. Orel SG, Mendonca MH, Reynolds C, et al. MR imaging of ductal carcinoma in situ. Radiology 1997;202:413–420.
9. Westerhof JP, Fischer U, Moritz JD, Oestmann JW. MR imaging of mammographically detected clustered calcifications: Is there any value? Radiology 1998;207:675–681.
10. Soderstrom CE, Harms SE, Copit DS, et al. Three-dimensional RODEO breast MR imaging of lesions containing ductal carcinoma in situ. Radiology 1996;201:427–432.
11. Müller-Schimpfle M, Ohmenhäuser K, Stoll P, et al. Menstrual cycle and age: Influence on parenchymal contrast medium enhancement in MR Imaging of the breast. Radiology 1997;203:145–149.
12. Ikeda DM, Baker DR, Daniel BL. Magnetic resonance imaging of breast cancer: Clinical indications and breast MRI reporting system. J Magn Reson Imaging 2000;12(6):975–983.
13. Morris EA. Illustrated breast MR lexicon. Semin Roentgenol 2001;36: 238–249.
14. American College of Radiology. Breast Imaging Reporting and Data System (BI-RADS), 3rd ed. Reston, VA, American College of Radiology, 1998.
15. Boetes C, Mus R, Holland R, et al. Breast tumors: Comparative accuracy of MR imaging relative to mammography and US for demonstration of extent. Radiology 1995;197:743–747.
16. Esserman L, Hylton N, Yassa L, et al. Utility of magnetic resonance imaging in the management of breast cancer: Evidence for improved preoperative staging. J Clin Oncol 1999;17:110–119.
17. Fischer U, Kopka L, Grabbe E. Breast carcinoma: Effect of preoperative contrast-enhanced MR Imaging on the therapeutic approach. Radiology 1999;213:881–888.
18. Harms SE, Flamig DP, Hesley KL, et al. MR imaging of the breast with rotating delivery of excitation off resonance: Clinical experience with pathologic correlation. Radiology 1993;187:493–501.
19. Heywang SH, Wolf A, Pruss E, et al. MR imaging of the breast with Gd-DTPA: Use and limitations. Radiology 1989;171:95–103.
20. Orel SG, Schnall MD, LiVolsi VA, Troupin RH. Suspicious breast lesions: MR imaging with radiologic-pathologic correlation. Radiology 1994;190:485–493.
21. Orel SG, Schnall MD, Powell CM, et al. Staging of suspected breast cancer: Effect of MR imaging and MR-guided biopsy. Radiology 1995;196:115–122.
22. Reiber A, Merkle E, Böhm W, et al. MRI of histologically confirmed mammary carcinoma: Clinical relevance of diagnostic procedures for detection of multifocal or contralateral secondary carcinoma. J Comput Assist Tomogr 1997;21:773–779.
23. Quan ML, Sclafani L, Heerdt AD, et al. Magnetic resonance imaging detects unsuspected disease in patients with invasive lobular cancer. Ann Surg Oncol 2003;10;1048–1053.
24. Veronesi U, Saccozzi R, Del Vecchio M, et al. Comparing radical mastectomy with quadrantectomy, axillary dissection, and radiation therapy in patients with small cancers of the breast. N Engl J Med 1981;305:6.
25. Winchester D, Cox J. Standards for breast conservation treatment. CA Cancer J Clin 1992;42:134.
26. Schmidt-Ullrich R, Wazer DE, Tercilla O, et al. Tumor margin assessment as a guide to optimal conservation surgery and irradiation in early stage breast carcinoma. Int J Radiat Oncol Biol Phys 1989;17:733–738.
27. Soderstrom CE, Harms SE, Farrell RS, et al. Detection with MR imaging of residual tumor in the breast soon after surgery. AJR Am J Roentgenol 1997;168:485–488.
28. Kaiser WA, Zeitler E. MR imaging of the breast: Fast imaging sequences with and without Gd-DTPA. Radiology 1989;170:681–686.
29. Liberman L, Morris EA, Lee MJ, et al. Breast lesions detected on MR imaging: Features and positive predictive value. AJR Am J Roentgenol 2002;179:171–178.
30. Liberman L, Morris EA, Dershaw DD, et al. Fast MRI-guided vacuum-assisted breast biopsy: Initial experience. AJR Am J Roentgenol 2003;181:1283–1293.
31. Morris EA, Liberman L, Dershaw DD, et al. Preoperative MR imaging-guided needle localization of breast lesions. AJR Am J Roentgenol 2002;178:1211–1220.
32. Boetes C, Strijk SP, Holland R, et al. False-negative MR imaging of malignant breast tumors. Eur Radiol 1997;7:1231–1234.
33. Warburg O. The metabolism of tumors. New York, Richard R. Smith, 1931, pp 129–169.
34. Avril N, Bense S, Ziegler SI, et al. Breast imaging with fluorine-18–FDG PET: Quantitative image analysis. J Nucl Med 1997; 38:1186–1191.
35. Nieweg OE, Kim EE, Wong WH, et al. Positron emission tomography with fluorine-18–deoxyglucose in the detection and staging of breast cancer. Cancer 1993;71:3920–3925.
36. Avril N, Rose CA, Schelling M, et al. Breast imaging with positron emission tomography and fluorine-18 fluorodeoxyglucose: Use and limitations. J Clin Oncol 2000;18(20):3495–3502.
37. Buck A, Schirrmeister H, Kuhn T, et al. FDG uptake in breast cancer: Correlation with biological and clinical prognostic parameters. Eur J Nucl Med Mol Imaging 2002;29(10):1317–1323.
38. Smith IC, Ogston KN, Whitford P, et al. Staging of the axilla in breast cancer: Accurate in vivo assessment using positron emission tomography with 2-(fluorine-18)-fluoro-2-deoxy-D-glucose. Ann Surg 1998;228(2):220–227.
39. Wahl RL, Siegel BA, Coleman RE, Gatsonis CG, for the PET Study Group. Prospective multicenter study of axillary nodal staging by positron emission tomography in breast cancer: A report of the staging breast cancer with PET Study Group. J Clin Oncol 2004;22(2):277–285.
40. Wahl RL, Cody RL, Hutchins GD, Mudgett EE. Primary and metastatic breast carcinoma: Initial clinical evaluation with PET with the radiolabeled glucose analogue 2-[F-18]-fluoro-2-deoxy-D-glucose. Radiology 1991;179:765–770.
41. Mortimer JE, Dehdashti F, Siegel BA, et al. Positron emission tomography with 2-[18F]Fluoro-2-deoxy-D-glucose and 16alpha-[18F]fluoro-17beta-estradiol in breast cancer: Correlation with estrogen receptor status and response to systemic therapy. Clin Cancer Res 1996;2:933–939.

42. Robson ME, Offit K. Breast MRI for women with hereditary cancer risk. JAMA 2004:292:1317–1325.
43. Kriege M, Brekelmans CT, Boetes C, et al. Magnetic Resonance Imaging Screening Study Group. N Engl J Med 2004;351:427–437.
44. Kuhl CK: Screening of women with hereditary risk of breast cancer. Clin Breast Cancer 2004;5:269–271.
45. Leach MO, Eeles RA, Turnbull LW, et al. The UK national study of magnetic resonance imaging as a method of screening for breast cancer (MARIBS). J Exp Clin Cancer Res 2002;21(3 Suppl):107–114.
46. Podo F, Sardanelli F, Canese R, et al. The Italian multi-centre project on evaluation of MRI and other imaging modalities in early detection of breast cancer in subjects at high genetic risk. J Exp Clin Cancer Res 2002;21(3 Suppl):115–124.

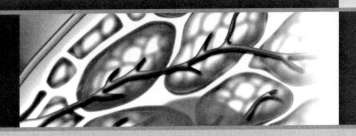

SECTION IV

STAGING AND PROGNOSIS

The number as well as the location of lymph nodes is critical to accurate staging. A high number of involved lymph nodes is a strong negative prognostic factor.[21] Patients with 1 to 3 positive axillary lymph nodes are classified as pN1a, patients with 4 to 9 positive axillary nodes are considered pN2a, and patients with 10 or more positive axillary nodes are considered pN3a. Metastasis to the infraclavicular lymph nodes is a significant adverse prognostic feature; thus, these nodes are also considered N3a.[22]

How are the internal mammary lymph nodes classified?

There is a synergistic effect on survival between the internal mammary (IM) and axillary lymph nodes, with disease to both nodal basins portending a poor prognosis. Additionally, the size of the metastatic deposit within the node is associated with survival.[23] IM nodes are classified based on how they were detected—SLN biopsy versus clinical exam or imaging—as well as on the number of positive axillary nodes. In a patient without axillary disease, IM lesions found with IHC are considered pN1b, whereas those detected clinically or radiographically are considered pN2b. In a patient with one to three involved axillary lymph nodes, IM lesions found with IHC are considered pN1c, whereas those detected clinically or radiographically are pN3b. Finally, all IM lesions associated with four or more involved axillary lymph nodes are considered pN3b.

How are the supraclavicular lymph nodes classified?

Historically, a dismal prognosis has been associated with disease in the supraclavicular lymph nodes (SCLNs). This has resulted in the M1 classification for these involved nodes in the past. However, recent data suggest that women with locally advanced breast cancer (LABC) and positive ipsilateral SCLN, but no other metastatic disease, have survival rates comparable to those seen in LABC patients without metastatic disease, and considerably better than those with stage IV disease who have metastases at distant sites.[24] Therefore, SCLN metastases have been reclassified as N3c or pN3c and are now placed in stage IIIC.

What are the five stages created with the TNM groupings?

Stage 0, defined as TisN0M0, affords a 10-year survival rate of 95%. Stage I is T1N0M0 and has an approximately 88% 5-year survival rate. Stage IIA is T0N1M0, T1N1M0, or T2N0M0 and has an overall survival rate of 81% at 10 years. Stage IIB can consist of T2N1M0 or T3N0M0 and has an overall survival rate of 70% at 10 years. Stage IIIA contains many permutations, including T0N2M0, T1N2M0, T2N2M0, T3N1M0, and T3N2M0, averaging a 59% 10-year overall survival rate. Stage IIIB encompasses all T4 tumors with N1 or N2 status that have not yet metastasized and demonstrates a 36% 10-year overall survival rate. Stage IIIC is any T stage combined with N3 status and also gives about a 36% 10-year overall survival

Table 19–3 Stage Groupings for Patients with Breast Cancer According to the TNM Classification

Stage 0	Tis	N0	M0
Stage I	T1	N0	M0
Stage IIA	T0	N1	M0
	T1	N1	M0
	T2	N0	M0
Stage IIB	T2	N1	M0
	T3	N0	M0
Stage IIIA	T0	N2	M0
	T1	N2	M0
	T2	N2	M0
	T3	N1	M0
	T3	N2	M0
Stage IIIB	T4	N0	M0
	T4	N1	M0
	T4	N2	M0
Stage IIIC	Any T	N3	M0
Stage IV	Any T	Any N	M1

From Greene FL, Page DL, Fleming ID, et al. AJCC Cancer Staging Manual, 6th ed. New York, Springer-Verlag, 2002.

rate. Evidence of distant metastases indicates stage IV and has an approximately 18% 10-year overall survival rate.[7,25] Table 19–3 lists the stages as determined by the TNM groupings.

Why is histologic grade not a factor in staging?

Even though the morphologic appearance of breast cancer and its degree of malignancy are likely to be related, histologic grading remains very subjective, and developing a uniform system to incorporate into staging has not been possible. Unfortunately, the available studies that link histologic grade to outcome in early breast cancers are both difficult to assess and variable in results. At this time, sufficient data are lacking to include this factor in a uniform staging system.[4]

Although histologic grade is not factored into the staging, all invasive breast carcinomas should be graded. The Nottingham combined histologic grade (Elston and Ellis modification of the Bloom-Richardson grading system) is the most commonly used.[26] Histologic grade is determined by assessing the tumor's morphologic features, including tubule formation, nuclear pleomorphism, and mitotic count. Each factor is then rated between favorable (1 point) and unfavorable (3 points). The scores for all three categories are added. Grade 1 is a combined score of three to five, grade 2 is a score of six or seven, and grade 3 is a score of eight or nine.[7]

Do all patients need to undergo a complete workup for distant disease?

The prevalence of detectable metastases at initial diagnosis is very low in the early stages of breast cancer. Nevertheless, their presence does significantly alter the course of treatment. Thus, it is important to distinguish patients with early distant disease. Unfortunately, widespread use of the entire gamut of

marrow include immunocytoc
cytometry.[38]

Numerous studies have eva
of BMM. A correlation has bee
breast cancer stage and a higl
tected.[39] BMM has also been sl
and grade of the primary tumo
42%, 62%, and 75% of T1, T2,
tively.[40] In grade I and II cance
of the patients had BMM, wh
52% had BMM.[40] There does
tionship between BMM and axi
BMM and axillary lymph node
sent independent routes of canc

Multiple studies have ider
between the presence of BMM
as decreased survival. In the fi
correlation, Cote and colleagu
distant recurrence rate for bor
was 3%, compared with 33% i
absolute number of malignant
also been shown to predict ear
survival.[37] In a study by Diel ar
with primary operable breast cai
developed distant recurrence ha
83% of those who died of their
of initial diagnosis.[40] Braun ar
women with stage I through III I
the presence of BMM was an inc
from breast cancer.[39]

From the data available, it is e
a breast cancer patient's bone ma
knowledge about the axillary I
research is necessary, however, tc
marrow status on outcome.

Are hormone receptors si even though they are not in the staging system?

Since the mid-1970s, estrogen rece
receptor (PR) status have been u
ment of breast cancer. They have
endocrine responsiveness and a
recurrence. Even though the horn
useful, their absolute prognostic p
fore they are not included in the s

ER positivity is known to be a f
tor, whereas PR positivity alone is i
indicator. Overall, about 58% of bi
positive. The next most frequently
ER positive, PR negative, which a
cancers. The least common group
accounts for only 4% of all canc
cancers show no hormone recepto
negative.[42]

ER-positive breast tumors hav
patients longer disease-free as well
of 1392 patients with early breast
determine whether hormone rece
independent prognostic informatic

Table 19–4 Sensitivity, Specificity, and Positive Predictive Value of Radiologic Staging Tests in Evaluating Asymptomatic Patients with Breast Cancer

	Sensitivity	Specificity	Positive Predictive Value
Chest radiograph	0.31	0.996	0.44
Bone radiograph	0.35	0.986	0.32
Bone scan	0.48	0.995	0.15
Liver ultrasound	0.29	0.995	0.33

From Ciatto S, Pacini P, Azzini V, et al. Preoperative staging of primary breast cancer: A multicentric study. Cancer 1988;61(5):1040.

staging tests is inaccurate, expensive, time-consuming, and anxiety provoking. Ideally, the subset of patients most likely to develop distant disease needs to be identified, allowing exhaustive workups to be performed appropriately. Patients with stage III disease merit a comprehensive workup.

The three most common sites of breast cancer metastasis are the bone, lung, and liver, in that order. A large study encompassing more than 3600 women with breast cancer who underwent preoperative metastatic workup with chest radiography, bone radiography or scintigraphy, and liver echography or scintigraphy revealed an abysmally low detection rate. It was concluded that this pattern of testing should not be recommended for asymptomatic women because of poor sensitivity and an extremely low detection rate of distant disease, as shown in Table 19–4.[27]

Who should be evaluated for bone metastases, and how should it be done?

Bone is the most frequent site of distant breast cancer spread, with about 25% of metastatic disease presenting at this site. Up to 70% of women who die from breast cancer will eventually have disease in the bony skeleton. The bones most commonly affected, in declining order, are the spine, ribs, pelvis, skull, and long bones of the extremities. Evaluation should commence with a history and physical examination aimed at eliciting osseous involvement. The patient should be questioned about bone pain, history of fractures, and possible symptoms of spinal cord compression such as lower extremity weakness with bowel or bladder dysfunction. If there is any suspicion of bony involvement, a workup may include measurement of serum alkaline phosphatase and serum calcium levels, technetium bone scan, computed tomography (CT), MRI, positron emission tomography (PET), or biopsy as appropriate.

The aforementioned multicenter review of more than 3600 patients demonstrated that preoperative evaluation of the skeleton, in the absence of symptoms, is not warranted because of low sensitivity and specificity. In this group, of 2450 stages I and II patients, only 22 (<1%) had a true-positive bone scan, whereas 125 had false-positive results. Further, there were no positive scans in patients without symptoms and with normal levels of alkaline phosphatase.[27] This supports the practice of performing radiologic or nuclear medicine studies only on patients with specific complaints or elevation of serum alkaline phosphatase.

More recently, PET scanning has been used to evaluate the entire body for metastatic tumor deposits. A study comparing whole-body PET scanning with traditional bone scintigraphy was performed on 51 women with breast cancer. With a specificity of 98%, PET scanning was superior to bone scintigraphy, which displayed only 81% specificity.[28] Additionally, compared with bone scintigraphy, MRI had a higher rate of skeletal metastases detection for the spine, pelvis, limb bones, sternum, scapula, and clavicle but a lower rate in the ribs and skull.[29]

Who should be evaluated for lung metastases, and how should it be done?

Up to 25% of patients with metastatic disease develop pulmonary metastases, with only a small percentage of these present at the initial breast cancer diagnosis. About two thirds of women who eventually die from breast cancer have evidence of disease in the lung. The initial evaluation for all breast cancer patients should begin with a history and physical examination directed at signs of pulmonary involvement, including fatigue, dyspnea, dry cough, and chest pain or a feeling of heaviness in the chest, even though most patients are asymptomatic. If there is suggestion of pulmonary involvement, the lungs may then be further studied with chest radiograph, CT, fluorodeoxyglucose (FDG)-PET scan, or bronchoscopy.

In a study of 3627 breast cancer patients undergoing preoperative staging by chest radiography, the detection rate of preclinical lung metastases was found to be 0.3%, with a sensitivity of 0.31 and positive predictive value of 0.44.[27] Clearly, the routine use of preoperative chest radiography for the detection of pulmonary involvement is neither clinically useful nor cost-effective because the false-positive results would necessitate further unnecessary testing. However, because of the age bracket of the women undergoing surgery for breast cancer, a preoperative chest radiograph is often required at many institutions. If there is an abnormal finding on the chest radiograph, a CT scan may help to delineate nodules as well as detect mediastinal disease. The presence of calcium in lung nodules indicates benign pathology.

To assess the utility of chest radiography in the long-term management of patients with breast cancer, 1161 chest radiographs of 141 patients were examined. Of the chest radiographs, 15% were clinically indicated, and the remaining 85% were undertaken as part of "routine" follow-up. Fewer than 0.4% of the routine chest radiographs demonstrated previously undiagnosed pulmonary disease. Thus, the use of routine chest radiography is not a viable method of monitoring asymptomatic breast cancer patients.[30] Finally, when FDG-PET was retrospectively compared with chest radiography for detection of metastatic disease, FDG-PET was found to be superior in the identification of pulmonary and lymph node metastases.[31]

Who should be evaluated for liver metastases, and how should it be done?

The liver is the third most common site of distant breast cancer metastases. Two thirds of patients with stage IV disease

will eventually sustain hepatic
ation for all breast cancer pati
and physical examination dire
right upper quadrant pain or f
hepatomegaly. It is exceedingl
early breast cancer to present
disease, such as portal hyperter
suggestion of hepatic involven:
with liver function tests and, p

Liver function testing in
enzymes alkaline phosphatase
ferase (AST), alanine aminot
dehydrogenase (LDH). The pe
patients with breast cancer at tl
very low yield. A study of 227 s
patients identified elevated live
33, only one enzyme was ele
Overall, the specificity of liver
detect hepatic metastases at the
sis. Including liver enzymes wi:
metastatic disease inevitably le:
and extensive evaluation, which
dict who will develop distant d
tion of most that only patient
liver enzymes or hepatomegaly
ographic evaluation of the liver.

Options for radiographic ev:
liver scan, CT, ultrasound, MRI,
scans cannot detect lesions sma
fore not very sensitive. A study :
revealed that screening liver ul
very low rates for detecting pre
tases, with positive predictive va
tively.[27] A study using a smaller s:
that preoperative ultrasound ma
of patients with markedly abno:
physical examination suggestive
not as a general screening tool.[28]
Kettering Cancer Center of 76 :
indeterminate liver lesions were
sound was a useful adjunct for
habitus in order to characteri
lesions.[33] CT and MRI are super
netium scanning for the identific:
in the liver; however, neither is
asymptomatic patients.[34] Finally,
spectively compared with chest 1
phy, and ultrasonography of the
metastatic disease, it was found t:
cation of pulmonary and lymph :
son with chest radiography, but it
of bone and liver metastases was
scintigraphy and liver ultrasonog:

In summary, because the perce
involvement at initial breast cance
screening tests are very nonspecifi
form routine screening in asympt
with right upper quadrant pain :
loss, or hepatomegaly, liver functi
ing studies are indicated.

Once hepatic involvement is p:
is between 1 and 14 months. F:

knowledge of genotype–phenotype correlations, including
penetrance estimates; cost; and the inconsistent willingness of
third-party payers, including Medicaid and Medicare, to pay
for the testing. A patient's decision to undergo genetic testing
is sometimes complicated by fear of the potential misuse of
genetic information by insurers.

What are the genes predisposing to breast and ovarian cancer?

Mutations in *BRCA1* and *BRCA2* are known to be major
causes of hereditary predisposition to breast cancer. The
BRCA1 gene was mapped in 1990 to 17q12 and cloned in
1994.[10,11] The *BRCA2* gene was mapped to chromosome
13q12-13 in 1994 and cloned in 1995.[12,13] Among the high-risk
families selected for mapping studies and subsequently used
for mutation analysis, these genes were thought to account for
about 90% of all hereditary breast cancer. *BRCA1* accounted
for 40% to 50% of hereditary breast cancer, and *BRCA2* for
about 35% to 45%. More recent studies have shown that
these contributions may have been overestimated.[14–20] The
distribution and frequency of mutations vary in diverse ethnic
populations.

Several hundred mutations distributed throughout
both genes have been identified. Readily available sources
of information about mutations include the Breast Cancer
Information Consortium (*http://research.nhgri.nih.gov/bic/*)
and Myriad Genetics (*http://www.myriad.com*). Mutations are
interpreted as deleterious if they prematurely terminate or
truncate the protein product of *BRCA1* at least 10 amino
acids from the C-terminal or the protein product of *BRCA2*
at least 110 amino acids from the C-terminal.[21] Specific
missense and noncoding intron mutations are interpreted as
deleterious on the basis of linkage analysis of high-risk
families, functional analysis, biochemical analysis, or demonstration of abnormal RNA processing. Genetic variants that
do not fulfill these criteria are reported as being of unknown
significance.

An inherited predisposition to the development of breast
cancer is also associated with germline mutations in *p53*
and may be seen in families with Li-Fraumeni syndrome,
characterized by an aggregation of soft tissue tumors and
hematologic tumors.[22,23] Likewise, breast (and thyroid) cancers are features of Cowden disease, an aggregation of hamar-
tomatous tumors that arise from mutations in the *PTEN*
gene.[24] Heterozygotes for the mutant allele causing ataxia-
telangiectasia, a recessively inherited syndrome predisposing
to cancer, have an increased risk for breast cancer, but these
genes contribute only marginally to the total number of
cases.[25,26] More recently, the variant 1100delC in CHEK2, a cell
cycle–checkpoint kinase, has been identified as a risk factor
for breast cancer.[27] In rare cases of male breast cancer, mutations in the androgen receptor gene may be contributory.[28] An
interesting recent finding is that biallelic mutations in *BRCA2*
contribute to the Fanconi anemia phenotype. As expected,
affected individuals have a familial aggregation of breast cancer.[29] All of these genes contribute only marginally to the total
number of cases with a hereditary predisposition; thus, an
unknown number of other predisposition genes have yet to be
identified.

What is the pattern of inheritance by which mutations in *BRCA1* and *BRCA2* are transmitted?

BRCA1 and *BRCA2* are transmitted as autosomal dominant
traits. Any carrier, female or male, has a 50% chance of transmitting the mutation to her or his offspring. The phenotype
of the carrier is gender dependent and variable, and penetrance for both breast and ovarian tumors is less than 100%.

What is the penetrance of predisposition genes?

Having a dominantly inherited breast cancer predisposition
gene is not sufficient to cause the development of breast cancer. Data obtained from the original families recruited for
the mapping studies demonstrated that the penetrance of
breast and ovarian cancer among mutation carriers of *BRCA1*
and *BRCA2* was high. These families were specifically selected
because they were large and had multiple affected family
members; thus, there was considerable bias of ascertainment.
Penetrance of breast cancer in *BRCA1* carriers in these high-
risk families was 51% by age 50 years and 85% by age 80
years.[6] The penetrance of ovarian cancer in these same families was lower, 23% by age 50 years and 63% by age 70 years.
Comparable risks applied to the occurrence of a second tumor
in the same individual. Penetrance estimates for breast cancer
among *BRCA2* carriers was equally high (87%), but the penetrance of ovarian cancer was considerably lower, about 6% to
10%. The penetrance of breast cancer in male carriers of
BRCA2 mutations was as high as 14%.[30]

Further studies in these high-risk families have confirmed
the high penetrance estimates and have also demonstrated
that the median age of onset of breast cancer in carriers of
BRCA2 mutations is higher than that in *BRCA1* carriers.[18]
BRCA2 is believed to confer about a 6% risk for breast cancer
to male carriers, and male carriers of *BRCA1* mutations are
also believed to be at increased risk for developing both
prostate cancer and breast cancer, but the exact risks have not
yet been determined.[31] Prostate cancer, pancreatic cancer, and
melanoma show increased frequency in carriers of *BRCA2*
mutations.[31] The frequency of other malignancies remains to
be defined. Recent studies have failed to identify an increased
frequency of colon cancer among carriers of mutations in
either of these genes.[32]

From the outset, investigators cautioned clinicians about
applying the penetrance values obtained from the high-risk
families to all carriers. Studies that were based on recall of
family history have demonstrated that penetrance of breast
and ovarian cancer among carriers may be significantly lower
in some families. However, a recent study based on genetic
analysis of the relatives of mutation carriers demonstrated
that the age-related penetrance by age 80 years was 82% for
breast cancer and 54% for ovarian cancer for *BRCA1* mutation carriers and 85% for breast cancer and 23% for ovarian
cancer for *BRCA2* mutation carriers.[33] A major determinant of
penetrance was birth year, with mutation carriers born after
1940 being at significantly higher risk for developing breast
cancer than mutation carriers born before 1940. This study
also showed that low prevalence within a family did not equal

low penetrance. Rather, the low-prevalence families could be explained on the basis of small family size or transmission through the paternal germline. This study was carried out exclusively among Ashkenazi Jews harboring one of the three founder mutations (discussed later), and it is unclear whether these penetrance values apply to other populations and mutations.

Have the same mutations been observed more than once?

Both *BRCA1* and *BRCA2* are large genes, and multiple mutations have been demonstrated in each gene, many of which occur in single affected families. Some mutations have been seen repeatedly, particularly among certain ethnic groups, indicating a historical progenitor or "founder." For example, among individuals of Ashkenazi Jewish origin, there are three recurrent common mutations: 185delAG and 5382insC in *BRCA1*, and 6174delT in *BRCA2*.[34,35] The 5382insC is common in other Eastern European groups, and the 185delAG mutation has been observed in Iraqi Jews, suggesting ancient origin.[36] The *BRCA1* 185delAG mutation has also been observed in groups that may have had historical Jewish links.[37] These three mutations account for more than 95% of all detectable mutations among Ashkenazi Jews. The frequency of nonfounder mutations detected among Ashkenazi families with a heritable predisposition is low, 2% to 4%.[38]

The prevalence of founder mutations is high in the unaffected Ashkenazi Jewish population. Among control populations, the frequency of 185delAG was about 1%, the frequency of 5382insC was 0.11%, and that of 6174delT was 1.36%.[15,34,39,40] Thus, 2.4% of all Ashkenazi Jews are carriers for at least one of these mutations, a rate at least eightfold greater than that in other populations. The cases that arise from the inherited mutations are thought to account for the excess of breast cancer among Ashkenazi Jewish women.[41] The founder mutations in this population group have provided the basis for many prevalence and penetrance studies.

There are multiple other populations in which founder mutations occur. In Iceland, a single *BRCA2* mutation, 999del5, accounts for all heritable cancer in the country.[42] The same mutation occurs in Finland. Founder mutations have been identified in other countries, regions, or ethnic groups, including those from Russia, Belarus, Poland, Norway, Sweden, Finland, the Netherlands, Belgium, France, Germany, England, Scotland, Wales, Northern Ireland, Spain, Italy, Sardinia, Hungary, Czech Republic, Slovenia, Greece, Turkey, Pakistan, India, Thailand, China, Mongolia, Japan, and the Philippines as well as African Americans and French Canadians (*http://research.nhgri.nih.gov/bic/*). Awareness of these founder mutations may facilitate testing because targeted mutation analysis may provide a more efficient approach to testing for a given individual with a known ethnic origin.

Is there a correlation between genotype and phenotype?

The clinical presentation depends on whether the patient is a *BRCA1* or *BRCA2* carrier. The frequency of mutations is inversely related to the age of onset, with a lower than expected contribution of *BRCA2* mutations in early-onset breast cancer.[14] The median age of onset of breast cancer among *BRCA1* carriers is 41 years, whereas that of *BRCA2* carriers is 45 years.[34] Mutations in *BRCA1* appear to be the major etiologic factor in breast-ovarian and site-specific ovarian cancer families.[17,43] Likewise, families in which there is an individual with both breast and ovarian cancer are far more likely to harbor mutations in *BRCA1*.[16] Mutations in *BRCA2* contribute to an increased risk for breast cancer in men and may account for almost 15% of the total cases of male breast cancers.[30] Some studies have suggested that there is a correlation between the presence of specific mutations and the risk for developing ovarian cancer. Some investigators have demonstrated that individuals carrying mutations in the first two thirds of the gene have a higher frequency of ovarian cancer than those carrying mutations in the terminal one third.[44,45] They have also reported that the occurrence of ovarian cancer is increased in *BRCA2* carriers in whom the mutation is found in exon 11.[46] Others have found no correlation.[16]

Who is at increased risk for developing breast cancer?

Women who present for breast cancer risk assessment may generally be divided into two groups, those at moderate risk and those at high risk.[47] Women at moderate risk have fewer affected family members, absence of a family history of ovarian cancer, and an older age at the time of diagnosis. The molecular basis of disease among such women may *not* be the result of inheritance of a single dominant susceptibility gene.

In contrast, women at high risk usually have multiple cases of breast cancer in close relatives or early age at diagnosis. The age of onset of disease tends to be one to two decades earlier than in the general population (frequently, ≤45 years of age). The affected relatives are often closely related, with one or more affected first-degree relatives, especially in succeeding generations, some with more than one primary tumor (i.e., bilateral breast cancer or breast and ovarian cancer). One or more affected individuals may have developed cancer before the age of 50 years, and some have a very early age of onset (<40 years of age). The earlier the age of onset, the more likely it is that a mutation will be identified. There may be one or more affected men in the family. The presence of a woman with ovarian cancer in a family of women with breast cancer or a woman with both breast and ovarian cancer significantly increases the risk for a familial predisposition mutation. The presence of any second primary tumor also supports the suspicion of an inherited predisposition mutation.[48] Any woman younger than 40 years, even in the absence of a family history, particularly if she comes from a high-risk group, should be considered to have a significant probability of being a mutation carrier. For women at moderate risk for developing breast cancer, the likelihood of developing disease has been determined empirically, based on observations from large numbers of individuals.

What are the statistical models used by genetic counselors and oncologists to estimate the probability that an individual will develop cancer?

Models of developing breast cancer used most frequently by risk assessment counselors on behalf of unaffected women are the Gail model and the Claus model (Table 20–1). These models of risk prediction were developed before genetic testing was available but are still useful for women who have not undergone genetic testing. Each of the models was based on a different study design and uses different factors for calculating risks. Hence, the estimates that are provided by each of these models may differ.

Gail Model

The Gail model is still used for unaffected individuals with a limited family history. Gail and colleagues based their model on data in the Breast Cancer Detection and Demonstration Project (BCDDP) of 2852 cases and 3146 matched controls.[49] Five variables were used to calculate risk ratios. These included current age, age at first live birth, age at menarche, number of first-degree relatives with breast cancer, and number of prior biopsies. The Gail model predicts cumulative risks from age 20 to 80 years and corrects for other causes of mortality. This model does not take into consideration the age at diagnosis of the relative's breast cancer, nor does it consider the occurrence of breast cancer in second-degree relatives, thereby overlooking the contribution of genetic mutations from the maternal grandparental generation as well from paternal relatives. Both tables and a computer program are available for estimating individual age-specific risks, based on this model.

Claus Model

The second model commonly used for unaffected women was derived by Claus and colleagues from data collected in the Cancer and Steroid Hormone (CASH) study on 4370 breast cancer cases in patients aged 20 though 54 years and 4688 controls.[5] This study provides age-related risks for breast cancer dependent on the presence of one or two affected first- or second-degree relatives together with their age at onset. These data were compiled to create lifetime risk tables based on family history of breast cancer (see Table 20–1).

Neither the Gail model nor the Claus model takes into consideration the carrier status of the proband or her affected relatives, the presence of affected men, or the occurrence of either bilateral breast cancer or ovarian cancer in family members. The lifetime estimate derived from these models for the proband remains the same, regardless of whether the proband or her relatives have been tested.

What are the statistical models used by genetic counselors and oncologists to estimate the probability that an individual will be a carrier?

BRCAPRO Model

Models have also been developed to estimate the likelihood that a woman carries a mutation in BRCA1 or BRCA2 (Table 20–2). BRCAPRO is a bayesian-based model that takes into account the prevalence of mutations in the population and the penetrance estimates that allows genetic counselors and oncologists to predict the likelihood that a given individual is a carrier of a BRCA1 or BRCA2 mutation[50] (see Table 20–2). It takes into account the affected or unaffected state of the proband,

Table 20–1 Parameters Included in Models for Estimating Risks of Developing Breast Cancer

Parameter	Gail	Claus	Tyrer-Cuzick
Personal Information			
Age	Yes	Yes	Yes
Body mass index	No	No	Yes
Hormonal factors	Yes	No	Yes
Age at menarche	Yes	No	Yes
Age at first live-born child	Yes	No	Yes
Age at menopause	No	No	Yes
Personal Breast Disease			
Breast biopsies	Yes	No	Yes
Atypical hyperplasia	Yes	No	Yes
Lobular carcinoma in situ	No	No	Yes
Ductal carcinoma in situ	No	No	Unknown
Family History			
First-degree relative with cancer	Yes	Yes	Yes
Second-degree relative with cancer	No	Yes	Yes
Age of onset in relatives	No	Yes	Yes
Age of onset in proband	N/A	N/A	Unknown
Bilateral breast cancer	No	No	Yes
Ovarian cancer	No	No	Yes
Male breast cancer	No	No	Yes
Genetic Testing			
Proband or relative had genetic testing	No	No	Unknown

Table 20–2 Parameters Included in Models for Estimating Risks for Carrying a BRCA1 or BRCA2 Mutation

Parameter	BRCAPRO	Frank[21]
Personal Information		
Age	Yes	Yes
Body mass index	No	No
Hormonal factors	No	No
Age at menarche	No	No
Age at first live-born child	No	No
Age at menopause	No	No
Personal Breast Disease		
Breast biopsies	No	No
Atypical hyperplasia	No	No
Lobular carcinoma in situ	No	No
Ductal carcinoma in situ	No	Yes
Family History		
First-degree relative with cancer	Yes	Yes
Second-degree relative with cancer	Yes	Yes
Age of onset in relatives	Yes	Yes
Age of onset in proband	Yes	Yes
Bilateral breast cancer	Yes	No
Ovarian cancer	Yes	Yes
Male breast cancer	Yes	No
Genetic Testing		
Proband or relative had genetic testing	Yes	No

whether she has unilateral or bilateral disease, and the presence or absence of breast and ovarian cancer and certain other cancers in all of her first- and second-degree relatives. Third-degree relatives are not included in this estimate, nor are men affected with breast cancer. The program provided by the developers of this model includes estimates from the Claus and the Gail models and from four other models. BRCAPRO is widely used by risk assessment counselors and, when compared with the estimates of experienced genetic counselors, was found to be slightly more sensitive in identifying carriers than were the counselors. Of note, 16% of carriers were not identified by this model when the cutoff for testing was set arbitrarily at 10% risk for harboring a mutation.

Many counselors use empirical data from Myriad Genetic Laboratories that reported their experience in identifying mutations in *BRCA1* or *BRCA2* in individuals submitting samples to their laboratory.[21] The patients were classified by their affected or unaffected status and by the presence of early-onset breast cancer or ovarian cancer in first- and second-degree relatives. The researchers divided their population of patients into 2233 Ashkenazi Jewish individuals and 4716 non-Ashkenazi Jewish individuals, because of the well-recognized greater frequency of founder mutations among Ashkenazi Jews. They took into consideration the type of tumor (breast, ovarian, or both), the age of onset, and the number of affected first- and second-degree relatives. These data did not recognize the presence of an affected male in the pedigree or the presence of bilateral breast cancer in either the proband or her relatives. In none of these models (Gail, Claus, or BRCAPRO) are third-degree relatives included. Estimates derived from these data may underestimate the a priori risk to be a carrier because male breast cancer was not included as a risk factor and all affected relatives older than 50 years were omitted from this model. In addition, the family history was derived from laboratory requisition forms and not confirmed independently. Some of these deficiencies have been addressed on Myriad's web-based compilation of data, but a drawback of the web-based data and the original study data is that the carrier status of affected relatives is not included in the calculations. Because some probands included in the web-based data came from families in which there was a known mutation, the estimates may be biased upward.

An important point of consideration is that all of these studies consider "affected" individuals to be only those with an invasive lesion. A limited study of probands affected by DCIS compared risk estimates for a small number of Ashkenazi women younger than 50 years with DCIS and those with invasive lesions. Further studies are required to elucidate these risks more fully. Another model includes women with DCIS but routinely adds 10 years to the age at diagnosis; for example, a woman diagnosed with DCIS at 45 years of age would be included as an affected subject diagnosed at 55 years of age.[51] This model has been weighted to include the possibility that DCIS may not always progress to an invasive lesion.

Tyrer-Cuzick Model

Lastly, a newer model, not presently available in a computerized version, includes many additional personal characteristics, including the presence of LCIS, height, weight, and body mass index (BMI).[52]

For clinical counseling, it is useful to calculate risks derived from several models and to offer these to patients as a range.

The experience and judgment of the genetic counselor are invaluable in applying the risk assessment models in the most appropriate way and in helping patients to understand their risks. The American Society of Clinical Oncology guidelines for genetic testing emphasize the importance of the clinical judgment in estimating these risks.[53]

Who should have genetic counseling for heritable risk for breast or ovarian cancer, and how is it undertaken?

Genetic counseling is appropriate for individuals who perceive themselves or their relatives to be at increased risk for breast or ovarian cancer (see Table 20–1). Generally, such perception is based on family history, although some individuals with early-onset or multiorgan disease perceive that *they and their family members* are also at risk for other malignancies. A genetic evaluation is a multistep procedure that may result in modifying risk. Because it is intended to be a service for each person who participates and because the implications of a positive test result can have profound ramifications for that person and the family, participation is always voluntary.

A detailed protocol that is used for counseling patients in the Human Genetics Program at New York University School of Medicine is presented in the appendix at the end of this chapter. An initial telephone contact by the genetic counselor will provide the patient with details about the overall consultation, and the counselor will obtain a preliminary family history. Some centers request that patients complete a written family history form before making an appointment. The counselor may suggest that more than one individual be involved in the counseling process, particularly if a relative is better suited to be tested initially. Arrangements are made to obtain relevant medical records and pathology reports. The patient will learn about the basic elements of the consultation, including the educational aspects of the genetic counseling session, the number of sessions to expect, and the way in which results will be communicated (almost always in person). Of considerable importance is communicating to the patient the nondirective stance of the counselor so that the patient is free, without coercion, to make a considered decision about whether to undergo genetic testing.

The first session lasts about 2 hours, during which the counselor obtains a detailed medical history and at least a three-generation family history with special attention to the history of cancer in the relatives. In addition, general medical and genetics histories are obtained to learn about other conditions about which the patient may be concerned. Based on this information, the genetic counselor or medical geneticist will identify the gene or genes most likely to account for the malignancies in the family or individual.

The educational aspects of the discussion include in-depth information about the testing protocol. This includes a discussion about the contribution of *BRCA1* and *BRCA2* (or other genes, if appropriate) to a hereditary predisposition to breast cancer, the genetics of cancer, an approximate estimate of the likelihood that the patient is a carrier, the likelihood of detecting a mutation, the frequency of variants of uncertain significance, the implications of both positive and negative results, the recommendations for surveillance and cancer prevention following testing, and the benefits and drawbacks of testing.[54] If the patient is part of a family group being tested, an opportunity is provided for each person to meet individually with the counselor or physician during this time.

The major reasons that individuals choose to be tested are (1) the results may modify medical care; (2) the results of testing may benefit relatives, especially daughters; and (3) just "to know." In conjunction with the first reason, there is considerable discussion about the options for medical care, which include (a) doing nothing differently because the patient is already following appropriate surveillance recommendations; (b) initiating more intensified surveillance, surgical intervention, or chemoprevention with referrals to appropriate specialists or a high-risk prevention clinic; or (c) reverting to surveillance appropriate for the general population because the patient has learned that she is not at high risk. With respect to the second reason, it is common that women seeking testing have not discussed the testing with their relatives, especially their daughters, with the intention of telling them the results after the testing has been completed. We routinely recommend that a woman inform her relatives of her intention to have genetic testing before undergoing the testing to learn whether those relatives want to learn the results. We encourage them to consider the rights of their relatives to make the same independent and autonomous decisions as they themselves have made.

At the conclusion of the first session, the patient has the choice of having blood drawn for testing, declining testing permanently, or deferring the decision about testing until a later time. Some patients defer testing until we can ascertain whether their testing will be covered by third-party payers. Others defer so that they can discuss the implications of testing with other family members and learn whether their family members want to have the information. Some defer because they determine that the information will not be useful to them personally. Still others feel so emotionally overburdened at the end of the session that they prefer to have their testing at a later time when they feel more comfortable.

Wherever possible, we make an effort to obtain pathology reports that document the malignancies in the patient and family members. This is particularly important with respect to gynecologic cancers. In a woman who has had endometrial or cervical cancer and not ovarian cancer, there is a significantly lower probability that she or a member of her family is a *BRCA1* or *BRCA2* carrier, compared with a woman who has had ovarian cancer. In addition, a woman who has had an in situ lesion has a lower probability of harboring a deleterious mutation.[21] If testing has been carried out in one or more family members, we request those results because they may allow us to interpret our patient's results with greater certainty or to estimate her risks to be a carrier with greater accuracy. When there is a question about the diagnosis, we may obtain slides for review by an in-house pathologist.

At the time that blood is drawn for testing, an appointment is made for the patient to return to learn the results in person. The results may be provided solely to the patient or in the presence of a relative or friend designated by the patient. If more than one member of a family is receiving results at the same session, we determine in advance whether they wish to receive their results separately or together. We have provided some anticipatory guidance about potential difficulties that may arise when one turns out to be a carrier and the other a noncarrier and in some instances have recommended

that they may wish to receive their results at individualized sessions.

An essential component of genetic counseling is a concern about the psychosocial issues surrounding illness, especially heritable disease. For the patient diagnosed with cancer or coming from a cancer-prone family, there may be a significant affective component. It is quite common that an individual coming for genetic counseling and testing has other stress-inducing events in her life that become even more burdensome in the context of dealing with cancer and its hereditary nature. She may be quite depressed or anxious.

Providing the patient with emotional support is a vital aspect of genetic counseling. One important element of this process is encouraging the patient to "tell her story," that is, to describe her experiences leading up to and following her diagnosis, to describe her support system and her response to her treatment, to provide her own evaluation of her emotional status, and to evaluate the impact of her disease on other family members such as her children, partner, and parents. There are many patients for whom recalling their experiences within a family with multiple affected members may be quite depressing and anxiety provoking. Many patients have not had an opportunity to discuss their experiences with a professional, and they express their appreciation at being given the opportunity to do so. Although it is ultimately beneficial to a patient to engage in this recollection, it can be emotionally exhausting, and the patient may not feel prepared to go ahead with the testing at that time. She may prefer to return to have her blood drawn.

The counselor or physician needs to be prepared not only for anger or depression among those who learn about an increased risk but also for paradoxical or perhaps unexpected responses. Patients who are told of positive results may express a sense of relief because the uncertainty with which they have lived has now been resolved. Patients who are told of negative results may experience a sense of "survivor's guilt," especially if other family members are told of positive results. Patients may be quite depressed and require a referral to a psychotherapist for psychotherapy or short-term use of antidepressants. Acute depressive reactions have been observed only rarely under such circumstances, although the physician or counselor should have made prior arrangements to obtain emergency psychiatric consultation, should this be required.

The indications and timing of surveillance by self-examination, physician examination, diagnostic imaging including digitized mammography, breast and pelvic sonography, magnetic resonance imaging (MRI), and tumor markers are reviewed. Use of risk-reducing surgery is an important subject for discussion, as is the potential role for chemoprevention.

How is genetic testing for *BRCA1* and *BRCA2* carried out?

Mutations in *BRCA1* and *BRCA2* can be detected with molecular techniques that use polymerase chain reaction, including direct DNA sequencing and single-stranded conformational polymorphism analysis together with targeted sequencing. Other methods are under development. For the individual being tested, only a small blood sample is required. Ideally, an individual in the family who is most likely to be a carrier should be tested first; that is, the youngest affected individual or an individual with multiple tumors. If a mutation is identified in this affected person, other family members wanting to know their carrier status may be tested. Any unaffected relative who does not have the family mutation is counseled that her chance of developing breast or ovarian cancer is no different from that of anyone else in the population. There may be exceptions to this in a given family, but this would be subject to a complete family and individual assessment.

If an affected individual from a high-risk family tests negative in the initial mutation analysis, it may be prudent to test another affected member because the first individual may constitute a sporadic case within a hereditary breast family. The estimate of risk for that first individual should be based on an assessment of the probability that breast cancer is heritable in the individual or family, together with an assessment of the sensitivity and specificity of the test.

What are the recommendations to people who are at high risk for developing breast cancer?

Although the complete implications of inheriting a mutation in either *BRCA1* or *BRCA2* are uncertain, it is still possible to provide some risk assessment to carriers. This should be individualized, taking into account the personal medical history of the patient, the family constellation of cancer, the ethnic origin, and the specific mutation. The care provider should investigate the latest studies and extrapolate from them information that is most relevant. He or she should provide a range of risks derived from multiple studies with an explanation of the limitations of these results with respect to the given individual. Patients should be educated about surveillance and about the possibility of reducing risk for disease by up to 95% by prophylactic mastectomy and oophorectomy.[55–57] These recommendations are applicable to patients who remain at high risk, even in the absence of a detectable mutation. In addition, risk assessment or testing and recommendations for screening may be applicable to other family members and should be offered.

Affected women with *BRCA1* mutations should be advised of their increased risk for a second primary tumor, either breast or ovarian, and referred for appropriate monitoring, as outlined below. Unaffected women who are carriers of the mutation should understand the range of risks to which they are subject, as discussed previously in the section on penetrance. Men carrying a *BRCA1* mutation should be monitored for prostate cancer and breast cancer, although it has not been demonstrated that there is an early age of onset.

Affected and unaffected women carrying the *BRCA2* mutation should be advised similarly as for *BRCA1* carriers, with the caveat that the probability of ovarian cancer, although higher than for the general population, is lower than for *BRCA1* carriers. Men who are carriers should also be examined regularly by their internists for signs of breast cancer. The benefit of mammography in men at high risk is unknown. Men and women should be screened for signs of melanoma and monitored for symptoms of pancreatic cancer (i.e., unexplained abdominal pain). Currently, there are no recommended screening tests for pancreatic cancer outside of an investigational protocol. In addition, men who are carriers should be monitored for signs of prostate cancer.

Breast Cancer

The major recommendations for increased surveillance for prevention of breast cancer are breast self-examination and mammography.[58] Monthly breast self-examination should begin in early adult life. The young woman should familiarize herself with the characteristics of normal breast tissue and should be instructed to palpate for lumps and to observe for unusual discharges or skin retraction. This should be supplemented by semiannual or annual clinical examination beginning at age 25 to 35 years. Up to 10% of breast cancers can be detected by clinical examination alone.[59]

Mammography, ultrasonography, and MRI are useful for identifying early cancers that may not be palpable by physical examination. For women who are at moderate or high risk, annual mammography is recommended beginning at age 25 to 35 years.[60] Whenever possible, the mammograms and sonograms should be performed at the same institution and with prior films and images available for comparison. Studies on the risks and benefits of mammography have been based on women with average risk; hence, the risks and benefits of mammography before age 50 years have not been established.[60] Although not proven, the estimated 20-fold increase in risk for developing breast cancer for *BRCA1* and *BRCA2* mutation carriers suggests that mammography and ultrasonography screening may be of benefit.

Two major concerns with early use of mammography have been expressed.[62,63] First, early and frequent exposure to radiation may, in fact, increase the risk for breast cancer, as discussed in Chapter 15. Second, mammography is less useful for identifying small masses in younger women, whose breasts are more dense than those of older women. Furthermore, clinical trials have provided preliminary reports of cases of breast cancer in women with increased genetic risk that were identified by MRI, but not by ultrasonography or mammography.[64,65] For carriers of mutations in these genes, because the risk for other malignancies is also increased, surveillance for carriers should include monitoring for ovarian and prostate cancer.

Ovarian Cancer

Two major screening methods are available for detection of early-stage ovarian cancer in *BRCA1* mutation carriers: vaginal ultrasound and measurement of the serum marker CA-125. Vaginal ultrasound can detect masses as small as 2 mm in diameter, that is, at a stage at which they may not be palpated during physical examination.[66,67] Two analytic methods have been applied to improve the discrimination between malignant and benign lesions: (1) application of a morphology index based on ovarian volume, cyst wall thickness, and septal structure; and (2) use of color-flow Doppler, which can reliably distinguish the lower impedance to blood flow of ovarian neoplasms.[68,69]

CA-125 is a glycoprotein that is shed into the blood by malignant cells, most commonly of ovarian epithelial origin.[70] After a baseline is established, elevation on a subsequent measurement may be indicative of the development of an ovarian cancer.[71] Unfortunately, both false-positive and false-negative results occur with a measurable frequency, suggesting that CA-125 is not a stand-alone technique to screen for early-stage ovarian cancer. In addition, clinical trials assessing a variety of techniques for early diagnosis of ovarian cancer are underway.

Risk-Reducing Surgery

Some individuals who are at increased genetic risk may choose to have risk-reducing surgery for prevention of breast and ovarian cancer. Bilateral salpingo-oophorectomy reduces the risk for ovarian cancer by 95% and for breast cancer by about 50%.[56] Bilateral prophylactic mastectomy reduces the risk for breast cancer by about 90%.[55,57] Residual breast or ovarian tissue following these operations provides the remaining risk.[72,73] For maximal reduction of risk, women might choose prophylactic oophorectomy and mastectomy. However, the single procedure that maximally reduces risk is prophylactic salpingo-oophorectomy.

Prostate Cancer

Screening for prostate cancer is endorsed by some professional groups but not by others.[74] The American Urological Association recommends that prostate-specific antigen (PSA) screening and digital rectal examination start at age 50 years in the general population and at age 40 years for men in high-risk groups (men with a positive family history and African American men).[75] The American Cancer Society similarly recommends that screening start at age 50 years for men in the general population, at 45 years for African American men and for men with one affected first-degree relative, and at 40 years for men at higher risk.[76] However, the American College of Physicians and the American College of Preventative Medicine recommend against the use of routine screening.[77,78] Those who are proponents of screening argue that since the widespread use of PSA testing there has been a migration to lower stages of disease at diagnosis, which would ultimately lead to an overall reduced cause-specific mortality rate.

What other social and psychological issues should be addressed with the patient?

Many individuals who are at high risk for hereditary cancer choose not to have such testing. Some may cite a desire "not to know," whereas others express concerns about potential misuse by third parties, including insurers and employers.[79] Given the sensitive nature of this information, there are several steps that the health care provider can take. First, he or she can provide the patient with a promise of confidentiality in compliance with federal and state regulations. These statutes include maintenance of the patient's record in a locked cabinet or within an electronic medical record that is not accessible to others. The patient's clinical information and test results can be disclosed to others only with the patient's written consent. The inpatient hospital record can be written so that only information necessary to the patient's care is provided. For example, it may be irrelevant to note that a patient is a *BRCA1* mutation carrier if she is being admitted for a routine pregnancy delivery. Obviously, the guarantee of confidentiality is waived by the patient when she signs a request directing her information to a third party.

Second, the provider can advise patients that several forms of legal protection exist on both the federal and state levels.[80] The major federal laws are the Health Insurance Portability and Accountability Act (HIPAA) of 1996 and the Americans with Disabilities Act (ADA) of 1990. HIPAA provides patients with the right to access their personal health information and to direct who else may have access. The Act also specifies the physical, procedural, and technologic security protections that health care providers must make to ensure the confidentiality of patients' medical information. The ADA provides a broad definition of disabilities, so that being perceived as having a disability is the same as actually having such a condition. This confers certain protections to employees or prospective employees with disabilities. For health care, the guiding principle is that employers cannot treat their disabled employees differently from other employees. Any requirements for pre-employment testing must be extended to all. Likewise, any limitations on health care benefits must be extended to all. In recent years, certain states have enacted protective legislation that limits the use of genetic testing by insurers and employers.[80] Nonetheless, individuals may still be coerced into having genetic testing.

Third, providers can anticipate adverse psychological interactions of family members. Although individuals may report no change of psychological state or may report resolution of anxiety, even when they learn about an adverse outcome, a few individuals may experience an acute depression. Learning of a favorable test outcome may trigger an adverse psychological response, including survivor's guilt, depression, or a manic attack. Before undertaking genetic testing, it is advisable to review how the patient may handle the results and to arrange for psychiatric support should an adverse psychological outcome occur.

The identification of genetic risks for development of breast and ovarian cancer has the potential to be a public health benefit by leading the identification of those at risk before the development of disease. Judiciously applied preventive strategies could have a major impact for those at highest risk. Significant changes are likely to occur with testing strategies and prediction of risks. Development in these areas is likely to occur during the next several years, and it may be necessary for health care providers to consult sources beyond this chapter.

REFERENCES

1. American Cancer Society. Cancer Facts and Figures: 2004. Atlanta, American Cancer Society, 2004.
2. Jemal A, Murray T, Ward E, et al. Cancer statistics, 2005. CA Cancer J Clin 2005;55:10–30.
3. Mettlin C, Croghan I, Nachimuthu N, Lane W. The association of age and familial risk in a case-control study of breast cancer. Am J Epidemiol 1990;131:973–983.
4. Broca P. Traites des tumeurs. Journal 1886;1:80.
5. Claus EB, Risch N, Thompson WD. Autosomal dominant inheritance of early-onset breast cancer. Cancer 1994;73:643–651.
6. Easton D, Ford D, Bishop DT, Consortium BCL. Breast and ovarian cancer incidence in BRCA1 mutation carriers. Am J Hum Genet 1995;56:265–271.
7. Antoniou AC, Gayther SA, Stratton JF, et al. Risk models for familial ovarian and breast cancer. Genet Epidemiol 2000;18:173–190.
8. Newman B, Austin MA, Lee M, King M-C. Inheritance of human breast cancer: Evidence for autosomal dominant transmission in high-risk families. Proc Natl Acad Sci U S A 1988;85:3044–3048.
9. Colditz GA, Rosner B. Cumulative risk of breast cancer to age 70 years according to risk factor status: Data from the Nurses' Health Study. Am J Epidemiol 2000;152:950–964.
10. Hall JM, Lee MK, Newman B, et al. Linkage of early onset breast cancer to chromosome 17q12. Science 1990;250:1684–1689.

11. Miki Y, Swensen J, Shattuck-Eidens D, et al. A strong candidate for the breast and ovarian cancer susceptibility gene, BRCA1. Science 1994;266:66–71.

12. Wooster R, Neuhausen SL, Mangion J, et al. Localization of a breast cancer susceptibility gene, BRCA2, to chromosome 13q12–13. Science 1994;265:2088–2090.

13. Wooster R, Bignell G, Lancaster J, et al. Identification of the breast cancer susceptibility gene BRCA2. Nature 1995;378:789–792.

14. Krainer M, Silva-Arrieta S, FitzGerald M, et al. Differential contributions of BRCA1 and BRCA2 to early onset breast cancer. N Engl J Med 1997;336:1416–1421.

15. Struewing JP, Hartge P, Wacholder S, et al. The risk of cancer associated with specific mutations of BRCA1 and BRCA2 among Ashkenazi Jews. N Engl J Med 1997;336:1401–1408.

16. Couch FJ, DeShano ML, Blackwood MA, et al. BRCA1 mutations in women attending clinics that evaluate the risk of breast cancer. N Engl J Med 1997;336:1409–1415.

17. Tonin P, Weber B, Offit K, et al. Frequency of recurrent BRCA1 and BRCA2 mutations in Ashkenazi Jewish breast cancer families. Nat Med 1997;2:1179–1183.

18. Schubert EL, Lee MK, Mefford HC, et al. BRCA2 in American families with four or more cases of breast or ovarian cancer: Recurrent and novel mutations, variable expression, penetrance, and the possibility of families whose cancer is not attributable to BRCA1 or BRCA2. Am J Hum Genet 1996;60:1031–1040.

19. Szabo CI, King MC. Population genetics of BRCA1 and BRCA2. Am J Hum Genet 1997;60:1013–1020.

20. Anglian Breast Cancer Study Group. Prevalence and penetrance of BRCA1 and BRCA2 mutations in a population-based series of breast cancer cases. Br J Cancer 2000;83:1301–1308.

21. Frank TS, Deffenbaugh AM, Reid JE, et al. Clinical characteristics of individuals with germline mutations in BRCA1 and BRCA2: Analysis of 10,000 individuals. J Clin Oncol 2002;20:1480–90.

22. Li FP, Fraumeni JF Jr. Soft-tissue sarcomas, breast cancer and other neoplasms. A familial syndrome? Ann Intern Med 1969;71:747–752.

23. Nichols KE, Malkin D, Garber JE, et al. Germ-line p53 mutations predispose to a wide spectrum of early-onset cancers. Cancer Epidemiol Biomarkers Prev 2001;10:83–87.

24. Waite KA, Eng C. Protean PTEN: Form and function. Am J Hum Genet 2002;70:829–844.

25. Swift M, Morrell D, Massey RB, Chase CL. Incidence of cancer in 161 families affected by ataxia-telangiectasia. N Engl J Med 1991;325:1831–1836.

26. Easton DF. Cancer risks in A-T heterozygotes. Int J Radiat Biol 1994;66:S177–S182.

27. Meijers-Heijboer H, van den Ouweland A, Klijn J, et al. Low-penetrance susceptibility to breast cancer due to CHEK2(*)1100delC in noncarriers of BRCA1 or BRCA2 mutations. Nat Genet 2002;31:55–59.

28. Wooster R, Mangion J, Eeles R. A germline mutation in the androgen receptor in two brothers with breast cancer and Reifenstein syndrome. Nat Genet 1992;2:132–134.

29. Wagner JE, Tolar J, Levran O, Scholl T, et al. Germline mutations in BRCA2: Shared genetic susceptibility to breast cancer, early onset leukemia and Fanconi anemia. Blood 2004;103:3226–3229.

30. Couch FJ, Farid LM, DeShano ML, et al. BRCA2 germline mutations in male breast cancer cases and breast cancer families. Nat Genet 1996;13:123–125.

31. Liede A, Karlan BY, Narod SA. Cancer risks for male carriers of germline mutations in BRCA1 or BRCA2: A review of the literature. J Clin Oncol 2004;22:735–742.

32. Kirchhoff T, Satagopan JM, Kauff ND, et al. Frequency of BRCA1 and BRCA2 mutations in unselected Ashkenazi Jewish patients with colorectal cancer. J Natl Cancer Inst 2004;96:68–70.

33. King MC, Marks JH, Mandell JB. Breast and ovarian cancer risks due to inherited mutations in BRCA1 and BRCA2. Science 2003;302:643–646.

34. Oddoux C, Struewing JP, Clayton CM, et al. The carrier frequency of the BRCA2 6174delT mutation among Ashkenazi Jewish individuals is approximately 1%. Nat Genet 1996;14:188–190.

35. Offit K, Gilewski T, McGuire P, et al. Germline BRCA1 185delAG mutations in Jewish women with breast cancer. Lancet 1996;347:1643–1645.

36. Bar-Sade RB, Kruglikova A, Modan B, et al. The 185delAG BRCA1 mutation originated before the dispersion of Jews in the Diaspora and is not limited to Ashkenazim. Hum Mol Genet 1998;7:801–805.

37. Ostrer H. A genetic profile of contemporary Jewish populations. Nat Rev Genet 2001;2:891–898.

38. Kauff ND, Perez-Segura P, Robson ME, et al. Incidence of non-founder BRCA1 and BRCA2 mutations in high risk Ashkenazi breast and ovarian cancer families. J Med Genet 2002;39:611–614.

39. Struewing JP, Abeliovich D, Peretz T, Avishai N. The carrier frequency of the BRCA1 185delAG mutation is approximately 1% in Ashkenazi Jewish individuals. Nat Genet 1995;11:113–114.

40. Roa BB, Boyd AA, Volcik K, et al. Ashkenazi Jewish population frequencies for common mutations in BRCA1 and BRCA2. Nat Genet 1996;14:185–187.

41. Egan KM, Newcomb PA, Longnecker MP, et al. Jewish religion and risk of breast cancer. Lancet 1996;347:1638–1639.

42. Thorcius S, Sigurdsson S, Bjanadottir H, et al. Study of a single BRCA2 mutation with high carrier frequency in a small population. Am J Hum Genet 1997;60:1079–1084.

43. Narod SA, Ford D, Devilee P. An evaluation of genetic heterogeneity in 145 breast-ovarian cancer families. Am J Hum Genet 1995;56:254–264.

44. Gayther SA, Warren W, Mazoyer S, et al. Germline mutations of the BRCA1 gene in breast and ovarian cancer families provide evidence for a genotype-phenotype correlation. Nat Genet 1995;11:428–433.

45. Risch HA, McLaughlin JR, Cole DE, et al. Prevalence and penetrance of germline BRCA1 and BRCA2 mutations in a population series of 649 women with ovarian cancer. Am J Hum Genet 2001;68:700–710.

46. Gayther SA, Mangion J, Russell P, et al. Variation of risks of breast and ovarian cancer associated with different germline mutations of the BRCA2 gene. Nat Genet 1997;15:103–105.

47. Hoskins KF, Stopfer JE, Calzone KA, et al. Assessment and counseling for women with a family history of breast cancer: A guide for clinicians. JAMA 1995;273:577–585.

48. Martin AM, Blackwood MA, Antin-Ozerkis D, et al. Germline mutations in BRCA1 and BRCA2 in breast-ovarian families from a breast cancer risk evaluation clinic. J Clin Oncol 2001;19:2247–2253.

49. Gail MH, Brinton LA, Byar DP. Projecting individualized probabilities of developing breast cancer for white females who are being examined annually. J Natl Cancer Inst 1989;81:1879–1886.

50. Euhus DM, Smith KC, Robinson L, et al. Pretest prediction of BRCA1 or BRCA2 mutation by risk counselors and the computer model BRCAPRO. J Natl Cancer Inst 2002;94:844–851.

51. Domchek SM, Eisen A, Calzone K, et al. Application of breast cancer risk prediction models in clinical practice. J Clin Oncol 2003;21:593–601.

52. Tyrer J, Duffy SW, Cuzick J. A breast cancer prediction model incorporating familial and personal risk factors. Statis Med 2004;23:1111–1130.

53. American Society of Clinical Oncology. Policy statement update: Genetic testing for cancer susceptibility. J Clin Oncol 2003;21:2397–2406.

54. Berry DA, Iversen ES Jr, Gudbjartsson DF, et al. BRCAPRO validation, sensitivity of genetic testing of BRCA1/BRCA2, and prevalence of other breast cancer susceptibility genes. J Clin Oncol 2002;20:2701–2712.

55. Rebbeck TR, Friebel T, Lynch HT, et al. bilateral prophylactic mastectomy reduces breast cancer risk in BRCA1 and BRCA2 mutation carriers: The PROSE Study Group. J Clin Oncol 2004;22:1055–1062.

56. Rebbeck TR, Lynch HT, Neuhausen SL, et al. Prophylactic oophorectomy in carriers of BRCA1 or BRCA2 mutations. N Engl J Med 2002;346:1616–1622.

57. Offit K, Robson M, Schrag D. Prophylactic mastectomy in carriers of BRCA mutations. N Engl J Med 2001;345:1498–1499; author reply, 1499–1500.

58. Reports of the Working Group to Review the National Cancer Institute—American Cancer Society Breast Cancer Detection Demonstration Project. J Natl Cancer Inst 19796;2:639–709.

59. Greenwald P, Nasca PC, Lawrence CE, et al. Estimated effect of breast self examination and routine physician examinations on breast cancer mortality. N Engl J Med 1978;299:271–273.

60. Burke W, Daly M, Garber J, et al. Recommendations for follow-up care of individuals with an inherited predisposition to cancer II. BRCA1 and BRCA2. JAMA 1997;277:997–1003.

61. Kerlikowske K, Grady D, Rubin SM, et al. Efficacy of screening mammography: A meta-analysis. JAMA 1995;273:149–154.

62. Fletcher SW, Black W, Harris R, et al. Report of the international workshop on screening for breast cancer. J Natl Cancer Inst 1995;85:1644–1656.

63. Mettler FA, Upton AC, Kelsey CA, et al. Benefits versus risks from mammography. Cancer 1996;77:903–909.

64. Kuhl CK, Schmutzler RK, Leutner CC, et al. Breast MR imaging screening in 192 women proved or suspected to be carriers of a breast cancer susceptibility gene: Preliminary results. Radiology 2000;215:267–279.

65. Podo F, Sardanelli F, Canese R, et al. The Italian multi-centre project on evaluation of MRI and other imaging modalities in early detection of breast cancer in subjects at high genetic risk. J Exp Clin Cancer Res 2002;21:115–124.

66. Higgins R, van Nagell J, Donaldson E, et al. Transvaginal sonography as a screening method for ovarian cancer. Gynecol Oncol 1989;34:402–406.

67. van Nagell J, Higgins R, Donaldson E, et al. Transvaginal sonography as a screening method for ovarian cancer. 1990;Cancer 65:573–577.

68. Kurjak A, Zalud I, Alfirevic Z. Examination of adnexal masses with transvaginal color ultrasound. J Ultrasound Med 1991;10:295–297.

69. Daly MB. The epidemiology of ovarian cancer. Hematol Oncol Clin North Am 1992;6:729–738.

70. Jacobs I, Bast RC Jr. The CA-125 tumor-associated antigen. Hum Reprod 1989;4:1–12.

71. Skates SJ, Feng-Ji X, Yin-Hua Y, et al. Toward an optimal algorithm for ovarian cancer screening with longitudinal tumor markers. Cancer 1995;76:2004–2010.

72. Bilimoria M, Morrow M. The woman at increased risk for breast cancer: Evaluation and management strategies. CA Cancer J Clin 1995;45:263–278.

73. Tobacman JK, Tucker MA, Kase R. Intraabdominal carcinomatosis after prophylactic oophorectomy in ovarian cancer prone families. Lancet 1982;2:795–797.

74. Nieder AM, Taneja SS, Zeegers MP, Ostrer H. Genetic counseling for prostate cancer risk. Clin Genet 2003;63:169–176.

75. Carroll P, Coley C, McLeod D, et al. Prostate-specific antigen best practice policy. Part I. Early detection and diagnosis of prostate cancer. Urology 2001;57:217–224.

76. Smith RA, Cokkinides V, von Eschenbach AC, et al. American Cancer Society guidelines for the early detection of cancer. CA Cancer J Clin 2002;52:8–22.

77. American College of Physicians. Screening for prostate cancer. Ann Intern Med 1997;126:480–484.

78. Zoorob R, Anderson R, Cefalu C, Sidani M. Cancer screening guidelines. Am Fam Physician 2001;63:1101–1112.

79. Lerman C, Narod S, Schulman K, et al. BRCA1 testing in families with hereditary breast-ovarian cancer. A prospective study of patient decision making and outcomes. JAMA 1996;275:1885–1892.

80. Ostrer H, Allen W, Crandall LA, et al. Insurance and genetic testing: Where are we now? Am J Hum Genet 1993;52:565–577.

Appendix: Genetic Counseling Protocol

TELEPHONE INTAKE

1. Ascertain the problem and concerns of the patient and source of referral.
2. Determine the affected or unaffected status of the patient and other family members by taking a brief family history.
3. Provide a short description of the evaluation process, to include
   a. The number and length of the sessions
   b. The elements of the evaluation
   c. The type of information that is to be obtained and given
   d. Who will accompany the patient to the meeting (partner, close friend, other relative, other)
4. Discuss fees and potential insurance issues.

5. Advise the patient about additional information or records that may be required.
6. Send release forms if necessary.

FIRST SESSION

1. Ascertain the motivation of the patient and others in seeking information and testing.
2. Determine the patient's understanding of what is to be learned and the patient's perception and that of others of the probability that cancer is heritable in the family or that the patient will develop cancer or have a recurrence.
3. Learn from the patient how the information is likely to be useful both personally and by other family members.
4. Learn whether the patient definitely wants testing, does not want it, or is uncertain, and learn what the factors that influence that opinion are.
5. Describe the elements of the consultation:
   a. The number of sessions (usually at least two)
   b. The content of the sessions
   c. Review of records and slides for confirmation of the diagnosis
   d. The time frame for the receipt of information and completion of testing
   e. How the patient will receive results (in person only, with occasional exceptions)
   f. The availability of other specialists (e.g., surgical, medical, and gynecologic oncologists, radiologists, other medical specialists, psychotherapists)
6. Obtain a detailed medical history, including the affected or unaffected status of the patient. If the proband is affected, find out the date and age of diagnosis; how the patient came to be diagnosed; the physicians providing care at each step of the diagnostic process; the treatment received, both surgical and medical; reproductive history; other medical history; exogenous hormone exposure; smoking history; alcohol consumption; dietary fat consumption; dietary supplements; and physical activity.
7. Obtain a detailed three-generation family history to include
   a. History of all maternal and paternal relatives, with information about as many relatives as possible from at least two antecedent generations (parental and grandparental) and relatives from all descendant generations (i.e., children, grandchildren, nieces, nephews)
   b. Ages of affected and unaffected relatives
   c. History of all malignancies in all recorded relatives and their ages at diagnosis and death
   d. Other genetic conditions in the family
8. Identify family members from whom confirmatory diagnostic information will be required and make arrangements to obtain records, slides, and other test results if possible.
9. Discuss a potential diagnosis and provide an estimate in qualitative and quantitative terms of the probability that there is a heritable cancer syndrome in the family and the probability that the patient and other family members are carriers. In discussing these issues, elicit whether the

patient has discussed testing with other family members and whether they want to receive results. Encourage the patient to inform relatives of the testing before it occurs, or at least before results are received.

10. Explain what testing or counseling may be applicable or appropriate to define the condition more precisely (this may not be possible until additional information and records are obtained).

If Family or Individual Wants to Consider Testing

1. Discuss the contribution of major genes to a hereditary predisposition to breast and ovarian cancer and describe the genetics of the applicable hereditary predisposition. Explain which gene or genes may be appropriate to test in the given family.
2. Give a full explanation of the testing procedures, including the identification of the individual within the family who may be most appropriate to test first (i.e., the youngest affected individual if possible).
3. Emphasize and quantify the accuracy and limitations of the diagnosis, including the sensitivity and the specificity of the testing.
4. Explain the implications of both positive and negative results.
5. Advise the patient that a specific diagnosis may not be possible.
6. Indicate whether the test is investigational and whether the laboratory is a research laboratory, is approved by the Clinical Laboratories Improvement Act, or is state licensed.
7. Indicate, before testing, the importance of obtaining medical records or other documentation of the diagnosis in relevant family members, with your understanding that it may not always be possible.
8. Discuss the emotional and psychological aspects of testing versus not testing.
9. Discuss the benefits and drawbacks of testing versus not testing for both affected and unaffected family members.

   a. Benefits of testing
      (1) Allows the patient to plan medical care
      (2) May be useful for other family members who want to learn their carrier status and risks and modify their health care
      (3) Allows unaffected family members to learn that they are not at increased risk or are at lower risk than anticipated
      (4) Alleviates the anxiety of not knowing
      (5) May improve family relationships
   b. Drawbacks of testing
      (1) May heighten anxiety in carriers
      (2) May interfere with family relationships
      (3) May produce guilt in parents who transmit the gene
      (4) May engender resentment among relatives, some of whom will learn they are carriers whereas others are noncarriers
      (5) Individuals choosing testing and carriers may encounter employment or insurance discrimination

      (6) Individuals choosing testing may, in the process, learn genetic information about relatives who choose not to be tested
      (7) Patient may encounter uncertainty because of the unknown efficacy of surveillance

10. Discuss issues of confidentiality; that is, results will be shared only with individuals identified by the patient, and the patient must provide written permission from these individuals to share the results with them
11. Discuss fees and insurance reimbursement; potential for insurance or employment discrimination.
12. Emphasize that testing will be limited to individuals who are of age to consent unless medical management is affected.
13. Remind the patient that testing is elective.
14. Tell the patient that he or she will receive the results in person only and may wish to be accompanied by a partner, relative, or friend.
15. Discuss the pros and cons of having individuals hear their results with other members of their family or separately.
16. If family members are being counseled as a group, provide adequate time for all individuals to meet privately with the counselor or physician.
17. Provide recommendations for surveillance and risk-reducing surgery following testing.
18. Provide to the patient a written summary of the content of the session summarizing the medical content of the session.
19. Draw blood for testing, sign consent form, complete insurance forms, or make arrangements for a second appointment.

If the Family Is Not a Candidate for Testing or Individuals Choose Not to Be Tested

1. Provide an estimate of the risks for recurrence or occurrence in affected and unaffected family members based on the family history, personal medical history, and data from current medical literature and risk assessment tools.
2. Offer DNA banking (tumor, lymphocytes, tumor block) for appropriate family members if indicated.
3. Discuss scheduling additional sessions if needed or indicated.
4. Provide the patient with a written summary and promise a copy of the letter to the physician.

   A patient may return to have blood drawn for testing at another time.

INTERIM

1. Collect medical records, pathology specimens.
2. Review the medical records, including review by the pathologist.
3. Update the literature search.
4. Conduct a multidisciplinary management conference.
5. Provide the referring physician with a summary of the evaluation to the patient and any other designated individual (written consent is required).

SECOND SESSION

1. Give results.

   a. Ascertain who is to be in the room (may be done before the appointment).

   b. Review the implications of diagnosis, giving individuals the opportunity not to learn their results, or to defer learning results.

   c. Provide results.

   d. Provide emotional support, especially for those learning of their at-risk status, or alleviate guilt for those not at risk, if appropriate.

   e. Reiterate the degree of accuracy and the limitations of the test.

   f. Review or explain how the risks were calculated.

   g. Discuss the patient's perception of the results and the alternatives.

   h. Discuss in greater detail preventive measures and surveillance and state that there is no clear evidence that surveillance improves outcome in breast cancer.

   i. Refer to other medical specialists, if indicated, including psychiatrist or psychotherapist.

   j. Discuss the availability of clinical trials.

   k. Discuss implications for other at-risk individuals in the family and offer testing if appropriate. If preventive measures should be performed before the legal age of consent, testing should be offered to children.

   l. After this session, write a letter to the patient summarizing the results of testing and risk assessment and include recommendations for surveillance. Provide a copy of the test report and obtain written consent to report results to any third party, including the physician.

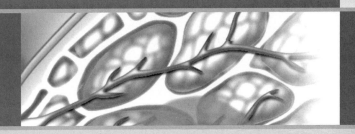

SECTION V

TREATMENT

CHAPTER 21

Development of Modern Breast Cancer Treatment

Daniel F. Roses

Breast cancer therapy has evolved through most of its long history without any verifiable understanding of the behavior of the disease, little technical means by which it could be studied, and limited diagnostic and therapeutic resources. By contrast, our present modern era of breast cancer treatment, beginning in the closing decades of the last century, has developed with increasing rapidity through the efforts of an extremely broad spectrum of basic research scientists and clinical investigators who have redefined our standards for developing, evaluating, and applying meaningful therapeutic strategies. Historically, the most important development in breast cancer treatment was the rise of modern surgery, which made careful and thorough ablation of local disease technically feasible and demonstrated to a skeptical medical world that breast cancer is a treatable disease. Paradoxically, this advance also made clear the limitations of therapy that was exclusively directed at the breast and its regional nodal drainage sites. As other therapeutic modalities were developed, the possibility of curing an ever-greater population of patients became a reality. At the same time, advances in radiographic and pathologic diagnosis also made clear the inappropriateness of overzealous and uniformly rigid efforts to extirpate local disease. As we enter into a new century, the intensity with which modern diagnostic and therapeutic strategies are assessed, and with which the molecular mechanisms of disease are being defined, carries the hope that we are on the threshold of a new era in which it will become possible to translate an enhanced understanding of oncogenesis and growth into universally effective treatment and even prevention.

Has breast cancer always been a major health problem?

Cases of breast cancer have been recorded in medical writings for more than 5000 years. In documents from the ancient world, they appear with perhaps greater frequency than any other form of cancer. This suggests that the incidence of breast cancer was significant, particularly considering that life expectancy in the ancient world was probably no more than 40 years. The first written evidence possibly indicating a breast cancer is from ancient Egypt and is found in the Edwin Smith Surgical Papyrus, a compendium of surgical cases and therapeutic recommendations, dating back from 3000 to 2500 B.C.E.[1] Although the patients referred to are to men, case 45 concerns a "bulging" tumor of the breast. Ancient Egyptian physicians are instructed to do nothing to such bulging tumors if they are hard and cool when touched—likely indicative of cancer. This is in contrast to case 39, a tumor that had "spread with pus over his breast" and had "produced redness, while it is very hot therein"—certainly indicative of an abscess. The recommended treatment here is incision with an instrument known as a "fire drill."

How did physicians in the ancient world view the etiology of cancer?

In ancient Greece, Hippocrates (circa 460–377 B.C.E.) set forth a humoral concept of cancer's origin, extending his belief that diseases were caused by imbalances in the four basic humors—blood, phlegm, and yellow and black bile—cancer being due to an excess of black bile. Before this, breast cancer was likely thought to be of supernatural origin. Clay models of breast tumors found in the remains of Greek temples suggest that remedies were sought through supernatural intervention.[2] Hippocrates wrote of "carcinoma apertus," which was a malignant ulcer, and "carcinoma occlusus," which was a nonulcerated, deep-seated tumor. Of the latter, he stated that it was better to omit treatment altogether, for, "if treated, the patients die quickly; but if not treated they hold out for a long time."[3] In the first century C.E., the teachings of the Roman scholar Celsus did suggest that efforts to extirpate malignant lesions early in their development might offer some hope of success, whereas treatment when the disease became more advanced might hasten its progression.[4]

Aglancon, by the second century C.E., embellished the humoral concept, teaching that when the temperature of the liver increased, it began to generate decomposed, thick blood,[5] which the spleen forced to various sites in the body. If this thick blood were to stagnate in an organ such as the breast, cancer would be produced. His student Galen, whose writings were destined to become the most authoritative therapeutic directive for centuries, expounded on such humoral theories of disease, also promoting the Hippocratic view that breast cancer, among other neoplasms, was due to an excess of black bile. The Greek surgeon and physician Paul of Aegina (625–690) again promoted the belief that cancer arose from thick overheated bile, which commonly affected the breast "due to its laxity which admitted humours."[6]

How was cancer treated in the ancient world?

The basic component of cancer therapy, according to Galen, was the use of purgatives, although he did recognize surgery as a form of therapy for accessible lesions. If surgery were resorted to, he advised that it be done "from the root," by which he meant encompassing the veins "full of the malignant matter."[7] Recorded clinical observations of progressive axillary nodal involvement, as well as descriptions of partial mastectomies by the Greek physician Leonides in the second century C.E., suggest that there existed a tension between the authoritative promotion of theories of humoralism on the one hand and the recognition that surgery, then a violent therapeutic intervention, might be required for a disease that so obviously did not respond to purgatives, bleeding, caustics, cauterization, or dietary manipulation.[8]

During the period from the fall of the Roman Empire to the Renaissance, medical progress remained stagnant as Christianity and Islam limited anatomic dissection and, in turn, surgical practice. The teachings of Galen were elevated to official doctrine, and efforts to question his dictates were viewed as heretical. Despite edicts to restrict the performance of surgery, eminent surgeons, such as Henri de Mondeville (1260–1320) and Guy de Chauliac (1300–1368), advocated surgery for breast cancers that could be completely excised. William of Salicet (1210–1277) and Lanfranc of Milan (?–1315) advocated extending surgery to complete removal of the breast. William of Salicet, in a synthesis of surgical and humoral thinking, stated that

the disease cannot be truly cured except by the amputation of the part, as I have said above, for its roots are imbedded in the veins which course about it, and which are full of melancholy blood [containing black bile]; and that it is necessary for the perfect cure that the veins be cut and the roots extracted in some fashion. This cannot be done except by removing the part in its entirety, and the disease cannot be cured by any other means. It appears to me that it is neither good, nor useful, nor honest for the physician to interfere with this cure. It would be better, to be sure, and I advise you, my friend, to decline.[9]

Medieval surgeons empirically recognized that inadequate excision was futile. It is understandable, therefore, that breast cancer, a disease that was likely to be locally advanced upon presentation to surgeons, was for the most part treated by attempts at local palliation using caustics. What was required to free breast cancer treatment conceptually, if not practically, from the dominance of folk wisdom and ancient medical dogma was anatomic observation and study.

When did anatomic concepts of breast cancer development appear?

Anatomic paradigms for breast cancer arose with the Renaissance and the renewed study of anatomy. The critical figure in the development of scientific anatomy based on observation and dissection was Andreas Vesalius (1514–1564). Vesalius was also a surgeon who is recorded as having operated for cancer of the breast, excising the lesion widely and achieving hemostasis by ligating blood vessels rather than by the brutal cauterization in common use during this era.[10] His

contemporary, Ambrose Paré (1510–1590), the most famous surgeon of the 16th century, described the swelling of axillary lymph nodes that he observed in patients with breast cancer.[11] Although he is recorded as having excised superficial lesions, for most patients he would compress the base of the breast between lead plates, the resulting ischemia hopefully arresting the progression of the disease.[8]

Several other surgeons of the 16th century described more surgically aggressive approaches to breast cancer, including Johannes Scultetus (1595–1645), who with great speed excised the breast after traction had been applied by heavy leather thongs threaded through its base, hemostasis being provided by a hot iron applied to the chest wall[12] (Fig. 21–1). Another surgeon, Wilhelm Fabry von Hilden of Germany (1560–1624), also developed a rapid technique using an instrument that lifted the breast away from the chest wall, its base then constricted with an iron ring, following which it was amputated. Guillaume de Houppeville incorporated the subjacent pectoralis major muscle in his mastectomies, and Marcus Aurelius Severino (1560–1634) first removed enlarged axillary lymph nodes.[13] Fabry von Hilden, however, observed that excising axillary tumors was difficult and dangerous because

the breast veins come together in that spot, bleeding from which must be controlled. Furthermore, also through contraction of such tumors, the breast muscles which aid in breathing might be injured, and for this reason there is danger of suffocation. Therefore it is necessary to proceed slowly, humbly, and gently with such parts.[14]

He recognized the futility of incomplete resection of fixed lesions, noting,

Above all things, one must inform himself carefully whether the tumor weaves about or moves from one place to another, or whether it can be removed from its base, including its roots. For all would be for naught if a part of the tumor, be it ever

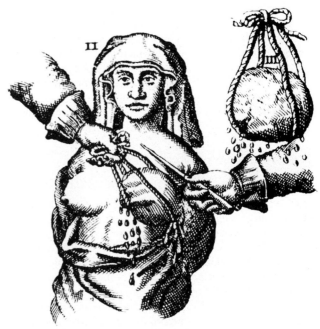

Figure 21–1   Mastectomy (breast amputation) for cancer.   (From Johannes Scultetus Armamentarium Chirurgicum, Amsterdam, 1741.)

so small, even a bit of membrane with which such tumors are generally surrounded, were to remain behind. Then it flames up again and becomes worse than ever before.[14]

Not surprisingly, he deferred treating ulcerating lesions and, believing cauterization incited further malignant growth, proposed the topical application of a distillate of suckling puppies boiled in wine.

Surgeons of the Renaissance were obviously frustrated by an inability to translate their new anatomic knowledge and more critical clinical observations into therapeutic progress. Despite their intentions, the extremes of disease continued to be managed by bizarre topical concoctions, such as those of Fabry von Hilden, and even by the application of animal feces to the tumor, excreta being frequently used medicinally during this era. Nevertheless, progress was clearly being made toward establishing an anatomic concept of the disease upon which a consistent therapeutic strategy could be constructed.

When was a local theory of breast cancer introduced?

The 18th century brought a new focus by surgeons on anatomic and experimental pathology. In France during this Age of Enlightenment, the ancient humoral theory of oncogenesis was discarded most forcefully by Henri François Le Dran (1685–1773) (Fig. 21–2). In a memoir published in 1757, he reasoned that because axillary nodal involvement in a patient with cancer of the breast was indicative of a worse prognosis, the disease must spread through the lymphatics to these lymph nodes and then into the general circulation after its origin in the breast. At its earliest phase of development, therefore, it was a local disease and might well be eliminated by surgery. If "cancer lymph" passed beyond the adjacent lymph nodes, the entire lymphatic system would become contaminated.[15] New theories on the lymphatic origins of cancer arose. At the University of Halle, Friedrich Hoffman (1660–1742) and Georg Ernst Stahl (1660–1734) espoused the view that cancer was composed of fermenting and degenerating lymph, a concept that was also proposed by John Hunter (1728–1793).[16]

When did a unified surgical approach to breast cancer arise?

The surgical application of Le Dran's conceptualization of breast cancer as a local disease found its most forceful advocate in Jean Louis Petit (1674–1750) of Paris (Fig. 21–3), a leading founder of the French Academy of Surgery. In Petit's book, *Traits des Maladies, Chirurgicales et des Operations*, published posthumously, he outlined a concept of ablative surgery that required excising the breast, palpable axillary lymph nodes, and underlying pectoralis major muscle if attached to the tumor. As he noted,

. . . the roots of cancer were the enlarged lymphatic glands; that the glands should be looked for and removed and that the pectoral fascia and even some fibers of the muscle itself should be dissected away rather than leave any doubtful tissue. The mammary gland too should not be cut into during the operation. . . . Where the integuments are also affected and strictly joined to the cancer there is little hope to expect a perfect cure if they are not both clearly extirpated together.[17]

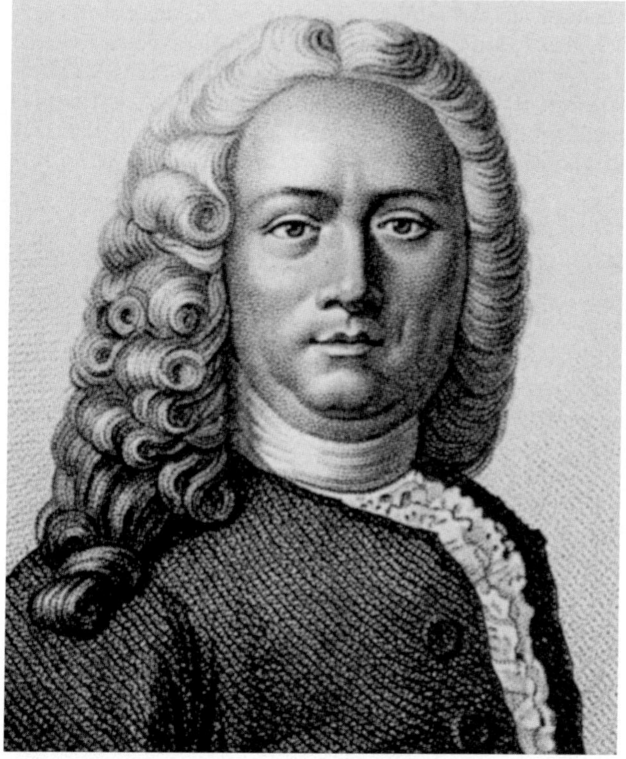

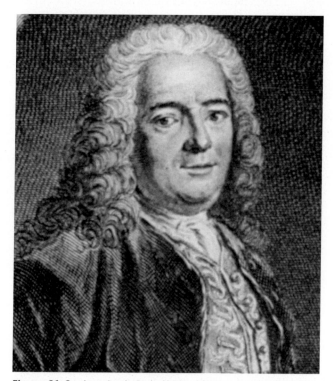

Figure 21–2   Henri François Le Dran (1685–1773), who developed a local theory of breast cancer. (Courtesy of New York Academy of Medicine.)

Figure 21–3   Jean Louis Petit (1674–1750), who developed an en bloc resection of the breast and palpable axillary lymph nodes. (Courtesy of National Library of Medicine, Washington, DC.)

Although Petit did not always encompass the nipple and areola in his procedures, he did clearly promote the concept of en bloc resection of cancer. Petit attracted students from many European surgical centers and certainly influenced the course of breast cancer surgery through the 18th and 19th centuries. Lorenz Heister (1683–1758) of Germany advocated mastectomy with the attached pectoralis major muscle and axillary nodes if necessary. However, his vivid description of a mastectomy performed in 1720 leaves no doubt as to the brutality of surgery at that time and the near impossibility of translating any detailed surgical concept into clinical reality.[18] Heister was able to report the surgical removal of cancers "bigger than one's fist" and one that weighed 12 pounds, reflecting the expanded advocacy of surgery as a therapeutic option.[18] Bernard Peyrilhe (1735–1804) in 1773 envisioned surgery that encompassed the entire breast, axillary nodes, and pectoralis major muscle.[19] Samuel Sharpe in England and Benjamin Bell (1749–1806) in Scotland also promoted mastectomy and the excision of palpable axillary lymph nodes. However, the limitations on surgery in the preanesthetic and preantiseptic era clearly continued to inhibit timely intervention and restrict its use except as a treatment of desperation. As a result, extreme pessimism regarding the curability of breast cancer persisted.

Did a local theory of breast cancer development result in any major change in treatment?

Despite the acceptance of Le Dran's local concept of breast cancer, surgery was still considered worse than the disease, and little advance in treatment resulted. A vivid account of a mastectomy performed on September 30, 1811, makes this clear. The patient, the novelist Fanny Burney, best known for her letters and diaries, was married to a French aristocrat, Alexander D'Ablay, and living in France when, in 1811, she noticed a lump in her breast. Cancer was diagnosed, and surgery was performed by the illustrious surgeon to Napoleon, Baron Dominique-Jean Larrey (1766–1842). In a letter to her sister on the ordeal, she wrote that she was given very little notice of her operation, only being informed that it would take place on the very morning of the day of the procedure. To gather up the necessary resolve, she was able to delay its commencement for several hours, at which time Larrey arrived with six assistants. After being prepared with wine she was laid down on a bedstead. A handkerchief was spread over her face to block her view, but it was thin, and she could make out what was about to take place. When the procedure commenced, she let out a scream, which, she wrote, "lasted unintermittently during the whole time of the incision," and when the instrument was withdrawn, the pain was undiminished. She recalled the "knife rackling against the breastbone—scraping it!" The operation lasted 20 minutes, during which time she fainted twice, and when the handkerchief was removed from her eyes, she "saw my good doctor Larrey, pale nearly as myself, his face streaked with blood, and its expression depicting grief, apprehension, and almost horror."[20] Madame D'Ablay lived another 30 years, which has even called into question the accuracy of the diagnosis. More typical of the results following surgery was the experience of 46-year-old Abigail Adams Smith, daughter of the second president of the United States. In the same year that Fanny Burney discovered

her tumor, she also felt a mass in her right breast and was advised by Dr. Benjamin Rush that the only remedy was "the knife." He wrote,

From her account of the moving state of the tumor, it is now in a proper situation for the operation. Should she wait until it superates or even inflames much, it may be too late. . . . I repeat again, let there by no delay. . . . Her time of life calls for expedition in this business, for tumors such as hers tend much more rapidly to cancer after 45 than more early in life.[21]

On October 8, 1811, in a bedroom next to that of John and Abigail Adams, a 25-minute mastectomy was performed by four surgeons. She recovered but died of her disease 2 years later. Even more typical of treatment during this era is a poignant account of an indigent patient having surgery for breast cancer that took place in a crowded amphitheater in Edinburgh in 1830, as recorded by an onlooking medical student, Dr. John Brown. The patient was brought into the amphitheater in her street clothes, accompanied by her husband and her dog, where she stoically withstood the painful procedure only to die of sepsis a few days later.[22]

Given the desperation of such therapy, it is no wonder that in the same year as the operations on Fanny Burney and Abigail Smith, the English surgeon Samuel Young again described treating breast cancer by compression, as had Paré 250 years earlier.[17] This technique was to prove no more successful than it had been when originally introduced. The problem of this era was best summarized by Henry Fearon (1750–1825), who noted that although surgery for breast cancer at an early time represented the most favorable opportunity for effecting a cure, it was unlikely that patients whose disease was creating few or any symptoms could be convinced of undergoing such painful and dangerous therapy.[23] In 1792, a cancer charity ward was established for the first time at Middlesex Hospital in London, where patients could be cared for and studied in an attempt to arrive at some new understanding of the natural history of a disease that so eluded comprehension and possible methods of treatment. In 1803, the first patient with breast cancer was admitted there for study.

Was breast cancer viewed as a curable disease at the beginning of the 19th century?

Such eminent English surgeons as James Syme (1799–1878), Sir James Paget (1814–1899), and Robert Liston (1794–1847) all wrote with skepticism on the possibility of effecting a cure for breast cancer through surgery.[24–26] Paget, who in 1874 was to describe one of the more favorable forms of carcinoma of the breast with which his name is attached, actually believed that women with what was described as "scirrhous carcinoma"—a generic category that encompassed any lesion with painless growth and a hard consistency—were less likely to have a prolonged survival if surgery were attempted rather than if the disease were allowed to progress unimpeded. In 1853, Paget wrote that "in deciding for or against the removal of a cancerous growth, in any single case, we may, I think, dismiss all hope that the operation will be a final remedy for the disease."[24] In 1856, citing his failure to have a disease-free survivor beyond 8 years among 235 patients on whom he had operated, he again wrote, "We have to ask ourselves whether it is probable that the operation will add to the length and comfort of life enough to justify incurring the risk for its own consequences."[25] In the United States, D. Hayes Agnew (1818–1892), ironically memorialized in the famous painting by Thomas Eakins depicting his supervision of a breast procedure at the University of Pennsylvania, wrote skeptically, "I do not despair of carcinoma being cured somewhat in the future, but this blessed event will never be wrought by the knife of the surgeon."[27]

What was the impact of microscopic pathology on breast cancer treatment?

The rise of microscopic pathology in the first half of the 19th century provided evidence for a verifiable and rational explanation on the natural history of breast cancer. Following the development of the achromatic microscope in 1830 by Joseph Jackson Lister (1786–1869), which enabled clear microscopic images to be studied without blurring, Johannes Müller (1801–1858) in 1838 was able to demonstrate the cellular structure of malignant growths, whereas Joseph Recamier (1774–1852) in 1829 first described "metastasis" as well as local infiltration of malignant tumors into surrounding tissues and veins.[28,29] Tumors were now clearly defined as lesions evolving from cells that could infiltrate and invade lymphatic and vascular structures. With the establishment of cellular pathology by Müller's student Rudolf Virchow (1821–1902) (Fig. 21–4), cancer was now viewed as evolving from normal cells.

The development of metastases, however, eluded pathologic observation and understanding. Virchow, for one, felt that metastatic spread occurred "by means of certain fluids, and these possessed the power of producing an infection which disposes different parts to a reproduction of a mass of the same nature as the one which originally existed."[30] Regional nodal metastases were viewed by Virchow as representing a temporary barrier to distant dissemination. Of axillary nodal metastases, Virchow stated in 1858,

When an axillary gland becomes cancerous, after previous cancerous disease of the mamma, and when during a long period only the axillary gland remains diseased without the group of glands next in succession or any other organs becoming affected with cancer, we can account for this upon no other supposition than that the gland collects hurtful ingredients absorbed from the breast and thereby for a time affords protection to the body, but at length proves insufficient, nay, perhaps at a later period itself becomes a new source of independent infection to the body, inasmuch as a further propagation of the poisonous matter may take place from the diseased parts of the gland.[31]

Karl Thiersch (1822–1893) and Wilhelm Waldeyer (1837–1921), by studying serial sections of cutaneous and gastrointestinal neoplasms, further established the epithelial origins of malignant growth. They believed that migration of cells, not the suffusion of "hurtful ingredients," through the lymphatic and circulatory system, led to metastases, agreeing that the regional lymph nodes served as a protective filter.[29] Virchow, like Paget before him, believed that cancer required a hereditary or constitutional predisposition. Both believed some inciting mechanism was required. For Virchow, the mechanism was chronic irritation; for Paget, it had been a

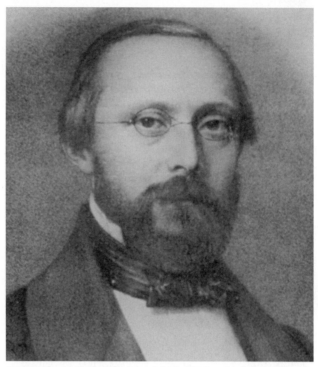

Figure 21–4   Rudolf Virchow (1821–1902), who believed lymph nodes to be a temporary barrier against breast cancer progression. (Courtesy of New York Academy of Medicine.)

humoral material that was spread throughout the vascular system.[32]

By the second half of the 19th century, therefore, the establishment of the cellular origins of disease and the local pattern of cancer's progression had provided a more rational framework on which to structure surgical treatment. If tumors expanded and infiltrated before spreading to other sites, then operations to encompass the disease widely, as originally proposed by Le Dran and Petit, were justified. Despite this rethinking, the constraints on surgical practice compelled surgeons in the mid-19th century to sympathize with even such a famously bold surgeon as Robert Liston of London, who wrote

Recourse may be had to the knife in some cases but the circumstances must be very favorable indeed to induce a surgeon to recommend or warrant him in undertaking any operation for removal of malignant disease of the breast. When the disease has been of some standing there is a considerable risk of the axillary glands having become contaminated. No one could now be found so rash or so cruel as to attempt the removal of glands thus affected whether primarily or secondarily.[26]

How did surgeons adapt the advances in cellular pathology to treatment?

The cellular basis of disease now began to permeate medical thought and emboldened many surgeons to advocate more thorough extirpation of the local origins of breast cancer. Joseph Pancoast (1805–1882) in the United States again advocated removal of the breast in continuity with involved axillary lymph nodes.[33] Writing in 1844, 2 years before the introduction of general anesthesia, he did urge careful selection of appropriate cases, noting the great likelihood of local recurrence "if it has involved the chain of axillary glands, and especially if it has become adherent to the pectoral muscles, or has formed an open ulcer," urging a candid discussion of such a risk with the patient.[33]

With the introduction of general anesthesia in 1846, a new window was opened on what might be attempted in the local extirpation of breast cancer. In 1869, Richard Sweeting in England advocated removing the lower portion of the pectoralis major muscle as well as a generous margin of skin, noting that if the cancer cells lie in the fascia, they are likely to embed themselves in the lower part of the pectoralis major muscle, "certainly not a vital organ that cannot safely be removed. The lower two-thirds of the muscle is more than occupied by the base of a large cancer."[34] Most influential was Charles H. Moore (1821–1870) (Fig. 21–5), a surgeon at the Middlesex Hospital, who in an 1867 article titled "On the Influence of Inadequate Operations on the Theory of Cancer" criticized the frequency with which the breast was only partly removed by other surgeons. He noted the tendency for cancer to recur centrifugally from the scar owing to inadequate removal. He stated that

local recurrence of cancer after operations is due to the continuous growth of fragments of the principal tumor. Such recurrences may take place also in a residual part of the organ respecting which it cannot be asserted that it is cancerous at the time of operation. . . .[35]

He urged wide resection around the tumor to avoid cutting through malignant tissue and directed surgeons to remove the entire breast as well as adjacent diseased tissue, including generous margins of skin and axillary lymph nodes to avoid "dividing the intervening lymphatics," a crucial concept in the development of surgical thinking.[35] This approach was supported by W. Mitchell Banks in London and in the United States by Samuel W. Gross (1837–1889), both of whom advocated the elective inclusion of an axillary dissection with the mastectomy.[36,37] Joseph Lister (1827–1912) detached the origins of both pectoral muscles to enhance his ability to dissect the axillary nodal contents. As he noted in an 1870 report on antiseptic surgery,

I have at present a patient about to leave the infirmary three weeks after the removal of the entire mamma for scirrhus, all the axillary glands having been at the same time cleaned out after division of both the pectoral muscles, so as to permit the shoulder to be thrown back and the axilla freely exposed, as is done in the dissecting room—a practice which I have for some years adopted where the lymphatic glands are affected in that disease.[38]

The surgical revolution brought about by general anesthesia, and then by antiseptic practice, proposed by Lister in 1867, led to an escalated effort to surgically treat breast cancer. In Germany, Ernst Küster (1838–1922) championed axillary dissection as a routine component of mastectomy, reporting on his experience in 1883.[39] Richard von Volkmann (1830–1889) (Fig. 21–6), writing in 1875, concluded that the fascia of the pectoralis major muscle could be infiltrated, and introduced a procedure to remove it along with the breast and axillary lymph nodes. As he explained,

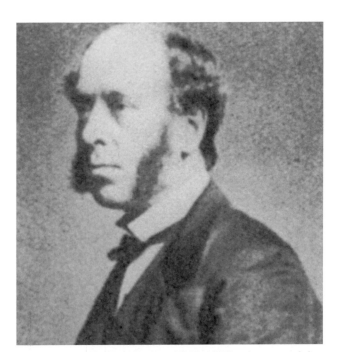

Figure 21–5   Charles H. Moore (1821–1870), who asserted that breast cancer evolved centrifugally and required wide resection en bloc with contiguous structures.   (Courtesy of National Library of Medicine, Washington, DC.)

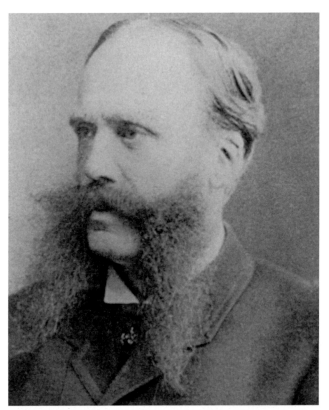

Figure 21–6   Richard von Volkmann (1830–1889), who advocated removal of the pectoralis major fascia along with the breast and axillary lymph nodes.   (Courtesy of National Library of Medicine, Washington, DC.)

I was led to adopt this procedure because, on microscopical examination, I repeatedly found when I had not expected it that the fascia was already carcinomatous whereas the muscle was certainly not involved.[40]

Lothar Heidenheim (1860–1940) provided support to Volkmann, reporting on the frequency of lymphatic metastases between the breast and pectoralis major muscle. In 1889, he reported on his experience of including not only the pectoralis major fascia but also a superficial layer of muscle or even the entire muscle for those instances in which the tumor was fixed to the underlying muscle.[41] The greater availability of surgical specimens enabled further detailed pathologic anatomic studies of breast cancer, many supporting a radiating pattern of lymphatic permeation.[42,43] A consolidation of the advances in surgery and the new conceptualization of breast pathophysiology into a dominant therapeutic doctrine was about to take place.

Why was Halsted so influential in the treatment of breast cancer?

William Stewart Halsted (1852–1922) (Fig. 21–7) had been raised in New York City and received his medical education and spent his early surgical career there. Like many well-to-do graduates of American medical schools, he had gone to Europe to immerse himself in the scientific medicine that was emerging in the great centers of European learning, particularly in Germany and Austria. Between 1878 and 1880, he traveled to Vienna, Berlin, Hamburg, Leipzig, Kiel, Halle, and Würzburg, where he was exposed to the modern advances in clinical investigation, antisepsis, microscopic anatomy, and pathology as well as to the great leaders of European surgery

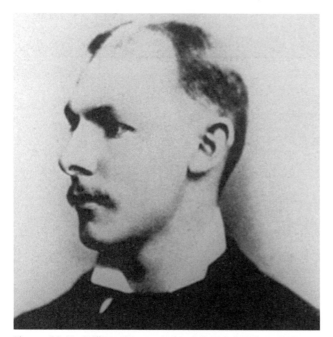

Figure 21–7 William Stewart Halsted (1852–1922), in 1889, at the time of his development of the radical mastectomy. (From Crowe SJ. Halsted of Johns Hopkins. The Man and His Men. Springfield, IL, Thomas, 1957.)

such as Theodor Billroth (1824–1887), von Volkmann, and Karl Thiersch (1822–1895).[44] His move to the new Johns Hopkins School of Medicine in 1888 and his subsequent appointment in 1889 as surgeon-in-chief to the outpatient clinic and appointment 2 years later as Professor of Surgery and Surgeon-in-Chief to the Johns Hopkins Hospital led to the establishment of a modern American school of scientific surgery and a surgical training system, greatly influenced by his European experience, that became the model for all those that were to follow in the United States. This position of influence contributed significantly to his impact on the treatment of cancer of the breast.

What was Halsted's contribution to breast cancer treatment?

Halsted extended the operation devised by von Volkmann. He believed that the Volkmann mastectomy was "obviously incomplete" because it failed to encompass fully the surrounding structures.[45] Halsted noted that von Volkmann's results, along with the results of his contemporaries, were dismal. Billroth, perhaps the most eminent surgeon of the era, had reported an operative mortality rate of 18.5% and an 82% local recurrence rate after only 3 years from treatment. Only 4.7% of Billroth's patients had survived more than 3 years. Halsted decided to include the entire pectoralis major muscle. Gross infiltration of the pectoralis major muscle was not uncommon, given the advanced presentations of many of the patients on whom Halsted operated.[46] This is clearly reflected by one hospital summary from 1905 in which Halsted describes an 8-cm cancer as "small" (Fig. 21–8).

In his first published reference to his operative approach to cancer of the breast in 1891, Halsted stated his reason for excising the pectoralis major muscle:

About eight years ago, I began not only to typically clean out the axilla in all cases of cancer of the breast but also to excise in almost every case the pectoralis major muscle, or at least a generous piece of it, and to give the tumor on all sides an exceedingly wide berth. It is impossible to determine with the naked eye whether or not the disease has extended into the pectoral muscle.

From the careful microscopical examination of many very small cancers of the breast, I am convinced that the pectoralis major muscle is usually, at the time of the operation, involved in the new growth. Strange to say, no authorities (to my knowledge) suggest the advisability of always removing the pectoralis major muscle or a portion of it in operations for the cure of cancer of the breast; and still stranger there are many surgeons of the first rank—surgeons in favor of methodically cleaning out the axilla—who instead of recommending the excision of the muscle advise the removal of the fascia only from the pectoral muscle. König, for example, in the fourth edition of his Surgery says: "When the fascia over the pectoralis major muscle is diseased, it [the fascia] must be removed." Surely it is absurd not to remove the muscle when its fascia is, even to the naked eye, diseased.[47]

The en bloc removal of the breast and pectoralis major muscle with wide resection of the skin and axillary nodes became known as the Halsted mastectomy.

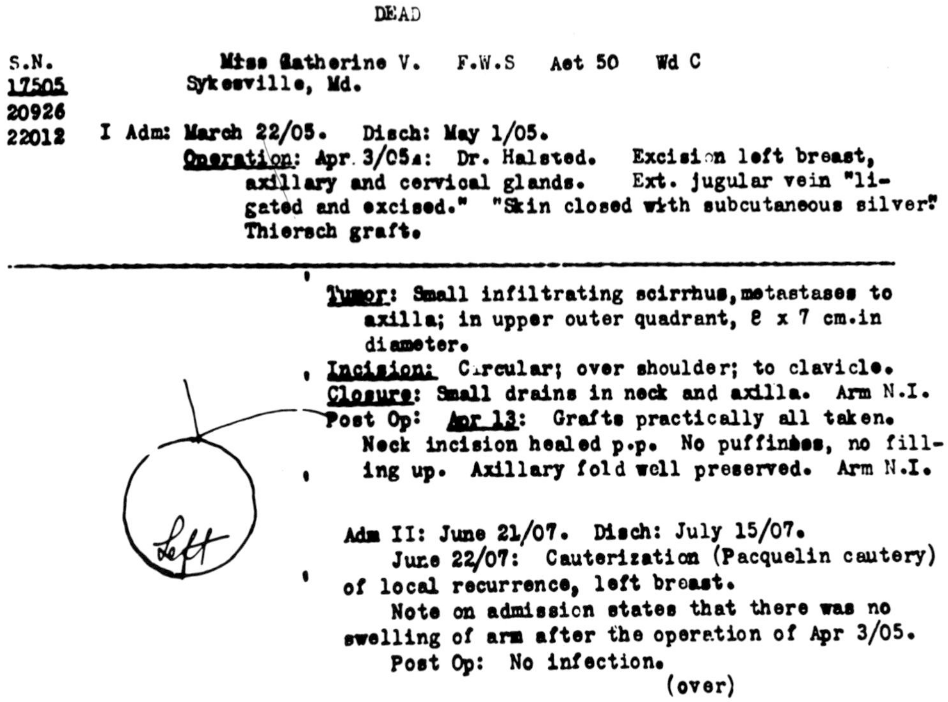

DEAD

```
S.N.        Miss Gatherine V.    F.W.S    Aet 50    Wd C
17505       Sykesville, Md.
20926
22012    I Adm: March 22/05.   Disch: May 1/05.
            Operation: Apr. 3/05a:  Dr. Halsted.   Excision left breast,
               axillary and cervical glands.    Ext. jugular vein "li-
               gated and excised."  "Skin closed with subcutaneous silver?
               Thiersch graft.
```

```
            Tumor: Small infiltrating scirrhus, metastases to
               axilla; in upper outer quadrant, 8 x 7 cm.in
               diameter.
            Incision:  Circular; over shoulder; to clavicle.
            Closure: Small drains in neck and axilla.   Arm N.I.
            Post Op:  Apr 13:  Grafts practically all taken.
               Neck incision healed p.p.  No puffiness, no fill-
               ing up.  Axillary fold well preserved.  Arm N.I.

            Adm II: June 21/07.  Disch: July 15/07.
               June 22/07:  Cauterization (Pacquelin cautery)
            of local recurrence, left breast.
               Note on admission states that there was no
            swelling of arm after the operation of Apr 3/05.
               Post Op:  No infection.
                                                   (over)
```

Figure 21-8 A summary report of a patient treated by Halsted in 1905 describing an 8-cm cancer as "small." (From Lewison EF, Montague AC [eds]. Current Concepts: Diagnosis and Treatment of Breast Cancer. Baltimore, Williams & Wilkins, 1981, p 7.)

Why was the Halsted mastectomy viewed as an advance in breast cancer treatment?

At first, the Halsted operation was called the complete operation, then the radical mastectomy. The original Halsted mastectomy consisted of en bloc removal of the entire breast and wide excision of the overlying skin, full dissection of the axilla, and resection of the pectoralis major muscle. In 1894, he wrote in the Johns Hopkins Hospital Reports,

The pectoralis major muscle, entire or all except its clavicular portion, should be excised in every case of cancer of the breast, because the operator is enabled thereby to remove in one piece all of the suspected tissues.

The suspected tissue should be removed in one piece, 1) lest the wound become infected by the division of tissues invaded by the disease or of lymphatic vessels containing cancer cells, and 2) because shreds or pieces of cancerous tissue might readily be overlooked in the piecemeal extirpation.[46]

In his 1894 paper, Halsted was able to report dramatic results with 50 patients who had been treated by his mastectomy since 1889. He maintained that "the efficiency of an operation is measured truer in terms of local recurrence than of ultimate cure."[46] Halsted compared the local recurrence rate in his patients with the results achieved by surgeons in Europe who were performing the von Volkmann mastectomy. In the European experience, local recurrence rates ranged from 51% to 82%, whereas Halsted was able to report an incidence of only 6% (Fig. 21–9).

Halsted's 6% local recurrence rate was particularly striking in light of his patients' advanced stages of disease. "The prognosis at the time of the operation was recorded as hopeless or unfavorable in 27 of the 50 cases of complete operation," he wrote. "In every one of the 50 cases, some or all of the axillary glands were cancerous."[46]

Local Recurrence Rates

Surgeon	Time Period	No. of Cases	Rate
Bergmann	1882–1887	114	51%–60%
Billroth	1867–1876	170	82%
Czerny	1877–1886	102	62%
Fischer	1871–1878	147	75%
Gussenbauer	1878–1886	151	64%
Halsted	1889–1894	50	6%
König	1875–1885	152	58%–62%
Küster	1871–1885	228	60%
Lücke	1881–1890	110	66%
Von Volkmann	1874–1878	131	60%

Figure 21-9 Halsted's report of his surgical experience compared with those of his European contemporaries. (Data from Halsted WS. The results of operations for the cure of cancer of the breast performed at the Johns Hopkins Hospital from June, 1889, to January, 1894. Johns Hopkins Hosp Rep 1894–1895;4:297–350.)

Halsted, in his analysis of the results, followed von Volkmann's definition of cure, which required patients to be disease free after 3 years. Halsted noted, "As to ultimate results, permanent cures effected by the operation—we again look to [von] Volkmann [who stated:] 'I unhesitatingly make this statement for all cancers, that when a whole year has passed and the most careful examination can detect neither a local recurrence nor swollen glands, nor any symptoms of internal disease, one may begin to hope that a permanent cure may be effected; but after two years, and after three years without exception, one may feel sure of the result.'"[45]

In 1898, Halsted reported to the American Surgical Association the results of 133 breast cancer operations performed at the Johns Hopkins Hospital over a 9-year period (1889–1898). Of the 133 patients, 13 (9%) had local

No one who h...
on a cancer of...
his extraordin...
and absorbed ...
directing his st...
delicate but fa...
disease relentl...
union; his mi...
infection and ...
point so that t...
negligible; his ...
autogenic skin...
and has never...
wound, coveri...
dressing, gave...
the performar...
minute labor ...
a master work...
discipline and...
was practicall...
invariably by ...

Halsted hi...

Operating for...
attempt more ...
including the ...
from two to f...
assistants; it i...
and the patie...

Halsted's i...
the "surgery ...
meticulous t...
surgeons wh...
similar resid...
As Samuel C...
and had dev...
1912,

The operatin...
1889–1890 v...
insisted on r...
tissues with ...
example, tha...
be subordin...

His techn...
surgeon in ...
Halsted stat...

I believe tha...
when opera...
might becon...
has passed t...
everywhere ...
liberation of ...
lymphatic v...
liberation of ...

In his 1...
Halsted not...

women are ...
examinatio...

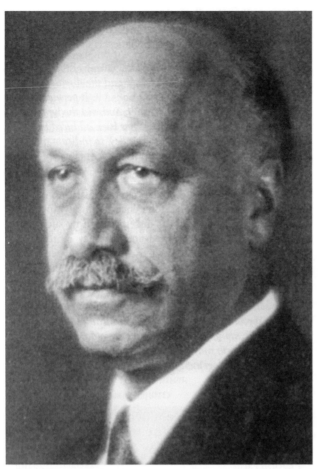

Figure 21–10 Willy Meyer (1858–1932), who reported on a radical mastectomy in 1894, the same year as Halsted. (From Walsh JJ. History of Medicine in New York, vol 4. New York, National Americana Society, 1919.)

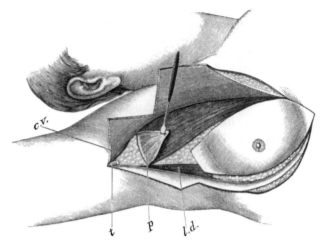

Figure 21–11 The mastectomy incision of Meyer.

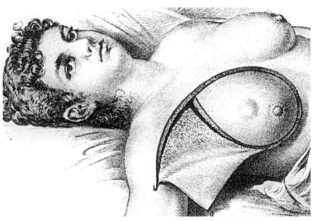

Figure 21–12 The mastectomy incision of Halsted. (From Halsted WS. The Surgical Papers, vol 2. Baltimore, Johns Hopkins Press, 1924.)

recurrences, and 22 (16%) had cervical or internal mammary regional recurrences. Of 76 patients who were operated on 3 or more years previously, 40 (52%) lived without signs of local recurrences or regional metastases for more than 3 years.[48] By contrast, the comparable disease-free survival statistics reported by Halsted from the European review of operations performed before the introduction of the radical mastectomy ranged from a low of 4.7% (Billroth) to a high of 30.2% (Bergmann).

Were there other surgeons proposing operations similar to Halsted's?

On September 19, 1894, the same year that Halsted reported on his initial 50 patients at the Johns Hopkins Hospital, Willy Meyer (1858–1932) (Fig. 21–10) of the New York Post-Graduate Medical School (now part of the New York University Medical Center) described a similar operation for breast cancer. Meyer, who had been born and educated in Germany before coming to the United States in 1884, developed his procedure independently of Halsted. It differed from Halsted's in certain details. First, Meyer made a diagonal incision (Fig. 21–11) in the breast rather than the teardrop incision preferred by Halsted (Fig. 21–12). Second, Meyer excised

the pectoralis minor muscle along with the pectoralis major, whereas Halsted divided the pectoralis minor but did not excise it.[49] Meyer's diagonal excision eventually came to be used more frequently than the teardrop incision, and Halsted himself later excised the pectoralis minor as well.

Both Halsted and Meyer emphasized the need to excise wide margins of skin and to immediately close the defect with a graft. In his 1898 report, Halsted noted, "We remove rather more skin than we did originally, and in all cases we graft the wound immediately. Grafts are cut from the patient's thighs large as or larger than one's hand. A single one of these large grafts may be enough to cover the raw surface."[48] Skin grafting, as practiced by Halsted, had originally been developed by 1886 by Thiersch, one of the surgeons whose clinic Halsted had visited on his tour of Germany.

For a time, Halsted extended the radical mastectomy to include routine removal of the ipsilateral supraclavicular nodes, viewing metastases to these nodes as equivalent to those in the axilla. The excision of anterior mediastinal nodes was first performed by one of his residents, Harvey Cushing (1869–1939), in cases of recurrent disease. Eventually, Halsted abandoned the practice of excising the supraclavicular nodes when he was unable to demonstrate an improvement in

outcome. He di
extension of hi
porated en bloc

Despite his ef
marks of his ra
early interventic
his 1894 paper,

*But now we can
curable disease i
emphasize too s
very early in cai
reason for not lc
operation.*[46]

Halsted was a
instances and
cancer by stage

*I know of no ve
of the breast wi
the importance
possible, is so e*

**What was
of cancer c**

In a 1907 rep
with the perm
by his Englisl
Sampson Ha

Figure 21–1
along with F
breast cance
Annals. Ann S

When was radiation introduced as a treatment of breast cancer?

In 1896, within one year after Roentgen reported on his discovery of x-rays using a cathode-ray tube, Emile Grubbe treated a woman with breast cancer. As he reported many years later, the patient survived only 1 month.[56] The biologic effects of radiation at that time were obviously untested. Soon thereafter, Marie and Pierre Curie, who discovered the emission of radiation by uranium crystals in 1896, noted inflammation and the shedding of skin at the ends of their fingers which had held radioactive materials. Henry Becquerel, after carrying in his vest pocket a small tube of radium given to him by the Curies wrapped in paper and a cardboard box for several hours, noted that a burn had developed on the underlying skin, the exact shape of the oblong tube. Subsequently, Pierre Curie observed that after strapping a radium fragment to his forearm for 10 hours, he also developed an area of inflammation which sloughed and subsequently healed. Furthermore, hair did not return to the healed skin. Becquerel and Pierre Curie reported these findings in 1901.[57] Soon thereafter, a number of investigators began attempting the use of radium in the treatment of benign cutaneous neoplasms. Alexander Graham Bell, for one, suggested in 1903 that radium be placed in a glass tube, which might then be inserted into a cancer.[58] Carcinoma of the cervix became an appropriate lesion upon which to initiate this new theory, and several dramatic responses were noted.

Breast cancer, an accessible lesion, became a target lesion early on in this effort. In 1906, there was a report from Boston on the use of radiation as primary therapy for breast cancer, and 2 years later a French physician, George Chicotot, attempted radiotherapy for breast cancer in Paris, memorializing his effort in a painting he did of himself and the patient[59] (Fig. 21–14). Not surprisingly, the often unrealistic expectations that had been generated by early enthusiasts inevitably gave way to pessimism as primitive equipment, the lack of ability to measure dose, and the general ignorance of the other biologic effects of radiation led to the use of massive radiation exposures aimed at eradicating tumors in one treatment. Significant morbidity and even mortality, let alone long-term complications and a high rate of recurrence, undermined the initial enthusiasm for the technique.

In 1919, Claude Regaud promoted the crucial concept of dose fractionation. He argued that malignant tumors mimicked the high cell turnover rate of spermatogenesis in the testes of experimental animals, which he was able to eliminate by sequential daily fractionated doses of radiotherapy. A single massive dose was not able to produce the same effect, while its toxicity to skin was prohibitive.[60] Similarly fractionated doses applied to cancer would be both more effective and safer. With Henri Coutard, a fellow worker at the Curie Foundation in Paris, efforts were initiated to treat head and neck cancer as well as cancer of the cervix.[61,62]

Although the treatment of breast cancer by radiotherapy became more common, its acceptance was limited to its use in treating local recurrences after surgery. The first major effort at primary radiation treatment for breast cancer was made by the English surgeon Geoffrey Keynes in 1922 using radium needles. Working at the St. Bartholomew's Hospital in London, he first applied this method without surgery, for

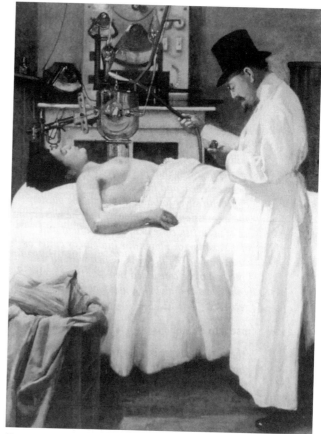

Figure 21–14   Painting by George Chicotot, *The First Trial of X-ray Therapy for Cancer of the Breast* (1908, Musée de l'Assistance Publique, Paris.) The physician pictured is Chicotot himself.

advanced and inoperable cases. In 1932, he was able to report a 77.1% 5-year survival in the absence of palpable nodes and a 33.6% survival with axillary metastases. Keynes extended his use of radiation therapy for more operable lesions, combining it with conservative surgery, having begun with very advanced inoperable tumors.[63] By 1937 he was able to report an 83.5% 3-year survival for patients whose lesions were confined to the breast treated by radium implants, and he suggested that the most effective therapy was the surgical excision of clinically obvious disease followed by radiation therapy to destroy any subclinical disease that may have remained.[64] Keynes proposed this treatment as an alternative to the radical mastectomy while recognizing that radiation was not without complications as a result of scarring and neurologic injury. His efforts were interrupted by the outbreak of World War II, when supplies of radium in London were dispersed because of the danger of air raids and when Keynes himself had joined the Royal Air Force.[65] In the United States, George E. Pfahler also reported in 1932 on an experience with the use of postoperative radiation, noting an improved survival in patients with axillary metastases.[66]

When was a systemic concept of disease treatment introduced?

Even before the emergence of radiation as a form of cancer therapy, hormonal manipulation had been recognized as influential in the progress of breast cancer. Sir Astley Cooper as early as 1835 had referred to observations he had made on size variations of tumors in pre- and postmenopausal patients as well as a greater frequency of the disease in nulliparous women.[67] In 1889, Albert Schinziger (1827-1911) proposed oophorectomy as a form of treatment based on his observation that the prognosis was worse in younger patients and the unlikely premise that this procedure might make women "a little bit older."[68] It was George Beatson (1848-1933) of Glasgow, however, who first performed a bilateral salpingo-oophorectomy on a 33-year-old woman with a chest wall metastasis from breast cancer in June of 1895. The dramatic response led him to treat two other similar patients, one of whom again demonstrated a response. He reported his experiences in 1896.[69] Other surgeons subsequently attempted oophorectomy in young patients with advanced disease. Subsequently, ovarian ablation by radiation was used by some as an alternative to surgical oophorectomy.

How was halstedian surgery extended?

The effort to follow halstedian principles was extended by the adoption of the frozen section technique for tissue preparation and rapid diagnosis by Rutherford in 1871[70] and promoted initially at the Johns Hopkins Hospital in 1895.[71] Frozen section preparation of biopsy tissue allowed surgery to be performed immediately after histologic diagnosis, a concept fully in keeping with the halstedian hypothesis of rapidly encompassing the disease process without delay or risking its dissemination through any surgical means. Most important, it withdrew any reservations about the histologic verification and study of disease, particularly as more patients were presenting with less advanced and clinically obvious disease. At the same time, halstedian principles were extended anatomically even further as attention was directed to internal mammary metastases. Richard S. Handley (1909–1984), stimulated by the observance of parasternal recurrences after radical mastectomy made by his father, W. S. Handley,[72] performed internal mammary node biopsies. In R. S. Handley's initial series of 50 patients, a significant 38% rate of metastases was demonstrated.[73] These observations suggested that the radical mastectomy was inadequate because it did not encompass this frequent site of regional metastases. W. S. Handley proposed treating the internal mammary nodes with interstitial radiation, but other surgeons began to develop surgical procedures that would encompass this drainage site en bloc with a radical mastectomy. Such an operation became formalized first by Mario Margottini (1898–1981) in Italy in 1948 and subsequently by Jerome Urban (1914–1991), among others.[74–76] Erling Dahl-Iversen (1892–1978) in Denmark again adopted Halsted's initial efforts to excise the supraclavicular as well as the internal mammary nodes as separate procedures at the time of radical mastectomy.[77] The most radical extension of halstedian doctrine was reported by Prudente in France, who treated advanced cases by a trans-scapulothoracic amputation of the upper extremity en bloc with the mastectomy.[78] Owen Wangensteen (1898–1981) also developed a "super-radical" mastectomy, which combined a radical mastectomy with resection of the supraclavicular, internal mammary, and mediastinal lymph nodes.[79] When an improvement in survival could not be demonstrated, and with an operative mortality

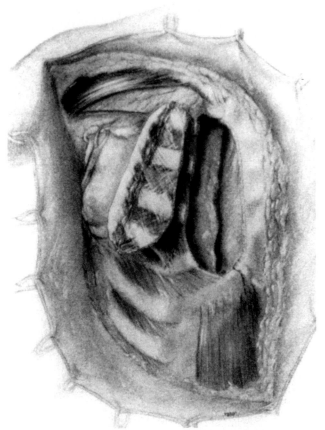

Figure 21–15 Extended radical mastectomy of Urban. The sternum has been split, and the chest wall is separated by cutting through the ribs and intercostal soft tissues just lateral to the costochondral junctions of the second through fifth ribs to achieve resection of the internal mammary chain in continuity with the overlying muscles and breast. (From Urban JA, Baker HW. Radical mastectomy in continuity with en bloc resection of the internal mammary lymph node chain. Cancer 1952;5:992–1008. Copyright © 1952 American Cancer Society. Reprinted by permission of Wiley-Liss, Inc., a subsidiary of John Wiley & Sons, Inc.)

of 12.5%, the procedure was abandoned.[80] An extended radical mastectomy continued to be advocated by Urban based on the premise that the lymphatic drainage of medial lesions was also to the internal mammary nodes (Fig. 21–15).

As extended radical procedures were attempted, there was a growing recognition of the multicentric evolution of breast cancer in many instances, an observation first made by G. L. Cheatle in England[81] in 1920, as well as the risk for contralateral breast cancer. This provided additional support for the basic concept of mastectomy, although conceptually detached from the lymphatic permeation theories that had been previously embraced, even for lesions far smaller than Halsted had encountered, and led some, such as New York surgeon George Pack (1898–1969), in 1951 to advocate bilateral mastectomies in the treatment of clinically unilateral disease.[82]

When did the radical mastectomy begin to lose favor?

While efforts were being made to encompass wider zones of local lymphatic permeation, evidence began to accumulate that lymphatic permeation could not be implicated in the dissemination of disease, as Halsted and Handley had proposed. The concept of en bloc resection was first called into question when J. H. Gray reported, in 1938, that lymphatic permeation was rarely observed through lymphatic channels extending from the primary lesion to the regional lymph nodes.[83] An alternative concept of lymphatic embolization was consistent with the concept of metastasis first established by the studies of Thiersch and Waldeyer. There also seemed to be a paucity of lymphatic vessels on or even approaching the deep fascia of the pectoralis major muscle, further undermining a basic premise of halstedian doctrine.

There also emerged the growing recognition of an intraepithelial phase in breast cancer evolution first recognized grossly by Joseph C. Bloodgood (1967–1935), who as an assistant to Halsted commented on the exudation from a clinically benign tumor "many grayish-white granular cylinders, which I called comedos."[84] Following further histologic observations by numerous investigators it was termed "in-situ" by Broders in 1932 and was notable for the absence of malignant cell migration beyond the ductal basement membrane[85] and for the absence of lymphatic permeation and lymph node involvement.[86] By the end of the 1930s, there began to emerge a reassessment of the concept of lymphatic permeation as a foundation for extensive surgery along with a growing appreciation of more favorable histologic characteristics for many cancers, which differed from those of the tumors for which radical procedures had been devised.

Halsted, as already noted, recognized that as many as 25% of his patients without lymph node metastases died of breast cancer. Furthermore, when his patients were followed for longer than 3 years, it became clear that the success of long-term cure diminished as even more time elapsed from the dates of initial treatment. As patients were followed to 5 and 10 years, there was a progressive decrease in survival, an observation also noted in series from the Massachusetts General Hospital, as reported by Greenough and colleagues in 1907,[87] and from the Mayo Clinic, as originally reported by Judd and Sistrunk in 1914[88] and then by Harrington in 1929.[89] In 1922, the eminent pathologist James Ewing (1866–1943) wrote,

From clinical and pathological studies I have drawn the impression that, in dealing with mammary cancer, surgery meets with more peculiar difficulties and uncertainties than with almost any other form of the disease. The anatomical types of the disease are so numerous, the variations in clinical course so wide, the paths of dissemination so free and diverse, the difficulties of determining the actual conditions so complex, and the sacrifice of tissue so great as to render impossible in a majority of cases a reasonably accurate adjustment of means to ends. The scope of the operative field having apparently reached a limit, the chief hope for a reduction in the mortality from mammary carcinoma lies in its prevention and earlier diagnosis.[90]

When was staging introduced?

As the surgical treatment of breast cancer expanded, Halsted's prophecy that women would present for treatment at earlier stages of disease was fulfilled. The broader spectrum of breast cancer faced by surgeons required appropriate prognostic criteria to enable meaningful study. The first attempt to establish a staging system based on clinical criteria is credited to Steinthal of Stuttgart[91] in 1905. More widely accepted was the clinical Manchester Staging System introduced in England in 1940[92] and the Portmann Classification introduced in Cleveland in 1943.[93]

However, it was Cushman Haagensen, a vigorous exponent of radical mastectomy, and Arthur Purdy Stout in the early 1940s who paradoxically signaled a retreat from the uniform application of the radical mastectomy by identifying those prognostic factors that made the procedure inappropriate. In reviewing more than 568 patients with breast cancer treated by the radical mastectomy at the Columbia-Presbyterian Hospital from 1915 to 1942, Haagensen and Stout defined three features that were associated with 100% mortality at 5 years and a 60% incidence of local recurrence despite treatment by radical mastectomy.[94,95] These features were edema of the skin that extended over one third of the breast, satellite nodules of cancer within the skin, and erythema and edema over one third of the breast indicative of inflammatory carcinoma. They also defined other features indicative of inoperability, which included internal mammary nodal metastases, supraclavicular nodal metastases, extensive axillary metastases leading to edema of the arm, and, of course, distant metastases. They further identified additional "grave signs," any two of which also placed the patient in the same inoperable category. These included edema of the skin over less than one third of the breast, skin ulceration, chest wall fixation, axillary lymph nodes greater than 2.5 cm in diameter, and fixation of the axillary lymph nodes to the skin or deep structures of the axilla. More prognostically favorable lesions were categorized by the size of the tumor or the presence or absence of movable axillary lymph nodes. The Columbia Clinical Classification (Table 21–1), dividing patients into stages A, B, C, and D, became the most important early classification system by which to stage patients for surgical treatment and to assess prognosis and long-term survival following treatment.[96]

What advances led to radiotherapy as a primary modality of therapy?

Between 1920 and 1940, kilovoltage therapy was developed. This was first introduced by William David Coolidge (1873–1977), who invented a vacuum x-ray tube that could produce energies as high as 200 kV.[97] Physicists studying the effects of radiation quantitated the radiation dose by identifying the first physical unit for measurement of radiation, the roentgen, which was replaced by the rad in 1956, as techniques for delivering radiation were refined. The physical dose distribution of 200 kV limited the use of kilovoltage therapy to superficial lesions. Higher beams of energy clearly had to be developed if greater cure rates were to be realized for deeper lesions.[98] Radioactive cobalt provided by nuclear fission soon after World War II provided a substitute for radium, which was extremely expensive. Concurrently, new electronic devices, such as the betatron and the linear electron accelerator, could provide beams of very high energy. Such megavoltage energies were able to produce their maximal ionization at levels much deeper than the skin, and the limitation of skin tolerance was no longer a major issue.[99]

Table 21–1   Columbia Clinical Classification

Stage A No skin edema, ulceration, or solid fixation of tumor to chest wall; axillary nodes not clinically involved
Stage B No skin edema, ulceration, or solid fixation of tumor to chest wall; clinically involved nodes, but <2.5 cm in transverse diameter and not fixed to overlying skin or deeper structures of axilla
Stage C Any of five grave signs of advanced breast cancer: • Edema of skin of limited extent (involving less than one third of the skin over the breast) • Skin ulceration • Solid fixation of tumor to chest wall • Massive involvement of axillary lymph nodes (measuring ≥2.5 cm in transverse diameter) • Fixation of the axillary nodes to overlying skin or deeper structures of the axilla
Stage D All other patients with advanced breast cancer, including • A combination of any two or more of the five grave signs listed under stage C • Extensive edema of the skin (involving more than one third of the skin over the breast) • Satellite skin nodules • The inflammatory type of carcinoma • Clinically involved supraclavicular lymph nodes • Internal mammary metastases, as evidenced by a parasternal tumor • Edema of the arm • Distant metastases

Adapted from Haagensen CD. Diseases of the Breast, 3rd ed. Philadelphia, WB Saunders, 1971, p 630.

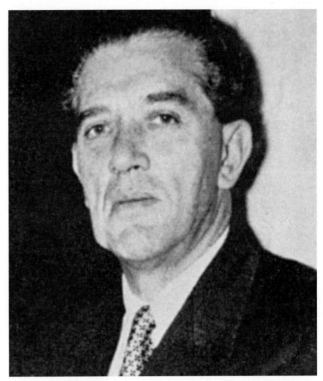

Figure 21–16   Robert McWhirter (1904–1994), who began to treat patients with radiation after total mastectomy as an alternative to radical mastectomy.   (Courtesy of New York Academy of Medicine.)

These advances made it possible to apply radiation therapy not only as a substitute for surgery for inoperable cases but also as an adjunct to the radical mastectomy for patients at high risk for local recurrence. In the 1930s, François Baclesse (1896–1967) administered radiation to 21 patients before surgery. Of note is the fact that in one third of the patients treated with preoperative radiation therapy, no tumor was found in the mastectomy specimens, with almost all of the others demonstrating marked changes in tumor morphology.[100] With larger series and longer follow-up, however, survival rates seemed the same, and there was a growing consensus that radiation therapy could be reserved for use following mastectomy, if necessary.

More significantly, some investigators began to use radiation as an adjunct to lesser surgical procedures. In 1941, Robert McWhirter (1904–1994) (Fig. 21–16) in Edinburgh began to perform mastectomy alone followed by postoperative irradiation of the axillary, supraclavicular, and internal mammary lymph nodes for patients with operable breast cancer, instead of a radical mastectomy, with comparable 5-year survival rates. For the first time, combining two modalities of therapy in the treatment of operable breast cancer was presented as a viable option.[101] In a trial conducted by Sigvaard Kaae and Helge Johansen[102] in Copenhagen between 1951 and 1957, patients were randomized to treatment with either extended radical mastectomy or total mastectomy and postoperative radiation therapy. Survival rates and local recurrence rates were equivalent, further supporting the use of

radiation therapy in the treatment of subclinical disease. This concept was extended to the breast itself by François Baclesse at the Curie Foundation, who began to treat patients with both operable and inoperable disease by radiotherapy, in most cases without excision of the tumor. Dosage was adjusted based on the size of the tumor, and the radiation portals were adjusted as well, based on the findings in the axilla. Although Baclesse concluded that this was not appropriate for all cases, he did suggest that in selected instances and for those who refused mastectomy, radiation was an alternative.[103] Sakari Mustakallio[104] in Finland initiated an effort to excise favorable lesions followed by radiation to the breast through tangential portals as well as axillary and supraclavicular radiation.

When was the radical mastectomy modified?

David H. Patey (1889–1977) and W. H. Dyson, of the Middlesex Hospital in London, began to question the appropriateness of routine removal of the pectoralis major muscle, particularly in instances in which there was no discernible involvement by the tumor. Because the original halstedian concept was based on large lesions often abutting or affixed to the pectoralis major muscle and the concept of continuous lymphatic tumor extension, removal of the pectoralis major muscle became increasingly questioned. While the pectoralis major was preserved in Patey's procedure, most of the other components of Halsted's procedure were left intact, including removal of the pectoralis minor, a complete axillary dissection, and excisions of wide margins of skin. Patey and Dyson first reported on their technique in 1948.[105] A subsequent analysis by Handley and Thackray of 143 patients treated with Patey's procedure at the Middlesex Hospital showed survival equivalent to that of radical mastectomy in patients classified as stage A by the Columbia Clinical Classification (see Table 21–1), with no recurrences in the pectoralis major muscle being noted.[106]

How did mammography alter therapeutic thinking?

Although efforts to detect breast cancer radiographically were made throughout the century, Jacob Gershon-Cohen in Philadelphia vigorously pursued this diagnostic technique and was able to demonstrate in 1948 the ability to detect nonpalpable carcinoma.[107] The feasibility of diagnosing breast cancer radiographically became increasingly evident through the efforts of Robert Egan[108] and others, and by the 1960s, strategies were proposed for evaluating asymptomatic patients in screening programs.[109] Initial data suggested that mortality could indeed be reduced by such an approach, and despite concern that mammography could itself induce breast cancer if used inappropriately and excessively, a concern largely abated by smaller radiation dosage, mammography became integrated into the diagnostic armamentarium of physicians.[110] This led to the detection of an increasing number of clinically occult and prognostically favorable cancers, providing even greater impetus to reducing the extent of surgery. If the radical mastectomy had demonstrated the feasibility of curing breast cancer and had encouraged women to seek treatment earlier, as Halsted had predicted, was it not equally appropriate to propose that a further inducement to earlier diagnosis would be a reduction not only in breast cancer mortality but also in the extent of surgery?

What led to a permanent withdrawal from radical mastectomy?

Increasingly, surgeons began to adopt the modification of the radical mastectomy proposed by Patey and Dyson, essentially the same prehalstedian operation that had been performed by Moore in 1867. In 1953, I. G. Williams and his colleagues[111] reviewed 1044 cases of breast cancer treated at St. Bartholomew's Hospital in London from 1930 to 1939. They found that the 10-year survival rates of patients treated by radical mastectomy, modified radical mastectomy, or simple mastectomy did not differ, with or without the use of additional radiation therapy. In the United States, the modified radical mastectomy was championed by such surgeons as John L. Madden[112] and Hugh Auchincloss.[113] The better cosmetic and functional results following the procedure were emphasized, and survival rates appeared comparable to those following Halsted's radical mastectomy. The extensive removal of skin advocated by Halsted, and even by Patey and Dyson in their modification, became questioned, and primary skin closures were increasingly achieved with reduced skin margins.

By 1972, the frequency with which the radical mastectomy was performed began to decline dramatically. Data developed by the Commission on Cancer of the American College of Surgeons revealed that between 1972 and 1981, use of the radical mastectomy had plummeted from 47.9% of operations for breast cancer to 3.4%. At the same time, the frequency with which the modified radical mastectomy—an often ill-defined designation—was performed had risen from 27.7% of operations for breast cancer to 73.2%.[114] By 1974, the modified radical mastectomy had eclipsed the radical mastectomy as the most widely performed procedure for breast cancer in the United States. During this time, reconstruction of the breast following mastectomy was introduced, first with implant placement techniques,[115,116] and then with autologous musculocutaneous flaps using the latissimus dorsi[117] or rectus abdominis muscles.[118]

The justification for lesser operative procedures was supported by the relative freedom from recurrence in the pectoralis major muscle following procedures in which it was preserved.[83] Evidence presented by Engell[119] that there was venous dissemination of cancer cells, not only in breasts but also in other solid tumor models, along with experimental evidence that cancer cells could bypass regional lymph nodes as well as extend from lymphatics to blood vessels, further undermined the concept of contiguous lymphatic permeation and even orderly embolization.[120,121] George Crile Jr., Oliver Cope, Vera Peters, and Bernard Fisher, among others, began to question not only the appropriateness of mastectomy in all instances but also, most important, the biologic principles used to support ablative surgery of the breast and regional lymph nodes. These questions coincided with the emergence of support for, and reliance on, prospective randomized trials to assess more objectively the comparative efficacy of different therapeutic options, not only surgical but also those directed at the increasingly perceived problem of early systemic dissemination. At the forefront of these efforts to carry out controlled clinical trials, with appropriate statistical power derived from the participation of multiple institutions, was the National Surgical Adjuvant Breast and Bowel Project (NSABP), initially founded as the Surgical Adjuvant Chemotherapy Breast Cancer Group, and directed by Bernard Fisher[122] (Fig. 21–17). These studies challenged physicians to prove or disprove clinical hypotheses by scientific methodology and to shun retrospective analyses that purported to support what might well be antiquated thinking that served as the biologic underpinning of surgical therapy.

How did multimodality therapy evolve?

Chemotherapy developed with great rapidity after World War II from several programs that dealt with such diverse goals as chemical warfare, nutrition, and research into basic biochemical mechanisms. The rapid development of chemotherapeutic agents and their potential applications to the treatment of solid tumors compelled the National Institutes of Health to organize national controlled studies to assess their efficacy. During this era as well, a renewed interest arose in the endocrine treatment of breast cancer as Charles B. Huggins (1901–1997) at the University of Chicago in 1941 demonstrated the efficacy of castration in the treatment of metastatic prostatic cancer and proposed that oophorectomy, as had originally been attempted in the late years of the 19th century,

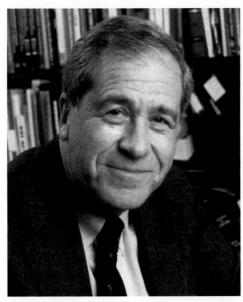

Figure 21–17 Bernard Fisher (1918–), whose championship and successful directorship of controlled clinical trials dramatically altered the direction of local and systemic therapy and led to a rethinking of breast cancer biology.

might be efficacious as well in the treatment of breast cancer.[123,124] The availability of corticosteroids made the prospect of adrenalectomy to further reduce endogenous hormones possible. Both testosterone and synthetic estrogen were used in the treatment of advanced breast cancer, provoking further investigation into the role of hormones in the etiology and promotion of the disease.[125] The demonstration of the estrogen receptor protein by Elwood V. Jensen and associates[126] and by Jack Gorski and associates in 1966[127] and its identification in human breast cancer by William McGuire,[128] and subsequently, the identification of progesterone receptors,[129] provided greater predictability to the impact of hormonal manipulation. The development of antiestrogen compounds, first described in 1971, provided another means of treatment for metastatic breast cancer.[130] Although such advances in chemotherapy and hormonal therapy were directed initially at metastatic disease, they refocused attention, with greater specificity, on the potential for systemic therapy of earlier stages of disease.

By the 1970s, the effectiveness of radiation therapy was becoming well established, and the increasing use of mammography had provided greater impetus toward early diagnosis and a possible reduction in the extent of surgery. The policy of screening populations of normal women with routine periodic mammography received a major impetus from the trial of the Health Insurance Plan (HIP) of Greater New York comparing 62,000 women randomized to have or not have annual mammography. In this trial, annual mammography detected a significant percentage of clinically occult cancers, with an associated 40% reduction in mortality.[131] The progressive realization that any efforts to improve survival might depend on the effective treatment of subclinical local and systemic disease led to a variety of trials initiated to assess the appropriateness of new approaches to local treatment and to assess what might be the impact of systemic drug therapy as

an adjunct to surgery in high-risk patients likely to harbor distant micrometastases.

A randomized trial using thiotepa as an adjuvant to surgical therapy was begun by the NSABP in 1958 under the direction and support of the National Institutes of Health. All patients were treated by a radical mastectomy with chemotherapy delivered at the time of surgery and for 2 days postoperatively so that cells that might have been disseminated at the time of surgery would be destroyed. When compared with patients receiving a placebo, a benefit was suggested for those receiving thiotepa who were premenopausal and had four or more lymph nodes containing metastases.[132] Subsequently, there were numerous trials of adjuvant chemotherapy based not on the presumption of tumor dissemination at the time of surgery but on the recognition of patients at high risk for harboring systemic micrometastases. Two such studies had a particularly strong impact on forming a consensus that adjuvant chemotherapy was of value, which in turn led to further study of a broader spectrum of patients. Between 1972 and 1975, the NSABP compared 349 patients randomized to receive L-phenylalanine mustard (L-PAM) for 2 years or placebo. All patients had been treated by radical mastectomy and had been demonstrated to have nodal metastases. L-PAM was chosen because of its relative lack of toxicity.[133] In another trial begun in 1973 by the Milan Cancer Institute, 386 patients treated with radical mastectomy and proved to have nodal metastases were randomized to receive a regimen of cytoxan, methotrexate, and 5-fluorouracil for 12 cycles given over the course of a year or placebo.[134] In the NSABP trial, a 9% improvement in recurrence-free survival for the treatment group was demonstrated, and in the Milan trial, a 12% improvement was seen, with subset analyses in both trials demonstrating a particularly significant improvement of 17% for premenopausal women. Such data clearly affected survival, a claim that advocates of differing approaches to local therapy could not make. These studies established the early systemic treatment of breast cancer as the linchpin of multimodality therapy and became the prototype for similar efforts with other solid malignant neoplasms.

When did molecular biology first affect breast cancer treatment?

A modern era of hormonal therapy was launched with the identification of estrogen receptor protein in breast cancer cells.[135] Subsequently, progesterone receptor assays became available, and it was shown that a high percentage of patients with advanced breast cancer responded to hormonal therapy when both the estrogen receptor and progesterone receptor were present. The level of hormone receptor and the positivity of only one of the two hormone receptors or the absence of both were directly related to the ability to elicit a response from hormonal ablation. Before then, trials of adjuvant oophorectomy, performed either surgically or by radiotherapeutic ablation, initiated in the 1950s and 1960s for premenopausal or early postmenopausal women, were equivocal. The development of antiestrogens, initially proposed as antifertility drugs, led to the use of one agent, tamoxifen, as a primary treatment option when antihormonal therapy was desired, and was applied to the adjuvant setting in several trials beginning in 1975 for both node-positive and node-negative patients.[136] The survival benefit to women receiving tamoxifen in the treatment of early breast cancer was supported in meta-analyses of adjuvant trials and, as expected, restricted to those with estrogen receptor–positive tumors.[137] An additional observation was a decrease in the development of contralateral breast cancer, particularly in those receiving prolonged therapy, prompting the initiation of the first randomized prevention trials using tamoxifen in women at high risk for developing breast cancer.[138–141] In the NSABP prevention trial (NSABP P-1), tamoxifen reduced breast cancer by 50% in high-risk patients, its effect also being limited to estrogen receptor–positive tumors.[141] The development of selective estrogen receptor modulators (SERMs), such as raloxifene, with potential preferential antiosteoporotic effects, but without undesired agonist effects in the uterus, and the development of aromatase inhibitors to selectively block estrogen production have further broadened the spectrum of antihormonal treatment and possible preventive strategies.

In 1997, Dennis Slamon and associates reported on the adverse impact on prognosis that tumor overexpression of *HER-2/neu*, an epidermal growth factor receptor, had in node-positive patients with breast cancer.[142] This led to the development of the monoclonal antibody trastuzumab[143] (Herceptin, Genentech, Inc., South San Francisco, CA) to interrupt *HER-2/neu* cancer cell growth stimulation.

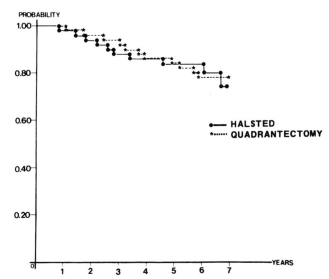

Figure 21–18   Actuarial disease-free survival from the National Tumor Institute of Milan trial comparing radical mastectomy with quadrantectomy, axillary dissection, and radiation. (Data from Veronesi U, Saccozzi R, DelVecchio M, et al. Comparing radical mastectomy with quadrantectomy, axillary dissection, and radiotherapy in patients with small cancers of the breast. N Engl J Med 1981;305:6–11. Copyright © 1981 Massachusetts Medical Society. All rights reserved.)

When was breast conservation established as an alternative to mastectomy?

As prospective randomized adjuvant systemic trials were increasingly applied in the effort to improve survival for high-risk patients, prospective randomized trials became applied as well to assess the efficacy of surgical therapy. Between 1971 and 1974, in 34 institutions participating in the NSABP protocol B-04, 1765 women with primary operable breast cancer and clinically negative axillae were randomized to radical mastectomy, total mastectomy followed by chest wall and regional nodal irradiation, or total mastectomy alone. Delayed axillary dissection was performed for the last group if their nodes became clinically positive. Women with clinically positive axillae were randomized to radical mastectomy or total mastectomy and locoregional radiation.[144] In the node-negative and node-positive groups, there was no difference in disease-free survival or overall survival in any of the treatment arms of the study. This consolidated the inappropriateness of radical mastectomy and provided support for those who viewed skeptically the therapeutic benefit of axillary dissection.

Two additional trials were of particular importance regarding mastectomy, then the foundation stone of surgical therapy. One, conducted by Umberto Veronesi and the National Cancer Institute of Milan between 1973 and 1980, compared 701 patients with lesions 2 cm in diameter or less and clinically negative axillae randomized to either radical mastectomy or quadrantectomy and axillary dissection followed by radiotherapy (QUART). Relapse-free survival and overall survival were the same[145] (Fig. 21–18). Between 1976 and 1984, a second trial begun in the United States by the NSABP (protocol B-06) randomized 1843 patients with lesions up to 4 cm in diameter to total mastectomy or segmental mastectomy (lumpectomy) with or without radiation

therapy.[146] This trial demonstrated that treatment with either total mastectomy or lumpectomy plus radiation was able to achieve equally effective local control of disease and that overall survival was equivalent in all three groups, although lumpectomy alone was significantly inferior to lumpectomy and radiation in achieving disease-free survival in the conserved breast (Fig. 21–19). Twenty-year follow-up of both trials has further confirmed the earlier findings and conclusions.[147,148]

Subsequent trials have been conducted to confirm and refine the appropriateness of breast-conserving treatment. The increasing use of mammography has led to the application of prospective randomized trials in the assessment of breast conservation for the expanding population of patients with noninvasive disease detected mammographically. When mastectomy is required or judged appropriate, reconstruction has been increasingly used with growing confidence that it does not adversely affect survival or the ability to detect recurrent disease.

The other foundation stone of surgical therapy, axillary dissection, has also been subjected to increased scrutiny because its direct therapeutic impact has remained unproven, whereas the prognostic significance of axillary metastases has been enhanced by effective adjuvant systemic therapy. Cabanas[149] introduced the concept that a specific cutaneous site—in the case he reported, a penile carcinoma—would drain not only to a specific nodal site but also to a specific sentinel node. Donald Morton[150] brought this concept into the operating room with great specificity in the treatment of melanoma using blue dye to map the lymphatic circulation and convincingly demonstrated that identifiable sentinel nodes were the first drainage sites not only of cutaneous lymphatics but also of nodal metastases. Armando Giuliano[151] applied this blue dye technique to the treatment of breast cancer to map the lymphatic drainage to the sentinel nodes,

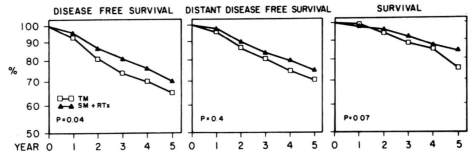

Figure 21–19   Life-table analysis showing disease-free survival, distant disease-free survival, and overall survival of patients treated by the National Surgical Adjuvant Breast and Bowel Project protocol B-06 comparing total mastectomy (TM) vs. segmental mastectomy plus radiation (SM + RTx).   (Data from Fisher B, Baver M, Margoles R, et al. Five-year results of a randomized clinical trial comparing total mastectomy and segmental mastectomy with or without radiation in the treatment of breast cancer. N Engl J Med 1985;312:666–673.)

a technique augmented by the use of radioisotope using a gamma probe as proposed by David Krag and others.[152] The nodal tumor status could thereby be evaluated by the selective assessment of this node or nodes while limiting the extent of surgery for those without nodal metastases. Sentinel lymphadenectomy has now become the focus of intense study and clinical application and is leading to a further redefinition of surgery for cancer of the breast.

SUMMARY

At the beginning of a new century, breast cancer treatment has shifted from a confident belief in the possibilities of improving survival with aggressive local treatment to a far broader effort to utilize the advances in diagnostic radiology, radiation therapy, and chemohormonal therapy to treat more appropriately both the local disease and the possible, often likely, systemic disease. Conservative and selective surgical approaches to the breast and axilla, once viewed as heretical, have become standard forms of therapy for most patients. Improved survival has been achieved for many patients with improvement in diagnostic imaging, technical advances in radiotherapy, the development of effective chemotherapeutic and pharmacologic hormonal agents, and the progressive ability to assay and develop therapies directed at the molecular components of the disease. This shift in treatment paradoxically reflects the still only vaguely understood origins and evolution of breast cancer. Certainly the advances in molecular biology, most significantly the identification of the susceptibility gene for early-onset breast cancer, *BRCA1*, by Mary-Claire King at the University of Washington,[153] followed by *BRCA2*, hold great promise for further directing studies to elucidate the basic mechanisms of breast cancer oncogenesis.

The modern advances in breast cancer treatment and basic research on the molecular biology of the disease have cast the often heroic efforts of our surgical ancestors as primitive, and even inhumane. Placed in a historical context, however, their efforts in the late 19th and early 20th centuries were quite the opposite, demonstrating that survival could be improved and, for the first time, providing evidence that breast cancer could be cured. After centuries of therapeutic nihilism that relegated women to an often painful existence and certain death, their

Table 21–2   Milestones in the Development of Modern Breast Cancer Treatment

Local origin of disease proposed (Henri François Le Dran), circa 1750
Principle of en bloc excision of breast and palpable axillary lymph nodes (Jean Louis Petit), circa 1750
Cellular origins of cancer (Johannes Müller), 1838
Axillary nodes barrier to dissemination (Rudolf Virchow), 1858
Centrifugal local dissemination encompassed by wide excision of breast, skin, axillary nodes, and, if necessary, pectoral muscles (Charles H. Moore), 1867
Inclusion of pectoralis major fascia in mastectomy (Richard von Volkmann), 1875
Radical mastectomy (William S. Halsted, Willy Meyer), 1894
Oophorectomy for metastatic breast cancer (George Beatson), 1896
Primary radiation treatment of breast cancer (Geoffrey Keynes), 1922
Total mastectomy and postoperative regional irradiation (Robert McWhirter),1941
Columbia Clinical Staging (Cushman Haagensen, Arthur Purdy Stout), 1943
Extended (internal mammary dissection) radical mastectomy (Mario Margottini, Jerome Urban), 1948
Mammographic detection of clinically occult breast cancer (Jacob Gershon-Cohen),1948
Modified radical mastectomy (David H. Patey, W. H. Dyson), 1948
Estrogen receptors (Elwood V. Jensen, Jack Gorski, William McGuire), 1950–1960
Excision and locoregional radiation (François Baclesse, Sakari Mustakallio), 1973
Adjuvant chemotherapy trials (Bernard Fisher, Gianni Bonadonna), 1975–1976
Breast conservation trials (Umberto Veronesi, Bernard Fisher), 1981–1985
Breast cancer susceptibility genes *BRCA1* and *BRCA2* (Mary-Claire King), 1990–1996
Sentinel lymphadenectomy (Donald Morton, Armando Giuliano, David Krag), 1991–1998

efforts to effectively ablate local disease, although significantly modified in recent decades, remain a critical component of modern therapy. Most important, their legacy provided the momentum for the present efforts made possible by modern technology, scientific methodology, and molecular biology to further improve survival and even to prevent breast cancer in the near future (Table 21–2).

REFERENCES

1. Breasted JH. The Edwin Smith Surgical Papyrus. Chicago, University of Chicago Press, 1930, pp 363–406.
2. Greaves M. Cancer, The Evolutionary Legacy. New York, Oxford Union Press, 2000, p 141.
3. Adams F, trans. The Genuine Works of Hippocrates. London, Sydenham Society, 1849, p 758.
4. Shimkin MB. Contrary to Nature. US Dept of Health, Education, and Welfare Publication No. (NIH) 76–720. Washington DC, Government Printing Office, 1977.
5. Said HM. Cancer: The last two and a half millennia of etiology and cure. In Twelfth International Cancer Congress, Buenos Aires, Oct 5–11, 1978. Karachi, Pakistan Hamdard Foundation, 1978.
6. Sebastian A. A Dictionary of History of Medicine. London/New York, Parthenon Publishing, 1999, p 147.
7. Galen C. Opera Omnia. Kuhn CG (ed)., Leipzig, 1824.
8. Robinson JO. Treatment of breast cancer through the ages. Am J Surg, 1986;151:317–333.
9. William of Salicet. On scrofula, induration, and cancer of the breast. In Zimmerman LM, Veith I (eds). Great Ideas in the History of Surgery. Baltimore, Williams & Wilkins, 1961, p 112.
10. Wagner FB. History of breast disease and its treatment. In Bland KI, Copeland EM III (eds). The Breast. Philadelphia, WB Saunders, 1991, p 5.
11. Wolff J. Die Lehre von der Krankenheit, vol. 1. Jena, G Fischer, 1907, p 42.
12. Scultetus J. Armamentarius Chirurgicum. Amsterdam, 1741.
13. Meade RH. An Introduction to the History of General Surgery. Philadelphia, WB Saunders, 1968, chap 13.
14. Hilden F von. How a cancer [of the breast] and other complications were caused by curdled milk. In Zimmerman LM, Veith I (eds). Great Ideas in the History of Surgery. Baltimore, Williams & Wilkins, 1961, p 246.
15. Kardinal CG, Yarbro JW. A conceptual history of cancer. Semin Oncol 1979;5:396–408.
16. King LS. The Philosophy of Medicine: The Early Eighteenth Century. Cambridge, MA, Harvard University Press, 1978.
17. Petit JL, cited by Power D. The history of amputation of the breast to 1904. Quoted by Robbins GF (ed). Silvergirl's Surgery: The Breast. Austin, TX, Silvergirl, 1984, p 35.
18. Heister L. General System of Surgery, vol II. London, Innys, 1745, p 14.
19. De Moulin D. A Short History of Breast Cancer. Boston, Martinus Nijhoff, 1983.
20. Burney F. Selected letters and journals. In Hembow J (ed). New York, Oxford University Press, 1986, pp 129–139.
21. Rush B. "Letters of Benjamin Rush." In Butterfield LH (ed). Princeton University Press, 1951, vol 2. Quoted in McCullough D. John Adams. New York, Simon & Schuster, 2001, p 602.
22. Yalom M. A History of the Breast. New York, Knopf, 1997, pp 225–226.
23. Frykberg ER, Bland KI. Evolution of surgical principles for the management of breast cancer. In Bland KI, Copeland EM III (eds). The Breast. Philadelphia, WB Saunders, 1991, pp 543–553.
24. Lewison EF. The surgical treatment of breast cancer: An historical and collective review. Surgery 1953;34:904–953.
25. Paget J. On the average duration of life in patients with scirrhous cancer of the breast. Lancet 1856;1:62–63.
26. Liston R. Elements of Surgery. With notes by Samuel D. Gross. Philadelphia, Barrington & Haswell, 1846, p 412.
27. Agnew DH, quoted in Donegan WL. An introduction to the history of breast cancer. In Donegan WL, Spratt JS (eds). Cancer of the Breast. Philadelphia, Elsevier Science, 2002, p 6.
28. Triolo VA. Nineteenth-century foundations of cancer research: Advances in tumor pathology, nomenclature, and theories of oncogenesis. Cancer Res 1965;25:75–106.
29. Wilder RJ. The historical development of the concept of metastasis. J Mt Sinai Hosp 1956;23:728–734.
30. Sugarbaker EV. Cancer metastases: A product of tumor-host interactions. Curr Probe Cancer 1979;3:7.
31. Virchow R. "Cellular Pathology". Chance F (trans). London, John Churchill, 1860, p 187.
32. Classics in oncology: Sir James Paget. CA Cancer J Clin 1971;21:302–304.
33. Pancoast J. Treatise on Operative Surgery. Philadelphia, Carey & Hart, 1844, p 269.
34. Sweeting R. On a new operation for cancer of the breast. Lancet 1869;1:323.
35. Moore CH. On the influence of inadequate operations on the theory of cancer. R Med Chir Soc Lond 1867;1:244–280.
36. Banks WM. A brief history of the operations practiced for cancer of the breast. Br Med J 1902;1: 5–10.
37. Gross SW. An analysis of two hundred and seven cases of carcinoma of the breast. Med News 1887;51: 413.
38. Lister J. Further evidence regarding the effects of the antiseptic system of treatment upon the salubrity of a surgical hospital. In Collected Papers, vol 2. Oxford, Clarendon Press, 1909, p 158.
39. Kuster E. Zur Behandlung des Brustkrebses. Arch Klin Chir 1883;29:723–735.
40. Haagensen CD. Diseases of the Breast, 3rd ed. Philadelphia, WB Saunders, 1986, chap 54.
41. Heidenheim L. Über die Ursachen der localen Krebsrecidive nach Amputation Mammæ. Arch Klin Chir 1889;39:97–166.
42. Rotter J. Concerning the topography of mammary carcinoma. Arch fur Klinische Chirurgie 1899;58: 346.
43. Stiles H. Contributions to the surgical anatomy of the breast. Edinb Med J 1892;37:1099
44. MacCallum WG. William Stewart Halsted, Surgeon. Baltimore, Johns Hopkins Press, 1930.
45. Halsted WS. The results of operations for the cure of cancer of the breast performed at the Johns Hopkins Hospital from June, 1889 to January, 1894. Johns Hopkins Hosp Rep 1894–1895;4:297–350.
46. Halsted WS. Operation report. In Lewison EF, Montague AC (eds). Current Concepts: Diagnosis and Treatment of Breast Cancer. Baltimore, Williams & Wilkins, 1981, p 7.
47. Halsted WS. The treatment of wounds with especial reference to the value of the blood clot in the management of dead spaces. Johns Hopkins Hosp Rep 1890–1891;2:255–280.
48. Halsted WS. A clinical and histological study of certain adenocarcinomata of the breast and a brief consideration of the supraclavicular operation and of the results of operations for cancer of the breast from 1889 to 1898 at the Johns Hopkins Hospital. Ann Surg 1898;28: 557–576.
49. Meyer W. An improved method of the radical operation for carcinoma of the breast. Med Rec 1894;46:746–749.
50. Halsted WS. The results of radical operations for the cure of cancer of the breast. Ann Surg 1907;46:1–19.
51. Bryant T. The Disease of the Breast. London, Casess & Co, 1887.
52. Matas R. In memoriam—William Stewart Halsted: An appreciation. Bull Johns Hopkins Hosp 1928;36:2–27.
53. Crowe SJ. Halsted of Johns Hopkins: The Man and His Men. Springfield, IL, Thomas, 1957.
54. Bland CS. The Halsted mastectomy: Present illness and past history. West J Med 1981;134:549–555.
55. Shield AM. A Clinical Treatise on Diseases of the Breast. London, Macmillan, 1898.
56. Grubbe EH. X-ray Treatment: Its Origin, Birth, and Early History. St Paul, MN, Blace, 1949.
57. Quinn S. Marie Curie. New York, Simon & Schuster, 1995, chap 8.
58. Bell AG, quoted by Lichter AS. Radiation therapy. In Abeloff MD, Armitage JD, Lichter AS, et al. (eds). Clinical Oncology. New York, Churchill Livingstone, 1995, p 221.
59. Williams FH. A further note on a new method of using roentgen rays: Consideration of primary treatment of some early cases of breast cancer by these rays. Boston Med Surg J 1906;154:641.
60. Regaud C, Ferroux R. Discordance des effets des rayons X, d'une part et la peau, d'autre part dans le testicule, par le fractionnement de la dose. Diminution de l'efficacité dans le peau, maintien d l'efficacité dans le testicule. C R Soc Biol (Paris) 1927;97:431–434.
61. Regaud C. Sur les principles radiophysiologiques de la radiothérapie des cancers. Acta Radiol 1930;11:456–486.
62. Regaud C, Coutard H, Hautant A. Contribution au traitement des cancers endolaryngés par les rayons-X. In Tenth International Congress of Otolaryngology, 1922, pp 19–22.
63. Keynes GL. The radium treatment of carcinoma of the breast. Br J Surg 1932;19:415–480.
64. Keynes GL. Conservative treatment of carcinoma of the breast. Br J Med 1937;2:643–647.
65. Ellis H. A History of Surgery. London, Greenwich Media, Ltd., 2001, p 179.

66. Pfahler GE. Results of radiation therapy in 1,022 private cases of carcinoma of the breast from 1902 to 1928. AJR Am J Roentgenol 1932;27:497.

67. Cooper A. The Anatomy and Diseases of the Breast. Philadelphia, Lea & Blanchard, 1845.

68. Wagner FB. History of breast disease and its treatment. In Bland KI, Copeland EM III (eds). The Breast. Philadelphia, WB Saunders, 1991, p 14.

69. Beatson GT. On the treatment of inoperable cases of carcinoma of the mamma: Suggestions for a new method of treatment, with illustrative cases. Lancet 1896;2:104–107.

70. Rutherford W, cited by Schofer AE. A Course of Practical Histology. London, Smith Elder, 1877, p 285.

71. Cullen TS. A rapid method of making permanent specimens from frozen section by the use of formalin. Bull Johns Hopkins Hosp 1895;6:67–73.

72. Handley WS. Cancer of the Breast and Its Treatment, 2nd ed. London, John Murray, 1922, p 256.

73. Handley RS, Thackray AC. The internal mammary lymph chain in carcinoma of the breast: Study of 50 cases. Lancet 1949;2:276.

74. Margottini M. Recent developments in the surgical treatment of breast cancer. Acta Union Int Contra Cancer 1952;8:176–178.

75. Sugarbaker ED. Radical mastectomy combined with incontinuity resection of the homolateral internal mammary node chain. Cancer 1953;6:969–979.

76. Urban JA. Surgical excision of internal mammary nodes for breast cancer. Br J Surg 1964;51:209–212.

77. Dahl-Iversen E, Tobiassen T. Radical mastectomy with parasternal and supraclavicular dissection for mammary carcinoma. Ann Surg 1969;170:889–891.

78. Prudente A. L'amputation inter-scapulo-mammothoracique (technique et résultats). J Chir (Paris) 1949;65:729.

79. Wangensteen OH. Carcinoma of the breast. Ann Surg 1950;132:833–843.

80. Wangensteen OH, Lewis FJ, Arhelger SW. The extended or super-radical mastectomy for carcinoma of the breast. Surg Clin North Am 1956;36:1051–1063.

81. Cheatle GL. Benign and malignant changes in the epithelium of the breast. Br J Surg 1920;8:21.

82. Pack GT. Argument for bilateral mastectomy. Surgery 1951;29:929–931.

83. Gray JH. The relation of lymphatic vessels to the spread of cancer. Br J Surg 1938;26:462–495.

84. Bloodgood JC. Comedo carcinoma (or comedo-adenoma) of the female breast. Am J Cancer 1934;22:842–853.

85. Broders AC. Carcinoma in-situ contrasted with benign penetrating epithelium. JAMA 1932;99:1670–1674.

86. Fechner RE. History of ductal carcinoma in situ. In Silverstein M (ed). Ductal Carcinoma in Situ. Philadelphia, Lippincott Williams & Wilkins, 2002, pp 3–11.

87. Greenough RB, Simmons CC, Barney JD. The results of operations for cancer of the breast at the Massachusetts General Hospital from 1894–1904. Surg Gynecol Obstet 1907;3:39–50.

88. Judd ES, Sistrunk WE. End-results in operation for cancer of the breast. Surg Gynecol Obstet 1914;28:289–294.

89. Harrington SW. Carcinoma of the breast: Surgical treatment and results. JAMA 1929;92:208–213.

90. Ewing J. Neoplastic Diseases. A Treatise on Tumors. Philadelphia, WB Saunders, 1940, p 598.

91. Steinthal CF, translated by Sugg SL. Staging and prognosis. In Donegan WL, Spratt JS (eds). Cancer and the Breast, 5th ed. Philadelphia, Elsevier, 2002, p 479.

92. Patterson R. The treatment of malignant disease by radium and x-rays. London, Edward Arnold, 1948.

93. Portmann UV. Clinical and pathologic criteria as a basis for classifying cases of primary cancer of the breast. Cleveland Clin J 1943;10:41.

94. Haagensen CD, Stout AP. Carcinoma of the breast. I. Criteria of operability. Ann Surg 1943;118:859–876.

95. Haagensen CD, Stout AP. Carcinoma of the breast. II. Criteria of operability. Ann Surg 1943;118:1032–1051.

96. Haagensen CD, Stout AP. Carcinoma of the breast: Results of treatment 1935–1942. Ann Surg 1951;134:151–172.

97. Coolidge WD. A powerful roentgen-ray tube with a pure electron discharge. Phys Rev 1913;2:409–413.

98. Buschke F. Radiation therapy: The past, the present, the future. Janeway lecture, 1969. AJR Am J Roentgenol 1970;108:236–246.

99. Schulz MD. The supervoltage story. Janeway lecture, 1974. AJR Am J Roentgenol 1975;124:541–559.

100. Baclesse F, Gricouroff G, Tailhefer A. Essai de roentgen-thérapie du cancer du sein suivie d'operation large: Résultat histologiques. Bull Cancer 1939;28:729–743.

101. McWhirter R. The value of simple mastectomy and radiotherapy in the treatment of cancer of the breast. Br J Radiol 1948;21:599–610.

102. Kaae S, Johansen H. Breast cancer: Five-year results. Two random series of simple mastectomy with postoperative irradiation versus extended radical mastectomy. AJR Am J Roentgenol 1962;87:82–88.

103. Baclesse F. Roentgen therapy done for cancer of the breast. Acta Union Intcontra Cancer 1959;15:1023.

104. Mustakallio S. Treatment of breast cancer by tumor extirpation and roentgen therapy instead of radical operation. J Fac Radiol 1954;16:23–26.

105. Patey DH, Dyson WH. The prognosis of carcinoma of the breast in relation to the type of operation performed. Br J Cancer 1948;2:7–13.

106. Handley RS, Thackray AC. Conservative radical mastectomy (Patey's operation). Ann Surg 1969;170:880.

107. Gershon-Cohen J. Atlas of Mammography. New York, Springer-Verlag, 1970.

108. Egan RL. Experience with mammography in a tumor institution. Radiology 1960;25:894–900.

109. Shapiro S, Venel W, Strax P, et al. Ten- to fourteen-year effect of screening on breast cancer mortality. J Natl Cancer Inst 1982;69:349–355.

110. Wald N, Frost C, Cuckle H. Breast cancer screening: The current position. BMJ 1991;302:845.

111. Williams IG, Murley RS, Curwen MP. Carcinoma of the female breast: Conservative and radical surgery. BMJ 1953;2:787–796.

112. Madden JL. Modified radical mastectomy. Surg Gynecol Obstet 1965;121:1221.

113. Auchincloss H. Modified radical mastectomy: Why not? Am J Surg 1970;119:506.

114. Report by the American College of Surgeons Commission on Cancer. Chicago, Oct 22, 1982. Cited by Frykberg ER, Bland KI. Evolution of surgical principles for the management of breast cancer. In Bland KI, Copeland EM III (eds). The Breast. Philadelphia, WB Saunders, 1991.

115. Bostwick J, Vasconez LO, Jurkiewicz MJ. Breast reconstruction after a radical mastectomy. Plast Reconstr Surg 1978;61:682.

116. Radovan C. Tissue expansion in soft-tissue reconstruction. Plast Reconstr Surg 1983;74:482.

117. Schneider WJ, Hill LH, Brown RG. Latissimus dorsi myocutaneous flap for breast reconstruction. Br J Plast Surg 1981;30:286.

118. Hartrampf CR, Scheflan M, Black PW. Breast reconstruction with a transverse abdominal island flap. Plast Reconstr Surg 1982;69:216.

119. Engell HC. Cancer cells in the circulating blood. Acta Chir Scand Suppl 1955;201:1–7a.

120. Fisher B, Fisher ER. The interrelationship of hematogenous and lymphatic tumor cell dissemination. Surg Gynecol Obstet 1966;122:791.

121. Fisher B, Fisher ER. Barrier function of lymph node to tumor cells and erythrocytes. I. Normal nodes. Cancer 1967;20:1907–1913.

122. Fisher B. From Halsted to prevention and beyond: Advances in the management of breast cancer during the twentieth century. Eur J Cancer 1999;35:1963–1973.

123. Huggins C, Hodges CV. Studies on prostatic cancer. I. The effect of castration, of estrogen, and of androgen injection on serum phosphatase in metastatic carcinoma of the prostate. Cancer Res 1941;1:293–297.

124. Huggins C, Doa TLY. Adrenalectomy and oophorectomy in the treatment of advanced carcinoma of the breast. JAMA 1953;151:1388–1394.

125. Muss HB. Endocrine therapy for advanced breast cancer: A review. Breast Cancer Res Treat 1992;21:15.

126. Jensen EV, Block GE, Smith S, et al. Estrogen receptors and breast cancer response to adrenalectomy. In Hall TC (ed). Prediction of Response to Cancer Therapy. Monogr Natl Cancer Inst 1971;34:55–70.

127. Toft D, Shyamala C, Gorski J. A receptor molecule of estrogens: Studies using a cell-free system. Proc Natl Acad Sci U S A 1967;57:1740–1743.

128. McGuire WI, Carbone PP, Vollmer EP. Estrogen Receptors in Human Breast Cancer. New York, Raven, 1975.

129. Allegra JC, Lippman ME, Thompson EB, et al. Distribution, frequency, and quantitative analysis of estrogen, progesterone, androgen, and glucocorticoid receptors in human breast cancer. Cancer Res 1979;39:1447.

precautions are warranted, but it is unusual for such conditions to be severe enough to preclude irradiation. When this is the case, a simple complete mastectomy is performed, often using regional and local anesthesia.

The risk to the heart is associated with the treatment of left-sided breast cancer. The left ventricle may receive irradiation from the tangential field, and an increase in left descending coronary artery disease has been reported.[154] The left ventricle is also at risk when the internal mammary chain of lymph nodes is treated. Large prospective randomized trials looking at the role of irradiation following mastectomy and as part of breast-conserving therapy (BCT) have shown a slight increase in the number of cardiac deaths in irradiated patients with left-sided breast cancer.[154] This is almost exclusively in stage I disease. Once these risks became known, changes in the technique of delivering the radiation using CT-directed conformal therapy appear to be eliminating cardiac damage. Endomyocardial injury has been reported when radiation was given while patients were receiving doxorubicin.[155]

Some lung tissue almost always receives low amounts of radiation, especially when the treatment plan includes the regional lymph nodes. Using electrons instead of photons, especially in the treatment of the supraclavicular nodes, may reduce the incidence of acute pneumonitis. Pulmonary fibrosis may occur in portions of the lung included in treatment fields because the lung is the most sensitive tissue.[156] This can result in some slight decline in pulmonary function but not enough to cause symptoms in a normal patient. The concern comes when there exists underlying chronic lung disease.

Rheumatologic Disorders

A history of one of the numerous rheumatologic diseases, although affecting only a relatively small number of patients with breast cancer, is not to be overlooked. Often, these diseases are associated with small vessel vasculitis or significant skin changes. The presence of such conditions obviously may complicate the use of radiation and affect the cosmetic results of BCT. Awareness of potential risks was initially noted in a report from the University of Texas M. D. Anderson Cancer Center,[157] where skin complications of moist desquamation, ulceration, and skin necrosis were observed in three patients.

It should be noted, however, that the number of instances of patients with connective tissue disorders reported to have had complications following breast-conserving radiation therapy is quite small.[158,159] Many of these earlier reports used techniques not used today, and rheumatologic diseases represent a spectrum of disorders that affect the vessels and connective tissues in different ways. Thus, the knowledge that a patient has such a disease should be considered on a case-by-case basis.[160] Recht[161] recommended that radiation in these patients be limited to a dose of 45 Gy given in 25 fractions using 6 MV or higher-energy photons. He emphasized that care should be taken to minimize any match-line overlap and not to combine radiation with chemotherapy.[161]

A number of rheumatologic diseases may be associated with dilated cardiomyopathy, including systemic lupus erythematosus, polyarteritis nodosa, and progressive systemic sclerosis. Heart disease is virtually never the presenting symptom in these patients, and persons with connective tissue disease may have a degree of cardiac involvement overlooked or underestimated when they present with breast cancer.

How does age affect the decision-making process?

Patient age as a factor in planning appropriate breast cancer therapy has been an area of some controversy. The question really concerns two patient groups, the very young (<35 years old) and the older group (>80 years old). In response to this question, one is tempted to state simply that age is not a factor and that patients are managed according to stage of disease, with exceptions in the very elderly based on significant comorbid disease.

This would, however, be an oversimplification, and it is important to review the issues that have been raised concerning the effect of age in the selection of therapies. Most debate has focused on patients younger than 35 years. A number of centers reported that patients younger than 35 years treated with breast conservation appeared to have a higher risk for recurrence of cancer within the treated breast than that observed for older patients.[162–172] Others have argued that improved patient selection, especially regarding the presence of extensive intraductal component (EIC) (Fig. 22–4), and insistence on good, histologically negative margins eliminated the observed increase in recurrence of cancer within the treated breast.[173–177] As a result, surgeons and radiation oncologists no longer dissuade young patients from breast conservation but pay careful attention to the histology and uniformly recommend re-excision of the biopsy site.[161] The re-excision is done to establish optimal margins and to be sure all EIC, if present, has been excised. Further, even if there is a slight increased risk for local recurrence, it is not at all clear that this would translate into a decrease in overall survival.[161]

At the other end of the age spectrum (patients in their eighth and ninth decades of life), there has been some sentiment that these elderly patients would not tolerate breast radiation well or that it was not necessary to achieve disease control. Clearly, there is no evidence that such patients cannot tolerate good radiotherapy.[162,178,179] What is not known is whether all such patients require radiotherapy for control. At this state of our knowledge, it is certainly best to include

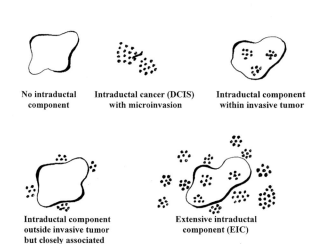

No intraductal component   Intraductal cancer (DCIS) with microinvasion   Intraductal component within invasive tumor

Intraductal component outside invasive tumor but closely associated   Extensive intraductal component (EIC)

Figure 22–4 Patterns of associated intraductal component, including extensive intraductal component. *Wavy lines* indicate the invasive tumor border, and *clusters of dots* show intraductal cancer.

radiation as part of the treatment. When early-stage disease is found in a patient in this advanced age group, a generous wide excision under local anesthesia with good follow-up is probably excellent treatment. Also, good physician–patient communication and solicitation of the patient's treatment preferences are critical to building a successful partnership with elderly patients. Spending the extra effort to do so will improve the quality of the treatment decisions by the elderly.[180]

Are there other medical conditions that affect treatment decisions?

Rarely, patients provide a history of prior high-dose irradiation for other malignancies—most commonly Hodgkin's lymphoma. It is best to recommend mastectomy for such patients. Low-dose irradiation, given in the past as treatment for infant thymic enlargement, is not considered a contraindication for breast conservation.

Some have argued that a strong family history is a risk factor for local failure if breast conservation is used.[161] Others have failed to show this, and in fact there are not enough data collected to provide a confident answer. At this time, the appropriate decision would rest significantly on the strength of the family history coupled with genetic testing, evidence regarding the overall risk for developing contralateral breast cancer, and of course, the patient's desire. If these factors, taken together, add up to a physician–patient decision to consider prophylactic mastectomy, then perhaps an optimal cosmetic result and overall risk reduction can be best achieved by bilateral mastectomies and transverse rectus abdominis myocutaneous (TRAM) reconstruction.

What about breast cancer occurring in the pregnant patient?

Since 1975, there has been a 60% increase of first full-term pregnancies in women older than 30 years of age.[181] As a result, there is an increase in the number of breast cancers diagnosed during pregnancy (about 1 to 3 per 10,000 pregnancies).[182] Mammograms are not routinely used as part of the initial evaluation in pregnant women presenting with breast symptoms, both to avoid radiation risk to the fetus during the first and second trimester and because mammography is less reliable as a diagnostic tool in the dense gestational breast. Ultrasound may be useful in differentiating cystic lesions from solid tumors. In addition, MRI is useful for evaluating the breast during pregnancy and can also be used to look for evidence of metastatic disease, if indicated.[183]

If the diagnosis is made early in pregnancy, a difficult decision must be made regarding a therapeutic abortion. Obviously, this would greatly simplify treatment decisions. However, recent evidence indicates that especially in early nondisseminated disease, there is no benefit to early abortion, survival being the same with or without abortion.[182] Breast cancer cells do not cross the placenta, as occurs with some cancers such as melanoma, lymphosarcoma, or leukemia, and therefore are not a direct threat to the fetus.[182]

Modified radical mastectomy is usually the treatment of choice for such patients. If the patient is in the third trimester, a decision can be made to seek early induced delivery and to hold the radiation for breast conservation until after delivery. In almost all cases, chemotherapy is not used during pregnancy but delayed until after delivery. The effect of chemotherapy on the fetus is directly related to gestational age and drug dosage. Certainly, cytotoxic therapy has been used after the first trimester without apparent damage to the fetus. Even so, the risk for complications such as sepsis and hemorrhage during unplanned delivery make the risk of chemotherapy during even the last trimester too great to justify its use in an adjuvant setting.[183,184]

What is meant by the term *multimodality therapy*?

When a patient is newly diagnosed with stage I or II breast cancer, she and her physician team are faced with a number of treatment decisions. The choices to be made depend heavily on the input of the radiologist evaluating the imaging of the tumor within the breast, the pathologist evaluating the tumor grade and the adequacy of the surgical margins, and the design of an appropriate treatment plan by the surgeon, radiation oncologist, and medical oncologist. When mastectomy is part of the treatment, a plastic surgeon experienced in breast reconstruction is also important to the multidisciplinary approach. It is this team of physicians that is best prepared to determine appropriate local therapy, management of regional nodes, selection of adjuvant therapy, and most important, the best sequencing of available treatment options.

The many decisions that need to be carefully considered and, to a great extent, the continued complexity of these decisions, in light of rapidly advancing new knowledge derived from laboratory investigations of the biology of cancer and from the results of clinical trials research, are the basis for a multidisciplinary team approach to both the diagnosis and the treatment of breast cancer. All members of the team contribute valuable knowledge and critical thinking to the sequencing of the various therapeutic options. This medical team is joined by psychiatrists and psychologists expert in working with cancer patients and their families and by social workers, genetic counselors, and support groups to help the patient through the difficult time of diagnosis and therapy. Providing an expert team is the best way to ensure having a patient prepared to continue a productive high-quality life at the completion of the treatment phase.

Even though the greater use of screening mammography is resulting in the detection of smaller and smaller cancers, the risk for developing a distant recurrence that ultimately leads to death has not been eliminated. As a result, there is an ongoing requirement to include systemic therapy in the management of the primary tumor. Strategies of clinical research that examine drug combinations, doses of drug, new agents, and endocrine therapies are now being applied to the treatment of newly diagnosed, early-stage, node-negative breast cancer as well as locally advanced disease. How these systemic therapies should be integrated with local therapies (surgery and radiation), the intensity of the systemic therapy to be used, and how such systemic treatment may alter local therapy are important questions for future study. Having a multidisciplinary team approach greatly facilitates the selection of clinical trials research to be made available to the group's patients and encourages physician and patient participation in these trials. Thus, the standard of care is raised to its highest level by the combined input of physicians with different areas of clinical expertise.

In the paragraphs that follow, the surgical, radiotherapeutic, and chemotherapeutic-hormonal options for treatment are examined for their specific indications and their sequencing in the overall plan.

What are the indications for breast conservation?

The 1990 National Cancer Institute Consensus Conference on the treatment of early-stage breast cancer stated that "breast conservation treatment is an appropriate method of primary therapy for most women with stage I and II breast cancer and is preferable because it provides survival rates equivalent to those of total mastectomy and axillary dissection while preserving the breast."[185] Given that BCT is an equivalent therapy when compared with mastectomy, the factors that become important to the patient in making this choice are the risk for local recurrence after BCT (vs. mastectomy) and the ability to achieve the desired cosmetic result. Thus, this question is not really "what are the indications for BCT," but instead "what are the factors, if any, that might be considered contraindications."

For example, the first step is a careful evaluation of preoperative breast images. These may need to be repeated before radiation following lumpectomy (tumorectomy) to ensure clearance of microcalcifications. Film-screen mammography must include magnification views for microcalcifications. These magnification imaging studies define the extent of the tumor and determine the status of the remainder of the involved breast as well as the contralateral breast.

In recent years, the additional images obtained by MRI have also been useful in defining the extent of tumor involvement. As noted earlier, in cases of malignancy, it is important that microcalcifications be surgically cleared from the region of the tumor to eliminate the possibility of multicentricity. The presence of extensive microcalcifications is often an indication of the presence of an EIC. The goals are to ensure, by imaging, that (1) the contralateral breast is clear of any mammographically suspicious areas that would require biopsy; (2) the involved breast has been cleared of all suspicious areas; and (3) if microcalcifications were a feature of the primary tumor, magnification views have documented their extent, and postsurgical films have confirmed that they were cleared.

The second step is a careful pathologic evaluation of the breast tissue removed. There is no substitute for a direct review of the gross specimen and histology by the surgeon sitting in consultation with the pathologist. The surgeon must be responsible for correct specimen orientation so that all sides can be inked using different colors. Gross tumor measurements are performed by the pathologist only after the gross intact specimen has been oriented and appropriately inked. Although inking is the preferred method for assessing margins, there are some problems with this technique that the surgeon should be aware of. For example, during the excision of the specimen and subsequent initial handling, some of the fatty tissue may be rubbed off the exterior surface. In addition,

the ink may seep into crevices in the margin surface, causing some microscopic confusion regarding the actual margin depth.

This discussion regarding specimen orientation and inking of margins underscores the importance of obtaining adequate tumor-free margins in determining the risk for local recurrence.[186] The best data and most frequently quoted studies are those of the National Surgical Adjuvant Breast and Bowel Project (NSABP) and the Joint Center for Radiation Therapy (JCRT).[178,187,188] In the JCRT study of 340 patients treated with 60 Gy, patients with EIC-negative tumors had a 5-year local recurrence rate of 1% if margins were negative and 2% if margins were negative but the carcinoma was within 1 mm of the ink but not at the ink.[188] If there was focal margin involvement (i.e., three or fewer low-power fields were positive), the risk for recurrence increased to 9%. When margins were more than focally involved, the risk was 19%. For patients with EIC-positive tumors, the risk for local recurrence in the JCRT patients with negative margins was 8%. This risk increased to 27% when EIC-positive tumors demonstrated histologically positive margins.[178,188]

In practice, it is best to obtain generous negative margins, especially when there is a significant EIC. Although the definition of a negative margin may differ among institutions, most breast cancer surgeons strive to achieve a margin of a minimum of 1 to 3 mm of normal tissue. In other institutions, the standard is a margin of 1 cm or greater.[189] When concerned about adequacy of margins, it is in the patient's best interest to re-excise the original biopsy site.

As suggested, the presence of EIC must be carefully considered. A re-excision of the tumor bed should be performed in all EIC-positive tumors to ensure the absence of multicentricity (skip areas of DCIS scattered among normal breast tissue in the areas around the primary tumor). If the re-excision specimen exhibits multiple areas of residual cancer, mastectomy is the preferred treatment (Table 22–3).

Table 22–3 Management of Patients with an Extensive Intraductal Component

Definition	Ductal carcinoma in situ (DCIS) inside *and* outside the index lesion *or DCIS* with minimal amounts of invasion.
Workup	Pay careful attention to the mammogram. EIC patients frequently have microcalcifications. Make sure all suspicious-looking microcalcifications are excised.
Primary excision	Should be wide; negative pathologic margins should be the goal.
Re-excision	Use liberally, especially if margin is positive or if residual microcalcifications are present.
Treatment	If margins are negative on first excision or re-excision shows minimal tumor with negative margins, treat with lumpectomy plus radiation. If new margins are positive, especially with widespread DCIS in the re-excision specimen, treat with mastectomy.

Modified from Abeloff MD, Lichter AS, Niederhuber JE, et al. Breast. In Abeloff MD, Armifage JO, Lichter AS, et al. (eds). Clinical Oncology. New York, Churchill Livingstone, 1995, p 1617.

What seems to be clear from all reports is the conclusion that the greater the extent of resection, the lower the risk for local failure. Thus, even when EIC is present, patients undergoing quadrantectomy have an acceptable failure rate, and those with EIC-negative tumors drop below a 1% risk.[190] The surgeon and the patient are faced with balancing the extent of breast resection with a desire for a favorable cosmetic outcome. The greater the resection, as in quadrantectomy, the worse the cosmetic result and the less the indication for breast preservation. The cosmetic result of a reconstructed breast may actually be preferred.

Smitt and colleagues[186] at Stanford University evaluated the impact of surgical margins on long-term local control. They found that truly negative margins (greater than 2 mm) resulted in 90% local control at 10 years, in contrast to 82% for patients with positive and close margins. Re-excision to a negative margin was important, providing a 97% 10-year local control rate. When tumors were EIC positive, the re-excision specimen demonstrated residual cancer 82% of the time, compared with only 31% for EIC-negative tumors.

In another report examining re-excision for EIC-positive tumors, residual DCIS was noted a minimum of 2 cm from the primary in at least 30% of EIC-positive tumor re-excision specimens. This finding confirmed that a wide excision such as segmentectomy or quadrantectomy is necessary to provide the lowest risk for local failure.[191] Younger patients (<40 years old) and those with comedo-type DCIS histology are reported to demonstrate a greater distance of spread within the adjacent ductal systems, perhaps accounting for the increased difficulty of truly clearing these lesions and the greater risk for local failure observed in EIC-positive tumors for young women and comedo histology.[192] Although the presence of EIC is not considered in itself a contraindication to breast preservation, it clearly demands an exacting approach to ensuring clear margins through a resection of greater volume. The importance of re-excision cannot be overemphasized.

Perez recently reported the experience of treating T1 and T2 breast cancer by breast preservation and radiation at Washington University School of Medicine in St. Louis.[193] He analyzed the records of 1347 patients treated with breast preservation between 1970 and 1997 at their institution. The 10-year incidence of local failure was 7% for T1 tumors and 11% for T2 tumors. It is important to note that Dr. Perez also found that patients younger than 40 years who had EIC had a greater risk for local relapse (17%) compared with a similar EIC-positive group of postmenopausal women, who had a relapse rate of 10%.

Although most invasive breast cancers are adenocarcinomas arising from the terminal ducts (about 80%), there are several less common histologic findings that have a better overall prognosis. The better prognosis of these tumors (mucinous, medullary, papillary, tubular, and adenoid cystic) is best seen in node-negative patients.[194] Other pathologic features, such as vascular-lymphatic invasion, inflammatory response, and degree of intratumor necrosis, have been less helpful in predicting risk. Eventually, genomic and proteomic profiling will provide more specific prognostic information.

The final determinant in selecting a woman for BCT has to do with the patient's desires and expectations. It requires a certain commitment of a surgeon's time to listen carefully to what the patient is saying and to ask appropriate nonleading questions that give an insight into the patient's wishes regarding cosmetic outcome. The size of the required breast resection compared with the breast size and the expected changes in the breast secondary to the radiation must be carefully evaluated to provide reasonable expectations of what the final cosmetic outcome might be.

From a technical standpoint, placement of the incision is important to the cosmetic outcome. It is best placed in a circumareolar position or in a line that runs parallel to the margin of the areola. It is essential to obtain optimal hemostasis of the cavity and to avoid closure of the deep tissues, letting the cavity fill with a small seroma that will gradually be reabsorbed during the healing process. Drains in the breast should be avoided. The placement of small titanium clips in the walls of the cavity will assist the localization of the radiation boost. Every effort is made to keep the site of the lumpectomy entirely separate from the site of the axillary surgery.

What are the contraindications to breast-conserving therapy?

Perhaps an easier way to approach the question of selecting patients for BCT is to review the absolute and relative contraindications or the reasons for choosing mastectomy. The Joint Committee of the American College of Surgeons, the American College of Radiology, the College of American Pathologists, and the Society of Surgical Oncology attempted to provide a consensus of standards, which was published in 1992.[195] Absolute contraindications to BCT are well established (Table 22–4). They include (1) prior therapeutic radiation to the involved breast, (2) a patient in the first or second trimester of pregnancy, (3) the presence of two or more distinct tumors present in different quadrants of the breast, and (4) the presence of diffuse, suspicious microcalcifications involving more than one quadrant of the breast.

Relative contraindications are, by their nature, somewhat controversial. They include (1) a large tumor volume–to–breast volume ratio precluding an acceptable cosmetic outcome; (2) a very large breast, which may present unacceptable difficulty in delivering a uniform radiation dose to the breast following tumorectomy; and (3) a history of collagen-vascular disease and primary lung disease.

The intensity of the skin reaction and fibrosis in patients with a collagen-vascular disorder such as scleroderma, cutaneous lupus, and active collagen disease may be related to

Table 22–4 Contraindications to Breast-Conserving Therapy

Absolute Contraindications
• Prior therapeutic radiation to the involved breast
• When the patient is in the first or second trimester of pregnancy
• The presence of 2 or more distinct tumors involving different quadrants of the breast
• The presence of diffuse, suspicious microcalcifications involving more than 1 quadrant of the breast

Relative Contraindications
• Large tumor volume-to-breast volume ratio precluding an acceptable cosmetic outcome
• Very large breast, which may present unacceptable difficulty in delivering a uniform radiation dose to the breast
• History of collagen-vascular disease and primary lung disease

how much their skin and subcutaneous tissues are clinically involved. This must be carefully evaluated before making a decision regarding radiation therapy. Although prior radiation to the chest wall is generally a contraindication to BCT, it is important to have the radiation oncologist assess the previous port sites, the dosage received, and the time lapse from prior treatment before arbitrarily excluding the patient. The issue of the large breast is not often a deterrent if methods are devised to immobilize the breast to ensure a homogeneous radiation dose. The problem with the very large, essentially fatty breast is not the ability to deliver the appropriate radiotherapy but the risk of the breast's developing marked fibrosis and retraction following radiotherapy. These patients often are better served by mastectomy and reconstruction with a TRAM flap accompanied by a significant reduction mastopexy of the contralateral breast.

In the past, patients with tumors located beneath the nipple–areolar complex were not considered good candidates for BCT. The concern was that such patients had a more extensive spread of tumor along the various branching ducts that would not be adequately excised by lumpectomy.[196] The extent to which such lesions should be resected (i.e., whether the nipple–areolar complex is excised) remains a contentious subject. Recent data suggest the nipple-areola may be left in place as long as an acceptable negative tumor margin is achieved. Even if one includes the nipple–areolar complex as part of the resection, the cosmetic result is actually quite acceptable, leaving a good breast mound with normal skin sensation and texture. There is no evidence that the incidence of local recurrence is higher when central lesions are treated by the same criteria used elsewhere in the breast.[197–199]

What is the current status of sentinel lymph node mapping and axillary node dissection?

The size of the primary tumor and the status of the axillary lymph nodes, although independent predictors, are additive and still remain the strongest prognostic factors in determining survival from breast cancer. Of these two staging features, physicians have, by tradition, placed a greater weight on the presence of tumor cells in axillary nodes as the more accurate predictor of systemic occult metastases. Thus, there are three important reasons to consider axillary dissection. The first is to determine whether the axillary nodes are positive or negative and to what extent they are involved. This knowledge provides essential information for the process of making sound therapeutic decisions. The second reason, although controversial, concerns the fact that positive nodes left untreated may later cause the patient to have significant local problems such as pain, impaired motion, ulceration with infection, and limb edema. The third reason is also controversial and concerns the risk that nodal disease may, in itself, be the source of distant spread. Although these three concepts have provided the rationale for node dissection, they must be considered, to some extent, the historical basis for this procedure.

To my best knowledge, Sir Charles Moore was the first, in 1867, to record a dissection of the axillary content when removing a cancerous breast.[200] Eventually, this concept led, in the United States, to the widely accepted Halsted radical mastectomy, which persisted as the primary treatment of breast cancer until appropriately tested by the surgeons of the NSABP in their B-04 trial.[201,202] This trial, which began in 1971, clearly demonstrated that breast cancer patients with clinically determined stage II disease had equal long-term outcome whether treated by radical mastectomy or by total mastectomy (without axillary node dissection) plus radiation to nodal areas.

For clinically determined stage I patients, the survival results were identical whether the patient had a radical mastectomy, total mastectomy plus nodal radiation, or total mastectomy with delayed nodal dissection when and if nodal disease developed. In the last group, only 20% of patients with clinical stage I disease went on to develop involved nodes despite the 40% rate of detecting positive nodes in the radical mastectomy group. This extremely important trial began to place in question the role of axillary dissection and most certainly began to eliminate arguments for even more radical surgery such as dissection of the internal mammary nodes and the supraclavicular nodes. The B-04 trial was followed by B-06, designed to evaluate the efficacy of breast-preserving surgery.[203] Like B-04, long-term follow-up of patients enrolled in B-06 has continued to add to our understanding of the role of axillary dissection.

Two factors have had a significant impact on the evolution of the approach to the axillary nodes. The first event was the introduction some 30 years ago of the concept of adjuvant chemotherapy.[204,205] The use of either chemotherapy or hormonal therapy has been shown to provide statistically significant benefits to most women with breast cancer. The decision to offer adjuvant therapy, as indicated earlier, initially was primarily based on nodal status. This fact accounts to a great extent for the ongoing practice of including axillary nodal dissection. What remains unclear is the impact of adjuvant therapy on occult nodal disease.

The second significant change has been the impact of screening and routine mammography on the stage of detected disease. As a result, today it is estimated that 80% of newly detected breast cancers each year represent early-stage disease.[185] Thus, when we answer the question implied in the title of this chapter, that is, "What is meant by the term *multimodality therapy?*," we do so today in the context of a very different set of parameters, which include more patients with noninvasive disease, smaller invasive cancers, more favorable histologic findings, and the increasing frequency of finding only microscopic minimal involvement of one or two axillary nodes.

Nevertheless, we are still left with a desire to know whether this extremely important prognostic indicator is positive or negative. One factor in the equation has been well documented over the years and demonstrated again in recent studies. This factor is the knowledge that we are not very successful at clinically assessing the axilla. In an analysis of 377 breast cancers of stage T1 to T4 tumors undergoing axillary dissection, 44% of those judged to have clinically negative axilla were actually pathologically positive, and 34% judged preoperatively as clinically positive proved at pathologic review to be negative.[206] In this study, the authors confirmed two other commonly held principles: (1) the rate of detecting involved nodes correlates with the risk for finding axillary metastases, and (2) there is only a 2% incidence of skipped metastases to level III nodes when levels I and II are negative. This latter finding supports the perception that resecting level I and II lymph nodes provides adequate staging.

Over the years, surgeons have noted that patients with palpable breast cancers were more likely to have positive axillary nodes. Silverstein and his colleagues[207] found evidence to support this axiom when they reviewed their practice experience. They compared the predictive value of using T stage in combination with the physical findings of either a palpable or nonpalpable tumor compared with using only the T stage to predict axillary stage. Their conclusions were based on 1554 axillary node dissections in which 551 (35.5%) were node positive. They found that even in early T-stage cancers (T1b, T1c, and T2), if the lesion could be palpated on breast examination, there was a significantly greater risk ($P < .002$) of finding involved axillary nodes than when the tumor was nonpalpable for the same T stage.

It is important to remember that multiple studies have reported axillary node involvement in 12% to 37% of patients whose tumors were 1 cm or smaller.[208] These numbers concerning the risk for axillary metastasis, however, may overstate the problem because of the dramatic downward slope of the maximum tumor diameter today. Cady,[209] in a review of cases at the New England Deaconess Hospital from 1989 to 1993, found 29% of all invasive cancers to be only T1a or T1b (1 cm or smaller). If this trend continues, the median diameter will be less than 1 cm within this decade. This clearly requires changes in the standard approach to surgical therapy.

Certainly there is no argument with the fact that surgical clearing of the axillary nodes provides excellent local control of the disease. The issues behind the controversy of providing such treatment for all patients are the increasing numbers of patients presenting with early-stage, nonpalpable cancers and the decreasing use of nodal status in deciding whether adjuvant therapy is to be used.[210] Couple these facts with the associated morbidity of axillary dissection arm edema, paresthesias, loss of shoulder mobility, and pain and the possibility that adjuvant therapy in itself may be adequate therapy for micrometastatic nodal disease, and one has the basis for the dilemma facing surgeon and patient. Is there a way to select patients who really need axillary staging?

Sentinel Lymph Node Mapping

The answer has come in a somewhat unexpected way—not through discovery of a prognostic marker[211–215] but through the development of a new surgical technique termed *sentinel lymph node* (SLN) *mapping*. SLN mapping has taken on the role of being the best current method for selecting clinical stage I patients for axillary dissection. The concept of SLN mapping dates back to work by Cabanas in 1977 describing the first draining lymph node in squamous cell carcinoma of the penis.[216] Morton and colleagues[217] applied this concept to melanoma staging, and in 1993, Krag[218] reported identification of the SLN in the axilla of breast cancer patients using radioisotope localization. This was almost simultaneously followed by a report by Giuliano and colleagues using the blue dye technique established by his colleague Morton for melanoma SLN mapping.[219,220] Giuliano and coworkers[221] were able to find a sentinel node in 114 of 174 lymphadenectomies and demonstrated that the sentinel node accurately predicted the status of the axillary nodes in 96% of the dissections.

This technique involved the injection of 3 to 5 mL of 1% isosulfan blue vital dye into the breast tumor and surrounding breast tissue or into the wall of the previous biopsy site. A small incision was placed in the low axilla, and the lymphatic channels stained by the blue dye were carefully identified and followed to the blue-stained sentinel node. In the hands of Giuliano and associates, a careful analysis of the sentinel node was more accurate in predicting a positive axilla than a standard level I and II dissection with routine histopathology of the identified nodes. It is important to note that in their investigation, T1 tumors had a somewhat higher-than-expected incidence of positive nodes, 20%. Other investigators have used ^{99m}Tc-labeled antimony sulfur colloid injected into the breast lumpectomy (biopsy) site to identify lymphatic drainage and a sentinel node.[222]

During the years since these initial reports, many technical advances have simplified the SLN mapping procedure and have resulted in even greater accuracy of SLN identification (now generally accepted to be >95%).[223] For example, anatomic studies demonstrated that lymphatic drainage in the breast occurs in a nonrandom fashion to the axillary SLN.[224] In addition, many studies showed that injecting the tracer into the dermis or subdermal skin and in a subareolar location was equal to or perhaps slightly better than peritumoral injection. Compared with the breast parenchyma, the skin around the areola has a much denser lymphatic network. Hand-held gamma probes have been specifically designed for SLN identification. They have a smaller probe head of 14 mm and more internal shielding to improve accuracy.

SLN mapping is a minimally invasive procedure and as such has rapidly gained popularity and acceptance by both surgeons and patients. In multiple nonrandomized studies, SLN mapping accuracy for predicting the status of the axillary nodes has been quite high, with an apparent false-negative rate of 2% to 3%. Thus, although not as yet confirmed by a randomized trial, SLN mapping has been widely adopted, and patients with a negative SLN are not subjected to an axillary dissection. It remains unclear whether patients with an SLN positive for microscopic disease need a completion axillary dissection. Several studies suggest that micrometastases detected only by immunohistochemistry in the SLN of patients with T1 tumors have a very low incidence of involvement of additional axillary nodes.

The important questions to validate SLN mapping are being addressed by two large phase III trials. The NSABP B-32 trial opened in 1999 randomizes clinically node-negative patients with T1-3 breast cancers to SLN mapping followed by axillary dissection or SLN biopsy alone. In the SLN biopsy alone group, if the SLN is positive, the patients go on to axillary dissection. All negative SLN patients are further assayed using immunohistochemistry (*www.nsabp.pitt.edu*). The second major trial is being conducted by the American College of Surgeons Oncology Group (ACOSOG) as protocols Z0010 and Z0011. Z0010 is attempting to determine whether SLN biopsy in T1-2, N0, M0 patients, including immunohistochemical assessment, is equal to or better than bone marrow aspiration for determining prognosis. The B-32 trial and Z0010 have reached accrual and await maturity. Z0011 randomizes SLN-positive patients (excluding those positive only by immunohistochemistry) to completion axillary dissection or to no immediate axillary dissection or axillary radiation (*www.acosog.org*).

Some surgeons recommend SLN mapping for patients with high-grade or extensive DCIS, where it is possible that occult microinvasion exists or has been documented but no clinical data exist to support SLN mapping in these cases. When, however, the DCIS is so extensive as to require mastectomy, SLN mapping can be used to avoid unnecessary axillary dissection.

There are several contraindications at present for doing SLN mapping and proceeding directly to axillary dissection. These include the clinically suspicious axilla and tumors located in the tail of the breast (tail of Spence). In addition, if the surgeon fails to identify with confidence an SLN, axillary dissection is required. Some debate continues about whether SLN mapping should be performed before beginning patients on neoadjuvant or induction chemotherapy, but the results of the NSABP B-27 trial indicate that SLN biopsy is a reliable staging procedure following chemotherapy.[225] There is a significant learning phase for surgeons, and initially an axillary dissection should be performed with the SLN mapping until confidence is established in the ability to identify the SLN accurately. It is not uncommon to find two and sometimes three nodes that qualify as the SLN, and interestingly, there is evidence that those with multiple negative SLNs have a better prognosis.[226]

Technical Aspects of Level I and II Node Dissection

The extent of axillary node dissection needed to accurately stage and treat the breast cancer patient has also been the subject of debate. From past experience, it is clear that when levels I and II are negative, it is rare that there will be skip metastasis to level III, the highest axillary nodes. The best estimate of the risk for such an occurrence is generally cited to be about 2%.[206] In recent years, this has led most surgeons to do at least a level I dissection and to include level II when the tumor size predicted a greater risk. By limiting the node dissection to only levels I and II (i.e., dissecting only to the medial border of the pectoralis minor muscle), the risk for associated long-term morbidity is virtually eliminated. A level I and II node dissection is associated with the lowest risk for subsequent axillary recurrence. Care is taken to preserve the lymphatic channels along the anterior surface of the axillary vein and overlying the brachial plexus. The lateral and medial pectoral nerves are avoided, as are the long thoracic nerve and the thoracodorsal nerve. Preserving the upper branches of the costobrachial sensory nerve avoids the dense and bothersome numbness along the upper inner arm.

Because screening has resulted in discovery of smaller and smaller tumors, the number of women being subjected to unnecessary node dissection is a concern. When no nodes were removed from the axilla, the Danish Breast Cancer Group recorded a 19% recurrence in the axilla in 5 years.[215] This contrasted with a 5-year risk of 5% when more than five negative nodes were resected.[215]

From this discussion, it seems safe to conclude that, based on present knowledge, axillary dissection of at least level I and II nodes is indicated for patients undergoing mastectomy (this also ensures removing all of the tail of the breast), patients for whom therapy would be changed by identifying whether the axilla was positive or negative and to what extent positive (i.e., number of nodes positive), and patients involved in clinical trials.

The essential question, which requires further testing, is whether the presence of micrometastases in axillary nodes requires primary resection in the setting of multimodality

therapy.[227] It is certainly possible that careful sentinel node analysis may provide the necessary prognostic information, but current trial results must be awaited. The approach to sentinel node evaluation may be further aided by use of reverse transcriptase polymerase chain reaction (RT-PCR) to detect the presence of tumor cell DNA in otherwise histologically negative sentinel nodes.[228] Proof of the efficacy of sentinel node staging should eliminate the need to evaluate the entire axilla and permit managing the axilla expectantly following adjuvant chemotherapy. Eventually, T1 tumors may all be managed expectantly for development of axillary metastases without even the sentinel node testing.

Which mastectomy patients benefit from radiation therapy?

Historically, postmastectomy radiation therapy was common practice in the management of breast cancer. The more advanced stage of disease at diagnosis and the high rate of development of local skin flap and chest wall recurrent disease accounted for this approach. The first trial to test this question was the Manchester, England, study of immediate compared with delayed postmastectomy chest wall radiation. This trial began in 1948, and in the intervening years, a number of randomized prospective trials were completed.[229–236] Although none of these early trials found a clear survival benefit, we now know that there is a significant decrease in chest wall relapse, approaching 5%, when postoperative irradiation is used.[237,238]

With the passage of time, an interesting conclusion from the analysis of the many adjuvant chemotherapy trails began to emerge. This conclusion indicated that chemotherapy failed to lower the risk for chest wall recurrence.[239–241] This was even true when high-dose polychemotherapy was used.[242] These perhaps surprising results have led to a re-evaluation of the indications for postmastectomy chest wall irradiation (Table 22–5). For example, the Danish Cooperative Breast Group published a report that in premenopausal women treated with mastectomy and CMF (cyclophosphamide, methotrexate, and 5-fluorouracil) adjuvant chemotherapy, the addition of chest wall irradiation not only improved disease-free survival but also improved disease-free survival when node-positive, premenopausal patients were analyzed.[243,244] These observations, plus the introduction of aggressive polydrug adjuvant chemotherapy for node-positive patients, led to the use of postmastectomy chest wall

Table 22–5 Indications for Postmastectomy Chest Wall Irradiation

Indicated
• Positive or close (1–2 mm) margins following mastectomy
• T3 tumors (especially stages T3, N1)
• All T4 tumors
• High-dose chemotherapy for cure in patients with extensive nodal involvement
• Extracapsular nodal disease
Considered
• ≥4 positive nodes, especially premenopausal

irradiation only in selected patients with stage II tumors having evidence or risk of internal mammary node involvement and/or local extension close to or into the chest wall.

Often, the question is raised concerning extending the irradiation to the axilla in breast conservation and in mastectomy patients. In node-positive patients, the incidence of recurrence in the axilla is less than 1% when a careful axillary dissection has been performed. Currently, radiation to the axilla is advised when there is extracapsular extension of the tumor in the involved nodes or when there are four or more involved nodes.

Who should receive adjuvant chemotherapy?

Even though the first randomized prospective clinical trials designed to determine the benefits of adjuvant chemotherapy began more than 30 years ago, questions persist regarding the choice of therapy, the intensity, and the duration of therapy. In addition, there has been great concern that every effort be made to identify risk factors that would better select patients for such treatment. The debate has focused on a real concern that many women were receiving potentially dangerous therapy unnecessarily. To address these issues, the Early Breast Cancer Trialists' Collaborative Group (EBCTCG) undertook a meta-analysis of all randomized trials conducted before 1985.[210] This analysis included 133 randomized prospective trials involving some 75,000 women.[210] This group convened again in 1995 and 2000 to update their analysis.[245–247] As a result, the EBCTCG overview analyses provide excellent support for several sound conclusions regarding the use of adjuvant therapy. These are as follows:

1. There is a significant survival benefit for women receiving polychemotherapy.
2. The survival advantages have been demonstrated in all age groups, but the magnitude of the benefit appears to be less in older women.
3. Polychemotherapy has been shown to be of greater benefit than single-agent chemotherapy.
4. Administering adjuvant chemotherapy for more than 6 months has not generally been of great benefit.
5. Adjuvant tamoxifen is of some benefit in all patient groups but appears to have a greater benefit in women older than 50 years.
6. Several years of tamoxifen treatment provides greater benefit than a single year.
7. The analysis appears to support the conclusion that combined chemoendocrine therapy is superior to either chemotherapy or endocrine therapy alone (the benefit appears greater in older women than younger).
8. Perhaps the most important and somewhat unexpected result of the analysis was evidence that gains in survival from adjuvant treatment were larger at 15 years than at 5 years.

Translating results of the EBCTCG meta-analysis into terms that are understandable for the patient is never easy. A woman with a T1 or T2 tumor that is node negative has a 10% to 20% risk for dying of breast cancer. The smaller the tumor and the more favorable the histology, the closer the risk is to 10% or even less (5%). Given the standard adjuvant treatment, she can expect an approximate benefit of 4% (a decrease of four deaths for 100 women treated). This translates to a persistent annual reduction in the odds of death of 30%. For node-positive patients, the benefit is 12%, with a reduction in annual risk for death of 15%. This is summarized in Table 22–6.

The benefit of adjuvant chemotherapy is certainly real, and because of the very large number of women affected by cancer worldwide, it is extremely valuable. The benefit, however, is only a modest change, and women at significant risk for developing recurrent disease continue to do so whether or not they have been treated with polychemotherapy with or without tamoxifen. Of great significance is the observation that the long-term (15-year) follow-up of these trials by the EBCTCG never shows a plateau in the curve, suggesting instead a prolongation in time to relapse rather than a true elimination of occult disease.[247] As a result, current interest has focused on dose intensity, scheduling of drug administration, sequencing of therapies (primary chemotherapy), and, of course, new agents.

Addressing the issue of dose intensity, Cancer and Leukemia Group B (CALGB) members reported a clinical breast trial comparing three dose levels of CAF—cyclophosphamide (Cytoxan), doxorubicin (Adriamycin), and 5-fluorouracil—for node-positive patients.[248] The two higher-dose arms had significantly better relapse-free and overall survival results than the low-dose arm. The highest-dose arm, however, was essentially what is commonly used in standard practice. This is consistent with the EBCTCG analyses[244,246] that found anthracycline-containing regimens to be better than standard CMF.

The Southwest Oncology Group (SWOG) reported in 2001 the results of comparing tamoxifen alone to CAF plus tamoxifen (CAFT) therapy in postmenopausal, node-positive, receptor-positive patients. The 5-year disease-free survival rate was 76% for CAFT and 67% for tamoxifen alone.[249] The NSABP B-20 trial showed that both premenopausal and postmenopausal women who were node negative but had hormonally dependent tumors benefited from the addition of

Table 22–6 Improvement in 10-Year Survival from Treatment of 100 Women with Stage II Breast Cancer

Treatment	Proportional Reduction in Annual Mortality Percentage (SD)	Absolute Reduction in 10-Year Mortality/ 100 Women Treated (SD)
Age <50 yr		
Polychemotherapy	25 (5)	10 (3)
Ovarian ablation	28 (9)	11 (4)
Polychemotherapy + ovarian ablation	? 30–40	? 12–16
Age >50 yr		
Polychemotherapy	12 (4)	5 (2)
Tamoxifen	20 (2)	8 (1)
Polychemotherapy + tamoxifen	30 (5)	12 (2)

Adapted from Early Breast Cancer Trialists' Collaborative Group. Systemic treatment of early breast cancer by hormonal, cytotoxic or immune therapy: 133 randomised trials involving 31,000 recurrences and 24,000 deaths among 75,000 women. Lancet 1992;339:71–85. © by The Lancet Ltd.

tamoxifen to their adjuvant chemotherapy.[250] The results of these trials suggest that receptor-negative tumors may be more responsive to chemotherapy.

Of the new drugs introduced in recent years, certainly the taxanes have been the most interesting.[251–254] These drugs act to disrupt microtubules. Other drugs include those that interfere with epidermal growth factor receptors on cancer cells, known as the *epidermal growth factor receptor inhibitors* (gefitinib, erlotinib, lapatinib), or agents that interfere with the capacity of cancer cells to invade (matrix metalloproteinase inhibitors), and inhibitors of angiogenesis. In a study of paclitaxel in an adjuvant setting, the CALGB conducted a trial that randomized women with node-positive breast cancer to four cycles of CA (Cytoxan [cyclophosphamide] and Adriamycin [doxorubicin]) given every 3 weeks with or without four additional cycles of paclitaxel given every 3 weeks.[255] The sequential treatment using paclitaxel resulted in an improved 5-year disease-free survival (65% without paclitaxel vs. 70% with) and an improved overall survival (77% without paclitaxel vs. 80% with). Of interest is the observation that the benefit of the additional paclitaxel was confined to women with ER-negative tumors. Similar results were found in the NSABP B-28 trial of similar design.[256,257]

The benefits of adjuvant chemotherapy and adjuvant hormonal therapy have also been shown to improve disease-free survival and overall survival in low-risk, node-negative patients. Because node-positive patients obviously suffer from a greater risk for treatment failure, the benefit, as expected, is not as great in the node-negative patients. As a result, there is considerable interest at present in searching for prognostic and predictive indicators that would better select node-negative patients for adjuvant therapy. Ideally, these markers of disease risk would also aid in selecting the type of adjuvant therapy most likely to be beneficial.

Many studies have been conducted to evaluate the value of *p53* as a prognostic indicator in node-negative patients. These studies in general have failed to document that *p53* expression has a predictive value.[258] About one fourth to one third of breast cancer specimens stain positive for *p53*.[258,259] It is possible that actual cDNA sequencing to identify *p53* gene mutations may identify a higher-risk group and be better than immunohistochemical identification of *p53*. Other markers being studied include those of microvessel density (angiogenesis), tumor invasion (urokinase plasminogen activator inhibitor-2), the presence or absence of telomerase activity, and expression of cathepsin, *erbB-2,* and *mdr-1*. Obviously, whether these or other markers prove useful will require considerably more study. The design of such studies is difficult because of their complexity.

For today's patient, with a low-risk, node-negative tumor, the risk markers of age, tumor size, hormone receptor level, and degree of tumor differentiation must still be used to decide whether adjuvant therapy is indicated and what therapy should be recommended. For a tumor that is 1 cm or less in diameter, a 95% to 99% relapse-free survival rate can be expected unless the histologic findings show a poor nuclear grade and lymphatic invasion. If this is the case, the relapse-free survival drops to 67%, similar to that of a node-positive tumor, and adjuvant therapy is certainly indicated.[260–262] Patients with node involvement or node-negative patients with tumors greater than 1 cm in diameter (T1c) are appro-

priate candidates for adjuvant chemoendocrine therapy. Patients with T1c-staged tumors that are node negative but ER negative receive CA. If they are younger than 50 years, such patients are also given tamoxifen if they are ER positive. Patients with T1c tumors who are ER positive and older than 50 years are treated with tamoxifen unless they are node positive, in which case they have an option for CA followed by tamoxifen.

Who should receive adjuvant hormonal therapy?

Clinical trials data, epidemiologic studies, and now molecular research support the role of estrogen in the initiation and development of hormonally dependent breast cancer.[263–268] As a result, antagonizing estrogen is a prime target to reduce the risk for recurrence of breast cancer following treatment of the primary tumor and for prevention of second breast cancers.[269,270] Receptors for estrogen were discovered in 1966, and within a few years, it became obvious that patients whose tumors lacked ER rarely responded to endocrine ablative surgery or hormonal therapy. The first SERM developed was the nonsteroidal tamoxifen.[271] Tamoxifen was approved by the FDA in 1986 for adjuvant treatment of postmenopausal women with node-positive disease and in 1990 for node-negative disease. Postmenopausal women have breast cancer that usually expresses ER and PR, and in such women, there are multiple sources of endogenous estrogen such as the skin, fat, muscle, and breast stromal cells. Breast cancer cells also can be shown to produce estrogen.[270]

Tamoxifen has been shown to reduce the development of recurrent disease by some 47% and overall mortality by 26% in ER-positive breast cancer patients.[272] Five phase III randomized trials comparing tamoxifen to placebo have been performed in women at risk for developing breast cancer. All trials were positive for tamoxifen, showing a 38% to 48% reduction in ER-positive breast cancers but no effect for preventing ER-negative cancers.[273] As a result, tamoxifen became the drug of choice for hormonal therapy of women with ER- or PR-positive tumors.

The EBCTCG reported a recent meta-analysis that provides an overview of the use of tamoxifen as adjuvant therapy either alone or in combination with chemotherapy.[210,273,274] In these trials, tamoxifen reduced the incidence of breast cancer by 38%. Although the incidence of breast cancer was reduced in all age groups, it was only the incidence of receptor-positive tumors that was reduced. Both this meta-analysis and a similar review of the NSABP prevention trials confirmed the risks associated with daily tamoxifen use.[275] These included endometrial cancer and thromboembolic occurrences as the most serious complications of therapy. Although serious and potentially life threatening, both were rare and almost never occurred in women younger than 50 years. Vasomotor symptoms and genitourinary effects were the most common toxicities—especially in women in their perimenopausal years.

Tamoxifen, however, is not the perfect SERM and exhibits partial estrogen-like actions as well. These are amply demonstrated by its toxicities, such as the development of endometrial polyps or cancer and the occurrence of thromboembolic disease. In addition, tamoxifen has an estrogen-like positive effect on reducing osteoporosis and the incidence of osteoporotic fractures.[276] In efforts to identify and synthesize more efficacious drugs for antagonizing estrogen, investigators have focused on the estrogen synthetase enzyme (aromatase), which is the rate-limiting enzyme catalyzing the conversion of androgens to estrogens. Highly specific aromatase inhibitors (AIs) that block total body estrogen production by more than 99% have been developed. When AIs have been compared with tamoxifen in direct comparison trials, they have appeared superior. As a result, efforts are now underway to compare third-generation AIs. There are two classes of AIs: steroidal (class I) and nonsteroidal (class II). The third-generation AIs are more effective and less toxic. Anastrozole (1 mg daily) is completely absorbed from the gastrointestinal tract and has a half-life of about 50 hours with steady-state serum concentrations achieved at about 7 days. Letrozole (2.5 mg daily) is also completely absorbed by the gastrointestinal tract and has a half-life of 2 to 4 days. Steady state is achieved at 2 to 6 weeks. Both are nonsteroidal AIs. Exemestane (25 mg daily) is a steroidal AI with nonreversible enzyme binding and, unlike the others, appears to also prevent bone loss. It is also readily absorbed and is about 90% protein bound. Exemestane reduces estrogen levels to a greater degree than anastrozol.[277]

The largest trial to evaluate the AIs for adjuvant treatment of breast cancer is the anastrozole (Arimidex), tamoxifen alone or in combination (ATAC) trial. The drugs are given for 5 years to 9366 postmenopausal women. The first analysis at 33.3 months (median) follow-up showed anastrozole to have a significantly better disease-free survival than tamoxifen (reduced by 17%; $P = .006$). There did not appear to be a benefit from combining the drugs at this early date of analysis.[278]

Thus, adjuvant treatment of postmenopausal women with invasive breast cancer with tamoxifen or an AI is indicated for all T1-3, N0, ER-positive, PR-positive tumors with unfavorable histology or associated risk factors such as angiolymphatic invasion, high nuclear grade, and HER-2 overexpression. For those patients who are perimenopausal (<60 years of age) with ER- or PR-positive tumors, adjuvant chemotherapy followed by 5 years of tamoxifen or AI is indicated for the additive effects. Of the available AIs, anastrazole continues to be the preferred agent, but there is increasing interest in exemestane because it is slightly more active and because it appears to prevent bone loss. Whenever possible, the AIs should be administered as part of a clinical trial. Of importance is the evidence that indicates that the steroidal AIs do not show cross-resistance with the nonsteroidal AIs, and vice versa. A single study (MA17 Intergroup) compared 5 years of letrozole versus placebo in postmenopausal women with hormone receptor–positive breast cancer who, after receiving 4.5 to 6 years of adjuvant tamoxifen, were still disease free.[279] The early results of this trial are strongly supportive of the continuation of endocrine therapy using an effective AI in sequence with the 5 years of tamoxifen. The estimated 4-year disease-free survival rate is 93%, compared with 87% for the placebo group ($P < .001$).

For premenopausal women, there is increasing evidence that ovarian ablation or suppression using luteinizing hormone–releasing hormone plus tamoxifen is equivalent to adjuvant chemotherapy.[23] Further research is needed to document this and to explore the potential benefit of timing the oophorectomy to occur during the luteal phase of the cycle.

How can the quality of life of breast cancer survivors be improved?

Patients who have been successfully treated for breast cancer make up the largest group of long-term cancer survivors. It is important to recognize that at least one fourth of these are women younger than 50 years. As a result, issues of quality of life (QOL) are an extremely important component of overall outcome assessment. The term QOL defines the physical, psychological, social, and spiritual aspects of everyday living—measured during active anti-cancer therapy or as a survivor without known disease. Studies of QOL in such patients are important to identify the specific needs of patients that could be addressed by medication, psychosocial intervention, and physical therapy and exercise.

Only a few studies have compared breast cancer survivors with noncancerous healthy women.[280,281] Arndt and colleagues in Germany reported the results of a study designed to describe the QOL of patients with breast cancer 1 year after diagnosis and compared them to women in the general population.[282] They concluded that overall the QOL, general health, and physical functioning of breast cancer survivors 1 year after diagnosis was comparable to that of women in the general population. This was not the case, however, when they evaluated the emotional, social, role, and cognitive functions. These assessed measures of QOL showed persistent deficits and were more likely to be found in young women. Bloom and colleagues at the University of California, Berkeley, conducted in-person interviews with 185 women younger than 50 years at diagnosis who were cancer free for 5 years.[283] They compared QOL in the physical, psychological, social, and spiritual aspects of daily living at 5 years with an assessment performed a few months after the diagnosis. They found that about 75% were now menopausal with an improved QOL. They did not find any significant changes in employment status, marital or partner status, sexual activity, sexual problems, self-esteem, and attendance at religious services or frequency of prayer. Greater improvement in their physical QOL was associated with having fewer chronic health conditions, being employed, and having been treated with chemotherapy.

One of the more bothersome problems for younger women who have been treated for breast cancer is the symptoms associated with therapy-induced menopause.[284] As a result, the surgeon is frequently consulted by such patients regarding estrogen replacement therapy. The safety of using hormone replacement therapy (HRT) in women with a history of breast cancer has always been questioned because of the possibility that these hormones would stimulate the growth of micrometastases or induce the development of new primary tumors. A retrospective analysis from the Royal Hospital for Women in Australia found that women given HRT following the diagnosis and treatment of breast cancer had 16 new or recurrent incidents of breast cancer, compared with 31 incidents in a matching group of breast cancer patients not given HRT.[285] It is highly likely that any differences in increased risk for patients receiving HRT would be small if risks do exist, and therefore large numbers of patients would need to be randomized to establish a clear answer. A National Cancer Institute workshop concluded that HRT users could be predicted to have survival decreases greater than 2 years. This decrease does not appear to be as great when progestin is used in combination with tamoxifen to alleviate unwanted symptoms. Users of tamoxifen plus progestin are projected to live more than 0.5 year longer than users of tamoxifen alone.[286]

There are other options for managing concerns regarding osteoporosis, such as alendronate (Fosamax), an aminobisphosphonate that acts as a specific inhibitor of osteoclast-mediated bone resorption. The bisphosphonates inhibit the recruitment function of osteoblasts to produce an inhibitor of osteoclast formation. Clinical trials involving postmenopausal women treated with alendronate showed a 9% increase in lumbar spine density over a 3-year span as well as a significant increase in hip, forearm, and total-body bone density.[287] This resulted in a 50% reduction in fractures.[288,289]

The ability of the bisphosphonates to increase bone density and their lack of significant risk have positioned them as the first alternative to HRT in dealing with postmenopausal osteoporosis. Evidence has suggested that they may be useful in delaying the development of bone metastases. This promises to be an important new area of investigation in the management of breast cancer.[290,291]

There has also been increased interest in the role of physical exercise as an intervention that could improve QOL in cancer patients. One of the difficulties has been in determining the type of exercise—aerobic versus strength training—and there is little information regarding the frequency, duration, and timing of exercise interventions. In a review of 12 published randomized trials, the authors found a positive effect of exercise on overall QOL in three studies, a positive benefit in terms of decreasing fatigue in three studies, an improvement in physical function in one study, and an improvement in physical capacity, muscular strength, or both, during and after cancer treatment in six studies.[292] It certainly appears that exercise can be an extremely important part of the therapy regimen, but almost certainly such interventions need to be specifically designed and in fact tailored to the individual. The program needs to be adjusted to meet specific needs of the individual patient during different phases of active anti-cancer therapy.

How should patients with stages I and II breast cancer be followed?

The standards for follow-up and surveillance of breast cancer patients whose primary tumors have been successfully treated for cure are well established.[293] Initially, patients are seen by a member of the treatment team for interview and examination every 4 months for the first 2 years. This frequency is chosen in part not so much for the risk for early recurrence as for the positive effect physician–patient interactions have on addressing psychological as well as physiologic issues that determine post-therapy QOL. The visits are scheduled every 6 months for the remainder of the first 5 years and then conducted on an annual basis. At the time of the visit, a CBC, platelet count, and general laboratory chemistries, including a liver function panel and prothrombin time, are drawn. Some reports suggest that routine laboratory testing is not justified and that a carefully conducted patient interview and physical examination is sufficient for the early discovery of recurrent disease.[294] A chest film and mammogram are obtained every 12 months. For patients treated by breast conservation, the first follow-up mammogram should be obtained 6 months after completion of the breast radiotherapy.

Women taking tamoxifen require close follow-up regarding the risk for endometrial carcinoma. A yearly pelvic examination is mandatory. Controversy exists regarding the value of yearly uterine ultrasound, but certainly any change in ultrasound pattern of the uterine lining or vaginal bleeding is indication for uterine lining biopsy. It must be remembered that women with a history of breast cancer are also at risk for developing second malignancies and that colon surveillance every 3 to 5 years is as important as yearly pelvic examination for ovarian cancer and endometrial cancer.

Signs and symptoms obtained by careful interview or laboratory findings suggestive of recurrent disease require immediate restaging. This is accomplished by obtaining a bone scan and CT imaging of the chest, abdomen, and pelvis. MRI is generally equivalent to CT imaging unless there are specific indications for MRI's use. For example, MRI is preferred for evaluation of the central nervous system and spine. Biopsy of accessible specific lesions may be helpful, providing confirmation of the metastatic disease and an opportunity to determine the receptor status and *HER-2* expression as it relates to the metastatic disease—even when this information is available concerning the primary tumor.

It is important that the patient be able to identify with one physician member of the multidisciplinary treatment team. This can be a very supportive relationship and reduces the number of visits for the patient while continuing to provide optimal coordinated follow-up.

What can be said in conclusion?

Looking back at the list of questions that compose the format of this chapter, I am reminded of the much longer list of questions and concerns brought by patient and family to the initial interview. I am convinced there is nothing more devastating to the people of our time than to hear the words—no matter how carefully delivered—that announce the diagnosis of cancer. Those words change forever one's life and his or her confidence about the future. For a woman who often has such awesome responsibilities to children, spouse, and extended family, I believe the words have an even greater weight. For most women today, breast cancer is their greatest fear. The physician should remember this when providing for her needs and should listen intently as her responsible physician and member of her team. Finally, the goal is to reduce or eliminate this list of questions. This can only be accomplished through more questions and the research to find their answers.

REFERENCES

1. Bloom HJ, Richardson WW, Harrier EJ. Natural history of untreated breast cancer (1805–1933). BMJ 1962;2:213–221.
2. Schipper H, Turley EA, Baum M. A new biological framework for cancer research. Lancet 1996;348:1149–1151.
3. Brinkley D, Haybrittle JL. The curability of breast cancer. Lancet 1975;2:95–97.

4. Mamby CC, Love RR, Heaney E. Metastatic breast cancer 39 years after primary treatment. Wisc Med J 1993;92:567–569.

5. Gershon-Cohen J, Berger SM, Klickstein JG, et al. Roetgenography of breast cancer moderating concept of "biologic predetermination." Cancer 1963;16:961–964.

6. Spratt JS, Kaltenbach ML, Spratt JA. Cytokinetic definition of acute and chronic breast cancer. Cancer Res 1977;37:226–230.

7. Fournier D, von Kubli F, Barth V. Growth rates of 147 mammary carcinomas. Cancer 1980;45:2198–2207.

8. Skehan P. Cell growth tissue neogenesis and neoplastic transformation. In Skehan P, Friedman SJ (eds). Growth, Cancer, and the Cell Cycle. Clifton, NJ, Humana Press, 1984.

9. Gompertz B. On the nature of the function expressive of the law of human mortality, and on a new mode of determining the value of life contingencies. Philos Trans R Soc Lond B Biol Sci 1825;115:513–583.

10. Norton L, Simon R. Tumor size, sensitivity to therapy, and design of treatment schedules. Cancer Treat Rep 1977;61:1307–1317.

11. Norton L. A Gompertzian model of human breast cancer growth (comment). Cancer Res 1988;48:7067–7071.

12. Goldie JH, Goldman AJ. The genetic origin of drug resistance in neoplasms: Implications of systemic therapy. Cancer Res 1984;44: 3643–3653.

13. Skipper HE. Kinetics of mammary tumor cell growth and implications for therapy. Cancer 1971;28:1479–1499.

14. Citron ML, Berry DA, Cirrincione C, et al. Randomized trial of dose-dense versus conventionally scheduled and sequential versus concurrent combination chemotherapy as postoperative adjuvant treatment of node-positive primary breast cancer: First report of the Intergroup Trial C9741/Cancer and Leukemia Group B Trial 9741. J Clin Oncol 2003;21:1431–1439.

15. Piccart-Gebhart MJ. Mathematics and oncology: A match for life? J Clin Oncol 2003;21:1425–1428.

16. Chavaudra N, Richard JM, Malaise EP. Labeling index of human squamous cell carcinomas. Comparison of in vitro and in vivo labeling methods. Cell Tissue Kinet 1979;12:145–152.

17. Tubiana M, Pejovie MH, Chavaudra N, et al. The long-term prognostic significance of the thymidine-labeling index in breast cancer. Int J Cancer 1987;33:441–445.

18. Bergers E, van Diest PJ, Baak JP. Tumour heterogeneity of DNA cell cycle variables in breast cancer measured by flow cytometry. J Clin Pathol 1996;49:931–937.

19. Plevritis SK. A mathematical algorithm that computes breast cancer sizes and doubling times detected by screening. Math Biosci 2001;171:155–178.

20. Jansen JT, Zoetelief J. MBS: A model for risk benefit analysis of breast cancer screening. Br J Radiol 1995;68:141–149.

21. Michaelson JS, Halpern E, Kopana DB. Breast cancer: Computer simulation method for estimating optimal intervals for screening. Radiology 1999;212:551–560.

22. Jacks T, Weinberg RA. Taking the study of cancer cell survival to a new dimension. Cell 2002;111:923–925.

23. Love RR, Niederhuber JE. Models of breast cancer growth and investigations of adjuvant surgical oophorectomy. Ann Surg Oncol 2004; 11:818–828.

24. Demicheli R, Retsky MW, Swartzendruder DE, Bonadonna G. Proposal for a new model of breast cancer metastatic development. Ann Oncol 1987;87:1075–1080.

25. Demicheli R, Terenziani M, Valagussa P, et al. Local recurrences following mastectomy: Support for the concept of tumor dormancy [comment]. J Natl Cancer Inst 1994;86:45–48.

26. Baum M. Keynote Address at San Antonio Breast Cancer Symposium, December 12, 2002.

27. Saphner T, Tormey DC, Gray R. Annual hazard rates of recurrence for breast cancer after primary therapy. J Clin Oncol 1996;14:2738–2746.

28. Demicheli R, Abbattista A, Miceli R, et al. Time distribution of the recurrence risk for breast cancer patients undergoing mastectomy: Further support about the concept of tumor dormancy. Breast Cancer Res Treat 1996;41:177–185.

29. Baum M, Badwe RA. Does surgery influence the natural history of breast cancer? In Wise L, Johnson Jr H (eds). Breast Cancer: Controversies in Management. Armonk, NY, Futura Publishing, 1994, pp 61–69.

30. Retsky MW, Demicheli R, Swartzendruber DE, et al. Computer simulation of a breast cancer metastasis model. Breast Cancer Res Treat 1997;45:193–202.

31. Retsky M, Demicheli R, Hrushesky W. Premenopausal status accelerates relapse in node positive breast cancer: Hypothesis links angiogenesis, screening controversy. Breast Cancer Res Treat 2001;65:217–224.

32. Yakovlev AY, Tsodikov AD, Boucher K, Kerber R. The shape of the hazard function in breast carcinoma. Cancer 1999;85:1789–1798.

33. Sugg SL, Donegan WL. Staging and prognosis. In Donegan WL, Spratt JS (eds). Cancer of the Breast. Philadelphia, WB Saunders, 2002, pp 491–506.

34. Yasui Y, Potter JD. The shape of age-incidence curves of female breast cancer by hormone-receptor status. Cancer Causes Control 1999;10: 431–437.

35. Rosner BA, Colditz GA, Chen WY, et al. Risk factors for estrogen receptor positive and estrogen receptor negative breast cancer [abstract 157]. Am J Epidemiol 2003;157:S40.

36. Spratt JS, Spratt JA. What is a breast cancer doing before we can detect it? J Surg Oncol 1985;30:156–160.

37. McGuire WL, Randon AK, Allred DC, et al. How to use prognostic factors in axillary node-negative breast cancer patients. J Natl Cancer Inst 1990;82:1006–1015.

38. Prichard KI, Trudeau ME, Chapman JW, et al. Prognostic variables in node-negative breast cancer: An all subset analysis [abstract]. Proc Am Soc Clin Oncol 1993;12:68.

39. Chapman JW, Murray D, McCready DR, et al. An improved statistical approach: Can it clarify the role of new prognostic factors for breast cancer? Eur J Cancer 1996:32A:1949–1956.

40. Gorman RP, Sejnowski TJ. Analysis of hidden units in a layered network trained to classify sonar targets. Neural Networks 1988;1: 75–89.

41. Ravdin PM, Clark GM. A practical application of neural network analysis for predicting outcome of individual breast cancer patients. Br Cancer Res Treat 1992;22:285–293.

42. Cameron DA, Gregory WM, Bowman A, et al. Mathematic modeling of tumor response in primary breast cancer. Br J Cancer 1996;73: 1409–1416.

43. Cady B, Stone MD, Schuler JG, et al. The new era in breast cancer: Invasion, size and nodal involvement dramatically decreasing as a result of mammographic screening. Arch Surg 1996;131:301–308.

44. Tabar L, Fagerberg G, Chen HH, et al. Efficacy of breast cancer screening by age. The results from the Swedish two-country trial. Cancer 1995;75:2507–2517.

45. Leitch AM, Garvey RF. Breast cancer in a county hospital population: Impact of breast screening on stage of presentation. Ann Surg Oncol 1994;1:516–520.

46. Burstein HJ, Polyak K, Wong JS, et al. Ductal carcinoma in situ of the breast. N Engl J Med 2004;250:1430–1441.

47. Stomper PC, Connolly JL, Meyer JE, Harris JR. Clinically occult ductal carcinoma in situ detected with mammography: Analysis of 100 cases with radiologic-pathologic correlation. Radiology 1989;172: 235–241.

48. Stomper PC, Connolly JL. Ductal carcinoma in situ of the breast: correlation between mammographic calcification and tumor subtype. AJR Am J Roentgenol 1992;159:483–485.

49. Newcomb PA, Lantz PM. Recent trends in breast cancer incidence, mortality, and mammography. Breast Cancer Res Treat 1993;29: 97–106.

50. Taplin SH, Ichikawa L, Buist DSM, et al. Evaluating organized breast cancer screening implementation: The prevention of late-state disease. Cancer Epidemiol Biomarkers Prevention 2004;13:225–234.

51. Ostbye T, Greenberg GN, Taylor DH Jr, Lee AM. Screening mammography and Pap tests among older American women 1996–2000: Results from the Health and Retirement Study (HRS) and Asset and Health Dynamics Among the Oldest Old (AHEAD). Ann Fam Med 2003;1:209–217.

52. Juster FT, Suzman R. An overview of the Health and Retirement Study. J Hum Resour 1995;30(Suppl):57–356.

53. Myers GC, Juster FT, Suzman RM. Asset and Health Dynamics Among the Oldest Old (AHEAD): Initial results from the longitudinal study. Introduction. J Geront B Psychol Sci Soc Sci 1997;52:v–viii.

54. Blustein J, Weiss LJ. The use of mammography by women aged 75 and older: Factors related to health, functioning and age. J Am Geriatr Soc 1998;46:941–946.

55. Howe HL. Annual report to the nation on the status of cancer (1973 through 1998), featuring cancers with recent increasing trends. J Natl Cancer Inst 2001;93:824.

56. Tabor L. Beyond randomized controlled trials: Organized mammographic screening substantially reduces breast carcinoma mortality. Cancer 2001;91:1724.

57. Baum M. Screening mammography re-evaluated. Lancet 2004;255:751.

58. Blanka RG. Effect of NHS breast screening programme on mortality from breast cancer in England and Wales, 1990–8: Comparison of observed with predicted mortality. BMJ 2000;321:665–669.

59. Duffy S, Tabor L, Chen HH, et al. The impact of organized mammographic service screening on breast cancer mortality in seven Swedish counties. Cancer 2002;95:458–469.

60. Breen N, Wagener D, Brown ML, et al. Progress in cancer screening over a decade: Results of cancer screening from 1987, 1992 and 1998 NHIS. National Health Interview Surveys. J Natl Cancer Inst 2001;93:1704–1713.

61. Olson O, Gotzsche PC. Cochrane review on screening for breast cancer with mammography. Lancet 2001;358:1340–1428.

62. Kopans DB. Breast cancer screening: Women 40 to 49 years of age. PPO Updates 1994;8:1–11.

63. Niederhuber JE. Seeking calmer waters in a sea of controversy. Oncologist 2002;7:172–173.

64. Swedish Cancer Society and the Swedish National Board of Health and Welfare: Breast-cancer screening with mammography in women aged 40–49 years. Int J Cancer 1996;68:693–699.

65. Nystrom L, Andersson I, Bjurstam N, et al. Long-term effects of mammography screening: Updated overview of the Swedish randomized trials. Lancet 2002;359:909–919.

66. Donegan WL. Tumor-related prognostic factors for breast cancer. CA Cancer J Clin 1997;47:28–51.

67. Kuiper GJM, Enmark E, Pelta Huikko M, et al. Cloning if a novel estrogen receptor expressed in rat prostate and ovary. Proc Natl Acad Sci U S A 1996;93:5925–5930.

68. Melvin VS, Harrell C, Adelman JS, et al. The role of the C-terminal extension (CTE) of the estrogen receptor alpha and beta DNA binding domain in DNA binding and interaction with HMGB. J Biol Chem 2004;279:14763–14771.

69. McInerney EM, Weis KE, Sun J, et al. Transcription activation by the human estrogen receptor subtype β (ERβ) studied with ERβ and ERα receptor chimeras. Endocrinology 1998;139:4513–4522.

70. Cheung E, Schwabish MA, Kraus WL. Chromatin exposes intrinsic differences in the transcriptional activities of estrogen receptors α and β. EMBO J 2003;22:600–611.

71. Cowley SM, Hoare S, Mosselman S, Parker MG. Estrogen receptors α and β form heterodimers on DNA. J Biol Chem 1997;272:19858–19862.

72. Loven MA, Wood JR, Nardulli AM. Interaction of estrogen receptors alpha and beta with estrogen response elements. Mol Cell Endocrinol 2001;181:151–163.

73. Hyder SM, Chiapetta C, Stancel GM. Interaction of human estrogen receptors α and β with the same naturally occurring estrogen response elements. Biochem Pharmacol 1999;57:597–601.

74. Nilsson S, Makela S, Treuter E, et al. Mechanism of estrogen action. Physiol Rev 2001;81:1535–1565.

75. Donegan WL. Prognostic factors. Stage and receptor status in breast cancer. Cancer 1992;70(Suppl 6):1755–1764.

76. Katzenellenbogen BS, Katzenellenbogen JA. Biomedicine. Defining the "S" in SERMs. Science 2002;295:2380–2381.

77. Heldring N, Nilsson M, Buehrer B, et al. Identification of tamoxifen-induced coregulator interaction surfaces within the ligand-binding domain of estrogen receptors. Mol Cell Biol 2004;24:3445–3458.

78. Hedley DW, Clar GM, Cornelius CV, et al. Consensus review of the clinical utility of DNA cytometry in carcinoma of the breast: Report of the DNA Cytometry Consensus Conference. Cytometry 1993;14:482–485.

79. Gerdes J, Lemke H, Baisch H, et al. Cell cycle analysis of a cell proliferation-associated human nuclear antigen defined by the monoclonal antibody Ki-67. J Immunol 1984;133:1710–1715.

80. Gasparine G, Pozza F, Meli S, et al. Breast cancer cell kinetics: Immunocytochemical determination of growth fractions by monoclonal antibody Ki-67 and correlation with flow cytometric S-phase and with some features of tumor aggressiveness. Anticancer Res 1991;11:2015–2021.

81. Veronese SM, Gambacorta M, Gottardi O, et al. Proliferation index as a prognostic marker in breast cancer. Cancer 1993;71:3926–3931.

82. Railo M, Nordling S, Von Boguslawsky K, et al. Prognostic value of Ki-67 immunolabelling in a primary operable breast cancer. Br J Cancer 1993;68:579–583.

83. Porter-Jordan K, Lippman ME. Overview of the biologic markers of breast cancer. Hematol Oncol Clin North Am 1994;8:73–100.

84. Colognato H, Yurchenco P. Form and function: The laminar family of heterotrimers. Der DYN 2000;218:213–234.

85. Ivaska J, Heino J. Adhesion receptors and cell invasion: Mechanism of integrin-guided degradation of extracellular matrix. Cell Mol Life Sci 2000;57:16–24.

86. Shen X, Qian L, Falzon M. PTH-related protein enhances MCF-7 breast cancer cell adhesion, migration, and invasion via an intracrine pathway. Exp Cell Res 2004;294:420–433.

87. Philbrick WM, Wysolmerski JJ, Galbraith S, et al. Defining the role of parathyroid hormone-related protein in normal physiology. Physiol Rev 1996;76:127–173.

88. Dales JP, Garcia J, Carpentier S, et al. Prediction of metastasis risk (11 year follow-up) using VEGF-R1, VEGF-R2, Tie-2/Tek and CD105 expression in breast cancer (n = 905). Br J Cancer 2004;90:1216–1221.

89. Lin P, Polverini P, Dewhirst M, et al. Inhibition of tumor angiogenesis using a soluble receptor establishes a role for Tie2 in pathogenic vascular growth. J Clin Invest 1997;100:2072–2078.

90. Matsuno F, Haruto Y, Kundo M, et al. Induction of lasting complete regression of preformed distinct solid tumors by targeting the tumor vasculature using two new anti-endoglin monoclonal antibodies. Clin Cancer Res 1999;5:371–382.

91. Siemeister G, Schriner M, Weindel K, et al. Two independent mechanisms essential for tumor angiogenesis: inhibition of human melanoma xenograft growth by entering either the vascular endothelial growth factor receptor pathway or the Tie-2 pathway. Cancer Res 1999;59:3185–3192.

92. Glukhova M, Koteliansky V, Sastre X, et al. Adhesion systems in normal breast and in invasive breast carcinoma. Am J Pathol 1995;146:706–716.

93. Rimm DL, Sinard JH, Morrow JS. Reduced a-catenin and E-cadherin expression breast cancer. Lab Invest 1995;72:506–512.

94. Blackwood MA, Weber BL. Recent advances in breast cancer biology. Curr Opin Oncol 1996;8:449–454.

95. Siitonen SM, Kononen JT, Helin JH, et al. Reduced E-cadherin expression is associated with invasiveness and unfavorable prognosis in breast cancer. Am J Clinic Pathol 1996;105:294–402.

96. Palacios J, Benito N, Pizarro A, et al. Anomalous expression of P-cadherin in breast carcinoma. E-cadherin expression and pathological features. Am J Pathol 1995;146:605–612.

97. Paredes J, Milanez F, Sergio Reis-Filho J, et al. Aberrant P-cadherin expression: Is it associated with estrogen-independent growth in breast cancer? Pathol Res Pract 2002;198:795–801.

98. Christofori G, Semb H. The role of the cell-adhesion molecule E-cadherin as a tumor suppressor gene. TI BS 1999;24:73–76.

99. Ronzitti G, Callegari F, Malaguti C, Rossini GP. Selective disruption of the E-cadherin-catenin system by an algal toxin. Br J Cancer 2004;90:1100–1107.

100. Stetler-Stevenson WG. Type IV collagenases in tumor invasion and metastasis. Cancer Metastasis Rev 1990;9:289–303.

101. Duffy MJ, Blaser J, Duggan C, et al. Assay of matrix metalloproteinases types 8 and 0 by ELISA in human breast cancer. Br J Cancer 1995;71:1025–1028.

102. Yu M, Sato H, Seiki, M, et al. Complex regulation of membrane-type matrix metalloproteinase expression and matrix metalloproteinase-2 activation by concanavalin A in MDA-MB-231 human breast cancer cells. Cancer Res 1995;55:3272–3277.

103. Okada A, Bellocq J-P, Rouyer N. Membrane-type metalloproteinases (MT-MMP) gene is expressed in stromal cells of human colon, breast and head and neck carcinomas. Proc Natl Acad Sci U S A 1995;92:2730–2734.

104. Sato H, Takimo T, Okada Y, et al. A matrix metalloproteinase expressed on the surface of invasive tumor cells. Nature 1994;370:61–65.

105. Polette M, Gilbert N, Stas I, et al. Gelatinase A expression and localization in human breast cancers. An in situ hybridization study and immunohistochemical detection using confocal microscopy. Virchows Arch 1994;424:641–645.

106. Ito A. Nakajima Y, Sasaguri Y, et al. Co-culture of human breast adenocarcinoma MCF-7 cells and human dermal fibroblasts enhances the production of matrix metalloproteinases 1, 2 and 3 in fibroblasts. Br J Cancer 1995;71:1039–1045.

107. Noel AC, Polette M, Lewalle JM, et al. Coordinate enhancement of gelatinase A mRNA and activity levels in human fibroblasts in response to breast-adenocarcinoma cells. Int J Cancer 1994;56:331–336.

108. Sledge GW, Qualali M, Goulet R, et al. Effect of matrix metalloproteinase inhibitor batimastat on breast cancer regrowth and metastasis in athymic mice. J Natl Cancer Inst 1995;87:1546–1550.

109. Sledge GW. Implications of the new biology for therapy in breast cancer. Semin Oncol 1996;23:76–81.

110. Aaltonen M, Lipponen P, Kosima V-M, et al. Prognostic values of cathepsin-D expression in female breast cancer. Anticancer Res 1995;15:1033–1038.

111. Bossard N, Descotes F, Bremond AG, Bobbin Y. Keeping data continuous when analyzing the prognostic impact of a tumor marker: an example with cathepsin D in breast cancer. Br Cancer Res Treat 2003;82:47–49.

112. Gion M, Mione R, Dittadi R. Relationship between cathepsin-D and other pathologic biochemical parameters in 1752 patients with primary breast cancer. Eur J Cancer 1995;31A:671–677.

113. Berns EM, Klijn JG, Van Staveren H, et al. Prevalence of amplification of the oncogenes c-myc, HER2/neu, and int-2 in one thousand human breast tumours: Correlation with steroid receptors. Eur J Cancer 1992;28:697–700.

114. Slamon DJ, Clar GM, Wong SG, et al. Human breast cancer: Correlation of relapse and survival with amplification of the HER-2/neu oncogene. Science 1987;235:177–182.

115. Seshadri R, Firgaira FA, Horsfall DJ, et al. Clinical significance of HER-2/neu oncogene amplification in primary breast cancer. The South Australian Breast Cancer Study Group. J Clin Oncol 1993;11:1936–1942.

116. Perren TJ. c-erb-2 Oncogene as a prognostic marker in breast cancer. Br J Cancer 1991;63:328–332.

117. Yu D, Hamada J, Zhang H, et al. Mechanisms of c-erb 2/neur oncogene-induced metastasis and repression of metastatic properties by adenovirus 5 EIA gene products. Oncogene 1992;7:2263–2270.

118. Press MF, Pike MC, Chazin VR, et al. HER-2/neu expression in node-negative breast cancer: Direct tissue quantitation by computerized image analysis and association of overexpression with increased risk of recurrent disease. Cancer Res 1993;53:4960–4970.

119. Gusterson VA, Gelber RD, Goldhirsch A, et al. Prognostic importance of c-erb-2 expression in breast cancer. International (Ludwig) Breast Cancer Study Group. J Clin Oncol 1992;10:1049–1056.

120. Muss HB, Thor AD, Bery DA, et al. c-erb-2 Expression and response to adjuvant therapy in women with node-positive early breast cancer. N Engl J Med 1994;330:1260–1266.

121. Berns EM, Klijn JG, Van Putten WI, et al. c-myc Amplification is a better prognostic factor than HER2/neu amplification in primary breast cancer. Cancer Res 1992;52:1107–1113.

122. Allred DC, Clar GM, Elledge R, et al. Association of p53 tumor suppressor gene protein: An independent marker of prognosis in breast cancers. J Natl Cancer Inst 1993;85:200–206.

123. Silvestrini R, Benini E, Daidone MG, et al. p53 As an independent prognostic marker in lymph node negative breast cancer patients. J Natl Cancer Inst 1993;85:965–970.

124. Thor AD, Moore DH, Edgerton SM, et al. Accumulation of p53 tumor suppressor gene protein: An independent marker of prognosis in breast cancers. J Natl Cancer Inst 1992;84:845–855.

125. Bieche I, Champeme MH, Matifas F, et al. Loss of heterozygosity on chromosome 7q and aggressive primary breast cancer. Lancet 1992;339:139–143.

126. Lindblom A, Rothstein S, Skoog L, et al. Deletions on chromosome 16 in primary familiar breast cancers are associated with development of distant metastases. Cancer Res 1993;53:3707–3711.

127. Peron CM, Sorlie T, Eisen MB, et al. Molecular portraits of human breast tumors. Nature 2000;406:747–752.

128. Hedenfalk I, Duggan D, Chen Y, et al. Gene-expression profiles in hereditary breast cancer. N Engl J Med 2001;344:539–548.

129. Sorlie T, Peron CM, Tibshirani R, et al. Gene-expression patterns of breast carcinomas distinguish tumor subclasses with clinical implications. Proc Natl Acad Sci U S A 2001;98:10869–10874.

130. Sotiriou C, Powles TJ, Corosett M, et al. Gene-expression profiles derived from fine needle aspiration correlate with response to systemic chemotherapy in breast cancer. Breast Cancer Res 2002;4:R3.

131. Amatschek S, Koenig U, Auer H, et al. Tissue-wide expression profiling using a cDNA subtraction and microarrays to identify tumor-specific genes. Cancer Res 2004;64:844–856.

132. Hu Y, Hines LM, Weng H, et al. Analysis of genomic and proteomic data using advanced literature minim. J Proteome Res 2003;2:405–412.

133. Sotiriou C, Neo S-Y, McShane LM, et al. Breast cancer classification and prognosis based on gene expression profiles from a population based study. Proc Natl Acad Sci U S A 2003;100:1059–10398.

134. Puszatai L, Ayers M, Stec J, et al. Gene-expression profiles obtained from fine-needle aspirations of breast cancer reliability identify routine prognostic markers and reveal large scale molecular difference between estrogen-negative and estrogen-positive tumors. Clin Cancer Res 2003;9:2406–2415.

135. Dwek MV, Alaiya AA. Proteome analysis enable separate clustering of normal breast, benign breast and breast cancer tissues. Br J Cancer 2003;89:305–307.

136. Adam PJ, Boyd R, Tyson KL, et al. Comprehensive proteomic analysis of breast cancer cell membranes reveals unique proteins with potential roles in clinical cancer. J Biol Chem 2003;278:6482–6489.

137. Rui Z, Vian-Gno J, Yuan-Peng T, et al. Use of serological proteomic methods to find biomarkers associated with breast cancer. Proteomics 2003;3:433–439.

138. Chakravarthy B, Pietenpol JA. Combined modality management of breast cancer: Development of predictive markers through proteomics [review]. Semin Oncol 2003;30(4 Suppl 9):23–36.

139. Sadowsky NL, Semine A, Harris JR. Breast imaging. A critical aspect of breast conserving treatment. Cancer 1990;65:2113–2118.

140. Teixdor HS, Chu FC, Kim YS, et al. The value of mammography after limited breast surgery and before definitive radiation therapy. Cancer 1992;69:1418–1423.

141. Hustin R, Bernard F, Alavi A. Whole-body FDG-PET imaging in the management of patients with cancer [review]. Semin Nucl Med 2002;32:35–46.

142. Goerres GW, Michel SC, Fehr MK, et al. Follow-up of women with breast cancer: Comparison between MRI and FDG-PET. Eur Radiol 2003;13:1635–1644.

143. Daniel BL. Breast cancer magnetic resonance imaging and magnetic resonance guided therapy. Presented at Stanford Advanced Breast Imaging Course, Carmel, California, June 29, 1997.

144. Boetes C, Mus RD, Holland R, et al. Breast tumors: Comparative accuracy of MR imaging relative to mammography and US for demonstrating extent. Radiology 1995;197:743–747.

145. Merchant TE, Obertop H, DeGraaf PW. Advantages of magnetic resonance imaging in breast surgery treatment planning. Br Cancer Res Treat 1993;25:257–264.

146. Liberman L, Morris EA, Dershaw DD, et al. MR imaging of the ipsilateral breast in women with percutaneously proven breast cancer. AJR Am J Roentgenol 2003;180:901–910.

147. Rodenko GN, Harms SE, Pruneda JM, et al. MR imaging in the management before surgery of lobular carcinoma of the breast: Correlation with pathology. AJR Am J Roentgenol 1996;167:1415–1419.

148. Rubio I, Hars S, Klinberg VS, et al. Role of MRI in assessment of the extent of infiltrating lobular carcinoma of the breast [abstract]. Proc Am Soc Clin Oncol 1997;16:131a.

149. Hancock SL, Tucker MA, Hoppe RT. Breast cancer after treatment of Hodgkin's disease. J Natl Cancer Inst 1993;85:25–31.

150. Yaholom J, Petrek JA, Biddinger PW, et al. Breast cancer in patients irradiation for Hodgkin's disease: A clinical and pathological analysis of 45 events in 37 patients. J Clin Oncol 1992;10:1674–1681.

151. Kriege M, Brekelmans CTM, Boetes C, et al. Efficacy of MRI and mammography for breast-cancer screening in women with a familial or genetic predisposition. N Engl J Med 2004;351:427–437.

152. Mussurakis S, Buckley DL, Horsman A. Prediction of axillary lymph node status in invasive breast cancer with dynamic contrast-enhanced MR imaging. Radiology 1997;203:317–321.

153. Mumtaz H, Hall-Craggs MA, Wotherspoon A, et al. Laser therapy for breast cancer: MR imaging and histopathologic correlation. Radiology 1996;200:651–658.

154. Rutqvist Le, Lax I, Formander T, et al. Cardiovascular mortality in a randomized trial of adjuvant radiation therapy versus surgery alone in primary breast cancer. Int J Radiat Oncol Biol Phys 1992;22:887–896.

155. Valagussa P, Zambetti M, Biasi S, et al. Cardiac effects following adjuvant chemotherapy and breast irradiation in operable breast cancer. Ann Oncol 1994;5:209–216.

156. Lingos TI, Recht A, Vicini F, et al. Radiation pneumonitis in breast cancer patients treated with conservative surgery and radiation therapy. Int J Radiat Oncol Biol Phys 1991;21:355–360.

157. Fleck R, McNeese MD, Ellerbroek NA, et al. Consequences of breast irradiation in patients with pre-existing collagen vascular diseases. Int J Radiat Oncol Biol Phys 1989;17:829–833.

158. Robertson JM, Clar DH, Pevzner MM, et al. Breast conservation therapy. Severe breast fibrosis after radiation therapy in patients with collagen vascular disease. Cancer 1991;68:502–508.

159. Ross JG, Hussey DH, Mary NA, et al. Acute and late reactions to radiation therapy in patients with collagen vascular disease. Cancer 1993; 71:3744–3752.

160. Pezner RD, Patterson MP, Lipsett JA, et al. Factors affecting cosmetic outcome in breast-conserving cancer treatment-object quantitative assessment. Breast Cancer Res Treat 1991;20:85–92.

161. Recht A. Selection of patients with early stage invasive breast cancer for treatment with conservative surgery and radiation therapy. Semin Oncol 1996;23(Suppl 2):19–30.

162. Recht A, Connolly JL, Schmitt SJ, et al. The effect of young age on tumor recurrence in the treated breast after conservative surgery and radiotherapy. Int J Radiat Oncol Biol Phys 1988;14:3–10.

163. Nixon AJ, Schnitt S, Connolly JL, et al. Relationship of patient age to pathologic features of the tumor and the risk of local recurrence for patients with stage I or II breast cancer treated with conservative surgery and radiation therapy. Int J Radiat Oncol Biol Phys 1992; 24(Suppl 1):221–222.

164. Fowble BL, Schultz DJ, Overmoyer B, et al. The influence of young age on outcome in early breast cancer. Int J Radiat Oncol Biol Phys 1994;30:23–33.

165. Borger J, Kempermann H, Hart A, et al. Risk factors in breast conservation therapy. J Clin Oncol 1994;12:653–660.

166. Kurtz JM, Jacquemier J, Amalric R, et al. Why are local recurrences after breast-conserving therapy more frequent in younger patients? J Clin Oncol 1990;8:591–598.

167. Fourquet A, Campana F, Zafrani B, et al. Prognostic factors of breast recurrence in the conservative management of early breast cancer. A 25-year follow-up. Int J Radiat Oncol Biol Phys 1989;17:719–725.

168. Matthews RH, McNeese MD, Montague ED, et al. Prognostic implications of age in breast cancer patients treated with tumorectomy and irradiation with mastectomy. Int J Radiat Oncol Biol Phys 1988;14: 659–663.

169. Muscolino G, Luini A, Bedini AV, et al. Impact of young age on local recurrence risk in patients with early breast cancer undergoing QUART [abstract]. Breast Cancer Res Treat 1988;12:106.

170. Sismondi P, Bordon R, Arisio R, et al. Local recurrences after breast conserving surgery and radiotherapy. Correlation of histopathological risk factors with age. Breast 1994;3:8–13.

171. Rambert P, Lasry S, Hennebelle F, et al. Recedives mammaites après traitement conservateur du cancer du sein: Facteurs de risqué, topographies des recidives, evolution. Bull Cancer 1994;81:616–624.

172. Touboul E, Belkacemi Y, Ozahin M, et al. Conservative surgery and radiation therapy in the treatment of stage I and II breast cancer: Radiation therapy in the treatment of stage I and II breast cancer; influence of type boost (electrons vs iridium 192 implant) on local control [abstract]. Int J Radiat Oncol Biol Phys 1994;30:(Suppl 1): 245.

173. Halverson KJ, Perez CA, Taylor ME, et al. Age as a prognostic factor for breast and regional node recurrence following breast conservative surgery and irradiation in stage I and II breast cancer. Int J Radiat Oncol Biol Phys 1993;27:1045–1050.

174. Murthy AK, Hartsell WF, Griem KL, et al. Effects of age on local control of carcinoma of the breast after conservative surgery and radiation therapy [abstract]. Radiother Oncol 1992;24(Suppl):S40.

175. Van Dongen JA, Bartelink H, Fentiman IS, et al. Factors influencing local relapse and survival and results of salvage treatment after breast-conserving therapy in operable breast cancer: EORTC Trial 10801, breast conservation compared with mastectomy in TNM stage I and II breast cancer. Eur J Cancer 1992;28:801–805.

176. Burke M-F, Allison R, Tripcony L. Conservative therapy of breast cancer in Queensland. Int J Radiat Oncol Biol Phys 1995;31:295–303.

177. Vicini F, Recht A, Abner A, et al. The association between very young age and recurrence in the breast in patients treated with conservative surgery (CS) and radiation therapy (RT) [abstract]. Int J Radiat Oncol Biol Phys 1990;19(Suppl 1):132.

178. Vicini FA, Recht A, Abner A, et al. Recurrence in the breast following conservative surgery and radiation therapy for early-stage breast cancer. Monogr Natl Cancer Inst 1992;11:33–39.

179. Wyxkoff J, Greenberg H, Sanderson R, et al. Breast irradiation in the older woman: A toxicity study. J Am Geriatric Soc 1994;42:150–152.

180. Macy, RC, Umezawa Y, Leake B, Silliman RA. Determinants of participation in treatment decision-making by older breast cancer patients. Breast Ca Res Treat 2004;85:201–209.

181. Titcomb CL. Breast cancer and pregnancy. Hawaii Med J 1990;49: 18–22.

182. van der Vange, van Dongen JA. Breast cancer and pregnancy. Eur J Surg Oncol 1991;17:1–8.

183. Petrek JA. Breast cancer during pregnancy. Cancer 1994;74(Suppl): 518–527.

184. Petrek J, Seltzer V. Breast cancer in pregnant and postpartum women. J Obstet Gynecol Canada 2003;25:994–950.

185. National Institute of Health Consensus Conference. Treatment of early-stage breast cancer. JAMA 1991;265:391–395.

186. Smitt MC, Nowels KW, Zdeblick MJ, et al. The importance of lumpectomy surgical margin status in long-term results of breast conservation. Cancer 1995;76:259–267.

187. Fisher B, Redmond C, Poisson R, et al. Eight-year results of a randomized clinical trial comparing total mastectomy and lumpectomy with or without irradiation in the treatment of breast cancer. N Engl J Med 1989;320;822–828.

188. Gage I, Nixon AJ, Schnitt SJ. Pathologic involvement and the risk of recurrence in patients treated with breast-conserving therapy [abstract]. Int J Radiat Oncol Biol Phys 1995;58:225–228.

189. Mokbel K, Ahmed M, Nash A, et al. Re-excision operation in nonpalpable breast cancer. J Surg Oncol 1995;58:225–228.

190. Veronesi U, Luini A, Del Vecchio M, et al. Radiotherapy after breast-preserving surgery in women with localized cancer of the breast. N Engl J Med 1993;328:1587–1591.

191. Connolly JL, Harris JE, Schnitt SJ. Understanding the distribution of cancer within the breast is important for optimizing breast-conserving treatment. Cancer 1995;76:1–3.

192. Ohtake T, Abe R, Kimijimi I, et al. Intraductal extension of primary invasive breast carcinoma treated by breast-conservative surgery. Computer graphic three-dimensional reconstruction of the mammary duct-lobular systems. Cancer 1995;76:32–45.

193. Perez CA. Conservatory therapy in T1-T2 breast cancer: Past, current issues, and future opportunities. Cancer J 2003;9:442–453.

194. Rosen PP, Groshen S, Kinne DW, et al. Factors influencing prognosis in node negative breast carcinoma: Analysis of 767 T1N0M0/T2N0M0 patients with long-term follow up. J Clin Oncol 1993;11:2090–2100.

195. Winchester DP, Cox JD. Standards for breast-conservation treatment. CA Cancer J Clin 1992;42:134–162.

196. Danoff BF, Pajak TF, Solin LJ, et al. Excisional biopsy, axillary node dissection and definitive radiotherapy for stages I and II breast cancer. Int J Radiol Oncol Biol Phys 1985;11:479–483.

197. Giard S, Vanderstitches S, Laurent JC, et al. Conservative surgery in central small size breast cancer. Eur J Cancer 1994;30A(Suppl 2): S41.

198. Haffty BG, Wilson LD, Smith R, et al. Subareolar breast cancer: Long-term results with conservative surgery and radiation therapy. Int J Radiat Oncol Biol Phys 1995;35:53–57.

199. Dale PS, Giuliano AE. Nipple-areolar preservation during breast-conserving therapy for subareolar breast carcinomas. Arch Surg 1996; 131:430–433.

200. Moore CH. On the influence of inadequate operations on the theory of cancer. R Med Chir Soc Lond 1867;1:244–280.

201. Fisher B. Ten-year results of a randomized clinical trial comparing radical mastectomy and total mastectomy with or without resection. N Engl J Med 1985;312:674–681.

202. Fisher B, Jeong J-H, Anderson S, et al. Twenty-five year follow-up of a randomized trial comparing radical mastectomy, total mastectomy and total mastectomy followed by irradiation. N Engl J Med 2002; 397:567–575.

203. Fisher B, Anderson S, Bryant J, et al. Twenty-year follow-up of a randomized trial comparing total mastectomy, lumpectomy and lumpectomy plus irradiation for treatment of invasive breast cancer. N Engl J Med 2002;347:1233–1241.

204. Bonadonna G, Brusamolino E, Valagussa P, et al. Combination chemotherapy as an adjuvant treatment in operable breast cancer. N Engl J Med 1976;294:405–410.

205. Fisher B, Carbone P, Ecnomou SG, et al. L-Phenylalanine mustard (L-PAM) in the management of primary breast cancer. A report of early findings. N Engl J Med 1975;292:117–122.

206. Van Lancker M, Goor C, Sacre R, et al. Patterns of axillary lymph node metastasis in breast cancer. Am J Clin Oncol 1995;18:267–272.

207. Silverstein MJ, Gierson ED, Wierson JR, et al. Predicting axillary node positivity in patients with invasive carcinoma of the breast by using a combination of T category and palpability. J Am Coll Surg 1995;180:700–704.

208. Chadha M, Chabon AB, Freidmann P, et al. Predictors of axillary lymph node metastases in patients with T1 breast cancer. A multivariate analysis. Cancer 1994;73:350–353.

209. Cady B. Traditional and future management of nonpalpable breast cancer. Am Surg 1997;63:55–58.

210. Early Breast Cancer Trialists' Collaborative Group. Systemic treatment of early breast cancer by hormonal, cytotoxic or immune therapy: 133 randomised trials involving 31,000 recurrences and 24,000 deaths among 75,000 women. Lancet 1992;339:71–85.

211. Leher S, Garey J, Shank B. Nomograms for determining the probability of axillary node involvement in women with breast cancer. J Cancer Res Clin Oncol 1995;121:123–125.

212. Menard S, Bufalinio R, Rilke F, et al. Prognosis based on primary breast carcinoma instead of pathological nodal status. Br J Cancer 1994;70:709–712.

213. Menard S, Cascinelli N, Rilke F, et al. Re: Prediction of axillary lymph node status in breast cancer patients by use of prognostic indicators. J Natl Cancer Inst 1995;87:607–608.

214. Ravdin PM, DeLaurentiis M, Vendely T, et al. Prediction of axillary lymph node status in breast cancer patients by prognostic indicators. J Natl Cancer Inst 1994;86:1771–1775.

215. Graversen HP, Blichert-Toft M, Andersen JA, et al. Breast cancer: Risk of axillary recurrence in node-negative patients following partial dissection of the axilla. Eur J Surg Oncol 1988;14:407–412.

216. Cabanas RM: An approach for the treatment of penile carcinoma. Cancer 1977;39:456–466.

217. Morton DL, Wen DR, Wong JH, et al. Technical details of intraoperative lymphatic mapping for early stage melanoma. Arch Surg 1992;127:392–399.

218. Krag ND, Weaver DL, Alex JC, et al. Surgical resection and radiolocalization of the sentinel lymph node in breast cancer using a gamma probe. Surg Oncol 1993;2:335.

219. Giuliano AE, Kirgan DM, Guenther JM, et al. Lymphatic mapping and sentinel lymphadenectomy for breast cancer: Ann Surg 1994;220:391–401.

220. Giuliano AE, Jones RC, Brennan M, et al. Sentinel lymphadenectomy in breast cancer. J Clin Oncol 1997;15:2345.

221. Giuliano AE, Dale PS, Turner RR, et al. Improved axillary staging of breast cancer with sentinel lymphadenectomy. Ann Surg 1995;222:394–401.

222. Uren RF, Howman-Giles RB, Thompson JF, et al. Mammary lymphoscintigraphy in breast cancer. J Nucl Med 1995;36:1775–1780.

223. Tuttle TM. Technical advances in sentinel lymph node biopsy or breast cancer. Am Surg 2004;70:407–413.

224. Turner RR, Ollila DW, Krasne DC, et al. Histopathologic validation of the sentinel node hypothesis for breast carcinoma. Ann Surg 1997;226:271–278.

225. Pimas EP. Sentinel lymph node biopsy after neoadjuvant systemic therapy. Surg Clin North Am 2003;83:931–942.

226. Pendas S, Giuliano R, Tourdner M, et al. Worldwide experience with lymphatic mapping for invasive breast cancer. Semin Oncol 2004;31:318–323.

227. Haffty BG, Ward B, Pathare P, et al. Reappraisal of the role of axillary lymph node dissection in the conservative treatment of breast cancer. J Clin Oncol 1997;15:691–700.

228. Noguchi S, Aihara T, Nakamori S, et al. The detection of breast carcinoma micrometastases in axillary lymph nodes by means of reverse transcriptase-polymerase chain reaction. Cancer 1994;74:1595–1600.

229. Bedwinek J. Adjuvant irradiation for early breast cancer. An ongoing controversy. Cancer 1984;53:729–739.

230. Lipsett MB. Postoperative radiation for women with cancer of the breast and positive axillary lymph nodes: Should it continue? N Engl J Med 1981;304:112–114.

231. Levitt SH, Potish RA. The role of radiation therapy in the treatment of breast cancer: The use and abuse of clinical trials, statistics and proven hypotheses. Int J Radiat Oncol Biol Phys 1980;6:791–798.

232. Cuzick J, Steward H, Peto R, et al. Overview of randomized trials comparing radical mastectomy without radiotherapy against simple mastectomy with radiotherapy in breast cancer. Cancer Treat Rep 1987;71:7–14.

233. Fletcher GH. History of irradiation in the primary management of apparently regionally confined breast cancer. Int J Radiat Oncol Biol Phys 1985;11:2133–2142.

234. Lichter AS. Is radiation therapy in conjunction with mastectomy indicated for the treatment of operable breast cancer? Cancer Invest 1987;5:243–261.

235. Edlund RW. Presidential address: Does adjuvant radiation therapy have a role in the post-mastectomy management of patients with operable breast cancer?—revisited. Int J Radiat Oncol Biol Phys 1988;15:519.

236. Fletcher GH, McNeese MD, Oswald MJ. Long-range results for breast cancer patients treated by radical mastectomy and postoperative radiation without adjuvant chemotherapy: An update. Int J Radiat Oncol Biol Phys 1989;17:11–14.

237. McCormick B. Radiation therapy for breast cancer. Curr Opin Oncol 1993;5:976–981.

238. Pierce LJ, Glatstein E. Post mastectomy radiotherapy in the management of operable breast cancer. Cancer 1994;74:477–485.

239. Stefanik D, Goldberg R, Byrne P, et al. Local-regional failure in patients treated with adjuvant chemotherapy for breast cancer. J Clin Oncol 1985;3:660–665.

240. Griem KL, Henderson IC, Gelman R, et al. The 5-year results of a randomized trial of adjuvant radiation therapy after chemotherapy in breast cancer patients treated with mastectomy. J Clin Oncol 1987;5:1546–1555.

241. Fowble B, Gray R, Gilchrist K, et al. Identification of a subgroup of patients with breast cancer and histologically positive axillary nodes receiving adjuvant chemotherapy who may benefit from postoperative radiotherapy. J Clin Oncol 1988;6:1107–1117.

242. Marks LB, Halperin EC, Posnitz LR, et al. Post-mastectomy radiotherapy following adjuvant chemotherapy and autologous bone marrow transplantation for breast cancer patients with greater than or equal to 10 positive axillary lymph nodes. Cancer and Leukemia Group B. Int J Radiat Oncol Biol Phys 1992;23:1021–1026.

243. Overgaard M, Christensen JJ, Johansen H, et al. Evaluation of radiotherapy in high-risk breast cancer patients: Report from the Danish Breast Cancer Cooperative Group (DBCG 82) Trial. Int J Radiat Oncol Biol Phys 1990;19:1121–1124.

244. Ragz J, Jackson SM, Plenderleith IH, et al. Can adjuvant radiation therapy (XRT) improve the overall survival (OS) of breast cancer (BRCA) in the presence of adjuvant chemotherapy (CT)? 10-year analysis of the British Columbia Randomized trial. 1993;12:60.

245. Early Breast Cancer Trialists' Collaborative Group. Polychemotherapy for early breast cancer: An overview of the randomized trials. Lancet 1998;352:930–942.

246. Early Breast Cancer Trialists' Collaborative Group. Ovarian ablation in early breast cancer: Overview of the randomized trials. Lancet 1996;348:1189–1196.

247. National Institutes of Health Consensus Development Panel: National Institutes of Health Consensus Development Conference Statement. Adjuvant therapy for breast cancer, November 1–3, 2000. J Natl Cancer Inst Monographs 2001;30:5–15.

248. Wood WC, Budman DR, Lorzun AH, et al. Dose and dose intensity of adjuvant chemotherapy for stage II, node-positive breast carcinoma. N Engl J Med 1994;330:1253–1259.

249. Albain K, Grean S, Rardin P et al. Overall survival after cyclophosphamide, Adriamycin, 6-FU, and tamoxifen (CAFT) is superior to T alone in postmenopausal receptor (+), node (+) breast cancer: New findings from Phase III Southwest Oncology Group Intergroup trial S8814 (INT-0100) [abstract 94]. Proc Am Soc Clin Oncol 2001;20.

250. Fisher B, Dignam J, Wolmamk N et al. Tamoxifen and chemotherapy for lymph node-negative, estrogen receptor positive breast cancer. J Natl Cancer Inst 1997;89:1673–1682.

251. Hudis C, Seidman A, Raptis G, et al. Sequential adjuvant therapy with doxorubicin (A), paclitaxel (T), and cyclophosphamide (C) in women patients with resected breast cancer (BC) and 4 (+) lymph nodes (LN): Preliminary results [abstract]. Proc Am Soc Clin Oncol 1995;14:113.

252. Latreille J. The role of docetaxel (Taxotere) in the management of breast cancer: A summary. Semin Oncol 1995;22:1–2.

253. Hudis CA, Seidman AD, Baselga J, et al. Sequential adjuvant therapy with doxorubicin/paclitaxel/and cyclophosphamide for resectable

breast cancer involving four or more axillary nodes. Semin Oncol 1995;22:18–23.

254. Ravdin P. Taxoids: Effective agents in anthracycline-resistant breast cancer. Semin Oncol 1995;22:29–34.

255. Henderson IC, Berry DA, Demetri GD, et al. Improved outcomes from adding sequential paclitaxel but not from escalating doxorubicin dose in an adjuvant chemotherapy regimen for patients with node-positive primary breast cancer. J Clin Oncol 2003;21:976–983.

256. Piccart MJ, Lohrisch C, Duchateau L, et al. Taxanes in the adjuvant treatment of breast cancer: Why not yet? J Natl Cancer Inst Monogr 2001;30:88–95.

257. Mamounas EP, Bryant J, Lembersky BC, et al. Paclitaxel (T) following doxorubinary cyclophosphamide (AC) as adjuvant chemotherapy for node-positive breast cancer. Results from NSABP B-28 [abstract 12]. Proc Am Soc Clin Oncol 2003;22:4.

258. Rosen PP, Lesser ML, Arroyo CD, et al. p53 In node-negative breast carcinoma: An immuhistochemical study of epidemiologic risk factors, histological features and prognosis. J Clin Oncol 1995;13:821–830.

259. MacGrogan G, Bonichon F, de Mascarel I, et al. Prognostic value of p53 in breast invasive ductal carcinoma: An immunohistochemical study on 942 cases. Breast Cancer Res Treat 1995;36:71–81.

260. Goldhirsch A, Wood WC, Senn JH, et al. Meeting highlights: International consensus panel on the treatment of primary breast cancer. J Natl Cancer Inst 1995;87:1441–1445.

261. Leitner SP, Swern AS, Weinberger D, et al. Predictors of recurrence for patients with small (1 cm or less) localized breast cancer (T1 a.b N0 M0). Cancer 1995;76:2266–2274.

262. Hudis CA, Norton L. Adjuvant drug therapy for operable breast cancer. Semin Oncol 1996;23:475–493.

263. Clemons M, Goss PE. Mechanisms of disease: Estrogen and the risk of breast cancer. N Engl J Med 2001;344:276–285.

264. Harvell DM, Strecker TE, Tochacek M, et al. Rat strain-specific actions of 17β-estradiol in the mammary gland: correlation between estrogen-induced lobuloalveolar hyperplasia and susceptibility to estrogen-induced mammary cancer. Proc Natl Acad Sci U S A 2000; 97:2779–2784.

265. Thomas HV, Key TJ, Allen DS, et al. A prospective study of endogenous serum hormone concentrations and breast cancer risk in postmenopausal women on the island of Guernsey. Br J Cancer 1997;76: 401–405.

266. The Endogenous Hormones and Breast Cancer Collaborative Group. Endogenous sex hormones and breast cancer in postmenopausal women: Reanalysis of nine prospective studies. J Natl Cancer Inst 2002;94:606–616.

267. Zhang Y, Kiel KP, Kreger BE, et al. Bone mass and the risk of breast cancer among postmenopausal women. N Engl J Med 1997;336:611–617.

268. Cummings SR, Duong T, Kenyon E, et al. Serum estradiol level and risk of breast cancer during treatment with raloxifene. The Multiple Outcomes of Raloxifene Evaluation (MORE) Trial. JAMA 2002;287: 216–220.

269. Clemens M, Gross PE. Estrogen and risk of breast cancer. N Engl J Med 2002;346:340–352.

270. Tilson-Mallet N, Santner SJ, Feil RD. Biological significance of aromatase activity in human breast tumors. J Clin Endocrinol Metab 1983;57:1125–1128.

271. Jordon VC. The development of tamoxifen for breast cancer therapy: A tribute to the late Arthur Walpole. Br Cancer Res Treat 1988;11: 197–209.

272. Early Breast Cancer Trialists' Collaborative Group. Tamoxifen for early breast cancer: An overview of randomized trials. Lancet 1998;351: 1451–1467.

273. Smith RE, Good BC. Chemoprevention of breast cancer and the trials of the national Surgical Adjuvant Breast and Bowel Project and others. Endocrine-Related Cancer 2003;10:347–357.

274. Cuzick J, Powles T, Veronesi U, et al. Overview of the main outcomes in breast cancer prevention trials. Lancet 2003;361:296–300.

275. Day R, Ganz PA, Constantine JP, et al. Health related quality of life and tamoxifen in breast cancer prevention: a report from the National Surgical Adjuvant Breast and Bowel Project NSABP Breast Cancer Prevention Trial (BCPT). Br Cancer Res Treat 2001;69:210.

276. Jordon VC. Selective estrogen receptor modulation: Concept and consequences in cancer. Cancer Cell 2004;5:207–213.

277. Arora A, Potter JF. Aromatase inhibitors: Current indications and future prospects for treatment of postmenopausal breast cancer. J Am Geriatrics Soc 2004;52:611–616.

278. The ATAC Trialists Group. Anastrozole alone or in combination with tamoxifen versus tamoxifen alone for adjuvant treatment of postmenopausal women with early breast cancer: first results of the ATAC randomized trial. Lancet 2002;359:2131–2139.

279. Goss PE, Ingle JN, Martino S, et al. A randomized trial of letrozole in postmenopausal women after five years of tamoxifen therapy for early-stage breast cancer. N Engl J Med 2003;349:1793–1802.

280. Dorval M, Manunsell E, Deschenes L, et al. Long term quality of life after breast cancer: Comparison of 8-year survivors with population controls. J Clin Oncol 1998;16:487–494.

281. Tomich PL, Helgeson VS. Five years later: A cross-sectional comparison of breast cancer survivors with healthy women. Psychooncology 2002;11:154–169.

282. Arndt V, Merx H, Sturmer T, et al. Age-specific detriments to quality of life among breast cancer patients one year after diagnosis. Eur J Cancer 2004;40:673–680.

283. Bloom JR, Stewart SL, Chang S, Banks PJ. Then and now: Quality of life of younger breast cancer survivors. Psychooncology 2004;13:147–160.

284. Couzi RJ, Helzlsouer KJ, Fetting JH. Prevalence of menopausal symptoms among women with a history of breast cancer and attitudes toward estrogen replacement therapy. J Clin Oncol 1995;13:2737–2744.

285. Gitsch G, Hanzal E, Jensen D, et al. Endometrial cancer in premenopausal women 45 years and younger. Obstet Gynecol 1995;85: 504–508.

286. Perlman JA, Parnes JL, Ford LG, et al. Projections of the longevity effects of tamoxifen (TAM) and progestin (T&P) versus hormone replacement therapy (HTR) in breast cancer survivors requiring hormone symptom relief [abstract]. Proc Am Soc Clin Oncol 1997;16: 131.

287. Liberman UA, Weiss SR, Broll J, et al. Effect of oral alendronate on bone mineral density and the incidence of fractures in postmenopausal osteoporosis. The Alendronate Phase III Osteoporosis Treatment Study Group. N Engl J Med 1995;33:1437–1443.

288. Black DM, Cummings SR, Karpf DB, et al. Randomised trial of effect of alendronate on risk of fracture in women with existing vertebral fractures. Fracture Interventional Trial Research Group. Lancet 1996; 348:1535–1541.

289. Tucci JR, Tonino RP, Emkey RD, et al. Effect of three years of oral alendronate treatment in postmenopausal women with osteoporosis. Am J Med 1996;101:488–501.

290. Hortobagyi GN, Theriault RL, Porter L, et al. Efficacy of pamidronate in reducing skeletal complications in patients with breast cancer and lytic bone metastases. N Engl J Med 1996;335:1785–1791.

291. Diel IJ, Solomayer EF, Goerner R, et al. Adjuvant treatment of breast cancer patients with the bisphosphonate clodronate reduces incidence and number of bone and non-bone metastases [abstract]. Proc Am Soc Clin Oncol 1997;461:130.

292. Oldervoll LM, Kaasa S, Hjermstad MJ, et al. Physical exercise results in improved subjective well-being of a few or is effective rehabilitation for all cancer patients? Eur J Cancer 2004;40:951–962.

293. National Comprehensive Cancer Network. Clinical Practice Guidelines in Oncology, Version 1, 2005, Breast Cancer http://www.necn.org/professional/physician_gls/PDF/breast.pdf.

294. Pivot X, Asmar L, Hortobagyi GN, et al. A retrospective evaluation of indicators of recurrent breast cancer [abstract]. Proc Am Soc Clin Oncol 1997;16:134.

CHAPTER 23

Treatment of In Situ Breast Cancer

Gordon Francis Schwartz

When our surgical predecessors more than two generations ago began to use the "in situ" label to describe an "earlier," noninvasive stage of breast malignancy, they never realized the controversy their contributions would create several decades later. Until recently, it was believed that success in breast cancer therapy was directly related to the magnitude of the operation the surgeon could perform. The term *radical* was virtually always part of the description of the operative procedure employed to "cure" patients. It was not until screening mammography to achieve earlier detection became ubiquitous in the 1970s that our patients first questioned the appropriateness of their reward, that is, mastectomy, for their diligence.

Lobular carcinoma in situ (LCIS) and ductal carcinoma in situ (DCIS) were first described and first named by Foote and Stewart in 1941 and 1946, respectively.[1,2] *Lobular neoplasia* was first suggested as an alternative term for LCIS by Lattes[3]; the term *carcinoma* was challenged by Haagensen[4] as being misleading because the disease was not considered malignant in its own right. The name itself often led to more aggressive procedures based only on this unfortunate designation and the anxiety it engendered, affecting both patients and their doctors. Within the past 2 decades, largely because of screening mammograms, DCIS has come to occupy its own place on the program of virtually every breast cancer conference. Moreover, the discussion changes from one program to the next, with enthusiastic and outspoken advocates of what appear to be widely disparate philosophies about diagnosis, classification, and treatment.

LOBULAR CARCINOMA IN SITU (LOBULAR NEOPLASIA)

The treatment of LCIS, or lobular neoplasia, as some breast specialists prefer to call this risk marker, has been the source of considerable controversy. It was initially thought that this lobular proliferation of the breast epithelium, if untreated, led to the development of invasive lobular carcinoma in that breast. Haagensen was among the first to challenge this shibboleth with studies that indicated that LCIS was only a marker of risk and not itself malignant in the customary sense of the term.[3,5] He considered it a benign pathologic-clinical entity when it occurred by itself, without a coexisting invasive carcinoma. Despite Haagensen's efforts to effect a name change for this condition, from the anxiety-invoking term "lobular *carcinoma* in situ" to the less awesome "lobular neoplasia," LCIS remains the most commonly used name.

How is lobular carcinoma in situ diagnosed?

LCIS is almost always an incidental finding in a breast biopsy specimen, the biopsy having been performed for another reason. Unlike DCIS, it does not form a mass, it does not produce nipple discharge, and there are no mammographic findings to signal its presence. It is often multicentric and occurs bilaterally. Metastasis does not occur in LCIS. The lesion often involves both the acini of the lobules and the terminal ducts, and within the ducts, its differentiation from DCIS is sometimes difficult.

The evolution of LCIS within the mammary acini remains controversial. Within the lobules are two types of cells: epithelial cells, and beneath them, lining the cell membrane, the myoepithelial cells. These latter cells are not regularly seen within the acini. The proliferating cells of LCIS arise from the epithelial cells, filling the lumina of the acini to form solid rounded structures. These neoplastic cells are only slightly larger than the normal acinar epithelial cells, and mitoses are unusual. As these cells increase in number, they fill the acini, and the lobules become enlarged and more obvious. However, the diagnosis is not dependent on the number or size of the affected acini; rarely, a single lobule may be involved. Although most of the acini involved by LCIS are crowded with these cells, the cells do not have to fill the lumina to merit the diagnosis of LCIS. Occasionally, if a group of isolated lobules of LCIS is seen within the fat of the breast, it may be mistaken for infiltrating carcinoma. However, normal lobules may also be seen similarly isolated in the mammary fat.[5]

How can one tell the difference between lobular carcinoma in situ extending into ducts and ductal carcinoma in situ extending into lobules?

LCIS often involves both the acini of the lobules and the terminal ducts, and within the ducts, its differentiation

383

from DCIS is sometimes difficult. The involvement of small ducts by LCIS at the ductulolobular junction is often confusing. LCIS cells may form buds around the periphery of a duct, displacing the glandular epithelium, in a pattern that resembles Paget's carcinoma of the nipple. These growth patterns are commonly called *pagetoid spread* because of the presumed extension of LCIS cells into the epithelium of the ducts. Whether this finding represents DCIS extending backward into the lobule or LCIS extending into the duct is often a difficult decision for a pathologist.[6]

These occasional findings at the ductulolobular junction have also led to the question of whether LCIS and DCIS have a common origin in a stem cell lesion capable of going in either direction, that is, ductal or lobular. If a common precursor cell for both DCIS and LCIS could be documented, this would in part explain why the invasive cancers that develop subsequently in women with LCIS may be of ductal or lobular character and occur in almost equal proportions.

When the terminal ducts of the breast are involved by LCIS—and this may occur even to the point of the ducts' being more extensively involved than the contiguous lobules—the stain for E-cadherin can help to distinguish between LCIS and DCIS.[7,8] E-cadherin is a transmembrane glycoprotein responsible for calcium-dependent cell-to-cell adhesion. This protein is usually absent in LCIS but not in DCIS. Thus, at least in theory, DCIS cells stain for E-cadherin, and LCIS cells do not. Studies to date support this hypothesis with reasonable accuracy. Because current treatment recommendations for LCIS and DCIS differ, this distinction does assume clinical significance. Because a difficult distinction between LCIS and DCIS implies that the DCIS is almost always small in volume and of low nuclear grade, however, many DCIS experts would not recommend any treatment more aggressive than local excision and surveillance anyway. The major question then becomes whether to re-excise the area encountered to examine the contiguous breast tissue for additional areas of disease. Re-excision is generally not indicated for LCIS, whereas DCIS usually requires wider excision.

Quite recently, staining for high-molecular-weight (HMW) cytokeratins has been added to staining for E-cadherin at the Armed Forces Institute of Pathology (AFIP) to help differentiate borderline lesions into lobular and ductal phenotypes. The staining characteristics for these two markers are reversed in LCIS and DCIS, compared with the staining for E-cadherin. The stains for HMW cytokeratin are negative in DCIS and positive for E-cadherin; the opposite is true in LCIS, namely (perinuclear) staining for HMW cytokeratins but absence of staining for E-cadherin.[9] This simple-sounding (if expensive) way to differentiate these two lesions from each other is complicated by two groups of hybrid cells: positive hybrids that exhibit both markers, and negative hybrids that exhibit neither. The AFIP uses a designation *mammary intraepithelial neoplasia (MIN)* for an intermediate proliferation that cannot be assigned to either ductal or lobular origin by light microscopy; these hybrids may represent as many as half of the lesions designated MIN. The other half of these can be separated into lobular or ductal origin by these staining characteristics.

For reasons that remain unexplained, LCIS most often occurs in premenopausal women, or in postmenopausal women who are using estrogen replacement therapy, with or without concurrent progestins.

What was the initial experience with surveillance alone for patients with lobular carcinoma in situ?

The early Columbia studies of Haagensen convinced that institution's surgeons to observe rather than treat these patients, so that long-term data are available in that patient population. Two of the largest series of such patients are from the Columbia-Presbyterian Medical Center and from Memorial Sloan-Kettering Cancer Center.[5,10] Observations at the two institutions were similar, with only a minority of patients developing a subsequent invasive cancer. Their treatment options were initially quite different, however—surveillance alone, versus mastectomy, often bilateral—and the differences in treatment were considered to be related to where in New York City the diagnosis was made—West Side (Columbia-Presbyterian) or East Side (Memorial).

How common is lobular carcinoma in situ?

Because LCIS occurs uncommonly and is generally an unforeseen finding in a breast biopsy specimen obtained for another reason, Haagensen reviewed almost 10,000 benign breast biopsies to determine the actual incidence of LCIS. He found that LCIS was identified in 2.7% of biopsies for benign breast lesions. However, Page and colleagues found LCIS in only 0.5% of more than 10,000 benign biopsies at Vanderbilt University.[11]

What has been the subsequent experience with surveillance alone for lobular carcinoma in situ?

That patients with LCIS are at increased risk for invasive breast cancer at some time in the future is not questioned. All major studies have made this observation, although the reported incidence of subsequent breast cancer varies, from a low of 4% to a high of 35%. In the longest follow-up series, the probability of a woman's developing an invasive carcinoma was 13% by 10 years after the diagnosis of LCIS, 26% after 20 years, and 35% by 35 years, roughly a 1% increase per year.[12] Of crucial importance is the observation that after an initial diagnosis of LCIS, both breasts are at the same risk. Therefore, there appears to be no logical reason to perform mastectomy of *only* the breast known to harbor LCIS. The appropriate prophylactic procedure would be *bilateral* total mastectomy.

Whether there is a quantitative risk relationship between the extent of LCIS in the biopsy specimen and the likelihood of a subsequent breast cancer is also uncertain. Although studies indicate a trend in this direction, it has not been proved. Bodian and associates noted a 1.6-fold greater risk if more than 10% of the total number of lobules in a specimen were involved by LCIS, compared with specimens that had less than 10% of the lobules involved.[12] This difference was not statistically significant.

Are there any other risk factors for the development of invasive cancer in the patient with lobular carcinoma in situ?

Family history of breast cancer in the mother or a sister of a woman with LCIS might convey additional risk; this is of most concern in women who are diagnosed with LCIS before age 40 years. From the reported experience of Haagensen, the breakpoint between an even greater risk than the risk usually associated with the diagnosis of LCIS occurred at age 40 years.

An understanding of the typical course of the breast cancer that may develop is also crucial to the formulation of a treatment plan when LCIS is encountered. Both breasts, not just the one in which the LCIS was detected, are at about the same long-term risk for subsequent breast cancer. This observation suggests that LCIS, if not excised, does not itself progress to invasive cancer. Moreover, such lack of progression may be inferred by the histology of the subsequent breast cancer. In the review by Bodian and associates, only 27% of the subsequent breast cancers were invasive lobular carcinomas; the remainder were invasive ductal carcinoma, with several subtypes of ductal carcinoma found.[12] If progression from LCIS to invasive cancer were the rule, it would be expected that the later invasive cancer would be of the same origin. (Although purely invasive lobular carcinoma constitutes only about 10% of all breast cancers, many cancers seem to have both lobular and ductal features in association with each other.)

How has the management of lobular carcinoma in situ evolved?

Despite the reluctance of the medical community to change the name of LCIS to lobular neoplasia or another less threatening term, the treatment of LCIS has undergone significant evolution as physicians have accepted the concept that what had initially been considered a "real" cancer was in fact a marker of increased risk. Before its recognition as a marker, rather than as being malignant in its own right, it was most often treated by mastectomy. As this disease became better understood, unilateral mastectomy was abandoned as treatment, in favor of surveillance alone. To be sure, there are women for whom the specter of a subsequent invasive breast cancer is too great to endure, and this increased risk for developing a potentially life-threatening cancer leads them to choose mastectomy, with or without reconstruction. However, it must be stressed that mastectomy, in this context, is a prophylactic, not therapeutic, procedure. If chosen, it should be bilateral because both breasts are at about equal risk. Unilateral mastectomy, even with so-called mirror-image biopsy of the opposite breast, is not a logical choice. If the diagnosis of LCIS is made on the basis of a biopsy of one breast for an unrelated benign finding, it should be accepted that LCIS may also be present in the contralateral breast as well, given its predilection for bilaterality and multicentricity. Radiation therapy for LCIS is never indicated.

It has been a major undertaking to convince many surgeons that observation alone is appropriate when LCIS is detected. As recently as 1988, surgical oncologists were surveyed about their approach to LCIS, and one third of the respondents still advocated mastectomy. A slim majority, 54%, advised observation alone. When a similar questionnaire was sent to the same physician groups in 1996, 10% of the respondents still recommended unilateral mastectomy, suggesting their lack of information about this disease or their conviction that LCIS is a premalignant lesion.[13]

What advice should be given to the patient who has a core biopsy that reveals lobular carcinoma in situ?

The difficulty in making the diagnosis of LCIS with certainty in borderline situations is magnified when the specimen is a core biopsy performed to explore a mammographic finding. This is often true whether the tissue is obtained with a standard core needle or a vacuum-assisted core device (Mammotome [Biopsys Medical Instruments, Irvine, CA]). What should the next recommendation be—surgical needle-guided biopsy to excise the area in its entirety, or careful follow-up, usually a 6-month-interval mammogram? This problem has been addressed by several teams of breast specialists with modestly different conclusions based on small series of patients.[14-16] Because the diagnosis of LCIS in these situations is probably an incidental finding, this decision should be made in part by reviewing the reason for the original recommendation for biopsy (e.g., mass, parenchymal distortion, calcifications). If the microscopic findings *in addition to* the LCIS are not concordant with the mammograms, a surgical procedure would be mandated. When a suitable explanation for the mammographic findings is documented by the core biopsy and the explanation would not itself demand a surgical procedure, the incidental finding of LCIS would not play a role in this decision, and open surgical biopsy would not be recommended based only on the finding of LCIS. This recommendation is not valid if the microscopic sections are equivocal (i.e., LCIS vs. DCIS, LCIS vs. ADH [atypical ductal hyperplasia]) or if the pleomorphic form of LCIS is the diagnosis. Because LCIS itself is not considered malignant and is known to be multicentric and bilateral, attempting to excise all of it from the breast is futile and unnecessary. The same recommendations are valid if a core biopsy reveals atypical lobular hyperplasia (ALH) only.

What advice should be given to the patient with lobular carcinoma in situ?

Patients whose otherwise benign breast biopsies reveal the presence of LCIS should be informed that a marker for increased risk has been detected. They should be aware of the nomenclature and of the inaccurate use of the word *carcinoma* in this diagnostic phrase as the term is customarily employed. Because mammography has become the mode of diagnosis for DCIS, the differences between DCIS and LCIS should be discussed with the patient. Even when DCIS is treated by observation alone, it requires clear surgical margins (see the discussion of DCIS that follows) and is considered a unilateral threat, unlike LCIS. The patient should be informed that LCIS is usually multicentric and bilateral but requires no further treatment after its diagnosis. However, the patient should be informed of her two options: either bilateral total mastectomy with or without reconstruction, or lifetime observation. If mastectomy is chosen, it must be done with the patient's understanding that it is a prophylactic, not therapeutic, procedure. When acquainted with the risk for subsequent invasive cancer, using an approximation of a 25% risk in the next 25 to 30 years, the patient's choice depends on her own perceptions of this risk. Is her glass 75% full or 25% empty?

The Society of Surgical Oncology (SSO) has addressed this subject, in part, in its position statement on prophylactic mastectomy, updated in 2001: "Clinicopathologic presentations that portend risk of cancer with a specific indication for bilateral prophylactic mastectomies include . . . atypical hyperplasia of lobular . . . origin," and indications for unilateral prophylactic (contralateral) mastectomy in patients with a diagnosis of the ipsilateral breast include "lobular carcinoma in situ in the remaining breast . . . and . . . development of either invasive lobular or ductal carcinoma in a patient who elected surveillance of lobular carcinoma in situ."[17] The SSO did not make a recommendation for mastectomy in these situations. Its statement was issued, at least in part, "to guide insurance programs in determining coverage and help patients (who elect prophylactic mastectomy) to obtain reimbursement."[17] In 1996, the National Surgical Adjuvant Breast Project (NSABP) findings, in their review of 182 women with LCIS (only) enrolled in Protocol B-17, concluded that there was no reason to perform mastectomy on women with LCIS.[18]

LOBULAR CARCINOMA IN SITU SUMMARY

Since its presence and significance were first understood about two generations ago, and its acceptance as a risk marker, rather than as cancer sui generis, has been almost universally adopted, research interest in LCIS as a separate proliferative lesion has waxed and waned. The origin, detection, treatment, and even prevention of other breast proliferations or neoplasms moved LCIS into the background, so that interest in LCIS is generally resurrected only when its diagnosis is in doubt or its presence in conjunction with other lesions mandates consideration of its coexisting effects as well. It has now been well accepted by most breast experts that the treatment of LCIS is based on the patient's perceptions of the risk-to-benefit ratio, choosing between the subsequent theoretical development of an invasive and, therefore, possibly life-threatening cancer and the immediate effects of bilateral mastectomy. Additionally, no correlation has yet been made between the known genetic mutations that increase the risk for invasive cancer (e.g., BRCA1, BRCA2) and the occurrence of LCIS, or whether the combination of any genetic mutation and a personal history of LCIS implies a greater risk than either of these factors alone.

If we could identify precisely which patients with LCIS today will develop a "real" cancer tomorrow, perhaps we could tailor treatment to fit the situation. Using today's knowledge, however, bilateral mastectomy is unnecessary surgery for most women with LCIS. In a specialty practice devoted to breast diseases for more than 25 years, I have not yet performed a bilateral mastectomy for LCIS.

DUCTAL CARCINOMA IN SITU

What was the initial treatment for ductal carcinoma in situ?

Although the initial descriptions of what we currently call DCIS may have been formulated in 1946, it was not until 2 decades later that the difference between its behavior and that of frankly invasive breast cancer was really considered. In 1956, in the first edition of his book, *Diseases of the Breast,* Haagensen noted the various subgroups of "intraductal" carcinomas (i.e., comedo, solid, cribriform, and low papillary—morphologic definitions that still partially survive).[19] His patients' cancers were found as palpable masses with a mean diameter of almost 5 cm, and most had axillary node metastasis. The 5-year survival rate for these women was 58%, leading him to comment that the pathologists' suggestion that these tumors were "noninfiltrating" did not take into account the small portion of the entire epithelium that could be examined in any individual case, irrespective of how many microscopic sections were studied. Haagensen thought these cancers should be treated no differently from other invasive breast cancers, which at that time were managed by radical mastectomy.

As initial experience with mammography was gained in the late 1960s and early 1970s, these smaller and entirely intraductal cancers were detected with increasing frequency, usually as tiny groups of clustered calcifications, not yet forming an actual mass. Nevertheless, the standard of care remained mastectomy. It was assumed that despite the absence of invasion in the sections studied, progression to invasive cancer would inevitably occur. This assumption was based, in general, on observations of the coexistence of DCIS with invasive carcinomas, as well as on studies of patients who subsequently developed breast cancer after prior biopsies for what was thought to be benign disease but that on review demonstrated DCIS. This led to the recommendation for mastectomy, albeit with the expectation that the likelihood of the patient's dying of breast cancer without mastectomy would be negligible.

What has led to a reassessment of the management of ductal carcinoma in situ?

It was not until the late 1970s that Betsill and his colleagues suggested that untreated DCIS did not necessarily progress to invasive cancer, at least in some patients.[20] That observation has, in part, led to the current controversy about the treatment of this disease, compounded by the increasing incidence of DCIS detected by mammograms. This has occurred as screening mammography for asymptomatic women has been embraced as a major advance in the discovery of earlier malignancies and as notable improvements in mammographic technique, such as magnification films, have detected tiny, subtle changes within the breast.

In the past several years, current experience, including our own data, indicates that as many as one fourth of nonpalpable breast cancers (those detected by mammography) will prove to be DCIS. As implied by the name, DCIS appears to arise within ducts of the breast that become greatly dilated as the process evolves. In the usual scenario, when necrosis occurs within the lumina of the ducts, the precipitation of radiographically opaque inorganic material, usually containing calcium, leads to the mammographic discovery of these areas of intraductal disease as areas of clustered "calcifications" on a mammogram. It had been assumed that if the process continues without interference, the involved ducts grow in number and volume until finally discovered by the patient or physician as a palpable mass. At some time in this process, the formerly intraductal, cytologically malignant but biologically noninvasive cells penetrate through the basement membrane of the ducts, and the disease becomes invasive, with all of the implications of any invasive carcinoma.

As this inevitable progression of DCIS to invasive carcinoma has been challenged, with a minimum risk to the patient of developing a subsequent, life-threatening cancer, the importance of the identification of DCIS at some early stage in its natural history that will obviate the obligatory treatment of the *entire* breast (whether by mastectomy or by irradiation) has become a topic of great debate. If, as now accepted, DCIS is not always accompanied by invasion or does not necessarily progress to this stage, to prescribe lesser treatment for DCIS—that is, excision—than for invasive carcinoma implies an obligation to recognize when simple identification and excision of DCIS at this one site constitutes adequate treatment. This premise, however, also implies that the eradication of DCIS at one location ensures that the site detected is no greater in significance than what might be a concurrent, as yet undetected but more important (e.g., invasive) finding at another location within the same breast. We have reported that in our own series of patients with mammographically detected malignancy, other (multicentric) foci of DCIS may occur in other quadrants of the breast, but the likelihood of an unsuspected *invasive* cancer is remote.

What is the significance of *clinical* ductal carcinoma in situ?

The separation of *clinical* from *subclinical* DCIS to permit a more careful comparison of equivalent diseases was first suggested by Gump and coworkers, and their distinction also has great implications for treatment.[21] DCIS presenting as a palpable mass, as nipple erosion (Paget's carcinoma), or as nipple discharge is not the same as DCIS presenting as an area of calcifications on a screening mammogram or discovered as an incidental finding in a specimen of breast tissue removed for another reason. Haagensen and his contemporaries detected cancer based on clinical findings, whether as mass, nipple erosion, or nipple discharge; the so-called intraductal cancers that he treated had a mean diameter of almost 2 inches!

Staging systems for breast cancer have not yet addressed the entire spectrum of DCIS, so that all DCIS is considered stage 0, Tis. This presumes the absence of any invasion, however microscopic. Microinvasion of any size changes the staging to stage I, T1mic. The subdivision of DCIS into categories for consideration is somewhat arbitrary. Therefore, it is easier from the treatment viewpoint to discuss *clinical DCIS* (vide infra) than *subclinical DCIS*, which is detected by mammography or as an incidental finding. Current data indicate that there are patients in whom DCIS is *not* inexorably followed by invasive cancer, but I do not consider most women with *clinical* DCIS among that group. Except for highly selected patients, until data are available that refute this recommendation, patients with clinically detected DCIS should continue to undergo treatment that includes the entire breast, that is, irradiation or mastectomy, and selected patients should undergo axillary sentinel node biopsy. Exceptions to this dictum might be made for those patients with small (<1 cm diameter), palpable, but biologically favorable types of DCIS.

Therefore, using these definitions, the term *palpable DCIS* is almost an oxymoron. A palpable mass, even if largely intraductal, should not be considered noninvasive. As already noted, the appropriate designation should probably be "no invasion documented in the sections studied." Except in the case of such specially selected patients, these allegedly intraductal but palpable lesions are often accompanied by microinvasion, even when not seen, and the appropriate treatment addresses the entire breast and, arguably, the axilla as well.

Some of these predominately intraductal but palpable lesions may achieve considerable size and may be accompanied by clinically involved axillary nodes. They are characterized by their firmness, their fairly well-delimited margins, and an abundance of malignant-appearing calcifications on mammography. Patients with these large lesions are usually not candidates for treatment by irradiation because of the difficulty of excising all of the calcifications that permeate the ducts contiguous to and even at great distance from the mass itself. The palpable masses called DCIS that radiotherapists currently seek to treat are small ones, amenable to wide local excision with clear surgical margins.

What is the major histopathologic dilemma in the diagnosis of ductal carcinoma in situ?

The controversy about DCIS begins with a more careful definition. As noted previously, Haagensen and others carefully separated the term *intraductal* from the term *noninfiltrating*. The terms were not then considered synonyms! As radiographic techniques improved and the mammographic detection of smaller masses, then areas of nonpalpable calcifications, became more common, the terms *noninvasive, in situ ductal, intraductal, noninfiltrating,* and *DCIS* have become interchangeable. As currently used, each of these defining terms confirms the absence of invasive carcinoma. Additionally, rather than each being an entity unto itself, there is probably a continuous spectrum of "neoplastic activity" from what pathologists currently call atypical ductal hyperplasia (ADH) through DCIS to invasive carcinoma. The sometimes subtle changes that characterize the differences between these lesions (i.e., from ADH to DCIS and from DCIS to microinvasive carcinoma) often confound the most experienced pathologists. When shown the same slides, even renowned pathologists often disagree among themselves when trying to distinguish among these borderline lesions.[22] For example, Page has stated that the lesion should be considered DCIS instead of ADH if at least two duct spaces are involved.[23] Other pathologists consider geometric size more important, 2.0 mm being the cutoff between ADH and DCIS.[24] Irrespective of this controversy, even if labeled as DCIS, the lesion described in this scenario would be considered low grade, and the diagnostic designation on the "bottom line" of the pathology report should not influence patient care. The recognition of these difficulties in distinguishing what might be called low-grade DCIS from ADH has even led to the suggestion for a new name to describe these borderline lesions—MIN, ductal type, or ductal intraepithelial neoplasia (DIN).[25] The only difference between this system and current ones is avoiding the use of the term *carcinoma* in the body of the report. Instead, the terms, *DIN 1-a, DIN 1-b, DIN 1-c, DIN 2,* and *DIN 3* are used to describe the progression of changes that start with ADH and end with the comedo type of DCIS. Changing the terminology in this manner only minimally addresses the major question of classification in general.

Within the past few years, differences in architecture or morphology have gradually assumed less significance than nuclear grade, the presence and amount of necrosis, and immunohistochemical findings such as steroid hormone receptors, proliferation markers (e.g., Ki-67), and gene products (e.g., *HER-2, p53*). Because no current system combines ease of use, clear prognostic value, and reproducibility well enough to be uniformly acceptable, the optimal combination of these factors to influence treatment recommendations remains elusive. At a conference on DCIS held in Philadelphia in April 1997, the classification of DCIS was a major topic of discussion. About 30 distinguished scientists, including 20 breast pathologists from the United States and Europe, gathered for a consensus conference to attempt to codify the microscopic features that distinguish subsets of DCIS from one another. The intent of this conference included the identification of specific morphologic features of DCIS subgroups that convey prognosis. The proceedings of this conference have been published and are summarized in the next section.[26]

Microscopic Considerations

How is ductal carcinoma in situ currently classified?

Although DCIS was considered a single entity until recently, it is perhaps the ubiquitous use of screening mammography and the exponential increase in its frequency that have changed the way in which DCIS is regarded by most pathologists. The heterogeneity of DCIS is now well accepted among pathologists, and cases of DCIS with comedo features are probably outnumbered by those without.[27] When DCIS is detected as a palpable mass in the breast, its comedo features are almost invariably present. Less universally accepted has been the system of classification that describes differences in architecture. The major and customary architectural patterns that have been popularized are the comedo, solid, cribriform, papillary, and micropapillary types, although only rarely do any of these exist alone. Often, the papillary and micropapillary types are grouped together, so that four, rather than five, major subsets of DCIS based on architecture may be enumerated by some investigators. Unfortunately, criteria for differentiating among these various patterns are not clearly defined, so that comparisons of different studies of DCIS are difficult. When such studies are reviewed by other pathologists, as many as one third of the cases are reclassified.[28] There is no current system of classification of DCIS used by pathologists that combines the three ingredients required to make clinicians

comfortable—ease of use, reproducibility among pathologists, and, most important, *clinical significance.*

Prior classifications emphasized morphology, dividing DCIS into two basic groups, comedo and noncomedo. In general, the comedo type of DCIS is described as composed of pleomorphic cells, usually with a high mitotic rate, accompanied by central ductal necrosis. The absence of these factors then defines the noncomedo type, whether solid, cribriform, or otherwise described. Implied in this two-tiered system is a greater degree of aggressiveness of the comedo form of DCIS and its putative greater likelihood of recurrence in patients treated by less than mastectomy.

Only recently have pathologists addressed other factors, such as cytonuclear differentiation and biologic markers. This classification separates DCIS into three categories on the basis of the first two of these factors, cytonuclear and architectural differentiation. These categories are *poorly differentiated, intermediately differentiated,* and *well-differentiated* DCIS, also described as nuclear grades III, II, and I, respectively. These differences are best described by pathologists as they view slides. Already, the prior system of classification used by many American pathologists (comedo and noncomedo) has been replaced by a system that stresses nuclear grade, necrosis, and cell polarity, with architecture a secondary consideration only. The report of the consensus conference in 1997 emphasized the importance of nuclear grade in stratifying DCIS, with less emphasis given to architectural patterns and to the presence of necrosis.[26] The most promising area of research into the prediction of outcome following treatment is the use of genomic markers to stratify breast cancers. Gene expression patterns analyzed by complementary DNA (cDNA) microarrays may provide a "molecular portrait" of each lesion that correlates with prognosis. If this were to become available, each patient's treatment could be individualized with much grater precision and certainty about outcome. These patterns are currently being explored in invasive cancers, with interesting relationships being observed, and it is not fanciful to assume that DCIS might ultimately be stratified in the same way.

Quantifiable biologic markers, such as steroid hormone receptors, measurements of proliferation rate (Ki-67), and identification of gene products (*p53, c-erbB-2*), are now always available because they may be retrieved from paraffin blocks of formalin-fixed tissue. (They no longer need to be retrieved from fresh specimens within minutes.) Their roles in differentiating ADH from DCIS, or in defining degrees of aggressiveness of DCIS to aid in therapeutic recommendations, are currently unclear. Whether they are independent variables or only mirror what the pathologist can describe is also controversial.

Because DCIS itself is not a threat to the patient's outcome, it is only those patients who will develop invasive cancer who theoretically require (prophylactic) treatment. It is now accepted that at least some patients, perhaps a majority, with DCIS will never develop invasive cancer. What is currently unclear is how to make this distinction and recommend appropriate therapy for those who are in jeopardy.

Therapeutic Considerations

If pathologists cannot agree about the very definitions of in situ carcinoma, and if at both ends of the spectrum the subtleties between ADH and DCIS and those between DCIS and microinvasive ductal carcinoma are even more contentious, it is not surprising that treatment recommendations for DCIS are equally controversial. Early in the days of its recognition, patients with DCIS underwent mastectomy, usually with axillary dissection. Treatment was based on the (incorrect) presumption that an earlier stage of an inexorable, obligatory progression from DCIS to invasive cancer had been detected. Treatment for this earlier stage was the same as for its invasive successor, but with a better outcome anticipated.

Only as screening mammograms detected DCIS as smaller and smaller clusters of calcifications did this almost universal recommendation for mastectomy begin to change. The spectrum of disease or diseases that is represented by the term *DCIS* influences differences in therapy as physicians review each patient's situation individually. As already noted, the term *subclinical DCIS* has evolved to describe these mammographic findings or the incidental finding of DCIS in a (benign) biopsy specimen, the procedure having been performed for another reason. Clinically evident DCIS is represented by Paget's carcinoma, the presence of nipple discharge as the presenting symptom, or a palpable mass that is called DCIS.

How is Paget's carcinoma treated?

Paget's carcinoma, presenting as nipple erosion, is a form of breast carcinoma that may be entirely noninvasive. It grows initially within the milk sinuses of the nipple and extends within the ducts beneath the nipple in an apparently intraductal, but not always in situ, manner. The development of the disease may be multicentric within the breast. Patients with Paget's disease rarely have axillary node metastasis, unless a mass representing invasive carcinoma accompanies the nipple and areolar findings. Tempting as it may be to consider less aggressive surgical procedures, mastectomy with axillary dissection or sentinel lymph node (SLN) biopsy has remained the treatment of choice except in unusual situations. The mammograms in Paget's disease may be helpful in defining the retroareolar spread of disease. Although not well described in the literature, it has been our observation that calcifications in a branching distribution in the retroareolar area may help outline the intraductal spread of Paget's disease, proving its widespread character and the need for mastectomy.[29]

Although it is not necessarily true that the absence of retroareolar calcifications proves a more limited distribution of disease, when the calcifications are seen to be distributed in this pattern, the failure of any procedure that does not treat the entire breast can be appreciated. Nevertheless, we have treated several women with Paget's carcinoma by irradiation only, *not* excising the nipple–areolar complex. This choice is tenable only when the biopsy of the nipple indicates a relatively confined distribution of disease. These several patients have also been quite vocal and unequivocal in their desire to retain their breast. Despite this limited success with what should be considered a quasi-experimental approach, Paget's carcinoma should be considered as clinical DCIS, at the least. Untreated, Paget's carcinoma is inevitably progressive, albeit slowly.

How is ductal carcinoma in situ presenting as nipple discharge managed?

Patients presenting with spontaneous nipple discharge due to intraductal carcinoma are tempting candidates for treatment by something less than mastectomy. Because the mammograms in these patients rarely show evidence of mass or calcifications, and the usual morphology of the malignant cells is less rather than more aggressive, why not consider these patients within the group to be followed by surveillance alone? That had been our initial query as we began to search for patients with DCIS who might be candidates for local excision alone. However, after the first two patients so treated experienced recurrence relatively promptly, and we then reviewed the mastectomy specimens in other patients with the same presenting symptoms, we became more convinced that nipple discharge as the first sign of DCIS implies an uncertain intraductal, usually multicentric, distribution peripherally. At least in the traditional sense, in these patients it is impossible to perform a local excision ("lumpectomy") that definitively circumscribes the macroscopic disease. Irradiation as an alternative to mastectomy is not usually suitable because, if one believes that the macroscopic extent of the disease must be excised before irradiation, the nipple and areola must be part of the tissue sacrificed. Additionally, if one also believes in additional radiation to the site of the primary lesion, there is no specific site to boost.

Within the past few years, ductal lavage and ductoscopy have emerged as techniques to gain less invasive access to the ductal system of the breast through cannulation of retroareolar ducts, by obtaining effluent from duct irrigation for cytologic examination or by direct visualization, respectively. Proponents of these techniques claim that the diagnosis and extent of intraductal lesions, including carcinoma, can be aided by one or both of them. At this time, both should be considered experimental techniques, subjects for clinical trials but not yet part of the standard surgical armamentarium. Neither is currently indicated to influence a therapeutic decision.

How is the axilla to be treated in patients with ductal carcinoma in situ presenting as nipple discharge?

Treatment of the axilla is more controversial in patients with clinical DCIS detected as nipple discharge than in patients with intraductal carcinoma detected as Paget's disease or as a palpable mass. If frank invasion is present, treatment includes the same attention to the axilla as for any other invasive cancer when invasion is questioned, even if the invasion is termed *focal* or *microinvasive*. At least a sentinel node biopsy is a reasonable recommendation, with a more extensive dissection if the sentinel nodes are positive for metastasis.

It is more difficult to justify treatment of the axilla in patients in whom microscopic sections fail to detect any question of invasion whatsoever. However, because most of these particular patients are currently treated by mastectomy, and a total mastectomy includes the removal of the axillary prolongation (tail of Spence) of the breast, the lowermost axillary lymph nodes—those in what would be called by anatomists

irradiated or the patient is merely observed after excision, appropriate attention should be paid to achieving clear margins. The careful excision of a small area of calcifications is more difficult than a breast biopsy performed for a palpable lesion, especially if the surgeon wishes to spare a small breast from a significant cosmetic deformity. Not infrequently, a second specimen may be required to ensure that the mammographic abnormality has been removed. Because most needle-guided biopsies are performed for benign disease (our current benign-to-malignant ratio is 3:2, 40.7% of needle-guided biopsies proving to be for malignant disease), the pathologist's enthusiasm for the appropriately defined specimen must be tempered by the surgeon's and the patient's concern about the total outcome, including cosmetic concerns.

How the margins are measured is also variable, with most pathologists relying on inking the edges of the specimen in different ways (e.g., applying different colored inks each 90 degrees around the periphery of the specimen). We have never accepted this technique as optimal. These specimens are not smooth marbles that lend themselves to being coated by India ink in a uniform way. The excised tissue contains "nooks and crannies" related to varying proportions of fat, stromal elements, and glandular breast tissue. Excision of the primary site with separate dissection of the margins and the base of the wound and the application of metallic clips to these sites is our preferred alternative. This part of the procedure is best described as trying to peel an onion from the inside out. After the "lesion" has been excised according to the surgeon's judgment (best guess), arcs of tissue are excised from the edges of the biopsy site—for example, the superior, inferior, medial, and lateral wound margins—and from the base of the wound (the deep margin). As many marginal biopsies may be taken as the surgeon feels is appropriate. Each of these specimens is submitted to the pathologist in formalin in a separate, labeled container. If a single margin is positive, the appropriate area in the breast can be re-excised. If multiple margins are involved, perhaps the patient would be better served by mastectomy. Although we do not perform frozen sections on these marginal biopsies, if one did so, a positive frozen section margin would allow the removal of additional tissue at that site before closing of the wound.

The importance of margins was also discussed at the Philadelphia DCIS Consensus Conference in April 1997. The surgeons present at this conference generally felt that this technique of assessing margins by their separate excision was at least equivalent to the pathologists' inking putative margins of an excised specimen.[26] What's been left behind is more important than what's been removed! This is especially appropriate for the many patients with DCIS who have been referred for treatment recommendations following initial biopsy and diagnosis elsewhere. Re-excision of the primary site and dissection of wound margins and base are more precise than inking the margins of the specimen because the specimen is almost never uniform in its consistency or shape.

How should the excision site be managed?

When the specimen is sent to the pathologist, grossly apparent areas of abnormality may be examined by frozen section, and if malignancy is confirmed, a portion of the specimen may be saved for receptor and cytometric studies. It is more important, however, to determine invasion, if present, because treatment decisions in these particular cases are more likely related to the presence of invasion than to the quantification of receptors. Moreover, these studies may be performed subsequently, with even more accuracy, by immunohistochemical assay on formalin-fixed tissue from the paraffin blocks.

The earlier detection of mammographic abnormalities has led to greater technical difficulties for the surgeon and surgical pathologists. More often than not, there are no grossly apparent abnormalities in the breast tissue even though the calcifications are known to be within the specimen. We rely on the radiologist to confirm the presence of the calcifications within the excised tissue by specimen radiography, and often a clip is placed at the exact site within the specimen, as small as it may be. Both the specimen and the specimen radiograph are sent to the surgical pathologists so that they can be alerted to the exact site of the area of greatest concern, even within an already small specimen.

Additionally, because the orientation of the intraductal disease is segmental and often follows the distribution of the ductal anatomy, there is justification for excision of DCIS with orientation of the specimen toward the nipple. This implies a pyramid-shaped specimen, the apex of this pyramid being toward the nipple. When feasible, it is helpful to the pathologist to tag the apex of this pyramid with a suture to orient the specimen more carefully.

The application of metallic clips to wound margins and base offers precise localization of this site on subsequent mammograms. Because recurrence is most commonly detected as new calcifications at or near the same site as the primary lesion, using these clips to demarcate this area on subsequent mammograms facilitates the radiologist's detection of a new problem. We have used this technique of clipping wound margins and base for almost 20 years to prepare patients for irradiation following local excision (and axillary dissection) for invasive carcinomas. Both radiation therapists and radiologists have found it helpful to determine the site of the previous lesion accurately in this way.

How should the operative specimen be handled?

As with most of the treatment algorithms for DCIS, we use size as a treatment criterion. It is relatively easy to measure the area of calcifications on the mammogram, but this measurement often underestimates the extent of the DCIS within the breast. Lagios has suggested that the pathologist cut and embed each specimen sequentially when DCIS is suspected to ensure the most accurate measurement of size.[35] This lengthy approach is probably the most accurate one, but it is rarely employed outside research protocols because it is so costly and labor intensive. The ideal surrogate for the measurement of size by step-sections has not been found. What is needed is a technique that is accurate, reproducible, and cost-effective. Many small areas of DCIS are not easily defined by a single dimension, that is, diameter. Some are rectangular or irregular as DCIS propagates along the course of intramammary ducts. Perhaps a preferable measurement should be the total area of DCIS, the greatest length times the greatest width, as

We do not believe that
should be dogmatically
believe that it represents
predict the behavior of D
In our own experience, f
be a factor that independ
not when we have divi
younger than 50 years a
that younger women ha
grade 3 disease than olde
chance of recurrence.

Molecular markers s
receptors, Ki-67, p53, HE
been explored as offering
likelihood of recurrence.
shown the ability to di
treatment recommendat
cases, unfavorable marke
higher nuclear grade. In
cal difference was noted
and HER-2. Patients ha
both markers were eleva
very early in this chapte
analyzed by cDNA mic
portrait" of each lesion t

Why is excision alo considering curren about ductal carci

Another major reason t
an option for many of
culty in diagnosis. Altho
to distinguish from each
ing borderline lesions is
pathologists often inte
Patients whose patholo
subtleties and merely st
(DCIS), without a mo
treatment recommenda
same nonspecific desi
to resist making an imr
subclinical DCIS and
specimen. For example,
specimens initially calle
senior surgical patholog
are appropriately treate
equivalently experienced
diagnosis.

What is the role o treatment of ducta

As tamoxifen has becon
ment of invasive cancer
tioned. Few studies, hc
effects of tamoxifen aft
B-24 trial did address t
to tamoxifen or placebo
radiation; local excision

have entirely noninvasive lesior
dence of recurrence and will
Failure to treat the entire breast
however "micro" it is descri
survival.

3. *Adequate local excision of the prii*
   tioned, this is the only criterion
   trol because tumor biology and s
   of the tumor itself. Attention to t
   specimen is the surgeon's respor
   sion is the best compromise bet
   and the widest possible local exci
   greater than 10-mm (1.0-cm) clea
   around the area of DCIS. A pa
   has little tolerance for a large ex
   patient can obviously lose mor
   the edges of her area of DCIS.
   the actual size of the measured are
   mammogram is only a relative
   surveillance as opposed to radiatie

4. *Localized disease.* Recurrence is mo
   tiple foci of DCIS within the bre
   also generally prefer not to treat t
   when the mammogram shows m
   malignant-appearing calcification
   considered. This admonition abou
   only a relative contraindication wh
   are small and near each other. If a
   of calcification can be excised th
   and clear margins are achieved aro
   surveillance remains an option to
   DCIS is proven at several areas of
   graphically unreachable through
   mastectomy is the most reasonab
   option.

5. *Nuclear grade or presence of come.*
   argued that patients with the come
   have recurrence if the whole breast
   observations do not support th
   although we do agree that the mo
   forms of DCIS are more likely to
   different architectural features. Th
   features alone is not enough to disq
   sideration of breast conservation if
   be achieved.

6. *Absence of residual malignant-appea*
   postexcision mammogram. Even if th
   shows that the calcifications prove
   been removed and match the preop
   an additional postoperative mar
   mended. This should include mag
   site. If this film must be postponed
   fortable enough to undergo the films
   jeopardy to breast or outcome is
   interval is required to ensure that a
   have been removed.

7. *A compliant, motivated patient.* The p
   breast conservation for DCIS, with
   must accept the lifetime need for c
   first mammogram of the affected
   months after treatment. Mammograr
   month intervals for 3 years, than an

measured by assessment of the area of calcifications on the
mediolateral or craniocaudal mammographic projection. If,
over time, we could assess more accurately the discrepancy
between the mammographically measured disease (calcifications) and the actual disease measured microscopically, an
appropriate algorithm could be generated that would be both
reproducible and valid. Currently, measurement of the mammographic findings is the most reproducible estimate of size.
The specimen radiograph should confirm the excision of the
area in question, or a postoperative mammogram is indicated
to substantiate this important criterion.

How should the axilla be treated in patients with subclinical DCIS?

Because DCIS is noninvasive, there should be no reason to
address the axillary nodes in these patients. Before the advent
of axillary sentinel node biopsy, this was not a major question
because even the few publications that noted an infrequently
encountered axillary metastasis in patients with DCIS did not
consider this justification for the routine dissection of the
axilla. Because SLN biopsy has so significantly decreased
the morbidity associated with axillary surgery, whether SLN
biopsy should be part of the treatment for DCIS has emerged
as a new question.

If the data about axillary metastasis in DCIS are analyzed
carefully, they are almost always associated with the presence
of microinvasion or occult invasion in the breast, or with
patients undergoing mastectomy because of the extent of
DCIS within the breast. The consensus conference in 1999, as
did the consensus conference on sentinel node biopsy in 2001,
concluded that SLN biopsy is not indicated in patients with
DCIS treated by breast conservation with or without radiation.[32,36] In patients undergoing mastectomy for DCIS because
of the wide extent of malignant-appearing calcifications in the
breast, SLN biopsy is an appropriate consideration for two reasons: (1) should there be unexpected invasion detected in the
specimen, a subsequent axillary procedure after mastectomy is
difficult; and (2) in the presence of widespread DCIS in the
breast, even the most careful microscopic examination of the
specimen might overlook a tiny area of invasion. In these cases,
the pathologist's diagnosis of noninvasive disease may be
entirely correct, but only for the sections studied, irrespective
of how carefully the specimen is dissected. It is virtually
impossible to serial-section the entire breast in these cases
to rule out the presence of invasion without equivocation, and
the negligible morbidity of SLN biopsy in these patients is warranted to gain the additional assurance of a negative axilla.

What has been the experience treating patients with ductal carcinoma in situ by irradiation?

Comparing treatment of DCIS by lumpectomy only and
lumpectomy and irradiation, the National Surgical Adjuvant
Breast Project (NSABP) has reported the results of
their Protocol B-17, initially in 1993 with an update in
1997[37,38] (Table 23–2). Radiation decreased the likelihood
of both invasive and noninvasive recurrence. Invasive
recurrence after radiation was 3.9%; after lumpectomy alone,
it was 13.4%; recurrence as DCIS only was 8.2% in the irradiated group and 13.4% in nonirradiated patients. On the basis
of this study, the NSABP recommended radiation therapy
for *all* women with DCIS when breast preservation was
employed.

The European Organization for Research and Treatment of
Cancer (EORTC) also carried out a prospective randomized
trial comparing radiation and local excision alone for DCIS.
In their preliminary reports, this group also noted a reduction
in the incidence of invasive and noninvasive recurrence in the
radiated patients.[39]

Solin and colleagues, in a multi-institutional study, followed a group of 418 women (442 cases of DCIS) treated by
breast conservation for a median follow-up time of 9.4 years.
All of these women underwent radiation therapy for DCIS. Of
this group, there were 48 local recurrences, with a 15-year
actuarial rate of local recurrence of 16%. These data supported their conclusion that irradiation was an appropriate
treatment for DCIS.[40]

Unfortunately, these widely read and accepted publications
failed to contain any subset analysis, based on morphologic or
biologic parameters, that might identify subgroups of the
DCIS population who might fare as well with local excision
alone. The NSABP recommendation was for irradiation for
all DCIS patients who have breast conservation. In some
respects, the NSABP reports, carrying the weight of a prospective clinical trial by a widely respected group of investigators,
were a giant leap backward in the treatment of DCIS. We
and others have strongly emphasized the importance of
multiple factors, such as tumor size, margin status, nuclear
grade, necrosis, steroid hormone receptors, growth rate, and
immunohistochemical markers, that may determine the likelihood of recurrence after breast conservation. Various combinations of these factors may predict more precisely which
patients may be treated by breast conservation alone, which
might require radiation, and which might be best served by
mastectomy.

Table 23–2 Results of Local Excision and Radiation Therapy for Mammographically Detected Ductal Carcinoma In Situ

Study	No. of Breasts	Follow-up Time (months)	Recurrence (%)	Invasive (%)
Silverstein et al., 1999[33]	237	106 (mean)	20	46
Fisher et al. (NSABP), 1999[38]	410	128 (mean)	15	48
Solin et al., 2001[40]	422	112 (mean)	16	53
Julien et al. (EORTC), 2000[39]	507	51 (median)	10	45

Table 23–3 Results of Treatment o

Study	No.
Schwartz, 2002[46]	
Schreer, 1996[45]	
Arnesson et al., 1989[43]	
Silverstein et al., 2003[51]	
Lagios et al., 2002[41]	

What is the contemporary
with treating selected pati
with DCIS by excision alor

In 1975, Lagios and coworkers beg
with DCIS the possibility of local
tectomy nor irradiation[41] (Table 2:
women have been the most elega
been the longest. Thus far, 22% o
oped local recurrence, either furtl
carcinoma, after a mean follow-up
cancer deaths have occurred in
influenced by similar observations
greater participation in their ow
began to offer highly selected patie
excision alone—with the caveat th:
to 40% (our initial estimates) of
develop a subsequent invasive carc

The surveillance option after loc:
LCIS having been championed by
olation of the same treatment from
standable, but not accurate The
Haagensen about LCIS provided
commitment to the surveillance op
this study was initiated, however, tl
of information available about pati
local excision alone. Since that tim
published, but they have almost i
generically, without separating ca:
from the others. Thus, it has been d
to glean meaningful information al
clinical DCIS from the extant litera
patients reported by Lagios, howev
and Swedish reports of patients
detected by mammographic scree
and surveillance alone. The group
Carpenter and colleagues from C
London included 28 women treatec
mean follow-up of about 3 years.[42]
subsequent local recurrence. The g
by Arnesson and associates from tl
Linkoping, Sweden, included 38
alone.[43] After a mean follow-up c
(13%) had recurrence.

In 1992, we reported our own i
cases of subclinical DCIS in 70 pati
sion and surveillance alone. The me
times for this group were 49 month
tively, with the longest follow-up
the lesions in this group, all were

If our observations a
ther, only about 10% o
invasive cancer followi
number is higher, shou
of women with radiati
proportion will deve
cancer subsequently? Sl
Additionally, because a
tion therapy usually cal
ation at the time of in
attempt at treatment b
patients who have exp
alone, several have ch
without radiation or r
with bilateral DCIS w
patients in this situatic
their concerns are no
younger.

Documenting these
rence is crucial. If caref
it is yet noninvasive, p;
this alternative to mas
implication that recurr
the patient. If a sizal
excision and surveilla
carcinoma as the first :
fraction of this group
disease, and for thos
surveillance alone was

What is necessar
confident recom
excision and sur
patients with du

The challenge to thos
sion and surveillance
subclinical DCIS is de
define precisely the ul
cer, not further DCIS
cancer might occur,
may occur. We must t
dict who is at greatest
nuclear grade are the c
patients with DCIS a
recurrence. For exam
specimen of tissue re
associated with either
no patient with inc

Table 23–4 University

Parameter
Size (mm)
Margin width (mm)
Pathologic classificatic
Age (yr)

---

options remain open. The patient may be treated again by local excision alone, by local excision and radiation, or by mastectomy, using the same criteria cited at the time of her initial diagnosis. Although there may be a greater risk for additional recurrence in these patients, there are no data to suggest that any of these choices is now associated with a greater threat to life. We have treated several patients with second, and even third, DCIS events in the ipsilateral breast by additional attempts at local excision alone. It has been our experience, however, that as additional events occur, patients become more willing to undergo mastectomy and reconstruction instead of waiting for the "next shoe to drop." Nevertheless, none of our patients has yet developed systemic metastasis, even when an invasive cancer has been the second event.

What is the threat to life from ductal carcinoma in situ?

Irrespective of the recommendations for treatment—mastectomy, breast conservation with radiation, or breast conservation alone—and with or without the addition of tamoxifen, the available data indicate that DCIS is rarely life-threatening, even when it recurs. Ten-year disease-specific survival is reported between 96% and 100%.[50] In our own practice, the only patient with DCIS who has died from breast cancer is an elderly woman who developed an invasive cancer of the contralateral breast about 5 years after her treatment for DCIS by local excision alone. The contralateral breast cancer was unrelated to the initial diagnosis of DCIS. She subsequently developed metastatic disease, presumably from the invasive cancer, without ever demonstrating evidence of local recurrence of the DCIS.

Because of the very small long-term threat associated with the diagnosis of DCIS, and because the publications that recommend radiation as the treatment for all patients with DCIS still recognize that as many as 80% of the patients will not develop a recurrence or a second event when treated by local excision alone, we must continue to search for the specific characteristics of DCIS that will permit us to separate precisely those destined to recur from those that will never be a threat to either breast or to life. Current information about nuclear grade and margins, for example, is but a crude basis on which to separate patients into treatment recommendation categories.

Our experience thus far has reinforced our own impression that for most patients with DCIS, wide local excision, with margins of at least 10 mm, is treatment enough, presuming that the local excision can be achieved with a cosmetically acceptable breast. Patients with large or multiple areas of DCIS are better treated by mastectomy, so that our own greatest dilemma is really which patients with DCIS are best served by radiation therapy after local excision. If one accepts the NSABP results (which is a significant leap, because not all investigators accept their data as totally valid), why should we irradiate 100 patients to benefit 10? Because 10% of DCIS events will recur even with radiation, and 80% will not recur even without radiation, should we not be searching for the characteristics of patients or disease that identify the 10% who truly benefit from radiation therapy? The same analysis applies to the addition of tamoxifen; our information about tamoxifen is even more speculative than that about radiation.

That the patient must recognize the limits of our current knowledge about this disease is implicit in the mutual agreement between patient and physician to choose breast conservation as an option. A clear understanding of the biology and natural history of the disease that we call subclinical DCIS still eludes us. As clinicians, we have been involved in the care of too many women with lethal breast cancers, so that reluctance to abandon traditional treatment in favor of lesser options is understandable. Our respect for breast cancer is too great! "Overkill" has always been assumed to be a more sound philosophy than "underkill" when dealing with malignancy. If we could be convinced that certain diseases that we currently call malignant, such as DCIS, are not inevitably followed by invasive, life-threatening cancers, and that even if recurrence does occur, there is a second opportunity for successful interference, perhaps there would be greater enthusiasm for less, rather than for more, treatment. Unless we can enroll our patients in protocols that observe rather than always treat this disease, we will never know which, if any, women with DCIS can be merely observed without facing the specter of subsequent invasive breast cancer.

REFERENCES

1. Foote FW, Stewart FW. Lobular carcinoma in situ. Am J Pathol 1941;17: 481–495.
2. Foote FW, Stewart FW. A histologic classification of carcinoma of the breast. Surgery 1946;19:74–79.
3. Haagensen CD, Lane N, Lattes R, et al. Lobular neoplasia (so-called lobular carcinoma in situ) of the breast. Cancer 1978;42:737–769.
4. Haagensen CD. Diseases of the Breast, 3rd ed. Philadelphia, WB Saunders, 1986, p 211.
5. Haagensen CD. Diseases of the breast, 3rd ed. Philadelphia, WB Saunders, 1986, pp 192–241.
6. Rosen PP. Rosen's Breast Pathology, 2nd ed. Philadelphia, Lippincott Williams & Wilkins, 2001, p 596.
7. Jacobs TW, Pliss N, Kouria G, et al. Carcinomas in situ of the breast with indeterminate features: Role of E-cadherin staining in categorization. Am J Surg Pathol 2001;25:229–236.
8. Goldstein NS, Kestin LL, Vicini FA. Clinicopathologic implications of E-cadherin reactivity in patients with lobular carcinoma of the breast. Cancer 2001;92:738–747.
9. Bratthauer GL, Moinfar F, Stamatakos MD, et al. Combined E-cadherin and high molecular weight cytokeratin immunoprofile differentiates lobular, ductal, and hybrid mammary, intraepithelial neoplasias. Hum Pathol 2002;620–627.
10. Rosen PP, Lieberman PH, Braun DQ, et al. Lobular carcinoma of the breast. Detailed analysis of 99 patients with average follow-up of 24 years. Am J Surg Pathol 1978;2:225–251.
11. Page DL, Kidd TE Jr, Dupont WD, et al. Lobular neoplasias of the breast: Higher risk for subsequent invasive cancer predicted by more extensive disease. Hum Pathol 1991;22:1232–1239.
12. Bodian CA, Perzin KH, Lattes R. Lobular neoplasias: Long-term risk of breast cancer and relation to other factors. Cancer 1996;78:1024–1034.
13. Gump FE, Kinne DW, Schwartz GF. Current treatment for lobular carcinoma in situ. Ann Surg Oncol, 1998;5:33–36.
14. Liberman L, Sama M, Susnik B, et al. Lobular carcinoma in situ at percutaneous breast biopsy: Surgical biopsy findings. AJR Am J Roentgenol 1999;173:291–299.
15. Berg WA, Morse HE, Ioffe OB. Atypical lobular hyperplasia or lobular carcinoma in situ at core-needle biopsy. Radiology 2001;218:503–509.
16. O'Driscoll D, Britton P, Bobrow L, et al. Lobular carcinoma in situ on core biopsy: What is the clinical significance? Clin Radiol 2001;56: 216–220.
17. Society of Surgical Oncology. Position statement on prophylactic mastectomy, August 11, 2002 [On-line]. Available: http://www.surgonc.org. sso/mastectomy/htm.

18. Fisher ER, Costantino J, Fisher B, et al. Pathologic findings of the National Surgical Adjuvant Breast Project (NSABP) Protocol B-17. Five year observations concerning lobular carcinoma in situ. Cancer 1996;78:1403–1416.

19. Haagensen CD. Diseases of the breast, 1st ed. Philadelphia, WB Saunders, 1956, pp 502–506.

20. Betsill WL Jr, Rosen PP, Lieberman PH, et al. Intraductal carcinoma: Long-term followup after treatment by biopsy alone. JAMA 1978;239: 1963–1967.

21. Gump FE, Jicha DL, Ozello L. Ductal carcinoma in situ (DCIS): A revised concept. Surgery 1987;102:790–795.

22. Rosai J. Borderline epithelial lesions of the breast. Am J Surg Pathol 1991;15:209–221.

23. Page DL, Rogers LW. Combined histologic and cytologic criteria for the diagnosis of mammary atypical ductal hyperplasia. Hum Pathol 1992; 23:1095–1097.

24. Connolly JL, Schnitt SJ. Benign breast disease: Resolved and unresolved issues. Cancer 1993;71:1187–1189.

25. Tavassoli F. Mammary intraepithelial neoplasias: A translational classification system for the Intraductal epithelial proliferations. Breast J 1997;3:48–58.

26. Consensus Conference on the Classification of Ductal Carcinoma in Situ. Cancer 1997;80:1798–1802.

27. Patchefsky AS, Schwartz GF, Finklestein SD, et al. Heterogeneity of Intraductal carcinoma of the breast. Cancer 1989;63:731–741.

28. vanDongen J, Holland R, Peters J, et al. Ductal carcinoma in situ of the breast: Second EORTC consensus meeting. Eur J Cancer 1992;28:626–629.

29. Schwartz GF, Carter WB, Finkel GC. Paget's carcinoma of the breast. Surg Oncol Clin North Am 1993;2:93–106.

30. International Breast Cancer Consensus Conference Committee. Image-detected breast cancer: State of the art diagnosis and treatment. J Am Coll Surg 2001;193:297–302.

31. Liberman L. Ductal carcinoma in situ: Percutaneous biopsy considerations. Semin Breast Dis 2000;3:14–25.

32. Schwartz GF, Solin LJ, Olivotto IA, et al. Consensus conference on the treatment of in situ ductal carcinoma of the breast, April 22–25, 1999. Cancer 2000;88:946–954.

33. Silverstein MJ, Lagios MD, Groshen S, et al. The influence of margin width on local control in patients with ductal carcinoma in situ (DCIS) of the breast. N Engl J Med 1999;340:1455–1461.

34. Boland GP, Chan KC, Knox WF, et al. Value of the Van Nuys Prognostic Index in prediction of recurrence of ductal carcinoma in situ after breast-conserving surgery. Br J Surg 2003;90:426–432.

35. Lagios MD. Duct carcinoma in situ: Pathology and treatment. Surg Clin North Am 1990;70:853–871.

36. Schwartz GF, Giuliano AE, Veronesi U, and the Consensus Conference Committee. Proceedings of consensus conference on the role of

37. Fisher B, Costantino J, Redmond C, et al. Lumpectomy compared with lumpectomy and radiation therapy for the treatment of intraductal breast cancer. N Engl J Med, 1993;328:1581–1586.

38. Fisher B, Dignam J, Tan-Chiu E, et al. Pathologic findings from the National Surgical Adjuvant Breast Project (NSABP) eight-year update of Protocol B-17: Intraductal carcinoma. Cancer 1999;86:429–438.

39. Julien JP, Bijker N, Fentiman IS, et al. Radiotherapy in breast conserving treatment for ductal carcinoma in situ: First results of the EORTC randomized phase III trial 10853. Lancet 2000;355:528–533.

40. Solin LJ, Fourquet A, Vicini FA, et al. Mammographically detected ductal carcinoma in situ of the breast treated with breast conserving surgery and definitive irradiation: Long-term outcome and prognostic significance of patient age and margin status. Int J Radiat Oncol Biol Phys 2001;50:991–1002.

41. Lagios MD. The Lagios experience. In Silverstein MJ, Recht A, Lagios MD, eds. Ductal Carcinoma of the Breast, 2nd ed. Philadelphia, Lippincott Williams & Wilkins, 2002, pp 302–307.

42. Carpenter R, Boulter PS, Cooke T, et al. Management of screen detected ductal carcinoma in situ of the breast. Br J Surg 1989;76:672–675.

43. Arnesson L-G, Smeds S, Fagerberg G, et al. Follow-up of two treatment modalities for ductal carcinoma in situ of the breast. Br J Surg 1989;76:672–675.

44. Schwartz GF, Finkel GC, Garcia JC, et al. Subclinical ductal carcinoma in situ of the breast: Treatment by local excision and surveillance alone. Cancer 1992;70:2468–2474.

45. Schreer I. Conservation therapy of DCIS without irradiation. Breast Dis 1996;9:27–36.

46. Schwartz GF. Treatment of subclinical ductal carcinoma in situ of the breast by local excision and surveillance alone: An updated personal experience. In Silverstein MJ, Recht A, Lagios MD, eds. Ductal Carcinoma of the Breast, 2nd ed. Philadelphia, Lippincott Williams & Wilkins, 2002, pp 309–321.

47. Silverstein MJ, Lagios MD, Craig PH, et al. A prognostic index for ductal carcinoma in situ of the breast. Cancer 1996;77:2267–2274.

48. Silverstein MJ. The University of Southern California/Van Nuys prognostic index for ductal carcinoma of the breast. Am J Surg 2003;186: 337–343.

49. Fisher B, Dignam J, Wolmark N, et al. Tamoxifen in treatment of intraductal breast cancer: National Surgical Adjuvant Breast and Bowel Project B-24 randomized control trial. Lancet 1999;353:1993–2000.

50. Morrow M, Strom EA, Bassett Law, et al. Standard for the management of ductal carcinoma in situ of the breast (DCIS). CA Cancer J Clinician 2002;52:256–276.

51. Silverstein MJ. The University of Southern California/Van Nuys prognostic index for ductal carcinoma in situ of the berast. Am J Surg 2003;186:337–343.

CHAPTER 24

Surgery for Breast Cancer

Daniel F. Roses and Armando E. Giuliano

The surgical options for the treatment of breast cancer have greatly broadened in recent decades as the acceptance of breast conservation and local radiotherapy, selective surgical approaches to axillary lymph nodes, reconstruction, and adjuvant systemic therapy, as well as the adoption of more precise approaches to radiographic and pathologic assessment, have made treatment far more selective. The retreat from a uniform reliance on mastectomy, however, has often blurred a definition of the appropriate extent of surgery. This lack of precision reflects in turn an uncertainty about the impact that different forms of local treatment may have on survival. Nevertheless, despite paradigms of breast cancer biology that emphasize the importance of systemic rather than local therapy, and therapeutic strategies that incorporate nonsurgical modalities for both local and systemic disease, modern breast cancer treatment continues to require, and has even amplified, the application of sound surgical principles and techniques for both the local control and the appropriate staging of disease.

DEVELOPMENT AND TOPOGRAPHIC ANATOMY OF THE BREAST

An appreciation of the topographic anatomy of the breast is essential not only for clinical and radiographic diagnosis but also for planning surgical strategies and delineating the optimal sites for incisions as well as the extent of the breast parenchyma and regional lymphatic drainage. An ever-increasing emphasis on the opportunities to achieve a satisfactory or even excellent aesthetic result through breast conservation or reconstruction, as well as an emphasis on more limited surgery for the axilla, has made topographic considerations in breast cancer surgery of particular importance.

How does breast topography develop embryologically?

Embryologically, the breast develops from an ectodermal ridge found in a 7-week embryo extending on each side from the base of the forelimb to the region of the hind limb.[1] This milk line persists by the ninth week only in the region of the future pectoral muscles, the remainder having involuted, although fragments may persist in a line from the axilla to the pubis. In a small percentage of women, this accessory tissue persists as accessory nipples, known as *polythelia,* or as accessory parenchyma in locations along this epithelial milk line, most commonly in the region of the axilla. Rarely, an ectopically located remnant may develop into a formed mammary gland, known as *polymastia.* Conversely, the breast may fail to develop completely, referred to as *hypomastia* or *micromastia;* may not develop at all, known as *amastia;* or may fail to develop with an intact nipple, known as *amazia.* Complete or incomplete development of the breast may also be associated with an absence of the pectoral muscles and syndactyly, referred to as *Poland's syndrome,* after its original recognition by Alfred Poland in 1841.[2,3] His original description followed an anatomic dissection of a cadaver with this anomaly that he observed while a medical student. Subsequent reports added the additional component of hypoplasia, or complete absence of the breast, as well as costal cartilage and rib defects.

In the third month of gestation, squamous epithelial cells infiltrate from the persistent ectodermal mass into the underlying mesenchyme in the pectoral region. The ductal epithelium develops from these invading epithelial buds, which further develop 16 to 24 secondary buds that will go on to develop into the lobes of the mature breast that radiate from the central nipple. Also in the third month, the original mesenchymal cells differentiate into the smooth muscle of the nipple and areola.

At the end of prenatal life, the epithelialized sprouts are canalized into the major lactiferous ducts, while secondary buds go on to form the small ducts leading to alveoli or terminal secretory ductules. Each of the lobes has excretory ducts and a single lactiferous duct, which opens into a lactiferous sinus situated beneath the nipple. Occasionally, the lactiferous duct terminates at the site of original epithelial invagination without development of an everted, formed nipple, which persists into adult life as an inverted nipple. At puberty, generally between the ages of 10 and 13 years, the lobes further develop their subdivisions, or lobules, which terminate in the alveoli or secretory units of the mature breast.

The mammary glands develop in much the same way as other apocrine glands, of which they are considered modifications. The glands of Montgomery around the areola, the secretion of which serves as a source of lubrication of the nipple during lactation, are considered as transitional between sweat and lactiferous glands. Sweat glands, as well as sebaceous glands and hair follicles, may also be found on the areola and periareolar skin. The connective tissue support for the mature breast, the suspensory ligaments first described by Sir Astley Cooper,[4] forms at puberty from the mesoderm, from which the dermis of the skin as well as the subcutaneous superficial fascia also develop (Fig. 24–1).

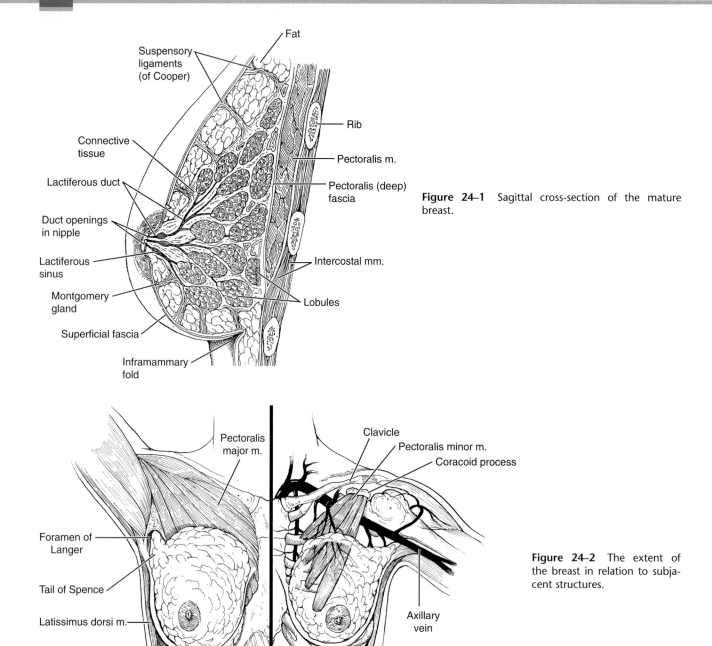

Figure 24–1 Sagittal cross-section of the mature breast.

Figure 24–2 The extent of the breast in relation to subjacent structures.

What is the anatomic extent of the normal adult breast?

The rudimentary structures found in both the male and prepubertal female increase in size in the female at puberty and extend radially into the underlying breast fat. While each breast has a defined appearance on the unilateral, anterior chest wall, extending from the edge of the sternum medially to the anterior border of the latissimus dorsi muscle laterally and from the second rib superiorly to the seventh rib inferiorly (Fig. 24–2), ductal tissue may be found extending to the

clavicle and below the inframammary crease, as well as overlying the sternum, where it may fuse with the contralateral breast. About two thirds of the breast overlies the pectoralis major muscle, whereas the inferior and lateral extension overlies the serratus anterior muscle. The greatest density of breast tissue is seen in the upper outer quadrant, where it extends toward the axilla and, in fact, enters that anatomic plane through a defect in the encasing fascia of the axilla, described by Langer.[5] The extension of breast tissue into the axilla through this foramen of Langer, an extension that disrupts the conical topography of the breast, was described by Spence.[6] A prominence or lesion in this axillary tail of Spence may be

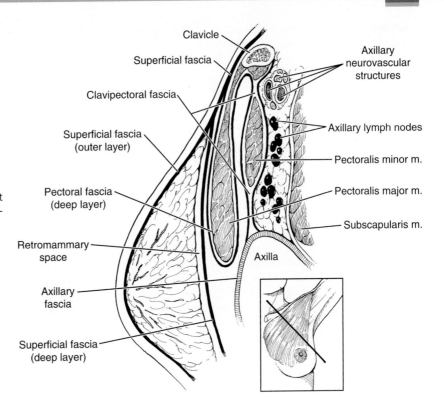

Figure 24–3 The fascial layers of the breast and axilla in a sagittal view through the mid-axillary region.

difficult to differentiate clinically from axillary lymphadenopathy. Discrepancy in breast size is common, as is the density of breast tissue in what appear to be topographically symmetrical breasts.

How is the axilla defined topographically?

The axilla is regarded topographically as the hair-bearing hollow below the shoulder, the anterior wall of which is made up of the fibers of the pectoralis major and minor muscles and whose posterior wall consists of the subscapularis, teres major, and tendon of the latissimus dorsi muscle. It is defined by an anterior axillary fold, which is formed by the lateral border of the pectoralis major muscle; a posterior axillary fold, which is formed by the lateral border of the latissimus dorsi muscle; and a medial border, which is formed by the serratus anterior muscle on the chest wall. The axilla is, of course, the location of the major depot of lymphatic drainage from the breast parenchyma. It is within the hollow of the axilla that lymph nodes are clinically palpated and surgically extirpated.

How are the breast and axilla separated from surrounding structures?

The fascial envelope of the breast consists of a fragile superficial layer that is continuous with the superficial abdominal fascia of Camper below and the superficial cervical fascia above. It is separated from the skin by a layer of subcutaneous fat of variable thickness. This fascial plane is relatively avascular, separating as it does the subdermal veins and arteries from larger vessels coursing over the superficial breast. Where the breast overlies the pectoralis major, the fascia is essentially

indistinct from the superficial fascia of the muscle, although a loose areolar plane, the retromammary space, separates the two. The deep fascia of the pectoralis major, like the superficial fascia of the breast, is continuous with the abdominal fascia below and the axillary fascia superiorly and laterally. It fuses with the sternum medially and the clavicle superiorly.

Another deep fascial layer, the clavipectoral fascia—a fusion of layers that are attached to the clavicle, the subclavius muscle, the pectoralis minor, and suspensory ligaments of the axilla, which are attached to the axillary fascia—is of particular surgical importance. Also known as the *costocoracoid fascia, the deep pectoral fascia,* or the *clavicoaxillary aponeurosis,* it encompasses the pectoralis minor muscle and attaches to and surrounds the subclavius muscle beneath the clavicle. Its most medial extent is a thickening referred to as *Halsted's ligament,* which traverses the tiny space separating the medial clavicle and the first rib where the subclavian vessels submerge. Laterally, the clavipectoral fascia unites with the anterior layer of the pectoralis major fascia and inferiorly with the axillary fascia, which forms the hollow of the axilla (Fig. 24–3). The fusion of the clavipectoral fascia and the pectoralis major fascia covers the serratus anterior muscle, whereas the axillary fascia continues laterally as the fascia of the latissimus dorsi. The surgical significance of the clavipectoral fascia derives from the access to the vascular and lymphatic anatomy of the axilla that its division allows for the surgeon.

The breast is essentially a subcutaneous structure with a significant component of fat. Its support comes largely from the fibrous bands linking the skin with the deep fascia over the underlying muscles, particularly the pectoralis major. These suspensory ligaments of Cooper are intact in young and nulliparous women but may become stretched and weakened with age, in obesity, or after multiple pregnancies. Although this may lead to an apparent distortion of the topographic landmarks in many patients, breast tissue continues to be confined to its normal anatomical landmarks.

How does topographic anatomy relate to the planning of incisions?

Topographic anatomy is relevant not only to the accurate clinical assessment of patients but also to planning surgical approaches to breast disease. The major topographic considerations in surgery for breast cancer relate to the appropriate placement of incisions in both the breast and axilla to provide optimal access and exposure of surrounding structures in order to allow appropriate extirpation of disease while at the same time achieving a satisfactory aesthetic result. In the past, incisions in the breast for cancer were largely limited to diagnostic biopsies, not definitive excisions. Their placement was considered almost exclusively in relation to the location of subsequent mastectomy scars, with little regard for cosmetic results or for appropriate surgery for cancer when breast conservation was planned, and certainly no regard for the use of adjuvant radiation therapy in conjunction with such breast-conserving surgery. The aesthetic consequences of where an incision in the breast was placed were invariably considered in the context of excisions for benign lesions. In this regard, periareolar incisions were used as often as possible. When this was not feasible, surgeons were directed to follow the direction of Langer's lines, originally described in the 19th century as the directions of least skin tension.[5] These were represented in diagrams emanating circumferentially from the central areolar edge. Incisions placed along Langer's lines were considered particularly appropriate in younger premenopausal patients without breast ptosis for whom the surgical excision of benign lesions, such as fibroadenomas, is common. They came to be regarded as the appropriate lines along which incisions should be placed in the breast to minimize the tension that might be exerted on the skin, thereby optimizing the resulting scar. Conversely, radially placed incisions were regarded as inappropriate for the excision of benign lesions.

In planning incisions for carcinomas already diagnosed by needle biopsy, however, other considerations become relevant. Although periareolar incisions and incisions along Langer's lines may be optimal, lines of least skin tension with the patient in an upright position may not always correspond to Langer's lines, particularly in the peripheral extensions of the medial and lateral breast. Certainly in older patients, the lines of least tension are likely to correspond to the more transversely oriented direction of collagen fibers described by Kraissl.[7] In certain instances, even radially placed incisions may be optimal, particularly if an elliptic skin resection with underlying breast parenchyma is required. For example, incisions placed medially along lines of skin tensions are often in a radial alignment. For centrally placed lesions, periareolar or para-areolar incisions conforming to Langer's lines may well be appropriate. However, in the inferior breast, a radial incision may exert less downward traction on the nipple–areolar complex, particularly when skin is elliptically removed along with underlying breast tissue, whereas incisions near or at the inframammary crease or high in the upper breast are best placed in a curvilinear transverse direction. Likewise, in the upper outer quadrant or tail of the breast near the axilla, a circumferential incision, along which both Langer's lines

and lines of resting skin tension coincide, may be optimal (Fig. 24–4).

As breast conservation has become increasingly used for ductal carcinoma in situ (DCIS), broader areas of extirpation may be required. In many instances, they are more optimally placed in radial directions, to both encompass the often radial, lobar distribution of disease and minimize distortion of nipple-areola symmetry with the contralateral breast that may result from a wide excision of breast parenchyma and overlying skin with resultant significant traction on the central breast. In planning incisions, it is often best to consider the direction of placement with the patient in an upright position, whereby the pectoralis major exerts traction on the breast and overlying skin to create lines of tension. This does not occur when the patient is supine and the breast is distorted by lateral and posterior gravitational pull. For carcinomas medial and lateral to the nipple–areolar complex in particular, major ductal segments may be better encompassed by transversely placed incisions, particularly when ellipses of skin, along with underlying parenchyma, are required, thereby preventing inversion of skin at the incision site. In all instances of segmental excisions for cancer, therefore, planning must consider the issues of encompassing the disease and maintaining breast symmetry as well as the issue of placement of the cutaneous scar.

In the axilla, incisions are optimally placed in lines of minimal skin tension. Natural skin lines can be demonstrated throughout the axilla, particularly below the hair-bearing

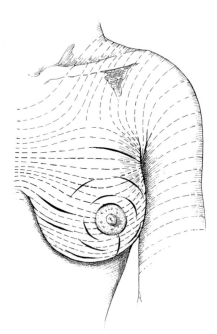

Figure 24–4 Skin incisions for breast cancer excisions, particularly in the older or ptotic breast, are best placed along lines of minimal skin tension. This is especially so in the medial breast. Inferiorly located lesions may even be best excised through radial incisions to avoid traction and distortion of the nipple–areolar complex, particularly when skin or significant segments of underlying breast parenchyma are included in the excision. In the central breast, periareolar or para-areolar incisions, conforming to Langer's lines, are appropriate.

area, where they provide excellent anatomic access and are largely unnoticeable within the confines of the axillary hollow (Fig. 24–5).

SURGICAL ANATOMY OF THE BREAST AND AXILLA

What is the arterial supply to the breast?

The breast receives its blood supply from the internal mammary artery; the highest (supreme) and lateral thoracic arteries; the pectoral branch of the thoracoacromial artery; the intercostal arteries in the third, fourth, and fifth intercostal spaces; and branches of the subscapularis and thoracodorsal

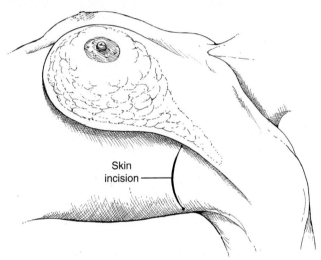

Figure 24–5 Skin incision placement in the axilla.

Skin incision

arteries. The perforating branches of the internal mammary artery supply the greatest source of blood to the breast through the fourth and fifth anterior intercostal branches, as well as through branches in the upper sixth intercostal spaces, all of which perforate the pectoralis major muscle (Fig. 24–6). The lateral thoracic artery of the axillary artery emerges lateral to the pectoralis minor muscle and then supplies the serratus anterior, pectoralis major and minor, and subscapularis muscles, giving off lateral mammary branches as well to the breast.

Although the major blood supply to the breast comes from the internal mammary and lateral thoracic arteries, branches to the breast may arise from the highest (supreme) thoracic artery, which arises at the highest point in the traversal of the axillary artery before it submerges beneath the subclavius muscle; from the thoracoacromial artery, which branches into the pectoral artery, supplying branches to both the pectoralis major and minor muscles; and from the subscapularis artery, which becomes the thoracodorsal artery and which may give branches to the breast. The intercostal perforating arteries of the fourth, fifth, and sixth intercostal spaces provide additional arterial blood to the central and lateral breast. The extensive anastomotic connections between these sources of arterial blood, particularly the internal mammary and lateral thoracic arteries, provide the breast with a rich arterial network. This allows great latitude in planning operative approaches and incisions in the treatment of breast cancer, provided there is careful adherence to basic surgical principles.

What is the venous drainage of the breast?

Venous drainage parallels the arterial supply to the breast. Medially, the perforating branches enter the internal mammary vein, which then joins the brachiocephalic vein. Laterally, the axillary vein, which lies medial to the axillary artery, receives one or two pectoral branches from the breast.

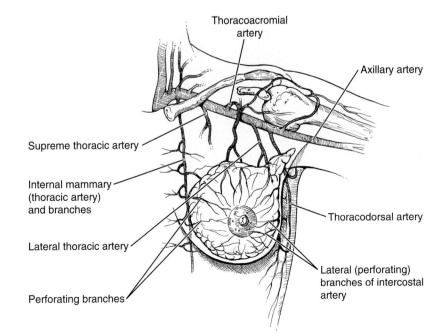

Figure 24–6 Arterial supply to the breast.

It is not uncommon to encounter a bifurcate axillary vein. To avoid division of the lower branch, or even both branches, it is obviously important to recognize this anomaly as being equivalent to a single axillary vein and not to mistake it for a branch or branches off the trunk of the major axillary vein. When its path continues proximal to the first rib, the axillary vein becomes the subclavian vein.

The intercostal veins communicate anteriorly with the internal mammary veins and thereby with the brachiocephalic vein and posteriorly with the vertebral veins, which enter the azygos veins and ultimately the superior vena cava. Venous drainage through the internal mammary vein and branches of the axillary vein has been cited as the route that leads to dissemination of breast cancer to the lungs and more distal systemic sites, whereas drainage through the intercostal veins, which communicate with the vertebral venous system, has likewise been cited as leading to dissemination to the vertebrae.[8]

How is the lymphatic drainage of the breast defined?

As discussed in Chapter 21, lymphatic anatomy and its relation to the spread of breast cancer has long been a focus of intense study. In recent decades, the principles that determine lymphatic flow have been reassessed as previous concepts on the centrifugal lymphatic dissemination of cancer by direct permeation have been largely disproved, and most recently, mapping of the lymphatics has become a widespread practice in the highly selective management of regional lymph nodes.

The lymphatics of the skin begin in a subepithelial plexus located in the papillary dermis, from which they communicate with a subdermal plexus. In the central breast, these cutaneous and subcutaneous lymphatics merge with the subareolar plexus of Sappey, which also receives lymphatic vessels from the nipple and areola. This subareolar plexus communicates with the lymphatics of the lactiferous ducts, which in turn flow to the perilobular and deep subcutaneous lymphatic plexus. Recent studies provide supportive evidence that the skin of the breast and the parenchyma of the breast share the same lymphatic drainage network.[9]

Lymph flows toward the regional lymph nodes and parallels the direction of blood flow in the major veins. The concept that lymphatic flow from the parenchyma of the breast moves centripetally toward the subareolar plexus has been largely refuted.[10] Lymphatic flow is unidirectional to regional lymph nodes, and the rich anastomotic connections between lymphatics enable areas of obstruction to be bypassed and thereby allow lymph to flow unimpeded through the other valveless lymphatics toward the regional lymph nodes. Early radioisotope studies using colloidal gold (^{198}Au) estimated that 97% of lymphatic flow is toward the axilla and the remainder to the internal mammary nodes.[11] Recent studies by Kern on both dye and radioisotope migration following subareolar injection have demonstrated that one or at most two major lymphatic channels carry the dye or isotope to the axilla.[12,13] Clearly, the lymphatic drainage pattern of the breast to the axilla is a unified system terminating in a very focal lymphatic channel or channels and anatomically focal lymph nodes.

How is the lymph node drainage of the breast defined?

The lymph node drainage of the breast has been subdivided by various methods for surgical, pathologic, and prognostic purposes. The classic reviews of Haagensen[14] and others, drawing on the studies of Poirier and Cunéo[15] as modified by Rouvière,[16] divided the lymph nodes anatomically into six groups (Fig. 24–7). The largest of these is the central group of

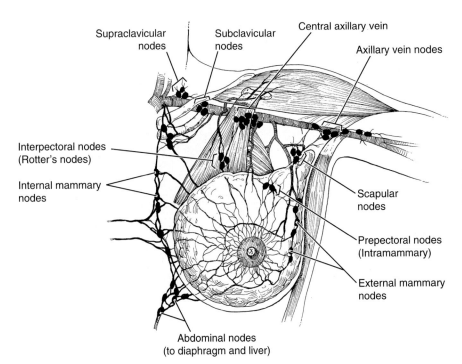

Supraclavicular nodes

Subclavicular nodes

Central axillary vein

Axillary vein nodes

Interpectoral nodes (Rotter's nodes)

Internal mammary nodes

Scapular nodes

Prepectoral nodes (Intramammary)

External mammary nodes

Abdominal nodes (to diaphragm and liver)

Figure 24–7 Anatomic distribution of venous circulation and lymph nodes draining the breast.

nodes located in the lateral hollow of the axilla and easily palpated against the chest wall. The second largest group is the axillary vein nodes lying on the caudal and ventral surfaces of the lateral axillary vein. The other groups are the scapular nodes along the thoracodorsal branches of the subscapular vessels, also in the lateral axilla; the external mammary nodes lying beneath the lateral edge of the pectoralis major muscle along the medial border of the axilla and following the lateral thoracic artery on the chest wall from the second to sixth ribs; the subclavicular nodes lying on the caudal and ventral surfaces of the medial axillary vein beneath the subclavius muscle; and the interpectoral nodes, also known as *Rotter's nodes*, located between the pectoralis major and minor muscles. In addition, a prepectoral lymph node or nodes may occasionally be found high in the upper outer quadrant of the breast, simulating a well-defined lesion on mammography. Intercostal lymph nodes may also be located along the posterior thoracic cavity within the intercostal spaces and may receive lymphatic drainage from the breast.

The internal mammary lymph nodes have historically been of particular surgical interest because their location sets them apart from traditional en bloc resections to encompass breast cancer. These nodes receive lymphatic flow from vessels that accompany the perforating blood vessels piercing the pectoralis major and intercostal muscles. These nodes also receive lymphatic vessels from the liver, diaphragm, rectus sheath, and upper rectus abdominis muscle.

The internal mammary nodes lie close to the internal mammary vessels in extrapleural fat in the first six intercostal spaces. Studies have demonstrated that the greatest concentration of nodes is in the first three intercostal spaces.[10] Although internal mammary lymph nodes have traditionally been regarded as receiving lymphatic drainage from the medial and central portions of the breast, studies have demonstrated that lymphatic drainage from any quadrant may go to the internal mammary lymph nodes[17] and, as noted, does so in less than 3% of instances in which patterns of lymphatic drainage have been studied.[11]

Rarer sites of lymphatic drainage, usually as a second-echelon site when direct nodal drainage sites are occluded, are the intercostal lymph nodes of the posterior chest wall near the termination of the ribs, the anteriorly located diaphragmatic nodes beneath the lower sternum at the xiphoid, and contralateral internal mammary nodes.

How are axillary lymph nodes defined for pathologic orientation?

For the purpose of pathologic analysis, axillary lymph nodes have been divided by anatomic levels reflecting the traditional concept that nodal metastases extend sequentially from lateral to medial[18] (Fig. 24–8). The greatest number of lymph nodes are contained in what has been referred to as level I, the grouping of nodes located below the axillary vein and between the lateral border of the pectoralis minor muscle and the anterior border of the latissimus dorsi muscle. Included in this group are the lower external or lateral mammary nodes, which follow the course of the lateral thoracic artery on the chest wall from the second to sixth rib. The level II lymph nodes are those that lie behind the pectoralis minor muscle, and the level III nodes are those nodes that lie below the axillary vein from the medial border of the pectoralis minor muscle to the submergence of the axillary vein below the subclavius muscle at the costoclavicular (Halsted's) ligament. When identifiable, Rotter's interpectoral nodes are apart from these divisions but may be dissected with the pectoralis minor fascial attachments and incorporated into the axillary nodal contents when an axillary dissection is performed. If excised, however, it is often as a separate specimen.

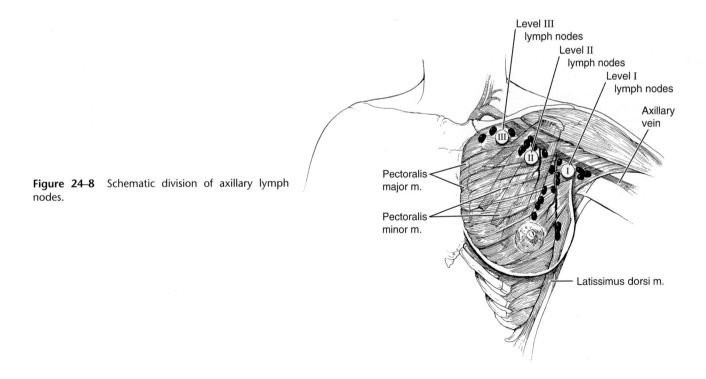

Figure 24–8 Schematic division of axillary lymph nodes.

What is the sentinel lymph node?

The most recent efforts to define the lymphatic drainage pattern of breast cancer have resulted in the concept of the sentinel lymph node. The sentinel node is that lymph node to which lymphatic drainage from the location of the cancer in the breast is directed. It is the node most likely to contain a metastasis if nodal dissemination has occurred. The concept originally evolved from an appreciation that areas of skin have patterns of drainage to specific lymph nodes within the regional nodal basin to which lymphatic vessels are directed, as first described by Cabanas for the treatment of penile cancer,[19] and most convincingly defined by the pioneer studies of Morton and colleagues, in the treatment of cutaneous melanoma, using vital blue or isosulfan blue dyes.[20] Subsequent applications to the breast using both dye and radioisotopes in conjunction with a gamma probe as lymphatic mapping agents confirmed the validity of the concept for mapping the potential specific location of lymph node metastases from breast cancer.[21,22]

What is the neural innervation of the breast?

The innervation to the skin and parenchyma of the breast occurs by way of the medial and lateral intercostal nerves, although a portion of the superior breast, as well as the upper chest wall, comes from branches of the supraclavicular nerve, which originates as a branch of the cervical plexus. Innervation to the nipple is from the lateral and medial branches of the fourth intercostal nerve. The lateral portions of the breast and chest wall receive sensory innervation from the lateral branches of the third through sixth intercostal nerves, whereas the medial aspect of the breast and sternal area receives its innervation from the medial branches.

What anatomically related neural structures are encountered in the axilla?

Several major nerves require identification during surgical procedures that include dissection of axillary lymph nodes (Fig. 24–9). Neuromuscular branches that are related anatomically to the axilla and underlying chest wall muscles include, most significantly, the brachial plexus, the divisions of which lie above and posterior to the axillary vein. In the lateral axilla, the brachial plexus has three divisions, or cords, which surround the axillary artery. Appreciation of the location of the brachial plexus is obviously basic to the surgical anatomy of the axilla, but in addition, it cautions the surgeon against undue stretching during efforts at positioning the arm to create exposure of the axillary contents. Rapid, forceful, or prolonged movement of the arm, superiorly and posteriorly in particular, may create excessive tension on the brachial plexus, creating brachial plexitis, a potential source of significant morbidity and even paralysis.

Traversing the axillary contents is a branch of the second intercostal nerve identified as the intercostobrachial nerve, which supplies sensory fibers to the medial aspect of the upper arm, axillary skin, and upper lateral breast. It arises as the lateral cutaneous branch of the ventral primary ramus of T2. It pierces the external intercostal muscle of the second intercostal space lateral to the lateral border of the pectoralis minor muscle and then the serratus anterior, before crossing through the lymphoadipose tissue of the axilla over the border of the latissimus dorsi muscle toward the medial upper arm. In its course through the posterior axilla, it joins with a filament of the medial brachial cutaneous nerve, the smallest branch of the medial cord of the brachial plexus. An additional contact has been described with the posterior brachial cutaneous branch of the radial nerve.[23] The size of the intercostobrachial nerve and the extent of its distribution appear to vary inversely with the size and distribution of the medial brachial cutaneous nerve. Anastomoses between the intercostobrachial and the lateral cutaneous branches of T1 and T3 have often been described. The anastomosis between intercostobrachial and medial brachial cutaneous nerves is rather constant and may be represented by two or more filaments connecting them. Anastomosis with branches of T1 and T3 and the posterior brachial cutaneous branch of the radial nerve appear to be occasional or inconstant findings. The intercostobrachial nerve may give off two or more branches as it traverses the axillary fat.

The medial brachial cutaneous nerve is the smallest branch of the medial cord of the brachial plexus. It is formed from fibers arising from cord segments C8 and T1 or from T1 alone. Descending through the axilla, it pierces the brachial fascia at about the middle of the arm. It innervates the skin and subcutaneous tissues of the posterior aspect of the lower third of the arm as far as the olecranon. The nerve may occasionally arise as a branch of the medial antebrachial cutaneous nerve, which also arises from C8 and T1. It may receive fibers from T2 or T3, or both, or it may be absent. Because the medial brachial cutaneous nerve frequently has direct contacts and varies inversely in size with the intercostobrachial nerve, it should be considered as often sensory to the axilla as well.

A second intercostobrachial nerve often arises from the lateral cutaneous branch of T3. It supplies the axilla and medial side of the arm.[24] The first intercostal nerve provides a lateral cutaneous branch, which supplies the skin of the axilla and may communicate with the intercostobrachial nerve and the medial brachial cutaneous nerve as well. Denervation or division of the intercostobrachial nerve will lead to numbness of the skin in the upper medial arm and axilla. The anesthesia that is produced is often interpreted by the patient as a sense of swelling in the upper medial arm. Paresthesias will be of varying degrees, distribution, and duration owing to the richness of the sensory nerve supply to the axilla and upper arm.[25]

The pectoral nerves are particularly relevant to the surgical treatment of breast cancer that requires axillary dissection. These nerves innervate the pectoral muscles, and denervation can lead to atrophy and a loss of muscle mass that can compromise the aesthetic benefits of breast conservation. Likewise, reconstructive procedures after mastectomy clearly benefit from an intact pectoralis major and the resulting normal chest wall and axillary contour as a foundation.

The lateral pectoral nerve arises medial to the pectoralis minor muscle, its designation as a lateral nerve deriving from its origin in the lateral cord of the brachial plexus. It can be clearly delineated when the pectoralis minor is divided, emerging medial to the muscle before it branches out to innervate the lower portion of the pectoralis major muscle. The medial pectoral nerve emerges lateral to the pectoralis

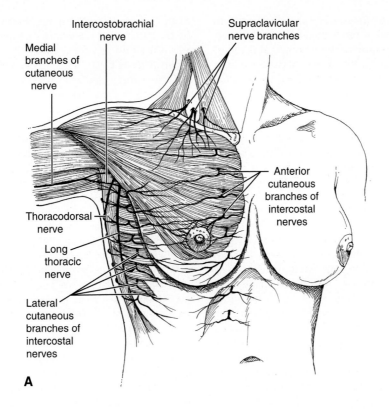

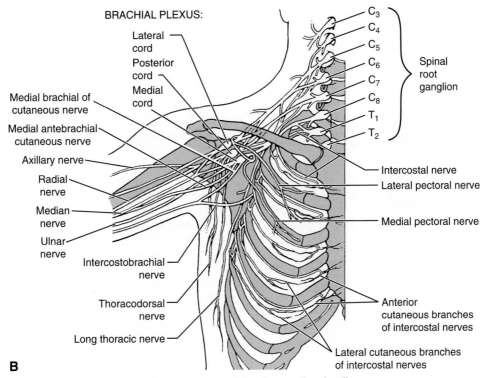

Figure 24–9   *A* and *B*, Neurologic structures of the chest wall and axilla.

minor muscle, the medial designation likewise deriving from its origin in the medial cord of the brachial plexus. It innervates the pectoralis minor muscle, but a branch also innervates fibers in the lateral border of the pectoralis major muscle. This branch is often accompanied by a small artery and vein. Its preservation ensures conservation of the lateral pectoralis major muscle.

The two additional nerves of importance in breast cancer surgery are the thoracodorsal nerve, or nerve to the latissimus dorsi muscle, and the long thoracic nerve. The thoracodorsal nerve lies on the subscapularis muscle accompanied by the thoracodorsal artery and vein. Preservation of the entire thoracodorsal neurovascular bundle maintains the viability of the latissimus dorsi muscle, which may be required for reconstructive purposes, as detailed in Chapter 25. Division of the nerve paralyzes the latissimus dorsi muscle and functionally weakens internal rotation and abduction of the arm, whereas no noticeable clinical deformity may result. Patients may complain of a limitation of backward rotation when attempting to touch the scapular region of the back. Of greater functional significance is the long thoracic nerve, which is formed over the most superior component of the serratus anterior from nerves arising in the fifth, sixth, and seventh roots of the brachial plexus. The long thoracic nerve lies superficial and lateral to the surface of the serratus anterior muscle, gradually moving medially to submerge below the fascia of the muscle at the fourth or fifth intracostal space. Division of this nerve creates a deformity that is commonly referred to as a "winged scapula" owing to paralysis of the serratus anterior muscle. This may be a source of significant cosmetic and functional morbidity. During efforts to raise or use the arm for pulling, the scapula, without tension exerted on it by a functioning serratus anterior, will no longer be drawn forward but will instead awkwardly rise outward.

PREOPERATIVE CONSIDERATIONS

What is the best timing for definitive breast cancer surgery?

The window of time between diagnosis and definitive surgery for breast cancer has widened as surgeons and patients in the last decades have expanded the opportunities for careful discussion and consideration of options in therapy. Initially there had been no evidence that two-staged procedures—with excision of the primary lesion preceding, by days or weeks, wider excisions, mastectomy, or axillary nodal procedures—adversely affected outcome, but with the availability of diagnostic strategies by needle biopsy instead of surgical biopsy, even this issue has been largely obviated. However, for lesions that are clinically occult and only detected mammographically, and for which needle biopsy is inconclusive either for a malignant diagnosis or to establish an entirely noninvasive or low-grade invasive diagnosis, or for lesions that are poorly defined by palpation, mammographically, or by additional radiographic criteria, excision as an initial procedure to allow full histopathologic assessment is often desirable. This information is essential before considering therapeutic options, in particular the appropriateness of breast conservation and

axillary staging. Furthermore, when a decision has been made by the patient and physicians that mastectomy is appropriate, reconstruction is often discussed and consultation with a reconstructive plastic surgeon encouraged.[26]

If the patient elects to have breast reconstruction, it is best performed at the same time as mastectomy. There is no evidence that this adversely affects the ability to detect recurrent disease.[27] Immediate reconstruction also may broaden the choice of reconstructive techniques, allow greater flexibility in reconstruction technique, optimize the aesthetic results, and eliminate an additional procedure also requiring general anesthesia. There is ample evidence as well that immediate reconstruction provides a positive psychological balance to the negative impact of mastectomy.[28,29] All of these decisions on surgical therapy are best made in a reasoned rather than a rushed and emotionally charged setting, which may be the case when an inappropriate emphasis is placed on the importance of making an immediate decision on treatment.

The identification of patients at risk for developing negative psychological sequelae after breast cancer surgery allows the employment of appropriate psychosocial support during the decision-making process before definitive therapy. Patients with an antecedent psychiatric history, those with little or no family or social support, those with a history of substance abuse, those who express excessive anxiety, fear, or depression, and certainly those expressing suicidal thinking should be helped and encouraged to seek appropriate consultation.[30,31] As discussed in Chapter 38, this information must often be sought by the initial consulting surgeons and physicians.

The influence of the menstrual cycle has entered the discussion of treatment because some studies purport to demonstrate that performance of surgery at certain times in the menstrual cycle may be an independent prognostic variable. Concern theoretically hinges on enhanced metastatic potential during phases of unopposed estrogen stimulation. Immune function may be reduced during this follicular phase of the cycle, whereas the increase in progesterone during the luteal phase (days 15 to 36) may down-regulate estrogen receptors and alter normal cell—and presumably cancer cell—proliferation. The first such report by Hrushesky and associates[32] suggested that surgery during the week before or just after menstruation was associated with increased survival, compared with surgery at other times in the menstrual cycle. Senie and associates[33,34] reported an improvement in survival for patients with nodal metastases if surgery was performed in the luteal phase, compared with the follicular phase, of the menstrual cycle. Other studies supported this observation for patients with metastases.[35–38] However, Spratt and associates[39] obtained a statistically significant improvement in survival when surgery was performed between days 7 and 20 of the menstrual cycle, although only 40 cases were reviewed. These were retrospective analyses, and since then, there have also been reports that were either inconclusive or failed to demonstrate any effect of the timing of surgery in the menstrual cycle on patient outcome.[40–48]

A prospective analysis of patients operated on at different times in the menstrual cycle and adjusted for multiple prognostic factors would be required to arrive at a reliable resolution of the issue of the timing of surgery in relation to menstruation. It would clearly require large numbers of patients. Ongoing studies may help resolve some of the conflicting conclusions and concerns expressed to date.[49,50] As the surgical treatment of breast cancer at the present time may be fragmented by multiple procedures that include needle biopsy, segmental excision, sentinel lymphadenectomy, axillary dissection, segmental re-excision, or mastectomy and reconstruction, the timing of surgical procedures based on the menstrual cycle may be logistically formidable. One study purporting to show a survival benefit from surgery performed in the progestogenic phase (days 0 to 2 and 13 to 35) found no such benefit if definitive surgery was performed in a single procedure.[51] Adjusting surgery to fit into a specific menstrual time frame requires a very clear definition of potential benefits from appropriately controlled studies that objectively assess the precise timing within the menstrual cycle and the uniformity of surgical treatment, staging, and adjuvant therapies.

SURGICAL BIOPSY

Heightened public awareness of breast cancer and mammographic screening, and a proliferation of radiographic techniques with increasing applicability to diagnosis, particularly sonography, have led to a tremendous increase in breast biopsies. More than 20 million women have mammography or sonography annually in the United States,[52] leading to more than 1 million breast biopsies for nonpalpable breast abnormalities.[52] For palpable lesions, as well as radiographically detected nonpalpable lesions, percutaneous needle biopsy, as discussed in Chapter 17, has become the preferred diagnostic approach for most breast lesions. Needle biopsy techniques fulfill the need for an expeditious diagnosis of the formidable numbers of detected findings with minimal invasiveness.

The two principal indications for breast biopsy are a dominant, palpable mass that is not a simple cyst on aspiration, or a suspicious lesion detected radiographically. Treatment of breast cancer requires an unequivocal cytologic or histologic diagnosis, and this can be accomplished by needle biopsy for palpable lesions as well as for most nonpalpable lesions with the appropriate use of radioguidance. The availability of needle biopsy has greatly expanded the indications for biopsy for many vaguely perceived dominant findings even in the absence of radiographic correlation. There are instances, however, in which surgical biopsy is indicated because of an inability to use needle biopsy techniques or because of inadequacies in the histologic material provided by needle biopsy techniques. Even when clinical impression, radiographic criteria, and fine-needle aspiration are used to assess a solid breast mass, physicians must be sensitive to the vagaries of clinical and radiographic criteria and the pitfall of hypocellular fine-needle aspiration biopsy results' leading to a failure to diagnose cancer.[53]

What are the indications for surgical breast biopsy?

Surgical biopsies are required if the location of the radiographic findings precludes or complicates needle biopsy, when the histologic material obtained by needle biopsy is inadequate for definitive diagnosis, and when physical findings warrant biopsy but there is no defined radiographic abnormality and needle biopsy has failed to establish a diagnosis concordant with the physical findings.

Excision with preoperative wire localization and specimen radiographic confirmation may be required for lesions in the immediate retroareolar region of the breast or posteriorly near the underlying chest wall. Inadequate compression of the breast in these locations and the associated technical limitations of core biopsy or vacuum-assisted core biopsy as a result often preclude the use of such needle biopsy techniques in these instances. Likewise, very faint clusters of microcalcifications may make stereotactic imaging and specimen radiographic correlation uncertain and therefore necessitate surgical excision for diagnosis.

Patients may also require surgical biopsy as a result of inadequate histologic sampling following core needle biopsy. Certain diagnoses require complete excision of the target lesion. Most important in this regard is the diagnosis of atypical ductal hyperplasia on large core needle biopsies that are most often performed for clustered microcalcifications, but occasionally for mass lesions. Numerous studies have shown in 13% to 50% of cases an upgrade from atypical ductal hyperplasia to DCIS and, rarely, to invasive cancer, when needle biopsy diagnosis is followed by surgical excisional biopsy.[54–58] The rates of upgrade from atypical ductal hyperplasia may well decrease as large core vacuum-assisted devices become standard for needle biopsy of clustered microcalcifications. Indications for surgical excision in these instances may be further altered in the future.[59,60] Certainly, patients demonstrating mild or focal atypia and those of advanced age may be appropriately managed with radiographic and clinical follow-up, whereas those with marked atypical ductal hyperplasia, particularly with a broader lesion less optimally sampled or with a past history or significant family history of breast cancer, are more safely assessed with surgical excision.

Other groups of lesions diagnosed by core needle biopsy for which surgical excision has been recommended are atypical lobular hyperplasias and lobular carcinomas in situ (LCIS). They are invariably diagnosed as incidental histologic findings on core biopsy for high-risk radiographic findings, and these diagnoses will likely become more frequent as vacuum-assisted techniques increase the tissue volume retrieved on core needle biopsy. The yield of subsequent carcinoma following core biopsy–diagnosed uncomplicated LCIS has been in the 5% to 10% range.[61] Decision making is often complicated by the coexistent mammographic lesion for which the core biopsy was performed as well as by other coexistent histologic findings.[62–67] Certainly, women at high risk, particularly with a personal history of breast cancer, and those with coexistent histologic findings that may put them at risk or with associated mammographic findings, might be prudently managed by surgical excision. Whether other patients diagnosed on core needle biopsy can be approached in the same way as patients with coincidentally diagnosed atypical lobular hyperplasia or LCIS on surgical excision remains unresolved.

Papillary lesions diagnosed by core biopsy represent another group for which excision has been recommended. Experience to date has been limited to almost anecdotal instances of carcinoma diagnosed by surgical excision after the diagnosis of a benign papillary lesion.[64,68,69] If there is a significant residual lesion or a discordance with a suspicious radiologic appearance, or if atypia is present, excision would seem prudent. With increasing sampling from vacuum-assisted core biopsies, this may become a less problematic issue.

Radial scars represent another group that, if diagnosed by core needle biopsy, is prudently followed by complete excision. The mammographic appearance may be indistinguishable from an infiltrating carcinoma.[70] The histologic features may be variable, with features of ductal hyperplasia with or without atypia, papillomatosis, and adenosis, leading to its other designation as a complex sclerosing lesion. Because of its histologic heterogeneity and the potential that DCIS may be a component of the entire lesion, as well as its significance as a potential marker lesion for increased risk for breast cancer, excision at the present time is prudent.[71,72]

Finally, surgical biopsy may be indicated for suspected Paget's disease of the nipple, skin changes suggestive of inflammatory carcinoma, and bloody or serous nipple discharge, all in the absence of any associated radiographic findings.

What is the appropriate biopsy for Paget's disease?

The changes noted in the nipple or nipple–areolar complex with Paget's disease may include erythema, scaling, crusting, or weeping, which may progress to ulceration with an underlying palpable mass. When the nipple–areolar changes are noted, Paget's disease must be suspected and a biopsy performed in conjunction with mammographic assessment for an underlying neoplasm. The biopsy should optimally include a full-thickness wedge of the nipple–areolar complex from an area demonstrating the clinical changes, including underlying ductal tissue. Histology of the crust on the nipple surface, touch preparations, or scrape cytology may fail to demonstrate the diagnostic Paget cells present in the basal epidermal layers.

What is the appropriate biopsy for inflammatory carcinoma?

In the presence of skin changes that suggest an inflammatory cancer, a sample of involved skin should be included for histologic study. Underlying breast tissue should be included as well. The diagnosis of inflammatory carcinoma is most often clinically suspected in the absence of any dominant palpable or radiographic breast density and is histologically established by the finding of dermal and subdermal lymphatic permeation by tumor emboli. Skin thickening may be evident mammographically, corresponding to areas of erythema and peau d'orange, and parenchymal thickening may be seen mammographically as well. As the skin changes reflect dermal lymphatic dilation and hypervascularity, not necessarily corresponding to the presence of carcinoma, areas of dermal tumor permeation may not always be evident on small punch biopsy or surgical skin biopsy specimens. Therefore, a more generous excision of skin may be required in the absence of any breast parenchymal changes, but from an area where the cutaneous evidence of disease is apparent. A high index of suspicion by clinical criteria and an assiduous effort to establish the diagnosis of primary inflammatory carcinoma histologically are required in the absence of any palpable or radiographic breast changes other than diffuse firmness or a vague diffuse mammographic density.

BREAST-CONSERVING SURGERY

What is the proper term for breast-conserving procedures?

Many terms have been applied to breast-conserving procedures for cancer. These include *lumpectomy, wide excision, tylectomy, segmentectomy, segmental excision of the breast, segmental mastectomy, partial mastectomy, tumorectomy,* and *quadrantectomy.* These terms may have different implications for the surgeon and patient. The absence of a uniform nomenclature reflects in turn the absence of a uniform anatomic definition of breast-conserving approaches to cancer. Even the term *quadrantectomy,* which implied removing an entire quarter of the breast, but originating from a desire to excise major lobular components, clearly lacked anatomic precision.

The major goal of breast-conserving surgery at the present time is to appropriately excise the entire lesion along with surrounding breast tissue, the margins of which are free of cancer histologically. The extent of resection surrounding the lesion to optimally achieve margins free of malignant change has not been defined and has great variability depending on the architectural and histologic characteristics of the specific tumor. For this reason, the generic phrases *segmental excision* and *partial mastectomy* would seem more appropriate. The former is likely preferable, as any phrase that includes *mastectomy* may be confusing to a patient desirous of breast conservation.

What is the goal of breast-conserving surgery?

Implicit in all breast-conserving procedures is the recognition that an effort will be made to balance the highest priority of complete excision of the cancer and tumor-free margins with the achievement of an excellent aesthetic result—the major reason for the patient to elect breast conservation. To achieve the proper balance, numerous variables must be considered, among which are tumor size, location, breast size, and the histopathology of the lesion. The failure to arrive at a precise descriptive title for such procedures is therefore understandable, given the potential spectrum in the extent of surgery that might be regarded as appropriate for any given tumor, based on these considerations. Furthermore, with few exceptions, radiation therapy is used as an adjunct to primary local treatment. Although radiation therapy may provide some additional latitude in planning the extent of surgery, it does not abrogate the major goals of surgical treatment. Efforts to avoid additional surgery for patients with close or positive margins using aggressive local radiotherapy as well as systemic adjuvant strategies have been associated with significant breast recurrences.

Recurrence-free survival following breast-conserving treatment therefore may depend on many factors, but available data support tumor-free margins as the benchmark for successful breast-conserving therapy.[73–77] The optimal extent of excision to achieve histologically clear margins may be further complicated by the limitations and lack of uniformity in histologic margin assessment from one pathologist to the next.[78,79] A specimen with tumor cells detected focally at a single site may be described as "positive," whereas one in which there is extensive gross tumor less than 1 mm away from histologically free margins in multiple areas may be described as "negative." These situations may have different implications for the adequacy of resection and are very different from an incomplete excision, which leaves gross tumor in the breast. The generic use of the terms *positive margins* and *negative margins* undoubtedly gives rise to conflicting views in the literature on the true importance of margin involvement. It is clear, however, that patients with margins histologically clear of invasive or in situ cancer have a lower incidence of recurrence after breast-conserving surgery and radiotherapy.[80–86] In a study by Frazier and associates[87] of patients having mastectomy or re-excision after a previous segmental excision, 52.5% of those who initially had involved margins had residual tumor, but, significantly, 26.3% of those who had been evaluated as having clear margins had residual tumor as well. A retrospective study by Smitt and associates[81] of 289 patients with 303 stage I and II invasive carcinomas of the breast treated by breast conservation and radiation found the achievement of negative margins either initially or with re-excision to be the most important predictor of local control. The probability of local control in patients with negative margins was 98% at 10 years, whereas it decreased to 82% in patients with non-negative margin status.[81] Similarly, a study by Mansfield and associates[88] of 1070 patients treated by breast conservation and radiation, when assessed by multivariate analysis, found positive margin status to be a significant risk factor for local recurrence. In a study from the Joint Center for Radiation Therapy in Boston, of 343 patients with stage I or II breast cancer having radiation therapy as part of breast-conserving treatment with a median follow-up of 10.8 years, 7% with negative or close margins treated with 60 Gy or greater to the tumor bed had a breast recurrence, compared with 14% with focally positive margins and 27% with more extensive margin involvement.[89] No difference was noted in patients with close margins of 1 mm compared with wider margins (greater than 1 mm). Although the extent of tumor-free breast tissue around a lesion is presently undefined, wider margins in several series have clearly been inversely related to recurrence.[90,91]

The relationship of positive surgical margins to systemic recurrence is less clear. Nevertheless, positive surgical margins are associated with, if not necessarily causative of, systemic relapse in several studies.[81–86,92–95] Certainly, efforts to minimize breast disease recurrence would appear self-recommending, and the most significant variable in achieving this goal is tumor-free margins of resection. Even advocates of boost radiation to the tumor bed to optimize tumor control in the preserved breast endorse the advisability of achieving tumor-free excision margins.[96] Although lesser margins are more likely to provide security for a well-defined, low-grade lesion than for a high-grade invasive lobular or ductal carcinoma surrounded by foci of intraductal carcinoma, for neither lesion has the appropriate margin been clearly defined. Furthermore, the contraction of surrounding tissue that may follow excision can create discordance in the objective assessment of the true extent of margins from the operating room to the pathology laboratory.

Until the issue of the appropriate extent of tumor-free margins is better resolved, an effort by the surgeon to achieve margins of 1 cm around the reference lesion would appear to provide confidence that histologically free margins, despite the inherent limitations of such histologic assessment, are an accurate reflection of the architectural configuration of the reference carcinoma to surrounding tissue. Adjustments in the extent of segmental excision of the breast can be made based on the palpable and radiographic characteristics of the tumor, the location of the lesion, the size and consistency of the breast, the histologic characteristics of the tumor, and the age of the patient. Objective data to provide reproducible guidelines on the appropriate extent of tumor-free margins are likely in the future. As will be discussed, there are several appropriate technical considerations for the surgeon and pathologist, as well as the radiologist, particularly with nonpalpable lesions, that have an impact on achieving complete tumor excision with histologically free margins. In most instances, this should be achievable without adversely affecting the aesthetic goals inherent in breast-conserving treatment.

BREAST CONSERVATION FOR IN SITU CANCER

As detailed in Chapters 21, 22, and 23, surgical approaches to breast cancer have undergone very significant changes in the last decades. This is true for invasive as well as for in situ carcinoma. LCIS, which had long been a source of controversy, in particular underwent reassessment. Such changes were, of course, stimulated both by the increasing support for breast conservation in the treatment of operable breast cancer and by the significant increased incidence of the diagnosis of DCIS, a result of widespread mammographic screening efforts at early detection.

For the treatment of LCIS, as detailed in Chapter 23, the most broadly acceptable approach is that originally proposed by Haagensen,[14] which is nonoperative observation, recognizing that LCIS represents a risk factor for the development of cancer in either breast but is not an obligate precursor lesion for invasive cancer in the reference breast. The reassessment of surgery for DCIS has certainly been more complex. For most of the time that DCIS was recognized as a separate pathologic entity, mastectomy was the standard form of therapy. It remained the gold standard, with disease-free survival approaching 100%. Even mastectomy, however, may be associated with local recurrence and mortality resulting from invasive disease undetected at the time of initial surgery or from residual breast tissue that has the potential for developing invasive cancer.[97,98] The incidence, however, is no more than 1% to 3%.[99]

Before the last 2 decades, there was no advocacy for treating DCIS by observation following excision, as there was for LCIS. Limited series of patients inadvertently given a benign misdiagnosis following biopsy were untreated for what was subsequently shown to be noncomedo DCIS, with breast recurrences in the 25% to 36% range.[100–102] Such experiences tend to inhibit enthusiasm for observation as a therapeutic option. Furthermore, as reconstruction became a widely accepted adjunct to mastectomy, it became particularly applicable to patients with DCIS, who represent a group with a very low risk for regional recurrence and, more recently, an optimal presentation for skin-sparing mastectomy incisions that further facilitate the aesthetic benefits of reconstruction using prosthetic implants or autologous tissue flaps. In earlier reports that considered treatment options, however, there was a lack of reference to the various histologic subtypes of DCIS,[103] let alone an appreciation of the focal presentation of disease in most patients. Because all DCIS was broadly categorized as one homogeneous group, there was uncertainty as to the appropriateness of breast conservation. Furthermore, patients in earlier series tended to have larger, sometimes palpable forms of the disease.[104,105] Such lesions would more often be associated with areas of microscopic or frank invasion, even if histologically undetected.[96]

Predictably, the equivalent results for breast conservation compared with mastectomy for stage I invasive cancer of the breast led to an interest in treating noninvasive cancer with breast conservation. The issue, of course, was whether the almost 100% survival with mastectomy could be matched by breast conservation, and, as with patients with stages I and II invasive cancers, to what extent patients should be selected. The answers hinged on several issues, among them the architectural pattern and pathologic characteristics of the noninvasive cancer, the effectiveness and appropriateness of adjuvant radiotherapy, and the impact of these variables on breast cancer recurrence and the natural history of the disease. Other related issues were, and continue to be, the extent of the excision and the ability to diagnose and successfully treat breast cancer recurrence.

What is the impact of multicentricity and multifocality on breast-conserving surgery for ductal carcinoma in situ?

DCIS had been associated with a higher incidence of multicentricity (i.e., DCIS in other quadrants of the breast) than are invasive lesions. As smaller foci of DCIS have been diagnosed, the incidence of multicentricity has been reassessed. The incidence of multicentricity in series that adhere to its definition as carcinoma in other quadrants is about one third.[98,106] Lagios (see Chapter 8) suggested that multicentricity be defined as a second, separate focus of DCIS at a distance of at least 5 cm from the primary focus. A major reason for reassessment of both the true incidence and the clinical significance of multicentricity is the observation that most recurrences after breast-conserving therapy for DCIS are in the immediate vicinity of the original cancer.[107–111] In the experience of Silverstein, 97 of 109 local recurrences (89%) were at or near the site of original surgery.[111] The clinical significance of possible occult multicentricity is therefore subject to debate, particularly because studies have failed to demonstrate any impact of these occult foci on survival. The pattern of breast recurrences after breast-conserving treatment of DCIS within the same quadrant as the primary lesion implicates what might more appropriately be regarded as "residual" disease, rather than multicentricity, in treatment failure.[112]

The issue of multifocality of DCIS in the same quadrant of the breast has similarly come under re-evaluation. In the studies by Holland and colleagues,[113] mastectomy specimens were serially sectioned at distances of 5 mm and radiographically imaged. Each suspicious finding was examined histologically along with an extensive sampling of the quadrant of the reference lesion as well as the other quadrants and the central nipple and subareolar region. The correlative radiologic-pathologic study of more than 150 such carefully evaluated specimens found that even with extensive lesions there was a unifocal pattern and suggested, as emphasized by Silverstein,[111] that presumed multifocality may represent an artifactual pattern resulting from inadequate histologic sampling of an arborizing pattern of distribution. This would lead to artificial skip areas as portrayed on two-dimensional histologic slides. The clear implication of a unifocal concept of the distribution of DCIS is that even what is inappropriately presumed to be multifocal disease may be encompassed by appropriately planned surgery. The possibilities for breast conservation with careful adherence to surgical principles to achieve appropriate tumor-free margins are certainly broadened by such a conceptual reassessment. The final determinant will be the long-term results of expanded efforts at breast conservation for DCIS.

What is the frequency of recurrence after breast conservation for ductal carcinoma in situ?

In series of patients in which breast-conserving treatment has been applied to the treatment of DCIS by wide local excision alone, recurrence rates averaging 26% with follow-up intervals exceeding 5 years have been documented.[114–120] Significantly, about half of these recurrences are invasive. Local recurrence rates have been greatest when the original lesion was palpable[120,121] and when pathologic confirmation of clear margins had not been assured.[96,122] Such lesions would be expected to be of higher nuclear and architectural grade, to demonstrate comedonecrosis, and even to have areas of microinvasion or frank invasion that might elude histologic detection. Furthermore, recurrences have occurred as late as 10 years after treatment. This suggests that at greatest risk for recurrence might be not only patients with larger lesions, but also young women, with their longer life expectancy, the application of potentially less stringent criteria for volume of excised breast or breadth of margins in an attempt to achieve optimal cosmesis, their inherently more aggressive histologic and biologic characteristics, and a different hormonal milieu.[123,124] Recent efforts at predicting the biologic behavior of DCIS using molecular markers may introduce additional significant variables into therapeutic decision making.[125] Still unresolved is the issue of the need for radiotherapy with excision and breast conservation. Certainly, patients with smaller lesions (<10 mm diameter), particularly those lesions incidentally noted on excision specimens for predominantly benign entities (and these are most often low-grade lesions), might appear to be those treated safely by excision alone with no radiotherapy. Several investigators have focused attention on criteria to select patients who might be safely treated without breast irradiation.[126,127] These efforts are detailed in Chapter 23. What is clear from a surgical perspective is the importance of achieving tumor-free margins independent of the issue of whether radiotherapy is used as an adjunct to breast conservation treatment for DCIS.[128] The difficulty in always defining the limits of ductal carcinoma, the extent of which may not always correspond to and which is often broader than the mammographic region of such microcalcifications, as well as the technical limits of histologic criteria for assessing margins, represents the major surgical challenge in treating DCIS.[126,129]

Is radiotherapy needed for the treatment of ductal carcinoma in situ when breast conservation is desired?

With the increasing appreciation of the histologic heterogeneity of DCIS and with the increasing ability to detect very small foci of DCIS mammographically, as well as situations in which foci of DCIS are detected incidentally in biopsy specimens obtained for a clinically benign lesion, the incidence of microinvasion and multicentricity is certainly low. As detailed in Chapters 8 and 23, recurrences seem to predominate in cases of larger lesions with high-grade histologic features, certainly when there is a question regarding involvement of the margins.

The addition of radiation therapy to segmental excision for DCIS results in high rates of local control. In series of patients with follow-up exceeding 5 years, breast recurrence rates average 11%.[112,130–137] The most comprehensive prospective randomized study of excision and radiation therapy for DCIS to date was Protocol B-17 of the National Surgical Adjuvant Breast Project (NSABP), which randomized 818 women with DCIS to undergo either excision alone or excision with radiation. The addition of radiation therapy after 8 years of follow-up reduced the incidence of local noninvasive breast recurrence by 15% (recurrence was 27% for excision alone vs. 12% for excision and radiotherapy).[74,138] The recurrences were more significant for invasive recurrences (10.5% vs. 3%) than for noninvasive recurrences (10% vs. 7.5%) when excision alone was compared with excision plus radiotherapy. A study by the European Organization for Cancer Research (EORTC) also randomized 1010 patients to either excision alone or excision and radiotherapy for DCIS up to 5 cm in size. After 4 years of follow-up, recurrence was higher in the excision-alone group than in the excision plus radiotherapy group (16% vs. 9%).[139] Thus, in the NSABP B-17 trial, radiotherapy reduced local recurrence by 59%; in the EORTC trial, by 38%.

The results of these randomized trials have led to a general recommendation for the use of radiotherapy after complete excision of DCIS. However, this tends to blur the distinctions in various subtypes of DCIS, in the varying breadth of architectural distribution, breast configuration, extent of excision, age, and other potentially relevant clinical variables. Furthermore, the impact of radiotherapy on the subsequent treatment of recurrence relevant to breast conservation or reconstruction and the potential long-term sequelae of radiotherapy have led clinical investigators to question a blanket recommendation and consider more selective approaches to the application of radiotherapy, as discussed in Chapter 23. Perhaps most compellingly, there remain no data in prospective randomized trials demonstrating an impact of breast recurrence on survival.

How should mammographically detected ductal carcinoma in situ be approached surgically?

The most common indicator of DCIS is the mammographically detected cluster of microcalcifications, which is almost always nonpalpable unless it is extensive and may, in fact, contain areas of microinvasion or frank invasion. Because the pattern of clustered microcalcifications may be varied and not reliably predictive of a benign or malignant diagnosis, as discussed in Chapter 15, an expeditious histologic diagnosis is appropriate. Diagnostic options are stereotactic fine-needle aspiration or core biopsy, vacuum-assisted core biopsy, or surgical biopsy with preoperative needle localization and specimen radiographic control. The optimal diagnostic strategy has yet to be assessed in a prospective controlled study. Certainly, if the mammographic finding is broad (occupying a segment exceeding 3 cm) and highly suggestive of carcinoma of the breast by the Breast Imaging Reporting and Data System (BIRADS V), a stereotactic core biopsy may be used to establish the diagnosis of intraductal carcinoma. If the patient were to then elect treatment by breast conservation, appropriate excision could be planned; if the breadth of the mammographic findings warranted mastectomy, this could be performed with optimal reconstruction if so elected by the patient, allowing for skin conservation and the best selection of reconstructive technique.

For faint clusters of microcalcifications not well seen on stereotactic imaging units and for microcalcifications in subareolar locations or locations close to the chest wall that may restrict the application of needle biopsy techniques, a segmental excision to incorporate the cluster with appropriate free margins is the initial diagnostic procedure that would most often translate to an appropriate therapeutic procedure as well, should carcinoma be diagnosed histologically. This requires preoperative needle localization and intraoperative specimen radiographic confirmation.

It has been argued that surgical excision of a cluster of indeterminate microcalcifications is unnecessarily burdensome, invasive, and costly for the approximately 75% of patients whose lesions will prove to be benign. In addition to stereotactic fine-needle and core biopsy, as well as vacuum-assisted core biopsies using the Mammotome (Biopsys Medical Instruments, Irvine, CA), these concerns were addressed by more complete sampling, and even excision has been achieved using needle technologies that extract larger volumes of the target tissue such as the ABBI (U.S. Surgical, Norwalk, CT).[140–142] Definitive excision of the cluster, if a malignant diagnosis has been established and a clip placed, enables optimal planning of the margins of excision. Because DCIS often extends beyond the confines of the area with the microcalcifications, definitive excision with appropriate attention to margins strengthens the chance for local control with breast conservation. Any ambiguity about the histology, or discordance between a benign needle biopsy diagnosis and suspicious radiographic appearance, should be followed by definitive surgical excision. Definitive excision abrogates repeated-interval radiographic evaluation. With current percutaneous biopsy techniques, patients with benign diagnoses can usually be spared a surgical biopsy, whereas patients with a malignant diagnosis may be further studied radiographically with magnetic resonance imaging (MRI) if appropriate, and a sound decision on appropriate treatment made in a carefully considered manner and followed by careful surgical planning.

An excision for clustered microcalcifications associated with malignant disease should enable a clear definition of margins. When the cluster of microcalcifications is mammographically subtle and tiny, diagnosis by multiple core biopsies runs the risk of significantly reducing or even completely removing the microcalcifications. Radiographic metallic clip placement is therefore essential because a definitive excision would be compromised or made unfeasible in the absence of any marker calcifications needed for localization.

When is mastectomy appropriate for ductal carcinoma in situ?

Consideration must be given to mastectomy if there is a diffuse pattern of comedonecrosis with significant extension to margins despite a broad excision or re-excision, if the microcalcifications are extensive in other areas of the breast as well, if the histologic pattern of the excised cancer is more diffusely malignant than mammographic patterns would have suggested, and if prior radiotherapy or conditions such as significant collagen-vascular disease contraindicate the use of radiation therapy. The risk for recurrence with breast conservation in these circumstances may be prohibitively high, particularly because available data suggest that half of the recurrences in the involved breast, even with radiation therapy, are invasive. Where involvement of margins is limited or focal, re-excision to achieve tumor-free margins without resorting to mastectomy is appropriate. MRI should be considered when the mammographic and sonographic assessment of extent of disease is uncertain. Although MRI may reveal unappreciated areas of invasive carcinoma, the reliability of assessing DCIS that may extend beyond areas of microcalcifications—the only marker of disease mammographically—remains unresolved. Finally, patient preference may dictate the choice of mastectomy.

When mastectomy is performed for high-grade DCIS that is extensive or multicentric, the possibility of microinvasion, and even lymph node micrometastases, has suggested that when excising the tail of the breast from the lateral axilla, the performance of a limited level I dissection is appropriate. This enables those lymph node micrometastases, most commonly located within the level I group of nodes, to be diagnosed and effectively ablated. Sentinel lymphadenectomy may well alter this approach to axillary lymph nodes for such high-risk DCIS, as will be discussed. Although the incidence of axillary metastases for pure DCIS is 0%, sentinel lymph node biopsy in selected series of patients with DCIS has revealed an incidence of nodal micrometastases of 6% to 13%,[143–145] highlighting the potential underappreciation of invasion in all instances of pathologically diagnosed DCIS. This would be particularly relevant for patients for whom mastectomy has been chosen because of the architectural extent and high-grade histologic characteristics.[146]

Mastectomy for DCIS presents an optimal setting for immediate reconstruction with skin-sparing techniques, as discussed in Chapters 23 and 25. This may particularly enhance the cosmetic results of autogenous transverse rectus abdominis myocutaneous (TRAM) flap reconstruction.[147]

SEGMENTAL EXCISION FOR NONPALPABLE CARCINOMA

The increasing use of stereotactic and sonographically directed biopsy techniques, using either fine-needle aspiration or core biopsy, has increased the number of patients with clinically occult cancers coming to definitive breast-conserving surgery. These patients tend to fall into three radiographically definable groups: (1) patients with a cluster of microcalcifications, (2) those with an area of architectural distortion, and (3) those with a mammographically or sonographically definable mass lesion. When breast conservation has been decided on after clinical and radiographic as well as medical and patient-related considerations, every effort should be made to achieve definitive excision with tumor-free margins in one procedure. In those instances when the decision for an axillary procedure, either sentinel lymphadenectomy or axillary dissection, requires more complete analysis of tumor size and histopathologic characteristics, the segmental excision is performed alone. When a definitive diagnosis of intermediate or high-grade invasive carcinoma has been established by stereotactic or sonographically directed core biopsy, and size is clearly evaluable mammographically or sonographically, sentinel lymphadenectomy or axillary dissection can be performed together with the definitive criteria. However, for noninvasive lesions or small (T1a) and selected T1b low-grade invasive lesions, deferring a possible axillary procedure until its appropriateness can be assessed on the basis of a full consideration of the relevant histopathologic information is advantageous, particularly because the segmental excision may be easily performed for the patient as an ambulatory surgical procedure and almost always using local anesthesia.

What preoperative measures ensure optimal excision of the lesion?

A nonpalpable lesion, or a clip indicating the site of a core biopsied lesion, should always be preoperatively localized using an appropriate hooked wire device. Preoperative localization based exclusively on mammographic views in the craniocaudal and mediolateral positions without such a localizer is unreliable. Distances measured from the nipple to the lesion in the superior to inferior and medial to lateral axes of patients in the sitting position may differ from the distances with the patient in the supine position required for surgical biopsy. In addition, the measured depth from the skin to the lesion may be different in these positions. Misguided excisions performed without preoperative wire localization may fail to include the lesion in the biopsy specimen. Furthermore, when the lesion is excised, the margins around the lesion may be inappropriately asymmetrical, with a margin in one plane excessively beyond the lesion, while a margin in another plane abuts the excised lesion or is grossly involved with a lesion that is incompletely excised.

After the radiologist places the hooked wire localizer by the shortest direct path from the skin to the lesion, as detailed in

Chapter 15, the site of the hooked wire placement in relation to the lesion and to the nipple should be clearly communicated. For example, the location of a nonpalpable lesion in the upper outer quadrant might be described as 5.5 cm lateral and 1.0 cm above the mid-nipple line, with the wire through and the hook 3.0 mm medial to the lesion (Fig. 24–10). For patients with sonographically but not mammographically detected lesions, the same mammographic description should be provided to the surgeon after the sonographically guided placement of the hooked wire. For patients with microcalcifications, particularly those that extend over a distance of several centimeters, framing the area with two or more wire localizers enables greater confidence that the entire breadth of the lesion will be excised.[148] The hooked wire localizers should be taped securely to the patient to minimize dislodgment during transport from the radiology suite to the operating facility.

Concerns about the frequency of positive margins after segmental excisions with preoperative wire localization, as well as patient discomfort and logistical issues and occasional wire displacement, have prompted efforts to seek alternative techniques. These include a variety of approaches, such as radioactive localization using a titanium seed containing ^{125}I deployed at the lesion site and identified intraoperatively using a gamma probe, carbon marking, methylene blue marking, and intraoperative ultrasound-guided excision of the hematoma within the core biopsy track or of a gel marker.[149,150] These techniques are being studied but have not displaced wire localization techniques at the present time.

What anesthesia is appropriate?

Although excisions performed without any axillary procedures are done in an ambulatory surgery setting, it is essential that optimal local anesthesia be employed. One percent lidocaine (0.5% when the need for large volumes is projected) without epinephrine is injected intradermally and into the perioperative field. Care should be taken to maintain a volume of anesthetic below the safety limit (<500 mg or 4.5 mg/kg of lidocaine). A small wheal should be raised first, and the remaining length of the incision injected subcutaneously with anesthetic using a long needle before completing the intradermal infiltration. The addition of 1 mL of 8.5% sodium bicarbonate to each 10 mL of 1% lidocaine without epinephrine neutralizes the pH and creates less of a burning discomfort at the onset of infiltrating the anesthetic. Excessive patient discomfort and anxiety may create an intraoperative environment that hinders the successful excision of the appropriate area with the care necessary to ensure both an optimal cancer operation and aesthetic result and may erode the patient's confidence in the surgeon. A nurse at the head of the table to reassure and engage the patient in conversation is an essential adjunct to the surgeon's own comforting narrative and efforts to maintain a calm ambience of professionalism. Supplemental sedation is advisable for the anxious patient, in whom pain may clearly be accentuated by stress, and for those patients having an excision of a deep lesion in a large breast. It should be recognized that anxiety is common even if

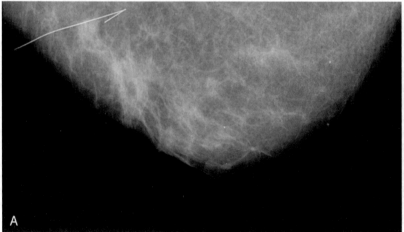
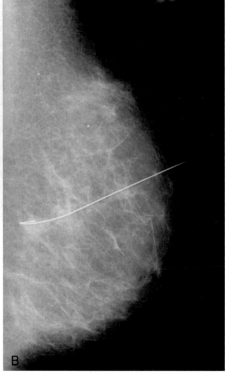

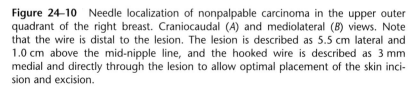

Figure 24–10 Needle localization of nonpalpable carcinoma in the upper outer quadrant of the right breast. Craniocaudal (*A*) and mediolateral (*B*) views. Note that the wire is distal to the lesion. The lesion is described as 5.5 cm lateral and 1.0 cm above the mid-nipple line, and the hooked wire is described as 3 mm medial and directly through the lesion to allow optimal placement of the skin incision and excision.

sion and magnification (Fig. 24–13). This may be particularly valuable in assessing the adequacy of an excision for clustered microcalcifications. If any margins are deemed too close to the lesion on gross inspection or specimen radiography, an additional segment from the excision bed at the site indicated by the orientation markers is best excised. To ensure that the lesion has been completely excised and to maximize the likelihood of free margins on final histopathologic assessment, particularly in the patient with a dense fibroglandular breast where margin involvement may not always be suspected by gross inspection or evaluation of the radiographs, it may be of value to excise an additional segment of the excision bed from any margin that on gross inspection or on specimen mammographic evaluation appears near a specimen margin or margins, and the new margin should be appropriately tagged for identification by the pathologist. Finally, the specimen is immediately conveyed to the pathologist for further assessment before the procedure is completed. It has been suggested that additional specimens be excised from each of the excision

bed margins (i.e., superior, inferior, medial, lateral, and posterior), which can then be further assessed to ensure that the margins are free of tumor.[154] Whatever the technique, efforts to achieve tumor-free margins while avoiding unnecessarily excessive excisions of tissue are appropriate and best performed at the time of initial definitive surgery.

How does the pathologist evaluate the specimen?

After specimen radiography has confirmed that the lesion, or clip, is well contained within the excised segment, the specimen is carefully oriented by the pathologist as indicated by the surgically placed marking sutures or clips. Every effort should be made to ensure that the communication in this regard between surgeon and pathologist is clear. The surface is then cleaned of blood with alcohol and blotted dry, and the margins are inked to allow appropriate evaluation on final histopathologic sections. Multicolored gelatin dye systems are most commonly used for color coding and identifying different margins. The dyes are applied with a small paintbrush and blotted dry again.

After the appropriate inking of the margins, the specimen is serially sectioned into 3- to 4-mm parallel slices. A definable lesion may be identified on examination and any specific proximity to a specific margin or margins communicated to the surgeon. Additional specimen radiographs of the sectioned tissue for detection of more subtle lesions, particularly clustered microcalcifications, are also obtained using a table-top unit (Faxitron X-ray Corp., Wheeling, IL) (Fig. 24–14). The slices on the specimen radiographs are labeled and placed in cassettes.

The potential pitfalls in pathologic margin assessment are evident to anyone viewing the technique, as dye works its way

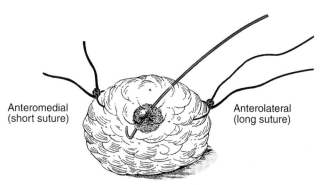

Anteromedial
(short suture)

Anterolateral
(long suture)

Figure 24–12 As it is excised, the specimen is appropriately tagged for orientation by at least two marking sutures or tags.

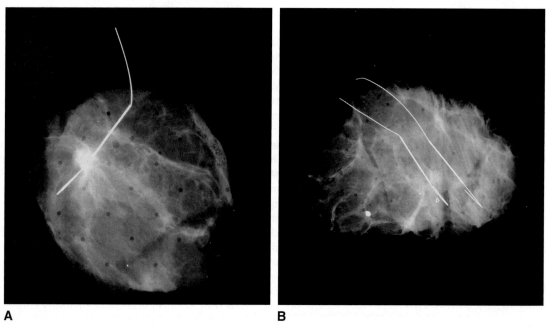

A   **B**

Figure 24–13 *A,* Magnification specimen radiography confirms the lesion centrally located in the specimen. *B,* Magnification specimen radiography confirms a Mammotome clip, the site of diagnosis of ductal carcinoma in situ, and additional microcalcification framed by two hooked wire localizers.

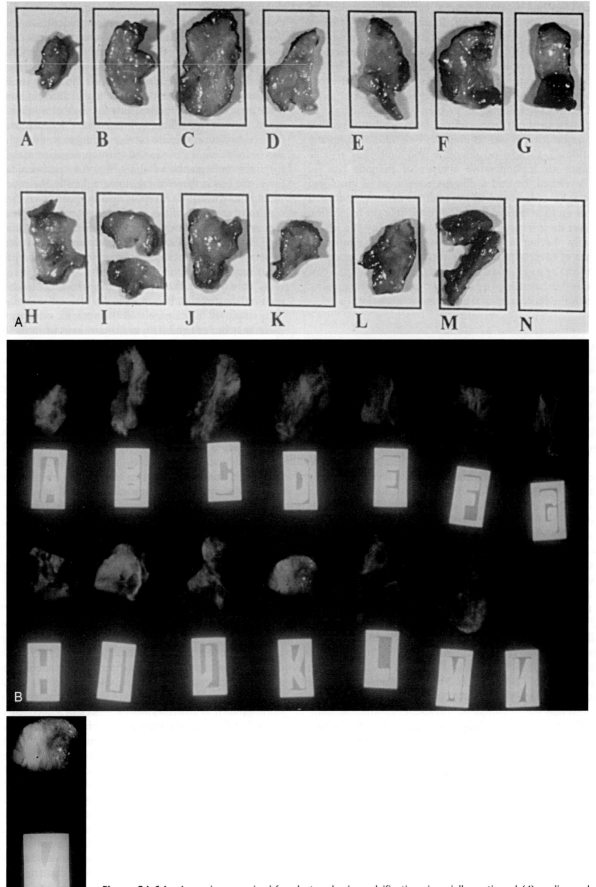

Figure 24–14 A specimen excised for clustered microcalcifications is serially sectioned (*A*), radiographs are obtained (*B*), and the major site of the microcalcifications is identified (*C*).

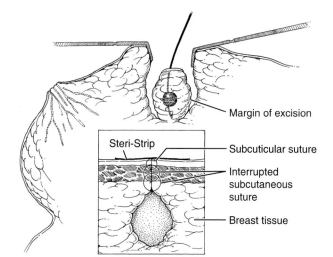

Figure 24–15   Closure of segmental excision.

is applied to the wound with a fluffed gauze dressing, but tape applied under tension to secure the dressing should be avoided because this may cause blistering and even full-thickness loss of skin if the tape is applied with significant stretching. Rather, the patient should be instructed to wear a brassiere postoperatively and certainly for the first evening to provide additional compression of the dressing and support of the surgical wound. A sports bra after the first day and even for weeks afterward is recommended as a further means of achieving comfort during the postoperative phase. Advance purchase of a sports bra that closes with hooks is recommended. Showering is permitted with appropriate wound protection, with a sealing dressing or impermeable cover placed in a bra worn in the shower.

SURGICAL MANAGEMENT OF THE AXILLARY LYMPH NODES

Does axillary dissection confer any survival advantage?

There is no convincing evidence that axillary dissection improves survival. In a meta-analysis of six clinical trials that randomized patients to breast cancer surgery by segmental excision and radiation with or without axillary dissection or to mastectomy with or without axillary dissection, Orr demonstrated an average survival advantage of 5.4% of those groups having axillary dissection.[168] However, these trials were from an era when far fewer patients received adjuvant systemic therapy and few were treated for nonpalpable lesions, an ever-increasing component of the present population of breast cancer patients. The two largest trials included in the analysis were those from the NSABP (B-04)[169] and the Institut Curie.[170] In the NSABP B-04 trial, 25% of patients with positive nodes were free of disease at 10 years, regardless of whether they had been treated by elective dissection or delayed dissection for clinically detected metastases. In the Institut Curie trial, there was a survival advantage of 4% for patients having axillary dissection. However, there was greater use of both adjuvant systemic therapy and radiation therapy in patients whose elective axillary dissection revealed metastatic disease. If a survival advantage did result from axillary dissection, it would clearly be limited to a small subset of patients. Accrual of clinical evidence that would either demonstrate or disprove a survival advantage for axillary dissection is even more unlikely as the use of adjuvant systemic therapy broadens for patients with invasive cancers and as the percentage of patients diagnosed with nonpalpable T1a and T1b lesions increases.

Is the evaluation of axillary lymph nodes important for staging?

The pathologic assessment of axillary lymph nodes remains the most important prognostic variable for the invasive breast cancer patient. In the absence of any evidence of distant metastases, the status of axillary lymph nodes has maintained its dominant influence, even with the trend toward earlier detection of clinically occult cancers and the proliferation of molecular assays of the primary tumor. No other factors, including size, either alone or in combination, are superior at predicting the potential for relapse.[171] Data from the NCI Surveillance and Epidemiology and End Results (SEER) program reporting on 5-year survival in 24,740 patients demonstrated a predictable increased risk for lymph node metastases as tumor size increased but demonstrated as well that size and nodal metastases are independent variables. Even for tumors equal to or greater than 5 cm, survival decreased from 82.2% if node negative to 45% if four or more nodes had metastases.[172] Furthermore, the extent of nodal involvement, the number of metastatic axillary nodes,[172–174] the size of metastases,[175,176] and the extension of metastases beyond the capsule[177] have demonstrated impact on survival, as detailed in Chapter 19. As further refinements in the pathologic evaluation of micrometastases evolves, including immuno-histochemical staining[178–182] and molecular assays such as polymerase chain reaction (PCR),[183] the importance of axillary nodal assessment may be enhanced. However, the true prognostic significance of nodal metastases consisting of small emboli of cells in the nodal sinuses, immunohistoclinically detected isolated cells, or PCR-positive assays, compared with true micrometastases (<2 mm), has yet to be reproducibly determined. Conversely, the widespread use of adjuvant systemic strategies may limit the importance of such assessment. It is for these reasons that more selective approaches to axillary surgical management have particular appeal.

Can the axilla be staged noninvasively?

No clinical or radiographic techniques have yet been demonstrated to have the sensitivity necessary to accurately stage the axilla. Physical examination can detect gross disease but has an unacceptable rate of false-positive as well as false-negative findings.[184–187] Mammography, ultrasound, power Doppler sonography, MRI, lymphoscintigraphy, and radiolabeled monoclonal antibody scanning have proved inadequate to date.[185,185–193] More recently, positron emission tomography (PET) has been evaluated, but this technique can detect only tumors that are about 1.0 cm or larger.[194]

Size and the histologic and molecular characteristics of the primary tumor, as well as patient age, have been analyzed as determinants of axillary metastases. The most accurate predictor remains primary tumor size.[172,195] The incidence of axillary involvement increases with the size of the primary tumor and may even exceed 20% for tumors smaller than 1 cm (T1a and b). In the experience of one of the authors, as noted, the rate of axillary metastasis associated with T1a tumors was 10% using hematoxylin and eosin (H&E) staining alone and 15% using immunohistochemical staining in addition to H&E staining.[196] As data have accrued on the more detailed pathologic analysis of sentinel nodes, the frequency of nodal metastases has increased. When investigators have looked at the incidence of nodal involvement as a function of tumor size as well as lymphatic or vascular invasion, histologic grade, laminin receptor and c-erb-2 overexpression, patient age, progesterone receptor status, and S-phase fraction,[197–199] they have concluded that analysis of the primary tumor could not replace histologic evaluation of the axillary nodes as an effective staging technique at the present time. Furthermore, the more detailed assessment of axillary nodes may shed increasing light on the biologic significance of micrometastases as well as on the group of patients heretofore considered node negative by traditional histologic analysis of the entire axilla but who experienced recurrence, despite a presumed favorable prognosis.

What is the role of axillary dissection in the treatment of breast cancer?

Axillary dissection has remained a component of the local treatment of invasive breast cancer but has been subjected to increasing scrutiny in recent years. For patients with palpable lymphadenopathy, it remains an essential component of surgical therapy. Of patients without lymphadenopathy, more than 70% will have no histologic evidence of nodal involvement, and this incidence will likely increase as the diagnosis of smaller and biologically more favorable lesions increases.[200]

The controversy relating to elective axillary dissection in the absence of palpable lymphadenopathy derives from a failure to demonstrate clearly an independent therapeutic value and from the perception that it should be applied only for patients in whom the histologic investigation of axillary nodes would alter adjuvant therapeutic strategies. This perception, however, may oversimplify the prognostic information that may be gained from axillary dissection and also undermine the potential for achieving effective local treatment of axillary metastases with minimal morbidity, thereby preventing axillary recurrence. Until recently, the alternative to elective axillary dissection has been surveillance or radiation. A more selective approach using intraoperative lymphatic mapping and sentinel lymphadenectomy has now gained hold as a means of both staging and directing the potential therapeutic benefits of axillary dissection. A detailed consideration of sentinel lymphadenectomy will follow. Suffice it to say at this point that sentinel lymphadenectomy circumvents the

limitations of surveillance and radiation, which fail to obtain the prognostic information provided by histologic assessment of the axillary lymph nodes, and it directs axillary dissection for those patients most likely to benefit from the procedure. This enables full assessment of the prognostic information the axillary nodes may provide, which is related not only to the presence or absence of axillary micrometastases but also to the extent of such micrometastases. Such information has been well demonstrated to correlate with survival.[201–203] In this sense, the detailed analysis of sentinel lymph nodes may allow even more specific prognostic information and effective therapeutic strategies.

How effective is axillary dissection in the local control of disease?

The rarity of axillary recurrence following a carefully performed axillary dissection is well established.[204,205] In the NSABP B-04 study, axillary recurrence was reported in only 1.4% of node-negative patients and in 1.0% of node-positive patients following axillary dissection, whereas 17.8% of patients with clinically negative axillae randomized to not have an axillary dissection developed clinically palpable nodal metastases.[206] Series of patients whose axillae were not treated have been reported by Cady and associates,[207] who found an axillary failure rate of 16%, and by Baxter and associates,[208] who found a 10-year actuarial axillary failure rate of 23%. Radiation is an effective alternative, as reported by Recht and associates,[209] who noted an 0.8% incidence of axillary recurrence following axillary radiation in 355 clinically node-negative patients. Wong and associates[210] reported on 92 patients with no lymphadenopathy treated with radiotherapy that included the level I nodes. A single axillary recurrence in association with a breast recurrence, but no isolated axillary recurrence, was noted.

Radiotherapy can decrease axillary recurrence in the absence of clinically diagnosed axillary metastases, but it does not yield prognostic information that might impact adjuvant therapy.[209] Furthermore, as reported in the NSABP B-04 study, the axillary recurrence rate in patients receiving axillary radiation rather than axillary dissection for palpable nodal disease was 12%. An even higher rate of 19% was reported in a series by Osborne and associates[211] from the Royal Marsden Hospital. It has not been feasible to date to segregate the impact that axillary dissection may or may not have on the natural history of breast cancer because any benefit is inextricably linked to the greater use of adjuvant therapy resulting from the information obtained from axillary dissection. Axillary dissection has therefore remained a component of the local treatment of invasive breast cancer, but it has appropriately come under intense scrutiny as the frequency of smaller, often nonpalpable and low-grade cancers has risen as a result of more widespread mammographic screening and as more refined sentinel lymphadenectomy techniques are developed. The issue of complications from axillary dissection will be discussed later in this chapter. While complications depend on a clear definition of the extent of surgery, the issue for our present consideration is whether the detection of axillary metastases might be optimized and axillary dissection limited to only those patients in whom a prognostic and possible therapeutic benefit might be realized.

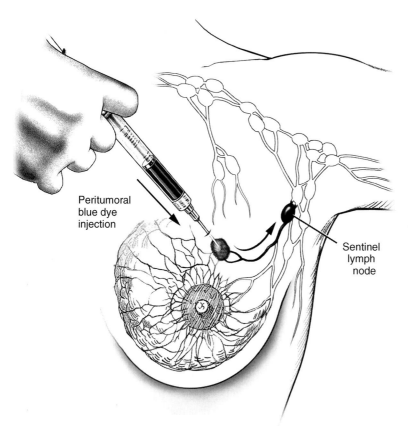

Peritumoral
blue dye
injection

Sentinel
lymph
node

Figure 24–16   Blue dye and/or radioisotope injection at site of cancer.

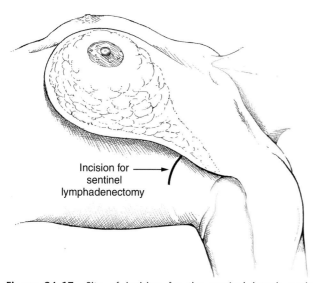

Incision for
sentinel
lymphadenectomy

Figure 24–17   Site of incision for the sentinel lymph node biopsy.

disruption of a blue lymphatic channel because this may result in inadequate staining of the sentinel node and unnecessary blue staining of the soft tissues. After the blue channel or channels are detected by careful dissection with a mosquito clamp and electrocautery, they are traced both proximally and distally to ensure that the first node in the chain is identified. Following identification of a blue node with appropriately high radioisotope counts, great care is exerted in handling the node. A traction suture may be placed adjacent to it, or a noncrushing Babcock clamp may also be used to

deliver the node into the field and allow its complete excision (Fig. 24–18).

After excision of the node or nodes, care must be taken to evaluate the specimen for its color and for its ex vivo radioactive counts. A potential pitfall of the use of radiocolloid and gamma detection of sentinel nodes is "shine-through" of radioactivity, not only from an injection site close to the axilla but also from a node or nodes behind or adjacent to the presumed sentinel node. The excised nodes should have the same ex vivo counts as recorded in vivo (Fig. 24–19). The nodes should be evaluated for radioactive counts away from the operative field. With a larger node, a specific focus of high radioisotopic counts may be identifiable and can be tagged with a suture to direct the pathologist to this potential site of metastatic disease. The site of excision should also be evaluated for residual background radioactivity, with the probe directed not only centrally but also in all directions around the periphery of the field of dissection except toward the site of injection. It has been suggested that nonsentinel node counts should be less than 10% of the sentinel nodes.[242] Certainly, if the ex vivo counts over the node are lower than the in vivo counts, if the concentration of the blue dye is uncertain, and if the background counts are not significantly lower than the reference nodes, further dissection is indicated. The proliferation of gamma detection instruments and collimators requires that the surgeon be familiar with the specifications and calibration of the specific instrument being used. Careful recording of the counts, not over-reliance on audible features, is essential. Inspection and palpation of the axilla may reveal a grossly involved node that has failed to concentrate dye or radioisotope, or a blue node that has been overlooked. These should be excised, because a node replaced by metastatic

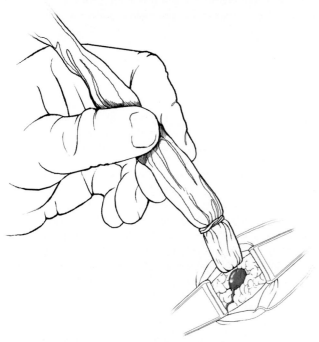

Figure 24–18 Blue-stained lymphatic channel coursing toward blue-stained lymph node is identified.

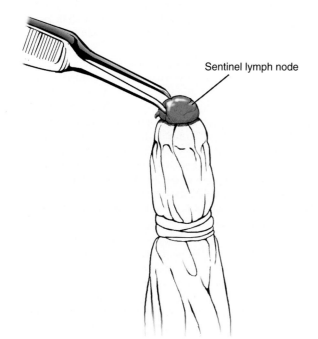

Sentinel lymph node

Figure 24–19 Sentinel lymph node or nodes, excised, and radioisotope counts confirmed ex vivo.

Table 24–2 Pitfalls of Sentinel Lymphadenectomy

1. Failure to inject dye intraparenchymally, favoring the axillary side of the intact lesion or segmental incision site.
2. Failure to inject isotope at least 1 to 2 hours prior to commencement of the procedure.
3. Failure to record time of injection of dye and/or isotope and time of commencement of the procedure.
4. Failure to massage the site of dye injection.
5. Failure to place the incision below the hair-bearing area of the axilla to allow extension to an axillary dissection incision, if necessary.
6. Failure to transect tissues directly down to the clavipectoral fascia.
7. Failure to carefully dissect until blue-stained lymphatic channel(s) are identified to avoid their disruption.
8. Failure to achieve meticulous hemostasis.
9. Failure to carefully review gamma probe settings and collimation characteristics.
10. Failure to direct gamma probe away from injection site, particularly to avoid "shine-through" with lesions in the upper outer quadrant.
11. Failure to check ex vivo counts of sentinel node(s), away from the operative field, to ensure that they approximate in vivo counts.
12. Failure to check background counts at excision site to ensure that there has been a reduction to less than one tenth of the hottest node.
13. Failure to inspect the excision site for any suspiciously enlarged or palpable nodes and failure to excise such nodes regardless of their failure to concentrate dye or radioisotope.

these situations, the more extended procedure may not be justified.

The pitfalls of sentinel lymphadenectomy are listed in Table 24–2.

How is the sentinel node examined?

The sentinel node is immediately conveyed to the pathology lab, where it is inspected. If there is any suspicion of metastatic disease by gross inspection or after the node is bivalved along the longitudinal axis, the sentinel node is examined by frozen section. If the sentinel node demonstrates metastasis on frozen section, a standard level I and II axillary lymph node dissection is performed at the initial surgical procedure. For nodes that are not suspicious by inspection, the issue of intraoperative evaluation is more controversial. There is certainly an advantage to establishing a diagnosis of metastatic carcinoma at the time of initial surgery, particularly in the setting of mastectomy and reconstruction. When breast conservation is planned the issue is not as compelling, given the limited extent of surgery and the frequently ambulatory setting for performing these procedures. This experience had led some to recommend sentinel node biopsy as an initial separate procedure for those having mastectomy and reconstruction.[253]

There are potential pitfalls in the routine use of frozen section analysis, including tissue loss, which occurs particularly with a small lymph node, and there are recognized limitations on the accuracy of frozen section diagnosis. When compared

carcinoma may direct lymphatic flow to other nodes and fail to take up dye or isotope.[251,252] Finally, failure to identify the sentinel nodes should be followed by an axillary dissection, except in those instances in which the probability of nodal metastases is low, there are relative contraindications to the procedure, or the potential for altering prognosis is small. In with permanent paraffin section results, frozen section analysis of sentinel nodes may have a false negative rate of 11% to 43%.[254–263] With more exhaustive intraoperative frozen section analysis this may be reduced, but micrometastases may continue to elude detection.[264,265]

Another intraoperative approach is the use of touch preparation analysis. Nodes are bisected, and after inspection, imprints are made for cytologic analysis.[266–269] As with touch preparation assessment of segmental excision margins, touch preparation of lymph nodes depends on available expertise in cytologic analysis, but in experienced centers it is an accurate means of assessment, with sensitivity as high as 94.4%.[267] Subsequent analysis of sentinel nodes by multiple sectioning and immunohistochemical staining for cytokeratins is detailed in Chapter 11.

Certainly, sentinel lymphadenectomy has resulted in increasing sensitivity in detecting nodal metastases. Frozen section detects about 70% of positive nodes that are eventually judged positive with H&E.[89] Immunohistochemical staining has detected an additional 10% to 20% of nodes that were thought to be negative by H&E.[270–273] Multiple sectioning with immunohistochemical analysis of the sentinel node is clearly a powerful means of detecting metastases but would be logistically formidable for the much larger axillary lymph node dissection specimen. In the study of Giuliano and associates, among patients with positive sentinel nodes, 32% were positive on routine histology, whereas immunohistochemical staining increased the yield of positivity to 42%.[228] The true significance of micrometastases detected by immunohistochemical staining alone or more recently by reverse transcription polymerase chain reaction (RT-PCR) remains to be determined.

To determine how sentinel lymphadenectomy compares with axillary lymphadenectomy as a staging technique, Giuliano and associates also examined the axillary nodes excised from 162 patients undergoing sentinel lymphadenectomy followed by complete axillary lymphadenectomy and 134 patients undergoing axillary lymphadenectomy alone.[274] Axillary lymph node dissection specimens were examined by H&E alone, and sentinel nodes by H&E and immunohistochemical staining. The rate of detection of axillary metastases was higher in the sentinel node dissection and axillary dissection group than in the group undergoing axillary dissection alone (42% vs. 28%, respectively; $P = .05$) This difference reflected the larger number of micrometastases (<2 mm) detected in the sentinel node group (16%) than in the exclusive axillary dissection group (3%). Using H&E only, micrometastases were found in 9% of the sentinel node group and in 3% of the axillary dissection group. When the sentinel nodes were examined with immunohistochemical staining, the incidence of micrometastases increased by 7%. This study highlighted the greater sensitivity of sentinel lymphadenectomy compared with axillary dissection in detecting nodal metastases. Veronesi and associates compared 516 patients with primary breast cancer in whom the tumor was equal to or less than 2 cm to sentinel node biopsy and axillary dissection or sentinel node biopsy alone followed by axillary dissection only if the sentinel node contained metastases.[275] The sentinel node was positive in 32.3% of the sentinel node and axillary dissection group and in 33.5% of the group having only sentinel node biopsy. There were no cases of overt axillary metastases in the sentinel node group evaluated as negative for metastasis and not having axillary dissection.

Should axillary dissection follow the detection of a sentinel node metastasis?

While the standard of care has been to perform an axillary dissection (the techniques of which will be detailed later in this chapter) for a confirmed axillary nodal metastasis, the sentinel node technique has focused attention on certain assumptions about the value of axillary dissection. Specifically, what is the significance of a micrometastasis (≤2 cm) or a "submicrometastasis" (≤0.2 cm) as a cluster or, even more problematically, as individual cells, often detected by immunohistochemical staining, not only for prognosis but surgically as an indication for completion axillary dissection? Prognostically, the issue has significant implications for adjuvant systemic therapy as well. Complicating the study of these questions are the limitations of pathologic assessment of completion axillary dissection specimens, which are rarely evaluated with the same exhaustive techniques as are sentinel nodes, making data on the likelihood of additional nodal disease imperfect. These issues were addressed in a consensus conference on sentinel lymph node biopsy.[241] At the present time, the issue of whether completion axillary dissection confers any advantage following the detection of a sentinel node metastasis is unresolved. In the previously cited study by Veronesi and associates, in 60 of 175 patients in whom only a micrometastasis (foci <2 mm diameter) was found in the sentinel nodes, 10 (17%) had another node involved.[275]

The use of immunohistochemical staining and the detection of submillimeter metastases present a dilemma for the surgeon outside of the clinical trial setting. Controversy persists, with some questioning the value of additional dissection in view of the low probability of additional nodal disease.[276–280] Jakub and associates[281] found that 14.5% of patients with metastases detected by positive immunohistochemical staining for cytokeratin in the sentinel node had additional nodal metastases in completion axillary dissection specimens, leading them to recommend consideration of the procedure. Studies that have considered variables that might affect the possible involvement of nonsentinel lymph nodes have demonstrated a greater likelihood with increasing tumor size[282] and the size of the metastasis (>2 mm).[283] Clearly, such decisions must weigh the impact that a completion axillary dissection would have on adjuvant therapeutic decisions and outcome as well as morbidity. A group of 46 women with sentinel node metastases who refused or were recommended to omit axillary dissection for comorbid conditions was studied by Guenther and associates.[284] After a mean follow-up of 32 months, none had developed an axillary recurrence, and one developed distant metastases.

An ongoing clinical trial by the American College of Surgeons Oncology Group (ACOSOG Z0011) randomizes patients with T1 or T2 tumors with clinically negative axillae and treated by breast conservation and who have a single sentinel lymph node metastasis on H&E to either have or not have a completion axillary dissection. Use of adjuvant breast radiotherapy and systemic therapy is the same for both groups.[285] This study should provide important data to help resolve the issue.

Are there any adverse reactions to lymphatic mapping?

The potential for allergic and anaphylactic reaction to isosulfan blue dye has now been documented. Montgomery and associates reviewed a series of 2392 patients having sentinel lymphadenectomy using isosulfan blue dye and reported allergic reactions in 1.6%, 69% of which were grade 1 (urticaria, blue hives, rash, or pruritus), 8% grade 2 (hypotension not requiring pressor support), and 23% grade 3 (hypotension requiring pressor support).[286] No cross-reactivity was found among patients having a sulfa drug allergy. Awareness of this potential for allergic reactions allows appropriate diagnosis and treatment with diphenhydramine as well as hydrocortisone for more severe reactions.

The patient's urine is frequently blue in the hours following the procedure, and the stool, through excretion of dye in the bile, may also be blue. During surgery, falsely decreased pulse oximeter readings may result from the circulating dye. Blue dye may suffuse into the surrounding breast not encompassed by the surgery. The resulting blue hue invariably dissipates with time, and the patient should be reassured in this regard.

Radioactive colloid use for sentinel lymphadenectomy is considered safe, with radiation exposure to the patient, surgeon, and staff a small fraction of the maximum allowable yearly dose.[241,287,288] The Consensus Conference on Sentinel Node Biopsy for Breast Cancer noted reassuringly that women who are potentially or actually pregnant are not exposed to any significant risk. Although local radiation safety precautions may differ, special precautions were not deemed necessary beyond the appropriate sealing and identification of waste materials according to institutional practice.[241]

The potential complications of axillary dissection will be discussed later in this chapter. Sentinel lymphadenectomy now has a documented and predictably lower incidence of pain, paresthesias, range-of-motion limitations, seroma formation, axillary web syndrome (a cordlike extension from the axilla down the arm), and arm edema.[289,290] A drain is not required, and arm mobility may resume immediately after surgery. Paresthesias and pain should be avoidable with careful dissection near the intercostobrachial nerve, although transient symptoms may be experienced.

Is lymphoscintigraphy required for sentinel lymphadenectomy?

Lymphoscintigraphy images lymphatic channels and lymph nodes using radioactive isotopes in the nuclear medicine department, after injection of the isotope around the tumor or biopsy cavity. The patient then lies on a scintiscanner, which tracks the radioactive isotope as it travels from the tumor site through the lymphatic channels to the sentinel node. A hard copy is made of this drainage pattern, and the sentinel node site may then be marked on the skin with ink.

The issue is whether this preoperative imaging is required in managing the breast cancer patient for whom the injection of isotope and sentinel lymphadenectomy with a gamma probe and blue dye is to be performed. When used for malignant melanoma, lymphoscintigraphy has been of particular value in delineating patterns of lymphatic drainage from ambiguous areas such as the trunk and the head and neck, where the direction of lymphatic flow may be variable, multiple, and even unpredictable. This is useful in planning intraoperative sentinel lymphadenectomy strategies for the melanoma patient. For breast cancer, the needs are less compelling. Many lesions arise in the upper outer quadrant, where the radioactive scatter may obscure the lymphatic channels and sentinel nodes, while the drainage pattern from all other sites is overwhelmingly to the axilla. Hence, the procedure has not been considered a requirement.[291,292] McMasters and associates found no advantage to the sentinel node identification rate, false-negative rate, or number of sentinel nodes removed if preoperative lymphoscintigraphy was performed.[292] Furthermore, the value of detecting occasional internal mammary node or supraclavicular node drainage patterns in altering management remains unclear at this time. Certainly, the sensitivity of intraoperative gamma probes largely obviates the information obtained by preoperative lymphoscintigraphy.

Is there an appropriate learning mechanism for sentinel lymphadenectomy?

Any institution considering the adoption of sentinel lymphadenectomy in the treatment of breast cancer patients must recognize the role not only of the surgical team but also of the pathology and nuclear medicine departments. For the procedure to have a meaningful impact on patient care, multidisciplinary cooperation and continued review and critical analysis of all components of lymphatic mapping, surgical technique, and histopathology should be in place. Traditional training in a surgical procedure relies on the expertise and experience of those transmitting the information to those being trained. The technique of sentinel lymphadenectomy, like laparoscopic surgery before, has been rapidly embraced, with few experienced surgeons to provide direct supervision. To adopt the technique appropriately and develop their competence, surgeons have been encouraged to perform the procedure and follow with an axillary dissection to protect against false-negative sentinel node biopsies by validating that nodes containing metastatic disease were indeed the sentinel nodes. Only in this way would the sentinel node reflect the status of the axilla. An area of discussion therefore became what number of such validating sentinel lymphadenectomies followed by axillary dissections should be required to ensure surgeon proficiency with the procedure.[234,293,294] Recommendations in general were that a volume in excess of 20 procedures and a rate of failure for identifying the sentinel nodes of less than 5% appeared appropriate.[295] Institutional experience and volume, and the level of expertise of those instructing others, would affect the appropriate number for a surgeon in a specific center. As the procedure continues to be adopted and taught in residency training and fellowship programs and as experience builds, specific issues in credentialing will be addressed.[296,297] As experience broadens, however, it may be inappropriate to ask patients to have completion axillary dissections for the purpose of developing surgeon proficiency with a technique that is being done largely to avoid axillary dissections.

Is internal mammary sentinel lymphadenectomy indicated?

Sentinel node identification has led to a reconsideration of the role of internal mammary node excision in the treatment of breast cancer. Isolated internal mammary nodal metastases in the absence of axillary nodal involvement have been seen in 5% to 10% of patients for whom both axillary dissection and internal mammary node dissection have been performed.[298–300] Isolated internal mammary nodal metastases carry the same prognostic implications as isolated axillary nodal metastases.[301,302] If the identification of such metastases would alter therapeutic management, then the determination by lymphoscintigraphy of those few patients with internal mammary drainage patterns, and sentinel lymphadenectomy of those nodes, would be justified. The presence of both internal mammary and axillary drainage has significant adverse prognostic significance, but because most patients with internal mammary drainage also have axillary drainage, an effort to map internal mammary sentinel nodes has the potential to benefit only a small number of patients.[303] An added concern is the technical limitation of mapping the nodes from medial lesions; this limitation is created by the proximity of radioisotope as well as blue dye at the primary site, both techniques obscuring the potential for isolating the site of sentinel node drainage. Incisions overlying the medial upper intercostal spaces may lead to visible scars, which may become hyperplastic near a midline location, a further consideration when weighing the possible benefits and risks of internal mammary sentinel lymphadenectomy.

Two recent studies on nonaxillary sentinel lymph node biopsy, including internal mammary sentinel nodes, indicated success rates for identifying internal mammary sentinel nodes of 63%[304] and 80%.[305] Isolated internal mammary metastases were detected in 7.3% and 3.1%[305] of patients. A study from Milan of sentinel lymphadenectomy for inner quadrant lesions with lymphoscintigraphic evidence of drainage to the internal mammary nodes found 12 (10%) with metastases in the internal mammary sentinel nodes. All patients had axillary dissections as well, of whom 18% (8 of 45) had axillary metastases and 5% (4 of 77) did not, the internal mammary sentinel node being the only nodal metastasis.[306] Ongoing studies may provide reproducible guidelines, but the issue of internal mammary sentinel lymphadenectomy remains unresolved until its therapeutic impact can be more clearly determined. Certainly, the capability of assessing internal mammary nodes, with far less morbidity than was previously the case in the era of extended radical mastectomy, despite the reservations noted, invites a reconsideration of potential benefits.

Is sentinel lymphadenectomy ever indicated for ductal carcinoma in situ?

Theoretically, DCIS does not metastasize, and therefore there is no rationale for any axillary surgery, regardless of how limited. However, sentinel lymph node biopsy for DCIS in four studies had a reported incidence of metastases of 3% to 13%.[307–310] These unexpected incidences highlight the paradoxical limitations of histologically designating all DCIS as categorically noninvasive, particularly when such designation is based on core biopsy or incisional surgical biopsy specimens. In view of the biologic heterogeneity of DCIS, it would appear reasonable to consider sentinel node biopsy in those patients with extensive high-grade DCIS, particularly when there is associated radiographic or clinical suggestion of a mass lesion in association with the DCIS, as well as in patients with extensive disease often necessitating mastectomy. In other instances, breast conservation does not preclude performing sentinel lymphadenectomy as a staged procedure if histologic assessment demonstrates unexpected invasion. Most sentinel nodal metastases in patients with DCIS have been detected by immunohistochemical staining alone.[309,310] With the increasing use of immunohistochemical staining of sentinel lymph nodes has come uncertainty about the biologic and prognostic significance of micrometastases detected by this technique, a group that may be expanded by routine sentinel lymphadenectomy for all DCIS.

What are the contraindications to sentinel lymphadenectomy?

Any attempt to establish restraints on the performance of sentinel lymphadenectomy runs the risk of being quickly refuted by newer data in this rapidly evolving area of investigation. Certainly, patients with palpable axillary disease or patients discovered at the time of surgery to have a palpable nonsentinel node are not candidates for initiating or continuing the procedure, respectively. Patients with T3 lesions (>5 cm) are not appropriate candidates, although it has been suggested that those whose cancers have been downstaged by neoadjuvant systemic therapy may be candidates.[311] Patients with multifocal and multicentric disease, previously considered not to be candidates for sentinel lymphadenectomy, are being reevaluated in this regard. Tousimis and associates reported no difference in the accuracy, sensitivity, or false-negative rate in sentinel lymph node biopsy for 70 patients having multifocal or multicentric breast cancer compared with literature validation studies of sentinel lymphadenectomy, most patients in those studies having single-site invasive breast cancer.[312,313] This experience supported previous observations that regardless of location, tumors drain through afferent lymphatic channels to a common axillary sentinel lymph node.[314,315] Whether the presently held belief that radiation to the breast or prior breast or axillary surgery is a contraindication to sentinel lymphadenectomy will be altered based on evolving experience remains to be seen.

When is axillary lymph node dissection appropriate?

Clearly, the introduction of sentinel lymphadenectomy has challenged the popular adherence to performing an axillary dissection as an essential component of the surgical treatment for most invasive carcinomas of the breast. Despite the caution that has been expressed against adopting sentinel lymphadenectomy as a standard of care until the technique and its impact on patient outcome have been validated in prospective trials as well as by individual surgeons and institutions critically assessing both their surgical and histopathological techniques, the trend is unquestionably toward abandoning elective axillary dissection in favor of sentinel lymph node biopsy.[316] In this regard, an ongoing randomized phase III clinical trial by the NSABP (Protocol B-32) assigns patients to sentinel lymphadenectomy with axillary dissection, or to sentinel lymphadenectomy alone if there is no evidence of metastases by intraoperative imprint cytology or permanent H&E-stained sections. If metastases are found in the sentinel nodes in the latter group, an axillary dissection is performed.[317] At the present time, for patients with metastases in the sentinel nodes, patients with clinically evident axillary metastases, patients with grossly apparent axillary metastases intraoperatively that may fail to absorb dye or radioisotope, selected patients with a very high risk for harboring axillary micrometastases, and those for whom sentinel lymphadenectomy would not be appropriate, axillary dissection remains a relevant component of primary surgery.

How is axillary dissection defined?

Axillary dissection for breast cancer was originally described as an integral part of radical mastectomy and remained an essential component of the various subsequent modifications of the radical mastectomy that preserved the pectoralis major muscle.[318,319] In that context, axillary dissection connoted a complete resection of the lymph nodes in the axilla at all three levels. Efforts were made as well to include all external mammary lymph nodes extending from the medial border of the axilla along the chest wall from the second to sixth ribs. When the pectoralis major was preserved, dissection of the level III apical nodes could be facilitated by transecting the attachment of the pectoralis minor muscle to the coracoid process. As described by one of the authors, dividing the sternal portion of the pectoralis major could further facilitate axillary exposure and dissection, following which the muscle would be reconstructed.[320]

When an axillary dissection is performed in conjunction with a breast-conserving procedure, the extent of dissection has often been modified. Data on elective axillary dissection for breast cancer suggest that in the absence of palpable or suspicious adenopathy encountered intraoperatively, axillary dissection most appropriately incorporates level I and II nodes because the incidence of micrometastases in level III in the absence of micrometastases in level I or II is less than 1%.[321,322] Metastasis to level II nodes is more frequent. Although the incidence of isolated metastasis to level II was still less than 2% in the series of Veronesi and associates[321,322] and Rosen and associates,[323] the incidence of "skip" metastases did exceed 20% in the reports of Pigott and associates[324] and of Danforth and colleagues.[325] Level I and II dissection now represents the anatomic extent of axillary dissection in most reports. Certainly, the inclusion of the lymph nodes beneath the pectoralis minor muscle is easily accomplished and would appear advisable based on these studies. In Giuliano's original sentinel lymph node description, 27% of sentinel nodes were in level II with or without a sentinel node in level I.[22]

The introduction of adjuvant systemic therapy heightened the importance of axillary nodes as a predictor of recurrence, even while the therapeutic role of axillary dissection was being questioned. Proposals that axillary "sampling" might provide the same prognostic information as a more complete axillary dissection, with less morbidity, failed to gain acceptance and were completely retired with the accurate identification and excision of intraoperatively mapped and dyed or radioisotopically labeled sentinel lymph nodes. The random sampling of lateral nodes without such efforts at precise delineation of the draining nodes from the specific site of the primary cancer has been associated with significant rates of axillary recurrence exceeding 10%, the recurrence rate being inversely related to the number of nodes sampled.[136] When axillary dissection is performed, it should be performed as a formal anatomic procedure to include nodes within defined boundaries. This further enables the accurate identification and preservation of related neurologic structures, injury to which could be a source of morbidity.

Despite refinements in indications for axillary dissection, the major issue of controversy remains the uncertainty of its therapeutic impact on survival. Recent attempts to refine the indications for axillary dissection have focused on whether the procedure is indicated (1) when the risk for additional micrometastases is low following a sentinel node biopsy and (2) when the results of axillary dissection are not likely to alter subsequent adjuvant therapy, particularly in postmenopausal patients.[326–328] Refinement of indications has been particularly important with more widespread adoption of breast-conserving procedures, whereby an axillary dissection for a sentinel micrometastasis is most often an additional surgical procedure, in contradistinction to when it is performed en bloc with a mastectomy, or when an axillary dissection following mastectomy, sentinel lymphadenectomy, and reconstruction can pose additional technical challenges. The adoption of induction systemic therapy for more locally advanced breast cancers and its application to trials of stage II and even stage I disease may significantly alter even the prognostic value of axillary staging.

Should an axillary dissection be performed at the same time as a segmental excision?

When a patient has a clearly defined lesion diagnosed as invasive cancer by needle biopsy and a demonstrable metastasis in the sentinel node or nodes at surgery, it is appropriate to perform an axillary dissection at the same time as segmental excision. When a metastasis is not demonstrable, and when a more diffuse malignant pattern not appreciated clinically or mammographically is demonstrated histologically in the segmental excision specimen, necessitating either re-excision or, in some cases, a recommendation for mastectomy, axillary dissection is obviously dependent on final sentinel node histopathology. An advantage of sentinel lymphadenectomy is that it allows better technical planning of mastectomy and axillary dissection if they are required. Furthermore, the issue of immediate reconstruction can also be more optimally approached with the knowledge that an axillary dissection will or will not be performed.

A common problematic patient in this regard is the woman with a palpable mass but ill-defined carcinoma in a fibro-nodular breast in which clear mammographic, sonographic, or even MRI assessment of the extent of the cancer may be compromised by the density and nodularity of surrounding breast parenchyma. Such ill-defined lesions in the patient desirous of breast conservation are best assessed by a staged procedure—performing the segmental excision and sentinel lymphadenectomy and then awaiting full histopathologic evaluation. If a more extensive infiltrative or intraductal component is found that could not be appreciated by palpation or radiographic evaluation, and the axilla is accurately staged by histologic study of the sentinel node, the issue of mastectomy can be more objectively discussed with the patient, as can immediate reconstruction. If the lesion has been histologically confirmed to be encompassed by appropriate tumor-free margins, breast conservation can be accepted with greater confidence. Sentinel lymphadenectomy provides accurate information on the appropriateness of a subsequent axillary dissection.

What is the appropriate incision for an axillary dissection?

An axillary dissection is best performed through a curvilinear incision that follows a natural skin crease placed below the hair-bearing area of the axilla. When it follows sentinel lymphadenectomy, it can encompass that incision with a skin ellipse. The medial extent of the incision is kept below the edge of the pectoralis major. Posteriorly, the incision extends to the posterior axillary line, although it can be extended more posteriorly to allow additional traction on the skin for better exposure of the axilla. Extending the incision posteriorly is preferable to extending the incision medially over the edge of the pectoralis major. The sentinel lymphadenectomy incision is best planned with a view to the possibility of extending it into a full axillary dissection incision.

For most lesions in the upper outer quadrant, it is aesthetically preferable to use a separate axillary dissection incision (Fig. 24–20). A second incision in the axilla is less likely to create a visible scar and defect than when an attempt is made to perform the segmental excision and sentinel lymphadenectomy and possible axillary dissection en bloc through a single

incision. An exception is a lesion high in the tail of the breast, where the incision used to perform the segmental excision through a natural skin crease below the hair-bearing area of the axilla would be directly contiguous with a sentinel lymphadenectomy and possible subsequent axillary dissection incision.

How is the patient positioned?

The patient is positioned with the posterior axillary line at the edge of the table. The breast and axilla are prepared and draped with the arm free and out on an armboard at a right angle to the patient. It is not necessary to place a pad beneath the shoulder to assist in exposure of the axilla. With slight rotation of the table toward the contralateral side and with the patient in the reverse Trendelenburg position, the axilla can be well positioned for dissection, with less posterior stretch on the shoulder girdle than if a pad were used to project the axilla anteriorly. Similarly, one should not position the arm superiorly at an oblique angle because unnecessary traction in that direction, particularly if done rapidly or for an extended period of time, may stretch the brachial plexus. As already discussed, undue traction on the arm, which may stretch the brachial plexus, may create a brachial plexitis with its attendant neurologic symptoms and even paralysis.[329] Prepared and draped, the arm free it can be gently positioned in a medially abducted direction, thereby facilitating retraction on the pectoralis major and minor muscles to enhance exposure of the medial axillary contents (Fig. 24–21).

What is the technique of axillary lymph node dissection?

The incision is outlined, and skin and subcutaneous tissue are transected with a thin ellipse encompassing the sentinel lymphadenectomy incision if this has been performed. Flaps are raised beneath the subcutaneous layer medially to the edge of

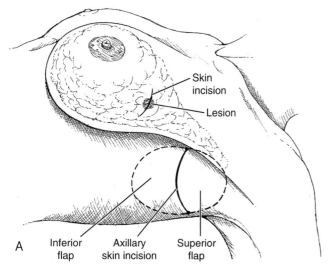
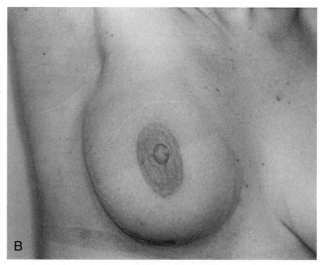

Figure 24–20   *A* and *B*, Separate incisions for segmental excision and axillary dissection for a lesion in the upper outer quadrant of the breast. In most instances, it is an extension of the sentinel lymphadenectomy incision following detection of sentinel node metastases.

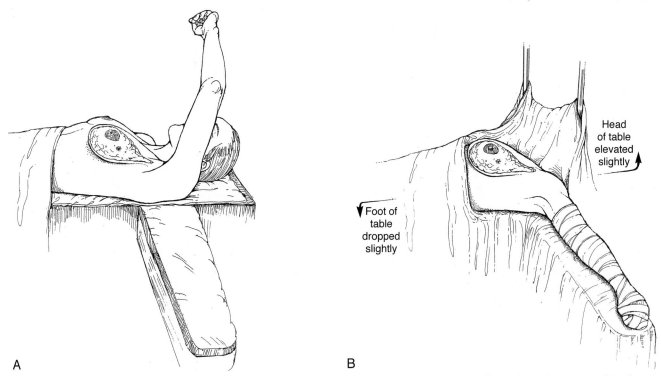

Figure 24–21   *A* and *B*, The breast and axilla are prepared and draped with the arm free and at a right angle to the patient. This allows arm mobility during the procedure, which facilitates exposure of the axillary contents.

the pectoralis major, superiorly to its tendinous insertion, inferiorly to the level of the sixth rib (to incorporate the external mammary nodes), and posteriorly to the edge of the latissimus dorsi, which is directly at the posterior limit of the skin incision. In an obese patient, the edge of the latissimus dorsi may be elusive at first, but unnecessary posterior dissection through the fat in an attempt at its identification should be avoided because this may be an additional source of seroma formation postoperatively. Clear definition of the edge of the latissimus dorsi, particularly at its tendinous insertion superiorly, ensures inclusion of the most lateral nodes in the lateral axillary group in the dissection specimen. Occasionally, a muscular band is encountered traversing the axillary vein, arching from the latissimus dorsi to the insertion of the pectoralis major. Dividing this muscular arch enables identification of the edge of the latissimus dorsi superiorly. In elevating the flaps, traction is placed superiorly and inferiorly with the use of sharp rake retractors. When the flaps are elevated, a self-retaining retractor may then be used to maintain exposure along this axis (Fig. 24–22).

After skin flaps have been elevated and the margins of the dissection have been defined, the thin fascial layer overlying the lateral pectoralis major muscle fibers is dissected laterally while the pectoralis major is easily retracted medially. With medial traction on the pectoralis major, the lateral edge of the pectoralis minor is defined. The medial pectoral nerve branches and vessels are preserved while the clavipectoral fascia contiguous with the pectoralis minor fascia is opened parallel to the lateral edge of the muscle. The clavipectoral fascia is further incised from the upper edge of the pectoralis minor proceeding laterally, thereby exposing the lymphoadipose

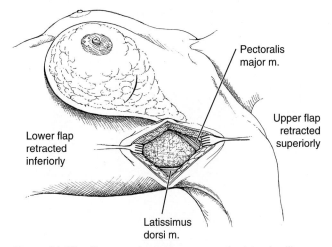

Figure 24–22   Flaps are elevated to expose the lateral axilla.

contents of the axilla (Fig. 24–23). With a right-angle retractor providing traction superiorly and medially on the upper portion of the pectoral muscles, and with gentle traction inferiorly on the lymphoadipose tissue, the axillary vein is identified. A plane of dissection is frequently easy to identify just above the axillary fat as it wraps itself just superior to the axillary vein, and this is divided. An exerted effort to dissect all of the soft tissue off the brachial plexus and the adventitia of the axillary vein is inappropriate. Although Rotter's nodes may be dissected free, care should be taken to protect the medial pectoral nerve and vascular bundle, which may be seen lateral to

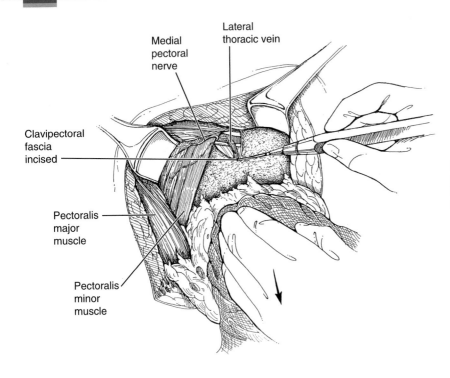

Figure 24–23 labels: Medial pectoral nerve, Lateral thoracic vein, Clavipectoral fascia incised, Pectoralis major muscle, Pectoralis minor muscle

Figure 24–23 Retraction is placed on the pectoral muscles, and the clavipectoral fascia is divided to expose the surgical anatomy of the axilla.

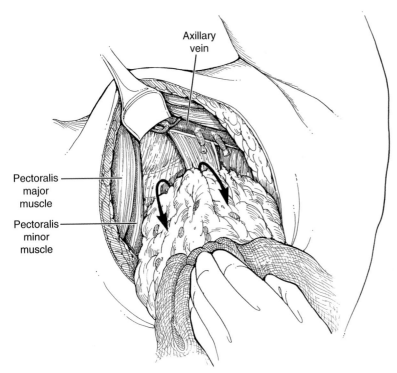

Figure 24–24 labels: Axillary vein, Pectoralis major muscle, Pectoralis minor muscle

Figure 24–24 Axillary dissection proceeds from level II laterally.

the pectoralis minor muscle but in some instances may enter the pectoralis minor before some of its fibers emerge to innervate the lateral pectoralis major muscle. Dividing the fascia lateral to the border of the pectoralis minor enables retraction medially and facilitates the dissection of level II nodes subjacent to the superior extension of the muscle (Fig. 24–24).

When nodes are palpable on preoperative evaluation and confirmed or noted to be enlarged at surgery, particularly if apparent enlargement extends just lateral to or beneath the pectoralis minor, it is appropriate to extend the axillary

dissection to include the nodes at the apex (level III). For this purpose, it may be helpful (although not always necessary) to divide the insertion of the pectoralis minor from the coracoid process after incising the fascia over the coracobrachial muscle. Division of the pectoralis minor will require division of branches of the medial pectoral nerve, but care should be taken to preserve the lateral pectoral nerve and thoracoacromial vessels, which emerge medial to the pectoralis minor (Fig. 24–25). Nevertheless, division or injury of branches of the medial and lateral pectoral nerves is likely when the

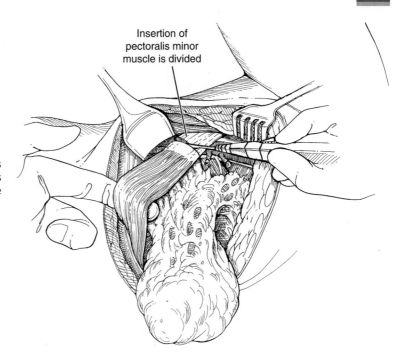

Insertion of
pectoralis minor
muscle is divided

Figure 24-25 When complete axillary dissection is performed, division of the insertion of the pectoralis minor from the coracoid process may facilitate the apical dissection.

interpectoral space is entered by division of the insertion of the pectoralis minor muscle, which in turn may lead to varying degrees of atrophy of the pectoralis major, particularly of its lateral border.[330] Division of the pectoralis minor to achieve a complete axillary dissection should therefore be applied selectively.

To allow clear access to the apex of the axilla, the pectoral branches of the thoracoacromial vessels are sacrificed. In dissecting free the level II or, when indicated, level III nodes, it is appropriate to have an assistant support the forearm in a position directed toward the contralateral side and parallel to the patient. This facilitates retraction of the pectoralis major and exposure of the nodes at this higher level. Although the use of an illuminated right-angle retractor may be of some value, with appropriate proper positioning of the arm, gentle lateral traction on the axillary contents, and medial retraction on the pectoral muscles, this has not been necessary in our experience. Lymphatic dissection then proceeds off the inferior axillary vein, dividing and ligating vascular tributaries as the procedure progresses laterally. All branches of the axillary vein and artery are divided and ligated from the level of the thoracoacromial vessels. Posteriorly directed subscapular vessels are not ligated.

In most instances in which the pectoralis minor is divided from the coracoid process to facilitate exposure of the apical lymph nodes, the thoracoacromial vessels and lateral pectoral nerves are preserved. The highest points in the dissection, either the apical nodes or the level II nodes, are tagged to facilitate orientation and identification by the pathologist. As the dissection proceeds laterally, the inferior axillary contents are dissected off the serratus anterior fascia. The intercostobrachial nerve is identified as it exits the second intercostal space and is preserved whenever possible. Preservation of this nerve is achieved by dissecting it from the surrounding axillary fat as it courses upward and lateral to innervate the axillary skin and medial upper arm. If the intercostobrachial

nerve is transected, paresthesias of the skin of the axillary and medial arm will result, although this may abate with time because of the richness of sensory innervation of the axilla and upper arm, as previously described.[331] Preservation of the intercostobrachial nerve or its superior fibers when it is arborized is clearly desirable, as has been well recognized,[332] but when it is sacrificed, sensation may be expected to return or improve in most patients. Clearly, temporary paresthesias in the early postoperative period may occur even with preservation, but sensation in such instances will more predictably return.[333] Certainly, the thoroughness of the lateral axillary dissection when grossly involved nodes are encountered should not be compromised by a compulsive effort to preserve anatomically the intercostobrachial nerve despite the desirability of keeping sensory innervation intact.

As the dissection moves to the junction of the serratus anterior and subscapularis muscles, the lateral intercostal perforating vessels and nerves are divided and ligated. The lymphoadipose tissue is continually retracted and swept laterally off the serratus anterior fascia. The fascia of the serratus anterior may coalesce in a line that may be mistaken for the long thoracic nerve. A gentle incision in the filmy adventitia about 1 to 2 cm lateral and parallel to the chest wall will facilitate clear visualization of the nerve throughout its course over the lateral chest to the fourth or fifth intercostal space. With lateral traction applied to the axillary contents that have already been freed, and after a sharp incision lateral to the long thoracic nerve throughout its visible length, the nerve is gently reflected and returned medially to its position along the chest wall, further securing its safe preservation (Fig. 24-26).

After the incision in the filmy adventitia overlying the axillary contents and the identification, gentle medial retraction, and preservation of the long thoracic nerve, another incision is made paralleling the chest wall into the thin subscapularis fascia. With the arm elevated slightly and with gentle traction exerted medially on the dissected axillary contents, the

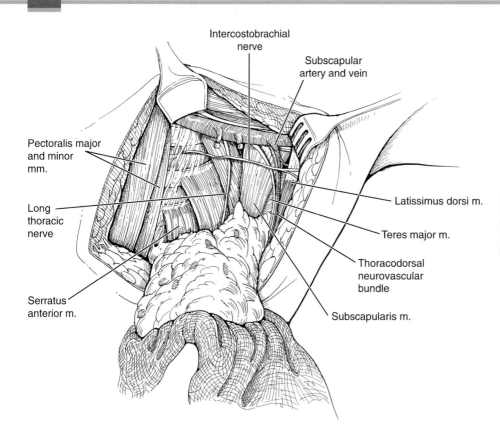

Figure 24–26 Dissection proceeds laterally to preserve the long thoracic nerve, while the intercosto-brachial nerve is preserved whenever possible throughout its length.

thoracodorsal nerve and vessels are easily identified. The arm is then again placed downward at a right angle to the patient, and by following the plane established by incision into the filmy subscapularis fascia and gentle traction laterally, the thoracodorsal nerve and vessels can be easily preserved and the axillary contents further dissected lateral to these structures. Adherence of grossly involved lateral axillary nodes to the thoracodorsal bundle may, in rare instances, necessitate its sacrifice with minimal discernible consequence.

Dissection is then completed to the edge of the latissimus dorsi and the lateral extent of the axillary vein where the specimen is transected (Fig. 24–27). Tagging the lateral margin of the axillary dissection further orients the specimen for the pathologist. The wound is irrigated with saline solution, and meticulous hemostasis is ensured.

Should the axilla be drained?

Controversy exists over the advisability of drainage following an axillary dissection. The hollow that exists after removal of the lymphoadipose contents, as well as the movements of the chest wall during respiration and of the arm, make the accumulation of serum, lymph, and inflammatory exudate inevitable. Although such fluid accumulation requiring aspiration is basically a source of annoyance without lasting sequelae, it may lead to secondary infection and a delay in initiating adjuvant therapy. Arm immobilization, flap-tacking sutures, and even bovine spray thrombin have been proposed to minimize this complication.[334] Closed-suction drainage, however, has been the mainstay of efforts to minimize this problem. Drainage is advisable not only to lessen fluid accumulation but also to provide appropriate negative pressure that allows the overlying skin to adhere to the newly formed hollow of the axilla. It has been noted that seromas requiring at least a single aspiration occur in about 30% of patients with drains left in place until the drainage has decreased to minimal levels (20 mL/day).[335] However, drainage exceeding 100 mL/day is common in the first 2 to 3 days after axillary dissection. Continued drainage of the axilla until the volume decreases to less than 20 mL/day, common by postoperative day 5, would seem judicious and certainly is easily managed on an ambulatory basis. A closed-suction or drainage system using a single-limb Jackson-Pratt drain or a double-limb Hemovac system brought out through separate stab wounds beneath the lower flap and secured to the skin is advisable, the drains being very gently held away from the neurovascular structures with loosely tied absorbable sutures placed in a site in the serratus anterior muscle. A subcutaneous closure of 2-0 or 3-0 absorbable sutures, followed by a subcuticular closure and the application of Steri-Strips to the skin, is then completed (Fig. 24–28). Efforts to minimize drainage and decrease the length of time closed-suction drainage is required have focused on the use of fibrin sealants, but concerns regarding cost, viral safety, and the need for closed-suction drainage despite their use have limited their widespread adoption despite favorable reductions in days to drain removal and fluid drainage in a prospective randomized trial.[336]

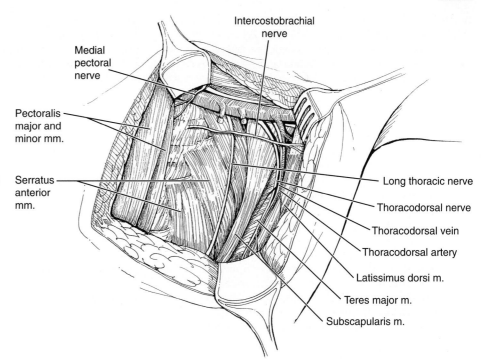

Figure 24–27 Completion of the axillary dissection.

Labels on figure:
Intercostobrachial nerve
Medial pectoral nerve
Pectoralis major and minor mm.
Serratus anterior mm.
Long thoracic nerve
Thoracodorsal nerve
Thoracodorsal vein
Thoracodorsal artery
Latissimus dorsi m.
Teres major m.
Subscapularis m.

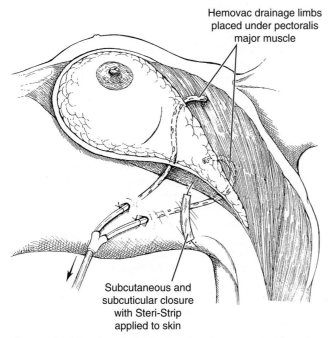

Labels on figure:
Hemovac drainage limbs placed under pectoralis major muscle
Subcutaneous and subcuticular closure with Steri-Strip applied to skin

Figure 24–28 The incision is closed over closed-suction drainage.

Is physical therapy required after axillary dissection?

Normal shoulder mobility is preserved when an axillary dissection is performed with the appropriate care to protect the neuromuscular structures as previously outlined. Shoulder immobilization has been advised to decrease postoperative seroma formation after axillary dissection, although the duration of such limitation of movement has not been defined.[337]

Certainly, vigorous physical therapy would seem inappropriate following an axillary dissection that anatomically preserves neuromuscular function. If closed-suction drainage is employed, modest mobility of the arm is advisable to minimize stiffness and the risk for a frozen shoulder if immobility is prolonged. On the first postoperative day, the patient is encouraged to elevate the arm so that the head can be touched. This allows any inhibition in mobilizing the arm to be overcome and reassures the patient that normal range of motion is intact. Vigorous arm motion is discouraged while closed-suction drainage is in place. When it is clear that adherence of the skin to the base of the underlying axillary hollow is ensured and that seroma formation is not occurring, the patient is encouraged to increase the use of the arm with full range-of-motion activity. Some serous accumulation may result, which is easily managed by simple aspirations until the space seals and fluid no longer collects. Particularly with older patients, prolonged arm immobilization, which may lead to a frozen shoulder that in turn requires physical therapy, should be discouraged. These guidelines are also appropriate after mastectomy, as will be discussed.

MANAGEMENT OF LOCAL AND REGIONAL RECURRENCE AFTER BREAST-CONSERVING SURGERY

Cancer recurrence after excision and radiation therapy is dependent on many variables, which include most significantly the extent of the initial surgery and margin status but also the adequacy of radiation dosage and the technique and timing of radiation; histopathologic characteristics and architectural pattern, including the extent of intraductal disease when an invasive cancer is being treated or the grade of histopathology when an exclusively intraductal cancer is being treated; lymphatic vessel invasion; and clinical factors such as age and even family history and *BRCA1* or *BRCA2* mutations. The potential role of molecular biologic markers as a predictor of risk for local recurrence remains to be defined. A recurrence near the original excision site, a brief time to recurrence, and an identical histologic pattern would suggest that it evolved from residual disease. As discussed in Chapter 26, 70% to 80% of the recurrences seen within 10 years of treatment are adjacent to or in the same quadrant as the original excision, which has prompted the application of boost doses of radiation to the site of tumor excision in selected instances.[338,339] The longer the time to recurrence, the greater the chance that the recurrence will be noted in another quadrant, although even with more prolonged disease-free intervals, most recurrences are in the vicinity of the initial excision. Whether the recurrence is viewed as the progression of residual disease or as a new primary lesion, reported incidences at 5 years double by 10 years.[340,341] In a review from the National Cancer Institute in Milan of 2233 women treated by breast-conserving therapy (quadrantectomy, axillary dissection, and radiotherapy), local failures occurred at a rate of about 1% per year for the first decade after treatment,[342] an incidence not dissimilar to the risk for contralateral breast cancer.[343] It might be expected that with the appropriate selection of patients for breast conservation based on reported experiences to date, as well as the application of surgery that optimizes tumor-free margins and improvements in radiation technique, the incidence of recurrence in the breast would decrease in future series. Whether breast cancer recurrence leads to decreased survival remains unanswered. Meric and colleagues, in a retrospective review of more than 1000 patients, identified positive surgical margins and breast cancer recurrence as independent variables of poor disease-specific survival.[95] Such an analysis, however, does not necessarily implicate breast cancer recurrence as the initiator of distant relapse.

Until the biologic significance of breast cancer recurrence is elucidated, efforts at optimal local treatment remain essential. It must be appreciated as well that effective surgery and radiotherapy do not eliminate the risk for a new cancer developing in the treated breast, and therefore continued surveillance of both the treated and the untreated opposite breast remains essential.

What is the treatment of recurrence after breast-conservation therapy?

Patients with a recurrence after breast-conservation therapy should be evaluated for concurrent distant metastases, which will be detected in about 10% of patients.[330,344,345] For the remaining 90% of patients, the issue will be whether breast conservation is still possible or whether mastectomy is mandatory. Clearly, evidence of inadequate initial surgery or radiotherapy in a patient who develops mammographically detected intraductal carcinoma adjacent to the site of initial surgery suggests that an additional attempt at breast conservation may be warranted. Kurtz and associates[346] reported on a selected group of patients treated by wide excision following ipsilateral breast recurrence. Patients were divided into those treated for recurrence before or after the first 5 years of initial treatment; the authors noted subsequent ipsilateral failure rates of 36% and 22%, respectively. Further, a breast failure

rate of 50% occurred in 14 patients reported by Dalberg and associates following wide excision for breast recurrences.[347] Until specific criteria are developed for selecting patients for whom continued breast conservation might be appropriate, these experiences warrant the continued recommendation of mastectomy as the procedure of choice for ipsilateral recurrence following breast-conserving surgery and radiation. Locoregional control rates of 85% at 5 years and disease-free survival rates exceeding 40% at 5 years have been reported.[348,349] Certainly, the recommendation for mastectomy is particularly compelling for patients whose initial surgery and radiation therapy were performed with techniques and precautions directed toward achieving maximal local disease control, for those whose recurrence is at a site in the breast clearly separate from the initial excision, for those whose initial treatment surgically encompassed a significant segment of breast, and for those whose recurrence demonstrates lymphatic permeation or a prominent intraductal component.

The local and regional recurrence rates reported after mastectomy following recurrence in the irradiated breast are, in most series, less than 10%.[330,335,337,339,350] Reconstruction in this setting should not be discouraged in most instances. Because irradiated tissue is less malleable and less likely to withstand the potential ischemia of tissue expansion and implant placement, autologous tissue transfer techniques are more appropriate, as discussed in Chapter 25.[351] The surgical management of the axilla is obviously dependent on whether a sentinel lymphadenectomy or axillary dissection was performed initially and also on the pathologic findings of the recurrent cancer. If the recurrence is an invasive lesion and the axilla was not previously dissected, a level I and II dissection is performed with the mastectomy, reserving a complete dissection to level III for patients with palpable or intraoperatively detected axillary metastases. Sentinel lymphadenectomy may be appropriate in the absence of clinical axillary metastases, but the impact of prior surgery and radiotherapy may preclude this technique. Certainly, the appropriateness of sentinel lymphadenectomy in this setting remains to be determined.

Survival rates following mastectomy for recurrence have been reported to be comparable to those following mastectomy for primary lesions. In the largest reported series of Kurtz and associates,[340] the 5-year survival rate was 69%, with a survival rate of 84% if the recurrence was more than 5 years after initial treatment, decreasing to 48% if the recurrence was within the first 2 years of initial treatment. Prognostic and adjuvant therapeutic considerations are being evaluated but are likely the same as with mastectomy for a primary carcinoma. The phrase "salvage mastectomy" in this setting may therefore inappropriately connote a situation of desperation that may not be justified.

What other malignant lesions can occur after breast-conservation and radiation therapy?

Angiosarcoma of the breast has been reported following breast-conserving surgery and radiation therapy. Lymphedema of the conserved breast has been implicated as a contributing cause.[352–354] A latency period of 4 to 7 years from primary therapy to presentation has been reported.[355–361] The patient may be noted to have a bluish or purple plaquelike eruption or nodules with surrounding erythema (Fig. 24–29),

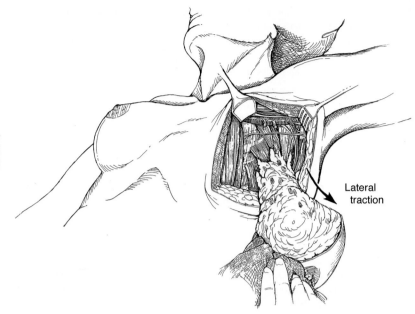

Figure 24–32 Total mastectomy and axillary dissection. The pectoral muscles are reflected medially, the clavipectoral fascia is incised, and the axillary contents are exposed.

Lateral traction

is as described for axillary dissection, and the highest level, be it level II or level III, is tagged to orient the specimen for the pathologist. The axillary contents are then dissected free from the chest wall, proceeding laterally. The intercostobrachial nerve is preserved whenever possible, and the long thoracic nerve as well as the thoracodorsal nerves and vessels are identified and preserved (Fig. 24–33). The thoracodorsal bundle is essential if a latissimus dorsi flap reconstruction is planned; thus, its preservation is particularly important if this option is selected or if it might be used in the future. The lateral margin of the axillary dissection is also tagged for orientation of the specimen by the pathologist.

After removal of the specimen and thorough irrigation of the wound, reconstruction is commenced, as discussed in Chapter 25. If immediate reconstruction is not planned, Hemovac catheters are placed through separate stab wounds at the lower margin of the inferior flap, and the lateral limb is guided to the axilla and carefully secured beneath the pectoralis major muscle and away from neurovascular structures with a carefully placed and loosely tied absorbable suture. The medial limb is similarly guided and secured over the pectoralis major. Tacking sutures may be placed, as discussed for total mastectomy, to minimize seroma formation, and the skin is closed, as also described for a total mastectomy.

The management of drains and the advisability of arm mobility are the same as discussed for axillary dissection. Concomitant reconstruction may alter the recommendations, as also discussed in Chapter 25.

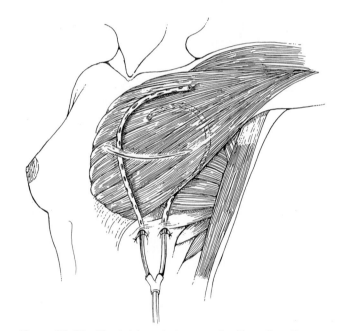

Figure 24–33 The total mastectomy and axillary dissection are completed.

RADICAL MASTECTOMY

Is a radical mastectomy ever indicated for operable breast cancer?

The performance of a radical mastectomy for operable cancer of the breast is rarely indicated. The 25-year follow-up of the NSABP (Protocol B-04) comparing radical mastectomy, total mastectomy without axillary dissection but with postoperative radiation, and total mastectomy with axillary dissection only if nodes became positive demonstrated no advantage over radical mastectomy.[74] Likewise, the 20-year follow-up of the World Health Organization study comparing radical mastectomy with breast-conserving therapy for patients with tumors 2 cm or smaller showed no advantage to radical mastectomy.[375] These reports have sealed the fate of radical mastectomy, a procedure that faded following the initial reports of these studies more than 2 decades earlier. In instances in which there is unexpected adherence or infiltration of the pectoralis major muscle by an overlying lesion, resection of this region of the muscle, followed by radiation therapy or resection of the entire sternal portion, if involved, may be performed. Inclusion of both pectoral muscles is reserved for more locally advanced disease refractory to neoadjuvant, systemic, and radiation therapy, but certainly not for earlier-stage breast cancer.

COMPLICATIONS OF MASTECTOMY AND AXILLARY DISSECTION

What are the complications of segmental or total mastectomy?

Complications of segmental or total mastectomy are infection and hemorrhage. Both are rarely encountered, although overly vigorous use of electrocautery to prevent hemorrhage may produce significant fat necrosis that may contribute to infection. Use of antibiotics prophylactically and while drains are in place is appropriate. Attention to flap viability further minimizes the risk for infection. Even with mastectomy, blood loss requiring transfusion should be very rarely required. Attention to drain function following mastectomy promotes flap adherence and prevents the accumulation of blood that may elevate the flap and potentiate further hematoma formation. Bleeding should be rapidly attended not only for hemodynamic reasons but also to prevent the wound complications from nonadherence of flaps, disruption of reconstruction when autologous tissue is used, or fluid accumulation and potential infections when prosthetic reconstructions are performed. Careful attention to a history of coagulopathies, anticoagulation, and the use of aspirin, vitamin E, anti-inflammatory medications, or any herbal use is essential in planning any surgical management.

How common is seroma formation?

Some serous collection is to be expected after mastectomy and axillary dissection. As previously discussed as it relates to axillary dissection, closed-suction drainage is advisable in the first postoperative week to minimize prolonged seroma formation, which, if undrained, would require repeated aspirations and could become secondarily infected. As noted, intraoperative antibiotic coverage, as well as the continued use of antibiotics when drains remain in place, is advisable. Prolonged seroma formation after drain removal is managed by aspiration but may rarely require reinsertion of a closed-suction drain if prolonged or excessive.

The influence of shoulder exercises on seroma formation has been assessed for axillary dissection performed with breast conservation or with total mastectomy. As also discussed, vigorous arm mobilization is not appropriate in the early postoperative period when drains are in place. Delaying shoulder exercises for a week postoperatively has not been associated with arm dysfunction in several studies and may diminish seroma formation.[376–378]

How common is lymphedema?

Lymphedema of the arm of any degree is often a cause of great concern and potential disability to the patient following breast cancer treatment. Despite its nonmalignant cause, even a minimal degree of swelling or a sense of arm heaviness may become a constant physical reminder of the original cancer. Although the initial presentation of lymphedema is often insidious and subtle, it can expand into more obvious and disabling enlargement because increased lymphatic pressure prevents diffusion of lipids and protein while promoting fibrosis and susceptibility to infection in a continued vicious circle of progressive stagnation and swelling. Although certain factors that contribute to lymphedema, including obesity and variations in lymphatic anatomy, are not readily controllable, some aspects of therapy and subsequent management should be appreciated as they relate to this problem.

The retreat from radical mastectomy, as well as the retreat from postoperative radiation therapy following mastectomy, significantly reduced the incidence of the severe lymphedema that was a feared long-term sequela of radical surgery in an earlier era. The risk for lymphedema is attributable to the extent of axillary dissection and the use of postoperative radiotherapy.[379] Although the degree of lymphedema varies in reported series and depends on the specific criteria used, as well as the time from surgery at which patients are assessed for this problem and the extent of the axillary dissection performed, the long-term risk following breast-conserving surgery with complete axillary dissection without axillary radiation was reported by Veronesi and associates[380] to be less than 5%.

Using objective criteria, Lin and associates[381] noted an increase in arm circumference on the operated side compared with the unoperated side in 16% of patients. In a study of 200 patients having a level I and II axillary dissection, 112 of whom had breast conservation and 88 of whom had total mastectomy, Roses and associates evaluated arm swelling 1 year or more after surgery.[333] All patients had arm circumference measurements at the same four sites on both the operated and nonoperated sides. No patient had an axillary recurrence. A difference in arm circumference of more than 2 cm in any of the four sites of the operated compared with the nonoperated side was 13%. Seven patients (3.5%) had mild swelling of the hand. Heavy and obese body habitus were the only significant predictors of edema on multivariate analysis. Other recently reported incidences of lymphedema after axillary dissection demonstrate a wide range, from 5% to 25.5%.[382–388] Meric and associates found an incidence of edema less than 3 cm below the elbow in 13 of 294 (4.5%) patients treated with breast conservation, 260 of whom had axillary dissection.[389] One hundred patients had nodal irradiation, including 10 of the 13 with significant edema. Limiting radiation to the axilla in only selected instances, as discussed in Chapter 26, has contributed to a decreased incidence of this complication.

The extent of axillary dissection with both mastectomy and breast-conserving surgery, not always precisely defined, no doubt influences the frequency of the complication, but the significant and debilitating lymphedema seen in previous eras, when radical mastectomy followed by chest wall irradiation was standard, has diminished. It will certainly diminish markedly as sentinel lymphadenectomy increases.[390] When axillary dissection is performed, long-term attention to minimizing the risk for cellulitis in the arm, which can lead to further inflammation and fibrosis of primary and collateral lymphatic channels, is also important in minimizing the risk for lymphedema. Patient education in this regard is essential, with particular attention to infection prevention, as discussed in more detail in Chapter 39. Physician measurement of arm circumference may also allow prompt identification of patients in whom changes identify the risk for progressive edema and therefore make them worthy of particular attention to minimize further change.[391] Older women may have a particular susceptibility to arm problems following axillary dissection, including swelling, with all of these changes amplified significantly by preexisting arthritis.[392]

How is lymphedema of the arm treated?

Lymphedema is best managed by arm elevation when the patient is in a recumbent position, elastic pressure-graded sleeves for daytime use when the arm is in a dependent position, and weight reduction and control whenever appropriate. Manual massaging to promote dilation of nonobstructed collateral lymphatics may further assist in reducing chronic lymphedema. Compression from the wrist to the upper arm is desirable, with the addition of a gauntlet extension for patients with hand swelling. Proper fitting of a sleeve with appropriate compression is necessary. Compression devices in the evening may be of some value for cases refractory to these initial measures. The use of such sequential-gradient compression devises in chronic situations should be extremely judicious because significant pressures applied for prolonged periods of time may be injurious, further traumatizing lymphatics and promoting the progression of lymphedema. The use of intermittent pneumatic compression has been recommended as an effective means of enhancing decompressive therapy.[393] All compression devices should be used with caution in patients with cardiovascular disease, active infection, or neurologic symptoms in the affected extremity.

Drug therapy, most commonly with diuretics, is of unproven efficacy. Diuretics do not affect the underlying osmotic pressure caused by the protein-rich lymphedema fluid. Casley-Smith and associates[394] have reported on the use of 5,6-benzo-α-pyrone to stimulate macrophage activity to eliminate stagnant proteinaceous material in lymphedema fluid, with mild improvement in a controlled trial. A variety of surgical approaches to managing severe chronic lymphedema, from excising deep fascia to improve lymphatic drainage, to omental transfer to create additional lymphatic drainage channels, to microsurgical lymphovenous anastomoses, to myocutaneous flaps, to liposuction, have failed to achieve reproducible satisfactory outcomes. Clearly, infections of the arm should be treated aggressively with antibiotics and elevation, and continuous, assiduous skin care for the affected arm should be encouraged. Early diagnosis and further efforts to minimize its progression are a major component of treatment of an often refractory and progressive problem.

How common is lymphangiosarcoma with chronic lymphedema?

A rare complication of chronic lymphedema is lymphangiosarcoma, first described in the postmastectomy patient by Stewart and Treves in 1948.[395] Vascular-appearing nodules in the edematous extremity are the hallmark. There is usually a prolonged interval between mastectomy and the development of lymphangiosarcoma, with mean intervals in the 10-year range. Despite vigorous efforts at local therapy, including amputation, reported survivors are rare, with a median survival of less than 2 years.[396]

What is the significance of edema of the breast?

Edema may be noted in the breast of the patient after treatment by breast conservation in conjunction with axillary dissection and radiation. This may be seen in the early posttreatment phase, with erythema of the skin often accompanying the edema. It may be particularly noted in a large pendulous breast with an added component of dependent edema. It may be confused with early recurrence or infection or with inflammatory breast cancer. Resolution is common, but it may take a prolonged period until collateral lymphatic drainage develops.

What are the complications resulting from nerve injury?

The nerves at risk in an axillary dissection, as discussed, are the intercostobrachial nerve, the long thoracic nerve, the thoracodorsal nerve, and the medial and lateral pectoral nerves. Division of the intercostobrachial nerve may create numbness or paresthesias of variable distribution in the upper medial arm and axilla, many of which resolve in the months after surgery on account of the richness of sensory innervation, as detailed earlier. A common complaint is a sense of swelling of the upper medial arm not dissimilar to the sense of swelling noted around the lips or cheek following the local anesthesia of dental procedures. Some element of numbness may persist. In a series of 200 patients previously cited,[333] numbness or paresthesias to the skin of the upper medial arm or axilla from intercostobrachial nerve sacrifice or injury occurred in 76.5% of patients in the initial postoperative period, but with prolonged follow-up, complete resolution was achieved in 22%, and the problems were improved in an additional 59%. This experience is similar to that reported by Salmon and associates.[331] In the study of Paredes and associates,[397] truncal section of the intercostobrachial nerve affected axillary and arm sensitivity in almost all patients when assessed after surgery; axillary anesthesia or analgesia persisted in more than 50% of patients. Most patients had a return of arm sensation after 12 months, 30% having complete return of sensation to both the axilla and arm. With nerve preservation, more than 50% of patients had early anesthesia or analgesia to the axilla and arm, almost all resolving after 12 months. Preservation of the intercostobrachial nerve fibers is therefore to be encouraged, but division of these fibers is not uniformly associated with long-term denervation.

Division of the thoracodorsal nerve is rarely associated with any deficiency noted by the patient, with the exception of a limitation of backward motion of the extended arm. The denervation of the latissimus dorsi, however, eliminates that structure from consideration as a method of reconstruction. As previously discussed, division of the long thoracic nerve creates a winged scapula resulting from denervation of the serratus anterior muscle. Division of branches of the medial pectoral nerve may result in atrophy of the lateral portion of the pectoralis major, whereas division of the lateral pectoral nerve, rarely encountered except if injured in detaching the insertion of the pectoralis minor, will create more significant atrophy of the sternal portion of the pectoralis major muscle.

Patients may experience a phantom breast phenomenon ranging from the perception of the presence of the breast to painful sensations that are not associated with the chest wall. Likewise, chest wall discomfort or itching or pain, often referred to as a tightening or spasmodic episodes of burning, may occasionally be experienced, particularly in the first year after surgery. Although pain after axillary dissection may be difficult to assess in the immediate postoperative period, of 2.5% of patients reporting pain requiring analgesia beyond the immediate postoperative period, none seen in long-term follow-up noted pain requiring analgesia attributable to the axillary dissection.[333] Nevertheless, the impact of axillary dissection may be additive to preexisting arthritis and can adversely affect quality of life.[392]

Are there any postoperative complications specific to mastectomy?

Although significant hemorrhage should be rare after mastectomy, failure to secure appropriate hemostasis of the medially located perforating branches that originate from the internal mammary artery, or the laterally located branches off the thoracodorsal vessels, may be a specific source of postoperative hemorrhage. A rare complication, even more uncommon now that radical mastectomy is rarely performed, is a pneumothorax from puncture of the pleura. This could result from a hemostat's being applied too vigorously when attempting to secure hemostasis on the chest wall, particularly hemostasis of medial perforating vessels from the internal mammary artery, which may retract out of direct vision. Recognition of the possibility of this occurrence in the postoperative patient who develops respiratory distress is obviously essential to a rapid diagnosis and expeditious management with closed-suction pleural drainage. Similarly, attributing sudden significant chest pain to the surgical incision is inappropriate because the discomfort of uneventful surgical procedures on the breast and axilla is usually minimal and clearly different from the pleural pain that may result from a pulmonary embolus.

What is the appropriate length of hospitalization following procedures that include mastectomy or axillary lymph node dissection?

The emphasis on the containment of escalating medical costs has focused attention on the length of hospitalization following surgical procedures for breast cancer, particularly mastectomy or lymph node dissection, with or without breast reconstruction. The medical issue is not whether a short length of hospitalization, often only 1 day or less, can be achieved, but whether this adversely affects patient care. Indeed, it has even been suggested that shortened hospitalization after breast surgery can improve patient care.[398]

The major indication cited for hospitalization in such patients is the management of drainage and pain. Less definable is the issue of emotional security and balancing the psychosocial support that may be facilitated by the hospital setting with the potential enhancement of confidence and sense of self-control that earlier discharge may give the patient. In a study of 208 patients discharged after a median length of stay of 1 day following axillary dissection, 0.6 day following segmental excision and axillary dissection, and 1 day following total mastectomy and axillary dissection, there was no apparent adverse effect resulting from early discharge. A readmission rate of 1.5% and infection rate of 1.5% were reported, but no dissatisfaction was noted from patients, and the authors reported a subjective sense of improved psychological and physical recovery.[376] Clearly, more data are required that address the emotional and physical issues.

Despite efforts to implement shortened length of hospital stay, dissatisfaction with a mandatory policy of early discharge following breast cancer surgery has prompted the passage of legislation by the New York State Assembly and Senate to lengthen the potential length of stay. The 1997 New York State Women's Health and Cancer Rights Act guarantees coverage of inpatient hospital care following mastectomy or segmental excision and axillary dissection for a period of time to be determined medically appropriate by the attending physician in consultation with the patient. The Act also covers reconstructive surgery for all stages of reconstruction.[399] The issue of length of stay is patient dependent and not rigid. Clearly, segmental excision and sentinel lymphadenectomy may be appropriately managed on an outpatient basis, but even in such instances, completion of an axillary dissection for operatively detected sentinel nodal metastases requires flexibility as to the need for limited hospitalization. The issue requires consideration of the age and the medical and psychological condition of the patient, which are further affected by the available family and social support, and the patient's geographic access to medical care. More data that address these questions are required before physicians and patients are coerced into a uniform policy of rapid discharge applied to all patients. At the present time, physician advocacy for the patient's physical and emotional needs is the highest priority. Nursing and psychosocial support and education should be instituted preoperatively and in the early postoperative period. This will facilitate the most appropriate and efficient use of the inpatient setting and lead to effective continuity of care as an outpatient. It will ensure that discharge from the hospital is accomplished safely and in the best interests of the patient with full patient and family confidence, rather than being perceived by them as based exclusively on reimbursement considerations.

LOCAL RECURRENCE FOLLOWING MASTECTOMY

How common is local recurrence following mastectomy?

Chest wall recurrences in the skin, subcutaneous fat, or muscles, as well as recurrences in the axilla if an axillary dissection was a component of the original mastectomy, are most appropriately referred to as *local* recurrences. Chest wall recurrences have a reported incidence of 6% following mastectomy.[400] In a recent series of 565 cases of skin-sparing mastectomy and immediate breast reconstruction, a local recurrence rate of 5.5% was reported, with a mean disease-free interval for those patients who experienced recurrence of 19.8 months (range, 2.9 to 61.6 months). In multivariate analysis, tumor grade and the presence of lymphovascular invasion were independent variables predictive of local recurrence.[401]

Recurrences in the supraclavicular or parasternal regions, emanating from nodal metastases beyond the field of initial surgical treatment, are best referred to as *regional*. The American Joint Committee on Cancer has reclassified proven metastases in supraclavicular nodes from distant metastatic disease (stage IV) to locally advanced breast cancer (stage IIIC) to reflect improved survival rates compared with patients with metastatic disease at distant sites.[402]

The frequency of local and regional recurrence for stages I and II breast cancer is clearly related to the stage of the original cancer.[403] The extent of axillary nodal involvement, specifically four or more positive nodes and extranodal extension of tumor, is a significant risk factor for locoregional recurrence.[404] Other biologic characteristics, such as hormone receptor status,[405] high-grade histologic characteristics,[406] and younger age of the patient,[407] as well as the use of adjuvant systemic therapy, are less well defined but may affect the incidence of local recurrence. The type of mastectomy (radical, total mastectomy with axillary dissection) has not been demonstrated to affect local recurrence.[408] Most local and regional recurrences present within the first 5 years after initial treatment, but 10% to 20% appear later.[409,410] The median time to recurrence in a series of 130 patients with chest wall recurrence after mastectomy at the University of Texas M. D. Anderson Cancer Center was 25.5 months.[411] Although recurrences after 10 years from initial treatment are uncommon, there are reports of local recurrences as late as 40 years after initial treatment.[412]

How is local recurrence diagnosed?

Any nodule or nodules presenting in the scar or in the skin, subcutaneous fat, or muscle should be suspected of being a local recurrence. Erythema presenting either focally or as a broad rash, sometimes with induration, should be suspected of representing a local recurrence as well. Supraclavicular or parasternal nodules should likewise be suspected of representing regional recurrences (Fig. 24–34). Although local recurrences are most common in the region of the scar or in the skin flaps, chest wall recurrences in skin or subcutaneous tissues beyond the periphery of initial surgery may occur. The possibility that these represent local recurrences must be appreciated. Not uncommonly, multiple nodules, as well as the synchronous presentation of both local and regional metastases, may be noted.[413]

Skin and subcutaneous nodules, as well as bulkier, deeper, or regional recurrences, can be expeditiously diagnosed by fine-needle aspiration biopsy. Because local and regional recurrences may be associated with synchronous distant metastases or the development of distant metastases at a later date, the assessment of distant metastases is mandatory before

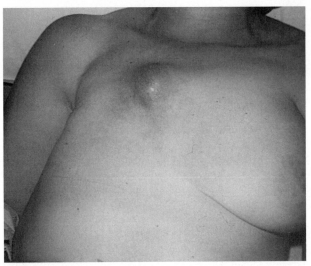

Figure 24–34 Parasternal recurrence in the second intercostal space from internal mammary nodal metastases following mastectomy.

embarking on therapy.[414] A bone scan and computed tomography (CT) scans of the head, chest, abdomen, and pelvis or PET scans are appropriate to establish the diagnosis of any distant disease as well as to provide a baseline for these patients who are at a particularly high risk for future systemic relapse. However, in the previously cited M. D. Anderson Cancer Center experience, of 130 patients with chest wall recurrence following mastectomy, with a median follow-up of 68.5 months after diagnosis of breast cancer and 37.4 months after diagnosis of chest wall recurrence, 51.5% had not developed distant metastases.[411]

How is local recurrence treated?

Local recurrence is best excised whenever possible. This is certainly true for small isolated lesions in the skin flaps, which may be excised with margins of at least 1 cm to achieve tumor-free margins and closed primarily. Prolonged local control may result from local surgery alone.[415] Except for these specific instances of solitary, easily resectable recurrences, particularly when they present after prolonged disease-free intervals from initial mastectomy, most patients will develop further local recurrence. Persistent, progressive local recurrence can be a source of significant morbidity, with ulceration, bleeding, pain, and extension around the chest wall through the soft tissues (carcinoma en cuirasse) that may restrict normal chest wall expansion. Extensive progression of local recurrence may be resistant to treatment. Therefore, additional local radiotherapy at the time of initial presentation and treatment should be considered. The use of radiotherapy has been associated with significantly improved prolonged survival.[411] Available data suggest that the entire anterior ipsilateral chest wall should be treated because more limited fields are associated with a high rate of progressive local recurrences.[416] The same principles should apply for recurrences in tissues surrounding an autologous breast reconstruction. Radiation following resection can be used, although fibrosis of the soft tissues in the reconstruction can alter the appearance of the reconstructed breast.[417,418]

The supraclavicular region is associated with about a 20% rate of regional recurrence that may progress to infiltrate the brachial plexus with significant motor function sequelae and pain, so that supraclavicular irradiation would seem appropriate. Internal mammary recurrence, however, is uncommon. If an axillary dissection was part of the initial treatment, axillary recurrence should also be uncommon. Furthermore, axillary radiation results in increasing rates of arm lymphedema. Irradiation of the internal mammary nodes and axilla, therefore, is best not included in treatment fields unless there is specific clinical or radiographic suspicion of recurrence at these sites. For bulky fixed disease, efforts at chemotherapy and radiotherapy may be successful, but failure to achieve a complete response may require chest wall resections, which are best closed by autologous myocutaneous flaps[419–424] (Fig. 24–35). Toi and associates[425] reported on 15 patients with full chest wall resections supported by perioperative and postoperative systemic treatment. Thirteen patients underwent combined resection of the sternum with defects ranging in size from 30 to 200 cm². Reconstruction was by transverse rectus abdominis myocutaneous flaps in 14 cases and by a latissimus dorsi myocutaneous flap in 1 case. In 4 cases, the chest wall was reinforced by Marlex mesh. The reported 5-year survival rate was 47.1%, with two patients surviving longer than 5 years without distant metastases. Three patients developed local recurrence, all having had microscopically positive margins, one responding to radiation therapy and surviving more than 5 years.

Is there a role for systemic therapy in the treatment of local or regional recurrence?

Available data demonstrate that systemic therapy improves 5-year survival for patients whose disease-free interval from mastectomy to recurrence exceeds 2 years; for those who had stage I disease compared with stage II at initial treatment; and for those with a single resectable site of recurrence compared with multiple sites or bulky or unresectable recurrent disease.[426] Nevertheless, most patients die from metastatic disease by 10 years. In a series from the Joint Center for Radiation Therapy, the 10-year survival rate for patients treated with radiation for locoregional recurrence after mastectomy was 36% if the recurrence had developed more than 2 years after mastectomy, and 7% if recurrence happened less than 2 years after mastectomy.[427] In a review of 69 patients from the M. D. Anderson Cancer Center having a locoregional relapse as their first evidence of recurrence following mastectomy and adjuvant chemotherapy, 19 (27.5%) were alive and free of disease at a median follow-up of 6.6 years. The two factors that significantly affected survival were whether recurrence was during or after adjuvant therapy, and whether the patient was

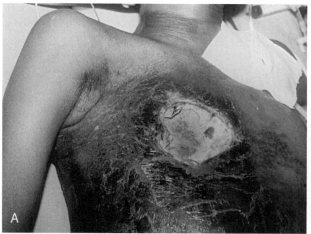

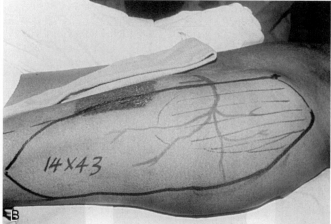

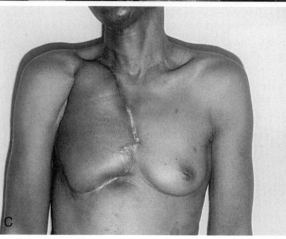

Figure 24–35 *A*, Patient with ulceration following chest wall radiation for bulky recurrence following mastectomy. *B*, A musculocutaneous free flap from the lateral thigh, incorporating portions of the rectus femoris, vastus lateralis, and tensor fasciae latae based on the lateral femoral circumflex artery, was used to reconstruct the defect. *C*, Postoperatively, following successful microvascular anastomosis between the lateral femoral circumflex artery and the right internal mammary artery with the venous anastomosis to the right external jugular vein, which was turned down over the clavicle.

rendered disease free after recurrence.[428] Factors that have also been implicated for improving survival after chest wall recurrence include a prolonged time to recurrence,[429–432] negative nodal status of the original cancer,[411,433,434] and a limited extent of recurrence by size and number of nodules.[435,436]

Although it would seem appropriate to treat patients with systemic therapy following local therapy for locoregional recurrence, there are no prospective controlled data to support this approach.[437,438] Given the dire prognostic implications of locoregional recurrence in patients with short disease-free intervals, particularly while receiving adjuvant systemic therapy, dose-intensive chemotherapy is a consideration for future investigation in such subsets of patients. The impact of antihormonal therapy is likewise unknown, although in the treatment of recurrences that are hormone receptor positive, systemic treatment plans that incorporate antihormonal strategies would seem appropriate. Appropriate molecular assays should obviously be obtained on all excised and resected recurrences. Certainly, prolonged survival for subgroups of patients with chest wall recurrence after mastectomy is achievable and fully justifies aggressive treatment, the foundation of which is complete surgical resection.[411,428–434]

REFERENCES

1. Langman J. Medical Embryology. Baltimore, Williams & Wilkins, 1963, pp 315–316.
2. Poland A. Deficiency of the pectoral muscles. Guys Hosp Rep 1841;6:191–193.
3. Mace JW, Kaplan JM, Schonberger JE, et al. Poland's syndrome: Report of seven cases and review of the literature. Clin Pediatr 1972;11:98–102.
4. Cooper A. The Anatomy and Diseases of the Breast, with Surgical Papers. Philadelphia, Lea & Blanchard, 1845.
5. Langer K. Zur Anatomie and Physiologie der Haut. Über die Spaltbarkeit der Cutis. Sb Akad Wiss Wien 1861;44:19–46.
6. Spence J. Lectures on Surgery. Edinburgh, 1871.
7. Kraissl CJ. The selection of appropriate lines for elective surgical incisions. Plast Reconstr Surg 1951;8:1–28.
8. Batson OV. The function of the vertebral veins and their role in the spread of metastases. Ann Surg 1940;112:138–149.
9. Nathanson SD, Wachna DL, Gilman D, et al. Pathways of lymphatic drainage from the breast. Ann Surg Oncol 2001;8:837–843.
10. Grant RN, Tabah EJ, Adair FF. The surgical significance of subareolar lymph plexus in cancer of the breast. Surgery 1953;331:71–78.
11. Hultborn KA, Larsen LG, Raghnult I. The lymph drainage from the breast to the axillary and parasternal lymph nodes: Studied with the aid of colloidal Au[198]. Acta Radiol 1955;43:52.
12. Kern KA. Sentinel lymph node mapping in breast cancer using subareolar injection of blue dye. J Am Coll Surg 1999;189(6):539–545.
13. Kern KA. Lymphoscintigraphic anatomy of sentinel lymphatic channels after subareolar injection of technetium 99m sulfur colloid. J Am Coll Surg 2001;193(6):601–608.
14. Haagensen CD. Diseases of the Breast, 3rd ed. Philadelphia, WB Saunders, 1986, p 240.
15. Poirier P, Cunéo B. Les lymphatiques. In Poirier P, Charpy A (eds). Traité d'anatomie humaine, vol 2, fasc 4. Paris, Masson, 1902.
16. Rouvière H. Anatomie des lymphatiques de l'homme. Paris, Masson, 1932.
17. Turner-Warwick RT. The lymphatics of the breast. Br J Surg 1959;46:574–582.
18. Berg JW. The significance of axillary node levels in the study of breast carcinoma. Cancer 1955;8:776.
19. Cabanas RM. An approach for the treatment of penile carcinoma. Cancer 1977;39(2):456–466.
20. Morton DL, Wen DR, Wong JH, et al. Technical details of intraoperative lymphatic mapping for early stage melanoma. Arch Surg 1992;127(4):392–399.
21. Krag DN, Weaver DL, Alex JC, et al. Surgical resection and radiolocalization of the sentinel lymph node in breast cancer using a gamma probe. Surg Oncol 1993;2(6):335–339; discussion, 340.
22. Giuliano AE, Kirgan DM, Guenther JM, et al. Lymphatic mapping and sentinel lymphadenectomy for breast cancer. Ann Surg 1994;220(3):391–398; discussion, 398–401.
23. Gardner E, Gray DJ, O'Rahilly R. Anatomy: A Regional Study of Human Structure, 4th ed. Philadelphia, WB Saunders, 1975.
24. Piersol GA. Human Anatomy, 6th ed. Philadelphia, JB Lippincott, 1918.
25. Maycock LA, Dillon P, Dixon JM. Morbidity related to intercostobrachial nerve damage following axillary surgery for breast cancer. Breast 1998;7:209–212.
26. Silverstein MJ, Murphy GP, Bostwick J, et al. Breast reconstruction: State of the art for the 1990s. Cancer 1991;68:1180.
27. Noone RB, Frazier JG, Noone GC, et al. Recurrence of breast carcinoma following immediate reconstruction: A 13-year review. Plast Reconstr Surg 1994;93:96.
28. Schain WS, Willish DK, Pasnau RO, et al. The sooner the better: A study of psychological factors in women undergoing immediate versus delayed breast reconstruction. Am J Psychiatry 1985;142:40.
29. Wilkins EG, Cederna PS, Lowery JC, et al. Prospective analysis of psychosocial outcomes in breast reconstruction: One-year postoperative results from the Michigan Breast Reconstruction Outcome Study. Plast Reconstr Surg 2000;106(5):1014–1025; discussion 1026–1027.
30. Massie MJ, Holland JC. Psychological reactions to breast cancer in the pre- and post-surgical treatment period. Semin Surg Oncol 1991;7:320–325.
31. National Comprehensive Cancer Network. NCCN practice guidelines for management of distress. Oncology 1999;13:113–147.
32. Hrushesky W, Bluning A, Gruber S, et al. Menstrual influence on the surgical care of breast cancer. Lancet 1989;2:949.
33. Senie R, Rosen P, Rhodes P, et al. Timing of breast cancer excision during the menstrual cycle influences duration of disease-free survival. Ann Intern Med 1991;115:337.
34. Senie RT, Tenser SM. The timing of breast cancer surgery during the menstrual cycle. Oncology 1997;11:1509.
35. Badwe RA, Gregory WM, Chaudary MA, et al. Timing of surgery during menstrual cycle and survival of premenopausal women with operable breast cancer. Lancet 1991;337(8752):1261–1264.
36. Gnant MF, Seifert M, Jakesz R, et al. Breast cancer and timing of surgery during menstrual cycle. A 5-year analysis of 385 pre-menopausal women. Int J Cancer 1992;52(5):707–712.
37. Kurebayashi J, Sonoo H, Shimozuma K. Timing of surgery in relation to the menstrual cycle and its influence on the survival of Japanese women with operable breast cancer. Surg Today 1995;25(6):519–524.
38. Veronesi U, Luini A, Mariani L, et al. Effect of menstrual phase on surgical treatment of breast cancer. Lancet 1994;343(8912):1545–1547.
39. Spratt J, Zirnheld J, Yancey J. Breast Cancer Detection Demonstration Project data can determine whether the prognosis of breast cancer is affected by time of surgery during the menstrual cycle. J Surg Oncol 1993;53:4–9.
40. Rageth J, Wyss P, Vorger C, et al. Timing of breast cancer surgery within the menstrual cycle: Influence on lymph node involvement, receptor status, postoperative metastatic spread, and local recurrence. Ann Oncol 1991;2:269.
41. Sigurdson H, Baldetorp B, Borg A, et al. Timing of surgery in the menstrual cycle does not appear to be a significant determinant of outcome in primary breast cancer. Proc Am Soc Clin Oncol 1992;11:62.
42. Goldhirsch A, Gelber RD, Forbes J, et al. Timing breast cancer surgery. Lancet 1991;338:691–692.
43. Nathan B, Bates T, Anbazhagen R, et al. Timing of surgery for breast cancer in relation to menstrual cycle and survival of premenopausal women. Br J Surg 1993;80:43.
44. d'Eridita G, DeLeo G, Punzo V, et al. Timing of breast cancer surgery during menstrual cycle. A 10-year analysis of 133 premenopausal women. Breast 1995;4:25–28.
45. Hagen AA, Hrushesky WJ. Menstrual timing of breast cancer surgery. Am J Surg 1998;104:245–261.
46. Pujol P, Daures JP, Brouillet JP, et al. A prospective prognostic study of the hormonal milieu at the time of surgery in premenopausal breast carcinoma. Cancer 2001;91(10):1854–1861.
47. Harlap S, Zauber AG, Pollack DM, et al. Survival of premenopausal women with breast carcinoma: Effects of menstrual timing of surgery. Cancer 1998;83(1):76–88.

48. Goldhirsch A, Gelber RD, Castiglione M, et al. Menstrual cycle and timing of breast surgery in premenopausal node-positive breast cancer: Results of the International Breast Cancer Study Group (IBCSG) Trial VI. Ann Oncol 1997;8(8):751–756.

49. Zurrida S, Galimberti V, Gibelli B, et al. Timing of breast cancer surgery in relation to the menstrual cycle: An update of developments. Crit Rev Oncol Hematol 2001;38(3):223–230.

50. Cooper LS, Gillett CE, Patel NK, et al. Survival of premenopausal breast carcinoma patients in relation to menstrual cycle timing of surgery and estrogen receptor/progesterone receptor status of the primary tumor. Cancer 1999;86(10):2053–2058.

51. Minckwitz G, Kaufmann M, Dobberstein S, et al. Surgical procedure can explain varying influence of menstrual cycle on prognosis of premenopausal breast cancer patients. Breast 1995;4:29–32.

52. Greenlee RT, Murray T, Bolden S, et al. Cancer statistics, 2000. CA Cancer J Clin 2000;50(1):7–33.

53. Osuch JR, Reeves MJ, Pathak DR, et al. BREASTAID: Clinical results from early development of a clinical decision rule for palpable solid breast masses. Ann Surg 2003;238(5):728–737.

54. Maganini RO, Klem DA, Huston BJ, et al. Upgrade rate of core biopsy-determined atypical ductal hyperplasia by open excisional biopsy. Am J Surg 2001;182(4):355–358.

55. Dershaw DD, Morris EA, Liberman L, et al. Nondiagnostic stereotaxic core breast biopsy: Results of rebiopsy. Radiology 1996;198(2):323–325.

56. Jackman RJ, Burbank F, Parker SH, et al. Atypical ductal hyperplasia diagnosed at stereotactic breast biopsy: Improved reliability with 14-gauge, directional, vacuum-assisted biopsy. Radiology 1997;204(2):485–488.

57. Liberman L, Cohen MA, Dershaw DD, et al. Atypical ductal hyperplasia diagnosed at stereotaxic core biopsy of breast lesions: An indication for surgical biopsy. AJR Am J Roentgenol 1995;164(5):1111–1113.

58. Liberman L, Smolkin JH, Dershaw DD, et al. Calcification retrieval at stereotactic, 11-gauge, directional, vacuum-assisted breast biopsy. Radiology 1998 l;208(1):251–260.

59. Adrales G, Turk P, Wallace T, et al. Is surgical excision necessary for atypical ductal hyperplasia of the breast diagnosed by Mammotome? Am J Surg 2000;180(4):313–315.

60. O'Hea BJ, Tornos C. Mild ductal atypia after large-core needle biopsy of the breast: Is surgical excision always necessary? Surgery 2000;128(4):738–743.

61. Dershaw DD. Does LCIS or ALH without other high-risk lesions diagnosed on core biopsy require surgical excision? Breast J 2003;9(1):1–3.

62. Shin SJ, Rosen PP. Excisional biopsy should be performed if lobular carcinoma in situ is seen on needle core biopsy. Arch Pathol Lab Med 2002;126(6):697–701.

63. Berg WA, Mrose HE, Ioffe OB. Atypical lobular hyperplasia or lobular carcinoma in situ at core-needle breast biopsy. Radiology 2001;218(2):503–509.

64. Irfan K, Brem RF. Surgical and mammographic follow-up of papillary lesions and atypical lobular hyperplasia diagnosed with stereotactic vacuum-assisted biopsy. Breast J 2002;8(4):230–233.

65. Renshaw AA, Cartagena N, Derhagopian RP, et al. Lobular neoplasia in breast core needle biopsy specimens is not associated with an increased risk of ductal carcinoma in situ or invasive carcinoma. Am J Clin Pathol 2002;117(5):797–799.

66. Pacelli A, Rhodes DJ, Amrami KK, et al. Outcome of atypical lobular hyperplasia and lobular carcinoma in situ diagnosed by core needle biopsy. Clinical and surgical follow-up of 30 cases. Am J Clin Pathol 2001;116:591–592.

67. Liberman L, Sama M, Susnik B, et al. Lobular carcinoma in situ at percutaneous breast biopsy: Surgical biopsy findings. AJR Am J Roentgenol 1999;173(2):291–299.

68. Liberman L, Bracero N, Vuolo MA, et al. Percutaneous large-core biopsy of papillary breast lesions. AJR Am J Roentgenol 1999;172(2):331–337.

69. Philpotts LE, Shaheen NA, Jain KS, et al. Uncommon high-risk lesions of the breast diagnosed at stereotactic core-needle biopsy: Clinical importance. Radiology 2000;216(3):831–837.

70. Adler DD, Helvie MA, Oberman HA, et al. Radial sclerosing lesion of the breast: Mammographic features. Radiology 1990;176(3):737–740.

71. Sloane JP, Mayers MM. Carcinoma and atypical hyperplasia in radial scars and complex sclerosing lesions: Importance of lesion size and patient age. Histopathology 1993;23(3):225–231.

72. Jacobs TW, Byrne C, Colditz G, et al. Radial scars in benign breast-biopsy specimens and the risk of breast cancer. N Engl J Med 1999;340(6):430–436.

73. Anscher MS, Jones P, Prosnitz LR, et al. Local failure and margin status in early stage breast carcinoma treated with conservation surgery and radiation therapy. Ann Surg 1993;218:22–28.

74. Fisher B, Anderson S, Bryant J, et al. Twenty-year follow-up of a randomized trial comparing total mastectomy, lumpectomy, and lumpectomy plus irradiation for the treatment of invasive breast cancer. N Engl J Med 2002;347(16):1233–1241.

75. Freedman GM, Hanlon AL, Fowble BL, et al. Recursive partitioning identifies patients at high and low risk for ipsilateral tumor recurrence after breast-conserving surgery and radiation. J Clin Oncol 2002;20(19):4015–4021.

76. Neuschatz AC, DiPetrillo T, Safaii H, et al. Long-term follow-up of a prospective policy of margin-directed radiation dose escalation in breast-conserving surgery. Cancer 2003;97(1):30–39.

77. Park CC, Mitsumori M, Nixon A, et al. Outcome at 8 years after breast-conserving surgery and radiation therapy for invasive breast cancer: Influence of margin status and systemic therapy on local recurrence. J Clin Oncol 2000;18(8):1668–1675.

78. Schnitt SJ, Connolly JL. Processing and evaluation of breast excision specimens. A clinically oriented approach. Anat Pathol 1992;98:126.

79. Gould EW, Robinson PG. The pathologist's examination of the "lumpectomy": The pathologists' view of surgical margins. Semin Surg Oncol 1992;8:129–135.

80. Anscher MS, Jones P, Prosnitz LR, et al. Local failure and margin status in early-stage breast carcinoma treated with conservation surgery and radiation therapy. Ann Surg 1993;218(1):22–28.

81. Smitt MC, Nowels KW, Zdeblick MJ, et al. The importance of the lumpectomy surgical margin status in long-term results of breast conservation. Cancer 1995;76(2):259–267.

82. Peterson ME, Schultz DJ, Reynolds C, et al. Outcomes in breast cancer patients relative to margin status after treatment with breast-conserving surgery and radiation therapy: The University of Pennsylvania experience. Int J Radiat Oncol Biol Phys 1999;43(5):1029–1035.

83. Fisher B, Anderson S, Redmond CK, et al. Reanalysis and results after 12 years of follow-up in a randomized clinical trial comparing total mastectomy with lumpectomy with or without irradiation in the treatment of breast cancer. N Engl J Med 1995;333(22):1456–1461.

84. van Dongen JA, Bartelink H, Fentiman IS, et al. Factors influencing local relapse and survival and results of salvage treatment after breast-conserving therapy in operable breast cancer: EORTC trial 10801, breast conservation compared with mastectomy in TNM stage I and II breast cancer. Eur J Cancer 1992;28A(4–5):801–805.

85. Dewar JA, Arriagada R, Benhamou S, et al. Local relapse and contralateral tumor rates in patients with breast cancer treated with conservative surgery and radiotherapy (Institut Gustave Roussy 1970–1982). IGR Breast Cancer Group. Cancer 1995;76(11):2260–2265.

86. Pittinger TP, Maronian NC, Poulter CA, et al. Importance of margin status in outcome of breast-conserving surgery for carcinoma. Surgery 1994;116(4):605–608; discussion, 608–609.

87. Frazier TG, Wong RW, Rose D. Implications of accurate pathologic margins in the treatment of primary breast cancer. Arch Surg 1989;124:37–38.

88. Mansfield CM, Komarnicky LT, Schwartz GF, et al. Ten-year results in 1,070 patients with stage I and II breast cancer treated by conservative surgery and radiation therapy. Cancer 1995;75:2328–2336.

89. Gage I, Schnitt SJ, Nixon AJ, et al. Pathologic margin involvement and the risk of recurrence in patients treated with breast-conserving therapy. Cancer 1996;78:1921–1928.

90. Ghossein NA, Alpert S, Barba J, et al. Importance of adequate surgical excision prior to radiotherapy in the local control of breast cancer in patients treated conservatively. Arch Surg 1992;127:411–415.

91. Vicini FA, Eberlein TJ, Connolly JL, et al. The optimal extent of resection for patients with stages I or II breast cancer treated with conservative surgery and radiotherapy. Ann Surg 1991;214:200–205.

92. Schnitt SJ, Abner A, Gelman R, et al. The relationship between microscopic margins of resection and the risk of local recurrence in patients with breast cancer treated with breast-conserving surgery and radiation therapy. Cancer 1994;74(6):1746–1751.

93. Voogd AC, Nielsen M, Peterse JL, et al. Breast Cancer Cooperative Group of the European Organization for Research and Treatment of Cancer. Differences in risk factors for local and distant recurrence after breast-conserving therapy or mastectomy for stage I and II breast

cancer: Pooled results of two large European randomized trials. J Clin Oncol 2001;19(6):1688–1697.

94. DiBiase SJ, Komarnicky LT, Heron DE, et al. Influence of radiation dose on positive surgical margins in women undergoing breast conservation therapy. Int J Radiat Oncol Biol Phys 2002;53(3):680–686.

95. Meric F, Mirza NQ, Vlastos G, et al. Positive surgical margins and ipsilateral breast tumor recurrence predict disease-specific survival after breast-conserving therapy. Cancer 2003;97(4):926–933.

96. Heimann R, Powers C, Halpern H, et al. Breast preservation in stage I and II carcinoma of the breast. Cancer 1996;78:1722–1730.

97. Kinne D, Petrek JA, Osborne MP, et al. Breast carcinoma in-situ. Arch Surg 1989;124:33–36.

98. Lagios MD, Westdahl, PR, Margolin FR, et al. Duct carcinoma in situ: Relationship of extent of noninvasive disease to the frequency of occult invasion, multicentricity, lymph node metastases, and short term treatment failures. Cancer 1982;50:1309–1314.

99. Montgomery RC, Fowble BL, Goldstein LJ, et al. Local recurrence after mastectomy for ductal carcinoma in situ. Breast J 1998;4:430–436.

100. Rosen PP, Braun DW Jr, Kinne DE. The clinical significance of pre-invasive breast carcinoma. Cancer 1980;46(4 Suppl):919–925.

101. Page DL, Dupont WD, Rogers LW, Landenberger M. Intraductal carcinoma of the breast: Follow-up after biopsy only. Cancer 1982;49(4):751–758.

102. Page DL, Dupont WD, Rogers LW, et al. Continued local recurrence of carcinoma 15–25 years after a diagnosis of low grade ductal carcinoma in situ of the breast treated only by biopsy. Cancer 1995;76(7):1197–200.

103. Lennington WJ, Jensen KA, Dalton LW, et al. Ductal carcinoma in situ of the breast: Heterogeneity of individual lesions. Cancer 1994;73:118–124.

104. Sunshine JA, Moseley HS, Fletcher WS, et al. Breast carcinoma in situ: A retrospective review of 112 cases with a minimum 10-year follow-up. Am J Surg 1985;150:44–51.

105. Asikari R, Hajdu SI, Robbins GF. Intraductal carcinoma of the breast. Cancer 1971;28:1182–1187.

106. Schwartz GF, Patchefsky AS, Finklestein SD, et al. Nonpalpable in-situ ductal carcinoma of the breast: Predictors of multicentricity and microinvasion and implications for treatment. Arch Surg 1989;124:29–32.

107. Fowble B. Overview of conservative surgery and radiation therapy for ductal carcinoma in situ. In Silverstein MJ (ed): Ductal Carcinoma In Situ of the Breast. Philadelphia, Lippincott Williams & Wilkins, 2002, pp 287–302.

108. Fisher B, Dignam J, Wolmark N, et al. Lumpectomy and radiation therapy for the treatment of intraductal breast cancer: Findings from National Surgical Adjuvant Breast and Bowel Project B-17. J Clin Oncol 1998;16(2):441–452.

109. Solin LJ, Fourquet A, Vicini FA, et al. Salvage treatment for local recurrence after breast-conserving surgery and radiation as initial treatment for mammographically detected ductal carcinoma in situ of the breast. Cancer 2001;91(6):1090–1097.

110. Holland R, Faverly DRG. The local distribution of ductal carcinoma in situ of the breast: Whole organ studies. In Silverstein MJ (ed): Ductal Carcinoma In Situ of the Breast. Philadelphia, Lippincott Williams & Wilkins, 2002, pp 240–248.

111. Silverstein MJ. Margin width as the sole predictor of local recurrence in patients with ductal carcinoma in situ of the breast. In Silverstein MJ (ed): Ductal Carcinoma In Situ of the Breast. Philadelphia, Lippincott Williams & Wilkins, 2002, pp 482–493.

112. Fowble B. In-situ cancer. In Fowble B, Goodman RL, Glick JH, et al. (eds). Breast Cancer Treatment. St Louis, Mosby–Year Book, 1991, pp 328–331.

113. Holland R, Hendriks JHCL, Verbeek ALM, et al. Extent, distribution, and mammographic/histological correlations of breast ductal carcinoma in situ. Lancet 1990;335:519–522.

114. Lagios MD. Duct carcinoma in situ: Pathology and treatment. Surg Clin North Am 1990;70:853–871.

115. Silverstein MJ, Cohlan BF, Gierson E, et al. Duct carcinoma in situ: 227 Cases without microinvasion. Eur J Cancer 1992;28:630–634.

116. Arnesson LG, Smeds, S, Fagerberg G, et al. Follow-up of two treatment modalities for ductal cancer in situ of the breast. Br J Surg 1989;76:672–675.

117. Gallagher WJ, Koerner FC, Wood WC. Treatment of intraductal carcinoma with limited surgery: Long-term follow-up. J Clin Oncol 1989;7:376–380.

118. Graham MD, Lakhani S, Gaazet JC. Breast conserving surgery in the management of in-situ breast carcinoma. Eur J Surg Oncol 1991;17:258–264.

119. Price P, Sinnett HD, Gusterson B, et al. Ductal carcinoma in situ: Predictors of local recurrence and progression in patients treated by surgery alone. Br J Cancer 1990;61:869–872.

120. Temple WJ, Jenkins M, Alexander F, et al. Natural history of in-situ breast cancer in a defined population. Ann Surg 1989;210:853–857.

121. Fisher ER, Sass R, Fisher B, et al. Pathologic findings from the National Surgical Adjuvant Breast Project (Protocol 6). 1. Intraductal carcinoma (DCIS). Cancer 1986;57:197–208.

122. Silverstein MJ. Can intraductal breast carcinoma be excised completely by local excision? Cancer 1994;73:2985–2989.

123. Vicini FA, Kestin LL, Goldstein NS, et al. Impact of young age on outcome in patients with ductal carcinoma-in-situ treated with breast-conserving therapy. J Clin Oncol 2000;18(2):296–306.

124. Goldstein NS, Vicini FA, Kestin LL, et al. Differences in the pathologic features of ductal carcinoma in situ of the breast based on patient age. Cancer 2000;88(11):2553–2560.

125. Hieken TJ, Farolan M, D'Alessandro S, et al. Predicting the biologic behavior of ductal carcinoma in situ: An analysis of molecular markers. Surgery 2001;130(4):593–600; discussion, 600–601.

126. Silverstein MJ, Lagios MD, Groshen S, et al. The influence of margin width on local control of ductal carcinoma in situ of the breast. N Engl J Med 1999;340(19):1455–1461.

127. Page DL, Lagios MD. Pathologic analysis of the National Surgical Adjuvant Breast Project (NSABP) B-17 Trial. Unanswered questions remaining unanswered considering current concepts of ductal carcinoma in situ. Cancer 1995;75(6):1219–1222; discussion, 1223–1227.

128. Neuschatz AC, DiPetrillo T, Steinhoff M, et al. The value of breast lumpectomy margin assessment as a predictor of residual tumor burden in ductal carcinoma in situ of the breast. Cancer 2002;94(7):1917–1924.

129. Faverly DR, Burgers L, Bult P, et al. Three dimensional imaging of mammary ductal carcinoma in situ: Clinical implications. Semin Diagn Pathol 1994;11(3):193–198.

130. Bornstein BA, Recht A, Connolly JL, et al. Results of treating ductal carcinoma of the breast with conservative surgery and radiation therapy. Cancer 1991;67:7–13.

131. Solin LJ, Recht A, Fourquet A, et al. Ten-year results of breast-conserving surgery and definitive irradiation for intraductal carcinoma of the breast. Cancer 1991;68:2337–2344.

132. White J, Lenne A, Gustafson G, et al. Outcome and prognostic factors for local recurrence in mammographically detected ductal carcinoma in-situ of the breast treated with conservative surgery and radiation therapy. Int J Radiat Oncol Biol Phys 1995;31:791–797.

133. Ray GR, Adelson J, Hayhurst E, et al. Ductal carcinoma in-situ of the breast: Results of treatment by conservative surgery and definitive irradiation. Int J Radiat Oncol Biol Phys 1994;28:105–111.

134. Solin LJ, Yeh I-T, Kurtz J, et al. Ductal carcinoma in-situ (intraductal carcinoma of the breast treated with breast conservation surgery and definitive irradiation). Cancer 1993;71:2532–2542.

135. Ringberg A, Andersson, J, Aspefren K, et al. Breast carcinoma in-situ in 167 women: Incidence, mode of presentation, therapy, and follow-up. Eur J Surg Oncol 1991;17:466–476.

136. Statter AT, McNeese M, Oswald MJ, et al. The flow of limited surgery with irradiation in primary treatment of ductal in-situ breast cancer. J Radiat Oncol Biol Phys 1990;18:283–287.

137. Delouche G, Bachelot F, Premont M, et al. Conservation treatment of early breast cancer: Long-term results and complications. Int J Radiat Oncol Biol Phys 1987;13:29–34.

138. Fisher ER, Dignam J, Tan-Chiu E, et al. Pathologic findings from the National Surgical Adjuvant Breast Project (NSABP) eight-year update of Protocol B-17: Intraductal carcinoma. Cancer 1999;86(3):429–438.

139. Julien JP, Bijker N, Fentiman IS, et al. Radiotherapy in breast-conserving treatment for ductal carcinoma in situ: First results of the EORTC randomised phase III trial 10853. EORTC Breast Cancer Cooperative Group and EORTC Radiotherapy Group. Lancet 2000;355(9203):528–533.

140. Cangiarella J, Waisman J, Symmans WF, et al. Mammotome core biopsy for mammary microcalcification: Analysis of 160 biopsies from 142 women with surgical and radiologic followup. Cancer 2001;91(1):173–177.

141. Ferzli GS, Puza T, Vanvorst-Bilotti S, et al. Breast biopsies with ABBI(R): Experience with 183 attempted biopsies. Breast J 1999;5(1):26–28.

142. Kelley W, Bailey R, Bertelson C, et al. Stereotactic automated surgical biopsy using the ABBI biopsy device: A multicenter study. Breast J 1998;4:302–312.

143. Pendas S, Dauway E, Giuliano R, et al. Sentinel node biopsy in ductal carcinoma in situ patients. Ann Surg Oncol 2000;7(1):15–20.

144. Cox CE, Nguyen K, Gray RJ, et al. Importance of lymphatic mapping in ductal carcinoma in situ (DCIS): Why map DCIS? Am Surg 2001;67(6):513–519; discussion, 519–521.

145. Klauber-DeMore N, Tan LK, Liberman L, et al. Sentinel lymph node biopsy: Is it indicated in patients with high-risk ductal carcinoma-in-situ and ductal carcinoma-in-situ with microinvasion? Ann Surg Oncol 2000;7(9):636–642.

146. Cody HS, Van Zee KJ. Sentinal lymph node biopsy is indicated for patients with DCIS. J Natl Comp Cancer Network 2003;1:199–206.

147. Slavin SA, Schnitt SJ, Duda RB, et al. Skin-sparing mastectomy and immediate reconstruction: Oncologic risks and aesthetic results in patients with early-stage breast cancer. Plast Reconstr Surg 1998;102(1):49–62.

148. Liberman L, Kaplan J, Van Zee KJ, et al. Bracketing wires for preoperative breast needle localization. AJR Am J Roentgenol 2001;177(3):565–572.

149. Smith LF, Henry-Tillman R, Rubio IT, et al. Intraoperative localization after stereotactic breast biopsy without a needle. Am J Surg 2001;182(6):584–589.

150. Gray RJ, Salud C, Nguyen K, et al. Randomized prospective evaluation of a novel technique for biopsy or lumpectomy of nonpalpable breast lesions: Radioactive seed versus wire localization. Ann Surg Oncol 2001;8(9):711–715.

151. Holland R, Hendriks JHCL. Microcalcifications associated with ductal carcinoma in situ: Mammographic-pathologic correlation. Semin Diagn Pathol 1994;11(3):181–192.

152. Faverly DR, Burgers L, Bult P, et al. Three dimensional imaging of mammary ductal carcinoma in situ: Clinical implications. Semin Diagn Pathol 1994;11(3):193–198.

153. Soni R, Silverstein MJ, Larsen L, et al. Breast biopsy and oncoplastic surgery for the patient with ductal carcinoma in situ: Surgical, pathologic, and radiologic issues. In Silverstein MJ (ed). Ductal Carcinoma of the Breast, 2nd ed. Philadelphia, Lippincott Williams & Wilkins, 2002, pp 190–191.

154. Schwartz GT. Ductal carcinoma in situ of the breast [commentary]. In Silberman H, Silberman AW (eds). Surgical Oncology. Oxford, UK, Arnold, 2002, pp 297–305.

155. Klimberg VS, Westbrook KC, Korourian S. Use of touch preps for diagnosis and evaluation of surgical margins in breast cancer. Ann Surg Oncol 1998;5(3):220–226.

156. Cox CE, Hyacinthe M, Gonzalez RJ, et al. Cytologic evaluation of lumpectomy margins in patients with ductal carcinoma in situ: Clinical outcome. Ann Surg Oncol 1997;4(8):644–649.

157. Weber S, Storm FK, Stitt J, et al. The role of frozen section analysis of margins during breast conservation surgery. Cancer J Sci Am 1997;3(5):273–277.

158. Niemann TH, Lucas JG, March WL. To freeze or not to freeze: A comparison of methods for the handling of breast biopsies with no palpable abnormality. Am J Clin Pathol 1996;106:225–228.

159. Ferreiro JA, Gisvold JJ, Bostwick DG. Accuracy of frozen-section diagnosis of mammographically directed breast biopsies in results of 1,490 consecutive cases. Am J Surg Pathol 1995;19:1267–1271.

160. Fessig L, Ghiriaghello B, Arisia R, et al. Accuracy of frozen-section diagnosis in breast cancer detection: A review of 4,436 biopsies and comparison with cytodiagnosis. Pathol Res Pract 1984;179:61–66.

161. Cheng L, Al-Kaisi WH, Lin AY, et al. The results of intraoperative consultation in 181 ductal carcinomas in-situ of the breast. Cancer 1997;80:75–79.

162. Burbank F. Stereotactic breast biopsy: Comparison of 14- and 11-gauge Mammotome probe performance and complication rates. Am Surg 1997;63(11):988–995.

163. Burbank F, Forcier N. Tissue marking clip for stereotactic breast biopsy: Initial placement accuracy, long-term stability, and usefulness as a guide for wire localization. Radiology 1997;205(2):407–415.

164. Kass R, Kumar G, Klimberg VS, et al. Clip migration in stereotactic biopsy. Am J Surg 2002;184(4):325–331.

165. Dale PS, Giuliano AE. Nipple-areolar preservation during breast-conserving surgery for subareolar breast carcinomas. Arch Surg 1996;131:430–433.

166. Hunter MA, McFall TA, Hehr KA. Breast-conserving surgery for primary breast cancer: Necessity for surgical clips to define the tumor bed for radiation planning. Radiology 1996;200:281–282.

167. Fein DA, Fowble BL, Hanlon AL, et al. Does the placement of surgical clips within the excision cavity influence local control for patients treated with breast-conserving surgery and irradiation? Int J Radiat Oncol Biol Phys 1996;34:1009–1017.

168. Orr RK. The impact of prophylactic axillary node dissection on breast cancer survival: A bayesian meta-analysis. Ann Surg Oncol 1999;6(1):109–116.

169. Fisher B, Redmond C, Fisher ER, et al. Ten-year results of a randomized clinical trial comparing radical mastectomy and total mastectomy with or without radiation. N Engl J Med 1985;312(11):674–681.

170. Cabanes PA, Salmon RJ, Vilcoq JR, et al. Value of axillary dissection in addition to lumpectomy and radiotherapy in early breast cancer. The Breast Carcinoma Collaborative Group of the Institut Curie. Lancet 1992;339(8804):1245–1248.

171. Whitworth P, McMasters KM, Tafra L, et al. State-of-the-art lymph node staging for breast cancer in the year 2000. Am J Surg 2000;180(4):262–267.

172. Carter CL, Allen C, Henson DE. Relation of tumor size, lymph node status, and survival in 24,740 breast cancer cases. Cancer 1989;63(1):181–187.

173. Wilking N, Rutqvist LE, Carstensen J, et al. Prognostic significance of axillary nodal status in primary breast cancer in relation to the number of resected nodes. Stockholm Breast Cancer Study Group. Acta Oncol 1992;31(1):29–35.

174. Fisher B, Bauer M, Wickerham DL, et al. Relation of number of positive axillary nodes to the prognosis of patients with primary breast cancer. An NSABP update. Cancer 1983;52(9):1551–1557.

175. Rosen PP, Saigo PE, Braun DW, et al. Axillary micro- and macrometastases in breast cancer: Prognostic significance of tumor size. Ann Surg 1981;194(5):585–591.

176. Huvos AG, Hutter RV, Berg JW. Significance of axillary macrometastases and micrometastases in mammary cancer. Ann Surg 1971;173(1):44–46.

177. Donegan WL, Stine SB, Samter TG. Implications of extracapsular nodal metastases for treatment and prognosis of breast cancer. Cancer 1993;72(3):778–782.

178. Hermanek P, Hutter RV, Sobin LH, et al. Classification of isolated tumor cells and micrometastasis. Cancer 1999;86(12):2668–2673.

179. Trojani M, de Mascarel I, Bonichon F, et al. Micrometastases to axillary lymph nodes from carcinoma of breast: Detection by immunohistochemistry and prognostic significance. Br J Cancer 1987;55(3):303–306.

180. Hainsworth PJ, Tjandra JJ, Stillwell RG, et al. Detection and significance of occult metastases in node-negative breast cancer. Br J Surg 1993;80(4):459–463.

181. Clare SE, Sener SF, Wilkens W, et al. Prognostic significance of occult lymph node metastases in node-negative breast cancer. Ann Surg Oncol 1997;4(6):447–451.

182. Sedmak DD, Meineke TA, Knechtges DS, et al. Prognostic significance of cytokeratin-positive breast cancer metastases. Mod Pathol 1989;2(5):516–520.

183. Verbanac KM, Fleming TP, Min CH, et al. RT-PCR increases detection of breast cancer sentinal lymph node micrometastases (abstract). Breast Cancer Res Treat 1999;57:41.

184. Ruffin WK, Stacey-Clear A, Younger J, et al. Rationale for routine axillary dissection in carcinoma of the breast. J Am Coll Surg 1995;180(2):245–251.

185. Recht A, Houlihan MJ. Axillary lymph nodes and breast cancer: A review. Cancer 1995;76(9):1491–1512.

186. Kinne DW. Controversies in primary breast cancer management. Am J Surg 1993;166(5):502–508.

187. Fisher B, Wolmark N, Bauer M, et al. The new era in breast cancer. Arch Surg 1996;131:301–307.

188. Dershaw DD, Panicek DM, Osborne MP. Significance of lymph nodes visualized by the mammographic axillary view. Breast Dis 1001;4:271–280.

189. Bruneton JN, Caramella E, Hery M, et al. Axillary lymph node metastases in breast cancer: Preoperative detection with US. Radiology 1986;158(2):325–326.

190. Mehta TS, Raza S. Power Doppler sonography of breast cancer: Does vascularity correlate with node status or lymphatic vascular invasion? AJR Am J Roentgenol 1999;173(2):303–307.

191. Allan SM, McVicar D, Sacks NPM. Prospects for axillary staging in breast cancer by magnetic resonance imaging. Br J Radiol 1993; 66(Suppl):15.

192. Black RB, Merrick MV, Taylor TV, Forrest AP. Prediction of axillary metastases in breast cancer by lymphoscintigraphy. Lancet 1980; 2(8184):15–17.

193. Tjandra JJ, Sacks NP, Thompson CH, et al. The detection of axillary lymph node metastases from breast cancer by radiolabelled monoclonal antibodies: A prospective study. Br J Cancer 1989;59(2):296–302.

194. Nieweg OE, Kim EE, Wong WH, et al. Positron emission tomography with fluorine-18-deoxyglucose in the detection and staging of breast cancer. Cancer 1993;71(12):3920–3925.

195. Fisher ER, Sass R, Fisher B. Pathologic findings from the National Surgical Adjuvant Project for Breast Cancers (Protocol no. 4). X. Discriminants for tenth year treatment failure. Cancer 1984;53(3 Suppl):712–723.

196. Giuliano AE, Barth AM, Spivack B, et al. Incidence and predictors of axillary metastasis in T1 carcinoma of the breast. J Am Coll Surg 1996;183(3):185–189.

197. Chada M, Chabon AD, Friedmann P, et al. Predictors of axillary lymph node metastases in patients with T1 breast cancer. Cancer 1994;73:350–353.

198. Menard S, Bufalino R, Rilke F, et al. Prognosis based on primary breast carcinoma instead of pathological nodal status. Br J Cancer 1994;70(4):709–712.

199. Ravdin PM, De Laurentiis M, Vendely T, et al. Prediction of axillary lymph node status in breast cancer patients by use of prognostic indicators. J Natl Cancer Inst 1994;86(23):1771–1775.

200. Bland KI, Menck HR, Scott-Conner CE, et al. The National Cancer Data Base 10-year survey of breast carcinoma treatment at hospitals in the United States. Cancer 1998;83(6):1262–1273.

201. Bali ABS, Waters R, Fish S, et al. Radical axillary dissection in the staging and treatment of breast cancer. Ann R Coll Surg Engl 1992;74:126–129.

202. Carter C, Allen C, Henson D. Relation of tumor size, lymph node status, and survival in 24,740 breast cancer cases. Cancer 1989;63:181–187.

203. Moffat FL, Senofsky GM, Davis K, et al. Axillary node dissection for early breast cancer: Some is good, but all is better. J Surg Oncol 1992;51:8–13.

204. Graverson HP, Toft MG, Andersen JA, et al. Breast cancer: Risk of axillary recurrence in node-negative patients following partial dissection of the axilla. Eur J Surg Oncol 1988;14:407–412.

205. Cabanes PA, Salmon RJ, Vilcoq JR, et al. Value of axillary dissection in addition to lumpectomy and radiotherapy in early breast cancer. Lancet 1992;339:1245–1248.

206. Fisher B, Redmond C, Fisher ER, et al. Ten-year results of a randomized clinical trial comparing radical mastectomy and total mastectomy with and without radiation. N Engl J Med 1985;312:674–681.

207. Cady B, Stone M, Wayne J. New therapeutic possibilities in primary invasive breast cancer. Ann Surg 1993;218:338–349.

208. Baxter N, McCready D, Chapman J-A, et al. Clinical behavior of untreated axillary nodes after local treatment for primary breast cancer. Ann Surg Oncol 1996;3:235–240.

209. Recht A, Pierce SM, Abner A, et al. Regional nodal failure after conservative surgery and radiotherapy for early-stage breast carcinoma. J Clin Oncol 1991;9:988–996.

210. Wong JS, Recht A, Beard CJ, et al. Treatment outcome after tangential radiation therapy without axillary dissection in patients with early-stage breast cancer and clinically negative axillary nodes. Int J Radiat Oncol Biol Phys 1997;39(4):915–920.

211. Osborne MP, Ormiston N, Harmer CL, et al. Breast conservation in the treatment of early breast cancer: A 20-year follow-up. Cancer 1984;53:349–355.

212. Berger AC, Miller SM, Harris MN, et al. Axillary dissection for tubular carcinoma of the breast. Breast J 1996;2:204–208.

213. Barth A, Craig PH, Silverstein MJ. Predictors of axillary lymph node metastases in patients with T1 breast carcinoma. Cancer 1997;79:1918–1922.

214. Pandelidis SM, Peters KL, Walusimbi MS, et al. The role of axillary dissection in mammographically detected carcinoma. J Am Coll Surg 1997;184:341–345.

215. Wazer DE, Erban JK, Robert NJ, et al. Breast conservation in elderly women for clinically negative axillary lymph nodes without axillary dissection. Cancer 1994;74:878–883.

216. Giuliano A, Barth AM, Spivack B, et al. Incidence and predictors of axillary metastasis in T1 carcinoma of the breast. J Am Coll Surg 1996;183:185–189.

217. White RE, Vezeridis MP, Konstadowlakis M, et al. Therapeutic options and results for the management of minimally invasive carcinoma of the breast: Influence of axillary dissection for treatment of $T1_a$ and $T1_b$ lesions. J Am Coll Surg 1996;183:575–582.

218. Cady D. The need to re-examine axillary lymph node dissection in invasive breast cancer. Cancer 1994;73:505–508.

219. Siegel BM, Mayzel KA, Love SA. Level I and II axillary dissection in the treatment of early-stage breast cancer: An analysis of 259 consecutive patients. Arch Surg 1990;125:1144–1147.

220. Petrek JA, Blackwood MM. Axillary dissection: Current practice and technique. Curr Probl Surg 1995;32:256–323.

221. Silverstein MJ, Gerson ED, Waisman JR, et al. Axillary lymph node dissection for $T1_a$ breast carcinoma: Is it indicated? Cancer 1994;79:664–667.

222. Chontos AJ, Maher DP, Ratzer ER, et al. Axillary lymph dissection: Is it required in $T1_a$ breast cancer? J Am Coll Surg 1997;184:493–498.

223. Norman J, Cruse CW, Espinosa C, et al. Redefinition of cutaneous lymphatic drainage with the use of lymphoscintigraphy for malignant melanoma. Am J Surg 1991;162(5):432–437.

224. Cabanas RM. An approach for the treatment of penile carcinoma. Cancer 1977;39(2):456–466.

225. Morton DL, Wen DR, Wong JH, et al. Technical details of intraoperative lymphatic mapping for early stage melanoma. Arch Surg 1992;127(4):392–399.

226. Morton DL, Wen DR, Cochran AJ. Management of early stage melanoma by intraoperative lymphatic mapping and selective lymphadenectomy: An alternative to routine elective lymphadenectomy or "watch and wait." Surg Oncol Clin North Am 1992;1:247–259.

227. Morton DL, Thompson JF, Essner R, et al. Validation of the accuracy of intraoperative lymphatic mapping and sentinel lymphadenectomy for early-stage melanoma: A multicenter trial. Multicenter Selective Lymphadenectomy Trial Group. Ann Surg 1999;230(4):453–463; discussion, 463–465.

228. Giuliano AE, Jones RC, Brennan M, et al. Sentinel lymphadenectomy in breast cancer. J Clin Oncol 1997;15(6):2345.

229. Veronesi U, Paganelli G, Viale G, et al. Sentinel lymph node biopsy and axillary dissection in breast cancer: Results in a large series. J Natl Cancer Inst 1999;91(4):368–373.

230. Borgstein PJ, Pijpers R, Comans EF, et al. Sentinel lymph node biopsy in breast cancer: Guidelines and pitfalls of lymphoscintigraphy and gamma probe detection. J Am Coll Surg 1998;186(3):275–283.

231. Krag D, Weaver D, Ashikaga T, et al. The sentinel node in breast cancer: A multicenter validation study. N Engl J Med 1998;339(14):941–946.

232. Bass SS, Cox CE, Ku NN, et al. The role of sentinal lymph node biopsy in breast cancer. J Am Coll Surg 1999;189:183–194.

233. Nwariaku FE, Euhus DM, Beitsch PD, et al. Sentinel lymph node biopsy, an alternative to elective axillary dissection for breast cancer. Am J Surg 1998;176(6):529–531.

234. Tafra L, Lannin DR, Swanson MS, et al. Multicenter trial of sentinel node biopsy for breast cancer using both technecium sulfur colloid and isosulfan blue dye. Ann Surg 2001;233(1):51–59.

235. McMasters KM, Wong SL, Martin RC 2nd, et al. Dermal injection of radioactive colloid is superior to peritumoral injection for breast cancer sentinel lymph node biopsy: Results of a multiinstitutional study. Ann Surg 2001;233(5):676–687.

236. Veronesi U, Galimberti V, Zurrida S, et al. Sentinel lymph node biopsy as an indicator for axillary dissection in early breast cancer. Eur J Cancer 2001;37(4):454–458.

237. Schrenk P, Hatzl-Griesenhofer M, Shamiyeh A, Waynad W. Follow-up of sentinel node negative breast cancer patients without axillary lymph node dissection. J Surg Oncol 2001;77(3):165–170.

238. Hansen NM, Grube BJ, Giuliano AE. The time has come to change the algorithm for the surgical management of early breast cancer. Arch Surg 2002;137(10):1131–1135.

239. Wong JH, Cagle LA, Morton DL. Lymphatic drainage of skin to a sentinel lymph node in a feline model. Ann Surg 1991;214(5):637–641.

240. Simmons R, Thevarajah S, Brennan MB, et al. Methylene blue dye as an alternative to isosulfan blue dye for sentinel lymph node localization. Ann Surg Oncol 2003;10:242–247.

241. Schwartz GF, Giuliano AE, Veronesi U, et al. Proceedings of the consensus conference on the role of sentinel lymph node biopsy in carcinoma of the breast, April 19–22, 2001, Philadelphia, Pennsylvania. Cancer 2002;94(10):2542–2551.

242. Martin RC 2nd, Edwards MJ, Wong SL, et al. Practical guidelines for optimal gamma probe detection of sentinel lymph nodes in breast cancer: Results of a multi-institutional study. For the University of Louisville Breast Cancer Study Group. Surgery 2000;128(2):139–144.

243. Derossis AM, Fey J, Yeung H, et al. A trend analysis of the relative value of blue dye and isotope localization in 2,000 consecutive cases of sentinel node biopsy for breast cancer. J Am Coll Surg 2001;193(5):473–478.

244. Cody HS 3rd, Fey J, Akhurst T, et al. Complementarity of blue dye and isotope in sentinel node localization for breast cancer: Univariate and multivariate analysis of 966 procedures. Ann Surg Oncol 2001;8(1):13–19.

245. Motomura K, Inaji H, Komoike Y. Combination technique is superior to dye alone in identification of the sentinel node in breast cancer patients. J Surg Oncol 2001;76(2):95–99.

246. Albertini JJ, Lyman GH, Cox C, et al. Lymphatic mapping and sentinel node biopsy in the patient with breast cancer. JAMA 1996;276(22):1818–1822.

247. Cox CE, Pendas S, Cox JM, et al. Guidelines for sentinel node biopsy and lymphatic mapping of patients with breast cancer. Ann Surg 1998;227(5):645–651; discussion, 651–653.

248. Shen P, Glass EC, DiFronzo LA, et al. Dermal versus intraparenchymal lymphoscintigraphy of the breast. Ann Surg Oncol 2001;8(3):241–248.

249. Smith LF, Cross MJ, Klimberg VS. Subareolar injection is a better technique for sentinel lymph node biopsy. Am J Surg 2000;180(6):434–437; discussion, 437–438.

250. Bass SS, Cox CE, Salud CJ, et al. The effects of postinjection massage on the sensitivity of lymphatic mapping in breast cancer. J Am Coll Surg 2001;192(1):9–16.

251. Boolbol SK, Fey JV, Borgen PI, et al. Intradermal isotope injection: A highly accurate method of lymphatic mapping in breast carcinoma. Ann Surg Oncol 2001;8(1):20–24.

252. Tousimis E, Van Zee KJ, Fey JV, et al. The accuracy of sentinel lymph node biopsy in multicentric and multifocal invasive breast cancers. J Am Coll Surg 2003;197(4):529–535.

253. Brady B, Fant J, Jones R, et al. Sentinel lymph node biopsy followed by delayed mastectomy and reconstruction. Am J Surg 2003;185(2):114–117.

254. Chao C, McMasters K. The current status of sentinel lymph node biopsy for breast cancer. Adv Surg 2002;36:167–192.

255. Giuliano AE, Kirgan DM, Guenther JM, et al. Lymphatic mapping and sentinel lymphadenectomy for breast cancer. Ann Surg 1994;220(3):391–398; discussion, 398–401.

256. Hingston GR, Cooke TG, Going JJ, et al. Accuracy of intraoperative frozen-section analysis of axillary nodes. Br J Surg 1999;86(8):1092; author reply, 1092–1093.

257. Turner RR, Hansen NM, Stern SL, et al. Intraoperative examination of the sentinel lymph node for breast carcinoma staging. Am J Clin Pathol 1999;112(5):627–634.

258. Zurrida S, Galimberti V, Orvieto E, et al. Radioguided sentinel node biopsy to avoid axillary dissection in breast cancer. Ann Surg Oncol 2000;7(1):28–31.

259. Canavese G, Gipponi M, Catturich A, et al. Sentinel lymph node mapping opens a new perspective in the surgical management of early-stage breast cancer: A combined approach with vital blue dye lymphatic mapping and radioguided surgery. Semin Surg Oncol 1998;15(4):272–277.

260. Van Diest PJ, Torrenga H, Borgstein PJ, et al. Reliability of intraoperative frozen section and imprint cytological investigation of sentinel lymph nodes in breast cancer. Histopathology 1999;35(1):14–18.

261. Rahusen FD, Pijpers R, Van Diest PJ, et al. The implementation of the sentinel node biopsy as a routine procedure for patients with breast cancer. Surgery 2000;128(1):6–12.

262. Weiser MR, Montgomery LL, Susnik B, et al. Is routine intraoperative frozen-section examination of sentinel lymph nodes in breast cancer worthwhile? Ann Surg Oncol 2000;7(9):651–655.

263. Chao C, Wong SL, Ackermann D, et al. Utility of intraoperative frozen section analysis of sentinel lymph nodes in breast cancer. Am J Surg 2001;182(6):609–615.

264. Veronesi U, Paganelli G, Galimberti V, et al. Sentinel-node biopsy to avoid axillary dissection in breast cancer with clinically negative lymph-nodes. Lancet 1997;349(9069):1864–1867.

265. Veronesi U, Zurrida S, Mazzarol G, et al. Extensive frozen section examination of axillary sentinel nodes to determine selective axillary dissection. World J Surg 2001;25(6):806–808.

266. Shiver SA, Creager AJ, Geisinger K, et al. Intraoperative analysis of sentinel lymph nodes by imprint cytology for cancer of the breast. Am J Surg 2002;184(5):424–427.

267. Henry-Tillman RS, Korourian S, Rubio IT, et al. Intraoperative touch preparation for sentinel lymph node biopsy: A 4-year experience. Ann Surg Oncol 2002;9(4):333–339.

268. Lee A, Krishnamurthy S, Sahin A, et al. Intraoperative touch imprint of sentinel lymph nodes in breast carcinoma patients. Cancer 2002;96(4):225–231.

269. Karamlou T, Johnson NM, Chan B, et al. Accuracy of intraoperative touch imprint cytologic analysis of sentinel lymph nodes in breast cancer. Am J Surg 2003;185(5):425–428.

270. Pendas S, Dauway E, Cox CE, et al. Sentinel node biopsy and cytokeratin staining for the accurate staging of 478 breast cancer patients. Am Surg 1999;65(6):500–505; discussion, 505–506.

271. Sabel MS, Zhang P, Barnwell JM, et al. Accuracy of sentinel lymph node biopsy in predicting nodal status in patients with breast carcinoma. J Surg Oncol 2001;77(4):243–246.

272. Turner RR, Giuliano AE, Hoon DS, et al. Pathologic examination of sentinel lymph node for breast carcinoma. World J Surg 2001;25(6):798–805.

273. Viale G, Maiorano E, Mazzarol G, et al. Histologic detection and clinical implications of micrometastases in axillary sentinel lymph nodes for patients with breast carcinoma. Cancer 2001;92(6):1378–1384.

274. Giuliano AE, Dale PS, Turner RR, et al. Improved axillary staging of breast cancer with sentinel lymphadenectomy. Ann Surg 1995;222(3):394–399; discussion, 399–401.

275. Veronesi U, Paganelli G, Viale G, et al. A randomized comparison of sentinel-node biopsy with routine axillary dissection in breast cancer. N Engl J Med 2003;349(6):546–553.

276. Hsueh EC, Turner RR, Glass EC, et al. Sentinel node biopsy in breast cancer. J Am Coll Surg 1999;189(2):207–213.

277. Reynolds C, Mick R, Donohue JH, et al. Sentinel lymph node biopsy with metastasis: Can axillary dissection be avoided in some patients with breast cancer? J Clin Oncol 1999;17(6):1720–1726.

278. Chu KU, Turner RR, Hansen NM, et al. Do all patients with sentinel node metastasis from breast carcinoma need complete axillary node dissection? Ann Surg 1999;229(4):536–541.

279. Turner RR, Chu KU, Qi K, et al. Pathologic features associated with nonsentinel lymph node metastases in patients with metastatic breast carcinoma in a sentinel lymph node. Cancer 2000;89(3):574–581.

280. Rahusen FD, Torrenga H, van Diest PJ, et al. Predictive factors for metastatic involvement of nonsentinel nodes in patients with breast cancer. Arch Surg 2001;136(9):1059–1063.

281. Jakub JW, Diaz NM, Ebert MD, et al. Completion axillary lymph node dissection minimizes the likelihood of false negatives for patients with invasive breast carcinoma and cytokeratin positive only sentinel lymph nodes. Am J Surg 2002;184(4):302–306.

282. Kamath VJ, Giuliano R, Dauway EL, et al. Characteristics of the sentinel lymph node in breast cancer predict further involvement of higher-echelon nodes in the axilla: A study to evaluate the need for complete axillary lymph node dissection. Arch Surg 2001;136(6):688–692.

283. McMasters KM, for the University of Louisville Breast Cancer Sentinel Lymph Node Study Group. Predicting the status of the nonsentinel axillary nodes: A multicenter study. Arch Surg 2001;136:563–568.

284. Guenther JM, Hansen NM, DiFronzo LA, et al. Axillary dissection is not required for all patients with breast cancer and positive sentinel nodes. Arch Surg 2003;138(1):52–56.

285. Wilke LG, Giuliano A. Sentinel lymph node biopsy in patients with early-stage breast cancer: Status of the National Clinical Trials. Surg Clin North Am 2003;83(4):901–910.

286. Montgomery LL, Thorne AC, Van Zee KJ, et al. Isosulfan blue dye reactions during sentinel lymph node mapping for breast cancer. Anesth Analg 2002;95(2):385–388.

287. Stratmann SL, McCarty TM, Kuhn JA. Radiation safety with breast sentinel node biopsy. Am J Surg 1999;178(6):454–457.

288. Waddington WA, Keshtgar MR, Taylor I, et al. Radiation safety of the sentinel lymph node technique in breast cancer. Eur J Nucl Med 2000;27(4):377–391.

289. Swenson KK, Nissen MJ, Ceronsky C, et al. Comparison of side effects between sentinel lymph node and axillary lymph node dissection for breast cancer. Ann Surg Oncol 2002;9(8):745–753.

290. Leidenius M, Leppanen E, Krogerus L, et al. Motion restriction and axillary web syndrome after sentinel node biopsy and axillary clearance in breast cancer. Am J Surg 2003;185(2):127–130.

291. Burak WE Jr, Walker MJ, Yee LD, et al. Routine preoperative lymphoscintigraphy is not necessary prior to sentinel node biopsy for breast cancer. Am J Surg 1999;177(6):445–449.
292. McMasters KM, Wong SL, Tuttle TM, et al. Preoperative lymphoscintigraphy for breast cancer does not improve the ability to identify axillary sentinel lymph nodes. Ann Surg 2000;231(5):724–731.
293. Morrow M, Rademaker AW, Bethke KP, et al. Learning sentinel node biopsy: Results of a prospective randomized trial of two techniques. Surgery 1999;126(4):714–720; discussion, 720–722.
294. Cox CE, Bass SS, Boulware D, et al. Implementation of new surgical technology: Outcome measures for lymphatic mapping of breast carcinoma. Ann Surg Oncol 1999;6(6):553–561.
295. McMasters KM, Wong SL, Chao C, et al. Defining the optimal surgeon experience for breast cancer sentinel lymph node biopsy: A model for implementation of new surgical techniques. Ann Surg 2001;234(3):292–299; discussion, 299–300.
296. Sanidas EE, de Bree E, Tsiftsis DD. How many cases are enough for accreditation in sentinel lymph node biopsy in breast cancer? Am J Surg 2003;185(3):202–210.
297. Tafra L, McMasters KM, Whitworth P, et al. Credentialing issues with sentinel lymph node staging for breast cancer. Am J Surg 2000;180(4):268–273.
298. Veronesi U, Cascinelli N, Greco M, et al. Prognosis of breast cancer patients after mastectomy and dissection of internal mammary nodes. Ann Surg 1985;202(6):702–707.
299. Morrow M, Foster RS Jr. Staging of breast cancer: A new rationale for internal mammary node biopsy. Arch Surg 1981;116(6):748–751.
300. Veronesi U, Cascinelli N, Bufalino R, et al. Risk of internal mammary lymph node metastases and its relevance on prognosis of breast cancer patients. Ann Surg 1983;198(6):681–684.
301. Noguchi M, Ohta N, Koyasaki N, et al. Reappraisal of internal mammary node metastases as a prognostic factor in patients with breast cancer. Cancer 1991;68(9):1918–1925.
302. Cody HS 3rd, Urban JA. Internal mammary node status: A major prognosticator in axillary node-negative breast cancer. Ann Surg Oncol 1995;2(1):32–37.
303. Veronesi U, Marubini E, Mariani L, et al. The dissection of internal mammary nodes does not improve the survival of breast cancer patients: 30-Year results of a randomised trial. Eur J Cancer 1999 Sep;35(9):1320–1325.
304. van der Ent FW, Kengen RA, van der Pol HA, et al. Halsted revisited: Internal mammary sentinel lymph node biopsy in breast cancer. Ann Surg 2001;234(1):79–84.
305. Tanis PJ, Nieweg OE, Valdes Olmos RA, et al. Impact of non-axillary sentinel node biopsy on staging and treatment of breast cancer patients. Br J Cancer 2002;87(7):705–710.
306. Galimberti V, Arnone P, Pesci Feltri A, et al. Stage migration in breast cancer after biopsy of the internal mammary lymph nodes. Eur J Cancer 2001;37(Suppl 6):S270.
307. Intra M, Veronesi P, Mazzarol G, et al. Axillary sentinel lymph node biopsy in patients with pure ductal carcinoma in situ of the breast. Arch Surg 2003;138:309–313.
308. Pendas S, Dauway E, Giuliano R, et al. Sentinel node biopsy in ductal carcinoma in situ patients. Ann Surg Oncol 2000;7(1):15–20.
309. Cox CE, Nguyen K, Gray RJ, et al. Importance of lymphatic mapping in ductal carcinoma in situ (DCIS): Why map DCIS? Am Surg 2001;67(6):513–519; discussion, 519–521.
310. Klauber-DeMore N, Tan LK, Liberman L, et al. Sentinel lymph node biopsy: Is it indicated in patients with high-risk ductal carcinoma-in-situ and ductal carcinoma-in-situ with microinvasion? Ann Surg Oncol 2000;7(9):636–642.
311. Stearns V, Ewing CA, Slack R, et al. Sentinel lymphadenectomy after neoadjuvant chemotherapy for breast cancer may reliably represent the axilla except for inflammatory breast cancer. Ann Surg Oncol 2002;9(3):235–242.
312. Tousimis E, Van Zee KJ, Fey JV, et al. The accuracy of sentinel lymph node biopsy in multicentric and multifocal invasive breast cancers. J Am Coll Surg 2003;197(4):529–535.
313. McMasters KM, Wong SL, Martin RC 2nd, et al. Dermal injection of radioactive colloid is superior to peritumoral injection for breast cancer sentinel lymph node biopsy: Results of a multiinstitutional study. Ann Surg 2001;233(5):676–687.
314. Tuttle TM, Colbert M, Christensen R, et al. Subareolar injection of 99mTc facilitates sentinel lymph node identification. Ann Surg Oncol 2002;9(1):77–81.
315. Chao C, Wong SL, Woo C, et al. Reliable lymphatic drainage to axillary sentinel lymph nodes regardless of tumor location within the breast. Am J Surg 2001;182(4):307–311.
316. Haddad FF, Shivers SC, Reintgen DS. Historical perspectives and future applications. Surg Clin North Am 1999;8:391–400.
317. NSABP Clinical Trials Overview. Protocol B-32 schema [Online]. Available: www.nsabp.pitt.edu. Accessed November 9, 2003.
318. Halsted WS. The results of operations for the cure of cancer of the breast performed at the Johns Hopkins Hospital from June, 1889 to January, 1894. Johns Hopkins Hosp Rep 1894–1895;4:297–350.
319. Patey DH, Dyson WH. The prognosis of carcinoma of the breast in relation to the type of operation performed. Br J Cancer 1948;2:7–13.
320. Roses DF, Harris MN, Potter DA, et al. Total mastectomy with complete axillary dissection. Ann Surg 1981;194:4–8.
321. Veronesi U, Rilke F, Luini A, et al. Distribution of axillary node metastases by level of invasion. Cancer 1987;59:682–687.
322. Veronesi U, Luini A, Galimberti V, et al. Extent of metastatic axillary involvement in 1,446 cases of breast cancer. Eur J Surg Oncol 1990;16:127–133.
323. Rosen PP, Lesser ML, Kinne DW, et al. Discontinuous or skip metastases in breast carcinoma. Analysis of 1228 axillary dissections. Ann Surg 1983;197:276–283.
324. Pigott J, Nichols R, Maddox WA, et al. Metastases to the upper levels of the axillary nodes in carcinoma of the breast and its implications for nodal sampling procedures. Surg Gynecol Obstet 1984;158:255–259.
325. Danforth DN, Findlay PA, McDonald HD, et al. Complete axillary lymph node dissection for stage I-II carcinoma of the breast. J Clin Oncol 1986;4:655–662.
326. Lin PP, Allison DC, Wainstock J, et al. Impact of axillary lymph node dissection on the therapy of breast cancer patients. J Clin Oncol 1993;11:1536–1544.
327. Chadha M, Chabon AB, Friedmann P, et al. Predictors of axillary lymph node metastases in patients with T1 breast cancer: A multivariate analysis. Cancer 1994;73:350–353.
328. Haffty BG, Ward B, Pathare P, et al. Reappraisal of the role of axillary lymph node dissection in the conservative treatment of breast cancer. J Clin Oncol 1997;15:691–700.
329. Griffin AC, Wood WG. Brachial plexitis: A rare and often misdiagnosed postoperative complication. Aesthetic Plast Surg 1996;20:263–265.
330. Merson M, Pirovano C, Balzarini A, et al. The preservation of minor pectoralis muscle in axillary dissection for breast cancer: Functional and cosmetic evaluation. Eur J Surg Oncol 1992;18:215–218.
331. Salmon RJ, Ansquer Y, Asselain B. Preservation versus section of intercostal-brachial nerve (IBN) in axillary dissection for breast cancer—a prospective randomized trial. Eur J Surg Oncol 1998;24(3):158–161.
332. Temple WJ, Ketcham AS. Preservation of the intercostobrachial nerve during axillary dissection for breast cancer. Am J Surg 1985;150(5):585–588.
333. Roses DF, Brooks AD, Harris MN, et al. Complications of level I and II axillary dissection in the treatment of carcinoma of the breast. Ann Surg 1999;230(2):194–201.
334. Burak WE, Goodman PS, Young DC, et al. Seroma formation following axillary dissection for breast cancer: Risk factors and lack of influence of bovine thrombin. J Surg Oncol 1997;64:27–31.
335. Harris MN, Gumport SL, Maiwandi H. Axillary lymph node dissection for melanoma. Surg Gynecol Obstet, 1972;135:936–940.
336. Moore M, Burak WE Jr, Nelson E, et al. Fibrin sealant reduces the duration and amount of fluid drainage after axillary dissection: A randomized prospective clinical trial. J Am Coll Surg 2001;192(5):591–599.
337. Knight CD, Griffen FD, Knight CD. Prevention of seromas in mastectomy wounds. The effect of shoulder immobilization. Arch Surg 1995;130:99–101.
338. Clarke DH, Le MG, Sarrazin D, et al. Analysis of local-regional relapses in patients with early breast cancers treated by excision and radiotherapy. Experience of the Institute Gustave Rousey. Int J Radiat Oncol Biol Phys 1983;71:137–145.
339. Recht A, Silen W, Schnitt SJ, et al. Time-course of local recurrence following conservative surgery and radiotherapy for early stage breast cancer. Int J Radiat Oncol Biol Phys 1988;15:255–261.
340. Kurtz JM, Amalric R, Brandone H, et al. Local recurrence after breast-conserving surgery and radiotherapy: Frequency, time course, and prognosis. Cancer 1989;63:1912–1917.

disease, the immediate reconstruction gives the patient added confidence that the cancer may be cured.

When is delayed reconstruction appropriate?

Despite the many positive aspects of immediate breast reconstruction, certain clinical situations are best treated with delayed reconstruction. When it is uncertain whether radiation therapy will be required, the reconstructive procedure may be delayed until the surgical pathology is reviewed and the radiation decision made. When radiation to the chest wall is required, the chance of achieving a cosmetically successful implant reconstruction is decreased, and these patients are often treated with flap reconstructions after radiation is completed.[21] Cordeiro and colleagues have shown that acceptable results can be achieved with tissue expander–implant reconstruction followed by postoperative radiation therapy when a specific protocol is followed.[22] Flap reconstructions that are subjected to radiation therapy often become suboptimal, with a loss of flap volume and an increased incidence of fat necrosis.

If the viability of the mastectomy skin flaps is questionable at the completion of the mastectomy, it is advisable to delay the reconstruction until healing is complete. This is especially important in patients undergoing tissue expander placement, because skin necrosis and expander exposure can result when necrosis of skin flaps occurs. In patients who smoke, are diabetic, or have collagen-vascular disease, assessment of skin flap viability at the time of mastectomy may be difficult, and great care and selection must be exercised before immediate tissue expander placement.

When there is questionable pathology in the contralateral breast or the patient is considering contralateral mastectomy, it is best to delay the reconstruction because bilateral reconstruction is most successful when both sides are reconstructed in the same operation.

Some patients simply cannot decide whether to undergo reconstruction or what type of reconstruction to have. These patients should be advised to defer reconstruction and be reassured that a successful reconstructive outcome is likely in the future.

What information should be reviewed with the patient before a decision regarding immediate reconstruction?

Often, the patient is referred to the plastic surgeon immediately after the diagnosis of breast cancer and recommendation for a mastectomy. This initial consultation, at which the patient is provided with information that will help her make an educated, informed decision, is very important. The patient is often under great psychological stress and must absorb a tremendous amount of information in a very short period of time. The plastic surgeon must make the breast reconstruction information concise and complete so that the patient can make an informed decision.

If the best choice for reconstruction is to be made, several key questions must be answered before the mastectomy.

1. *What is the risk for cancer's developing in the contralateral breast? Does the contralateral breast require biopsy to* resolve the pathologic issues, which would determine the need for contralateral mastectomy? These issues are important because the approach to bilateral reconstruction might be quite different from the approach to unilateral reconstruction.
2. *Is it feasible to alter the contralateral breast to obtain symmetry, or will the oncologic surgeon or mammographer object, feeling it will interfere with future monitoring?* This decision may alter the technique of breast reconstruction.
3. *Will postoperative chest wall radiation be required?* Radiation can significantly compromise the likelihood of success with reconstruction.
4. *Has the patient definitely decided on mastectomy, or is breast conservation an alternative?* When the reconstructive process is perceived as very complicated, the patient may choose breast conservation.

At the initial consultation, the patient must be given all information about alternatives and expected outcome. Patients undergoing immediate breast reconstruction usually follow the referral guidance of their oncologic surgeon and rarely seek second opinions. Showing the patient photographs of average as well as excellent reconstructions helps the patient understand the spectrum of surgical outcomes. It is also helpful to review diagrams of the surgical procedures with the patient so that she can better comprehend the scope of the surgery.

Facilitating discussion with other patients who have gone through the reconstruction process and the associated decision making is often the most helpful service one can provide. Only when all issues are addressed will the correct reconstructive decision be made. When there is significant uncertainty by either the reconstructive surgeon or the patient, reconstruction should be deferred.

What issues should be discussed with the oncologic surgeon before mastectomy?

During the past 10 years, techniques for breast reconstruction have been refined so that results are better and more reliable. By far, the biggest step toward achieving superior results in breast reconstruction has resulted from the more common use of the skin-sparing mastectomy. Maintaining the intrinsic shape of the breast at the time of mastectomy by sacrificing minimal skin and maintaining the envelope of the breast has allowed the reconstructive surgeon to achieve superior results by all techniques.

Skin-sparing mastectomy has made immediate breast reconstruction a more viable choice for the patient considering mastectomy as the method of treatment for breast cancer. Toth and Lappert in 1991 were the first to report the use of skin-sparing mastectomy with superior aesthetic results.[23]

The goal of a skin-sparing mastectomy is to remove the entire breast parenchyma as well as the nipple–areolar complex while preserving as much breast skin as possible. Because existing biopsy scars must also be removed, it is advisable for the oncologic surgeon to keep these biopsy incisions as close to the areola as possible so as not to require additional skin excision at the time of the mastectomy. Appropriate sentinel lymph node biopsy or axillary lymph node dissection can be performed through either the skin-sparing mastectomy incision or a separate axillary incision.

When the existing skin envelope shape is preserved during the skin-sparing mastectomy, symmetry with the contralateral breast is facilitated. When bilateral mastectomy is performed, removing equal and minimal amounts of skin facilitates symmetry. Carlson and associates in 1998 showed that skin-sparing mastectomy significantly reduced the need for contralateral symmetry procedures in the other breast.[24]

Various types of skin incisions are used to perform a skin-sparing mastectomy. Considerations in choosing the type of incisions include the size of the areola, the size of the breast, the presence of previous biopsy scars, the need to modify the other breast, the type of reconstruction chosen, and the presence of diabetes or a history of cigarette smoking.

The periareolar incision removes the entire nipple–areolar complex as well as a few millimeters of surrounding skin because ductal tissue can extend into the surrounding skin. This incision is ideal when an autologous reconstruction has been chosen and the areola is of adequate size. Care should be taken when using this incision in diabetics or smokers because the viability of the long skin flaps can be compromised. Periareolar incisions with lateral extension can facilitate axillary dissection when additional exposure is required. The modified ellipse incision converts the periareolar incision into an ellipse and is useful when the areola is relatively small, a tissue expander reconstruction has been chosen, or the contralateral breast will be reduced (Fig. 25–1). It is our opinion that the reduction mammoplasty or anchor incisions should be avoided because of the increased incidence of skin flap necrosis. Slavin and coworkers reported using periareolar incisions in 55% of their patients, the periareolar with lateral extension in 27%, the periareolar with medial and lateral extensions in 10%, and the ellipse in 8%.[25] Many of the series reporting on incision selection show a tendency to use the periareolar incision later in their series, as surgeons become more skilled in this technique.[26]

All techniques of breast reconstruction can be used after skin-sparing mastectomy. When tissue expander or implant reconstruction is chosen, the mastectomy incision must be closed primarily, making the modified ellipse the incision of choice. Both TRAM flap and latissimus dorsi flap reconstructions allow closure of the incision using the skin paddle of the flap. Mastectomy skin flap problems are easier to manage with autologous reconstruction than with implant reconstruction.

Studies in the literature show no difference in local recurrence in patients undergoing skin-sparing mastectomy when compared with patients who have undergone non–skin-sparing mastectomy.[27]

The coordinated effort of the oncologic and reconstructive surgeon to preserve native breast skin by performing skin-sparing mastectomy produces superior cosmetic reconstructions without increased oncologic risk or morbidity.

What issues should be considered in determining the type of reconstruction?

Several factors must be considered when selecting the type of breast reconstruction to be performed. When recommending a specific reconstructive technique to the patient, the basic body anatomy, general medical condition, age, risks for contralateral disease, and patient preference as well as expectations all must be evaluated.

Anatomic considerations must include the necessity of altering the contralateral breast with reduction, mastopexy, or augmentation as well as the availability of tissues at the various donor sites. Patients undergoing a long surgical procedure and recovery must be in good general health to minimize operative and postoperative morbidity. Smoking limits the success rates of certain flap techniques for breast reconstruction. A history of diseases, such as diabetes and collagen-vascular disease, that result in microcirculatory impairments may also compromise the success rates of certain flap techniques.

Previous radiation to the chest wall is another important variable because any technique that involves implants has a high failure rate in irradiated tissues.[28] Flap reconstruction is more prone to complications in irradiated tissues, but a satisfactory result is usually possible.[29] Any patient with significant back problems should not undergo a TRAM flap because weakening of the abdominal wall musculature may exacerbate existing dormant back problems. In young patients, an increased risk for contralateral breast cancer over the life span influences the choice of procedure because bilateral reconstructions are best when the same technique has been used on both sides. Certain flap techniques (including TRAM flap) cannot be done a second time if contralateral reconstruction becomes necessary. Older patients do not tolerate complex flap reconstructions as well as younger patients. The patient's expectations for achieving symmetry with a contralateral breast often make certain techniques preferable in specific situations. Ultimately, if the patient is given enough information by the reconstructive surgeon, her preference will be a large factor in technique selection.

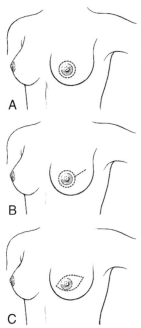

Figure 25–1   Three types of skin-sparing mastectomy incisions. *A,* Periareolar. *B,* Periareolar with lateral extension. *C,* Elliptic.

Recovery time and her feelings about the use of implants may be significant issues.

What are the two basic forms of breast reconstruction?

Techniques for breast reconstruction can loosely be divided into two basic categories: autologous techniques and implant techniques. Autologous, or flap, procedures include TRAM flaps, latissimus dorsi flaps, gluteus maximus flaps, or lateral thigh flaps. All have specific advantages and disadvantages. Implant procedures may be simple implant, tissue expander techniques, or latissimus dorsi flap with implant or tissue expander placement. In general, flap techniques have longer operative times, greater perioperative morbidity, longer recovery time, and more postoperative pain. Flap techniques are basically one-stage procedures, whereas tissue expander procedures involve two stages. Flap techniques are true immediate reconstructions. The patient undergoing simultaneous mastectomy and reconstruction with a flap never experiences the anatomic defect resulting from mastectomy, whereas the patient receiving a tissue expander after a mastectomy is just starting the reconstructive process. The final result of an implant reconstruction is never as soft and pliable as an autologous tissue reconstruction.

Ultimately, all reconstructions are judged on the degree of symmetry with the contralateral breast. A patient with large, ptotic breasts almost always requires reduction or mastopexy of the contralateral breast because the available donor site tissue or the ability to expand the mastectomy site is limited when size and ptosis are the predominant goals. Autologous tissue reconstructions more readily allow for precise symmetry at the expense of additional scars and donor site morbidity. Despite initial concerns, patients reconstructed with flap tissue do not appear to have delayed diagnosis of local or regional recurrence of their breast cancer.[30]

Implant reconstructions tend to have minimal ptosis and often produce a reconstruction that assumes the shape of the implant. These limitations of implant reconstructions may require augmentation of the contralateral breast. Implants may result in interference with future mammograms, a long-term risk in the contralateral breast. In addition, the implants may develop capsular contractures, deflate, or rupture. When mastectomy flaps are thin, the implant may be palpable, or rippling may be visible. The use of the latissimus dorsi myocutaneous flap may add additional camouflage to the implant as well as increased ptosis and shaping not possible with implant reconstructions alone.

The immediate latissimus dorsi flap and implant reconstruction essentially skips the expansion phase with its inherent delay and morbidity. The latissimus dorsi is often an excellent choice when previous radiation has been administered or the patient has underlying microcirculatory problems.

Understanding the patient's goals and priorities is essential. Often, patients will compromise their expectations in favor of a simple, less complicated technique. Defining the patient's needs is an important part of the reconstructive surgeon's evaluation. Understanding the limitations and expected results of the techniques available is important so that the patient can make an informed decision.

IMPLANT BREAST RECONSTRUCTION

What are the limitations of one-stage implant reconstruction?

The simple placement of an implant for breast reconstruction, either as an immediate procedure or as a delayed procedure, is a one-stage technique with minimal morbidity. The indications for this procedure were reduced significantly with the development of textured, anatomically shaped tissue expanders. Freeman in 1962 and 1969[31,32] and Snyderman and Guthrie in 1971[33] described the subcutaneous placement of an implant after mastectomy. In 1981, Gruber[34] reported that submuscular breast reconstruction significantly lowered the risk for capsular contracture. The development of the Becker expander-implant facilitated a one-stage implant reconstruction technique.[35] The Becker device can serve as both an expander and a final implant, making it possible to offer a one-stage procedure to a larger percentage of patients.

In the immediate breast reconstruction setting, several factors may make simple implant placement difficult. The immediate placement of an implant of adequate size to achieve symmetry with the contralateral breast may be impossible because of soft tissue deficiency or questionably viable skin flaps. It may be necessary to place a smaller implant initially and later exchange it for a larger one. This approach offers minimal, if any, benefit over two-stage tissue expander techniques.

In the delayed reconstruction setting, it may be easier to place an implant of adequate size. The ultimate result, however, is often inferior to a two-stage expander-implant reconstruction. Creation of a well-demarcated inframammary fold and maintaining adequate breast projection at the correct level may be difficult. When any degree of ptosis is present, the ability to simulate this ptosis is enhanced by placing a tissue expander low and then, at the second stage, creating a properly positioned inframammary fold while maintaining adequate breast projection. In selected cases in which the contralateral breast is small, there is no ptosis, and the inframammary fold is indistinct, simple implant placement may be adequate. Often, even in these cases, too much upper-pole breast fullness is created on the reconstructed side after the implant is placed.

Most one-stage implant breast reconstructions, whether done using the Becker implant-expander or simple implant, would benefit from a second procedure to reposition the implant and create a more distinct inframammary fold.

When previous chest wall radiation has been given or is planned postoperatively, achieving a long-term successful reconstruction by implant placement techniques is less likely.[21]

Early experience in breast reconstruction with smooth-surfaced tissue expanders demonstrated a high incidence of capsular contracture during the expansion phase that ultimately limited full expansion. During the period of time that these devices were used, simple implant reconstruction offered several theoretical advantages because capsular contracture rates were initially much lower when simple implants were placed submuscularly. The development of textured, anatomically shaped tissue expanders and implants decreased the risk for capsular contracture.[36] The improved contour has made simple implant reconstruction an infrequent procedure.

TISSUE EXPANDER–IMPLANT TECHNIQUE

What are the advantages of tissue expander–implant reconstruction?

In 1957, Charles G. Neumann, while working in the Department of Surgery at New York University, fashioned a balloon to a polyethylene tube and expanded the scalp to reconstruct the upper two thirds of a traumatically avulsed ear.[37] This single case report documents the first clinical use of tissue expansion, but the era of tissue expansion in breast reconstruction did not begin until more than 20 years later, when Chadomer Radovan presented his experience with this technique.[38] At about the same time, William Grabb[39] performed clinical studies using the breast tissue expander device. Since that time, numerous laboratory and clinical studies have helped to define the role of tissue expansion in both general reconstructive surgery and breast reconstruction.[37,40–42]

Trends toward more conservative mastectomies create new challenges for the reconstructive surgeon. Basic principles of reconstruction always favor the use of autologous tissues with similar color, texture, and subcutaneous fat. The postmastectomy defect lacks both skin and underlying breast mound. The skin envelope must have adequate laxity to allow the breast mound to project sufficiently and remain soft in consistency. When possible, careful planning with the oncologic surgeon, at the time of the mastectomy, makes the achievement of these goals easier. The smaller mastectomy defect and the ability to begin reconstruction at the time of mastectomy make tissue expansion a prime method to reconstruct the absent breast. The tissue expander is an ideal tool to prepare the remaining mastectomy skin to receive a permanent prosthesis.

Advances in tissue expander design have simplified the expansion procedure and made it more predictable and successful. Complete expansion has become easier; with the development of textured surfaces on the expander, the capsular response has been decreased during the expansion phase.[36] The texture also helps to prevent expander movement or migration during expansion. This allows for maximum expansion in precise areas. The introduction of an anatomic shape to the expander allows preferential expansion of the lower pole of the breast skin.

Who are appropriate candidates for tissue expansion reconstruction?

In general, patients with small, minimally ptotic breasts who have undergone a total mastectomy are good candidates for tissue expander reconstruction. Patients with large, ptotic breasts will require significant modification of the contralateral breast to achieve symmetry. Furthermore, recurrence of ptosis in the larger breast may make an initial good result deteriorate over time.

Which patients are not candidates for tissue expansion reconstruction?

Patients who have inadequate soft tissue after mastectomy to cover the tissue expander are not candidates for tissue expander–implant reconstructions. The radical mastectomy patient, with thin flaps and absent pectoralis major muscle, requires the addition of soft tissue and is not a candidate for tissue expander–implant reconstruction. Other patients who have undergone extensive skin excisions with tight closure and thin flaps are also better treated with flap reconstructions. Patients who have undergone previous breast-conserving surgery with radiation therapy as part of their treatment and patients who require postoperative chest wall radiation following a mastectomy also are less ideal candidates for tissue expander–implant reconstructions. Radiation injury to the chest wall tissues makes adequate expansion difficult and increases the risks for expander or implant complications, such as infection, implant exposure, rib fracture, and capsular contracture.[21,28] Alternative, usually autologous, reconstructive techniques are chosen for these patients. If one chooses to use tissue expansion in irradiated patients, both patient and surgeon must be prepared to abandon the technique if complications occur. A secondary plan should be available for completion of the reconstruction. Many of these cases can be successfully salvaged with a latissimus dorsi flap or other autologous reconstruction.

To achieve maximum symmetry with an implant reconstruction may require significant alteration of the contralateral breast by mastopexy, augmentation, or reduction. These issues must be considered and discussed with the patient, oncologic surgeon, and mammographer before reconstruction.

What issues in operative planning for immediate implant reconstruction should be considered by the oncologic surgeon?

Every effort should be made to develop healthy skin flaps, of uniform thickness, during the mastectomy. Ischemic flaps will delay healing of the incision and limit the uniform skin expansion required to achieve a good result. As discussed in Chapter 24, very long flaps, created to preserve large amounts of native breast skin, should be avoided. Rather, the goal should be to provide enough skin to comfortably close the incision without redundancy. Traditional guidelines for skin excision should be followed, adhering to standard oncologic principles. When bilateral mastectomy is being performed, every effort should be made to perform symmetrical skin excisions. Careful preoperative discussion with the oncologic surgeon is essential to achieve good results using this technique of reconstruction (Fig. 25–2).

What are the considerations in choosing the type of expander?

An anatomically shaped tissue expander with a textured surface and integrated port is desirable. Previous experience with smooth-surface expanders resulted in capsular contracture in

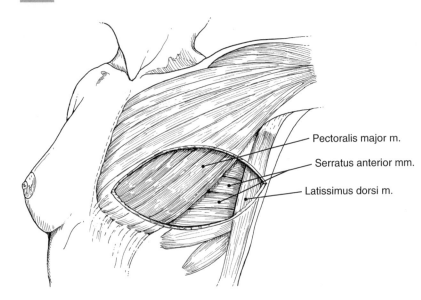

Pectoralis major m.

Serratus anterior mm.

Latissimus dorsi m.

Figure 25–2   Chest wound after mastectomy.

a significant number of patients,[40–43] which limited full expansion and the creation of a soft, pliable skin envelope of adequate size to accept the final implant. The anatomic shape allows for preferential expansion of the lower pole skin, thus achieving adequate anterior projection in the reconstructed breast. The use of an expander with an integrated port, rather than a remote port, makes the expansion process less painful because the skin over the integrated port is usually anesthetic, whereas the skin over a remote port has sensibility. Complications of port malfunction are also less likely with the integrated port.

The primary consideration when choosing the size of the tissue expander to be used is the width of the contralateral breast. One should always choose a tissue expander at least as wide as the contralateral breast. Smaller expanders are used in patients with narrow breasts, and larger sizes are used in patients with wider breasts. When bilateral mastectomy has been or is being performed, the size of the tissue expander is based on the preexisting base width, unless the patient prefers to have smaller or larger breasts. This discussion is part of the preoperative consultation with the patient.

What preoperative measures are taken with tissue expansion reconstruction?

With the patient standing, the inframammary fold position of the contralateral breast is marked, and a line is drawn to the middle of the chest. With the patient standing and examined from the side, the point of maximum breast projection is noted, as well as the breast's position relative to the inframammary fold. In the immediate reconstruction patient, alteration of the contralateral breast by mastopexy, reduction, or augmentation is performed during the implant exchange procedure. When a delayed reconstruction is being performed, the symmetry procedure may be performed at the time of the initial tissue expander placement. The future expected position of maximum breast projection is planned at the time of the expander placement. The location of the point of maximum breast projection is important because the tissue expander will be positioned so that the maximum anteroposterior expansion will be achieved to correspond to the point of

maximum breast projection on the unoperated breast. This may require positioning the expander several centimeters below the inframammary fold during the initial procedure. The single most important determinant for ultimate success of breast reconstruction using these techniques is achieving maximum anteroposterior expansion at the point of maximum breast projection. The end point of the expansion process is when adequate projection, rather than a specific volume, is achieved.

What intraoperative measures are taken with tissue expansion reconstruction?

Positioning of the expander must allow for maximum expansion at the desired level as well as the ultimate achievement of a normal inframammary fold. To achieve these two goals, the lower flap must frequently be undermined in the subcutaneous plane to a level inferior to the inframammary fold of the contralateral breast. This position is determined as discussed previously. To achieve a normal inframammary fold, the lower one third of the tissue expander is usually not covered with muscle. Close approximation of the dermis of the lower flap to the chest wall may be required at the second-stage operation to achieve a normal inframammary fold; therefore, any extra thickness of tissue in the inframammary fold should be avoided. The upper two thirds of the tissue expander are placed subpectorally. Other authors prefer total muscle coverage of the expander.[44] We have found that total muscle coverage is unnecessary and often does not allow complete expansion, resulting in a poor aesthetic result.

In the immediate-reconstruction setting, if the skin flaps are questionably viable, the placement of the expander is aborted and performed as a delayed procedure. This avoids the postoperative complication of tissue expander exposure and infection.

When an immediate reconstruction is being performed, the pectoralis major muscle is divided transversely where it joins the anterior rectus sheath. This division is continued medially and superiorly along the origin of the pectoralis major muscle to allow for adequate medial expansion (Fig. 25–3A and B). Most often, the tissue expander is filled with

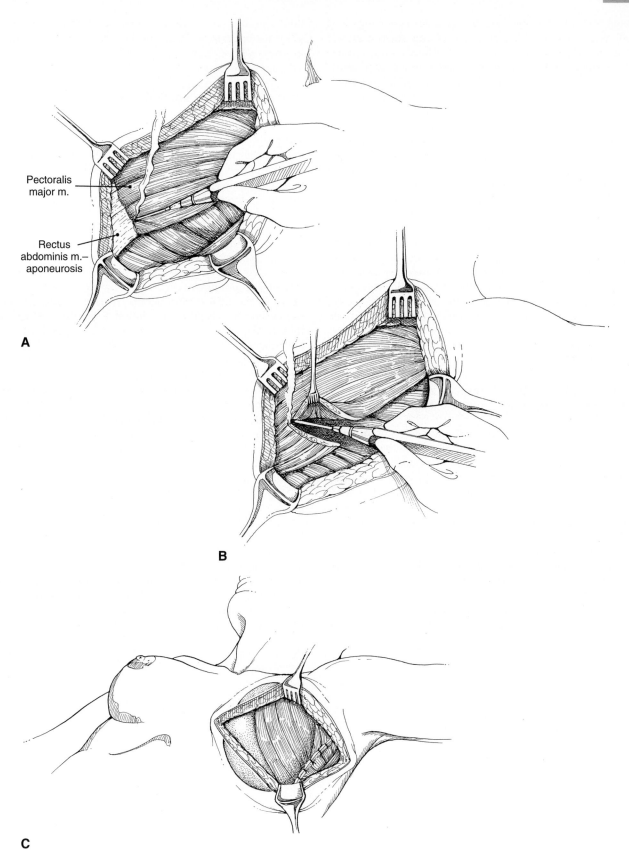

Pectoralis
major m.

Rectus
abdominis m.–
aponeurosis

A

B

C

Figure 25–3   *A* and *B,* Transection of the medial pectoralis major muscle to place the tissue expander. *C,* Pectoralis major muscle sutured to the serratus anterior muscle over the tissue expander.

about 100 mL of saline, and the pectoralis major muscle is redraped and sutured lateral to the serratus anterior muscle using absorbable sutures (Fig. 25–3C). These sutures stabilize the expander in its position, prevent lateral migration of the expander, and reestablish the anterior axillary fold. If an axillary dissection has been performed, two closed-suction drains are used. Otherwise, only one drain is used. Skin closure is performed in two layers using interrupted buried dermal sutures and interrupted or intracuticular skin sutures. Aggressive postoperative trimming of questionable skin edges will minimize the risk for expander exposure as well as allow for expansion to begin as early as possible.

When a tissue expander is being placed as a delayed procedure, the same technique of muscle covering the upper two thirds of the expander is employed. The lower flap, in the region of the inframammary crease, is frequently thinned by either direct vision or liposuction. More fluid is placed into the tissue expander than in the immediate-reconstruction setting, and expansion is begun earlier. Wound closure is more often done with a subcuticular suture after reapproximation of the deeper tissues. A drain is usually placed for 24 to 48 hours to minimize fluid collection and maximize the chances for tissue adherence to the tissue expander.

What postoperative measures are taken with tissue expansion reconstruction?

When a tissue expander is placed immediately, the patient is usually sent home with the drains in place, and the drains are removed in the office in 5 to 7 days. Repeated aspiration of postoperative seromas is to be avoided whenever possible because this will increase the risk for infection and possible expander perforation. The only seromas aspirated are axillary seromas, and this is done following immediate reconstruction. All patients receive 1 week of antibiotics. Limited use of the ipsilateral arm is allowed during the first 2 weeks, and all range-of-motion exercises are delayed for this period of time. Skin sutures are removed in 2 weeks, and expansion is usually begun at that time.

When a tissue expander is being placed as a delayed procedure, a drain is usually placed for 24 to 48 hours to minimize

fluid collection and maximize the chances for tissue adherence to the tissue expander. Range-of-motion exercises are begun 5 to 7 days after surgery.

What guidelines are followed for the expansion phase?

The goals of expansion are to achieve an adequate skin envelope for the permanent implant. This will result in a soft, pliable, natural-appearing breast. The amount of overexpansion must be adjusted based on the thickness of the skin flaps and the type of implant that will ultimately be used. All implants may ripple, and this may be visible through the skin. The tendency for rippling is greater with saline implants, especially when placed under thin flaps. When saline implants are used and the flaps are thick, overexpansion by 25% to 30% is recommended. This allows for trimming of excess skin at the exchange procedure, potentially creating a better-shaped breast in the final reconstruction. When the flaps are thin, overexpansion is kept to a minimum. Expansion will tend to thin the flaps further and accentuate visible rippling. In general, silicone implants have less rippling than saline implants, but the same general principles for overexpansion apply to patients receiving silicone implants.

In the immediate setting, when chemotherapy is being given, the exchange procedure is not done until the chemotherapy has been completed and the patient's laboratory values have returned to normal. In these cases, the final stages of expansion are delayed until chemotherapy is nearly completed. If an expander has been placed and the patient must receive chest wall radiation, the expander is usually fully expanded before radiation treatments begin. The patient's local response to radiation is followed closely. Removal of saline should be considered if the local reaction is severe and the health of the expanded skin is jeopardized.

In most circumstances, expansion is done weekly in the office using sterile technique and a 23-gauge butterfly needle. The end point for expansion is achievement of adequate anteroposterior projection (or slight overprojection) (Fig. 25–4). The patient's breast is allowed to remain fully expanded for 1 month before the exchange procedure.

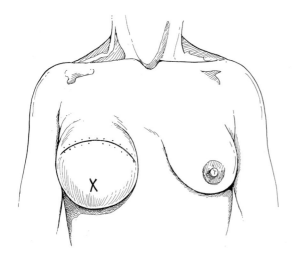
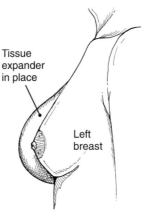

Tissue expander in place

Left breast

Figure 25–4 Appearance of the chest after completion of the tissue expansion process.

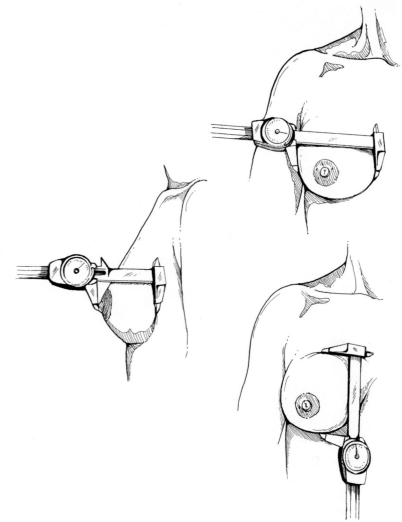

Figure 25–5 Measurement of the contralateral breast before selection of the permanent breast implant.

How is the appropriate implant selected for the exchange procedure?

The first consideration in planning the exchange procedure is choosing the appropriate implant. Available implants are either round or anatomically shaped. Anatomic implants are available in numerous shapes that vary in width, height, and projection. Evaluation of the contralateral breast is key to choosing an implant for exchange. When previous modification of the contralateral breast has been performed by reduction or mastopexy, the exchange procedure should be done only after enough time has elapsed to allow the modified breast to settle into a stable position. If modification of the normal breast is planned at the time of implant placement, its final shape and volume must be predicted at this stage to facilitate implant selection. The goals at placement of the permanent implant are to match the width, height, projection, and volume of the contralateral breast (Fig. 25–5). A general idea of the volume can be estimated by knowing the volume in the expander that matched the volume of the existing breast. Width, height, and projection are measured and the appropriate implant selected from available charts. One should always have many different-sized implants available at the exchange procedure. Saline implants look best when they are slightly overfilled, thus minimizing rippling. Often, the asymmetrical orientation of an anatomic implant will help match the contralateral breast shape.

What are the guidelines for inserting the implant?

Creation of an appropriately positioned and contoured inframammary fold is important. Preoperatively, the inframammary fold position of the contralateral side is marked with the patient standing. These marks are transferred to the expanded side. The expander is removed through the mastectomy incision, and the new inframammary fold position is liposuctioned through two or three small access incisions in the future inframammary crease. This removes any excess subcutaneous tissue, facilitating close approximation of dermis to chest wall. Several 1½-inch, 25-gauge needles are passed through the skin into the expanded pocket at the inframammary fold position (Fig. 25–6A). Using the needles as a guide, the operator sutures the capsule on the anterior surface of the pocket to the capsule on the chest wall with monofilament sutures. An effort is made to attach the dermis of the anterior flap to the chest wall. Although this maneuver often produces

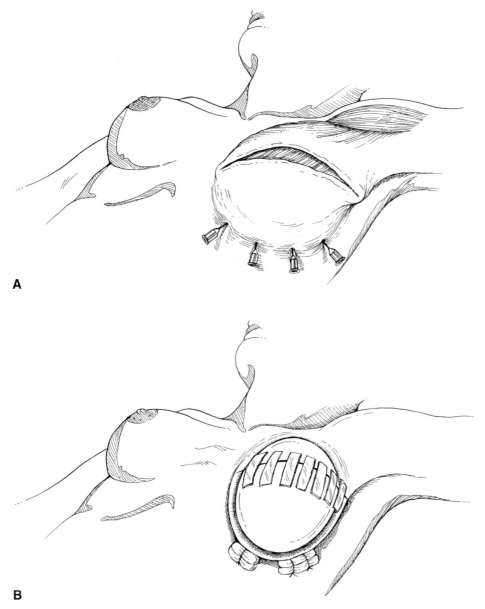

A

B

Figure 25–6 *A*, Marking the inframammary fold with needles as a guide to suturing the anterior and posterior capsules together. *B*, Appearance of the chest after placement of the permanent breast prosthesis.

dimpling of the skin, this dimpling ultimately resolves in 3 to 6 months. Multiple sutures are placed internally, and often external bolsters are added to reinforce the attachment of the anterior capsule to the chest wall (Fig. 25-6B). Capsulotomy and capsulectomy are performed whenever and wherever necessary, and the implant is filled to the appropriate volume with the patient in the sitting position on the operating table. Excess skin is then trimmed along the mastectomy incision to enhance shape and maximize projection. Final shape is more a function of the shape of the implant than the shape of the skin envelope. Overexpansion facilitates the ability to trim skin at the second procedure. When extensive capsulotomy or capsulectomy has been necessary, a closed-suction drain is placed.

Postoperatively, activity is restricted for 2 weeks, and the patient receives prophylactic antibiotics for 7 days. External bolsters are removed after about 5 to 7 days. The skin under the external bolsters must be monitored frequently to avoid pressure necrosis during the immediate postoperative period.

When extensive contralateral breast reduction surgery is performed, an adjustable implant should be considered on the reconstructed side to facilitate future size changes postoperatively. The ports on these adjustable implants are easily removed in the office (Fig. 25–7).

What are the potential complications of tissue expansion reconstructions?

In the immediate breast reconstruction setting, assessment of skin flap viability at the completion of the mastectomy is very important, especially in smokers, in whom microcirculatory compromise is likely. Any marginally perfused tissues should be trimmed to healthy tissue. In rare situations, fluorescein can be helpful to assess questionable areas of viability. If the plastic surgeon is still unsure about the viability of the skin flaps, immediate placement of a tissue expander should be abandoned and delayed reconstruction planned after primary

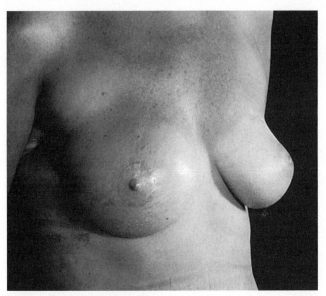

Figure 25–7 A patient after reconstruction with a tissue expander and breast prosthesis.

healing has occurred. Aggressive skin edge trimming, early in the postoperative period, will prevent expander exposure as well as minimize the time for wound healing. This allows inflation of the expander to begin as early as possible. If the expander is exposed in the early postoperative period, removal is recommended to avoid infection and potential systemic complications.

The early diagnosis and treatment of a hematoma is essential. If left untreated, a hematoma will increase the risk for capsular contracture and infection and make adequate expansion difficult.

When infection becomes apparent, antibiotic therapy should be instituted as soon as possible. Initial infection most often presents as cellulitis of the breast skin and only secondarily involves the expander pocket. Once the expander pocket is involved, the infection behaves like an abscess and requires removal of the expander, drainage of the space, and antibiotics. Replacement of the expander is delayed for 3 to 6 months until the tissues are soft and freely moveable over the chest wall. When the expander is replaced, organism-specific antibiotics are used. The risk for infection is increased in patients who have had prior radiation therapy or lymph node dissection.[45]

Capsular contracture during the expander phase can prevent full expansion. In the past, expansion with smooth expanders often resulted in significant capsular response. Expansion often needed to be abandoned because of discomfort and the inability to create a soft skin envelope of adequate size and projection to receive the final implant. At the time of implant placement, near-total capsulectomy was required to obtain a good result. The development of textured expanders has significantly decreased the incidence of capsular contracture during expansion. The tissue adherence between the expander surface and the envelope results in a thin, pliable capsule, making capsulectomy unnecessary at the time of implant placement. Infection, hematoma, and seroma are still significant causes of increased capsular response and contracture, despite the textured surface on the expanders.

Seroma formation may occur after mastectomy with or without axillary dissection. Proper drain placement at mastectomy and proper management of these drains can minimize seroma formation. Drains should remain in place long enough to minimize seroma formation. Nevertheless, seroma formation will occur in a significant number of cases following immediate placement of tissue expanders. Careful aspiration of the seroma by the plastic surgeon will be required. When a tissue expander is present, the risk for perforation with aspiration requires careful technique away from the expander surface. Repeated aspirations also increase the risk for infection within the expander envelope, which can result in an increased capsular response or even abscess formation.

Using small-gauge needles during inflation and carefully aspirating any seroma can minimize loss of volume in the expander during the expansion phase. Significant deflations require replacement of the tissue expander. Permanent saline implants may deflate at any time after their placement. These deflations are most often due to valve malfunction. Tissue ingrowth into the implant valve can make the implant valve incompetent, allowing for slow loss of saline from the implant. Newer valves are being developed to make deflations less likely. Care must be taken to ensure that the valve is sealed after the implant is filled.

Rib fracture is a rare complication of tissue expansion and most often occurs if the chest wall has been irradiated. Avoidance of tissue expanders in irradiated patients, as well as slow expansion and careful monitoring in nonirradiated patients, should eliminate this complication. If significant localized pain develops during expansion, the status of the underlying rib should be evaluated by radiographs. If a rib fracture is present, the tissue expander should be removed and other reconstructive techniques offered to the patient.

LATISSIMUS DORSI MYOCUTANEOUS FLAP RECONSTRUCTION

Initial attempts to reconstruct the radical mastectomy defect using silicone implants were often unsuccessful because of the absent pectoralis major muscle and thin skin. In 1976, the pedicled latissimus dorsi musculocutaneous flap was used for the treatment of radiation necrosis of the chest wall.[46] In 1977, the latissimus dorsi was used as an island pedicle flap for breast reconstruction.[47,48] The large, fan-shaped muscle could be completely transposed anteriorly to replace the absent pectoralis major muscle and re-create the anterior axillary fold, as well as provide a well-vascularized muscle and skin envelope to receive an implant. The skin island, when properly designed, could replace the skin removed at mastectomy. Initially, a smooth silicone implant was placed under the latissimus dorsi muscle, and significant incidence of capsular contracture resulted.[36,49,50] With the development of the TRAM flap, which did not require an implant, the latissimus dorsi flap became a secondary reconstructive choice. The development of textured implants, as well as expanders, has decreased the incidence of capsular contracture significantly.[36,50] In selected cases, when adequate subcutaneous fat is available over the latissimus dorsi muscle, no implant is required, and a total autologous breast reconstruction is possible.[51–54] Despite the trend toward less radical cancer surgery, the latissimus dorsi myocutaneous flap still plays a significant role in breast reconstruction.

Who is a candidate for latissimus dorsi flap reconstruction?

Patients who require the addition of autologous tissue to achieve breast symmetry with implants or who are not good candidates for TRAM flap reconstruction may benefit from the latissimus dorsi flap. The patient who has a large skin requirement at the mastectomy site and ptosis in the contralateral breast is usually best treated by autologous tissue techniques rather than by tissue expander and implant techniques. When the TRAM flap or another autologous tissue donor site is not an option because of lack of tissue, previous surgery, smoking, obesity, diabetes mellitus, or collagen-vascular disease, then the latissimus dorsi flap can be reliably used. The blood supply to the latissimus dorsi flap is excellent, even in patients with a compromised microcirculation. It is rare to have total or partial loss of a latissimus dorsi flap.

What are the advantages of latissimus dorsi flap reconstruction?

The latissimus dorsi flap and implant offers several advantages over tissue expander–implant techniques. The latissimus dorsi skin component replaces the skin removed at mastectomy and avoids the morbidity of tissue expansion. The latissimus dorsi flap provides a true, immediate breast reconstruction completed in one stage at the time of mastectomy. The latissimus dorsi muscle provides an envelope of tissue under the mastectomy skin. Ripples are less visible when a latissimus dorsi flap is used. This technique can often salvage a cosmetically poor tissue expander–implant reconstruction. When a tissue expander has been placed and chest wall radiation is required postoperatively, adequate expansion is often difficult to achieve.[21,28] In these cases, the addition of a latissimus dorsi flap can salvage a reasonable cosmetic result. Patients who have undergone breast conservation and develop tumor recurrence require total mastectomy. If the TRAM flap donor site is not available, the latissimus dorsi flap with an implant is a good second choice.

What are the anatomic considerations in latissimus dorsi flap reconstruction?

The latissimus dorsi muscle receives its primary blood supply from the thoracodorsal artery, a branch of the subscapular artery (Fig. 25–8). This single vessel runs deep to the insertion of the muscle, freely separated from the muscle at this level. The artery enters the muscle at the mid-scapular level and quickly branches within the muscle.[55] Musculocutaneous perforators provide blood supply to the skin over the muscle. A branch from the proximal thoracodorsal artery supplies the serratus muscle. When the proximal thoracodorsal vessel has been divided, the serratus branch will usually provide adequate blood supply to the latissimus dorsi muscle through retrograde flow from the intercostal vessels.[56,57] The abundant blood supply to both the muscle and the overlying skin allows for numerous flap design options to solve many clinical problems in breast reconstruction.

What are the preoperative considerations in planning a latissimus dorsi flap reconstruction?

A complete evaluation of the reconstructive requirements of the chest wall is an essential part of the planning of all types of breast reconstruction. It is especially important when a latissimus dorsi myocutaneous flap is being used. The volume of autologous tissue available with this flap is limited, and its positioning on the chest wall is critical to achieve a good cosmetic result.

The upper chest wall contour depends primarily on the adequacy of the pectoralis major muscle. The pectoralis major muscle is absent in the radical mastectomy patient, and even in the modified radical mastectomy patient, pectoralis major atrophy can occur secondary to denervation during axillary dissection. Reestablishment of a symmetrical upper chest wall contour takes high priority and may require de-epithelialization and subcutaneous placement of the skin flap paddle. Anterior axillary fold contour may need reconstruction. Transposition of the entire latissimus dorsi muscle with anterior positioning of its insertion enables reconstruction of the anterior axillary fold. The location and orientation of the mastectomy scar should be noted. The preferred final position of the skin island is in the lower lateral aspect of the reconstructed breast. High incisions and vertical incisions are best left alone when planning the flap inset. In these cases, a new incision should be planned so that an inferolateral inset is possible. When the chest wall has been irradiated, the skin requirements may be significantly greater than expected preoperatively. In situations in which the skin requirements are greater than can be provided by the latissimus dorsi skin island, a tissue expander, rather than an implant, should be placed at the time of flap transfer.

Evaluation of the latissimus dorsi muscle, subcutaneous tissue, and skin laxity is important. When the examination reveals that the latissimus dorsi muscle has been denervated at the time of axillary dissection, the thoracodorsal vessels have most likely been divided. Transfer of the musculocutaneous unit must then be based on the serratus branch of the thoracodorsal vessels, which will perfuse the flap through the intercostal vessels.[57] The need to base the flap on serratus vessels may limit the arc of rotation of the muscle and the ability to transfer the entire muscle anteriorly. This will limit the amount of tissue available for reconstruction, and an alternative reconstruction might be considered. The vascularity of the flap may also be significantly less when the flap is transferred on these secondary vessels. If a patient is a smoker, is diabetic, or has any other systemic microcirculatory disorders, partial or complete flap loss is more likely.

The laxity of the skin on the back is quite variable, as is the orientation of the greatest skin-laxity axis. When designing the skin island, these factors must be considered. Some patients have large amounts of subcutaneous fat, either just below the posterior axillary fold or lower on the back. Incorporating the subcutaneous fat excess under the skin island can add a large amount of autologous tissue to the flap and simplify the reconstruction.

Th
free
doub
flap
well
smol
may
TRA
doub
rectu
abdc
patie
prev
This
musc

**WI
in**

The
fat p
supe
rior
and
size
and
fron
and
thre
of tl
the
is cl
of tl

Fig
mu:

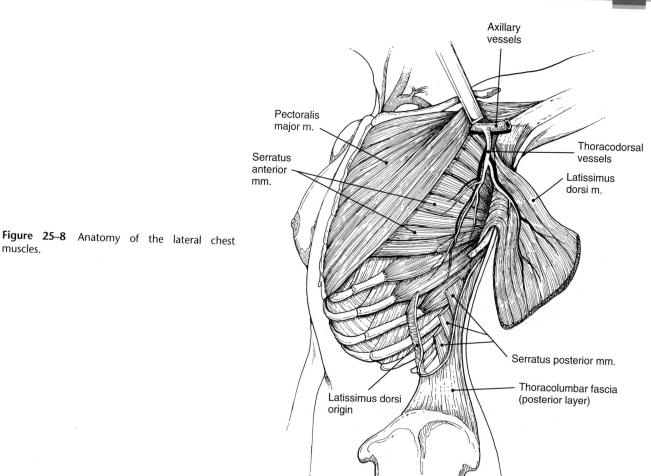

Figure 25–8 Anatomy of the lateral chest muscles.

(labels on figure: Axillary vessels; Pectoralis major m.; Serratus anterior mm.; Thoracodorsal vessels; Latissimus dorsi m.; Serratus posterior mm.; Thoracolumbar fascia (posterior layer); Latissimus dorsi origin)

What guidelines are followed when designing the skin island?

Various skin island designs are possible (Fig. 25–9). The orientation of the skin island is based on several variables. The best cosmetic scar is obtained when the long axis of the flap follows the natural lines of the skin of the back (see Fig. 25–9A). Frequently, a wide skin paddle with generous subcutaneous tissue can be obtained by this design. When there is excess skin and subcutaneous tissue at the posterior axillary fold, a fleur-de-lis pattern over this site will maximize the transfer of autologous tissue[58] (see Fig. 25–9B). Another useful skin island position is a vertically oriented skin paddle placed laterally on the back. This design allows for easy inset of the skin island lateral to and low on the anterior chest wall (see Fig. 25–9C). Complete muscle coverage both above and below the implant is possible, and a visible scar directly on the back is avoided. One must be prepared to modify any of these designs based on the reconstructive objectives. When elevating the latissimus dorsi myocutaneous flap, additional subcutaneous tissue can be harvested by beveling the incision through the subcutaneous tissue to incorporate large amounts of fat over the entire muscle surface. When this is performed over extensive areas of the back, consideration must be given to the effect on the subcutaneous tissue blood supply and ultimate healing of the donor site scar. With extensive harvest of tissue, donor site healing may be compromised.[54] A true autologous breast reconstruction, not requiring an implant, can sometimes be achieved by including extensive subcutaneous fat with the muscle flap.[51–54] Usually, a small implant is still required to assist with breast projection.

In general, the donor site from a latissimus dorsi skin island 10 cm in width or less can easily be closed primarily without undue skin tension. If a larger skin island is required, a tissue expander may be required under the latissimus dorsi muscle before flap elevation to facilitate primary closure of the donor site. When a tissue expander is placed under the transposed musculocutaneous flap, a textured expander is preferable because it will allow for less capsular response and ultimately a softer, more pliable skin envelope. When a permanent prosthesis is placed, an adjustable implant is sometimes preferable to allow for small postoperative adjustments of implant volume and to maximize symmetry. This is especially important if a symmetry procedure is done on the contralateral breast at the same time as flap placement.

What are the intraoperative considerations before commencing the latissimus dorsi flap reconstruction?

When a latissimus dorsi myocutaneous flap is being used for immediate reconstruction, the width of the skin removed at mastectomy is noted, and an attempt to replace this exact

mastectomy specimen can also be measured. All data that are available should be used to try to match the defect that is created. The skin replacement must be as close to exact as possible. If an inappropriate amount of skin is present in the mediolateral dimension, the breast will appear too wide or too narrow. If the amount of skin in the superoinferior dimension is wrong, the breast will have either too much or too little ptosis. It is always helpful if the oncologic surgeon saves as much skin as possible in the medial portion of the breast. This will allow preservation of the cleavage fold.

After the defect and the chest wall are assessed, the abdomen must be evaluated. The location of scars, the amount of fat, and the abdominal wall strength need to be noted. Pedicled TRAM flap is not possible if the patient has had bilateral subcostal incisions. A unilateral subcostal scar will prevent the use of a pedicle from that side. The presence of a unilateral subcostal scar does not preclude the use of the muscle on the other side. Patients who have undergone abdominoplasty surgery are not candidates for TRAM flaps.

The amount of fat available in the abdomen must be evaluated. The patient should be asked to tighten the abdominal wall to assess how much of the abdominal fat is extrafascial. The amount of fat present on one side of the abdomen must be estimated. Is this fat enough to reconstruct the breast with a single pedicle? If there is not enough fat available on one side of the abdomen, consideration must be made for a double-bipedicled TRAM flap reconstruction or a microvascular free flap. The strength of the abdominal wall must be assessed. If the abdominal wall is weak and lax, particularly below the arcuate line, then the TRAM flap should be placed higher on the abdomen. In addition, the weaker the abdomen, the more likely that the patient will require closure of the wound with prosthetic material. All patients should be told about the possibility that prosthetic material may be used for abdominal wall closure. Many patients who are undergoing TRAM flap reconstruction expect a totally autologous reconstruction. These patients should be aware that prosthetic material is frequently used to close the abdomen.

Are all abdominal scars a contraindication to TRAM flap reconstruction?

If bilateral subcostal scars are present, a microvascular free TRAM flap should be considered. Midline scars are not a contraindication to the TRAM flap. The presence of a midline scar will make the tissue contralateral to the pedicle unusable for the reconstruction. If more tissue than is available on one side of the abdomen is needed for breast reconstruction, then either a double-pedicled or free TRAM flap should be considered.

Appendectomy scars are usually not a contraindication to TRAM flap breast reconstruction. The position and length of appendectomy scars vary among patients. For right breast reconstruction, using a TRAM flap with a left rectus abdominis pedicle, there is usually sufficient tissue for the reconstruction, with all tissue lateral to the appendectomy scar discarded. For left breast reconstruction, there occasionally are problems with the right rectus abdominis pedicle after appendectomy. One might consider using a left rectus abdominis pedicle. If a right rectus abdominis pedicle is used, the appendectomy scar must be very lateral. All tissue lateral to

the appendectomy scar must be considered to be unreliable. A double-bipedicled or microvascular TRAM flap may be indicated in this situation.

What are the considerations in selecting the location of the TRAM flap on the abdomen?

The lower abdominal fat is the ideal tissue to be used in TRAM flap reconstruction. This is the area where most women have a fatty deposit. Also, the lower TRAM flap provides the ideal scar and the ideal abdominal aesthetic result. In cases in which unilateral tissue is adequate to reconstruct the breast, the lower abdominal TRAM flap is usually satisfactory.

Unfortunately, the lower abdominal TRAM flap is the most poorly vascularized in a single superior pedicled TRAM formation. When the patient is obese, smokes, or has complicated medical problems, one should consider placing the pedicled TRAM flap in either the mid-abdominal position or the upper abdominal position. Raising the TRAM flap on the abdomen increases the vascularity of the pedicled flap. However, as one raises the TRAM flap on the abdomen, the most useful infraumbilical fat is more likely to be excluded from the flap.

Another consideration is that as the TRAM flap is raised on the abdomen, the rotation of the pedicle and therefore the flap onto the chest becomes more difficult. In the mid-abdominal or upper abdominal position, ipsilateral flaps rotate onto the chest more easily than contralateral flaps because there is a shorter distance to travel. Therefore, when the TRAM flap is placed higher on the abdomen, an ipsilateral pedicle should be considered.

What determines the number and choice of TRAM flap pedicles?

The single-pedicled TRAM flap offers less destruction and subsequent weakness to the abdominal wall than the double-pedicled TRAM flap.[62] The single-pedicled TRAM flap is limited by the amount of tissue that can be carried for breast reconstruction. This tissue becomes more limited when the patient has additional risk factors, such as smoking, obesity, or other medical problems, that may decrease the vascularity of the flap, resulting in partial flap loss.[67] In these patients, or when the volume of tissue required to fill the mastectomy defect is greater than can be carried with a single-pedicled TRAM flap, a double-pedicled or microvascular free TRAM flap is indicated. Patients who have had chest wall radiation should have the best-vascularized tissue used for breast reconstruction: double-pedicled TRAM flap or microvascular free flap. The double-pedicled TRAM flap causes much more weakness to the abdominal wall,[62,70] and prosthetic closure is needed in most cases.

What determines the choice of an ipsilateral versus contralateral pedicle for TRAM flap reconstruction?

The contralateral TRAM flap pedicle offers the advantage of an easier flap rotation than the ipsilateral pedicle. In the

natura
must l
enough
and he
rior fla
and ke
The ur
flap co
to the n
the nur
the ped
to the f
strip of
carefull
The ent
eral por
sected t

Later
the abde
of musc
rators. I
the resp
rated fro
of the s
within t
muscle
cases ar
muscle r
muscle c
nervated
The late
innervat

If ther
blood su
inferior
(Fig. 25–
the flap i
Hemosta
the skin
chest. Th

How i

The abde
ally does
closed w
sutures. I
release ca
to decrea
second la
the side
cated to
line. Thi
monofila
pleted, an

How is

The TRA
planning

ipsilateral TRAM, the pedicle tends to sit on top of itself and rotate on itself. The muscle will often defold under the flap, which can cause kinking and decreased blood supply. The contralateral single-pedicled TRAM flap is rotated 90 degrees (Fig. 25–15A). This is clockwise for right breast reconstruction and counterclockwise for left breast reconstruction. In most cases, this is the superior method for reconstructing the breast. Rotating the contralateral pedicle 180 degrees (Fig.

25–15B) is safe and should be considered when the defect is wide and extends onto the chest or axilla. The ipsilateral pedicle (Fig. 25–15C) is indicated when the pedicled TRAM flap is carried high on the abdomen and the contralateral pedicle may not reach the mastectomy wound. The most favorable rotation for a double-pedicled TRAM flap is 90 degrees (Fig. 25–15D). This is counterclockwise for a left defect and clockwise for a right defect.

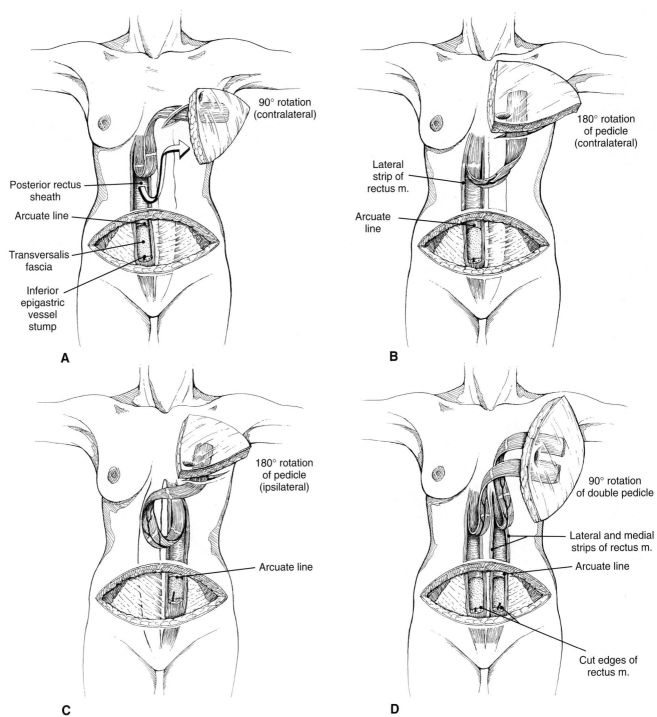

Figure 25–15 *A,* Contralateral single-pedicled TRAM flap with 90-degree rotation. *B,* Contralateral single-pedicled TRAM flap with 180-degree rotation. *C,* Ipsilateral single-pedicled TRAM flap with 180-degree rotation. *D,* Double-pedicled TRAM flap with 90-degree rotation.

**What
in pla**

The pat
marking
by Hartr
mastecto
point is
fold is
medial a
compari
reconstr
should b
TRAM f
dimensic
the flap
demonst
normal l
the diffe
be requi
superior
inferior
along a r
in the ar
the two
patient's
sible so
clothes. /
to be ir
required
extend o
cle. If m

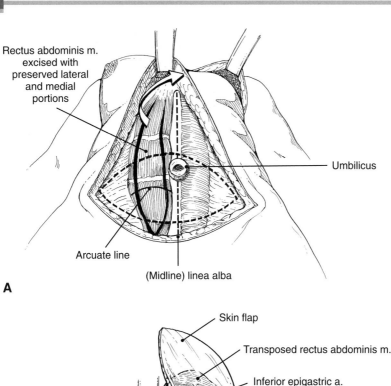

Rectus abdominis m. excised with preserved lateral and medial portions

Umbilicus

Arcuate line

(Midline) linea alba

A

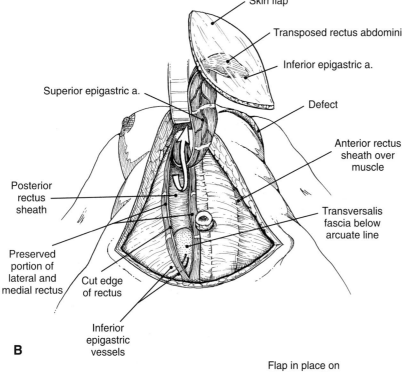

Skin flap

Transposed rectus abdominis m.

Inferior epigastric a.

Superior epigastric a.

Defect

Anterior rectus sheath over muscle

Posterior rectus sheath

Transversalis fascia below arcuate line

Preserved portion of lateral and medial rectus

Cut edge of rectus

Inferior epigastric vessels

B

Figure 25–17 *A,* Elevation of the abdominal skin and subcutaneous tissue flap and development of the subcutaneous tunnel. *B,* Elevation and rotation of the TRAM flap. *C,* Inset of the TRAM flap and closure of the abdominal wall fascia.

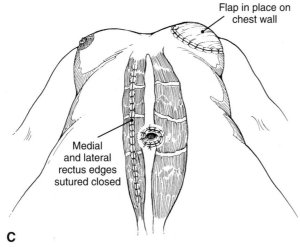

Flap in place on chest wall

Medial and lateral rectus edges sutured closed

C

Figure 25

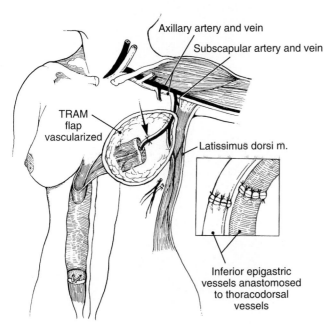

Figure 25–18 "Supercharging" the pedicled TRAM flap by microvascular anastomosis to the thoracodorsal vessels.

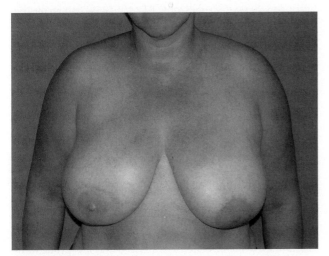

Figure 25–19 Unilateral TRAM flap breast reconstruction.

What are the preoperative considerations in delayed bilateral TRAM reconstruction?

When evaluating a patient for bilateral reconstruction after mastectomies, one must take note of the locations of the incisions. In addition, some patients have had a modified radical mastectomy on one side and a radical mastectomy on the other side. Even if the same mastectomy operation was performed on both sides, the volume requirements are sometimes different. All factors must be noted in the initial consultation before the onset of reconstruction. It is the goal of the reconstructive surgeon to make the breasts as symmetrical as possible. If more tissue is needed on one side for reconstruction, the TRAM flap can be asymmetrically split in such a way that this is accomplished.

What determines the choice of ipsilateral versus contralateral pedicled TRAM flaps for bilateral reconstruction?

When performing bilateral pedicled TRAM flaps, the flaps can be rotated either ipsilaterally or contralaterally. As in unilateral breast reconstruction, the contralateral pedicle technique (Fig. 25–20A) is the safest way to position the breast flaps because it results in a very direct route for vascular inflow and outflow to the flap. With 90-degree flap rotation and a contralateral pedicle, the thickest portion of the breast flap tends to be in the superior pole of the pocket. This may be a difficult problem to deal with at the time of inset. Using a contralateral pedicle with a 180-degree rotation can solve this problem (Fig. 25–20B). In addition, the use of contralateral pedicles results in minimal disruption of the inframammary folds. Ipsilateral pedicles at 90-degree rotation are possible in bilateral breast reconstruction. The same problems that exist with unilateral reconstruction are present with bilateral reconstruction, that is, the pedicle tends to fold under the flap.

How is the abdominal defect closed after bilateral TRAM elevation?

The abdominal wall closure is much more difficult in bilateral breast reconstruction than in unilateral single-pedicled reconstruction.[72] The closure of both sides of the abdomen should be performed simultaneously. If one side is closed before the other side, it may be difficult to close the second side. Either running or interrupted sutures may be used. In almost all cases, mesh will be needed either to reinforce the closure or to complete it. Lateral external oblique myofascial release may be performed to decrease the tension on the fascial closure.

How is the breast shaped after bilateral TRAM reconstruction?

The breast is shaped similarly to unilateral reconstruction. The superior portion of the flap is inset first. The tissue is again sutured superiorly and allowed essentially to hang. If contralateral pedicles are used, there is usually minimal disruption in the inframammary fold. If the inframammary fold needs to be created, this can be done using monofilament sutures. Obviously, symmetry should be as close as possible (Fig. 25–21).

MICROVASCULAR FREE FLAP BREAST RECONSTRUCTION

Microvascular Free TRAM Flap

The microvascular free TRAM flap offers improved flap blood supply and less abdominal wall trauma than the single-pedicled TRAM flap.[62,73,74] Abdominal wall function improves faster after a free TRAM flap than after a single-pedicled TRAM flap, but 6 months after surgery, the difference becomes insignificant.[75] The free TRAM flap is ideally suited for immediate breast reconstruction when the subscapular

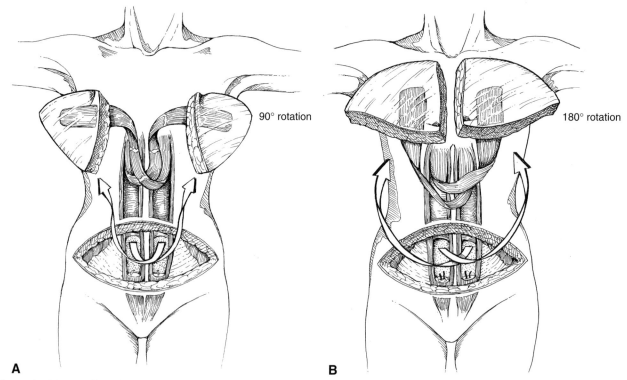

Figure 25–20   *A,* Bilateral TRAM flap reconstruction with contralateral flaps and 90-degree rotation. *B,* Bilateral TRAM flap reconstruction with contralateral flaps and 180-degree rotation.

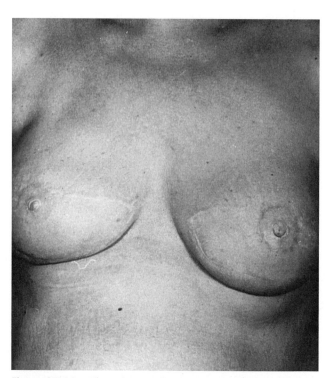

Figure 25–21   Bilateral TRAM flap breast reconstruction.

trunk is exposed during the mastectomy and is easily available for microvascular anastomosis.

The disadvantages of the free TRAM flap are the requirement that the surgeon be proficient in microsurgery and the rare risk for total flap loss.[76–78] Pedicled TRAM is almost never complicated by total flap loss but is more frequently complicated by fat necrosis and partial flap loss.[67,78] The cost of performing free TRAM flaps is not significantly higher then that of pedicled flaps in experienced hands.[79]

What are the contraindications to free TRAM flap reconstruction?

Although any kind of TRAM flap is relatively contraindicated in patients who smoke, are obese, or have severe medical problems, the relative contraindication is less for the free TRAM flap, which is better vascularized and less prone to tissue loss. Smokers are asked to stop smoking for at least 2 weeks before surgery and for 4 to 6 weeks afterward. In patients who require a large amount of tissue for breast reconstruction or who have had chest wall irradiation, the free TRAM flap and the bipedicled TRAM flap are the best options for reconstruction.

What are the preoperative considerations with free TRAM flap reconstruction?

Most free TRAM flaps are performed for immediate reconstruction. The incisions for the mastectomy are planned with the oncologic surgeon. Although oncologic considerations always take precedence over aesthetic ideals, an effort should be made to spare as much skin as possible. The flap can be elevated either simultaneously with the mastectomy or afterward, depending on the level of comfort the oncologic surgeon and the reconstructive surgeon have with simultaneous operating room logistics. The operating room logistics and patient positioning are similar to that for a pedicled TRAM flap.

What are the considerations when sentinel lymph node evaluation is performed at the same time as the mastectomy and reconstruction?

As more breast oncologic surgeons become comfortable with sentinel lymph node biopsy, the use of this technique will increase. If the sentinel lymph node evaluation is positive for metastatic disease, the recommendation is to perform a completion axillary lymph node dissection. If the diagnosis is established intraoperatively by frozen section or touch prep, and then the axillary dissection is completed, reconstruction may proceed using the thoracodorsal vessels as possible microvascular recipient vessels. If the diagnosis of axillary metastatic disease is established postoperatively, the subsequent axillary lymph node dissection could endanger the blood supply to the free flap if the thoracodorsal vessels were used as recipient vessels.

Kronowitz and coworkers[80] showed that 35% of patients with clinically negative axillae at initial presentation have axillary lymph node involvement at the time of mastectomy and free flap breast reconstruction. In their study, patient age younger than 50 years, tumor size greater than 2 cm, and lymphovascular invasion on the initial biopsy were independent predictors of axillary metastasis in the clinically node-negative patients.[74]

If sentinel lymph node evaluation is to be performed, particularly in higher risk patients, a nonaxillary site should be considered for recipient vessels for microvascular breast reconstruction. If a sentinel lymph node is found to have metastatic disease and a free flap reconstruction was performed using axillary based vessels, a reoperation will have to be performed with both the oncologic and reconstructive surgeon present. The risks and timing of this operation have to be discussed carefully with the patient.

What is the initial assessment intraoperatively?

In the case of delayed breast reconstruction, the chest incision should initially be reentered and the recipient vessels assessed for the possibility of microvascular anastomosis. Either the internal mammary or thoracodorsal vessels are usually used. If the thoracodorsal vessels are very scarred or were previously injured, then either the internal mammary vessels should be evaluated as recipient vessels or a pedicled TRAM flap should be performed.[81] At the level of the third interspace, the internal mammary vessels have been shown to be reliable.[82,83]

In immediate reconstruction, the thoracodorsal vessels are used more commonly. The more proximal vessels are larger and offer easier microvascular anastomosis. Usually, an area proximal to the serratus branch is comparable in size to the deep inferior epigastric vessels. The communication between the serratus branch and the thoracodorsal vessels should be left intact to allow potential latissimus dorsi elevation, based on retrograde blood flow, if such a need should arise.

How is the free TRAM flap prepared?

The upper incision of the free TRAM flap is usually at or just above the umbilicus, and the inferior incision is about 2 cm above the pubis. The upper incision is made first, and the abdominal flap is elevated proximally as far as is necessary to allow abdominal wall closure. The incision is beveled to include as much fat and periumbilical perforators as possible. The skin flap is redraped and the site of the inferior incision confirmed. The inferior incision is then opened and beveled inferiorly to include as much fat as possible. The contralateral deep inferior epigastric pedicle is usually used because this appears to provide the best flap lie. Others[84] use the ipsilateral pedicle. The skin flap on the side opposite the inferior epigastric flap pedicle is elevated past the midline to the medial row of perforators on the pedicled side. The pedicled side flap is elevated to the lateral row of perforators. Inferiorly, the flap is elevated to the most inferior perforator. The anterior rectus sheath is incised lateral to the lateral row of perforators. The inferior epigastric pedicle is identified and dissected proximally and distally. The pedicle is dissected to near its origin. The intercostal neurovascular bundles are left intact to preserve innervation to the portion of rectus abdominis muscle that is not taken with the flap. The point of entry of the inferior epigastric pedicle into the rectus abdominis muscle is identified, and the muscle lateral to this point is separated longitudinally using scissors. A similar procedure is performed medially to preserve a medial strip of muscle. The amount of medial muscle left intact is less important because the muscle is not innervated.[71] The inferior and superior portions of the muscle are then transected, and the flap is connected only by the pedicle (Fig. 25–22). The deep inferior epigastric pedicle is transected, and the flap is brought to the chest wall. Although minimal rectus abdominis muscle is taken with the flap, the function of the entire rectus muscle is affected by the surgery.[85]

How are the microvascular anastomoses performed?

The rectus abdominis muscle is sutured to the chest wall, and the vessels are aligned. The patient is tilted away from the side of the breast reconstruction. Self-retaining retractors are placed in the wound, and the operating microscope is brought into the field. The vein or veins are usually anastomosed with a microvascular coupler, and the artery is sutured with 9-0 microvascular sutures. The TRAM flap is reperfused, and attention is placed to the abdominal wall closure (Fig. 25–23).

How is the abdominal defect closed?

The anterior rectus sheath is closed with running or interrupted permanent sutures, and the opposite rectus fascia is plicated to centralize the umbilicus. Any supraumbilical laxity may be plicated at this time if indicated. The superior abdominal flap is closed over suction drains, and the patient is flexed as needed. Prosthetic material is almost never used.

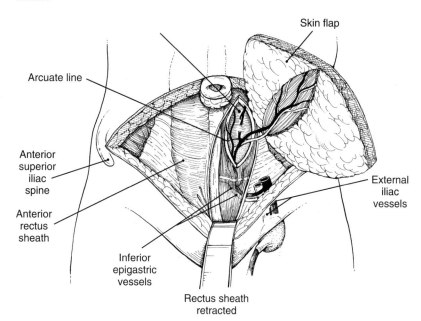

Figure 25–22 Mobilization of the free TRAM flap.

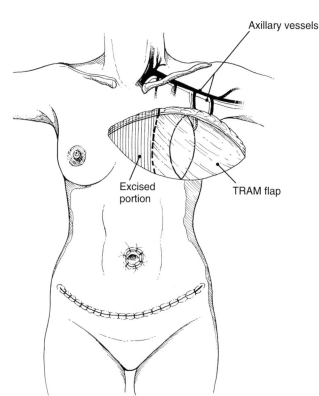

Figure 25–23 Inset of the free TRAM flap.

How is the TRAM flap inset performed?

The flap is inset with the patient in the sitting position. The rectus muscle is sutured to the chest wall in the appropriate position. The pedicle is evaluated for kinking, and the muscle position is adjusted as needed. The rectus muscle should be stable on the chest to minimize motion in the pedicle and lateral migration of the flap. A suction drain is placed in the axilla and under the flap. The flap is temporarily sutured or stapled in place and inset in a manner similar to a pedicled TRAM flap (see Fig. 25–23).

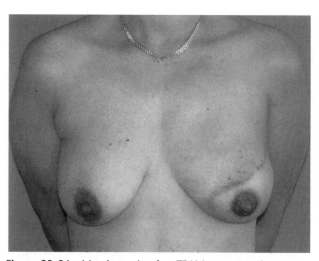

Figure 25–24 Muscle-sparing free TRAM reconstruction.

How is the patient managed postoperatively?

Postoperatively, the flap is minimally dressed and is monitored with visual inspection, temperature monitoring, or Doppler evaluation. The patient is allowed out of bed on the first postoperative day. Arm motion is limited, and abduction is discouraged. One aspirin is given daily for 30 days. No other anticoagulation is used. The patient is allowed to begin arm exercises 2 to 3 weeks postoperatively. Abdominal exercise is limited for 2 months (Fig. 25–24).

What are the complications of microvascular versus pedicled TRAM flaps?

The most devastating complication of microvascular free TRAM flap surgery is total flap loss from microvascular thrombosis in the early postoperative period. The incidence varies from about 1% to 4% in experienced hands, whereas total flap loss occurs in less than 1% of pedicled TRAM cases. However, the incidence of fat necrosis and partial flap loss is substantially less in microvascular free TRAM cases than in pedicled TRAM cases. The incidence of abdominal wall complications (hernia and bulging) also is less in microvascular free TRAM cases than in pedicled TRAM cases. The cost of surgery and the length of hospitalization are not substantially different for microvascular free TRAM and pedicled TRAM cases.

Deep Inferior Epigastric Artery Perforator Flap

What are advantages of the deep inferior epigastric artery flap compared with a microvascular TRAM flap?

The deep inferior epigastric perforator (DIEP) flap is similar to a TRAM flap, but no muscle is harvested with the flap.[86–88] The flap is based on the perforating vessels originating from the deep inferior epigastric vessels and traversing through the rectus abdominis muscle to supply the skin and fat of the abdomen. Because no muscle is taken with the flap, there is a decreased incidence of abdominal weakness, bulging, and hernias.[80,82]

What are the anatomic considerations in perforator flap reconstruction?

The microvascular free TRAM generally incorporates three to six perforators in the flap design. The DIEP flap usually incorporates one to three perforators. The anatomy of the perforators has been extensively studied in humans with Doppler ultrasound, and all patients have been found to have at least two perforators.[89] The perforator course through the rectus abdominis muscle varies. In 65% of cases, the perforator has a short intramuscular course. In other cases, the perforator may go through a tendinous intersection, have a long intramuscular course, or have a subfascial course.[90]

How is the flap harvest different in DIEP flaps compared with muscle-sparing free TRAM flaps?

The harvest of the DIEP flap is similar to that of the muscle-sparing free TRAM flap until the point that the medial and lateral rows of perforators are exposed. At that point, the largest perforator is chosen, and the anterior rectus sheet is opened around this neurovascular bundle. The muscle is split in the direction of the fibers to expose the DIEP. A second or third perforator is kept with the flap if it is aligned with the first perforator. Branches from the pedicle are divided, and the flap is now a skin and fat flap based on the deep inferior epigastric vessels. The microsurgery and flap inset are performed in a manner similar to a microvascular free TRAM flap (Fig. 25–25).

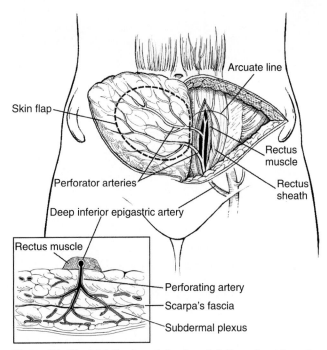

Figure 25–25   Mobilization of the deep inferior epigastric perforator (DIEP) flap.

What are the results of the DIEP flap?

The DIEP flap has a lower incidence of abdominal complications, such as hernia and bulging. Patients are able to achieve abdominal function near or at preoperative levels within 6 months.[91,92] The incidence of total flap loss and technical problems with the microsurgical anastomosis is similar to that of free TRAM flap cases.

There is a greater incidence of fat necrosis in DIEP flaps than in microvascular TRAM flaps. This is thought to be due to the less robust blood supply of the DIEP flap when compared with the microvascular TRAM flap.[93]

As with pedicled and microvascular free TRAM flaps, DIEP flaps have an increased incidence of fat necrosis, fibrosis, and flap contracture with postoperative radiation therapy.[94]

Gluteal Free Flaps

The superior gluteal flap was first reported by Fujino[95] and then popularized by Shaw.[96,97] This flap is typically considered a secondary or tertiary choice for free tissue reconstruction of the breast because of the increased operative time, complexity, and morbidity associated with the procedure. The patient considered for free gluteus microvascular transfer is usually not a candidate for TRAM flap (insufficient tissue or abdominal scars) but desires an autologous breast reconstruction.

What are the advantages and disadvantages of a superior gluteal flap?

The advantages of the superior gluteal free flap include abundant tissue for reconstruction, inconspicuous donor site, and minimal functional loss. Shaw and colleagues have

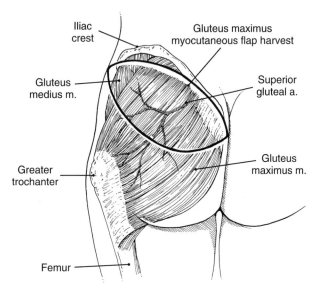

Figure 25–26   Anatomy of the superior gluteal flap.

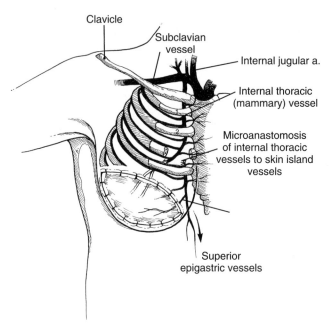

Figure 25–27   Inset and microvascular anastomosis of the superior gluteal flap.

demonstrated the spontaneous restoration of sensation in the flap without nerve reconstruction.[98]

The disadvantages of the superior gluteal free flap include the risk for total flap loss and greater operative time common to all free flap procedures. In addition, the superior gluteal flap is technically much more difficult to harvest than the TRAM flap, and the recipient vessel dissection (usually internal mammary) is more difficult than dissection of the thoracodorsal vessels.

What are the anatomic considerations in a free superior gluteal flap reconstruction?

The gluteus maximus muscle originates from the posterior third of the iliac crest, sacrum, sacrotuberous ligament, and coccyx. The muscle inserts on the gluteal tuberosity of the femur. The superior gluteal artery, vein, and nerve course between the gluteus medius and piriformis muscles. The origin of these vessels is 5 cm inferior to the posterior superior iliac spine and 2 to 3 cm lateral to the sacrum. The vessel supplies a cutaneous territory that exceeds the size of the gluteus maximus muscle. The skin island (Fig. 25–26) can be made anywhere over the gluteal area as long as it includes a cuff of muscle that includes the pedicle. The upper half of the muscle is vascularized by the superior gluteal vessels. The lower half of the muscle is vascularized by the inferior gluteal vessels. These vessels pass through the space between the piriformis and superior gemellus muscles along with the internal pudendal vessels and the sciatic nerve, inferior gluteal nerve, and posterior femoral cutaneous nerve. The dual vascularity of the gluteus muscle allows splitting of the muscle and preservation of blood supply.

Typically, a flap with a skin width of 8 to 10 cm can be harvested from the buttocks with primary closure of the donor site wound. This is usually sufficient to provide the necessary volume and ptosis to an average-sized breast. The length of the flap is usually 20 to 30 cm. The flap is much thicker in depth than the TRAM flap, usually 10 to 15 cm.

The pedicle of the myocutaneous gluteus flap is usually very short, and the internal mammary vessels are chosen as recipient vessels in most cases (Fig. 25–27). Usually, the third costal cartilage is removed to provide access to the vessels. Harvest of the flap using the superior gluteal artery perforators, not taking any muscle with the flap, provides a longer flap pedicle and easier microsurgical anastomosis.[99]

In these cases, the thoracodorsal vessels may be used for microanastomosis. The thickness of the flap and the central pedicle position may make vascular anastomosis difficult. The internal mammary artery is more reliable than the vein. In cases in which the vein is too small for microanastomosis, the cephalic vein or external jugular vein may be rotated down to become the recipient vein.[100] Vein grafts may also be used. The internal mammary vein becomes more reliable proximally.[81–83]

What are the advantages of an inferior gluteal free flap?

The inferior gluteal free flap offers the following advantages over the superior gluteal free flap: a longer pedicle, greater volume of tissue, and a lower incision that may be less conspicuous. The main disadvantages of the inferior gluteal flap are exposure of the inferior gluteal nerve, of the motor nerve to the gluteus maximus muscle, and of the sciatic nerve in the dissection.[101,102] Postoperatively, there is some discomfort with sitting related to the scar in the inferior gluteal fold. The longer pedicle allows the use of the thoracodorsal vessels for microvascular anastomosis. In addition, the pedicle in the inferior gluteal flap is located more toward the edge of the flap when compared with the superior gluteal flap. This allows more straightforward microvascular anastomosis. With either gluteal flap, positioning of the patient on the operating table is difficult. A corkscrew-type position usually makes simultaneous dissections possible.

After the microsurgery is completed, the flap is inset and the muscle used to fill out the infraclavicular hollow, and the lateral portion of the flap is used to re-create the anterior axillary fold or is folded on itself to enhance projection.

How is the patient managed postoperatively?

The postoperative care of the patient with a gluteal free flap involves maintaining the hip in extension over the first few postoperative days. The patient is gradually allowed to sit in a chair and then to ambulate. The patient is usually discharged 5 to 7 days after surgery. There is minimal functional deficit because only a small portion of the muscle is sacrificed. Seromas are the most common donor site complication and either resolve spontaneously or require aspiration.

Transverse Lateral Thigh Flaps

The lateral thigh flap was developed as an alternative site for harvest of autogenous tissue for breast reconstruction. The same patient who is a candidate for the gluteal flap is often a candidate for the lateral thigh flap. There often is significant redundant tissue in the thigh area compared with the abdomen or buttock. Like the gluteal area, the fat in the lateral thigh tends to be more rigid than the fat in the abdomen. This tends to result in a more projecting, youthful breast.

What are the anatomic considerations in a lateral thigh flap?

The vascular pedicle of the lateral thigh flap is the lateral femoral circumflex vessels that perfuse the skin through the musculocutaneous perforators of the tensor fascia lata. The axis of the flap (Fig. 25–28) is a line that goes from a point 10 cm inferior to the anterior superior iliac spine to the gluteal fold. This is the location of the pedicle. The axis of the flap may not coincide with the location of the greatest amount of fat in the thigh. The decision on the exact site of the skin island should be made with the patient. As long as a portion of the flap is over the pedicle axis, the tissue will be vascularized. The width of the skin island is about 7 to 8 cm. The size depends on the ability to close the wound. The length is usually 20 to 25 cm. The skin incisions are made, and the subcutaneous tissues are beveled for 4 to 5 cm. This creates extra fat for upper and lower pole fullness. Simultaneous chest vessel dissection and flap harvest is usually possible. The thoracodorsal vessels are usually used as recipient vessels for microsurgical anastomosis.

What are the intraoperative and postoperative considerations for a lateral thigh flap?

The flap is positioned in the chest pocket to attain the appropriate shape. The lateral position of the pedicle makes flap inset easier than in the gluteal flaps. The pedicle length is always longer than the superior gluteal pedicle and usually at least as long if not longer than the inferior gluteal pedicle. There usually is good vessel size match, although occasionally the flap vein is 6 to 7 mm in size. The risk for donor site hematoma may be reduced by prolonged closed-suction drainage and suture closure of the defect to obliterate as much of the dead space as possible. The main drawback to this flap is the visible location of the scar and the contour deformity that usually results. The contour deformity may be improved with liposuction of the contralateral unoperated side.[64]

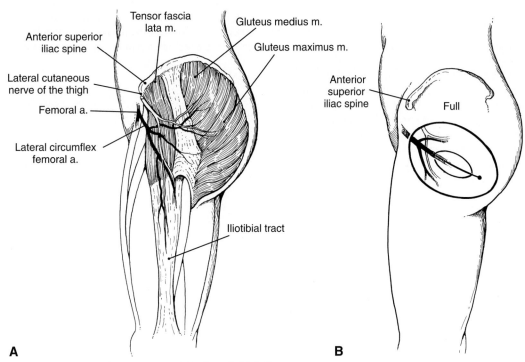

Figure 25–28   *A* and *B,* Anatomy of the lateral thigh flap.

NIPPLE-AREOLA RECONSTRUCTION

Breast mound reconstruction improves the patient's body image after mastectomy. Nipple-areola reconstruction allows closer symmetry and increases patient acceptance of the reconstructed breast. The nipple-areola is the initial focus of attention when visualizing the breast. In cases in which the mound reconstruction is slightly less than optimal, an excellent nipple-areola reconstruction may make the reconstructed breast look much more like the normal breast. Wellisch and colleagues[103] found that patients who had nipple-areola reconstruction had greater satisfaction than those who did not. The nipple-areola reconstruction should be considered a normal step in the process of total breast reconstruction. The patient should be aware of all stages in the reconstructive process before the initial procedure. If this is done, nipple-areola reconstruction will be accepted as a logical step in the reconstructive process.

What are the anatomic considerations in nipple-areola reconstruction?

The nipple-areola should be located on the most prominent portion of the breast. This will be the first area seen when the reconstructed breast is visualized. The nipple should point slightly upward and outward. There is significant variation in the shape and size of the nipple–areolar complex. The average nipple projects 3 to 7 mm. The average areola diameter is 35 to 45 mm.[64] The surface of the areola varies from smooth to rough. The number and prominence of the Montgomery glands is variable. The goal in nipple-areola reconstruction is to match the unoperated, normal breast. The nipple position should be marked with the patient in the upright position. Ideally, the patient should be sitting or standing in front of a mirror and participate actively in the planning process.

What are the choices for nipple reconstruction?

The most realistic nipple reconstruction is from the contralateral nipple. This is the only site that can perfectly match the color of the normal nipple.[104] The areola may be tattooed at a later date. The shape of the contralateral nipple is very important in the decision-making process. There must be enough nipple available to remove about 50% of the donor nipple and result in normal-appearing donor and recipient nipples. Unfortunately, the nipple is a sensitive donor site. This is particularly true in the mastectomy patient for whom nipple sensibility is of sexual importance. Aside from oncologic concerns, most patients reject the normal nipple as a donor site for nipple reconstruction.

Local flaps are reliable donor tissues that are accepted by most patients. These flaps can be created with or without skin graft reconstruction of the areola.[105–108] Skin graft reconstruction of the areola may be performed using axillary or abdominal "dog ears" if available. Labia donor sites are avoided because of increased patient morbidity. In general, skin grafts are avoided if a new scar would be created to harvest the graft. If a skin graft is to be used for areola reconstruction, and no previous incision site is available for graft harvest, the groin is used.

Tattooing may be used to match the color of the contralateral areola.[109–111] This is a particularly good method in patients who have smooth areolas. Patients with coarse areolas will do better with grafts. Tattooing may still be required to match the color. Prominent Montgomery glands may be matched with cartilage grafts.

What is the nipple-sharing technique?

The nipple-sharing technique is essentially a composite graft. The success of such a graft depends on meticulous preparation of the recipient site with absolute hemostasis. The larger the area of contact with the graft, the greater the chance of graft takes. If the patient has a long nipple, the tip of the nipple can be amputated as a cap and placed as a graft on the recipient site. The donor site will close primarily. The nipple may also be harvested as a wedge or as a transverse slice[64] (Fig. 25–29). Postoperative care is the same for all three procedures. A protective dressing is left in place for 7 to 10 days before its removal and the assessment of graft take.

What is the Skate-type flap?

The Skate-type flap raises a local flap from the breast mound that is wrapped upon itself to produce a nipple. The donor site will require skin graft reconstruction. The procedure is demonstrated in Figure 25–30. The nipple position is marked as previously described. The size of the areola is determined by comparing with the normal breast. A transverse line is marked across the areola at the superior base of the flap. The section above this line is de-epithelialized. A circle is drawn in the center of the areola to represent the proposed nipple diameter. Lines are drawn from the medial and lateral edges of this nipple site to the most inferior point of the areola (the 6-o'clock position). The medial and lateral wings of the flap are dissected in a deep dermal plane. The dissection

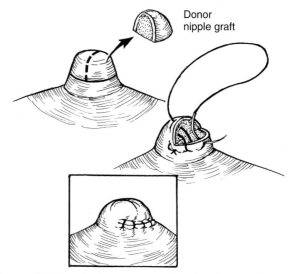

Donor nipple graft

Figure 25–29 Nipple reconstruction by the nipple-sharing technique.

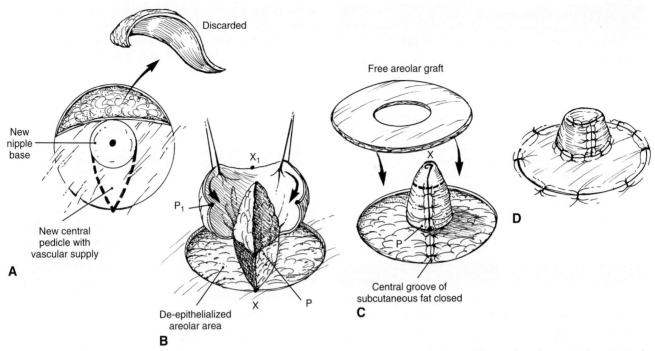

Figure 25–30 Skate-type nipple-areola reconstruction. *A,* Markings. *B,* Flap elevation. *C,* Flap rotation and graft preparation. *D,* Final appearance.

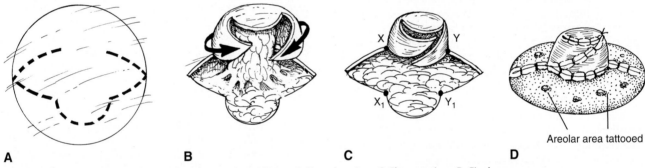

Figure 25–31 Local flap nipple reconstruction. *A,* Markings. *B,* Flap elevation. *C,* Flap rotation. *D,* Final appearance.

goes into the subcutaneous plane in the area directly inferior to the nipple. The flap is mobilized and elevated, and the skin flaps are wrapped around the central subcutaneous pedicle. The flaps are sutured together with absorbable sutures, and the tip of the flap is shortened to the appropriate length. The inferior-central exposed subcutaneous fat is closed with absorbable sutures, and a full-thickness skin graft is harvested from a previously determined area. The dressing consists of Telfa and a plastic syringe hub fashioned into a nipple splint that is held in place with Steri-Strips. The dressing is left in place for 7 to 10 days. If the graft is too pale after complete healing, it may be tattooed at a later date.

When is a local flap without areola skin graft indicated?

In patients who either are not good candidates for skin graft areola reconstruction or do not want additional scars associated with skin graft harvest, a local flap and areola tattooing is

a good option for nipple-areola reconstruction.[110,112] The local flap is raised for nipple reconstruction, and the donor sites are closed primarily without the need for skin grafts. The procedure is demonstrated in Figure 25–31. The nipple position is carefully marked as previously discussed. The diameter and height of the normal nipple are carefully measured. The nipple reconstruction should be made larger than the other side to allow for some contraction of the flap. Two triangular flaps are marked medially and laterally from the nipple base. The width of the triangles should be equal to the proposed height of the nipple. The flaps are raised initially in the deep dermal plane going into the subcutaneous tissue as the nipple area is approached. A semicircular flap is raised at the inferior edge of the flaps to make a nipple cap. The entire flap is elevated to an erect position, and the triangular flaps are wrapped around the base and sutured in place with absorbable sutures. The semicircular flap is sutured to the top of the nipple. The donor sites are closed directly. The areola is usually tattooed postoperatively after the wounds are completely healed.

What is the advantage of nipple-areola tattooing?

Areola tattooing offers several advantages over skin grafts. There is no donor site. The color can be controlled and modified with time. The nipple can be made darker than the areola. The procedure can be performed in the office with minimal anesthesia and no sedation. When a skin graft is present, tattooing can improve the nipple color even if the graft is the appropriate color. Tattooing may also camouflage poor take of a graft or a shape of a graft that is not optimal. The tattoo color should probably be made slightly darker than the normal nipple-areola to allow for normal fading. Nipple-areola tattooing is usually performed after healing is complete.

SYMMETRY PROCEDURES

When symmetry procedures are necessary, all issues must be discussed with the patient and other treating physicians. The need for contralateral breast surgery may alter the choice of technique chosen for breast reconstruction.

When choosing a method of breast reconstruction, it is often possible to select a technique that will closely match the contralateral breast in size and shape. Other times, the method chosen will require alteration of the contralateral breast to achieve symmetry. Some patients may even request surgery on the normal breast for either cosmetic or functional reasons. In patients with very large breasts, mammograms following breast reduction surgery will be easier to interpret. The timing of the symmetry procedure and the technique chosen should not interfere with either the patient's cancer treatment or future monitoring of the contralateral breast.

Available techniques include augmentation, reduction, mastopexy, or a combination of these techniques. Not only is the selection of technique important, but its timing is also critical to achieving the best cosmetic results.

What are the potential problems of augmentation?

Usually, augmentation is useful in small-breasted women who have undergone implant reconstruction and need additional upper breast fullness in the normal breast to achieve symmetry.

Studies have documented the interference an implant can cause to proper mammographic interpretation.[113-117] When the implant is small, placed subpectorally, and remains soft, the degree of mammographic distortion is minimal. The use of saline implants placed underneath the pectoralis muscle has significantly reduced the incidence of capsular contracture and subsequent firmness of the breast. Most often, the implants have been large silicone implants placed in a subglandular position with the expected 30% to 40% incidence of capsular contracture and subsequent hardening of the breast. This makes mammography both difficult and painful to perform. Often, several additional views are required to maximize parenchymal visualization. Long-standing implants can develop calcifications in the surrounding capsule that can also interfere with mammographic interpretation.

When augmentation is being considered, carefully documented consultations with the oncologic surgeon and mammographer are important. Augmentation is best performed at the time of final implant placement to achieve best symmetry.

When is contralateral breast reduction indicated?

Contralateral breast reduction is most often required when patients have breasts larger than a C cup. It is extremely difficult to achieve symmetry in these large, usually ptotic breasts by any reconstructive technique. If tissue expansion were chosen, the degree of expansion required would often result in extreme thinning of the overlying skin, and sufficient ptosis is usually impossible to attain. In the ptotic patient, autologous tissue reconstructive techniques are preferable, assuming there is adequate donor site tissue available.

Breast reduction is best performed at the time of flap reconstruction or tissue expander placement, especially in the delayed setting. Over several months, the reduced breast will develop ptosis, allowing for an accurate implant placement when a tissue expander has been placed in the contralateral breast. Breast reduction techniques all result in some internal breast scarring postoperatively. These mammographic changes are well understood and do not interfere with interpretation.[118] When breast reduction is performed, it is important to choose a technique that has a low risk for fat necrosis. When fat necrosis occurs within the breast, it can pose diagnostic problems, usually requiring biopsy. In selected cases, free nipple graft techniques are preferable to pedicle techniques. This technique results in the lowest risk for fat necrosis postoperatively. The long-term stable contour achieved with free nipple graft techniques is also preferable in very large-breasted older women. Free nipple graft techniques also allow for removal of all subareolar ductal tissue, theoretically potentially reducing the possible development of breast cancer. Liposuction is avoided in breast reduction owing to potential distortion of the internal architecture of the breast, which may make future mammographic interpretation more difficult.

When is mastopexy indicated?

Mastopexy is often required when significant ptosis exists in the contralateral breast and symmetry is the goal of reconstruction. Mastopexy, similar to breast reduction, is best performed at the time of the initial reconstructive procedure because some recurrence of ptosis is common over 6 months to 1 year postoperatively. Available mastopexy procedures either reshape the skin or internally reshape the breast mound. Internal architectural distortion should be minimized in these patients. It is best to avoid mastopexy techniques that extensively reshape the breast gland. In general, long-term results have been very similar for both internal reshaping procedures and dermal procedures.

BREAST RECONSTRUCTION AFTER BREAST-CONSERVING SURGERY AND RADIATION THERAPY

Increasingly, segmental excision and radiation therapy have become the established treatment for many patients with breast cancer. The aesthetic result after breast-conserving surgery is affected by the extent of surgical resection of the tumor, the location of the tumor, and the orientation of the skin incisions.[119,120] An unsatisfactory aesthetic result is related most commonly to poorly designed skin and parenchymal resections and the failure to reapproximate breast tissue when closing. Significant resection (quadrantectomy) is more likely to result in aesthetic problems than are more limited segmental excisions.[120] The size of the breast compared with the size of the excision is critical in determining the likelihood of distortion. The larger the excision relative to the breast size, the more likely that there will be cosmetic problems.

Radiation therapy often results in tissue erythema and edema that is followed with time by fibrosis, contracture, and telangiectasia formation. The decreased vascularity of the irradiated tissue may result in fat necrosis and diffuse calcification. The breast may develop retraction and contracture that superiorly dislocates the breast relative to the chest wall.

Berrino and associates[120] noted an incidence of unsatisfactory outcomes after lumpectomy and radiation therapy of 16% to 22%. They developed a classification system to describe the various types of deformity that occur after breast conservation and radiotherapy, among which the most difficult to correct was cutaneous parenchymal deficiency with or without subcutaneous tissue loss.

How can deformities in the conserved breast be treated?

Minimal deformities may be treated with local flaps, scar release, or tissue rearrangement. More extensive defects require release of all scar contracture and replacement with new tissue.

The risk for locally recurrent cancer in patients treated with breast-conserving surgery and radiation therapy has been reported as high as 10% to 20% in 10 years.[121–123] Any reconstructive technique that might interfere with surveillance of the breast is unacceptable. The use of breast prostheses could potentially obscure the visualization of small lesions mammographically. Even with specialized mammographic techniques, portions of the breast are likely to be missed.

Myocutaneous flaps will provide sufficient tissue to correct almost any tissue defect. Slavin and coworkers[124] reported that these tissues do not compromise mammographic interpretation. The muscle flap tissue becomes fibrofatty as soon as about 6 months after surgery and eventually becomes radiolucent.[124] Adjacent breast tissues are not concealed or obscured mammographically. In addition, the myocutaneous flap tissues are well vascularized and improve blood supply to the surrounding tissues. This produces a less dense breast than in irradiated breast tissue without muscle flap augmentation. The flap reconstruction of the breast should be delayed for 2 to 3 years after the surgical procedure until the erythema, edema, fibrosis, and contracture have stabilized.

Most defects after lumpectomy or quadrantectomy and radiation therapy are easily treated with latissimus dorsi myocutaneous flaps. This flap is well tolerated and has minimal donor site morbidity. The rectus abdominis myocutaneous flap is reserved for larger defects. The rectus abdominis flap donor site is associated with more donor site morbidity than the latissimus dorsi. In addition, if there is a breast cancer recurrence, the rectus abdominis will not be available for salvage reconstruction.

At the time of the reconstruction, the breast tissue must be assessed. This consists of evaluating the missing cutaneous component, the parenchymal volume loss, and the nipple malposition. The skin loss usually is greater than expected as a result of shrinkage from the radiation therapy. The flap skin island should be made slightly larger than the anticipated defect. In addition, there is likely to be some muscle atrophy, and the overall flap volume should be slightly larger than appears to be needed.

PSYCHOLOGICAL IMPACT OF BREAST RECONSTRUCTION

Today, almost all women with breast cancer are likely to be offered either breast-conserving surgery or mastectomy and reconstruction. The options for reconstruction have increased as the surgery for breast cancer has decreased. Most patients have multiple options available to reconstruct the breast. The gross distortion associated with the radical mastectomy is very rare. Most patients who choose breast reconstruction are satisfied with the surgery.[125]

Various studies[126–128] have shown that up to one third of patients who undergo mastectomy have significant emotional distress and sexual dysfunction. Clifford and colleagues,[129] in a study of women undergoing delayed breast reconstruction, showed that women who sought reconstruction were exhibiting positive coping and assertive, effective problem-solving behavior. Teimourian and Adham[130] showed that reconstruction was like a "reverse mastectomy" and neutralized the destructive effect of the loss of the breast.

What is the psychological benefit of breast reconstruction?

There is no dispute that breast reconstruction is beneficial to the patient. In the early days of breast reconstruction, the timing of the reconstruction (immediate vs. delayed) was of some dispute. The earlier advocates of breast reconstruction[131,132] felt that the patient should cope with the defect created by the mastectomy and the use of a prosthesis before reconstruction, assuming that the patient would value the reconstruction more after having to deal with the ablation. In addition, there was a fear that the reconstruction would delay detection of recurrence of the breast cancer. Dowden and associates[133] helped allay fears that the reconstruction adversely affected the outcome after recurrence. Johnson and coworkers[134] showed that the outcome in breast cancer patients depended on the biology of the tumor and not on the presence of a breast prosthesis. The satisfaction rates with the reconstructions were similar in delayed-reconstruction patients and in immediate-reconstruction patients. Schain and colleagues[135] noted that women who had immediate reconstruction were less anxious, less depressed, and less hostile than those who had delayed reconstruction.

Breast reconstruction after mastectomy has been shown to increase sexual responsiveness.[130,135] Gerard[136] showed that women who have breast reconstruction are more easily sexually aroused than women who have had mastectomy alone.

Wellisch and colleagues[103] studied the psychosexual impact of nipple-areola reconstruction after breast reconstruction. They found that the group that had nipple-areola reconstruction had increased satisfaction with the overall reconstruction, nude appearance, size, softness, and sexual sensitivity compared with patients who had reconstruction without creation of the nipple-areola.

Women who feel that they will be psychologically, socially, or sexually improved with breast reconstruction should be offered the procedure at the earliest possible time after mastectomy.

REFERENCES

1. Jurkiewicz MJ, Krizek TJ, Mathes SJ, Ariyan S. Plastic Surgery Principles and Practice. St. Louis, CV Mosby, 1990.
2. Alexander JE, Block LI. Breast reconstruction following radical mastectomy. Plast Reconstr Surg 1967;40:175.
3. Pontes R. Single stage reconstruction of the missing breast. Br J Plast Surg 1973;26:377.
4. Millard DR. Reconstruction mammaplasty using an economical flap from the opposite breast. Ann Plast Surg 1981;6:374.
5. Marshall DR, Anstee EJ, Stapleton MJ. Postmastectomy breast reconstruction using breast sharing technique. Br J Plast Surg 1981;34:426.
6. Gillies HD, Millard DR. Principles and Art of Plastic Surgery. Boston, Little Brown, 1957, pp 297–300.
7. Cronin TD, Gerow FJ. Augmentation mammaplasty: A new "natural feel" prosthesis. In Transactions of the Third International Congress of Plastic and Reconstructive Surgery. Amsterdam, Excerpta Medica, 1963.
8. Snyderman RK, Guthrie RH. Reconstruction of the female breast following radical mastectomy. Plast Reconstr Surg 1971;47:565.
9. Guthrie RH. Breast reconstruction after radical mastectomy. Plast Reconstr Surg 1976;57:14.
10. Birnbaum L, Olsen JA. Breast reconstruction following radical mastectomy, using custom designed implants. Plast Reconstr Surg 1978;61:355.
11. Hueston JT, McKenzie G. Breast reconstruction after radical mastectomy. Aust N Z J Surg 1970;39:367.
12. Frazier TG, Noone RB. Immediate reconstruction in the treatment of primary carcinoma of the breast. Surg Gynecol Obstet 1983;157:413.
13. Noone RB, Murphy JB, Spear SL, et al. A six-year experience with immediate reconstruction after mastectomy for cancer. Plast Reconstr Surg 1985;76:258.
14. Frazier TG, Noone RB. An objective analysis of immediate simultaneous reconstruction in the treatment of primary breast cancer. Cancer 1985;55:1202.
15. Rosato FE, Fink PJ, Horton CE, et al. Immediate post-mastectomy reconstruction. J Surg Oncol 1976;8:277.
16. Georgiade GS, Georgiade NG, McKarty KS Jr, et al. Modified radical mastectomy with immediate reconstruction for carcinoma of the breast. Ann Surg 1981;193:565.
17. Webster DJT, Mansel RE, Hughes LE. Immediate reconstruction of the breast after mastectomy: Is it safe? Cancer 1984;53:1416.
18. Noone RB, Frazier TG, Noone GC, et al. Recurrence of breast carcinoma following immediate reconstruction: A 13-year review. Plast Reconstr Surg 1994;93:96.
19. Kroll SS, Coffey A, Winn RJ, Schusterman MA. A comparison of factors affecting aesthetic outcomes of TRAM flap breast reconstructions. Plast Reconstr Surg 1995;96:860.
20. Elkowitz A, Colen S, Slavin S, et al. Various methods of breast reconstruction after mastectomy: An economic comparison. Plast Reconstr Surg 1993;92:77.
21. Rosato RM, Dowden RV. Radiation therapy as a cause of capsular contracture. Ann Plast Surg 1994;32:342.
22. Cordeiro PG, Pusic AL, Disa JJ, et al. Irradiation after immediate tissue expander/implant breast reconstruction: Outcomes, complications, aesthetic results, and satisfaction among 156 patients. Plast Reconstr Surg 2004;113:877–881.
23. Toth BA, Lappert P. Modified skin incision for mastectomy: The need for plastic surgical input in preoperative placing. Plast Reconstr Surg 1991;87:1048–1053.
24. Carlson GW, Bostwick J, Styblo TN, et al. Skin-sparing mastectomy oncologic and reconstructive considerations. Ann Surg 1998;225:570–578.
25. Slavin SA, Schmitt SJ, Duda RB, et al. Skin-sparing mastectomy and immediate breast reconstruction: Oncologic risk and aesthetic results in patients with early-stage breast cancer. Plast Reconstr Surg 1998;102:49–62.
26. Simmons RM, Kersey Fish S, Gayle L, et al. Local and distant recurrence rates in skin-sparing mastectomy compared with non-skin-sparing mastectomies. Ann Surg Oncol 1999;6:676–681.
27. Kroll SS, Khoo A, Singletary S, et al. Local recurrence after skin-sparing and conventional mastectomy: A 6-year follow-up. Plast Reconstr Surg 1999;104:421–425.
28. Evans GRD, Schusterman MA, Kroll SS, et al. Reconstruction and the radiated breast: Is there a role for implants? Plast Reconstr Surg 1995;96:1111.
29. Kroll SS, Schusterman MA, Reece GP, et al. Breast reconstruction with myocutaneous flaps in previously irradiated patients. Plast Reconstr Surg 1994;93:460.
30. Slavin SA, Love SM, Goldwyn RM. Recurrent breast cancer following immediate reconstruction with myocutaneous flaps. Plast Reconstr Surg 1994;93:1194.
31. Freeman BS. Subcutaneous mastectomy for benign breast lesions with immediate or delayed prosthetic replacement. Plast Reconstr Surg 1962;30:676.
32. Freeman BS. Techniques of subcutaneous mastectomy with replacement: Immediate and delayed. Br J Plast Surg 1969;22:161.
33. Snyderman RK, Guthrie RH. Reconstruction of the female breast following radical mastectomy. Plast Reconstr Surg 1971;47:565.
34. Gruber RP, Kahn RA, Lash H, et al. Breast reconstruction following mastectomy: A comparison of submuscular and subcutaneous techniques. Plast Reconstr Surg 1981;67:312.
35. Becker H. Breast reconstruction using an inflatable breast implant with detachable reservoirs. Plast Reconstr Surg 1984;73:678.
36. Maxwell GP, Falcone PA. Eighty-four consecutive breast reconstructions using a textured silicone tissue expander. Plast Reconstr Surg 1992;90:77.
37. Neumann CG. The expansion of an area of skin by progressive distention of a subcutaneous balloon. Use of the method for securing skin for subtotal reconstruction of the ear. Plast Reconstr Surg 1957;19:124.
38. Radovan C. Breast reconstruction after mastectomy using a temporary expander. Plast Reconstr Surg 1982;69:195.
39. Argenta LC, Marks MW, Grabb WC. Selective use of serial tissue expansion in breast reconstruction. Ann Plast Surg 1983;11:188.
40. Cohen IK, Turner D. Immediate breast reconstruction with tissue expanders. Clin Plast Surg 1987;14:491.
41. Becker H. The permanent tissue expander. Clin Plast Surg 1987;14:519.
42. Versaci AD. Reconstruction of a pendulous breast utilizing a tissue expander. Clin Plast Surg 1987;14:499.
43. Gibney J. The long-term results of tissue expansion for breast reconstruction. Clin Plast Surg 1987;14:509.
44. Spear S, Stefan MM. Breast reconstruction with tissue expanders and implants. Op Tech Plast Reconstr Surg 1994;1:13.
45. Nahabedian MY, Tsangaris T, Momen B, Manson PN. Infectious complications following breast reconstruction with expanders and implants. Plast Reconstr Surg 2003;112:467–476.
46. Olivari N. The latissimus flap. Br J Plast Surg 1976;29:126.
47. Schneider WJ, Hill HL, Brown RG. Latissimus dorsi myocutaneous flap for breast reconstruction. Br J Plast Surg 1977;30:277.

48. Muhlbauer W, Olbrisch R. The latissimus dorsi myocutaneous flap for breast reconstruction. Chir Plast (Berlin) 1977;4:27.
49. McCraw JB, Maxwell GP. Early and late capsular "deformation" as a cause of unsatisfactory results in the latissimus dorsi breast reconstruction. Clin Plast Surg 1988;15:717.
50. Barone FE, Perry L, Maxwell GP. The biomechanical pathological effects of surface texturing with silicone and polyurethane and tissue implantation and expansion. Plast Reconstr Surg 1992;90:77.
51. Hokin JA. Mastectomy reconstruction without a prosthetic implant. Plast Reconstr Surg 1983;72:810.
52. Hokin JA, Silverskoild KL. Breast reconstruction without an implant: Results and complications using an extended latissimus dorsi flap. Plast Reconstr Surg 1987;79:58.
53. Germann G, Steinau H-U. Breast reconstruction with the extended latissimus dorsi flap. Plast Reconstr Surg 1996;97:519.
54. Barnett GR, Gianoutsos MP. The latissimus dorsi added fat flap for natural tissue breast reconstruction: Report of 15 cases. Plast Reconstr Surg 1966;97:63.
55. Bartlett SP, May JW, Yaremchuck MJ. The latissimus dorsi muscle: A fresh cadaver study of the primary neurovascular pedicle. Plast Reconstr Surg 1981;67:631.
56. Fisher J, Bostwick J. Evaluation of the blood supply to the latissimus dorsi muscle after thoracodorsal vessel interruption. Surg Forum 1981;32:576.
57. Fisher J, Bostwick J, Powell RW. Latissimus dorsi blood supply after thoracodorsal vessel division: The serratus collateral. Plast Reconstr Surg 1986;72:502.
58. McGraw JB, Papp C, Edwards A, McMellin A. The autogenous latissimus breast reconstruction. Clin Plast Surg 1994;21:279.
59. McGraw JB, Arnold PG. McGraw and Arnold's Atlas of Muscle and Musculocutaneous Flaps. Norfolk, VA, Hampton Press, 1986.
60. Spear SL, Stefan MM. Breast reconstruction with expanders and implants. Oper Tech Plast Reconstr Surg 1994;1:13.
61. Place MJ, Song T, Hardesty RA, Hendricks DL. Sensory reinnervation of autogenous tissue TRAM flaps after breast reconstruction. Ann Plast Surg 1997;38:19.
62. Kroll SS, Schusterman MA, Reece GP, et al. Abdominal wall strength, bulging and hernia after TRAM flap breast reconstruction. Plast Reconstr Surg 1995;96:616.
63. Williams P, Warwick R. Gray's Anatomy, 36th ed. Edinburgh, Churchill Livingstone, 1980.
64. Hartrampf CR. Breast Reconstruction with Living Tissue. New York, Raven Press, 1991.
65. Moon HK, Taylor GI. The vascular anatomy of the rectus abdominis musculocutaneous flaps based on the deep superior epigastric system. Plast Reconstr Surg 1988;82:815.
66. Taylor GI, Palmer JH. The vascular territories (angiosomes) of the body: Experimental study and clinical applications. Br J Plast Surg 1987;40:113–141.
67. Watterson PA, Bostwick J, Hester R, et al. TRAM flap anatomy correlated with a 10-year clinical experience in 556 patients. Plast Reconstr Surg 1995;95:1185.
68. Karanas YL, Santoro TD, Da Lio AL, Shaw WW. Free TRAM flap breast reconstruction after abdominal liposuction. Plast Reconstr Surg 2003;112:1851–1854.
69. Singletary SE. Skin-sparing mastectomy with immediate breast reconstruction: The M. D. Anderson Cancer Center experience. Ann Surg Oncol 1996;3:411–416.
70. Mizgala CL, Hartrampf CR, Bennett GK. Assessment of the abdominal wall after pedicled TRAM flap surgery: 5 to 7 Year follow-up of 150 consecutive patients. Plast Reconstr Surg 1994;93:988.
71. Hammond DC, Larson DL, Severinac RN, Marcias M. Rectus abdominis muscle innervation: Implications for TRAM flap elevation. Plast Reconstr Surg 1995;96:105–110.
72. Kroll SS, Marchi M. Comparison of strategies for preventing abdominal-wall weakness after TRAM flap breast reconstruction. Plast Reconstr Surg 1992;89:1045.
73. Grotting JC, Urist MM, Maddox WA, Vasconez LO. Conventional TRAM flap versus free microsurgical TRAM flap for immediate breast reconstruction. Plast Reconstr Surg 1992;90:553.
74. Schusterman MA, Kroll SS, Weldon ME. Immediate breast reconstruction: Why the free TRAM over the conventional TRAM flap? Plast Reconstr Surg 1922;92:255.
75. Kind GM, Rademaker AW, Mustoe TA. Abdominal-wall recovery following TRAM flap: A functional outcome study. Plast Reconstr Surg 1997;99:417.
76. Kroll SS, Schusterman MA, Reece GP, et al. Choice of flap and incidence of free flap success. Plast Reconstr Surg 1996;98:459.
77. Banic A, Boeckx M, Greulich P, et al. Late results of breast reconstruction with free TRAM flaps: A prospective multicentric study. Plast Reconstr Surg 1995;95:1195.
78. Baldwin BJ, Schusterman MA, Miller MJ, et al. Bilateral breast reconstruction: Conventional versus free TRAM. Plast Reconstr Surg 1994;93:1410.
79. Kroll SS, Evans GRD, Reece GP, et al. Comparison of resource costs of free and conventional TRAM flap breast reconstruction. Plast Reconstr Surg 1996;98:74.
80. Kronowitz SJ, Chang DW, Robb GL, et al. Implications of axillary sentinel lymph node biopsy in immediate autologous breast reconstruction. Plast Reconstr Surg 2002;109:1888.
81. Feng LJ. Recipient vessels in free-flap breast reconstruction: A study of the internal mammary and thoracodorsal vessels. Plast Reconstr Surg 1997;99:405.
82. Clark CP, Rohrich RJ, Copit S, et al. An anatomic study of the internal mammary veins: Clinical implications for free-tissue transfer breast reconstruction. Plast Reconstr Surg 1997;99:400.
83. Dupin CL, Allen RJ, Glass CA, Bunch R. The internal mammary artery and vein as a recipient site for free-flap breast reconstruction: A report of 110 consecutive cases. Plast Reconstr Surg 1996;98:685.
84. Elliot LF. Free TRAM flap. Oper Tech Plast Reconstr Surg 1994;1:39–45.
85. Souminen S, Tervahartiala P, Von Smitten K, Asko-Seljavaara S. Magnetic resonance imaging of the TRAM flap donor site. Ann Plast Surg 1997;38:23.
86. Koshima I, Soeda S. Inferior epigastric artery skin flap without rectus abdominis muscle. Br J Plast Surg 1989;42:645.
87. Blondeel PN. One hundred free DIEP flap breast reconstructions: A personal experience. Br J Plast Surg 1999;52:104.
88. Nahabedian MY, Momen B, Galdino G, Manson PN. Breast reconstruction with the free TRAM or DIEP flap: Patient selection, choice of flap, and outcome. Plast Reconstr Surg 2002;110:466.
89. Allen RJ, Treece P. Deep inferior epigastric perforator flap for breast reconstruction. Ann Plast Surg 1994;32:32.
90. Vandevoort M, Vranckx JJ, Fabre G. Perforator topography of the deep inferior epigastric flap in 100 cases of breast reconstruction. Plast Reconstr Surg 2002;109:1912.
91. Hamdi M, Weiler-Mithoff EM, Webster MH. Deep inferior epigastric perforator flap in breast reconstruction: Experience with the first 50 flaps. Plast Reconstr Surg 1999;103:86.
92. Blondeel PN, Vanderstraeten GG, Monstrey SJ, et al. The donor site morbidity of the free DIEP flaps and free TRAM flaps for breast reconstruction. Br J Plast Surg 1997;50:322.
93. Kroll SS. Fat necrosis in free transverse rectus abdominis myocutaneous and deep inferior epigastric perforator flaps. Plast Reconstr Surg 2000;106:576.
94. Rogers N, Allen RJ. Radiation effects on breast reconstruction with the deep inferior epigastric perforator flap. Plast Reconstr Surg 2002;109:1919.
95. Fujino T, Harashina T, Enomoto K. Primary breast reconstruction after a standard radical mastectomy by a free tissue transfer. Plast Reconstr Surg 1976;58:372.
96. Shaw WW. Breast reconstruction by superior gluteal microvascular free flaps without silicone implants. Plast Reconstr Surg 1983;72:490.
97. Shaw WW. Microvascular free flap breast reconstruction. Clin Plast Surg 1984;11:333.
98. Shaw WW, Orringer JS, Ko CY, Ratto LC. The spontaneous return of sensibility in breasts reconstructed with autologous tissues. Plast Reconstr Surg 1997;99:394.
99. Allen RA, Tucker C. Superior gluteal artery perforator free flap for breast reconstruction. Plast Reconstr Surg 1995;95:1207.
100. Barnett GR, Carlisle IR, Gianoutsos MB. The cephalic vein: An aid in free TRAM flap breast reconstruction. Report of 12 cases. Plast Reconstr Surg 1996;97:71.
101. Palletta CE, Bostwick J III, Nahai F. The inferior gluteal free flap in breast reconstruction. Plast Reconstr Surg 1989;89:875–883.
102. Eaves FF, Codner MA, Nahai F. The inferior gluteal free flap in breast reconstruction. Oper Tech Plast Reconstr Surg 1994;1:58–65.
103. Wellisch DK, Schain WS, Noone RB, Little JW. The psychological contribution of nipple addition in breast reconstruction. Plast Reconstr Surg 1987;80:699.

104. Little JW. Nipple-areola reconstruction. Clin Plast Surg 1984;11: 351.
105. Chang WH. Nipple reconstruction with a T-flap. Plast Reconstr Surg 1984;73:140.
106. Cronin ED, Humphreys DH, Ruiz-Razura A. Nipple reconstruction: The S-flap. Plast Reconstr Surg 1988;81:783.
107. Kroll SS, Hamilton S. Nipple reconstruction with the double-opposing-tab flap. Plast Reconstr Surg 1989;84:520.
108. Little JW III, Munasifi T, McCulloch D. One-stage reconstruction of a projecting nipple: The quadrapod flap. Plast Reconstr Surg 1983;71: 126.
109. Rees TD. Reconstruction of the breast areola by intradermal tattooing and transfer: Case report. Plast Reconstr Surg 1986;77:673.
110. Anton MA, Eskenazi LB, Hartrampf CR Jr. Nipple reconstruction with local flaps. Perspect Plast Surg 1991;5:67.
111. Little JW Jr, Spear SL. The finishing touches on nipple-areolar reconstruction. Perspect Plast Surg 1988;2:1.
112. Eskenazi L. A one-stage nipple reconstruction with the "modified star" flap and immediate tattoo: A review of 100 cases. Plast Reconstr Surg 1993;92:671.
113. Brody GS. The effect of breast implants on the radiographic detection of microcalcifications and soft-tissue masses [discussion]. Plast Reconstr Surg 1989;84:779.
114. Dunn KW, Hall PN, Khoo CTK. Breast implant materials: Sense and safety. Br J Plast Surg 1992;45:315.
115. Hayes H, Vandergrift MS, Diner WC. Mammography and breast implants. Plast Reconstr Surg 1988;82:1.
116. Dershaw DD, Chaglassian TA. Mammography after prosthesis placement for augmentation or reconstructive mammaplasty. Radiology 1989;170:69.
117. Silverstein MJ, Handel N, Gamagami PG. The effect of silicone gel-filled implants on mammography. Cancer 1991;68(Suppl):1159.
118. Monsees BS, Destouet JM. Mammography in aesthetic and reconstructive breast surgery. Perspect Plast Surg 1991;5:103.
119. Matory WE Jr, Wertheimer M, Fitzgerald TJ, et al. Aesthetic results following partial mastectomy and radiation therapy. Plast Reconstr Surg 1990;85:739–746.
120. Berrino P, Campora E, Santi P. Postquadrantectomy breast deformities: Classification and techniques of surgical correction. Plast Reconstr Surg 1987;79:567–572.
121. Fisher B, Anderson S, Fisher ER, et al. Significance of ipsilateral breast tumor recurrence after lumpectomy. Lancet 1991;338:327.
122. Fisher B, Redmond C, Poisson R, et al. Eight-year results of a randomized clinical trail comparing total mastectomy and lumpectomy with or without irradiation in the treatment of breast cancer. N Engl J Med 1989;320:822.
123. Stotter AT, McNeese MD, Ames FC, et al. Predicting the rate and extent of locoregional failure after breast conservation therapy for early breast cancer. Cancer 1989;64:2217.
124. Slavin SA, Love SM, Sadowsky NL. Reconstruction of the radiated partial mastectomy defect with autogenous tissues. Plast Reconstr Surg 1992;90:854–853.
125. Asplund O, Korlof B. Late results following mastectomy for cancer and breast reconstruction. Scand J Plast Reconstr 1984;18:221–225.
126. Maguire GP, Lee EG, Bevington EJ, et al. Psychiatric problems in the first year after mastectomy. Br Med J 1978;1:963–965.
127. Morris T, Greer HS, White P. Psychosocial and social adjustment to mastectomy: A two year follow-up. Cancer 1977;40:2381–2387.
128. Jamison KR, Wellisch DK, Pasnau RO. Psychosocial aspects of mastectomy: The women's perspective. Am J Psychiatry 1978;235:432–436.
129. Clifford E, Clifford M, Georgiade NC. Breast reconstruction following mastectomy: II. Marital characteristics of patients seeking this procedure. Ann Plast Surg 1980;5:343–346.
130. Teimourian B, Adham MN. Survey of patients: Responses to breast reconstruction. Ann Plast Surg 1982;9:321–325.
131. Holland JC, Rowland JH. Psychological care of the patient with cancer. Handbook of psycho-oncology. New York, Oxford University Press, 1989, pp 188–208.
132. Lester LJ. A critical viewpoint by a general surgeon toward reconstructive surgery after mastectomy. Clin Plast Surg 1979;16:15.
133. Dowden RV, Blanchard JM, Greenstreet RL. Breast reconstruction, timing and local recurrence. Ann Plast Surg 1983;10:265–269.
134. Johnson C, Van Heerden JA, Donohue JH. Oncological aspects of immediate breast reconstruction following mastectomy for malignancy. Arch Surg 1989;124:819–823.
135. Schain WS, Wellisch DK, Pasnau RO, et al. The sooner the better: A study of psychological factors in women undergoing immediate versus delayed breast reconstruction. Am J Psychiatry 1985;142:40–46.
136. Gerard D. Sexual functioning after mastectomy: Life vs lab. J Sex Marital Ther 1982;8:305–315.

CHAPTER 26

Radiotherapy for In Situ, Stage I, and Stage II Breast Cancer

Randy E. Stevens

Radiation therapy has an integral role in the curative treatment of breast cancer. After conservative surgery for ductal carcinoma in situ (DCIS) or invasive carcinoma, radiation therapy of the breast improves the likelihood of locoregional freedom from disease and thereby enhances the long-term possibility of breast preservation. After mastectomy, in carefully selected patients, locoregional radiation therapy reduces the risk for recurrence and possibly prolongs survival. Therefore, clinicians caring for patients who have breast cancer require a clear understanding of the pertinent principles of radiation therapy: selection criteria, techniques of treatment, beneficial results, and side effects.

BASICS OF RADIATION BIOLOGY

How does radiation cause changes in the patient's tissues?

X-rays, gamma rays, electrons, and heavy particles (neutrons, protons) are believed to produce cell damage by indirectly or directly forming irreparable double-stranded DNA breaks.[1] When the cell next enters mitosis, it cannot divide, and cell death occurs (reproductive death).[1,2] One exception to this process is the interphase death of lymphocytes.

The precise mechanism of DNA damage is different for x-rays, gamma rays, and electrons (low linear energy transfer [LET] radiation) than for heavy particles (high LET radiation).[1] Low LET radiation results in sparse electron–tissue interaction. It is unlikely to deposit two electrons in the same DNA molecule. Rather, a single-stranded DNA break may occur. A second "hit" is required to yield a double-stranded DNA break. Both hits are likely to occur by an indirect mechanism: the result of an electron ionizing a water molecule and yielding a hydroxyl radical. Hydroxyl radicals can migrate a short distance (100 Å, or 10 nm) and, if near a DNA molecule, result in an interaction that produces a single-stranded break. The hydroxyl radical has a half-life, in microseconds, that can be prolonged by oxygen or electron-affinic compounds and shortened by free radical scavengers.[3] In contrast, high LET radiation deposits energy densely over a short distance. If it

happens to pass through a DNA molecule, two hits that produce double-stranded damage may occur.[1] Consequently, high LET radiation produces DNA damage independent of oxygen concentration.[1]

Regardless of the mechanism of DNA damage, the end result, reproductive cell death, explains the variation in rapidity of cell death (whether normal or malignant tissue). More rapidly dividing tissues display the effects of radiation, including cell death, faster than slowly dividing tissues.[4] The mucosa of the oral cavity, for example, shows damage sooner than does neural tissue.

Radiation sensitivity (see later) also varies with cell cycle.[5] Cells in the G_2 and M phases are more sensitive to ionizing radiation than cells in the G_0, G_1, or S phases.[5] Rapidly dividing neoplastic or normal tissues (e.g., skin, gastrointestinal mucosa, bone marrow) pass through mitosis more often, and radiation effects are seen sooner, than in more slowly dividing systems (e.g., subcutaneous tissues, kidney, brain). For the most part, neoplastic tissue behaves more like rapidly dividing (acute-responding) tissue than more slowly dividing (late-responding) tissue.[6,7]

What factors alter normal or tumor tissue response to radiation?

Time–Dose–Volume Relationships

Long-term or late effects are those detected more than 6 months after completion of radiation therapy. As the volume of normal tissue irradiated to a given dose increases, the risk for long-term damage increases.[8] A small volume can be treated to a higher total dose (compared with a larger volume and lower total dose) while maintaining the same risk for long-term effects. With the availability of modern computer-generated dose–volume histograms (percentage of organ treated vs. dose), the wealth of human data being collected is yielding an improved understanding of dose–volume relationships. This improved understanding should translate into reduced normal tissue toxicity in the future.

Dose fractionation (dose per time) is intimately related to radiation effects on normal and neoplastic tissue.[9] For example, 7000 cGy given continually over 7 weeks in 200-cGy fractions often cures squamous cell carcinoma of the supraglottic larynx. The same 7000 cGy in 200-cGy fractions but delivered with a 2-week interruption will yield a lower local control rate.[10] Total dose, dose per fraction, and overall time are interrelated and critical to the likelihood of tumor control and normal tissue effects.

Radiation sensitivity refers to the fraction of cells surviving after exposure to a given dose of ionizing radiation. Dose (energy per unit mass) is reported in gray (1 Gy = 1 J-kg^{-1}) or centigray (100 cGy = 1 Gy). Before use of standard international units, dose was recorded in rad (radiation absorbed dose; 1 rad = 1 cGy). In addition to cell cycle, variables affecting radiation sensitivity include the type of stem cell,[1] oxygen,[11] heat,[12] and certain chemotherapeutic agents.[13–15]

Oxygen is important to permit low LET radiation to produce double-stranded DNA breaks.[11] However, it remains controversial as to whether supplemental oxygen, hyperbaric oxygen, electron-affinic agents, or transfusions to increase oxygen-carrying capacity can improve cell kill. In hypoxic tumors, reoxygenation is postulated to occur spontaneously. After the oxygenated periphery of the tumor has been irradiated and cell death occurs, the previously hypoxic segments have less competition from other tumor cells for available oxygen. The newly reoxygenated tumor can effectively be damaged by subsequent ionizing radiation.

Chemotherapeutic agents may be used before, during, or after radiation therapy. They may be used to decrease the number of clonogens that the ionizing radiation must eliminate (e.g., doxorubicin or cyclophosphamide, methotrexate, 5-fluorouracil [CMF]) or synchronize cells in more sensitive phases of the cell cycle (e.g., paclitaxel [Taxol], which arrests cells in mitosis), yielding improved cell kill for a given dose of ionizing radiation.

Radioresponsiveness is the observable response of the malignancy to ionizing radiation, a combination of radiation sensitivity and cell loss due to the kinetics of the cell system. The overall likelihood of death is also dependent on fractionation, the percentage of organ irradiated or the size of the tumor (for tumor response), total dose prescribed, radiation sensitizers, ability to repair sublethal DNA damage, role of potentially lethal damage, and, in tumors, ability to repopulate during radiation.

Normal rates of cellular proliferation of non-neoplastic and neoplastic tissues may continue during irradiation. However, irradiation of tissues may induce some cells to accelerate their growth rate to replace cells destroyed by radiation. In normal tissue, this recruitment repopulates early-responding tissues to a greater extent than late-responding tissues. Therefore, long-term damage in skin and bone marrow, which are early-responding tissues, is minimized. In neoplastic tissue, accelerated repopulation may begin while the tumor appears grossly to be shrinking.[7–9] The surviving neoplastic clonogens proliferate faster than at the beginning of radiation. This accelerated regeneration may be important in inflammatory carcinoma of the breast, as well as other malignancies, and appears to act as an impediment to cure of disease.

How do a patient's normal tissues heal after radiation therapy?

Nonlethal cellular damage (DNA breaks) after radiation therapy may be repaired. Further ionizations may result in cell death. Two types of cell injury, called *potentially lethal* and *sublethal*, do not immediately lead to cell death. Potentially lethal damage requires the cellular environment to be modified for repair. If the required condition (e.g., a change in temperature, oxygen) can be met, the cell can survive. Repair of sublethal damage occurs, and is clearly demonstrated, when radiation is fractionated (divided into many small doses) and several hours intervene between doses (fractions). For many stem cells, sublethal damage repair has occurred after 6 to 8 hours. Fractionated radiation therapy exploits the difference in the ability of normal and malignant tissues to repair damage caused by ionizing radiation. After a multiweek course of radiation therapy, the damage is greater in the neoplastic tissue (optimally resulting in neoplastic cell kill) than in the normal tissue, or the damage is in the process of being repaired, thus allowing ionizing radiation to be an effective and well-tolerated therapeutic modality in the eradication of neoplasms.

BASICS OF THE PHYSICAL CONSIDERATIONS OF RADIATION THERAPY

What is ionizing radiation?

Ionizing radiation may be either electromagnetic or particulate packages of energy. The electromagnetic spectrum ranges from low-frequency (long-wavelength) radio waves, to intermediate-frequency visible and ultraviolet light, to high-frequency (short-wavelength) x-rays and gamma rays. X-rays and gamma rays, by virtue of their greater frequency, have relatively higher energy and are more penetrating in tissue, a property that is useful therapeutically. X-rays and gamma rays differ in the way they are formed. Gamma rays are emitted from the nucleus during decay of a radioactive isotope. X-rays are produced extranuclearly, usually by a machine that accelerates electrons, which bombard a heavy-metal target, releasing energy as heat and x-rays.

Particulate radiation includes electrons, protons, neutrons, negative pi mesons, alpha particles, and atomic nuclei. All of these examples of particulate radiation have been used in radiation therapy. Electrons are the most frequently employed, especially in the treatment of malignancies of the breast. Because these types of radiation have physical mass and charge, they do not penetrate tissues as easily as x-rays or gamma rays, a property that can be exploited clinically. Whether electromagnetic or particulate, ionizing radiation travels as a packet of energy (photon), which, when absorbed in tissue, results in ionization and, ultimately, in biologic damage.

Three mechanisms of ionization are possible, depending on the energy involved: (1) the photoelectric process, (2) the Compton effect, and (3) pair production.[16] The photoelectric process is the most common mechanism of x-ray interaction in diagnostic radiology because the equipment generally operates in the kilovoltage energy range. The likelihood of absorption of the ray is proportional to the cube of the atomic number (Z^3) of the tissue it encounters. This explains the whiter appearance of bone and the gray or blackish appearance of air on a diagnostic radiograph (Fig. 26–1). By contrast

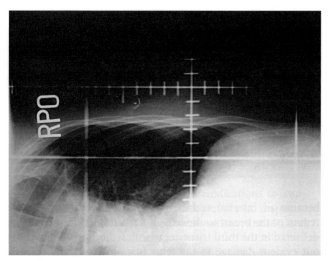

Figure 26–1 Radiograph of the breast and chest wall. The x-ray beam is tangential to the chest wall. This film was taken using a simulator that generates x-rays in the kilovoltage range, similar to diagnostic x-ray units. The bones (ribs) appear white; the lung appears black.

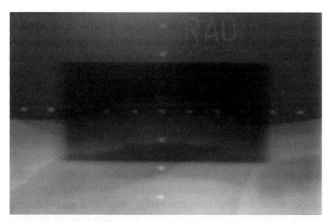

Figure 26–2 Port film of a breast treatment portal. Because this film was taken using a linear accelerator (megavoltage-range x-rays), the contrast between the bone and lung is muted, demonstrating the relative independence of the Compton effect on atomic number.

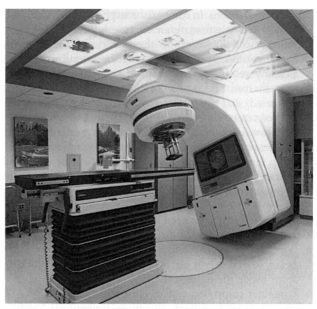

Figure 26–3 Linear accelerator. This Varian 2300 C linear accelerator can produce 6- and 18-MV photons as well as several energies of electron beam.

What is the hallmark of modern radiation therapy? What is a linear accelerator? How does it work?

"Modern radiotherapy" refers to the era of megavoltage treatment and was not widely available in the United States until the 1960s. Radiation therapy delivered before the megavoltage era used energy in the orthovoltage (150 to 500 kV) or supervoltage (500 to 1000 kV) range. Many undesirable effects resulted from treatment with the lower-energy machinery. Because of the importance of the photoelectric effect and the increased absorption of radiation in bone compared with soft tissue, orthovoltage radiation therapy could not effectively reach tumors behind bones and inflicted unnecessary injury in the bone. In addition, orthovoltage machinery lacked skin sparing; therefore, redness and reaction of the skin frequently limited the dose that could be delivered to the underlying tumors.

Currently, the most common machines providing megavoltage radiation therapy are linear accelerators (Fig. 26–3). A linear accelerator has several advantages over orthovoltage and cobalt 60 therapy:

1. It produces a higher-energy x-ray beam that enables greater skin sparing and more effective treatment of deep-seated lesions.
2. In addition to the x-ray beam, linear accelerators can provide a therapeutically useful high-energy electron beam. Electrons have a discrete range and, relative to photons, have most of their tissue interactions within a small distance. Therefore, there is a more abrupt falloff of dose beyond the electron's range of penetration. The range is proportional to the energy of the electron, and most modern linear accelerators produce a number of selectable electron energies that can be customized to the individual patient's anatomy and needs. Electrons, in general, are less skin sparing than photons and are useful for treating

with the photoelectric process, modern radiation therapy employs beams in the megavoltage range (at least 1 million volts). The Compton effect, the prevailing mechanism of x-ray interaction with tissue at megavoltage energies, is not dependent on atomic number but on the density of the absorbing medium (electrons per gram). Therefore, the differential absorption of bone compared with that of soft tissue is much less. This property helps create far more homogeneous radiotherapy than could be produced by older equipment. When comparing a port film (a localizing film taken using a treatment beam) to a diagnostic energy x-ray from a treatment simulator, the relative difference in the importance of atomic number and density of the two processes is apparent (Fig. 26–2). A practiced eye and extreme care are therefore required to ensure that treatment fields are precisely aimed throughout a course of treatment.

homogeneity of dose distribution usually is improved for the patient of average or larger breast size.

Should the entire breast be treated uniformly, or is a boost dose important?

After completion of whole-breast radiotherapy to a dose of 4500 to 5000 cGy, a boost to the area of the original tumor generally is employed (Figs. 26–14 and 26–15). The boost is used for two reasons. First, the area of the original lesion has been shown to have the highest bulk of microscopic residual disease.[49] Clinically, this correlates with the observed patterns of recurrence—mostly at or near the index lesion.[50–56] Second, hypoxia from surgically disturbed vasculature in the tumor bed may also require an increased dose to eradicate microscopic residual disease[11] (see prior discussion regarding oxygen effect). Therefore, a higher total dose to the initial tumor bed decreases recurrence rates.[57] The higher dose is limited to a small volume (the volume at highest risk for recurrence)

because doses above 5000 to 6000 cGy to the whole breast result in an increased incidence of breast edema and poor cosmesis.[58–60] The boost may be delivered using external-beam techniques (most commonly electron-beam therapy from a linear accelerator, as shown in Fig. 26–14), three-dimensional conformal therapy using photons or IMRT, or brachytherapy or intraoperative radiotherapy.[55,56,61–64] Electrons, as opposed to photons, have a discrete range that is dependent on their energy. Beyond their useful range, the dose falls off abruptly. Thus, they can be selected to treat the desired tumor volume homogeneously yet spare underlying normal tissues.

Brachytherapy is the placement of radioactive material into or next to the tumor or tumor bed. In breast radiotherapy,

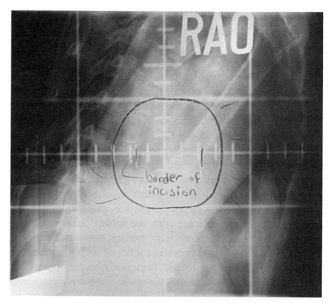

Figure 26–14   Simulation film of a boost portal for use in radiation therapy of the breast. Radiopaque clips were placed in the tumor bed at the time of surgery. A 1-cm margin is usually placed around the clips. The incision is also included in the field. Only the area within the circle will be treated. The hatched area outside the circle is not treated.

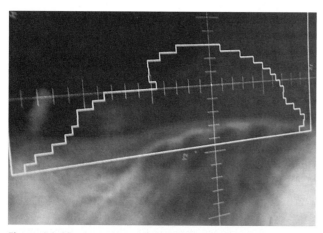

Figure 26–13   Intensity-modulated breast field showing the multileaf collimation (*jagged lines*) to modulate areas of the breast (decrease the dose) in the thinner areas that would otherwise receive a higher dose.

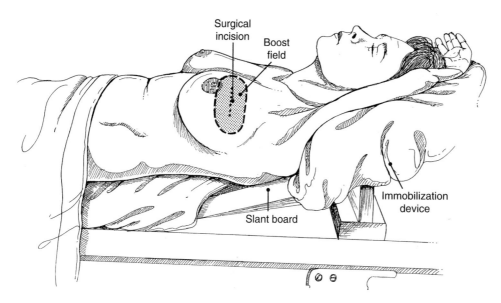

Figure 26–15   Diagram of an electron boost portal as viewed on the skin. If clips have not been placed in the tumor bed, a 3-cm margin is placed around the incision, as shown here. If CT scan planning is used; the tumor bed (boost portal) is localized from the postoperative changes in the tumor bed on CT scan.

temporary single- or double-plane implants of iridium 192 can be placed into the tumor bed to deliver the intended dose, 1500 to 2000 cGy over $1\frac{1}{2}$ to 2 days (low-dose-rate brachytherapy) or about 680 cGy divided between two brief treatments 6 hours apart using a high-dose-rate remote after-loader. Low-dose-rate brachytherapy requires local anesthesia, patient hospitalization, limited visitors, and precise identification of the tumor bed (because the dose falls off very rapidly in proportion to the inverse square of distance). The high-dose-rate brachytherapy avoids hospitalization and personnel exposure and provides similar control rates. When performed by an experienced radiation oncologist, interstitial brachytherapy and electron-beam therapy boost result in similar local control.[64–68] The electron-beam technique is more commonly used for the boost portion of the treatment because the patient remains an outpatient, the procedure is not invasive, and cosmesis is as good or superior.[26, 64–68]

Treatment planning for the electron-beam boost can be accomplished clinically with ultrasound guidance or CT scan planning.[69–71] First, the surgical tumor bed must be localized. This is most accurately accomplished if clips have been placed in the biopsy cavity at the time of surgery[72] (see Fig. 26–14). If surgical clips, ultrasound guidance, or CT scanning is not available, the clinician must use the incision in combination with the preoperative mammogram or ultrasound (see Fig. 26–15). Therefore, the radiation oncologist must know the position of the surgical incision relative to the location of the preoperative tumor. The treatment angle is then chosen (clinically or with ultrasound or CT) to provide the shortest path to the tumor bed and the incision. For electron-beam therapy, the depth from the skin surface to the base of the tumor bed is measured to determine the appropriate electron energy because the range of penetration varies with the energy of the electrons. (See prior discussion of electrons.) Although theoretically the most accurate,[73] CT scan–based planning has not been shown to reduce the local recurrence rates compared with the other planning methods.

Cerrobend blocking can be used to individualize the shape of the treatment portal and prevent treatment of more breast tissue than is medically necessary (Fig. 26–16). Cerrobend, a combination of cadmium, bismuth, and tin, has the ability to attenuate a treatment beam almost as effectively as lead and melts when heated to moderate temperatures. It can be poured into molds (and hardened) into any shape desired, further customizing treatment.

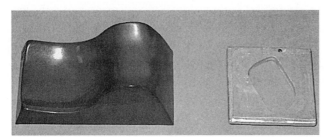

Figure 26–16 *Left,* Headrest used for patient positioning, reproducibility, and comfort. *Right,* Cerrobend has been poured and cut to the customized shape for the patient's boost portal. Only the oval area inside (not covered by) the Cerrobend will receive the prescribed dose.

Is the volume to be treated always the same?

For patients who have DCIS or stage I invasive carcinoma, the risk for a regional nodal recurrence is 0% to 5%,[51,63,74–76] and only the breast is treated (most commonly, two portals whose central axes are aimed tangential to the chest wall). For stage II invasive carcinoma, whether after conservative surgery or mastectomy, each patient's risk for regional nodal recurrence is evaluated individually. If the risk for nodal recurrence is greater than 10% to 15% or regional nodal irradiation may result in clinical benefit, simulation of the breast or chest wall and relevant nodal region is advised. The specific indications for regional nodal irradiation are considered in the discussions of invasive carcinoma and the postmastectomy patient.

If regional nodal irradiation is to be delivered in addition to whole-breast radiotherapy, treatment planning becomes a more complex process. Lack of attention to precise matching of the nodal and breast portals can result in underdosing or overdosing of a region. Overlap at the skin surface has resulted in classic "matchline fibrosis," a ridge of fibrosis that may be associated with telangiectases and impaired cosmesis.[58–60,77]

If the supraclavicular region is to be treated, usually the superior border of the breast tangents is lowered to the angle of Louis. The medial, inferior, and lateral tangent borders generally are unchanged. The inferior border of the supraclavicular field is the superior border of the breast portal. The medial border usually is placed at the ipsilateral pedicles. The lateral border is generally at the medial edge of the humeral head. Superiorly, the field is usually placed at the inferior aspect of the cricoid cartilage (Fig. 26–17).

If the axillary apex is to be treated, the lateral border of the supraclavicular field is generally extended to cover the posterior axillary skin fold. The lateral and inferior borders of the axillary field are those of the supraclavicular field. The medial border includes the chest wall and 1 cm of lung (to allow for respiratory movement), and the superior border is placed along the clavicle.

The internal mammary field is usually 6 cm in width. The medial border extends 1 cm past midline (toward the contralateral breast). Laterally, it abuts the medial edge of the tangential breast field. Usually, it extends superiorly and inferiorly to cover the first through third intercostal spaces. The medial border of the breast tangents and inferior border of the supraclavicular fields are determined by the borders of the internal mammary field.

Several technical discussions of the simulation for regional nodal irradiation have been published.[78–80] Inclusion of the nodal region at simulation and treatment increases the length of time required for simulation, daily setup, and treatment. (See the discussion of the indications for regional nodal irradiation in the invasive carcinoma and postmastectomy portions of this chapter.)

Does the entire breast require treatment?

Whole-breast radiation therapy is the standard of care for treatment of DCIS and early invasive carcinoma after lumpectomy or wide excision. For selected patients with early invasive ductal carcinoma, partial-breast irradiation may yield similar

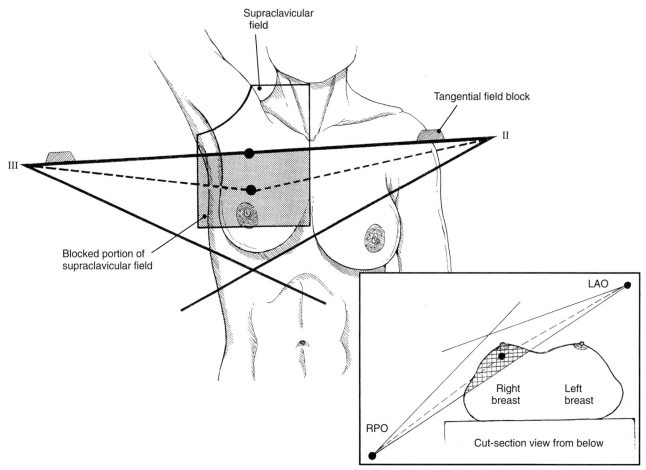

Figure 26–17   Schematic diagram of radiotherapy portals when irradiation of the supraclavicular lymph nodes is planned. The supraclavicular portal (*shaded region*) is treated from an anterior or anterior oblique approach. Note that the superior edge of the breast tangent portals is straight (horizontal) so that there is no overlap between the supraclavicular and breast portals. LAO, left anterior oblique; RPO, right posterior oblique.

local control and survival with greater convenience, similar or improved cosmetic result, and similar or reduced side effects. Partial-breast irradiation can be delivered with three-dimensional conformal radiation therapy,[81] IMRT, or low-dose-rate or high-dose-rate interstitial brachytherapy using multiple catheters or using a newer single catheter with a balloon placed into the tumor bed. Partial-breast irradiation can also be delivered by intraoperative radiation therapy (IORT) using electron-beam therapy or x-rays. Each technique has its own advantages and disadvantages.

IMRT is the most recent and most sophisticated version of three-dimensional conformal radiation therapy.[48] Using advanced computerized treatment planning software, a target or treatment volume is delineated, and dose limitations are prescribed to the adjacent normal tissues. A treatment plan is constructed to deliver the prescribed dose to the tumor or tumor bed precisely while meeting the usual tissue constraints. To accomplish true IMRT to a breast tumor bed, additional fields and longer treatment times are used than with the standard two tangential fields. The potential advantages include more even dose distribution across the intended target, lower dose to the presumed normal surrounding breast tissue, and therefore, possibly better cosmesis and decreased acute toxicity (i.e., erythema and edema). The potential

disadvantages include a larger volume of adjacent normal tissue exposed to a lower dose of radiation and more leakage radiation, which could yield a higher risk for later nonbreast cancer malignancies.

Interstitial breast brachytherapy can be performed at the completion of the lumpectomy or up to several weeks later. A series of catheters are implanted into the breast tumor bed, and radioactive material is subsequently placed into the catheters based on the treatment plan so that the tumor bed with a 1- to 2-cm margin is irradiated.[82] Low-dose-rate brachytherapy delivers a slow continuous dose of radiation, usually with iridium 192 implanted in the catheters over about 96 hours.[83] The patient is in the hospital in an "isolation room" during this time. The entire course of treatment is delivered in 4 days and, including surgery and planning, can be completed within 10 days to 2 weeks of surgery. Because of the isolation during treatment, the cost of hospitalization, and the development of high-dose-rate brachytherapy, low-dose-rate therapy is less frequently performed.

High-dose-rate brachytherapy uses a radioactive source (most often iridium 192) with a higher activity and delivers therapy in multiple short treatments on an outpatient basis. The source remains in a lead-lined container, usually in the radiation therapy department. The breast catheters are

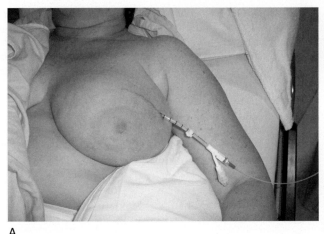

A

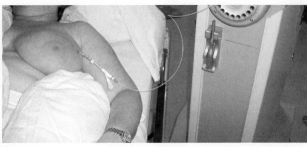

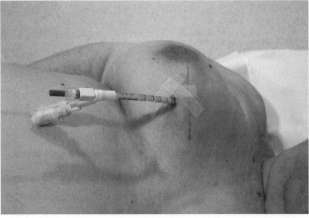

B

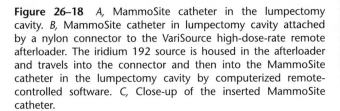

C

Figure 26–18 *A,* MammoSite catheter in the lumpectomy cavity. *B,* MammoSite catheter in lumpectomy cavity attached by a nylon connector to the VariSource high-dose-rate remote afterloader. The iridium 192 source is housed in the afterloader and travels into the connector and then into the MammoSite catheter in the lumpectomy cavity by computerized remote-controlled software. *C,* Close-up of the inserted MammoSite catheter.

connected to the high-dose-rate machine, and treatment is delivered in about 10 minutes. For partial-breast therapy, an average of 10 treatments are prescribed and delivered as 2 treatments per day, separated by 6 hours. The total treatment course is completed in 5 days.[83,84] Advantages of high-dose-rate brachytherapy include the shorter course of therapy compared with conventional external-beam radiation therapy, the lack of hospitalization required, and lack of personnel exposure.

Balloon catheter–based brachytherapy using the Mammo-Site device (Proxima Therapeutics, Marietta, GA) is a subset of high-dose-rate brachytherapy.[85] The dose and treatments are similar to those described earlier.[86] The applicator is a single catheter with an expandable balloon at one end. The applicator may be placed into the tumor bed at lumpectomy or about 2 weeks later once the final margins and pathology are available (Fig. 26–18). The balloon is inflated to fill the cavity and create a uniform spherical dose distribution providing a full dose at 1 cm beyond the edge of the balloon.

IORT uses a mobile linear accelerator to deliver electron-beam therapy[87,88] or uses a mobile x-ray device. The applicator can be placed directly into the tumor bed after lumpectomy, and the surrounding normal tissue (i.e., skin and chest wall) can be displaced or shielded to improve the therapeutic ratio. A single relatively high-dose treatment is performed. The advantages include accurate localization of the tumor bed, the ability to shield adjacent tissue, and the short treatment course. The disadvantages include the lack of final pathology and margin status, the possible fibrosis after a single high dose, and the potential impact on wound healing. In one series, the entire quadrant was treated after quadrantectomy, which was shown to reduce optimal cosmetic result in a randomized trial; hence, the primary end point in this series is not cosmesis.

The limiting step for partial-breast treatment is appropriate patient selection. A discussion of the selection criteria and available results is provided in the section on invasive breast cancer.[89]

What does the patient experience during each fraction of radiation?

Patients typically spend about 15 to 20 minutes in the treatment room. Most of that time is spent in placing the patient in the identical position she was in at simulation. Each treatment room should have overhead, left, and right lateral lasers. With the patient in the supine treatment position (on a slant board or resting in a polystyrene or other mold, if used at simulation) and with the ipsilateral arm abducted, the lasers (calibrated each morning) are aligned with the tattoos placed on the patient's skin at simulation. The linear accelerator is then rotated to the treatment angles determined at simulation. The light field is aligned with the field borders placed on the patient's skin at the conclusion of simulation (tattoos or carbolfuchsin). Before the first treatment, and then weekly, a verification film or digital image is taken on the treatment unit to confirm that the treated field internally matches (and continues to match) the simulated field. The treating radiation oncologist verifies, in the treatment room, the field set by the technologist and subsequently views and approves the verification films. Before treatment is delivered, the parameters set by the technologists operating the treatment unit (e.g., angles of the fields, appropriate field dimensions, and treatment time) are verified by a computer-based quality assurance system. For breast therapy, treatment takes about 1 minute per field. With IMRT or more than two fields, the treatment and setup time increase. After the first field is treated, the technologists reenter the treatment room and set the angles for the second field. The quality assurance steps in the treatment room and at the computer console are repeated.

While treatment is in progress, the technologists are outside of the treatment room at the computer console. Audio and video monitors allow constant observation of and communication with the patient. During treatment, the patient will not experience any treatment-specific sensations. She will hear mechanical noises from the machine. When she leaves the treatment room, she will feel no different than when she entered.

How precise is radiation therapy and how is its quality ensured?

Radiation therapy is extremely precise, generally to within 2 mm in both length and width. To ensure this precision, in addition to physicians and technologists, a complement of physics staff should always be on site: medical physicists, dosimetrists, and block cutters. All equipment, including the linear accelerators, simulators, and lasers, should undergo rigorous daily calibration and quality assurance testing before treatment of the first patient.

Weekly verification films confirm the precision of the machine and the proper positioning of the patient. Facilities that adhere to meticulous technique review their quality assurance processes in regularly held meetings attended by clinicians, physicists, dosimetrists, technologists, and nurses.

DUCTAL CARCINOMA IN SITU

What treatment options are available for ductal carcinoma in situ?

Until relatively recently, the recommended treatment option for DCIS—mastectomy—created a paradox of logic. Certainly, mastectomy yielded local control rates of 96% to 100%.[90–94] The cosmetic and psychological cost of the procedure, however, seemed unnecessarily high, especially when more aggressive invasive carcinomas were being cured by conservative surgery and radiation therapy. Yet, progress was stymied by two misperceptions: (1) DCIS was thought to be inherently radioresistant, and (2) the occasional pathologically observed microscopic multicentricity of DCIS was thought to preclude local control using radiation therapy.[92,93,95–98] However, as the routine use of mastectomy was re-evaluated, the presentation of DCIS also was changing. Carcinoma in situ is now the most frequently detected breast cancer presenting as a nonpalpable radiographic abnormality. The smaller volume of disease at diagnosis and increasing demand for breast preservation has allowed the option of breast-conserving surgery with or without radiation therapy to expand to DCIS.

The intent of radiation therapy in addition to excision is to improve local control by eradicating any occult residual microscopic in situ or invasive carcinoma left behind after

cosmetically optimal local excisions. The wide range in recurrence rates[93,96,99–111] after conservative surgery or radiation therapy, or both, shows that the term *ductal carcinoma in situ* encompasses a spectrum of diseases. As discussed in Chapters 8 and 23, several investigators have worked to restratify and classify in situ lesions into prognostically useful groups intended to help guide therapy. Currently, three treatment options may be offered, depending on the perceived biologic aggressiveness of the lesion: (1) wide excision alone, (2) wide excision followed by breast radiotherapy, or (3) mastectomy with or without reconstruction.

Which patients benefit from radiation after breast-conserving surgery?

Although there probably is a subgroup of small, biologically less aggressive, well-defined, unifocal lesions of DCIS that can be adequately treated with wide excision alone (without radiotherapy), the specific criteria to define them have yet to be unambiguously established.[95,99,112–116] In the literature, depending on the patient population studied, recurrence rates may approach 16% to 59% at 3 to 7 years after excision alone.[95,99,111,117–120] Lagios and colleagues,[107,121] based on a nonrandomized prospective series, and Silverstein and coworkers,[122,123] based originally on a retrospective series, have proposed prognostic criteria for treatment recommendations.

In 1989, Lagios and colleagues[107] described the care of 79 selected women who underwent wide excision alone for treatment of nonpalpable mammographically detected microcalcifications no larger than 25 mm that proved histologically to be DCIS. The margins of resection had to be free of disease. A postexcision mammogram documenting complete excision of microcalcifications was mandatory. The patient had to be compliant with follow-up evaluation and the breasts considered "favorable for clinical and mammographic evaluation." Meticulous step-section processing, not sampling, of the resected breast tissue was performed. The average lesion measured only 6.8 mm. At 4 years, 10% of patients had developed a local (in the same quadrant as the index lesion) recurrence; in half of this 10% the recurrence was invasive, and in the other half it was noninvasive. The authors retrospectively stratified the lesions based on grade and presence or absence of comedonecrosis. At 2 years, high-grade lesions with comedonecrosis had a 19% risk for recurrence. None of 33 low-grade lesions of the non-necrotic cribriform or micropapillary types had recurred.

Silverstein and coworkers used size, grade, and presence or absence of necrosis and retrospectively developed the Van Nuys Prognostic Index (VNPI) to guide treatment decisions for DCIS.[122,123] One to three points each for size, grade, and necrosis and width of the surgical margin are combined to achieve a score ranging from 3 to 9. The higher score portends a higher risk for recurrence, and the score is used to assess risk and propose therapy. In 2001, the VNPI was expanded to include age. The University of Southern California (USC) VNPI score now ranges from 4 to 12 points (Table 26–2). The risk for recurrence increases with the number of points. Based on this retrospectively devised scoring system, Silverstein and coworkers recommend radiation therapy after wide local resection, or the preferred oncoplastic resection, for patients with USC VNPI scores of 7, 8, or 9.[123] Excision alone is

Table 26–2 University of Southern California Van Nuys Prognostic Index Scoring System

Score	Pathology	Margin Width (mm)	Tumor Size (mm)	Age (yr)
1	Not high grade No necrosis	≥10	≤15	>60
2	Not high grade Necrosis	1–9	16–40	40–60
3	High grade	<1	>40	<40

Data from Silverstein MJ. An argument against routine use of radiotherapy for ductal carcinoma in situ. Oncology 2003;17:1511–1533.

recommended for scores of 4, 5, or 6. Mastectomy is recommended for scores of 10, 11, or 12.

The prospective randomized clinical trials described below do not agree with the Van Nuys recommendations. A benefit in risk for recurrence is demonstrated in all of the groups with DCIS compared with excision alone. There are several valid criticisms of the USC VNPI recommendations. First, the study began as a retrospective analysis and spans 30 years, 1972 to 2003, a time when many changes in the details of breast surgery, mammography, and radiation therapy occurred. The treatment options (i.e., wide excision or wide excision and radiation therapy) were not used equally throughout the study. Radiation therapy was delivered more often earlier in the study years when diagnostic (including mammography) and therapeutic technologies were less advanced.[113] Post-biopsy mammography or specimen radiography, routine margin assessment, and re-excision when necessary have lessened the burden of carcinoma remaining after excision.[97,124,125] With these technologic and clinical advancements, current VNPI 8 and 9 lesions, for example, might have the volume of microscopic residual disease following surgery lowered to a level that can be controlled with wide excision and radiotherapy.

Second, the meticulously detailed sectioning method used by Silverstein and Lagios and their coworkers yields a more highly selected group of specimens compared with the more common standard sampling methods. Applying the VNPI criteria to lesions processed by standard methods could understage a lesion and lead to undertreatment, a higher recurrence rate, and an increased risk for invasive carcinoma at recurrence.

Third, size, grade, and margin width are difficult to reproducibly assess.[111,113,115,116] At present, interobserver variability may result in disparate treatment recommendations for a given specimen. Only one study has applied the Van Nuys criteria prospectively.[126] Thus, although it is possible that the factors delineated by Silverstein and colleagues are predictive, a prospective randomized trial is needed to validate the ability of the VNPI to guide treatment recommendations. Compiling the data from all patients with DCIS treated with breast-conserving surgery, those with the least risk for recurrence after excision alone have the following:

• Nonpalpable DCIS
• Low-grade DCIS
• Free margins, generally at least 1 cm
• Small lesions, less than 1.5 to 2.5 cm, depending on the study and the pathologic technique

Additional selection criteria for wide excision alone include the following:

• A lesion detected radiographically, usually as microcalcifications that, if recurrent, would theoretically be detected more easily and earlier
• A compliant patient who will undergo serial screening and clinical follow-up evaluations as prescribed

However, even in this best prognostic group, the studies described subsequently continue to show a statistically significant improvement in local recurrence with postoperative radiation therapy.

What evidence is there that breast-conserving surgery and radiation therapy are effective treatment for DCIS?

Four published prospective randomized trials and numerous retrospective studies support the use of limited surgery and radiation therapy for DCIS.[98,99,117–120,127–133]

The National Surgical Adjuvant Breast Project (NSABP) Protocol B-17 randomized the care of 818 women who had DCIS to wide excision alone or wide excision and radiation therapy. Patients were accrued from 1985 to 1990.[99] Stratification variables included age, axillary dissection, histology (DCIS or DCIS with lobular carcinoma in situ [LCIS]), and method of detection (palpation, mammography, or both). All patients had free surgical margins. With a median follow-up of 57 months, the results indicate a statistically significant decrease in any type of breast cancer recurrence in the treated breast at 5 years for women receiving radiation therapy: 7% versus 16% (P < .001). Noninvasive recurrences were reduced from 10.4% to 7.5% (P = .055), and invasive recurrences were reduced from 10.5% to 2.9% (P < .001) with radiation therapy. Updated results, now with 12 years of follow-up, confirm the reduction in recurrence when radiation therapy follows wide excision. Patients who received wide excision followed by radiation therapy had an overall recurrence rate of 16% at 12 years, compared with 32% at 12 years for patients who did not receive radiation therapy.[131] A retrospective subset analysis of pathologic features including grade, size, and margin status documented the benefit of radiation therapy for *all* groups in the NSABP study.[112] However, this study has been criticized for its lack of prospective pathologic stratification, mammographic-pathologic correlation, and serial subgross sectioning.[116]

The European Organisation for Research and Treatment of Cancer (EORTC) 10853 trial randomized 1010 women with DCIS to wide excision alone or wide excision followed by radiation therapy. The design was similar to that of the

Probably the most influential trial, the NSABP B-06 trial,[51,144–146] conducted from 1983 to 1987, accrued 2105 women and randomized one third to treatment by lumpectomy alone, one third to lumpectomy and breast radiotherapy, and one third to mastectomy. After 15 years of follow-up, and after a National Cancer Institute audit, 1039 patients remained eligible and analyzable.[144,146] Requirements of the trial included an invasive carcinoma of up to 4 cm in diameter. Axillary lymph nodes may have been involved or uninvolved. Levels I and II of the axilla had to be dissected. Importantly, the margins of resection were required to be free of carcinoma (in the lumpectomy groups) on microscopic examination. If the margins were involved, the protocol recommended that the patient undergo mastectomy. In the radiation therapy arm, 5000 cGy was delivered to the whole breast, without wedges (generally considered essential today to produce homogeneity of dose) or a boost. Regional lymph nodes were not irradiated. 5-Fluorouracil and melphalan were prescribed for all patients who had pathologically involved axillary lymph nodes. No significant difference was observed in either overall survival or disease-free survival between the lumpectomy plus radiation therapy group and the mastectomy group.[144,146]

The five other prospective randomized series[52–56] confirmed the NSABP conclusions and provided additional information regarding breast preservation therapy and survival:

1. The type of conservative surgical procedure, whether segmental excision,[51] tumorectomy,[53,55,56] or quadrantectomy,[52] when followed by breast irradiation, does not affect survival.
2. Delivery of inadequate radiotherapy doses may compromise survival. In two trials from Guy's Hospital in London, wide excision (without axillary dissection) and radiation therapy were compared with mastectomy.[147–149] Following wide excision, patients received 3800 cGy to the breast and 2700 cGy to the axilla. The breast-preservation group experienced a higher rate of ipsilateral breast and axillary recurrence, systemic failure, and death. In contrast, prospective randomized trials (see Table 26–3) that prescribed 4500 to 5040 cGy to the whole breast[51–56] (and, in most trials,[52–56] a 1500- to 2500-cGy boost to the tumor bed) demonstrated no difference in survival between the mastectomy and breast-preservation groups.
3. Routine indiscriminate administration of regional nodal irradiation does not improve survival. Early on in the Milan trial (a study in which women with invasive carcinomas 2 cm or smaller were randomized to quadrantectomy, axillary dissection, and breast radiotherapy or radical mastectomy), patients with involved axillary lymph nodes received regional nodal irradiation.[52] In the EORTC trial, patients with tumors up to 5 cm were randomized to mastectomy or tumorectomy with a 1- to 2-cm margin of normal-appearing breast tissue.[53] One half of the patients with involved axillary lymph nodes were randomized to receive regional nodal irradiation. In both the Milan and the EORTC trials, regional nodal irradiation did not improve survival. Better selection of the patient population for regional nodal irradiation (see later) *may* affect survival, but regional nodal irradiation for all patients who have involved axillary lymph nodes does not.

What factors affect the risk for local recurrence after conservative breast surgery and radiation therapy?

Variables that appear to affect local control include the residual tumor burden (as represented by the volume of tissue resected),[150] the presence of multifocal or multicentric disease,[151–154] the margin status,[151,155–165] the use of radiation therapy,[144,146,166–168] the presence of an extensive intraductal component,[159,163,169–171] the dose of radiation therapy,[57,147–149,158,169,172–174] the timing of radiation therapy,[164,165,172,175–178] the use of chemotherapy,[51,179–181] and patient age.[57,144,151,155,163,166,182–186] Factors that are more debatable but that may affect local control include the presence of lymphovascular or perineural invasion,[184,187–189] the presence of necrosis,[183,189,190] the presence of an inflammatory infiltrate,[144,188,191] and the ER and progesterone receptor (PR) status.[161,192,193] Factors that do not appear to affect the rate of ipsilateral breast recurrence include tumor size (T1 vs. T2),[51,177,193,194] the location of the carcinoma within the breast,[195,196] the histology,[197–200] and the presence or absence of microscopic involvement of the axillary lymph nodes.[51,56,177,194,201]

What data suggest that radiation therapy lowers local recurrence rates?

In the NSABP B-06 trial, after 15 years of follow-up, patients randomized to lumpectomy plus radiation therapy had a statistically significant reduction in ipsilateral breast recurrence compared with patients treated by lumpectomy alone (12% vs. 36%; $P < .001$).[51,144] This reduction in risk for local recurrence with use of radiation therapy after breast-conserving surgery has been confirmed in all six prospective randomized studies.[52–56,144] This statistically improved benefit in ipsilateral breast tumor recurrence persists in studies selecting the patients with the most favorable breast tumors in whom it was thought radiation therapy might have no benefit.

Is radiation therapy always necessary?

Some investigators have attempted to define a "good" subset of patients who have a very small risk for experiencing a local recurrence, even without radiation therapy.[166,172,202] The most likely population should theoretically be those patients who have small, low-grade, well-differentiated (including pure tubular and medullary) invasive ductal carcinomas resected with wide margins, and, possibly, older patients who have ER-positive lesions who have undergone quadrantectomy.[166] However, four prospective randomized series of selected women who had invasive breast carcinomas smaller than 2.5 cm treated with or without radiation therapy demonstrate a statistically significant improvement in ipsilateral breast recurrence rates with the use of radiation therapy, regardless of the surgical procedure used (lumpectomy, sector resection, or quadrantectomy).[166–168,203–207] A retrospective subset analysis of one series revealed that women older than 65 years who had quadrantectomy (with removal of skin and pectoralis fascia) and axillary dissection did not have a further reduction in risk for local recurrence with the addition of radiation therapy.[166,203] A survival benefit was seen for women with involved lymph nodes who received postoperative radiation therapy compared with those women with involved lymph nodes who did not receive postoperative radiation therapy and for those women with an extensive intraductal component on pathology who received radiation therapy.[203] (See later discussion of the impact of age on recurrence rates.)

The NSABP completed a prospective randomized trial of 1009 women with invasive carcinoma 1 cm or smaller after lumpectomy, randomized to radiation therapy and placebo (RT), tamoxifen (tam), or both (RT/tam).[168] At 8 years, the risk for ipsilateral breast tumor recurrence was statistically significantly reduced in patients who received postoperative radiation therapy (2.8% RT/tam; 9.3% RT; 16.5% tam).

In a similarly designed prospective randomized trial conducted in Germany, 361 patients with pT1pN0, receptor-positive, grades I and II tumors were randomized to no further therapy, tamoxifen, radiotherapy, or both tamoxifen and radiotherapy. At 6-year follow-up evaluation, patients receiving breast-conserving surgery alone had a threefold greater incidence of local recurrence than patients who received radiation therapy. The authors concluded that even these heavily selected patients benefit from tamoxifen and breast radiotherapy.

Several single-arm prospective and heavily selected retrospective series document statistically increased or unacceptably high rates of local recurrence[202,208–212] after breast conservation surgery alone (with or without hormonal therapy), whereas a few investigators recommend accepting the higher recurrence risk and withholding radiotherapy, most frequently in "elderly" patients.

At present, after segmental excision or lumpectomy for invasive carcinoma, radiation therapy is generally recommended. Given that postoperative radiation therapy affects local recurrence more than survival, the impact of local recurrence, both medically and emotionally, needs to be considered. Withholding radiation therapy is most appropriate for the physiologically elderly (as opposed to the chronologically elderly) patient. Data are maturing for two prospective randomized series and will help to better define those patients whose risk of recurrence may be only minimally acceptably increased with conservative surgery without radiation therapy.

What is the effect of multicentricity and multifocality?

Gross *multifocal* disease is defined as areas of macroscopic carcinoma separated by small amounts of normal breast tissue. Depending on the investigator's definition, the lesions must be either in the same quadrant or within 5 cm of each other. Gross *multicentric* disease, in contrast, reflects gross lesions in two distinct quadrants or separated by more than 5 cm. Despite wide excision of all macroscopic disease and radiation therapy, multifocality or multicentricity may impose a higher local recurrence rate.[151–154,213,214]

The increased recurrence rate most likely reflects the greater burden of microscopic disease remaining after resection of multicentric or multifocal carcinoma, as compared with the burden of microscopic residual disease after resection of a macroscopically unifocal carcinoma. Even if the residual microscopic carcinoma could be controlled, the larger (or multiple physically distinct) segmental excisions required to obtain tumor-free margins will likely compromise cosmesis. One small series reports adequate control and acceptable cosmesis for multiple ipsilateral synchronous carcinomas.[23] Therefore, for cosmesis as well as control, mastectomy with or without reconstructive surgery generally is the preferred surgical option for multicentric disease. Similarly, diffuse malignant-appearing microcalcifications seen on mammography are often associated with diffuse carcinoma[213–215] and should be treated as gross multicentric disease.

What is the effect of margin status?

The status of the margin of resection has been correlated with the risk for recurrence and should be assessed on all specimens. A margin may be classified as free (uninvolved or clear), close (within 1 or 2 mm), or focally or diffusely involved.[157,158] Gross involvement is that which is apparent before microscopic examination. Both the EORTC[159] and Milan[160] breast conservation trials, as well as single-institution data,[57,151,155,157,161–163] demonstrate a twofold to fivefold increase in local recurrence rates if microscopically involved margins exist. For example, in the data of Veronesi and colleagues,[160] involved margins, after tumorectomy, correlated with a 17% 5-year recurrence rate, compared with an 8.6% rate with free margins.

In some cases, greater doses of radiation therapy may compensate for involved margins of resection.[158,169,174] Solin and associates[158] used a sliding-scale radiotherapy dose based on margin status and found no increase in recurrence rates with involved margins. Patients who had microscopically involved margins received a total dose of 6500 to 6600 cGy to the tumor bed, whereas patients who had free margins of resection received a total tumor bed dose of 6000 to 6400 cGy. The EORTC randomized women with a microscopically involved margin to a 10- or 26-Gy boost dose.[57] Because the tolerance of normal breast tissue sets the upper limit of the dose that can be delivered and still produce acceptable long-term effects and cosmesis, and because involved margins require a higher dose for optimal local control, free margins of excision should be obtained whenever possible. An increased boost dose appears capable of controlling a slightly higher volume of microscopic residual disease, such as a focally or microscopically involved margin of resection.

What is the effect of an extensive intraductal component?

The original definition of an *extensive intraductal component* (EIC), by Schnitt and coworkers in 1984,[170] required an invasive ductal carcinoma with (1) at least 25% of the primary tumor consisting of intraductal carcinoma and (2) intraductal carcinoma beyond the primary invasive carcinoma. The 5-year rate of ipsilateral breast cancer recurrence after radiation therapy in lesions with EIC was 23%, compared with 6% without EIC.[170] However, on subsequent reanalysis of the specimens with EIC, margin status was shown to be the overriding prognostic factor.[158,216] (Many of the patients were treated before our current appreciation of the importance of margin status.) Patients whose tumors had EIC but uninvolved final margins of resection had recurrence rates similar to patients without EIC. In contrast, patients who had intraductal carcinoma at the resection margin *and* EIC experienced up to a 50% recurrence rate. Thus, EIC in association with involved margins appears to be a marker for extensive microscopic residual intraductal carcinoma. Holland and associates[217] have provided detailed clinicopathologic data that explain the implications of EIC. The authors reviewed mastectomy specimens and simulated a lumpectomy; in cases in which EIC would have been diagnosed by lumpectomy, the residual microscopic disease was greater in amount and extended farther from the primary tumor mass.

Although the precise definition of EIC varies among other studies, Bartelink and associates,[159] Kurtz and colleagues,[163] and Smitt and coworkers[171] confirm the increased recurrence rates after conservative surgery and radiation therapy for tumors that have EIC and involved margins. In contrast, the NSABP B-06 study,[51] the Joint Center for Radiation Therapy study,[170] the EORTC series,[161] and others[218,219] document the efficacy of conservative surgery and radiation therapy in EIC-containing tumors if clear margins of resection are obtained. The work of Kurtz and colleagues[163] supports an increased risk for recurrence despite final clear margins. Their study, however, did not employ inked margins for pathologic analysis. Veronesi and associates found a statistically significant impact of EIC on local recurrence even in patients undergoing quadrantectomy.[203]

Preoperative and postoperative mammograms, as well as specimen radiography, are particularly valuable in the management of EIC. Because patients who are found to have EIC frequently have microcalcifications extending beyond the reference lesion on mammography, the distribution of the microcalcifications can be framed preoperatively by needle localization to guide the surgical resection. Postoperatively and before radiation therapy, mammography can be repeated to confirm total clearance.[159,214] If mammographic and pathologic analyses reveal an optimal resection (no residual suspicious microcalcifications and free margins of resection), the patient is likely to have a salutary outcome from conservative surgery and radiation therapy. Re-excision should be employed if residual disease is suspected based on margin status or mammography if breast-conserving therapy is still desirable.

How does the volume of resection affect outcome?

Resection of larger volumes of breast tissue may result in lower rates of local recurrence,[57,220] potentially at the cost of cosmetic appearance.[221] Veronesi and colleagues,[150,203] in a prospective study, randomized 148 women to treatment by (1) quadrantectomy, axillary dissection, and radiation therapy (QUART) or (2) tumorectomy with an intended 1-cm margin followed by radiation therapy (TART). At 39 months, 13% in the tumorectomy group, compared with 5% in the quadrantectomy group, had developed a local recurrence. However, an analysis by actual margin status was not described. In contrast, Vicini and associates[222] analyzed rates of recurrence by extent of resection and found that tumorectomy with a 1- to

2-cm margin yielded recurrence rates similar to those seen with larger volumes of resection if the margins of resection were uninvolved and EIC was not present.

What is the effect of radiotherapy dose and the use of a boost on local control?

The dose per fraction, dose per week, and total dose affect local control. A minimum of 800 cGy per week should be delivered. Kurtz and colleagues[163] and Osborne and co-workers[223] each reported increased local recurrence rates with delivery of less than 800 cGy per week. Fraction sizes less than 180 cGy may also increase the risk for local recurrence. Local control (and cosmesis) are optimized with conventional fractionation of 180 to 200 cGy per fraction, 5 days per week (greater doses per fraction often lead to impaired cosmetic outcome).[224] Inadequate total doses delivered to the breast or regional lymph nodes, as shown in the Guy's Hospital series, resulted in an increased incidence of recurrence.[147-149] The minimum dose to the whole breast should be 4500 to 5000 cGy. The role of and appropriate dose of additional radiotherapy localized to the tumor bed only (boost) is dependent on the use of re-excision and the presence or absence of residual carcinoma, the final margin status, and possibly the radiation therapy technique used for the whole-breast portion of the treatment. The rationale for the local boost at the primary tumor site is based on histopathologic and clinical findings. Holland and colleagues[49] have shown that microscopic residual carcinoma is most likely to occur within 2 cm of the margins of resection and is progressively less likely to occur with increased distance. The clinical correlate is reproduced in many series: 60% to 95% of recurrences occur at the site of the index lesion.[177,187,225,226]

Although the NSABP series achieved a high local control rate without using a boost, free microscopic margins of resection were required, and the lack of wedges gave parts of the breast a dose considerably higher than the 5000 cGy prescribed and thereby risked diminished cosmesis. Series using wedged compensation techniques typically prescribe 4500 to 5000 cGy to the whole breast, and most deliver a boost to the tumor bed of 1000 to 2500 cGy.[52-56] Extrapolation from series in which final margin status determines the total dose supports the ability of a graded boost dose to control a higher bulk of residual microscopic disease.[57,64,162,192]

The absolute necessity of a boost in patients who have free margins of resection is less than clear.[227] In the EORTC "boost–no boost" trial designed to clarify the role of the boost, 5569 patients with tumors up to 3 cm and free margins after tumorectomy and lymph node dissection were randomized to receive (1) 16 Gy as either an electron or an iridium boost or (2) no boost after 50 Gy to the whole breast.[57,228] At 5-year follow-up, use of a boost significantly improved local control.[57] The magnitude of the benefit was greatest in patients 40 years of age or younger, in whom local recurrence was halved by the addition of a boost dose.[57]

Who can receive partial-breast irradiation?

Selection criteria for partial-breast irradiation are continuing to evolve. The data with longest-term follow-up use interstitial brachytherapy. The acceptance of balloon catheter–based brachytherapy extrapolates from interstitial brachytherapy. Only time will show whether treatment using a single catheter and a radioactive source in a single position yield results equal to treatment with an interstitial planar implant with sources in multiple locations. Three-dimensional conformal treatment has short follow-up, as does intraoperative radiotherapy. In the interim, physicians should remain meticulous in their selection of patients for partial-breast brachytherapy.

Vicini and colleagues[229] treated 199 patients with interstitial partial-breast brachytherapy using low- or high-dose-rate therapy. The inclusion criteria required free surgical margins (≥2 mm), infiltrating ductal carcinoma less than 3 cm, patient age older than 40 years, and uninvolved lymph nodes. Patients with infiltrating lobular carcinoma, an extensive intraductal component, DCIS, or "clinically significant" areas of lobular carcinoma in situ were excluded. The incidence of local recurrence at 5 years was 1%. Additional series confirm these good results.[230,231] Series documenting either increased recurrence[232] or increased toxicity[233,234] require careful study to better define patient selection, dose fractionation, and technique.

Early results with the MammoSite balloon catheter brachytherapy device (approved by the U.S. Food and Drug Administration in 2002) show acceptable toxicity, feasibility, and at 2 years, adequate cosmesis and control[235,236] (see Fig. 26–18A and B). Longer follow-up is clearly necessary. A national registry, initially industry sponsored, opened in 2002 and closed in July 2004, will provide a wealth of data for MammoSite-based partial-breast brachytherapy. On protocol, eligibility included an infiltrating ductal carcinoma 2 cm or smaller, free surgical margins, negative axillary lymph nodes, and patient age at least 47 years. Patients with infiltrating lobular carcinoma or DCIS were not eligible. Additional technical factors were required, including minimum and maximum balloon size, shape and conformity of the balloon, and a minimum distance from the surface of the balloon to the skin of 7 mm (but ideally 1 cm or more)[237] (Fig. 26–19). A National Cancer Institute–funded clinical trial in development will compare partial-breast and whole-breast irradiation.

IORT may be another acceptable approach to partial-breast radiotherapy. After a dose-escalation trial,[238] a single relatively large fraction of electron-beam therapy is delivered in the operating room after the breast surgery.[239,240] Two hundred thirty-seven patients with tumors smaller than 2 cm underwent breast-conserving surgery with sentinel lymphadenectomy.[241] The median age was 59 (range, 33 to 80) years. At 19 months of median follow-up, 1.4% had an ipsilateral breast recurrence, 0.5% supraclavicular recurrence, and 0.5% distant failure. Longer follow-up is required for clinical control, recurrence rates, and longer-term cosmetic results.

External-beam–based partial-breast irradiation using three-dimensional conformal treatment planning or IMRT is also being investigated to treat the tumor bed and a margin of normal tissue. The dose and fractionation have been extrapolated from brachytherapy series. One group has performed a dose-escalation feasibility assessment.[242] Again, the tumor bed must be precisely delineated, and care must be taken to limit the integral dose to the surrounding normal tissues. Several techniques have been proposed.[242–243] Acute toxicity appears acceptable.[242,244] Follow-up, again, is short.

At present, unless the patient is participating in a clinical trial, partial-breast irradiation should be carefully used. Meticulous radiographic screening is necessary preoperatively to exclude patients who may have multifocality or multicentricity. Patients who have a stage 1 infiltrating ductal carcinoma, free margins, no extensive intraductal component, and nonlobular histology may be candidates. A discrete age criterion is not defined, but young patients may be at increased risk for recurrence based on existing breast-conserving therapy data.

The potential advantages of partial-breast irradiation may be numerous. In addition to convenience and a cosmetic improvement for the patient with a large pendulous breast (smaller-breasted patients have a high likelihood of good to excellent cosmetic outcome with standard therapy), re-irradiation and repeat breast-conserving surgery may be possible for the patient with a new primary tumor in a discrete quadrant many years after her first surgery and partial-breast irradiation. This is an active and exciting time for breast specialists and their patients as improved screening and improved technologies are leading the way toward refinements and reductions in therapy with similar control rates and similar or improved cosmetic results.

Ideally, when should radiotherapy begin?

Theoretically, the longer the delay between surgery and the institution of radiation therapy, the higher the risk for local recurrence because residual tumor cells are allowed to proliferate.[245] However, several variables, including margin status, axillary lymph node status, and chemotherapy, may modify the risk. Nixon and associates[246] retrospectively analyzed 591 patients who had pathologically uninvolved lymph nodes and did not receive chemotherapy. No difference in recurrence rates was found in patients starting radiation therapy 5 to 8 weeks after surgery, as compared with 0 to 4 weeks after surgery. However, other series[157,178] found an increased recurrence rate if radiotherapy was delayed beyond 7 weeks after surgery.

In patients receiving chemotherapy, deferring radiation therapy until the completion of chemotherapy may result in a delay of up to 4 to 8 months, depending on the chemotherapy regimen. Recht and colleagues[164] found that local recurrence rates were higher in patients who received 4

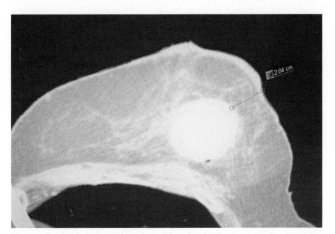

Figure 26–19 Computed tomography scan slice of a breast with the MammoSite balloon inflated with diluted Hypaque. The desired spherical shape of the balloon and the acceptable distance from the surface of the balloon to the skin are shown.

months of CMF followed by radiotherapy, as compared with radiotherapy first. On subset analysis, the local recurrence rate was most increased in patients who had involved or unknown margins of resection. At 5 years, the local recurrence rate was 26% when radiation therapy was delivered after chemotherapy and 14% when radiation was delivered before chemotherapy. Although two series[247,248] have found no difference, several others[165,249,250] also have found an increase in local recurrence with delayed radiotherapy. Thus, if unknown or involved margins exist, re-excision should be considered prior to the initiation of chemotherapy. If re-excision is not or cannot be performed, radiotherapy may be interdigitated into the treatment plan before the completion of chemotherapy.

Concomitant chemoradiotherapy avoids delaying either modality and potentially minimizes systemic and local failure. However, some investigators have commented that patients treated by concurrent therapy may tolerate less dose-intensive chemotherapy because of an increase in bone marrow suppression[251,252] and have an increase in side effects and a suboptimal cosmetic result[251-255] (see discussion of cosmesis). If radiation therapy is to be delayed until the completion of chemotherapy, clear margins of resection must be ensured.

What is the effect of chemotherapy on local control?

Chemotherapy, when added to conservative surgery and radiation therapy, further reduces the risk for local recurrence.[51,144,179-181] This reduction, however, does not compensate for the effect of radiation therapy. Despite chemotherapy, if radiation therapy is delayed for 4 or more months (or withheld[51]),[164,165] there is an increase in risk for local recurrence, especially in patients who have microscopically involved margins.[164,181]

Tamoxifen, in patients who have ER-positive tumors, may also lower local recurrence rates after conservative surgery and radiation therapy.[168,181] However, tamoxifen alone does not provide optimal local control even in small tumors with uninvolved lymph nodes.[168,207] The NSABP randomized 1009 women with invasive carcinoma and uninvolved lymph nodes to receive tamoxifen, radiation therapy, both, or neither. Patients receiving radiation therapy, as compared with tamoxifen alone, had a 50% reduction in risk for ipsilateral breast tumor recurrence. The recurrence rate at 8 years was 9% with radiation therapy but 3% with radiation therapy and tamoxifen.[168]

Results from the recently published German prospective randomized trial of 360 patients with pathologic stage I invasive cancers corroborate the NSABP results. Tamoxifen further lowers the risk for ipsilateral breast tumor recurrence provided by breast radiotherapy.[207] Aromatase inhibitors should have a similar effect, although long-term data are not yet available.

Are any other additional histopathologic factors associated with local recurrence?

An increased risk for local recurrence has been reported after conservative surgery and radiation therapy (and after mastectomy) for lesions that do not express ER (ER-negative tumors)[161,183,228] and for those that have a high nuclear grade,[168,177,182,188,190,191,256,257] lymphovascular invasion,[144,177,184,188,189] tumor necrosis,[185,188,191] or an inflammatory infiltrate.[144,168,188-191] These histopathologic factors are more commonly associated with young age.[168,185,186,258]

Is there an effect of age on local recurrence?

Young age (usually defined as younger than 40 years) is frequently associated with other factors that predict for local recurrence: EIC, ER-negative lesions, lymphovascular infiltrate, high histologic grade, inflammatory infiltrate,[186,258] and involved margins.[57,151,155] However, reports exist both supporting[151,155,182,184,203] and refuting[259,260] the increased risk for recurrence in younger patients. Smaller volumes of resected breast tissue and involved margins may have contributed to the higher local recurrence rates seen in these series.[57,258] Analyses of associated factors have not been performed routinely and may confound the importance of age as an independent prognostic factor for ipsilateral breast recurrence. With optimal surgery and correction for additional prognostic factors, Kurtz and colleagues[183] reported that age younger than 32 years imparted an increased local rate of recurrence (34% at 8.5 years).

In one prospective randomized series, older age (over 55 years) in patients undergoing quadrantectomy was associated with a lower risk for recurrence.[166]

Does family history of breast cancer or detection of genetic mutation preclude breast-conserving therapy and increase local recurrence?

Neither a family history of breast or ovarian carcinoma nor the detection of a *BRCA1* or *BRCA2* deleterious mutation precludes breast-conserving surgery and radiation therapy.[163,183,217,261-266] However, genetic carriers, while obtaining similar local control rates[266] as patients who do not express a *BRCA1* or *BRCA2* mutation, are at increased risk for subsequent, new breast tumors in the ipsilateral or contralateral breast.[267]

For these patients, we recommend genetic counseling, testing, and breast MRI before radiation therapy and, ideally, before surgery. Many *BRCA1* and *BRCA2* carriers, once they understand their risk for a second ipsilateral or contralateral breast cancer, opt for unilateral mastectomy or bilateral mastectomies with or without reconstruction.

Does tumor size influence local recurrence?

Local recurrence rates are not increased for T2 lesions as compared with TI lesions when controlled for final margin status.[51,177,192,194] Rosen and colleagues[195] assessed microscopic residual disease in mastectomy specimens in patients with T1 and T2 tumors after reproducing a wide excision. No statistically significant difference paralleling clinical results was found in the literature.

Does the location of the primary lesion influence local recurrence?

The location of the index carcinoma per se is not predictive of local recurrence[195,268] when controlled for other factors. On the other hand, tumors within 2 cm of the nipple–areolar complex[157,158,193] and those involving the nipple[196,269] have a higher incidence of multicentricity than do tumors distant from the nipple–areolar complex.[177] Therefore, specimens from central lesions should be reviewed particularly carefully and re-excision employed, if necessary, to obtain microscopically free margins.

Does histopathologic subtype influence local recurrence?

Invasive lobular, medullary, colloid, and tubular carcinoma all can be effectively treated with conservative surgery and radiation therapy.[197–200] The principles of mammographic-pathologic correlation are especially important in invasive lobular carcinoma, which frequently presents as a vague thickening, and often is more extensive microscopically than mammographically.

Does lymph node status influence local recurrence?

As shown in prospective randomized trials[51–56] and retrospective reports,[177,194] involvement of the axillary lymph nodes does not increase the risk for ipsilateral breast cancer recurrence after conservative surgery and radiation therapy. In the NSABP series, radiation therapy improved the rate of local control in both patients with uninvolved (12% vs. 32%) and patients with involved (5% vs. 41%) axillary lymph nodes. Patients who had involved lymph nodes actually had a lower local failure rate with radiation therapy than those who had uninvolved lymph nodes and received radiation therapy. The improved local control rate likely reflects synergy between the radiation therapy and the chemotherapy that was delivered to patients who had involved axillary lymph nodes. If radiation therapy to the breast is withheld, involvement of the axillary nodes is prognostic for ipsilateral breast tumor recurrence.[144,203]

Does regional nodal irradiation affect local and regional control?

Regional nodal irradiation has been shown to lower regional nodal failure but not ipsilateral breast tumor recurrence.[55] As with all medical therapy, the potential benefits (in this case, regional nodal control) are compared to the potential side effects of treatment. In an unselected population suitable for conservative surgery and radiation therapy, regional nodal failures (axillary, supraclavicular, and internal mammary) may be as low as 2% to 5% without regional nodal irradiation.[51,52,225,270,271] However, for selected patients who are at increased risk of disease recurrence (see later) in the regional lymph nodes, regional nodal irradiation becomes appropriate.

Recurrent disease in the supraclavicular region occurs in 10% to 26% of patients who have pathologically involved axillary lymph nodes.[225,271–273] Regional nodal irradiation should primarily be reserved for patients at substantial risk for developing a supraclavicular recurrence—that is, patients with four or more involved axillary lymph nodes or involved apical (level III) lymph nodes. It is not yet clear whether the survival benefits seen in premenopausal women undergoing regional nodal and chest wall irradiation after mastectomy[274,275] will apply to postmenopausal women or women undergoing breast-conserving therapy (see section on postmastectomy radiation therapy).

Irradiation of the dissected axilla is indicated less often because of the low incidence of axillary recurrence after dissection and the risk for arm edema after axillary dissection and full axillary irradiation.[225,276,277] Indications for axillary irradiation include lack of an axillary dissection (unless the risk for involvement is less than 10% to 15%) and gross residual axillary tumor after dissection. Microscopic extranodal extension and involvement of more than four axillary lymph nodes are more controversial indications for axillary irradiation.[278] Pierce and colleagues[201] have suggested that it is not necessary to irradiate the axilla in patients who have extracapsular microscopic extension of axillary nodal disease. They observed only a 5% rate of axillary recurrence in such patients, but caution in uniformly adopting this policy seems warranted given the small number of patients studied.

Indications for irradiation of the internal mammary chain are controversial. The risk for recurrence in the internal mammary lymph nodes is as low as 0% to 2% in some series.[270–273,277] The incidence of toxicity from treatment (hematologic suppression, pneumonitis, and cardiotoxicity), although minimized with modern radiotherapeutic technique, may be greater than the incidence of recurrence.

Using electrons or a combination of electrons and photons, symptomatic pneumonitis can be lowered to 2%, but some amount of lung must be irradiated to treat the internal mammary lymph nodes.[278,279] Irradiation of the internal mammary lymph nodes generally is recommended for patients with known microscopic involvement of the internal mammary lymph nodes and for patients who require total regional nodal irradiation (i.e., for bone marrow or stem cell transplantation protocols). For patients at high risk—those with inner quadrant or central lesions and involved axillary lymph nodes—positron emission tomography (PET) scan may be used before chemotherapy to evaluate the internal mammary chain. The role of adjuvant internal mammary nodal irradiation for women with stage II or III carcinoma of the breast undergoing breast conservation is not clearly delineated. In the two randomized trials of regional nodal irradiation after mastectomy, internal mammary nodal (IMN) irradiation was not randomized, and the impact of the IMN field versus the chest wall/supraclavicular fields is not clear. Given the toxicity, especially with increased use of anthracyclines and Herceptin and the potentially synergistic effects, extrapolation from the postmastectomy series[274,275] should be undertaken with caution until further data are available.

Summary

Most patients with stage I or II invasive carcinoma of the breast are candidates for conservative surgery and higher dose to the tumor bed with acceptable acute and late toxicity to the breast, could paradoxically result in an increase in second malignancies in the surrounding normal structures.[329]

What kind of cosmetic result is likely?

Overall, more than 85% of patients and their physicians rate the final cosmetic result as good to excellent[27,58,66,246,330] (Fig. 26–20). The outcome is a result of a multidisciplinary effort and is contributed to by specific attention to the details of surgery and radiation therapy. As discussed later, chemotherapy also can have an impact on the cosmetic result.

How can the surgeon help?

The size of the tumor, the necessary amount of tissue resected to obtain free margins, the location of the tumor, the location and size of the scar, and the patient's preoperative breast size affect the postoperative, preradiotherapy cosmetic result.[60,150,220,221,331,332] For example, in a small-breasted woman, resection of a 3.5-cm lesion (with free margins) may affect cosmesis more than the identical resection in a large-breasted woman. Because there is generally less breast tissue in the upper inner quadrant, resection of a lesion from this region may leave a more noticeable defect than an identical resection from the upper outer quadrant. Resection of a lesion inferior to the nipple may cause more disparity between the levels of the ipsilateral and contralateral nipples and yield poorer cosmesis.[220] Although the size and location of the lesion cannot be controlled by the surgeon, the placement of the incision and the additional volume of tissue resected (beyond that required for free margins) are within the surgeon's control and are important for cosmesis. Although a quadrantectomy, as opposed to a segmental excision, seemed to result in a small improvement in local control in the Milan QUART-TART trial,[150] it also resulted in a statistically significant decrease in a satisfactory cosmetic result.[26,29] If the patient does not have an optimal cosmetic result before radiation therapy, the long-term cosmesis is unlikely to improve after radiation therapy.

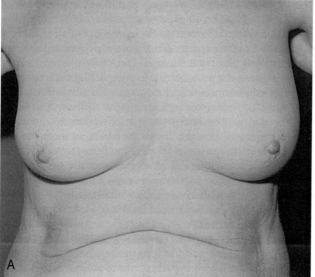
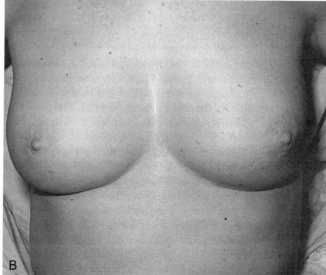
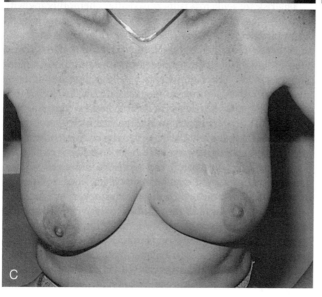

Figure 26–20 Examples of the cosmetic result in three patients who received conservative surgery and radiotherapy. *A,* Six months after radiation therapy (4600 cGy to the whole breast; 6000 cGy boost portal) to the left breast. The incision is at the anterior axillary line in the upper outer quadrant. *B,* Three months after radiation therapy to the left breast. The incision, with surrounding barely perceptible hyperpigmentation (6000 cGy to the boost portal), is seen in the upper inner quandrant. *C,* Two weeks after completing radiation therapy to the left breast. Residual hyperpigmentation is seen in the boost portal. The hyperpigmentation will fade with time.

Finally, the surgeon can aid the radiation oncologist by placing radiopaque clips in the tumor bed at the time of segmental excision. This enables the radiation oncologist to accurately place the boost, while minimizing its amount. The placement of surgical clips in the tumor bed is extremely helpful to the radiation oncologist and to the accuracy of the boost field placement when a reconstructive procedure is performed with the lumpectomy. Because treating a larger volume of tissue with a higher total dose may impair cosmesis, the smaller-volume boost is desirable.

What can the radiation oncologist do to maximize the cosmetic result?

The radiation oncologist can optimize the cosmetic outcome by choosing the proper machinery, energy of the beam, dose per fraction, total dose, and optimal treatment plan with the use of wedged compensators individually chosen for the patient. Inhomogeneity of dose across the breast and resultant hot spots may be seen with use of low-energy and nonlinear accelerator equipment and a beam energy that is too low for the patient's breast width. The resultant inhomogeneity increases the possibility of compromised cosmesis. As mentioned previously, the use of IMRT and additional fields may decrease inhomogeneity and improve cosmesis in selected patients.

Delivery of conventional fractionation of 180 to 200 cGy per fraction, as compared with doses above 250 cGy per fraction, minimizes reaction of the skin and breast tissue and optimizes the possibility of a good cosmetic result while effectively eradicating residual neoplastic cells.[24,25,58,60] A higher dose per treatment may be delivered with acceptable toxicity when the volume is small. Therefore, when treatment encompasses the tumor bed only or "partial breast," a shorter fractionation schema (fewer treatments, larger dose per treatment) may result in satisfactory cosmesis. However, when larger doses per fraction are delivered to the entire breast, patient selection is critical. The factors shown to lower the ultimate cosmetic outcome (i.e. large breast, large separation, width of chest wall) may result in a decline in cosmesis. If future or salvage mastectomy with reconstruction is performed and there has been an increase in fibrosis or subclinical cutaneous or vascular damage because of the larger dose per fraction, the reconstruction may be suboptimal. If the dose to the whole breast surpasses 5000 to 6000 cGy, an increased rate of long-term breast edema and compromised cosmesis are risked.[58] At doses above 7000 cGy, fibrosis, pain, and retraction may be seen.

The radiation oncologist should also keep the boost volume to the minimum required to encompass the tumor bed and, if using electron-beam therapy, should choose the appropriate energy. Using the clips placed in the tumor bed at surgery or using a CT scan or ultrasound[69] to localize the tumor bed, the radiation oncologist can accurately localize the volume and avoid excessive margins that may be required when the tumor bed is estimated from mammography and placement of the incision. If clips have not been placed and CT scan or ultrasound is not available or did not delineate the surgical bed, a 3-cm margin is placed around the incision. In comparisons of the two methods, placement of clips resulted in a smaller and more accurate boost volume.[71–73] Again directed by

radiopaque surgical clips, the radiation oncologist can choose the optimal electron energy required to reach the tumor bed while minimizing dose to the overlying (skin) and underlying (chest wall and lung) anatomy.[70] Using an iridium (brachytherapy) boost has resulted in worsened cosmesis in a few reports.[66,67,70] Intraoperative radiotherapy and balloon catheter brachytherapy have also been used to deliver the boost treatment.

Can systemic therapy recommendations affect cosmesis?

Chemotherapy may worsen the cosmetic result after conservative surgery and radiation therapy.[77,188,251–255] Both the timing of chemotherapy in relation to radiation therapy and the specific chemotherapeutic agents delivered affect the ultimate result.[26,333–335] General, concurrent chemoradiotherapy results in a worse cosmetic result than sequential therapy.[252,255] Impaired cosmesis has been documented with concurrent CMF.[252,255] Cytoxan and 5-fluorouracil concurrent with radiation therapy, in several series, did not affect the appearance of the breast.[26,333–335] Doxorubicin sensitizes the skin and, when given concurrently with radiation therapy, can result in an unacceptably brisk erythema. Paclitaxel and docetaxel arrest cells in mitosis (an extremely radiosensitive phase of the cell cycle) and increase the reaction to radiation therapy if given concurrently.[333,336] Gemcitabine is also a potent radiosensitizer and, when delivered concurrently with chest wall radiotherapy, commonly results in skin desquamation.[337]

The medical oncologist and radiation oncologist should work together to minimize the risk for relapse and toxicity while maximizing the cosmetic result.

What is the role of radiation therapy after mastectomy?

The goals of postmastectomy radiotherapy are to prevent locoregional recurrence and improve survival. Premenopausal or postmenopausal patients at substantial (i.e., greater than 10%) risk for locoregional recurrence (after mastectomy) should be considered. Patients who may have a survival benefit after postmastectomy radiation therapy are discussed next.

Is there any value to postmastectomy radiotherapy?

Radiation therapy may be delivered in the postmastectomy setting, usually in addition to chemotherapy, to eradicate micrometastatic deposits and thereby improve local control and survival. Because of the relationship of dose and tumor volume, radiotherapy delivered after development of a locoregional recurrence results in a complete response rate in only 50% of patients.[338] The morbidity from an uncontrolled recurrence has been well documented and includes ulceration, bleeding, pain, infection, lymphedema, and brachial plexopathy. Given the severity of symptoms and difficulty achieving palliation, the best treatment is prevention of the recurrence. Moreover, if recurrence is prevented in a patient with a low risk for distant failure, survival could potentially be improved.

Which patients are at high risk of locoregional recurrence?

Patients who have disease in their axillary lymph nodes have a relatively high risk for locoregional recurrence. Within this subset, the risk for recurrence rises with increasing numbers of involved lymph nodes.[141,339] To estimate the risk for locoregional recurrence and the value of postmastectomy radiation therapy, the axillary dissection should contain at least 10 lymph nodes. When an adequate axillary dissection has been performed, the risk for recurrence increases with increasing numbers of involved axillary nodes. In patients who do not receive radiation therapy after mastectomy and axillary dissection, the incidence of chest wall recurrence rises from 5% in patients who do not have involvement of their axillary lymph nodes, to 9% in those with one to three involved lymph nodes, to at least 20% in those with four or more involved nodes.[268,272,277,340-343]

The risk for locoregional recurrence also rises with enlarging primary tumor size from less than 10% in patients having tumors larger than 2 cm to 25% to 35% in patients having tumors larger than 5 cm.[268,277,340,344,345,346]

The risk for a supraclavicular lymph node recurrence also rises as the number of involved axillary nodes increases and may predict for distant dissemination.[339] The supraclavicular and infraclavicular regions should be included when postmastectomy radiation therapy is delivered.

Other factors that *may* be associated with locoregional recurrence include an involved surgical margin, high histologic grade,[347,348] age younger than 40 years,[268,349,350] pectoralis major fascia involvement,[345] ER-negative tumor,[345,351] and presence of tumor necrosis.[345]

The risk for an axillary recurrence is generally low, and the toxicity of irradiation to the full axilla is not justified when an adequate axillary dissection is performed.[339] If a more limited axillary dissection is performed and less than 10 lymph nodes are removed in a patient with axillary lymph node involvement, several studies have reported an increased risk for axillary recurrence.[275,339] Therefore, when an axillary dissection (and not sentinel lymphadenectomy) is indicated, an adequate dissection should be intended to avoid an increased risk for recurrence or the morbidity of axillary radiation therapy superimposed on the surgical morbidity.

Does chemotherapy prevent local recurrence and obviate the need for radiation therapy?

In most studies, chemotherapy does not significantly reduce the risk for locoregional failure.[345,347,352,353] Despite therapy with CMF, for example, patients who have primary tumors 5 cm or larger *and* four to seven involved axillary lymph nodes have a 20% to 30% risk for locoregional failure.[345,352,353] In one series of patients who had 10 or more lymph nodes involved and received high-dose chemotherapy and bone marrow transplantation, Marks and colleagues[354] reported a 30% chest wall recurrence rate. Although there are no prospective

randomized data investigating postmastectomy radiation therapy after adjuvant chemotherapy with anthracyclines or taxanes, the available data and ongoing adjuvant chemotherapeutic trials continue to use postmastectomy radiation therapy if the risk for locoregional recurrence is about 20% or greater.

Can radiation therapy decrease locoregional recurrence?

Radiation therapy clearly decreases the rate of locoregional recurrence, whether or not chemotherapy is used.[277,340,354-358] In most prospective and retrospective series, with or without chemotherapy, radiation therapy reduces the risk for locoregional failure from between 20% and 30% to less than 10%.[278,351,358-367]

Should the role of postmastectomy radiotherapy in the modern era be reassessed?

Several prospective randomized series that failed to find a benefit were conducted in the 1950s and 1960s and must be viewed in their proper perspective because they were done before the development of modern linear accelerators, electron therapy, and the current understanding of dose-response relationships in tumor and normal tissues.[272,368-370] Although locoregional recurrences were lowered, toxicity compromised the benefit. The lessons learned from these early studies are as follows:

1. Orthovoltage therapy (250 kV) increases complications in the skin, soft tissue, and heart because of relatively poor depth-dose profiles and resulting inhomogeneity of dose. In at least two trials, orthovoltage therapy likely contributed to increased mortality.[371,372]
2. The amount of heart and lung in the treatment portals should be kept to the minimum amount possible.[324,343,373-375]
3. Omission of postmastectomy radiation therapy to the chest wall (treating peripheral lymphatics only) results in an increased risk for chest wall recurrence and lower survival rates.[272,368,370]
4. Doses below 4500 cGy are not adequate to sterilize microscopic disease and result in increased recurrence rates.[272,368,370]
5. Increasing the daily dose per fraction increases long-term complications. A daily fraction size of 180 to 200 cGy is recommended.[368-370]
6. Patients who have uninvolved axillary lymph nodes and primary tumor size of less than 5 cm have a low risk for locoregional recurrence.[277,370]
7. If internal mammary lymph nodes are to be treated, direct photon fields should be avoided because of increased dose to the heart and increased cardiotoxicity.[369,370,372-376]

With modern technology and meticulous technique, optimal treatment to the desired sites (chest wall with or without regional lymph nodes) can be delivered, keeping the dose to normal tissues to a minimum. In summary, patients who should receive radiation therapy after mastectomy are (1) those with a tumor size of 5 cm or greater or four or more involved axillary lymph nodes and (2) those who have locally advanced disease undergoing up-front chemotherapy followed by surgery. Possible indications include involved surgical margins, suboptimal axillary dissection in a patient with stage II disease (i.e., three of a total of six lymph nodes involved), multiple risk factors that individually do not yield a 15% risk for locoregional recurrence (i.e., gross multicentric disease, extensive lymphovascular invasion, ER negativity), and microscopic disease in an internal mammary lymph node.

Does postmastectomy radiation therapy affect survival?

This has been and remains a difficult question to answer. Certainly, patients who have a high risk for distant failure (in general, 10 or more involved axillary lymph nodes) or a low (less than 10%) risk for locoregional recurrence (e.g., no involved axillary lymph nodes and tumor size less than 5 cm) would not be expected to have a survival benefit. Clinical experience verifies this.

In the early trials of regional radiation following mastectomy, all patients, regardless of tumor size and axillary nodal status, received postmastectomy radiation therapy.[272,368–370,373] These results were not analyzed by lymph node status or tumor size, and combined with the poor technique (by modern standards), resultant excessive morbidity, and small sample size, no difference in overall survival was seen. Two series reported a benefit in disease-free survival at 10 years.[378,379] On subset analysis of two additional trials, the Stockholm[142,365] and Oslo trials,[368] a benefit in disease-free survival at 10 years was noted for stage II patients.

In contrast, more recent studies[274,380,384] of radiation therapy in selected subsets of patients who had mastectomies have shown improved disease-free survival. Ragaz and colleagues[274,380,381] reported a study of premenopausal women who had involved axillary nodes and were randomized after mastectomy to CMF either with or without radiation therapy to the chest wall and regional lymph nodes. At 15 years, survival was improved in the women who received radiation therapy in addition to chemotherapy. The largest benefit was seen in the patients who had four or more lymph nodes involved, although given the small sample size and the 29% reduction in mortality from breast cancer, all groups experienced benefit from the addition of radiation therapy. The women who received radiation therapy also had a statistically significant 33% reduction in recurrence.

The Danish Breast Cancer Group has also shown improved survival attributable to the use of postmastectomy radiation therapy in patients who had T3 or T4 tumors or involved lymph nodes.[370,383] At 10 years, with the addition of radiation therapy, overall survival (54% vs. 45%; $P < .001$), disease-free survival (48% vs. 34%; $P < .001$), and locoregional recurrence (9% vs. 32%; $P < .001$) were all improved. Postmenopausal women received tamoxifen with or without radiation therapy, and at 5 years they experienced a statistically significant improvement in disease-free survival related to radiation therapy. Both premenopausal and postmenopausal groups had marked reductions in local recurrence rates with

radiation therapy (28% vs. 9% premenopausal [$P < .0001$]; 36% to 5% postmenopausal [$P < .0001$]). Van der Hage and colleagues, in a retrospective series of 3648 patients, also found a survival benefit for postmastectomy radiation therapy in women with one to three positive lymph nodes.[359]

Although many other series show no improvement in survival, these experiences raise the possibility of improved survival from radiation therapy when appropriate patient selection is employed. A North American intergroup trial was designed to better answer this question but was not completed. As increasingly effective cytotoxic and biologic therapies are employed, the role of locoregional recurrence and its potential contribution to overall survival may be increasingly meaningful. Premenopausal women with one to three involved axillary lymph nodes should consult with a radiation therapist. Until more data are available, selected premenopausal patients with one to three positive lymph nodes should be evaluated for radiation therapy. Factors that will influence the decision for or against radiation include tumor size, number of lymph nodes removed, the presence or absence of lymphovascular invasion, ER status, and possibly *HER-2* status.

In addition to the chest wall, should regional lymph nodes be irradiated?

It is my belief that, in general, patients who have T3 or T4 lesions and four or more involved lymph nodes should receive radiation therapy not only to the chest wall but also to the supraclavicular lymph nodes. As described earlier, the risk for recurrence in the chest wall and supraclavicular regions with a primary carcinoma larger than 5 cm and four or more axillary lymph nodes involved ranges from 10% to 45%. In addition, using meticulous technique, treatment of these sites is accomplished with acceptable toxicity (see earlier discussions of technique and late effects).

Because axillary recurrences are rare following adequate dissection, and because irradiation of the dissected axilla increases the risk for lymphedema, treatment of the axilla is generally reserved for patients who have suspected gross residual disease or an undissected axilla.[201,384,385]

Treatment of the internal mammary region remains controversial. The series reporting benefits in disease-free and overall survival included the internal mammary lymph nodes in the irradiated volume; however, it is not at all clear that treatment of the internal mammary region per se is critical. Surgical series document the greatest likelihood of microscopic involvement of the internal mammary chain in patients who have inner quadrant tumors and involved axillary lymph nodes. The data of Tubiana and associates[386] support a survival benefit for chest wall and regional lymph node irradiation (including the internal mammary nodes) in patients with central inner quadrant lesions and involved axillary nodes. However, the development of an internal mammary recurrence is rare after mastectomy (with or without chemotherapy), and given the synergistic cardiotoxicity of doxorubicin and irradiation,[274,387] when undertaken, irradiation of the internal mammary region should be performed with meticulous technique to minimize short- and long-term morbidity.

REFERENCES

1. Hall EJ. Radiobiology for the Radiologist. Philadelphia, JB Lippincott, 1994.
2. Thompson LH, Suit HD. Proliferation kinetics of x-irradiated mouse L cells studied with time-lapse photography. II. Int J Radiat Oncol Biol Phys 1969;15:347–362.
3. Boag JW. The time scale in radiobiology. In Radiation Research. Proceedings of the Fifth International Congress of Radiation Research. New York, Academic Press, 1975, pp 9–29.
4. Fowler JF. The second Klaas Breur memorial lecture. La Ronde radiation sciences and medical radiology. Radiother Oncol 1983;1: 1–22.
5. Sinclair WK, Morton RA. X-ray sensitivity during the cell generation cycle of cultured Chinese hamster cells. Radiat Res 1966;29: 450–474.
6. Fowler JF. The linear-quadratic formula and progress in fractionated radiotherapy. Br J Radiol 1989;62:679–694.
7. Withers HR, Taylor JM, Maciejewski B. The hazard of accelerated tumor clonogen repopulation during radiotherapy. Acta Oncol 1988; 27:131–146.
8. Withers HR, Taylor JM, Maciejewski B. Treatment volume and tissue tolerance. Int J Radiat Oncol Biol Phys 1988;14:751–759.
9. Withers HR. Biologic basis for altered fractionation schemes. Cancer 1985;55:2086–2095.
10. Parsons JT, Bova FJ, Million RR. A reevaluation of split-course technique for squamous cell carcinoma of the head and neck. Int J Radiat Oncol Biol Phys 1980;6:1645–1652.
11. Gray LH, Conger AD, Elbert M. The concentration of oxygen dissolved in tissues at the time of irradiation as a factor in radiotherapy. Br J Radiol 1953;26:638–648.
12. Haveman J. Enhancement of radiation effects by hyperthermia. In Anghileri JD, Robert J (eds). Hyperthermia in Cancer Treatment. Boca Raton, FL, CRC Press, 1986, pp 169–182.
13. Greco FA, Brereton HD, Kent H, et al. Adriamycin and enhanced radiation reaction in normal esophagus and skin. Ann Intern Med 1976;85:294–298.
14. Schilsky RL. Biochemical pharmacology of chemotherapeutic drugs used as radiation enhancers. Semin Oncol 1992;19:2–7.
15. Tannock IF. Combined modality treatment with radiotherapy and chemotherapy. Radiother Oncol 1989;16:83–101.
16. Khan FM. The Physics of Radiation Therapy. Baltimore, Williams & Wilkins, 1994, pp 78–90.
17. Winchester D, Cox J. Standards for breast conservation treatment. CA Cancer J Clin 1992;42:134–162.
18. Recht A. Patient selection for treatment with conservative surgery and radiation therapy. Cancer Invest 1992;10:471–476.
19. Moore GH, Schiller JE, Moore GK. Radiation-induced histopathological changes of breast: The effects of time. Am J Surg Pathol 2004;28: 47–53.
20. Racadot S, Marchol C, Charra-Brunaud C. Re-irradiation after salvage mastectomy for local recurrence after a conservative treatment: A retrospective analysis of 20 patients. Cancer Radiother 2003;7:369–379.
21. Deutsch M. Repeat high dose external beam irradiation for in-breast tumor recurrence after previous lumpectomy and whole breast irradiation. Int J Radiat Oncol Biol Phys 2002;53:687–691.
22. Intra M, Leonardi MC, Gatti G, et al. Intraoperative radiotherapy during breast conserving surgery in patients previously treated with radiotherapy for Hodgkin's disease. Tumor 2004;90:13–16.
23. Kaplan J, Giron G, Tartter PI, et al. Breast conservation in patients with multiple ipsilateral synchronous cancers. J Am Coll Surg 2003;197: 726–729.
24. Clarke D, Martinez A, Cox RS. Analysis of cosmetic results and complications in patients with stage I and II breast cancer treated by biopsy and irradiation. Int J Radiat Oncol Biol Phys 1983;9:1807–1813.
25. Ray GR, Fish VJ. Biopsy and definitive radiation therapy in stage I and II adenocarcinoma of the female breast: Analysis of cosmesis and the role of electron beam supplementation. Int J Radiat Oncol Biol Phys 1983;9:813–818.
26. Wazer DE, DiPetrillo T, Schmidt-Ullrich R, et al. Factors influencing cosmetic outcome and complication risk after conservative surgery and breast radiotherapy for early-stage breast carcinoma. J Clin Oncol 1992;10:356–363.

27. Pezner RD, Patterson MP, Lipsett JA, et al. Factors affecting cosmetic outcome in breast conserving cancer treatment—objective quantitative assessment. Breast Cancer Res Treat 1991;20:85–92.
28. Gray J, McCormick B, Cox L, et al. Primary breast irradiation in large-breasted or heavy women: Analysis of cosmetic outcome. Int J Radiat Oncol Biol Phys 1991;21:347–354.
29. Chin L, Cheng C, Siddon R. Three-dimensional photon dose distributions with and without lung corrections for tangential breast intact treatments. Int J Radiat Oncol Biol Phys 1989;17:1327–1335.
30. Chen AM, Obedian E, Haffty BG. Breast-conserving therapy in the setting of collagen vascular disease. Cancer J 2001;91:1191–1200.
31. De Naeyer B, De Meerleer G, Braems S, et al. Collagen vascular diseases and radiation therapy: A critical review. Int J Radiat Oncol Biol Phys 1999;44:975–980.
32. Fleck R, McNeese MD, Ellerbroek NA, et al. Consequences of breast irradiation in patients with pre-existing collagen vascular diseases. Int J Radiat Oncol Biol Phys 1989;17:829–833.
33. Robertson J, Clarke D, Peyzner M, et al. Breast conservation therapy: Severe breast fibrosis after radiation in patients with collagen vascular disease. Cancer 1991;18:502–508.
34. Ransoma D, Cameron F. Scleroderma: A possible contraindication to lumpectomy and radiotherapy in breast carcinoma. Australas Radiol 1987;31:317–318.
35. Urtasun R. A complication of the use of radiation for malignant neoplasia in chronic discoid lupus erythematosus. J Can Assoc Radiol 1971;22:168–169.
36. Matthews RH. Collagen vascular disease and irradiation. Int J Radiat Oncol Biol Phys 1989;17:1123–1124.
37. Solan AN, Solan MJ, Bednarz G, et al. Treatment of patients with cardiac pacemakers and implantable cardioverter-defibrillators during radiotherapy. Int J Radiat Oncol Biol Phys 2004;59:897–904.
38. Last A. Radiotherapy in patients with cardiac pacemakers. Br J Radiol 1998;71:4–10.
39. Thomas D, Becker R, Katus HA, et al. Radiation therapy-induced electrical reset of an implantable cardioverter defibrillator device located outside the irradiation field. J Electrocardiol 2004;37:73.
40. Mouton J, Haug R, Bridier A, et al. Influence of high-energy photon beam irradiation on pacemaker operation. Phys Med Biol 2002;47: 2879–2893.
41. Walz BJ, Reder RE, Pastore JO, et al. Cardiac pacemakers: Does radiation therapy affect performance? JAMA 1975;234:72–73.
42. Adamec JR, Haeflinger JM, Kellish JP, et al. Damaging effect of therapeutic radiation on programmable pacemakers. PACE 1982;5:146.
43. Katzenberg CA. Marcus FL, Heusinkveld RS, et al. Pacemaker failure due to radiation therapy. PACE 1982;5:156.
44. Quertermons T, Megahy M, Das Gupta S, et al. Pacemaker failure resulting from radiation damage. Radiology 1983;148:257–258.
45. Marbach JR, Sontag MR, Van Dyk J, et al. Management of radiation oncology patients with implanted cardiac pacemakers: Report of AAPM task group no. 34.   Med Phys 1994;24:85–91.
46. McFarland BJ. The effect of the dynamic wedge in the medial tangential field upon the contralateral breast dose. Int J Radiat Oncol Biol Phys 1990;19:1515–1520.
47. Fraass BA, Roberson PL, Lichter AS. Dose to the contralateral breast due to primary breast irradiation. Int J Radiat Oncol Biol Phys 1985; 11:485–497.
48. Leibel SA, Fuks Z, Zelefsky MJ, et al. Intensity-modulated radiotherapy. Cancer J 2002;8:164–176.
49. Holland R, Veling SHJ, Mravunac M, et al. Histologic multifocality of Tis, T1-2 breast carcinomas: Implications for clinical trials of breast-conserving surgery. Cancer 1985;56:979–990.
50. Kurtz JM, Spitalier J-M. Local recurrence after breast conserving surgery and radiotherapy. What have we learned? Int J Radiat Oncol Biol Phys 1990;19:1087–1089.
51. Fisher B, Redmond C, Poisson R, et al. Eight year results of a randomized clinical trial comparing total mastectomy and lumpectomy with or without irradiation in the treatment of breast cancer. N Engl J Med 1989;320:822–828.
52. Veronesi U, Saccozzi R, Del Vecchio M, et al. Comparing radical mastectomy with quadrantectomy, axillary dissection and radiotherapy in patients with small cancers of the breast. N Engl J Med 1981;305: 6–11.
53. Von Dongen J, Bartelink H, Fentimen I, et al. Randomized clinical trial to assess the value of breast conserving therapy in stage I and II breast cancer: EORTC 10801 trial 1. Monogr Natl Cancer Inst 1992;11:15–18.

54. Blichert-Toft M, Brincker H, Andersen J, et al. A Danish randomized trial comparing breast preserving therapy with mastectomy in mammary carcinoma. Acta Oncol 1988;27:671–677.

55. Sarrazin D, Le M, Arriagada R, et al. Ten-year results of a randomized trial comparing a conservative treatment to mastectomy in early breast cancer. Radiother Oncol 1989;14:177–184.

56. Lichter A, Lippman M, Danforth D, et al. Mastectomy versus breast conserving therapy in the treatment of stage I and II carcinoma of the breast: A randomized trial at the National Cancer Institute. J Clin Oncol 1992;10:976–983.

57. Vrieling C, Collette L, Fourquet A, et al. Can patient-treatment- and pathology-related characteristics explain the high local recurrence rate following breast-conserving therapy in young patients? Eur J Cancer 2003;39:932–944.

58. Harris JL, Levene MB, Svensson G. et al. Analysis of cosmetic results following primary radiation for stages I and II carcinoma of the breast. Int J Radiat Oncol Biol Phys 1979;5:257–261.

59. Olivotto IA, Rose MA, Osteen RT, et al. Late cosmetic outcome after conservative surgery and radiotherapy: Analysis of causes of cosmetic failure. Int J Radiat Oncol Biol Phys 1989;17:747–752.

60. Van Limbergen E, Rijnders A, Van der Schueren E, et al. Cosmetic evaluation of breast conserving treatment for mammary cancer. 2. A quantitative analysis of the influence of radiation dose, fractionation schedules and surgical treatment techniques on cosmetic results. Radiother Oncol 1989;16:253–267.

61. Reitsamer R, Peintinger F, Sedlmayer F, et al. Intraoperative radiotherapy given as a boost after breast-conserving surgery in breast cancer patients. Eur J Cancer 2002;38:1607–1610.

62. Harris JR, Botnick L, Bloomer WD, et al. Primary radiation therapy for early breast cancer: The experience at the Joint Center for Radiation Therapy. Int J Radiat Oncol Biol Phys 1981;7:1549–1552.

63. Fowble B, Solin L, Schultz D, et al. Ten year results of conservative surgery and irradiation for stage I and II breast cancer. Int J Radiat Oncol Biol Phys 1991;21:269–277.

64. Fowble B, Solin L, Martz K, et al. The influence of the type of boost (electron vs implant) on local control and cosmesis in patients with stage I and II breast cancer undergoing conservative surgery and radiation. Int J Radiat Oncol Biol Phys 1986;12(Suppl):150.

65. Kuske R, Compaan P, Cross M, et al. Breast conservation therapy: 417 breast cancers with a minimum follow-up period of five years. Int J Radiat Biol Phys 1989;17:235–236.

66. Triedman S, Boyages J, Silver B, et al. A comparison of local control and cosmetic outcome in patients boosted with electrons or implant in the conservative management of early breast cancer. In Proceedings of the 17th International Congress of Radiation Oncology, Paris, July 1989, p 48.

67. Gerard JP, Montbarbon JF, Chassard JL, et al. Conservative treatment of early carcinoma of the breast: Significance of axillary dissection and iridium implant. Radiother Oncol 1985;3:17–22.

68. Nobler MP, Venet L. Prognostic factors in patients undergoing curative irradiation for breast cancer. Int J Radiol Oncol Biol Phys 1985;11:123–133.

69. Smitt MC, Birdwell RL, Goffinet DR. Breast electron boost planning: Comparison of CT and US. Radiology 2001;219:203–206.

70. Solin LJ, Chu JCH, Larsen R. et al. Determination of depth for electron breast boosts. Int J Radiat Oncol Biol Phys 1987;13:1915– 1919.

71. Solin LJ, Danoff BF, Schwartz GF, et al. A practical technique for the localization of the tumor volume in definitive irradiation of the breast. Int J Radiat Oncol Biol Phys 1985;11:1215–1220.

72. Kokubo M, Mitsumori M, Yamamoto C, et al. Impact of boost irradiation with surgically placed radiopaque clips on local control in breast-conserving therapy. Breast Cancer 2001;8:222–228.

73. Benda RK, Yasuda G, Sethi A, et al. Breast boost: Are we missing the target? Cancer 2003;97:905–909.

74. Recht A, Pierce SM, Abner A, et al. Regional nodal failure after conservative surgery and radiotherapy for early-stage breast carcinoma. J Clin Oncol 1991;9:988–996.

75. Solin LJ. Radiation treatment volumes and doses for patients with early stage carcinoma of the breast treated with breast conserving surgery and definitive irradiation. Semin Radiat Oncol 1992;2:82–93.

76. Hetelekidis S, Schnitt S, Morrow M, et al. Management of ductal carcinoma in situ. CA Cancer J Clin 1995;45:244–253.

77. Rose MA, Olivotto I, Cady B, et al. Conservative surgery and radiation therapy for early breast cancer: Long-term cosmetic results. Arch Surg 1989;124:153–157.

78. Lichter AS, Fraass BA, van de Geijn J, et al. A technique for field matching and primary breast irradiation. Int J Radiat Oncol Biol Phys 1983;9:263–273.

79. Chu JCH, Solin LJ, Hwang CC, et al. A non-divergent three field matching technique for breast irradiation. Int J Radiat Oncol Biol Phys 1990;19:1037–1040.

80. Svensson GK, Chin LM, Siddon RL, et al. Breast treatment techniques at the Joint Center for Radiation Therapy. In Harris JR. Hellman S, Silen W (eds). Conservative Management of Breast Cancer. Philadelphia, JB Lippincott, 1983, pp 239–255.

81. Baglan KL, Sharpe MB, Jaffray D, et al. Accelerated partial breast irradiation using 3D conformal radiation therapy (3D-CRT). Int J Radiat Oncol Biol Phys 2003;55:302–311.

82. Nag S, Kuske RR, Vicini FA, et al. Brachytherapy in the treatment of breast cancer. Oncology 2001;15:195–202.

83. Vicini FA, Kestin L, Chen P, et al. Limited-field radiation therapy in the management of early-stage breast cancer. J Natl Cancer Inst 2003;95:1205–1211.

84. Wazer DE, Berle L, Graham R, et al. Preliminary results of a phase I/II study of HDR brachytherapy alone for T1/T2 breast cancer.

85. Streeter OE Jr, Vicini FA, Keisch M, et al. MammoSite radiation therapy system. Breast 2003;12:491–496.

86. Pawlik TM, Perry A, Strom EA, et al. Potential applicability of balloon catheter-based accelerated partial breast irradiation after conservative surgery for breast carcinoma. Cancer 2004;100:490–498.

87. Orecchia R, Ciocca M, Lazzari R, et al. Intraoperative radiation therapy with electrons (ELIOT) in early-stage breast cancer. Breast 2003;12:483–490.

88. Intra M, Gatti G, Luini A, et al. Surgical technique of intraoperative radiotherapy in conservative treatment of limited-stage breast cancer. Arch Surg 2002;137:737–740.

89. Wallner P, Arthur D, Bartelink H, et al. Workshop on partial breast irradiation: State of the art and the science, Bethesda, MD, December 8–10, 2002. J Natl Cancer Inst 2004;96:175–184.

90. Kinne DW, Petrek JA, Osborne MP, et al. Breast carcinoma in situ. Arch Surg 1989;124:33–36.

91. Sunshine JA, Moseley MS, Fletcher WS, et al. Breast carcinoma in situ. A retrospective review of 112 cases with a minimum 10 year follow-up. Am J Surg 1985;150:44–51.

92. Silverstein MJ, Waisman JR. Gamagami P, et al. Intraductal carcinoma of the breast (208 cases): Clinical factors influencing treatment choice. Cancer 1990;66:102–108.

93. Schuh ME, Nemoto T, Penetrante RB, et al. Intraductal carcinoma: Analysis of presentation, pathologic findings and outcome of disease. Arch Surg 1986;121:1303–1307.

94. von Rueden D, Wilson RE. Intraductal carcinoma of the breast. Surg Gynecol Obstet 1984;158:105–111.

95. Fisher E, Leeming R, Anderson S, et al. Conservative management of intraductal carcinoma (DCIS) of the breast. J Surg Oncol 1991;47:139–147.

96. Schwartz GF, Finkel GC, Garcia JC, et al. Subclinical ductal carcinoma in situ of the breast: Treatment by local excision and surveillance alone. Cancer 1992;70:2468–2474.

97. Holland R, Hendriks JH. Vebeek AL, et al. Extent distribution and mammographic/ histologic correlations of breast ductal carcinoma in situ. Lancet 1990;335:519–522.

98. Fisher ER, Sass R, Fisher B, et al. Pathologic findings from the National Surgical Adjuvant Breast Project (Protocol 6): I. Intraductal carcinoma (DCIS). Cancer 1986;57:197–208.

99. Fisher B, Constantino J, Redmond C, et al. Lumpectomy compared with lumpectomy and radiation therapy for the treatment of intraductal cancer breast cancer. N Engl J Med 1993;328:1581–1586.

100. Silverstein MJ, Cohlan BF, Gierson ED, et al. Duct carcinoma in situ: 227 cases without microinvasion. Eur J Cancer 1992;28:630–634.

101. Solin LJ, Yeh IT, Kurtz J, et al. Ductal carcinoma in situ (intraductal carcinoma) of the breast treated with breast conserving surgery and definitive irradiation. Cancer 1993;71:2532–2542.

102. McCormick B, Rosen PP, Kinne DW, et al. Ductal carcinoma in situ of the breast: An analysis of local control after conservation surgery and radiotherapy. Int J Radiat Oncol Biol Phys 1991;21:289–292.

103. Stotter AT, McNeese M, Oswald MJ, et al. The role of limited surgery with irradiation in primary treatment of ductal in situ breast cancer. Int J Radiat Oncol Biol Phys 1990;18:283–287.

104. Hiramatsu H, Bornstein BA, Recht A, et al. Local recurrence after conservative surgery and radiation therapy for ductal carcinoma in

Table 28–3   Cancers Detected by Selective Biopsy of the Opposite Breast in 258 Patients

Biopsy	No.	Pathologic Findings (No.)
Clinical or radiographic suspicion	11	Infiltrating (11)
Random biopsy	32	Infiltrating (4) Noninfiltrating (28)
Patients eligible for biopsy	258	
Total cancers detected	**43**	

Data from Pressman PI. Selective biopsy of the opposite breast. Cancer 1986;57:577–580.

Table 28–4   Calculated Cumulative Risk for Bilateral Disease by Age at First Diagnosis

Age at First Diagnosis (yr)	Incidence		
	Unilateral	Bilateral	Cumulative Risk (%)
<40	52	5	9.6
40–49	166	24	14.5
50–59	243	10	4.1
60–69	347	16	4.6
70–79	319	8	2.5
80+	158	3	5.9
Total	**1285**	**66**	**5.1**

Data from Adami HO, Bergstron R, Hansen J. Age at first primary as a determinant of the incidence of bilateral breast cancer. Cancer 1995;55: 643–647.

Generally, the technique of contralateral biopsy is to be discouraged. On the other hand, if biopsy of the opposite breast is to be tried, the most productive area is tissue from the central or upper outer quadrants of the breast because these are the most common sites of carcinoma. It is for this reason that a mirror-image biopsy can be productive. However, if the presenting malignancy is in the medial or inferior quadrants, biopsy is not performed only in the mirror image because breast parenchyma is relatively sparse in these areas. The random biopsy is carried out to include tissue from the central or upper outer quadrants and is designated as a contralateral biopsy. Because the findings will mainly be benign, circum-areolar, or laterally placed, incisions in skin lines are used to procure suitable specimens (at least 2 cm) while avoiding breast deformity. Occasionally, depending on breast volume, a triangular segment of tissue can be obtained to include central ducts in a radial orientation as well as tissue of the upper outer quadrant.

Reduction Mammoplasty with Primary Cancer (Opposite Breast). To achieve symmetry after unilateral breast reconstruction, reduction mammoplasty is sometimes carried out. An incidence of unsuspected carcinoma of 34% has been reported in the tissues removed at reduction surgery of the opposite breast in a series of 41 patients.[46] Another group showed analysis of reduction mammoplasty tissue to have a 0.7% rate of clinically occult malignancy in a random series of patients with an otherwise negative workup.[47]

Prophylactic Mastectomy. In a study in which prophylactic contralateral mastectomies were performed in a series of 126 patients selected because they were considered to be at high risk, the yield was 19.7%, of which 56% were LCIS or DCIS and 44% were invasive carcinomas.[20] In an older study, in which subcutaneous contralateral mastectomies were carried out as a part of breast reconstruction to achieve symmetry, 42.5% of the specimens examined in 3- to 5-mm serial sections contained either invasive carcinoma or in situ carcinoma.[14] Other studies have not supported these findings, but there is no question that concurrent malignancies or atypical lesions can be found with closer scrutiny of the tissues. It is also clear that with high-risk groups such as genetically positive patients, higher rates of contralateral disease can be found. These topics, as well as technical considerations of prophylactic mastectomy, are discussed later in this chapter.

What are the risk factors for contralateral breast cancer?

It is estimated that women who have had a breast cancer have a lifetime risk for a second primary tumor about five times that of women who have not had a first breast cancer.[48] This is therefore the single most important risk factor, but there are other major risk factors, as discussed subsequently.

Age
Age at time of the initial diagnosis of breast cancer is a major determinant of the risk of developing a second, metachronous breast cancer. Long-term survival presumably provides a longer exposure to pathogenic factors. In an epidemiologic study, it was calculated that the cumulative risk for a second, metachronous lesion in women younger than 50 years is 13.3% and in women older than 50 years is 3.5%, with an overall estimated 5% to 6% lifetime risk for both groups[49] (Table 28–4). For women with premenopausal familial breast cancer, there is a cumulative risk of 37% for the development of a new primary cancer in the contralateral breast over a 20-year period of survival.[50]

Family History
In all series, the risk for developing bilateral breast cancer is higher among women with a family history of the disease,[50,51] and this is typically expressed at an early age.[52] In addition, the yield of contralateral biopsies is twofold greater in women with a family history of breast cancer. The relative risk is reported as a fivefold increase in the lifetime incidence of bilateral breast cancer in familial versus nonfamilial patients.[53]

Genetics
Among *BRCA1* and *BRCA2* gene carriers, the cumulative lifetime risk for developing breast cancer by age 70 years is estimated to be 87%. For these women, there are only three approaches:[54,55] (1) intensified screening, (2) chemoprevention, and (3) prophylactic mastectomy.

Regular clinical examinations, mammography, sonography, and MRI for women in their 20s and 30s aids in early detection. The only available chemopreventive agent that has undergone long-term trials is tamoxifen. It reduces the occurrence of secondary primary breast cancers in the opposite breasts of postmenopausal woman.[56] Its value for such prophylaxis in younger women has also been demonstrated in a randomized trial.[57] Recently, other hormonal agents have shown similar and, in some cases, improved prophylaxis and may eventually supplant tamoxifen.[58] Women with BRCA mutation who undergo bilateral prophylactic oophorectomy decrease their risk for developing breast cancer.[59,60] Previously, bilateral prophylactic mastectomy was the only truly preventive strategy available for these women, but the true predictive risk for bilaterality based on having a defective gene is yet to be determined. The incidence of simultaneous occult carcinoma in the prophylactically removed breasts of these BRCA-positive women has yet to be reported.

The p53 gene is probably one of the genes responsible for an inherited susceptibility to various cancers. Abnormalities of p53 have been detected in 50% of bilateral and 25.8% of unilateral cases studied. The percentage of patients with a p53 gene abnormality and positive family history was higher for those with bilateral than with unilateral breast cancer, and in metachronous cases the incidence of p53 gene abnormalities was particularly high. These findings may suggest that the genetic changes and the mechanism of carcinogenesis in bilateral and unilateral breast cancer may be different.[61]

Recent work with other genetic factors, such as the ataxia-telangiectasia mutation (ATM), has looked at the incidence of both synchronous and metachronous breast cancer without showing any increase.[62]

Previous Radiation Therapy

There is no apparent risk to the contralateral breast in women whose breast cancer is treated by quadrantectomy, axillary dissection, and radiation therapy when compared with women treated by the Halsted radical mastectomy and no radiation therapy.[63] This is fortunate because breast conservation using radiation therapy has become the treatment of choice for early breast cancer.

There is considerable risk, however, for the development of bilateral breast cancer in young female patients successfully treated with mantle irradiation for Hodgkin's disease. Tumors tend to be bilateral and medially located within 10 years of initial radiation exposure.[64,65] In these patients, the actuarial incidence of developing breast cancer approaches 35% by 40 years. In children, older age (10 to 16 years vs. less than 10 years) at the time of radiation treatment and higher dose are associated with even higher risks.[66] In adults, younger age at time of treatment for Hodgkin's disease was associated with high risk. This risk decreased to average if the radiation was given over the age of 30 years.[67,68] This suggests that radiation exposure on the adolescent's developing breast tissue poses a significantly greater risk. Bilateral breast cancer has also been reported after whole-lung irradiation in osteosarcoma treatment.[69] We have personally observed bilateral breast cancers in patients whose skin had been irradiated for childhood acne and in those who had mastitis associated with breast-feeding.

Identification of High-Risk (Pathologic) Features in the Ipsilateral Breast

According to Foote and Stewart, "the most frequent antecedent of cancer in one breast is the history of having had cancer in the opposite breast."[70] The predictive value of examining the first breast histologically has been studied exhaustively, and as many as 38 pathologic factors have been assessed.[44,71,72] There is no correlation of bilateral breast cancer with tumor size, histologic differentiation, hormone receptor content, or the magnitude of lymph node involvement, except as these factors affect survival after the initial breast malignancy. However, there are a few truly predictive pathologic factors.

Lobular Carcinoma in Situ. LCIS has a bilaterality rate as high as 30% to 40%.[73] The highest incidences are reported when elective contralateral breast biopsy is performed. Investigators generally agree that patients who have histologic evidence of LCIS alone have a 25% chance of developing an infiltrating carcinoma, usually of the ductal type, in either breast within a period of 25 years. Patients with coexisting invasive lobular carcinoma have an even higher risk of developing a second breast cancer.[74] When LCIS coexists with infiltrating ductal cell carcinoma, the bilaterality rate has been reported to be as high as 57%.[75] The finding of LCIS alone in a breast biopsy is correctly called a marker of risk for the future development of an infiltrating breast carcinoma—a risk shared equally by both breasts. When it is found in association with an infiltrating carcinoma, it confers an even greater risk on the opposite breast. Recently, a high-grade pleomorphic variant of LCIS that has a higher incidence of both coexistent and subsequent development of invasive disease has been identified.[76,77]

Ductal Carcinoma in Situ. Mammographically detected DCIS now accounts for more than 20% of the breast cancers treated today, and there are no long-term statistics comparable to those for LCIS as regards the long-term risk for bilaterality. It is clear that, unlike LCIS, bilateral synchronous presentation is uncommon with DCIS, with an incidence of less than 5%.[78] In a carefully studied series of 1140 patients with pure DCIS, there was a 7.9% incidence of subsequent contralateral cancers with a median follow-up time of 78 months.[79] These findings are highly significant, and DCIS may be more important than LCIS as a marker of risk for the development of a metachronous contralateral breast carcinoma.

Infiltrating Lobular Carcinoma. Infiltrating lobular carcinomas are frequently large when detected clinically and account for many false-negative mammograms because they tend not to incite the desmoplastic reactions of ductal carcinomas. Although they may be isolated and discrete and behave like ductal cancers, they are frequently multicentric, particularly when associated with LCIS. A 25% incidence of either synchronous or metachronous carcinomas in the contralateral breast of patients with infiltrating lobular carcinoma has been reported.[80] In 419 patients with infiltrating lobular carcinoma, the incidence was 10%.[81] As previously noted, however, the incidences in association with LCIS are considerably higher.[74]

Multicentricity. A common denominator in the growth patterns of most of the high-risk histologic diagnoses discussed—LCIS, DCIS, and infiltrating lobular carcinoma—is multicentricity.[75] In an analysis of all the possible variables, the only factor with a statistically significant association with bilateral breast cancer was a histologic diagnosis characterized by multicentricity.[82,83] It is pertinent to repeat the initial premise of this chapter—that the breasts are paired organs and that whatever pathologic processes evolve in one breast are likely be reflected in the other.

What is the prognosis of bilateral breast cancer?

Survival of women with bilateral breast carcinoma is determined by the more advanced of the two malignancies. A clear example is a woman who has an invasive carcinoma in one breast and carcinoma in situ in the other. It is the invasive carcinoma that will determine the prognosis. When both of the carcinomas are at an in situ stage, the chance of cure is close to 100%. When both carcinomas are invasive, however, the patient is at an unpredictable risk with regard to survival. It has been reported that patients with metachronous breast cancer have a poorer prognosis than those with unilateral disease.[84–90] It is likely that this poorer prognosis depends on the impact of the stage of the second carcinoma rather than any influence of the first malignancy. On the other hand, patients with synchronous disease have been identified to overexpress high levels of *HER-2/neu*, raising the possibility that this may be the cause of higher mortality.[91] With vigilant follow-up of the opposite breast, the second cancers are discovered at an earlier stage than the first, and the prognosis can be highly favorable.[92]

It was observed in the National Surgical Adjuvant Breast Project (NSABP) Protocol B-04 that women with contralateral carcinomas presenting within 2 years of the first fared much worse than those whose tumors were discovered later.[51] This has been confirmed in another study in which it is clear that the interval between the discovery of the carcinomas is important. The recurrence-free survival rate of patients with second carcinomas diagnosed within 5 years was 58%, compared with 95% for patients diagnosed more than 5 years after the first carcinoma.[93]

The second lesions that occur within a 2-year period are probably synchronous, and these bilateral carcinomas have a poorer prognosis because the cancers are frequently more advanced. An exception is opposite cancers that are detected by true random biopsy on new diagnostic imaging. These are more likely to be at an in situ stage and theoretically should have a better prognosis by avoiding the risk of development of an invasive carcinoma.

Is there a role for contralateral prophylactic mastectomy?

A clinically and radiographically apparent unilateral carcinoma is investigated and treated according to the known pathologic findings. Contralateral biopsies, reduction mammoplasty, and opposite prophylactic mastectomy are elective means by which a second cancer may be discovered. Although it is natural to focus on the presenting unilateral problem, it is important to consider bilaterality and to carefully examine the opposite breast clinically just as the radiologist scrutinizes the mammogram. Pursuing subtle abnormalities with stereotactically, ultrasound-, or MRI-guided biopsy may provide useful information about the opposite breast.[94]

With the advent of breast-conserving therapy, there is a reluctance to recommend a true random biopsy of the opposite breast. As we have previously seen, a positive biopsy usually discovers LCIS, a lesion for which additional treatment is not mandated.

With an increased awareness of risk factors and the availability of good breast reconstruction, opposite prophylactic mastectomy is being offered in specific instances. Although there has not been a randomized or convincing nonrandomized trial to prove that contralateral prophylactic mastectomy improves survival, the issue may be compelling in certain situations. Because the malignancies encountered in the opposite breasts are mainly at an in situ or early invasive stage, in these women this procedure reduces the risk to that of the stage of the initial unilateral breast cancer and can improve survival.

Women who might be considered for contralateral prophylactic mastectomy may be those who have a constellation of factors, which include the following:

- Young age
- Hereditary breast carcinoma
- First-degree relatives with bilateral carcinoma
- LCIS in addition to infiltrating ductal or lobular carcinoma
- Multicentric lobular carcinoma
- Cancerophobia
- A planned transverse rectus abdominis muscle (TRAM) flap reconstruction
- *BRCA1* and *BRCA2* gene mutation

Other than having a known genetic abnormality, none of the above is an absolute indication. Together, the risks may seem acceptable to a woman who has a justified fear about developing a cancer in her opposite breast, particularly when surveillance has failed in her own case or with family members or friends. These women who elect to have a contralateral prophylactic mastectomy are extremely grateful and relieved.

Another consideration (not a risk factor) is the type of breast reconstruction planned for the initial mastectomy. An implant can always be matched at a future date with a second implant with the expectation of accomplishing good symmetry (Fig. 28–2). However, when a unilateral TRAM flap reconstruction has been used and a second mastectomy needs to be reconstructed (for a metachronous carcinoma), an entirely different technique is required, and the appearance is usually poor (Fig. 28–3). Because it cannot be repeated, whenever a TRAM flap reconstruction is planned, the risk for developing a second breast cancer needs to be evaluated and the role of a contralateral (prophylactic) mastectomy considered.[95] The best cosmetic result can be accomplished when the TRAM flap is used to reconstruct both breasts following simultaneous bilateral mastectomy (Fig. 28–4).

Prophylactic mastectomy can successfully prevent the development of a breast cancer.[96] A central ellipse of skin including the nipple–areolar complex is removed. This is an excellent setting for skin-sparing mastectomy (SSM). The incision can be planned with cosmetic intent and can be preservative of skin.[97] This is not a subcutaneous mastectomy that is performed through an inframammary incision and in which the nipple–areolar complex remains intact, which would virtually imply that residual breast parenchyma will remain on superficial deep planes. Recently, a modification of this original SSM has shown that the areolar skin can be preserved as well.[98,99]

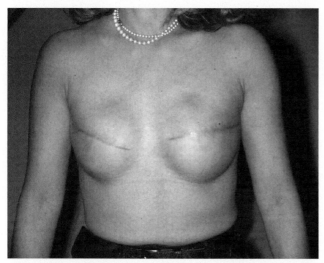

Figure 28–2 Bilateral tissue expander reconstruction. A 51-year-old woman initially underwent a right modified radial mastectomy for an invasive ductal carcinoma and breast reconstruction with an expander. An invasive carcinoma of the opposite breast was detected by random biopsy, and a second mastectomy with a similar reconstruction was subsequently carried out.

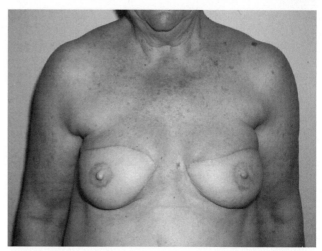

Figure 28–4 A 52-year-old woman with bilateral infiltrating breast carcinoma underwent modified radical mastectomies and immediate transverse rectus abdominis flap reconstruction.

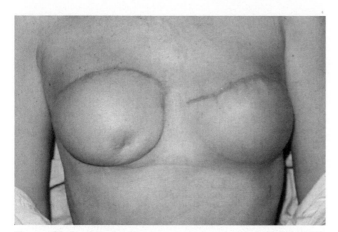

Figure 28–3 At age 42 years, a transverse rectus abdominis muscle flap reconstruction was used to reconstruct a right modified radical mastectomy. Five years later, a carcinoma in the left breast required a modified radical mastectomy and reconstruction with a tissue expander and saline implant.

This results in a more satisfactory cosmetic outcome, with a nipple reconstruction carried out secondarily. It must be stressed that the skin flaps should be developed with the same factors as for invasive disease with oncologic intent. In similar fashion, because the intent is to remove all underlying breast tissue, the nipple must be removed.

What are the treatment options for synchronous bilateral breast cancers?

Each breast cancer ideally should be treated according to its individual characteristics; however, the presence of a second cancer may dictate different priorities. The stage of the more advanced cancer (usually the presenting lesion) has greater

impact on the choice of treatment. When synchronous cancers are detected, it is necessary to make decisions about both breasts. Patients have been likely to have had treatment consistent with the approach preferred at the time. This would have been bilateral radical mastectomy in the 1960s or bilateral modified radical mastectomy in the 1970s. The option of implant breast reconstruction was added to the modified radical mastectomy in the 1980s, and myocutaneous flaps are now more frequently being used. Presently, breast-conserving surgery and radiation therapy have become the preferred approach. Some patients, however, are not candidates for breast conservation. Whether the cancers are infiltrating or at an in situ stage, a mastectomy can be performed with or without reconstruction. The necessity for an axillary dissection is based on sentinel lymph node biopsy. More recently, sentinel lymph node biopsy has also been used at the time of prophylactic surgery because the morbidity is low, and the possibility of finding invasive disease in the prophylactically removed breast tissue provides valuable information about the need for subsequent full axillary dissection.

Breast-conserving therapy is a successful and preferred approach to treating unilateral breast cancer. When bilateral synchronous infiltrating cancers are each amenable to breast conservation, this is also successful and can be advised.[100,101]

It is reasonable to use the same approach for both breasts to provide the best possible symmetry. Considerations in selection of management approaches include some of the following:

- The prolonged treatment (10 to 12 weeks) required for bilateral radiation therapy may motivate mastectomy, particularly in elderly women.
- Bilateral breast reconstruction may not be an option because of age or concurrent medical problems.
- Younger women may feel more secure with bilateral mastectomy and reconstruction because the risk for recurrence, which is acceptable with unilateral breast conservation (radiotherapy), is increased with two breasts treated. Also, a breast recurrence after radiation therapy usually mandates myocutaneous flap reconstruction, and this does not remain an option if the recurrence appears at an older age.

- Although radiation therapy may be optimal for an infiltrating cancer of one breast, it may not be appropriate for an in situ cancer of the opposite breast such as diffuse DCIS.
- Radiation therapy cannot be used where prior irradiation may have played an etiologic role.

What are the treatment options for metachronous contralateral cancer?

When the second cancer has been detected in the opposite breast in the follow-up of a woman who previously had a breast cancer, the treatment is inevitably influenced by a constellation of factors:

- The interval between the discovery of the new cancer and the first breast cancer
- The treatment approach used for the initial malignancy
- The success of the first breast cancer treatment and the stage of the new carcinoma
- The age of the patient at the time of the second diagnosis
- The method to accomplish the best symmetry
- Concurrent medical conditions
- The patient's personal choice

Reduction mammoplasty of the opposite breast is frequently performed as a secondary operation to improve symmetry after mastectomy when implant reconstruction has been carried out in the site of the initial cancer. Carcinoma may be found in the tissues removed.[37] If it is an infiltrating carcinoma, mastectomy with a lymph node dissection and expander reconstruction is usually indicated. If the malignancy encountered is LCIS, a simple mastectomy with similar reconstruction can be carried out. The option of observation without additional surgery also exists. The reduced breast, however, is more difficult to follow mammographically. If the finding is DCIS, the same considerations may apply as with LCIS.

The major problem with an unexpected finding of malignancy in the tissues removed during a reduction mammoplasty is that the exact location of the carcinoma in the breast is usually uncertain. Performing a mastectomy obviates the need to know the location of the malignancy, which would be important if radiation therapy were to be employed. The use of an implant can often accomplish better symmetry than the reduction procedure.

When the second breast cancer occurs many years later, the patient's perception of the outcome of the first cancer treatment has an impact on how the second malignancy will be managed. For example, a woman who was successfully treated 25 years earlier with a radical mastectomy with skin grafting and a 10-day hospitalization may feel secure only with another mastectomy, so that a modified radical mastectomy without reconstruction and 1 to 2 days in the hospital is an improved approach for her. Yet, with an identical prior history of treatment and outcome, another woman may be emphatic about saving her remaining breast and not mind the several weeks of radiation therapy involved following excision and axillary surgery. A woman with a metachronous cancer frequently has acquired more knowledge than when she was first treated, and a newer modality may be an option (Fig. 28–5).

When the first breast cancer was treated conservatively using lumpectomy and radiation therapy, it is appropriate for

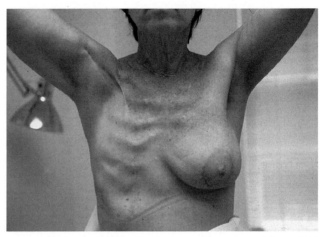

Figure 28–5   A 65-year-old woman underwent a right radical mastectomy when she was 35 years old. She elected to treat her second breast carcinoma with radiation therapy following a lumpectomy and axillary dissection.

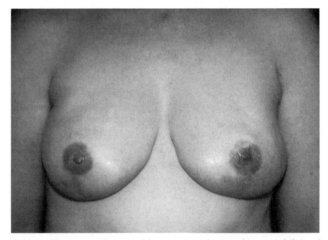

Figure 28–6   A 50-year-old woman who underwent bilateral skin-sparing mastectomies with bilateral free transverse rectus abdominis flap reconstruction—one therapeutic and one prophylactic.

the metachronous malignancy to be similarly treated using radiation therapy because the results are as good with unilateral as with bilateral disease.[102] Some women facing a second cancer are very happy to proceed with this similar approach. However, others may opt for bilateral mastectomy, removing the initially conservatively treated breast so as not to be concerned about the potential additional risks for bilateral local recurrence (Fig. 28–6).

SUMMARY

Most women treated for a unilateral breast carcinoma will not develop a malignancy of the opposite breast, and routine clinical and mammographic follow-up surveillance is appropriate. However, the possibility of bilaterality must always be considered. Because younger women are diagnosed more frequently with early-stage disease, the lifetime risk for developing a second breast cancer is greater. An awareness of genetic and pathologic risk factors makes it possible to make recommendations prospectively for appropriate investigative biopsies. This affects decisions regarding therapeutic and prophylactic mastectomy, reconstruction, and breast conservation. For the many reasons described, mastectomy is more frequently used for treating bilateral breast cancer. Although the risk of developing a contralateral primary carcinoma diminishes as women get older, new cancers continue to occur. There are special problems in management because some choices are not available related to age. A woman who develops a second breast cancer has acquired more information based on her experience and may be more proactive in making decisions about her care.

REFERENCES

1. Robbins GF, Berg JW. Bilateral primary breast cancers: A prospective clinicopathologic study. Cancer 1964;17:1501–1527.
2. Nielsen M, Christens L, Andersen J. Contralateral cancerous breast lesions in women with clinical invasive breast carcinoma. Cancer 1986;57:897–903.
3. Leis HP. Managing the remaining breast. Cancer 1980;46:1026–1030.
4. Pressman PI. Bilateral breast cancer: The contralateral biopsy. Breast 1986;5:29–33.
5. Urban JA, Papachristou D, Taylor J. Bilateral breast cancer. Cancer 1977;40:1968–1973.
6. Intra M, Rotmensz N, Viali G, et al. Clinicopathologic characteristics of 143 patients with synchronous bilateral invasive breast carcinomas treated in a single institution. Cancer 2004;101(5):905–912.
7. Slack NH, Bross IDJ, Nemoto T, et al. Experiences with bilateral primary carcinoma of the breast. Surg Gynecol Obstet 1973;136:433–440.
8. Rissanen TJ, Makarainen HP, et al. Mammography and ultrasound in the diagnosis of contralateral breast cancer. Acta Radiol 1995;36(4):358–366.
9. Cody HS. The impact of mammography on 1096 consecutive patients with breast cancer, 1979–1993. Cancer 1995;76:1579.
10. Hungness ES, Safa M, Shaughnessy FA, et al. Bilateral synchronous breast cancer: Mode of detection and comparison of histologic features between the 2 breasts. Surgery 2000;128(4):702–707.
11. Pressman PI. Selective biopsy of the opposite breast. Cancer 1986;57:577–580.
12. Lee SG, Orel SG, Woo IJ, et al. MR imaging screening of the contralateral breast in patients with newly diagnosed breast cancer: Preliminary results. Radiology 2003;226(3):773–778.
13. Slanetz PJ, Edmister WB, Yeh ED, et al. Occult contralateral breast carcinoma incidentally detected by breast magnetic resonance imaging. Breast J 2002;8:145–148.
14. Ringberg A, Palmer B, Linell F. The contralateral breast at reconstructive surgery after breast cancer operation: A histopathological study. Breast Cancer Res Treat 1982;2:151–161.
15. Khurana KK, Loosmann A, Numann PJ, et al. Prophylactic mastectomy: Pathologic findings in high-risk patients. Arch Pathol Lab Med 2000;124(3):378–381.
16. Hoogerbrugge N, Bult P, de Widt-Levert LM, et al. High prevalence of premalignant lesions in prophylactically removed breasts from women at hereditary risk for breast cancer. J Clin Oncol 2003;21(1):41–45.
17. Charache H. Metastatic tumors in the breast. Surgery 1953;33:385–390.
18. Pressman PI. Malignant melanoma and the breast. Cancer 1973;57:897–903.
19. Egan RL. Multicentric breast carcinomas: Clinical-radiologic-pathologic whole organ studies and 10-year survival. Cancer 1982;49:1123–1130.
20. Lesser ML, Rosen PP, Kinne DW. Multicentricity and bilaterality in invasive cancer. Surgery 1982;91:234.
21. Gallager HS, Martin JE. The study of mammary carcinoma by correlated mammography and subserial whole organ sectioning. Early observation. Cancer;1969;23:855–873.
22. Sterns EE, Fletcher WA, et al. Bilateral cancer of the breast: A review of clinical, histologic, and immunohistologic characteristics. Surgery 1991;110(4):617–622.
23. Tse GM, Kung FY, Chan AB, et al. Clonal analysis of bilateral mammary carcinomas by clinical evaluation and partial allelotyping. Am J Clin Pathol. 2003;120(2):168–174.
24. Agelopoulos K, Tidow N, Korsching E, et al. Molecular cytogenetic investigations of synchronous bilateral breast cancer. J Clin Pathol 2003;56(9):660–665.
25. Khafagy MM, Schottenfield D, Robbins GF. Prognosis of the second breast: The role of previous exposure to the first primary. Cancer 1975;35:596–599.
26. Leis H, Commarato A, La Raja R, et al. Bilateral breast cancer. Breast 1981;7:13–17.
27. Harrington SW. Survival rates of radical mastectomy for unilateral and bilateral carcinoma of the breast. Surgery 1946;19:154–166.
28. McSweeney MB, Egan RL. Bilateral breast carcinoma. Recent Results Cancer Res 1984;90:41–48.
29. Breslow A. Occult carcinoma of the second breast following mastectomy. JAMA 1973;226:1000–1001.
30. Jaffer SS, Goldfarb AB, Gold JE, et al. Contralateral axillary metastasis as the first evidence of locally recurrent breast carcinoma. Cancer 1995;75:2875–2878.
31. Senofsky GM, Wanebo HW, Wilhelm MC, et al. Has monitoring of the contralateral breast improved the prognosis in patients treated for primary breast cancer? Cancer 1986;57:597–602.
32. Lee JS, Grant CS, Donohue JH, et al. Arguments against routine contralateral mastectomy or undirected biopsy of invasive lobular breast cancer. Surgery 1995;118(4):640–647; discussion, 647–648.
33. Roubidoux MA, Helvie MA, Wilson TE, et al. Women with breast cancer: Histologic findings in the contralateral breast. Radiology 1997;203(3):691–694.
34. Thomas DB, Gao DL, Ray RM, et al. Randomized trial of breast self-examination in Shanghai: Final results. J Natl Cancer Inst 2002;94(19):1445–1457.
35. Wagman LD, Sanders RD, Terz JJ, et al. The value of symptom directed evaluation in the surveillance for recurrence of carcinoma of the breast. Surg Gynecol Obstet 1991;172:191–196.
36. Kolb T, Lichy J, et al. The impact of bilateral whole breast ultrasound in women with dense breasts and recently diagnosed breast cancer. Radiology Supplement 2000.
37. Moon WK, Noh DY, Im JG. Multifocal, multicentric, and contralateral breast cancers: Bilateral whole-breast ultrasound in the preoperative evaluation of patients. Radiology 2002;224(2):569–576.
38. Flobbe K, Bosch AM, Kessels AG, et al. The additional diagnostic value of ultrasonography in the diagnosis of breast cancer. Arch Intern Med 2003;163(10):1194–1199.
39. Hata T, Takahashi H, Watanabe K, et al. Magnetic resonance imaging for preoperative evaluation of breast cancer: a comparative study with mammography and ultrasonography. J Am Coll Surg 2004;198:190–197.
40. Morris EA, Liberman L, Ballon DJ, et al. MRI of occult breast carcinoma in a high risk population. AJR Am J Roentgenol 2003;181(3):619–626.
41. Adem C, Reynolds C, Soderberg CL, et al. Pathologic characteristics of breast parenchyma in patients with hereditary breast carcinoma, including BRCA1 and BRCA2 mutation carriers. Cancer 2003;97(1):1–11.
42. Kauff ND, Brogi E, et al. Epithelial lesions in prophylactic mastectomy specimens from women with BRCA mutations. Cancer 2003;97(7):1601–1608.
43. Wanebo HJ, Senofsky GM, Fechner RE, et al. Bilateral breast cancer: Risk reduction by contralateral biopsy. Ann Surg 1985;201:667–677.
44. Tulusan AH, Ronay G, Egger H, et al. A contribution to the natural history of breast cancer. Arch Gynecol 1985;237:85–91.
45. Staren ED, Robinson DA, Witt TR, et al. Synchronous, bilateral mastectomy. J Surg Oncol 1995;59(2):75–79.
46. de Mascarel M, Trojani JM, Coindre JM, et al. The incidence of cancer in contralateral reduction mammoplasty after mastectomy and reconstruction of the removed breast. Tumori 1986;72:183–186.
47. Ishag MT, Bashinsky DY, Beliaeva IV, et al. Pathologic findings in reduction mammoplasty specimens. Am J Clin Pathol 2003;120(30):377–380.
48. Robbins GF, Berg JW. Bilateral primary breast cancers. A prospective clinicopathological study. Cancer 1964;17:1501–1527.

49. Adami H, Bergstrom R, Hansen J. Age at first primary as a determinant of the incidence of bilateral breast cancer. Cancer 1985;55:643–647.

50. Harris RE, Lynch HT, Guirgis HA. Familial breast cancer: Risk to the contralateral breast. J Natl Cancer Inst 1978;60:955–960.

51. Fisher ER, Fisher B, Sass R, et al. Pathologic findings from the National Surgical Adjuvant Breast Project (Protocol No. 4). XI. Bilateral breast cancer. Cancer 1984;54:459–465.

52. Hislop TG, Worth AJ, Ellison LG. Secondary primary cancer of the breast: Incidence and risk factors. Br J Cancer 1984;49:79–85.

53. Lynch HT, Guirgis H, Lynch J, et al. Genetic factors in breast cancer. In Lynch HT (ed). Cancer Genetics. Springfield, IL, Charles C Thomas, 1975, pp 389–423.

54. Anderson DE. Genetics and the etiology of breast cancer. Breast 1977;3:37–41.

55. Weber BL, Giusti RM, Liv ET. Developing strategies for intervention and prevention in hereditary breast cancer. Mongr Natl Cancer Inst 1995;17:99–102.

56. Early Breast Cancer Trialists' Collaborative Group. Systemic treatment of early breast cancer by hormonal cytotoxic or immune therapy—133 randomized trials involving 31,000 recurrences and 24,000 deaths among 75,000 women. Lancet 1992;339:1–15

57. Fisher B, Costantino JP, Wickerham DL, et al. Tamoxifen for prevention of breast cancer: Report of the National Surgical Adjuvant Breast and Bowel Project P-1 Study. J Natl Cancer Inst 1998;90:1371.

58. The ATAC (Arimidex, Tamoxifen Alone or in Combination) Trialists' Group. Arimidex with tamoxifen versus tamoxifen alone for adjuvant treatment of postmenopausal women with early-state breast cancer. Cancer 2003;98:1802–1810.

59. Kauff ND, Satagopan JM, Robson ME, et al. Risk-reducing salpingo-oophorectomy in women with a BRCA1 or BRCA2 mutation. N Engl J Med 2002;346:1609–1615.

60. Rebbeck TR, Lynch HT, Neuhausen SL, et al. Prophylactic oophorectomy in carriers of BRCA1 or BRCA2 mutations. N Engl J Med. 2002;346:1616–1622.

61. Kinoshita T, Veda M, Bnomoto K, et al. Comparison of p53 gene abnormalities in bilateral and unilateral breast cancer. Cancer 1995;76:2504–2509.

62. Bernstein JL, Bernstein L, Thompson WD, et al. ATM variants 7271T>G and IVS10-6T>G among women with unilateral and bilateral breast cancer. Br J Cancer 2003;89(8):1513–1516.

63. Veronesi U, Banfi A, Salvadori E, et al. Breast conservation is the treatment of choice in small breast cancer: Long term results of a randomized trail. Eur J Cancer 1990;26:668–670.

64. Kurtz JM, Amalric R, Brandone H, et al. Contralateral breast cancer and other second malignancies in patients treated by breast-conserving therapy with radiation. Int J Radiat Oncol Biol Phys 1988;15:277.

65. Healey E, et al. Contralateral breast cancer: Clinical characteristics and impact on prognosis. J Clin Oncol 1993;11:1545.

66. Bhatia S, Robison L, Oberlin O, et al. Breast cancer and other second neoplasms after childhood Hodgkin's disease. N Engl J Med 1996;334:745–751.

67. Hanckock SL, Tucker MA, Hoppe RT. Breast cancer after treatment of Hodgkin's disease. J Natl Cancer Inst 1193;85:25.

68. Yahalom J, Petrick JA, Biddinger PW, et al. Breast cancer in patients irradiated for Hodgkin's disease: A clinical and pathologic analysis of 45 events in 37 patients. J Clin Oncol 1992;10:1674.

69. Ivins JC, Taylor WF, Wold LE. Elective whole-lung irradiation in osteosarcoma treatment: Appearance of bilateral breast cancer in two long term survivors. Skeletal Radiol 1987;16:133–135.

70. Foote FW, Stewart FW. Comparative studies of cancerous versus non cancerous breasts. Ann Surg 1945;131:197–222.

71. Fisher ER, Fisher B, Sass R, et al. Pathological findings from the National Surgical Adjuvant Breast Project (Protocol No. 4). Cancer 1954;54:3002–3011.

72. Hislop TG, Elwood JM, Coldman AJ, et al. Second primary cancers of the breasts: incidence and risk factors. Br J Cancer 1984;49:79.

73. Urban JA. Biopsy of the "normal" breast in treating breast cancer. Surg Clin North Am 1969;49:291–301.

74. Davis N, Baird RM. Breast cancer in association with lobular carcinoma in situ. Am J Surg 1984;147:641–645.

75. Lesser MI, Rosen PP, Kinne DW. Multicentricity and bilaterality in invasive breast carcinoma. Surgery 1982;91:234–240.

76. Middleton LP, Palacios DM, Bryant BR, et al. Pleomorphic lobular carcinoma: Morphology, immunohistochemistry, and molecular analysis. Am J Surg Pathol 2000;24(12):1650–1656.

77. Sneige N, Wang J, Baker, BA, et al. Clinical, histopathologic and biologic features of pleomorphic lobular (ductal-lobular) carcinoma in situ of the breast: A report of 24 cases. Mod Pathol 2002;15(10):1044–1050.

78. Schwartz G. Personal communication, January 2004.

79. Silverstein M. Personal communication, January 2004.

80. Baker RR, Kuhajda FP. The clinical management of a normal contralateral breast in patients with lobular breast cancer. Ann Surg 1989;210:444–448.

81. Lee JS, Grant CS, Donohue JH, et al. Arguments against routine contralateral mastectomy or undirected biopsy for invasive lobular breast cancer. Surgery 1995;118:640–648.

82. Pomerantz RA, Murad T, Hines JR. Bilateral breast cancer. Am Surg 1989;55:441–444.

83. Newman LA, Sahin AA, Cunningham JE, et al. A case-control study of unilateral and bilateral breast carcinoma patients. Cancer 2001;91(10):1845–1853 [published erratum I Cancer 2002;94(4):1191.

84. Fracchia AA, Robinson D, Legaspi A, et al. Survival in bilateral breast cancer. Cancer 1985;55:1414–1421.

85. Polednak AP. Bilateral synchronous breast cancer: A population-based study of characteristics, method of detection, and survival. Surgery 2003;133(4):383–389.

86. Brenner H, Engelsmann B, Stegmaier C, et al. Clinical epidemiology of bilateral breast cancer. Cancer 1993;72(12):3629–3635.

87. Heron DE, Komarnicky LT, Hislop T, et al. Bilateral breast carcinoma: Risk factors and outcomes for patients with synchronous and metachronous disease. Cancer 2000;88(12):2739–2750.

88. Burns PE, Dabbs K, May C, et al. Bilateral breast cancer in northern Alberta: Risk factors and survival patterns. CMAJ 1984;130(7):881–886.

89. Kollias J, Ellis IO, Elston CW, et al. Prognostic significance of synchronous and metachronous bilateral breast cancer. World J Surg 2001;25(9):1117–1124.

90. Carmichael AR, Bendall S, Lockerbie L, et al. The long-term outcome of synchronous bilateral breast cancer is worse than metachronous or unilateral tumors. Eur J Surg Oncol 2002;28(4):388–391.

91. Safal M, Lower EE, Hasselgren PO, et al. Bilateral synchronous breast cancer and HER-2/neu overexpression. Breast Cancer Res Treat 2002;72(3):195–201.

92. Singletary SE, Taylor SH, Guinee VF, et al. Occurrence and prognosis of contralateral carcinoma of the breast. J Am Coll Surg 1994;178:390–396.

93. Gustafsson A, Tarter PI, Brower ST, et al. Prognosis of patients with bilateral carcinoma of the breast. J Am Coll Surg 1994;178:111–116.

94. Mitnick JS, Vazquez MF, Pressman PI, et al. Stereotactic fine-needle aspiration biopsy for the evaluation of nonpalpable breast lesions: Report of an experience based on 2,988 cases. Ann Surg Oncol 1996;3:185–191.

95. Kroll SS, Miller MJ, Shuisterman MA, et al. Rationale for elective contralateral mastectomy with immediate breast reconstruction. Ann Surg Oncol 1994;1:457–461.

96. Pressman PI. Prophylactic mastectomy. Surg Oncol Clin North Am 1993;2:145–154.

97. Hidalgo DA, Borgen PJ, Petrick JA, et al. Immediate reconstruction after complete skin-sparing mastectomy with autologous tissue J Am Coll Surg 1988;187:17–21.

98. Patel M, Swistel A, Adamovich T, et al. Areolar-preserving skin-sparing mastectomy: An aesthetically and oncologically sound option for a subset of breast cancer patients. Plast Reconstr Surg 2005, in press.

99. Simmons RM, Brennen M, Christor P, et al. Analysis of nipple/areolar involvement with mastectomy: Can the areolar be preserved? Ann Surg Oncol 2002;9(2):165–168.

100. De La Rochefordiere A, Asselain B, Scholl S, et al. Simultaneous bilateral breast carcinomas: A retrospective review of 149 cases. Int J Radiat Oncol Biol Phys 1994;30:35–41.

101. Gollamudi RS, Gelman RS, Piero G, et al. Breast conserving therapy for stage I–II synchronous bilateral breast carcinoma. Cancer 1997;79:1362–1369.

102. Healey EA, Cook EF, Orav J, et al. Contralateral breast cancer: Clinical characteristics and impact on prognosis. J Clin Oncol 1993;11:1545–1552.

CHAPTER 29

Treatment of Locally Advanced Breast Cancer

Matthew Volm and Silvia Formenti

How is locally advanced breast cancer defined?

The definition of locally advanced breast cancer (LABC) has evolved during the past 50 years. Historically, the definition of LABC was based on work by Haagensen and Stout published in 1943 that described physical tumor characteristics associated with local and distant failure rates so high that surgery was strictly contraindicated: fixation of the tumor to skin or chest wall, skin edema (peau d'orange), skin ulceration, satellite nodules, fixed or matted axillary lymph nodes, supraclavicular lymphadenopathy, or arm edema.[1] Before Haagensen and Stout identified criteria of inoperability, en bloc radical mastectomy was the standard treatment for locally advanced breast cancer. After their publication, the term *locally advanced breast cancer* was associated with disease deemed inoperable based on their criteria.

Haagensen and Stout's work has withstood the test of time, and their observations remain the basis of the T4 and N2-3 categories in the current clinical staging system of the American Joint Committee on Cancer (AJCC), as shown in Table 29–1. The criteria of inoperability they identified are still used to select patients who are not candidates for surgery unless the local tumor burden can be successfully decreased with chemotherapy or radiation, as described later.

In the 1970s and 1980s, clinical practice progressed to include the option of breast-conserving surgery, lumpectomy, or segmental excision, followed by radiation as primary treatment for most patients with breast cancer. At the same time, the average tumor size decreased because of improved mammographic detection. As less extensive surgery became commonplace, the definition of *locally advanced disease* evolved to include tumors that are operable by the criteria of Haagensen and Stout, but that require mastectomy for a successful surgical outcome. Thus, an expanded definition of LABC now commonly includes large operable breast cancers, often those larger than 5.0 cm (T3 tumors in the AJCC system), in addition to inoperable T4 disease. This has led to a heterogeneous population of patients in many reported series of LABC, with many series including both T3 and T4 tumors.

The definition of LABC continues to evolve. In the past, ipsilateral infraclavicular or supraclavicular nodal involvement was considered to be distant metastatic disease (M1, stage IV), and patients were treated with largely palliative intent. More recently, however, the AJCC recognized clinical data showing that some of these patients achieve long disease-free survival and are possibly cured with contemporary multimodality therapy.[2,3] These patients are now classified as having N3 disease and are now often included in clinical trials for patients with LABC.

Some series in the LABC literature include patients with inflammatory breast cancer (IBC), an unusual, aggressive form of breast cancer presenting with inflammatory skin changes that reflect dermal lymphatic involvement (AJCC T4d tumors). IBC has a distinct biologic behavior that warrants considering it separately from other forms of locally advanced disease.[4] This chapter first discusses the approach to patients with noninflammatory LABC and then reviews the unique features and management of IBC.

Who gets locally advanced breast cancer?

LABC is the most common presentation of breast cancer worldwide. This is because of the high percentage of patients who present with locally advanced disease throughout the developing world. In India, for example, 50% to 70% of all breast cancer patients present with locally advanced disease.[5] Although LABC is less common in the developed world, where there is access to mammography and where breast cancer awareness in the medical community and general population is high, it remains a significant medical problem. In the United States, about 5% to 6% of patients present with locally advanced disease.[6] As expected, LABC is more common in poor, minority, and immigrant communities; in some medically underserved areas in the United States, up to one third of breast cancer patients present with LABC.[7]

How is locally advanced breast cancer diagnosed?

The diagnosis of LABC is usually straightforward in that most patients present with a large, firm, palpable breast mass. The differential diagnosis includes benign cysts, hematomas, fat necrosis, fibroadenomas, and phyllodes tumors. Diagnostic mammography, ultrasound, and magnetic resonance imaging (MRI) can assist in the diagnosis and help to delineate the extent of disease, but ultimately a suspicious lesion requires tissue sampling. A fine-needle aspirate can demonstrate the

Table 29–1   Primary Tumor (T) and Clinical Regional Lymph Node (N) Categories Comprising Locally Advanced Breast Cancer in the Current American Joint Committee on Cancer Classification System*

T3: Tumor more than 5 cm in greatest diameter
T4: Tumor of any size, with direct extension to chest wall or skin, as described below
T4a: Extension to chest wall, not including pectoralis muscle
T4b: Edema (including peau d'orange) or ulceration of the skin of the breast or satellite nodules confined to same breast
T4c: Both Ta and Tb
T4d: Inflammatory carcinoma
N2: Metastasis in ipsilateral axillary nodes fixed or matted, or in clinically apparent ipsilateral internal mammary nodes in the absence of clinically evident axillary node metastases
N3: Metastasis in ipsilateral infraclavicular or supraclavicular lymph nodes or in clinically apparent internal mammary nodes in the presence of clinically evident axillary node metastases

*In earlier editions of the American Joint Committee on Cancer Staging Handbook, stage III was confined to T4 or N2-3 disease (i.e., locally advanced, inoperable tumors). In the current system, in addition to locally advanced breast cancer, stage III includes tumors at high risk for systemic relapse because of involvement of four or more axillary nodes.
From Greene FL, Page DL, Fleming ID, et al. AJCC Cancer Staging Manual, 6th ed. New York, Springer-Verlag, 2002.

Table 29–2   Summary of the Management of Locally Advanced Breast Cancer

Clinical Diagnosis
Physical examination, mammogram, ultrasound
Pathologic Diagnosis
Core biopsy to confirm diagnosis of invasive carcinoma and to obtain estrogen receptor, progesterone receptor, and HER-2 status
Staging
Bone scan, computed tomography scans, routine laboratory studies
Neoadjuvant Chemotherapy
Use of an anthracycline and a taxane is recommended, e.g., four cycles of AC (doxorubicin, cyclophosphamide) followed by four cycles of paclitaxel or docetaxel; patients who would not tolerate chemotherapy and have hormone receptor–positive disease may be considered for treatment with tamoxifen or an aromatase inhibitor
Local Therapy
For patients who are surgical candidates after neoadjuvant chemotherapy, surgery (lumpectomy or mastectomy) followed by radiation
For patients who are not surgical candidates after neoadjuvant chemotherapy, radiation alone
Adjuvant Therapy
All patients with hormone receptor–positive disease should receive adjuvant hormonal therapy for 5 years or longer

presence of malignant cells but does not provide information about the architecture of the lesion (intraductal versus invasive carcinoma). A core biopsy, performed with local anesthesia, is usually sufficient to document the presence of invasive carcinoma and provides adequate tissue for assays for hormone receptors and HER-2, which may help to guide therapy.

Before therapy is initiated, an evaluation for metastatic disease is appropriate. At our institution, this includes laboratory work, computed tomography (CT) scans of the chest and abdomen, and a bone scan. An MRI of the brain is indicated when there are symptoms of central nervous system involvement. Despite the presence of locally extensive disease, it is unusual for patients to have clinically detectable metastases at presentation.

How is locally advanced breast cancer treated?

Contemporary management of LABC is a collaborative effort involving surgical, medical, and radiation oncologists. In order to be successful, the treatment of LABC must both achieve local control and eradicate any disseminated microscopic metastases. Although chemotherapy alone results in high overall response rates, it rarely eradicates the tumor in the breast and axilla. Radiation and surgery, on the other hand, improve local control but do not treat distant microscopic metastases. An outline of the contemporary multimodality treatment for patients with LABC is shown in Table 29–2. Treatment is initiated with chemotherapy, which provides early treatment of microscopic metastases and facilitates subsequent local therapy, which is usually surgery followed by radiation.

The importance of multimodality therapy is underscored by the historical experience demonstrating that the use of single-modality treatment results in poor local control and inferior survival.

What is the role of chemotherapy in the treatment of locally advanced breast cancer?

In the setting of LABC, systemic chemotherapy is given before local therapy and is referred to as *primary, induction,* or *neoadjuvant* therapy. Neoadjuvant chemotherapy has response rates in the primary tumor substantially higher than those seen when chemotherapy is given for metastatic disease, and it provides early systemic treatment for disseminated microscopic metastases. In addition, the downstaging achieved with neoadjuvant chemotherapy can often allow tumors that were inoperable at presentation to be removed by mastectomy and can allow breast-conserving surgery for some tumors that would otherwise have required mastectomy.

How does the response to neoadjuvant chemotherapy affect outcome?

Important prognostic information can be obtained by assessing the tumor's response to neoadjuvant therapy. The *clinical assessment* of response to neoadjuvant chemotherapy can be difficult: tumor measurements based on physical examination often overestimate or underestimate the degree of response and are less reliable than either mammographic or ultrasound measurements.[8] The ultimate *pathologic assessment* of treatment effect is determined after surgery. Clinical evidence indicates that the degree of pathologic response after primary chemotherapy can be used as a surrogate end point for survival. Despite differences in the methods used to measure and report the pathologic findings after neoadjuvant chemotherapy, all investigators have reported a similar correlation between the amount of residual disease found at surgery and patient outcome.[9–12] As expected, patients with complete clearance of tumor from the breast and axilla have the best outcome, and the degree of nodal involvement after neoadjuvant chemotherapy retains significant prognostic importance.

What are the results of multimodality treatment with neoadjuvant doxorubicin-based chemotherapy?

Although there is not a standard neoadjuvant chemotherapy regimen for LABC, it is possible to draw conclusions about the regimens that appear to be most effective. Results from anthracycline-based regimens are shown in Table 29–3. Several conclusions can be drawn about induction chemotherapy with an anthracycline-containing regimen. First, the response rates achieved with neoadjuvant chemotherapy for LABC are substantially higher than when similar regimens are given to treat metastatic disease. Second, although disease progression on chemotherapy is common in the setting of metastatic disease, it is rare for the patient on neoadjuvant chemotherapy, less than 5% in all reported series. Third, despite the high response rates achieved with conventional anthracycline-based neoadjuvant therapy, a pathologic complete response (i.e., no residual invasive tumor

in the breast or axilla) is unusual, occurring in 10% to 15% of patients in most series, and prolonged survival remains limited to about 50% of patients. Although it is difficult to make comparisons among trials with varied eligibility requirements and treatments, longer duration of neoadjuvant therapy appears to result in higher pathologic complete response rates.

How has the experience with neoadjuvant chemotherapy for locally advanced breast cancer affected the treatment of smaller tumors?

The safety and high response rates observed when neoadjuvant chemotherapy has been administered for LABC have encouraged the investigation of the neoadjuvant approach in patients with smaller operable tumors. To test the hypothesis that the administration of chemotherapy before surgery could improve relapse-free survival in patients with palpable, operable breast tumors, the National Surgical Adjuvant Breast and Bowel Project (NSABP) (B-18) conducted a large randomized trial comparing four cycles of neoadjuvant doxorubicin and cyclophosphamide (AC) to the same treatment provided after surgery.

Table 29–3 Anthracycline-Based Chemotherapy for Locally Advanced Breast Cancer

Study	No. of Patients and Tumor Characteristics	Treatment Regimen	Response	Breast Conservation	Survival
Schwartz et al., 1994[35]	158 patients with tumor > 5 cm	Doxorubicin-based chemotherapy given until response plateau → surgery → RT	Overall RR 85%; pCR in 10%	Breast-conserving surgery in 36% of responding patients	5-yr OS 69% for responding patients (67% for mastectomy patients; 80% for lumpectomy patients)
Merajver et al., 1997[36]	89 patients with 1997 AJCC stage III (tumor > 5 cm or N2 disease)	27 weeks of anthracycline-based chemohormonal therapy → patients with negative biopsy had RT only; all others had mastectomy followed by RT → additional chemohormonal therapy	Overall RR 97%; pCR in 28%	28% of patients with no tumor after neoadjuvant therapy had RT alone	5-yr DFS 44%, OS 54%; local control 82% in RT patients and 78% in patients with mastectomy and RT
Morrell et al., 1998[37]	55 patients with LABC or IBC	MVAC chemotherapy until maximal clinical response → surgery → MVAC × 6 cycles RT	Overall RR 89%; pCR in 27%	All patients had mastectomy	5-yr DFS 51%; 5-yr OS 63%
Kuerer et al., 1999[38]	372 patients with tumor > 4 cm	4 cycles of doxorubicin-based chemotherapy → surgery → additional chemotherapy → RT	pCR in 12%	Breast conservation in 29% of patients	5-yr DFS 89% for patients with pCR, 64% for patients with residual tumor
Zambetti et al., 1999[39]	88 patients with LABC (1997 AJCC T3 or T4a-c)	3 cycles of doxorubicin or epirubicin → surgery → CMF → RT	Overall RR 70%; pCR in only 2%	Breast conservation in 32% of patients	At 52 mo, DFS 52%, OS 62%
Therasse et al., 2003[40]	448 patients with T4 tumors	Patients randomized to 6 cycles of CEF or 6 cycles of dose-intense EC → surgery ± RT	Overall RR >90% in both groups; pCR in 14% for CEF and 10% for EC	Not reported	5-yr OS 51% for CEF, 53% for EC

AJCC, American Joint Committee on Cancer; CEF, cyclophosphamide, epirubicin, 5-fluorouracil; DFS, disease-free survival; EC, epirubicin, cyclophosphamide; IBC, inflammatory breast cancer; LABC, locally advanced breast cancer; MVAC, methotrexate, vinblastine, doxorubicin, cisplatin; RR, response rate; RT, radiation therapy; OS, overall survival; pCR, pathologic complete response.

The study demonstrated a high response rate for neoadjuvant chemotherapy (80%) but few pathologic complete responses (9%).[13] Although there was no difference in disease-free or overall survival between the two groups, the neoadjuvant group achieved a higher rate of breast conservation (67% vs. 60%). Neoadjuvant therapy has been incorporated into more clinical trials of systemic therapy for patients with operable breast cancer, in whom differences in response rates and especially pathologic complete response rates can provide useful information before survival data are available.

What is the effect of adding a taxane to the neoadjuvant therapy regimen?

The taxanes have recently become a part of standard postoperative adjuvant therapy for many patients with node-positive breast cancer. Their use has been investigated as neoadjuvant therapy in a more limited fashion in patients with LABC, as shown in Table 29–4. The results of these trials indicate that the taxanes, especially docetaxel, have good activity in patients with LABC. Although the NSABP B-27[14] and the German Preoperative Adriamycin Docetaxel Study Group (GEPAR-DUO)[15] studies were not limited to patients with LABC, the average tumor size was large in these randomized trials, and along with results of the study from the Aberdeen group,[16] the results support the use of four cycles of anthracycline-based therapy followed by four cycles of a taxane as a reasonable neoadjuvant regimen for LABC.

How are hormonal agents integrated into the treatment of locally advanced breast cancer?

Hormonal therapy with 5 years of tamoxifen was typically given to patients with hormone receptor–positive LABC after completion of all other treatment, including chemotherapy, surgery, and radiation. This practice is based on extensive data from adjuvant (i.e., postoperative) trials in the general breast cancer population that demonstrated an approximate 50% reduction in the annual odds of relapse for patients receiving tamoxifen. In the neoadjuvant setting, responses to tamoxifen appear to be slower and less complete than those achieved with chemotherapy, and tamoxifen has most often been administered to postmenopausal women considered poor candidates for chemotherapy.

More recently, with the development of a new class of hormonal agents, the aromatase inhibitors, there has been increased interest in neoadjuvant hormonal therapy. These agents, anastrozole (Arimidex), letrozole (Femara), and exemestane (Aromasin), inhibit the aromatase-dependent production of estrogen in postmenopausal women. They have largely replaced tamoxifen as front-line therapy for hormone receptor–positive disease in postmenopausal women with metastatic breast cancer and are being incorporated into the adjuvant setting. Several studies have investigated the use of an aromatase inhibitor in postmenopausal women with LABC. In the largest study, Ellis and associates randomized 250 postmenopausal patients with hormone receptor–positive breast cancer deemed ineligible for breast-conserving surgery to either tamoxifen or letrozole for 4 months before surgery.[17] The clinical response rate favored letrozole (60% vs. 41%), as did the rate of breast-conserving surgery (48% vs. 36%). A planned subset analysis showed a striking difference between the two treatments when tumors with HER-2 gene amplification were identified: the response rate was 88% for letrozole versus 21% for tamoxifen. This finding supports retrospective data from several adjuvant trials indicating that HER-2 amplification is associated with tamoxifen resistance. Of note, only 1% of patients in this study achieved a pathologic complete response, a rate significantly lower than is usually achieved with neoadjuvant chemotherapy regimens. In addition,

Table 29–4 Taxanes in the Neoadjuvant Treatment of Breast Cancer

Study	No. of Patients and Tumor Characteristics	Treatment Regimen	Response	Survival
Swain, 2003[41]	45 patients with tumor > 5 cm (median size, 9 cm)	DOC × 4 → surgery → AC × 4	Overall RR 58%; pCR 10%, residual disease < 5 mm 7%	5-yr OS 80%
Smith, 2002;[42] Hutcheon et al., 2003 (Aberdeen study)[16]	162 patients with tumor > 3 cm	Randomized to CVAP × 8 vs. sequential CVAP × 4 → DOC × 4	Clearance of tumor from the breast: 16% for CVAP vs 34% for CVAP → DOC	OS 78% for CVAP vs. 93% for CVAP → DOC ($P = 0.04$)
Ezzat et al., 2000[43]	72 patients with tumor > 4 cm	Paclitaxel and cisplatin for 3–4 cycles before surgery	Overall RR 90%, pCR in 22%	Projected DFS 74% at 3 yr
Bear et al., 2003 (NSABP B-27)[14]	2411 patients with palpable tumor > 1cm (mean, 4.5 cm)	Randomized to AC × 4 vs. AC → DOC × 4	Clinical CR 40.1% for AC vs. 63.6% for AC → docetaxel; pCR in the breast 14% for AC vs. 26% for AC → DOC	Not available
von Minckwitz et al., 2002 (GEPAR-DUO)[15]	913 patients with tumor > 2 cm (median, 4 cm)	Randomized to dose-dense ADOC × 4 (8 wk) vs. AC × 4 → 4 DOC × 4 (24 wk)	Overall RR for ADOC 77% vs. 87% for AC → DOC; pCR for ADOC 11% vs. 22% for AC → DOC	Not available

AC, doxorubicin, cyclophosphamide; ADOC, doxorubicin, docetaxel; CVAP, cyclophosphamide, vincristine, doxorubicin, prednisone; DFS, disease-free survival; DOC, docetaxel; OS, overall survival; pCR, pathologic complete response; RR, response rate.

disease progression was observed in 8% of patients taking letrozole and in 12% of patients taking tamoxifen (no statistically significant difference), a rate higher than is observed in neoadjuvant chemotherapy trials.

Although the effectiveness of adjuvant hormonal therapy is well established for hormone receptor–positive breast cancers of all stages, the role of neoadjuvant hormonal therapy for patients with LABC remains to be better defined. At present, neoadjuvant hormonal therapy can be considered a standard only for patients with hormone receptor–positive disease and relative or absolute contraindications to chemotherapy.

What is the best local therapy for patients with locally advanced breast cancer: radiation, surgery, or both?

Historically, after Haagensen and Stout's article defining inoperable breast cancers, radiation was used for palliation. In the absence of surgery or systemic therapy, standard doses of radiation provided poor local control for patients with inoperable disease, with local relapse rates of 30% to 70% and 5-year survival rates of 10% to 40%.[18,19] Higher doses of radiation could improve local control, but with increased toxicity.[20,21] As reports of high response rates and improved survival with chemotherapy were presented in the literature, neoadjuvant chemotherapy became the standard primary treatment for patients with LABC, and the question became, what is the optimal local therapy—surgery, radiation, or both? This question pertains to large operable tumors and to inoperable tumors that become technically resectable after responding to neoadjuvant chemotherapy. Patients with inoperable disease and a limited response to chemotherapy are treated with radiation.

Surgery Versus Radiation

Two clinical trials have compared radiation with surgery following neoadjuvant chemotherapy. The Cancer and Leukemia Group B (CALGB) treated 113 patients with LABC or IBC with three cycles of induction CAFVP (cyclophosphamide, doxorubicin [Adriamycin], 5-FU, vincristine, and prednisone).[22] Of the 113 patients, 91 (81%) were judged to have operable disease following neoadjuvant chemotherapy and were randomized to either mastectomy or radiotherapy. Of the initial disease relapses in each treatment arm, about half were local (27% in the radiotherapy arm and 19% in the surgery arm). Median survival for both groups was about 39 months. Similarly, an Italian study comparing radiation with mastectomy after three cycles of doxorubicin-based chemotherapy showed local control in about 70% of patients in both groups and equivalent survival.[23]

Surgery Followed by Radiation

There are no randomized studies comparing triple-modality therapy (neoadjuvant chemotherapy, surgery, and radiation) with dual-modality therapy (chemotherapy plus surgery or radiation). The current standard practice of incorporating surgery into multimodality treatment plans for LABC is based on retrospective data and indirect comparisons indicating higher local failure rates when surgery is omitted. Radiotherapy alone following neoadjuvant chemotherapy is associated with local recurrence rates of about 30% to 50%; when both modalities are used, the rate of local failure is reduced to about 10% to 20%.

Can patients with locally advanced breast cancer safely undergo breast-conserving surgery?

Data on breast-conserving surgery for patients with LABC come from a variety of nonrandomized clinical trials that differ significantly in tumor characteristics and treatment regimens. These studies support the concept that selected patients with LABC can safely forgo mastectomy in favor of less extensive surgery. Investigators at University of Texas M. D. Anderson Cancer Center systematically studied patients with LABC to answer this question. They first reviewed histologic findings in mastectomy specimens from LABC patients who received neoadjuvant chemotherapy to identify factors associated with multiquadrant involvement that would preclude breast conservation.[24] They established the following criteria for breast conservation and applied them to 362 patients who had received neoadjuvant anthracycline-based chemotherapy:

- No skin or chest wall involvement
- Lack of multicentric disease or extensive microcalcifications
- Tumor smaller than 5.0 cm
- Ability to localize primary tumor
- No contraindications to radiation
- Patient desire to preserve breast

The outcome of these patients has been reported.[25] At presentation, about one fourth of the patients had tumors smaller than 5.0 cm; the remaining three fourths had tumors greater than 5.0 cm or were otherwise locally advanced. With a median follow-up of 65 months, survival rates without local regional recurrence, with breast tumor recurrence, and with distant metastases were 91%, 94%, and 86%, respectively. Notably, the pretreatment tumor size did not predict for local recurrence, whereas pretreatment clinical N2 or N3 node status was associated with a higher rate of local failure. Pathologic findings at surgery associated with an increased risk for local failure included residual tumor mass greater than 2.0 cm, a multifocal pattern of residual disease, and lymphovascular space invasion.

Other groups have reported their experience with breast conservation for patients treated with neoadjuvant chemotherapy. The largest reported experience is that of Bonadonna and colleagues in Milan.[11] They reported their institution's experience with 536 patients considered ineligible for breast conservation because of tumor size greater than 2.5 cm. (The threshold for recommending mastectomy is frequently lower in Europe than in the United States.) After neoadjuvant chemotherapy, 85% of patients were able to have breast-conserving surgery. With a median follow-up of 65 months, 6.8% of patients have experienced an isolated local relapse.

Although these series support the safety of breast conservation for patients following successful neoadjuvant chemotherapy for LABC, they are not randomized, and the decision to proceed with mastectomy versus breast conservation may be subject to considerable selection bias, with more favorable tumors treated with breast conservation.

Could some patients with locally advanced breast cancer be treated effectively without surgery?

Based on nonrandomized, retrospective reviews of data, several investigators have questioned the need for surgery, especially when neoadjuvant chemotherapy achieves a complete clinical response. Ring and coworkers recently reported on 136 patients with operable breast cancers greater than 3.0 cm who achieved a clinical complete response following neoadjuvant chemotherapy.[26] Patients were offered the option of radiation alone or radiation and surgery. With a median follow-up of 7 years, disease-free and overall survival rates are the same for the two groups, which appeared to be well matched in terms of tumor characteristics. In the 69 patients who elected not to have surgery, there have been 16 local-only relapses, whereas of the 67 patients who had surgery (10 mastectomy, 57 breast conservation), 7 patients have had local-only relapses. In a similar retrospective review, Favret and colleagues reported on a group of 64 patients with IBC or LABC treated with neoadjuvant chemotherapy followed by either radiation alone or surgery and radiation, depending on the response of the tumor to chemotherapy and the patient's preference.[27] Forty-four patients received radiation alone, and 20 patients received radiation followed by surgery. With a mean follow-up of 51 months, no difference in local control, disease-free survival, or overall survival has been observed. Note that both of these series are nonrandomized and may be subject to substantial selection bias, with patients with more favorable tumors or better responses to neoadjuvant chemotherapy forgoing surgery.

What new approaches to locally advanced breast cancer are being investigated?

A variety of investigational approaches to the treatment of LABC are the subject of clinical trials and may lead to more effective treatments for LABC in the future. Experience from the treatment of locally advanced cancers in other anatomic sites suggests that combining chemotherapy and radiation currently may provide better local control and improved survival than providing the treatments in sequence. In breast cancer, concurrent chemotherapy and radiation has been investigated with 5-fluorouracil (5-FU) and paclitaxel. Formenti and associates reported a pathologic response rate (defined as fewer than 10 microscopic foci of disease in the resected breast) of 34% and a 5-year disease-free survival of 58% in patients with inoperable LABC treated with concurrent 5-FU and radiation.[28] A follow-up study using concurrent chemotherapy with paclitaxel and radiation also achieved a pathologic response rate of 34%.[29]

In addition to looking at novel ways of combining chemotherapy and radiation, new agents are being incorporated into the treatment of LABC. The most important of these is trastuzumab (Herceptin), a humanized monoclonal antibody directed at the membrane-bound HER-2 growth factor receptor, which is overexpressed in about one fourth of breast cancers. A phase II study of trastuzumab given in combination with paclitaxel for four cycles before surgery for tumors greater than 2.0 cm with HER-2 overexpression yielded a pathologic complete response rate of 18% in a group of patients that included many patients with large tumors.[30]

What is inflammatory breast cancer?

The classic presentation of inflammatory breast cancer is that of a younger patient who presents with recent onset of diffuse erythema and edema of the breast, frequently with peau d'orange skin changes and the absence of a palpable mass. The condition is often first treated as mastitis and recognized as IBC after antibiotics have failed and a biopsy demonstrates tumor emboli in dermal lymphatics. In the AJCC classification system, IBC comprises T4d tumors, a subset of stage III disease. The AJCC manual points out that IBC is a clinical rather than a pathologic entity: involvement of dermal lymphatics alone does not define IBC in the absence of the clinical syndrome, and a neglected noninflammatory LABC that has progressed to create edema and erythema should not be considered IBC. Although some cases may be difficult to classify as IBC versus an aggressive LABC, a recent review of data from the Surveillance, Epidemiology, and End Results (SEER) breast cancer registry confirmed that IBC is a distinct clinicopathologic entity with average age of onset 10 years before that for LABC, a lower rate of hormone receptor positivity, and a markedly poorer survival.[31] Laboratory evidence suggests that the diffuse involvement of dermal lymphatics and aggressive course of IBC may be related to overexpression of genes involved in angiogenesis: interleukin-8 (IL-8), vascular endothelial growth factor (VEGF), basic fibroblast growth factor (b-FGF), and others.[32] These mechanisms could be therapeutic targets for the treatment of IBC in the future.

How is inflammatory breast cancer treated?

Although IBC is a distinct clinical entity, it is treated in much the same manner as noninflammatory LABC: induction chemotherapy followed by local therapy with radiation and surgery. As with noninflammatory LABC, response rates to neoadjuvant anthracycline-based chemotherapy are high, on the order of 70% to 90%,[32,33] and rapid resolution of erythema and edema are commonly seen in the clinic. Despite high response rates to chemotherapy, however, survival remains poor, with median survival only 3 to 4 years. Investigators at M. D. Anderson Cancer Center have retrospectively reviewed the effect of adding paclitaxel to the neoadjuvant regimen in IBC and found significantly improved survival for patients with hormone receptor–negative disease.[34]

REFERENCES

1. Haagensen C, Stout A. Carcinoma of the breast: criteria of operability. Ann Surg 1943;118:859–868.
2. Brito RA, Valero V, Buzdar AU, et al. Long-term results of combined-modality therapy for locally advanced breast cancer with ipsilateral supraclavicular metastases: The University of Texas M. D. Anderson Cancer Center experience. J Clin Oncol 2001;19:628–633.
3. Olivotto IA, Chua B, Allan SJ, et al. Long-term survival of patients with supraclavicular metastases at diagnosis of breast cancer. J Clin Oncol 2003;21:851–854.

4. Anderson WF, Chu KC, Chang S. Inflammatory breast carcinoma and noninflammatory locally advanced breast carcinoma: Distinct clinico-pathologic entities? [see comment]. J Clin Oncol 2003;21:2254–2259.

5. Chopra R. The Indian scene. J Clin Oncol 2001;19:106S–111S.

6. Surveillance, Epidemiology, and End Results (SEER) Program. SEER*STAT Database: Incidence—SEER 11 Regs. Nov 2001 Sub (1973–1999), National Cancer Institute, DCCPS, Surveillance Research Program, Cancer Statistics Branch, released April 2002, based on the November 2001 submission. 2002; November 2001. Available: *www.seer.cancer.gov.*

7. Newman LA, Alfonso AE. Age-related differences in breast cancer stage at diagnosis between black and white patients in an urban community hospital. Ann Surg Oncol 1997;4:655–662.

8. Fornage BD, Toubas O, Morel M. Clinical, mammographic, and sono-graphic determination of preoperative breast cancer size. Cancer 1987; 60:765–771.

9. Feldman LD, Hortobagyi GN, Buzdar AU, et al. Pathological assessment of response to induction chemotherapy in breast cancer. Cancer Res 1986;46:2578–2581.

10. Buzdar A, Singletary S, Booser D, et al. Combined modality treatment of stage III and inflammatory breast cancer. M. D. Anderson Cancer Center experience. Surg Oncol Clin North Am 1995;4:715–734.

11. Bonadonna G, Valagussa P, Brambilla C, et al. Primary chemotherapy in operable breast cancer: Eight-year experience at the Milan Cancer Institute. J Clin Oncol 1998;16:93–100.

12. Kuerer HM, Newman LA, Buzdar AU, et al. Residual metastatic axillary lymph nodes following neoadjuvant chemotherapy predict disease-free survival in patients with locally advanced breast cancer. Am J Surg 1998;176:502–509.

13. Fisher B, Bryant J, Wolmark N, et al. Effect of preoperative chemother-apy on the outcome of women with operable breast cancer. J Clin Oncol 1998;16:2672–2685.

14. Bear HD, Anderson S, Brown A, et al. The effect on tumor response of adding sequential preoperative docetaxel to preoperative doxorubicin and cyclophosphamide: Preliminary results from National Surgical Adjuvant Breast and Bowel Project Protocol B-27. J Clin Oncol 2003; 21:4165–4174.

15. von Minckwitz G, Costa SD, Raab G, et al. Dose-dense doxorubicin, docetaxel, and granulocyte colony-stimulating factor support with or without tamoxifen as preoperative therapy in patients with operable carcinoma of the breast: A randomized, controlled, open phase IIb study. J Clin Oncol 2001;19:3506–3515.

16. Hutcheon AW, Heys SD, Sarkar TK, et al. Neoadjuvant docetaxel in locally advanced breast cancer. Breast Cancer Res Treat 2003;79:S19–24.

17. Ellis MJ, Coop A, Singh B, et al. Letrozole is more effective neoadjuvant endocrine therapy than tamoxifen for ErbB-1- and/or ErbB-2-positive, estrogen receptor–positive primary breast cancer: evidence from a phase III randomized trial [see comment]. J Clin Oncol 2001;19:3808–3816.

18. Perez CA, Graham ML, Taylor ME, et al. Management of locally advanced carcinoma of the breast. I. Noninflammatory. Cancer 1994; 74:453–465.

19. De Lena M, Zucali R, Viganotti G, et al. Combined chemotherapy-radiotherapy approach in locally advanced (T3b-T4) breast cancer. Cancer Chemother Pharmacol 1978;1:53–59.

20. Arriagada R, Mouriesse H, Sarrazin D, et al. Radiotherapy alone in breast cancer. I. Analysis of tumor parameters, tumor dose and local control: The experience of the Gustave-Roussy Institute and the Princess Margaret Hospital. Int J Radiat Oncol Biol Phys 1985;11: 1751–1757.

21. Chu AM, Cope O, Doucette J, Curran B. Non-metastatic locally advanced cancer of the breast treated with radiation. Int J Radiat Oncol Biol Phys 1984;10:2299–2304.

22. Perloff M, Lesnick GJ, Korzun A, et al. Combination chemotherapy with mastectomy or radiotherapy for stage III breast carcinoma: A Cancer and Leukemia Group B study. J Clin Oncol 1988;6:261–269.

23. De Lena M, Varini M, Zucali R, et al. Multimodal treatment for locally advanced breast cancer. Result of chemotherapy-radiotherapy versus chemotherapy-surgery. Cancer Clin Trial 1981;4:229–236.

24. Singletary SE, McNeese MD, Hortobagyi GN. Feasibility of breast-conservation surgery after induction chemotherapy for locally advanced breast carcinoma. Cancer 1992;69:2849–2852.

25. Chen AM, Meric F, Hunt KK, et al. Breast-conserving therapy after neoadjuvant chemotherapy: The M. D. Anderson Cancer Center experience. San Antonio Breast Cancer Conference 2003, Abstract #6.

26. Ring A, Webb A, Ashley S, et al. Is surgery necessary after complete clinical remission following neoadjuvant chemotherapy for early breast cancer? J Clin Oncol 2003;21:4540–4545.

27. Favret AM, Carlson RW, Goffinet DR, et al. Locally advanced breast cancer: Is surgery necessary? Breast J 2001;7:131–137.

28. Formenti SC, Dunnington G, Uzieli B, et al. Original p53 status predicts for pathological response in locally advanced breast cancer patients treated preoperatively with continuous infusion 5-fluorouracil and radiation therapy. Int J Radiat Oncol Biol Phys 1997;39:1059–1068.

29. Formenti SC, Volm M, Skinner KA, et al. Preoperative twice-weekly paclitaxel with concurrent radiation therapy followed by surgery and postoperative doxorubicin-based chemotherapy in locally advanced breast cancer: A phase I/II trial. J Clin Oncol 2003;21:864–870.

30. Burstein HJ, Harris LN, Gelman R, et al. Preoperative therapy with trastuzumab and paclitaxel followed by sequential adjuvant doxoru-bicin/cyclophosphamide for HER2 overexpressing stage II or III breast cancer: a pilot study. J Clin Oncol 2003;21:46–53.

31. Chang S, Parker SL, Pham T, et al. Inflammatory breast carcinoma incidence and survival: The surveillance, epidemiology, and end results program of the National Cancer Institute, 1975–1992. Cancer 1998;82: 2366–2372.

32. Cristofanilli M, Buzdar AU, Hortobagyi GN. Update on the manage-ment of inflammatory breast cancer. Oncologist 2003;8:141–148.

33. Low JA, Berman AW, Steinberg SM, et al. Long-term follow-up for inflammatory (IBC) and non-inflammatory (NIBC) stage III breast cancer patients treated with combination chemotherapy. Proc Am Soc Clin Onc 2002;21:63a.

34. Cristofanilli M, Buzdar AU, Sneige N, et al. Paclitaxel in the multi-modality treatment for inflammatory breast carcinoma. Cancer 2001; 92:1775–1782.

35. Schwartz GF, Birchansky CA, Komarnicky LT, et al. Induction chemotherapy followed by breast conservation for locally advanced carcinoma of the breast. Cancer 1994;73:362–369.

36. Merajver SD, Weber BL, Cody R, et al. Breast conservation and pro-longed chemotherapy for locally advanced breast cancer: the University of Michigan experience. J Clin Oncol 1997;15:2873–2881.

37. Morrell LE, Lee YJ, Hurley J, et al. A phase II trial of neoadjuvant methotrexate, vinblastine, doxorubicin, and cisplatin in the treatment of patients with locally advanced breast carcinoma. Cancer 1998;82: 503–511.

38. Kuerer HM, Newman LA, Smith TL, et al. Clinical course of breast cancer patients with complete pathologic primary tumor and axillary lymph node response to doxorubicin-based neoadjuvant chemother-apy [comment]. J Clin Oncol 1999;17:460–469.

39. Zambetti M, Oriana S, Quattrone P, et al. Combined sequential approach in locally advanced breast cancer. Ann Oncol 1999;10: 305–310.

40. Therasse P, Mauriac L, Welnicka-Jaskiewicz M, et al. Final results of a randomized phase III trial comparing cyclophosphamide, epirubicin, and fluorouracil with a dose-intensified epirubicin and cyclophos-phamide + filgrastim as neoadjuvant treatment in locally advanced breast cancer: An EORTC-NCIC-SAKK multicenter study. J Clin Oncol 2003;21:843–850.

41. Swain SM, Jahanzeb M, Erban JK, et al. Neoadjuvant docetaxel followed by adjuvant doxorubicin and cyclophosphamide for stage III breast cancer: Clinical response and long-term survival. Proc Am Soc Clin Oncol 2003;22:36 [abstract 143].

42. Smith IC, Heys SD, Hutcheon AW, et al. Neoadjuvant chemotherapy in breast cancer: Significantly enhanced response with docetaxel. J Clin Oncol 2002;20:1456–1466.

43. Ezzat AA, Ibrahim EM, Ajarim DS, et al. High complete pathological response in locally advanced breast cancer using paclitaxel and cis-platin. Breast Cancer Res Treat 2000;62:237–244.

CHAPTER 30

Emerging Local Treatment Modalities for Breast Cancer

Tara L. Huston and Rache M. Simmons

As biologic therapies for breast cancer evolve, the need for minimally invasive surgical intervention as part of a multidisciplinary approach to its treatment grows. This chapter discusses a number of ablative and percutaneous techniques for the treatment of breast cancer, including radiofrequency ablation, cryoablation, interstitial laser therapy, microwave thermotherapy, focused ultrasound ablation, stereotactic excision, and vacuum-assisted core biopsy. These modalities are guided by ultrasound, stereotactic mammography, or magnetic resonance imaging (MRI) and can be performed in the office or ambulatory surgery setting.

ABLATIVE TECHNIQUES

For many years, ablative techniques have been successfully used to treat metastatic hepatic tumors. More recently, they have been applied to malignancies in the breast, lung, bone, central nervous system, kidney, and prostate.[1] The breast is an ideal model for ablative therapies owing to its superficial location on the thorax and lack of intervening organs between it and the skin.

Most current and historical studies of breast cancer ablation include postprocedure resection of the specimen in order to evaluate the level of pathologic tumor destruction. A standard prerequisite, for any of the ablative techniques, is a core biopsy of the breast tumor to determine the presence of estrogen and progesterone receptors, *HER-2/neu*, and markers of proliferation, apoptosis, differentiation, and cell regulation. Once the tumor has been destroyed, none of these markers can be reliably assessed.[2]

Radiofrequency Ablation

How does radiofrequency ablation work?

Radiofrequency (RF) ablation accomplishes tissue destruction through heat. High-frequency alternating current flows from an electrode on the tip of the RF probe into surrounding tissue. This results in ions in close proximity oscillating at applied frequencies and creating friction. Cell death occurs at sustained temperatures above 40°C to 50°C.[3]

How is radiofrequency ablation performed?

In order to perform RF ablation on a breast cancer, the tumor must be identifiable by stereotactic mammography or ultrasound imaging.[4,5] The skin overlying the tumor is injected with local anesthetic, and then an insulated 15-gauge probe is inserted. Once the probe is in proper position, a starlike array of prongs is deployed to allow even distribution of the thermal energy[2,6] (Fig. 30–1). Temperature sensors are located within the prongs to monitor the temperature of the surrounding breast tissue. The usual RF ablation procedure achieves a target temperature of 95°C within 5 to 7 minutes; the temperature is maintained for 15 minutes and is followed by a 1-minute cool-down period.[2]

With varying deployment of the starlike array of prongs, a spherical ablation zone anywhere between 3 and 5 cm in diameter can be created.[5] To protect the patient from an electrical shock, a grounding pad must be applied to the patient's skin.[2,6] Most RF ablation procedures have been performed under monitored sedation or general anesthesia in the operating room and followed by previously planned standard surgical resection.[7,8]

What effect does radiofrequency ablation have on breast tissue?

Microscopically, RF ablation induces coagulative necrosis and protein denaturization.[4] Even though the basic architecture of the ablated tumor can be discerned, the assessment of tumor grade and lymphovascular invasion is hindered by the heat destruction.[9] At gross sectioning, the ablated region exhibits a firm, chalky, yellow-white center surrounded by a hyperemic red ring marking the edge of tissue destruction (Fig. 30–2). The tissues often do not show these changes for 48 hours; thus, examining a sample that was resected immediately after ablation may not reveal this characteristic pattern. To evaluate cell viability, nicotinamide adenine dinucleotide-diaphorase (NADH) staining is used in addition to the hematoxylin and eosin (H&E). With the NADH stain, an oxidation reaction in the cytoplasm of viable tissue stains dark blue, and the nonviable tissue stains pale gray.[1,2]

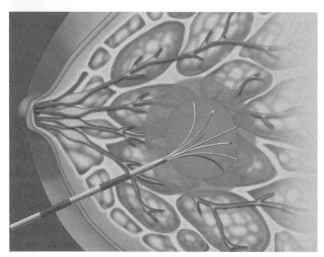

Figure 30–1 Radiofrequency ablation demonstrating deployment of the prongs within a breast tumor and even distribution of thermal energy.   (From Simmons R. Ablative techniques in the treatment of benign and malignant breast disease. J Am Coll Surg 2003;197[2]:334–338.)

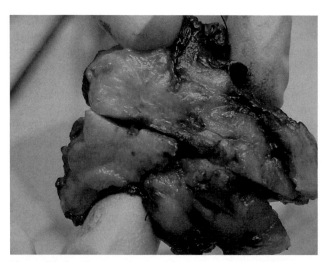

Figure 30–2 Gross sectioning of a tumor after radiofrequency ablation. The ablated region exhibits a firm, chalky, yellow-white center and is surrounded by a hyperemic red ring, which marks the edge of tissue destruction.   (From Simmons R. Ablative techniques in the treatment of benign and malignant breast disease. J Am Coll Surg 2003;197[2]:334–338.)

What are the data to support radiofrequency ablation?

In 1999, a pilot study to evaluate RF ablation as a treatment for breast cancer was undertaken by Jeffrey and colleagues.[8] Five women with locally advanced breast cancer, and tumors ranging from 4 to 7, underwent RF ablation in the operating room immediately before planned mastectomy. Histologically, all tumors showed some degree of cell death. The ablated zone extended between 0.8 and 1.8 cm around the tip of RF probe. NADH staining revealed complete cell death within the ablated zone in four of the patients. The fifth tumor harbored a single focus of viable cells smaller than 1 mm

partially lining a cyst. There were no perioperative complications related to the RF ablation.

Ultrasound-guided RF ablation was successfully performed on 26 women with needle core biopsy–proven T1 and T2 invasive breast cancers. The tumor size ranged between 0.7 and 3.0 cm, with a mean of 1.8 cm. All of the participants had RF ablation followed immediately by resection of the primary tumor. NADH staining revealed cell viability in only one of the 26 patients (4%). One woman sustained a full-thickness burn in the skin overlying the treatment zone, which was excised during the subsequent mastectomy without further complication.[10]

Another series of RF ablation of breast cancer in 17 women demonstrated that 94% of patients had complete tumor cell death at microscopic examination of the resected specimen. The single unsuccessful ablation was in a patient who had undergone neoadjuvant chemotherapy before ablation, which had resulted in nonconcentric tumor regression.[2,7]

Hayashi and associates studied 22 postmenopausal women with clinical T1N0 breast cancers and tumors smaller than 3 cm.[9] Tumors were initially thermally ablated and then surgically resected within the following 2 weeks. In three cases, residual disease was found at the ablation zone margin. One patient had dense breast tissue that bent the probe tips, another's tumor was too close to the chest wall, and in the third, ultrasound had significantly underestimated the size of the tumor. In five patients, the tumor was found to be multifocal distant to the ablation zone. A retrospective review of these five preprocedure mammograms had failed to identify the sites of multifocal disease. RF ablation alone would have been insufficient and would have led to a high rate of local failure in these five cases, equaling 23% of this study group. Overall, patient satisfaction was high, with minimal pain noted during the procedure itself, and 95% of women said they would be willing to have RF ablation again.

RF ablation has been successfully performed with the assistance of stereotactic guidance. A 71-year-old woman with a 1.6-cm infiltrating ductal carcinoma, diagnosed by stereotactic core needle biopsy, underwent RF ablation with an average temperature of 75°C for 20 minutes, after which a metallic clip was left in place. One month later, needle-localized surgical resection was performed with successful retrieval of the clip. The patient tolerated the procedure well, and no viable tumor was found. This case highlights a promising use for RF ablation in early breast cancers mammographically detected and then diagnosed with stereotactic core needle biopsy.[11]

As a result of these successful treatments with RF ablation, a few trials are now investigating the use of RF alone, not followed by resection. These protocols will likely exclude patients with large tumors or those with a high likelihood of harboring multifocal disease. The natural history of RF-treated breast tumors without resection remains unknown and justifies further evaluation.

Cryoablation

How does cryoablation work?

With cryoablation, tissue is destroyed through localized freezing. Cryoablation involves multiple freeze–thaw cycles to

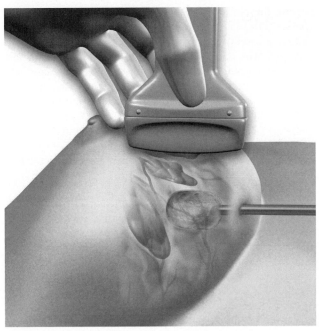

Figure 30–3 Demonstration of cryoablation showing sonographic probe placement and frozen ablation zone. (From Simmons R. Ablative techniques in the treatment of benign and malignant breast disease. J Am Coll Surg 2003;197[2]:334–338.)

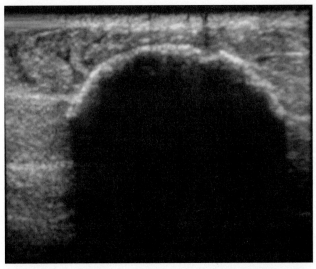

Figure 30–4 Image of sonographic freezeball during cryoablation. (From Simmons R. Ablative techniques in the treatment of benign and malignant breast disease. J Am Coll Surg 2003;197[2]: 334–338.)

achieve maximum tissue destruction. The size of the tumor determines the number of cycles that will be necessary.[2,4,12–14] The target temperature has been shown to be between −160°C and −190°C.[2,12,13] Gross determination of tissue destruction is very difficult for up to 1 week after cryoablation; thus, a delay is recommended before resection for adequate resection margins and histologic analysis.[2]

How is cryoablation performed?

The tumor is located by ultrasound probe and the overlying skin numbed with a local anesthetic. A small skin incision is then created through which the cryoprobe is inserted. No anesthesia is needed for the remainder of the procedure, as the freezing procedure itself acts as an anesthetic on the breast tissue. Patients stay completely awake for the procedure, and many view their procedure on the ultrasound monitor.[4]

The cryoprobe itself is entirely insulated except for a small area at the tip that is placed directly into the tumor (Fig. 30–3). While observing the ultrasound, one can visualize the generation of a sonographic freezeball from the liquid nitrogen or argon gas. With real-time ultrasound, the freezeball can be seen encompassing the tumor because a highly echogenic interface exists between frozen and unfrozen tissue (Fig. 30–4). The skin can sustain a thermal burn if the freezeball is too close. Therefore, to maintain a suitable distance, saline can be injected into the breast tissue between tumor and skin to create a separation. Alternatively, room-temperature saline or water can be dripped directly onto the skin's surface to protect it.[4]

Are there data to support cryoablation?

In 1985, Rand and colleagues produced one of the first pilot studies using cryoablation to treat breast cancer. The initial patient was a 77-year-old woman with a 1×2 cm palpable mass, which had malignant characteristics on mammogram. Using sonographic guidance aided by direct vision, a 5-mm cryoprobe was inserted into the lesion. The tumor underwent five freeze cycles and was then resected. No viable tumor cells were identified in the pathologic specimen. The patient had an uneventful recovery and, at a 2-year follow-up, was clinically and mammographically disease free.[15]

More recently, Staren and colleagues used cryoablation to treat a 76-year-old woman with two foci of infiltrating lobular carcinoma (0.5 and 0.8 cm) in the same quadrant, diagnosed by ultrasound-guided core needle biopsy. Cryoablation was performed separately on both tumors using sonographic guidance, and the masses were not resected. Core needle biopsy at 4 weeks and 12 weeks postablation revealed tissue necrosis, inflammatory cells, and cellular debris but were negative for persistent tumor. Shortly after the procedure, the patient developed a vague 2-cm firmness in the area between the two cryoablation zones, but this spontaneously resolved within 12 weeks.[13]

Stocks and associates[16] performed cryoablation on 11 women with core needle biopsy–proven breast cancer and then resected the specimens within 1 to 3 weeks. The mean tumor size was 13 mm, with a range of 7 to 22 mm. The sonographic freezeball was generated to surround the tumor as well as a 1-cm margin of normal-appearing breast parenchyma. Ten of the tumors showed complete ablation. The one tumor with residual malignant cells revealed ductal carcinoma in situ (DCIS) at the border of the ablation zone. Two of the women sustained minor dermal injuries before the use of saline injection for tumors near the skin.

Pfleiderer and coworkers[17] studied 15 women with 16 breast tumors, averaging 21 mm, to further investigate the potential of ultrasound-guided cryotherapy in breast cancer. Under ultrasound guidance, a 3-mm cryoprobe was inserted into each tumor. Two freeze–thaw cycles of 7 to 10 minutes and 5 minutes, respectively, were performed. Within 5 days after the cryoablation, all tumors were resected. The mean diameter of the freezeball was 28 mm. No severe side effects were observed. The five tumors smaller than 16 mm had no evidence of invasive cancer after treatment. However, two of these five had DCIS in the surrounding tissue. In the 11 tumors 23 mm or larger, histologic examination revealed incomplete necrosis. These authors concluded that the invasive components of small tumors can be treated using cryotherapy, but DCIS components that may not be detected before ablation represent a challenging problem.

The previously described studies indicate that cryoablation of breast cancers is a promising technique; however, more research needs to be done. In two of the studies, the presence of DCIS at the margin of the ablation zone resulted in incomplete tumor necrosis; thus, patients with DCIS may not be good candidates for cryotherapy. Major advantages to this technique are the obviation of anesthesia because the freezing numbs the breast, and the ability to perform this procedure in the office under real-time ultrasound guidance. Prospective randomized trials are needed to determine the long-term effectiveness of cryotherapy on breast cancer.

Interstitial Laser Ablation

How does interstitial laser ablation work?

Interstitial laser ablation (ILA) uses heat to destroy tissue. To perform the procedure, the lesion must be visualized by mammogram, MRI, or ultrasound. Mammographic guidance is used for microcalcifications or tumors seen solely on mammogram, whereas MRI tends to be used for other lesions. Ideally, the lesion should be well circumscribed and measure less than 1.5 cm in diameter.[18]

How is interstitial laser ablation performed?

No general anesthetic is necessary, but the skin overlying the cancer is numbed and a field block is performed directly at the site.[5,19] A small skin incision is made, through which a hollow stereotactic needle is inserted. Through the stereotactic needle, a 16- to 18-gauge laser-emitting optic fiber is deposited.[2,19] Parallel to the stereotactic needle, about 1 cm away, a multisensing probe is placed to monitor the temperature of the surrounding breast tissue. Laser coagulation cannot be monitored by real-time digital images, although continuous recording of the temperature grids can guide adequacy of treatment. The target temperature at the center is between 80°C and 100°C, which correlates to about 60°C registered on the probes at the periphery.[19] Contrast-enhanced Doppler can be used to see the loss of blood flow to the ablated area.[18]

Within 20 minutes, about 1400 joules of laser energy per cubic centimeter of calculated tissue are delivered at a rate of 5 to 7 watts/second.[5,18] The volume of tissue sphere encompassing the entire ablation zone is calculated by $V = 4/3\pi$ (radius)^3; thus, for the average 1-cm tumor with 0.5 cm surrounding cover of parenchyma, the volume is 4 cm^3, and 5600 joules of laser energy are needed for its complete ablation. Saline is continuously dripped from the tip of the laser to prevent overheating.[5] Using MRI, detailed temperature grids can be generated to outline the area of ablation and help to monitor the temperature of the surrounding breast tissue.[20]

What does interstitial laser ablation do to tissue?

Bloom and colleagues[21] reported a series of 40 patients with mammographically detectable T1 breast cancers treated by interstitial laser therapy. All tumors were excised within 5 to 42 days and examined to detail the pathologic changes induced by interstitial laser therapy. Upon evaluation, all revealed a characteristic series of concentric rings surrounding the laser needle tip cavity. Zone 1 was charred tissue within the cavity; zone 2 was coagulated with "wind-swept" nuclei similar to those seen in cautery artifact; zone 3 was a gray-tan ring that histologically showed recognizable tumor but did not express cytokeratin 8/18 (a viability marker) and was thus not viable; zone 4 was a ring of red-tan tissue in which the tumor architecture was evident but the cytoplasm and nuclear characteristics had been erased; and zone 5 was grossly hyperemic while histologically consisting of a rim of vascular proliferation with fat necrosis interspersed with aggregates of inflammatory cells and macrophages (Fig. 30–5). The classic zones were present in all patients regardless of the time that had elapsed between ablation and resection. Thus, it is the outer zone of fat necrosis that delineates the actual area of effective ablation.

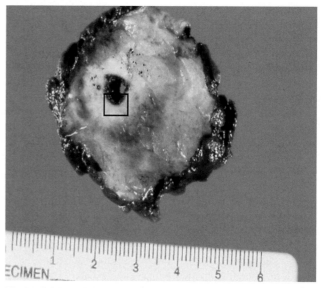

Figure 30–5   Resected tissue specimen following interstitial laser ablation. *Box* highlights pseudoviability zone, which is structurally and histologically intact but is composed of nonviable cells. (Courtesy of Dr. Kombiz Dowlatshahi.)

What are the data to support interstitial laser ablation?

Dowlatshahi and colleagues[19] studied the effect of laser therapy on 56 women with breast cancers smaller than 23 mm. Within 8 weeks of the ablation, the tissue was resected in all but 2 of these patients, both of whom were treated outside of the protocol. Sixteen of the 54 patients harbored residual tumor following ablation: 4 cases were early (learning phase) and not given sufficient laser energy; 2 patients were oversedated and moved involuntarily; 4 cases failed because of technical problems with the equipment; 5 cases had suboptimal target visualization because of excessive fluid infusion or needle biopsy hematomas; and 1 patient had a tumor larger than 2 cm. Difficult target visualization was overcome by inserting metallic markers around the tumor after numbing the skin but before the infusion of peritumoral anesthesia. The 2 patients who did not undergo resection were monitored by mammogram, ultrasound, and needle core biopsy for 2 years. This is of note because it is one of the only human demonstrations of the short-term natural history of interstitial therapy. In both patients, the laser-treated tumors first became smaller and were then replaced by a 2- to 3-cm oil cyst. After resolution of the cysts, fibrosis was identified on core biopsies.[18]

Laser ablation of breast cancers can also be done with MRI guidance. When compared with traditional MRI, rotating delivery of excitation off-resonance (RODEO) breast MRI affords higher contrast and improved spatial resolution in visualizing breast cancers. Using gadolinium further helps to locate the lesion. With RODEO MRI, an MRI-compatible needle is stereotactically placed within the lesion. The laser ablative therapy is then interactively controlled by continuous MRI with energy delivery correlated to tumor dimensions. The appearance of a hypointense zone on the image correlates with the effectiveness of the treatment.[20]

Harms and associates[22] performed MRI-guided laser ablation on 22 invasive cancers in 12 patients to test the feasibility of this approach. In 3 patients with tumors smaller than 3 cm, the goal was total ablation, whereas in the other 9 patients, only portions of large tumors were ablated. The laser-treated area was resected in all patients. The zone of ablation was measured as the greatest distance between two points on the hyperemic ring and was subjected to standard H&E as well as proliferation cell nuclear antigen (PCNA) staining for tumor viability. Pathologic analysis confirmed complete destruction in tumors smaller than 3 cm. The most frequent complaint, discomfort from compression of the MRI coils, was not related to the laser itself. An advantage of MRI-guided laser ablation is the ability to determine lesion margins precisely.

Microwave Ablation

How does microwave ablation work?

Microwave ablation involves thermal tissue destruction through two microwave phased array wave guide applicators. Because breast cancers have higher water content than surrounding normal breast tissue, the cancer should heat more rapidly than healthy tissue during microwave ablation. During the procedure, the breast is compressed between two acrylic plates to allow penetration of microwave energy and to minimize patient movement. The microwaves are focused at the center of the tumor, where a temperature probe is placed to regulate the target temperature of 43°C. To avoid heat injury to the overlying skin, noninvasive skin surface temperature probes are applied to the skin, and fans provide constant air cooling.[23]

What are the data to support the use of microwave ablation?

Gardner and colleagues[23] performed a pilot study using focused microwaves to achieve breast cancer thermoablation in 10 women planning to undergo mastectomy. The microwave treatment time averaged 34.7 minutes, with a range of 12 to 40 minutes. The mean peak temperature was 44.9°C and varied between 43.3°C and 47.7°C. All of the specimens were surgically resected as mastectomy specimens within 18 days. These data showed tumor size reduction averaging 41% (29% to 60%) on the basis of sonographic measurements before and after microwave therapy. On pathologic analysis, tumor necrosis was noted in 4 of 10 specimens and apoptosis was seen in 6. Three of the 10 women suffered flap necrosis following mastectomy that may have been associated with the elevated skin temperature during the laser therapy.

Can microwave ablation be used as a preoperative adjunct?

A group of nine patients with advanced breast carcinoma underwent hyperthermic tumor ablation (HTA) as a preoperative adjunct to determine whether tumor volume could be decreased. An 8-MHz radiofrequency heating device (Thermotron RF-8, Yamamoto Vinita, Japan) was combined with a grounded needle electrode to achieve a target temperature above 50°C. Tumor size was decreased from a mean of 122 cm^3 to 82.2 cm^3. Histologic examination of the primary focus showed total coagulation necrosis encompassing a sphere between 3.5 and 5.0 cm in diameter. The authors concluded that preoperative HTA is safe and well tolerated and results in a large volume of destruction of breast cancer tissue.[24]

Can microwave ablation be used with chemotherapy?

Heat treatment can be used alone to kill tumor cells but has also been shown to enhance chemotherapy's tumoricidal effects. An ongoing phase II trial of focused microwave thermotherapy in women with locally advanced breast cancer is comparing neoadjuvant chemotherapy to neoadjuvant thermochemotherapy. Specifically, this two-armed randomized trial is comparing neoadjuvant focused 915-mHz microwave energy treatment with neoadjuvant doxorubicin (Adriamycin) plus cyclophosphamide (Cytoxan) chemotherapy. By examining the thermal cell kill in resulting lumpectomy specimens, researchers hope to assess the added benefit of microwave thermotherapy to neoadjuvant chemotherapy.[25]

Focused Ultrasound Ablation

What is focused ultrasound ablation?

Focused ultrasound (FUS) ablates tumor tissue with heat, resulting in protein denaturation and tissue necrosis. The ultrasound beams penetrate soft tissue and can be directed at tissue volumes as small as a few cubic millimeters. The absorbed energy causes an elevated temperature in the breast tissue with such a high thermal gradient that the boundaries of the treatment area are sharply demarcated without damage to the surrounding parenchyma. In seconds, a target temperature between 55°C and 90°C is attained. MRI is ideal for guiding FUS ablation because it yields excellent anatomic resolution, is highly accurate in the detection of tumors, and allows the physician to monitor the ultrasound ablation in real time.[26] Dose calculations are based on tumor size and the length of the ultrasound pathway as measured by MRI.[27]

How is focused ultrasound ablation performed?

The patient is placed prone on a FUS table inside an MRI magnet. An anxiolytic is administered to reduce movement inside the MRI tube, and an analgesic is given to reduce the associated discomfort. No skin incision is needed. The transducer is positioned such that the ultrasound beam is focused directly on specific points within the tumor. At these focal points, the beam produces temperature elevations and coagulation necrosis. The treatment consists of a series of sonications throughout these points within the tumor itself plus a surrounding margin. At histologic assessment of resected specimens, the treated areas show a yellow-white area of central necrosis surrounded by a red hemorrhagic ring.[26]

What are the data to support focused ultrasound ablation?

In a pilot study of MRI-guided focused ultrasound ablation, Gianfelice and associates[26] treated 12 women with invasive breast cancer consisting of tumors smaller than 3.5 cm. The treatment was composed of multiple sonications at targeted points, which were monitored with temperature-sensitive MRI followed by surgical resection. The effectiveness was determined by comparing the volumes of necrosed and residual tumor in the resected specimen. The procedure was well tolerated, with two minor skin burns as the sole complications. In three patients treated with the first ultrasound system (InSightec-TxSonics Mark 1 InSightec TxSonics, Dallas, TX), a mean of 46.7% of the tumor was within the targeted zone, and a mean of 43.3% of the cancer tissue was necrosed. In nine patients treated with the more advanced second ultrasound system (InSightec-TxSonics Mark 2), a mean of 95.6% of the tumor was within the targeted zone, and a mean of 88.3% of the cancer tissue was necrosed. Residual tumor was identified predominantly at the periphery of the tumor mass. By increasing the total targeted area, such as with an increased number of sonications, a greater tumor volume could be destroyed. The authors' conclusion was that thermal coagulation of small breast tumors by means of MRI-guided focused ultrasound is a promising noninvasive ablation procedure for which further study is warranted.

Huber and colleagues performed a single-patient pilot study of a woman with a 2.2-cm centrally located invasive ductal carcinoma. The therapy involved 80 single ultrasound pulses of 9 seconds each at 30 to 50 watts of acoustic power. Immediately after the treatment, the patient was evaluated with gadolinium-enhanced MRI to determine the extent of tissue destruction. The images demonstrated a zone without contrast in the targeted area, suggesting a complete interruption of the blood supply. No anesthesia was needed, and the patient did not note any discomfort during the procedure. A lumpectomy was performed 5 days after the focused ultrasound ablation procedure. Histologic examination revealed both lethal and sublethal damage to the tumor. The authors concluded that noninvasive MRI-guided therapy of breast cancer is feasible and effective and that MRI-guided FUS may represent a new strategy for the neoadjuvant, adjuvant, or palliative treatment in selected breast cancer patients.[27]

Advantages of focused ultrasound ablation include the fact that no skin incision needs to be made, the focal point is continually changeable throughout the treatment, and there is great flexibility in matching the size of the treatment zone to the targeted volume of the tumor in three dimensions.[26]

PERCUTANEOUS TUMOR EXCISION: STEREOTACTIC EXCISION AND VACUUM-ASSISTED CORE BIOPSY

How does stereotactic excision work?

Stereotactic excision of small breast cancers is possible using the Advanced Breast Biopsy Instrumentation system (ABBI, U.S. Surgical Corporation, Norwalk, CT). It was originally introduced in 1996 as a diagnostic tool that incorporates large-bore cannulas within the stereotactic table and can remove mammographic breast tumors as a nonfragmented single-core specimen. A surgical cannula, up to 20 mm wide, is inserted along a stereotactically positioned axial wire in the center of the tumor. Tissue cylinders encompassing the entire tumor are then extracted in amounts significantly larger than those obtained by core biopsy.

What are the data on the use of stereotactic excision?

In 50 patients with in situ and invasive breast cancer, positive margins and residual tumor rates were similar to those seen with needle-localized excisional biopsy when compared by mammographic lesion size and ABBI cannula size.[28,29] As expected, there was a higher rate of positive margins when larger lesions were excised with smaller cannulas. Even though small tumors can be successfully excised with negative margins, there are limitations regarding incision placement and an increased incidence of wound hematoma compared with other methods.

How does the vacuum-assisted core biopsy work?

The two vacuum-assisted systems currently in use are the Mammotome (Biopsys Medical, Cincinnati, OH) and the Minimally Invasive Breast Biopsy (MIBB, U.S. Surgical Corporation, Norwalk, CT). Both techniques use a vacuum to pull tissue into a sampling chamber, where it is removed with high-speed rotating knives and then suctioned into an external chamber for harvest. This method avoids multiple passes, compared with a standard core biopsy, and allows the retrieval of contiguous samples. The Mammotome functions with internally rotating knives. The MIBB uses an externally oscillating knife that is capable of sampling larger specimens.[30,31]

What are the data to support the use of the vacuum-assisted core biopsy?

Fine and coworkers[32] published a multicenter nonrandomized study evaluating 124 women with low-risk palpable breast lesions resected using the Mammotome under ultrasound guidance. The 75 lesions 1.5 cm or smaller were removed with an 11-gauge probe, whereas the 49 lesions between 1.5 and 3.0 cm were removed using an 8-gauge probe. Follow-up evaluation was performed 10 days after the biopsy. Complete removal of the imaged lesion was similar between groups: 99% with the 8-gauge and 96% with the 11-gauge. Most complications were mild and anticipated. Ninety-seven percent of patients were satisfied with the appearance of the incision, and 98% would recommend the procedure to others. Thus, percutaneous removal of palpable benign breast masses using the Mammotome system is feasible, is safe, and yields high patient satisfaction.

The complete removal of small lesions under ultrasonographic guidance in an outpatient setting using the multidirectional hand-held vacuum-assisted biopsy device was also demonstrated by Johnson and associates.[33] One hundred one breast lesions in 81 patients were excised through 3-mm incisions using a hand-held 8-gauge or 11-gauge Mammotome. The average lesion size was 1.15 cm. Ninety-four (93%) of the lesions were benign, five (5%) were malignant, and two (2%) showed atypical hyperplasia. At subsequent excisional biopsy of the malignant lesions, only one was found to harbor residual disease. Of the two lesions with atypical hyperplasia, no evidence of malignant disease was noted in either excisional biopsy specimen. This study concluded that vacuum-assisted excisional breast biopsy under ultrasound guidance is an effective technique for the management of benign lesions.

CONCLUSION

Numerous methods of image-guided percutaneous breast cancer ablation and percutaneous tumor excision are currently being investigated in clinical trials. Long-term follow-up data regarding local effects on the surrounding breast tissue or recurrence rates are not yet available. There are limited data suggesting the possibility of fat necrosis within the unresected tissue.[2] Local breast changes may pose diagnostic dilemmas in future ablation-only trials, making it difficult to distinguish recurrent cancer from scar or fat necrosis.

We are cautiously optimistic that ablative and percutaneous excisional therapies will be used as a routine adjunct in the future to treat selected breast cancers. The challenge in the success of these techniques will lie in the ability to identify multifocal disease and to ensure complete and effective eradication of the breast cancer.

REFERENCES

1. Mirza AN, Fornage BD, Sneige N, et al. Radiofrequency ablation of solid tumors. Cancer J 2001;7:95–102.
2. Simmons RM, Dowlatshahi K, Singletary SE, Staren ED. Ablative therapies for breast cancer. Contemp Surg 2002;58:61–72.
3. Dickson J, Calderwood S. Thermosensitivity of neoplastic tissue in vivo. In Storm F (ed). Hyperthermia in cancer therapy. Boston, GK Hall Medical, 1983:63–140.
4. Kaufman CS, Bachman B, Littrup PJ, et al. Office based ultrasound-guided cryoablation of breast fibroadenomas. Am J Surg 2002;184: 394–400.
5. Edwards MJ, Dowlatshahi K, Robinson D, et al. 2001 Image-guided percutaneous breast cancer ablation meeting at the American Society of Breast Surgeons. Am J Surg 2001;182:429–433.
6. Dowlatshahi K, Francescatti D, Bloom KJ, et al. Image guided surgery of small breast cancers. Am J Surg 2001;182:419–425.
7. Singletary SE, Fornage BD, Sneige N, et al. Radiofrequency ablation of early-stage invasive breast tumors: An overview. Cancer J 2002;8: 177–180.
8. Jeffrey SS, Birdwell RJ, Ikeda DM, et al. Radiofrequency ablation of breast cancer. Arch Surg 1999;134:1064–1068.
9. Hayasi A, Silver SF, van der Westhuizen NG. Treatment of invasive breast carcinoma with ultrasound-guided radiofrequency ablation. Am J Surg 2003;185:429–435.
10. Izzo F, Thomas R, Delrio P, et al. Radiofrequency ablation in patients with primary breast carcinoma—a pilot study of 26 patients. Cancer 2001;92:2036–2044.
11. Elliot R, Rice PB, Suits JA, et al. Radiofrequency ablation of a stereotactically localized nonpalpable breast carcinoma. Am Surg 2002;68: 1–5.
12. Rand RW, Rand RP, Eggerding FA, et al. Cryolumpectomy for breast cancer: An experimental study. Cryobiology 1985;22:307–318.
13. Staren ED, Sabel MS, Gianakakis LM, et al. Cryosurgery of breast cancer. Arch Surg 1997;132:28–33.
14. Rui J, Tatsutani KN, Dahiya R, Rubinsky B. Effect of thermal variable on human breast cancer in cryosurgery. Breast Cancer Res Treat 1999;53: 185–192.
15. Rand RW, Rand RP, Eggerding FA, et al. Cryolumpectomy for carcinoma of the breast. Surg Gynecol Obstet 1987;165:392–396.
16. Stocks LH, Chang HR, Kaufman CS, et al. Pilot study of minimally invasive ultrasound-guided cryoablation in breast cancer [abstract]. Am Soc Breast Surg 2002.
17. Pfleiderer SO, Freesmeyer MG, Marx C, et al. Cryotherapy of breast cancer under ultrasound guidance: Initial results and limitations. Eur Radiol 2002;12:3009–3014.
18. Dowlatshahi K, Francescatti D, Bloom KJ. Laser therapy for small breast cancers. Am J Surg 2002;184:359–363.
19. Dowlatshahi K, Fan M, Gould VE, et al. Stereotactically guided laser therapy of occult breast tumors, work in progress. Arch Surg 2000;135: 1345–1352.
20. Harms S. Percutaneous ablation of breast lesions by radiologists and surgeons. Breast Dis 2001;13:67–75.
21. Bloom KJ, Dowlatshahi K, Assad L. Pathologic changes after interstitial laser therapy of infiltrating breast carcinoma. Am J Surg 2001;182: 384–388.
22. Harms S, Mumtaz H, Hyslop B, et al. RODEO MRI guided laser ablation of breast cancer. Society of Photo-Optical Instrumentation Engineers Proceedings 1999;3590:484–489.
23. Gardner RA, Vargas HI, Block JB, et al. Focused microwave phased array thermotherapy for primary breast cancer. Ann Surg Oncol 2002;9: 326–332.

24. Fujimoto S, Kobayashi K, Takahashi M, et al. Clinical pilot studies on pre-operative hyperthermic tumour ablation for advanced breast carcinoma using an 8 MHz radiofrequency heating device. Int J Hyperthermia 2003;19:13–22.

25. Gardner RA, Heywang-Kobrunner SH, Dooley WC, et al. Phase II clinical studies of focused microwave phased array thermotherapy for primary breast cancer: A progress report [abstract]. Am Society Breast Surg 2002.

26. Gianfelice D, Khiat A, Amara M, et al. MR imaging-guided focused US ablation of breast cancer: histopathologic assessment of effectiveness—initial experience. Radiology 2003;227:849–855.

27. Huber PE, Jenne JW, Rastert R, et al. A new noninvasive approach in breast cancer therapy using magnetic resonance imaging-guided focused ultrasound surgery. Cancer Res 2001;61:8441–8447.

28. Velanovich V, Lewis FR, Nathanson SD. Comparison of mammographically guided breast biopsy techniques. Ann Surg 1999;229:625–630.

29. Schwartzberg BS, Frager D, Choi P. Experience with breast biopsies using the advanced breast biopsy instrumentation while performing stereotactic breast biopsies: Review of 150 consecutive biopsies. J Am Coll Surg 2000;191:625–630.

30. Bassett LW, Caplan RB, Dershaw D. Stereotactic core needle biopsy of the breast. A report of the Joint Task Force of the American College of Radiology, American College of Surgeons and the College of American Pathologists. Cancer J Clin 1997;47:171–190.

31. Wong AY, Salisbury E, Bilous M. Recent developments in stereotactic breast biopsy methodologies: An update for the surgical pathologist. Adv Anat Pathol 2000;7:26–35.

32. Fine RE, Boyd BA, Whitworth PW, et al. Percutaneous removal of benign breast masses using a vacuum-assisted hand-held device with ultrasound guidance. Am J Surg 2002;184:332–336.

33. Johnson AT, Henry-Tillman R, Smith LF, et al. Percutaneous excisional breast biopsy. Am J Surg 2002;184:550–554.

Surveillance Following Breast Cancer Treatment

Tracey O'Connor and Stephen B. Edge

In the United States, there were more than 200,000 new cases of invasive breast cancer in 2003, with an additional 55,000 cases of carcinoma in situ,[1] making breast cancer the most common malignancy in American women. The increased incidence and improved mortality rate have resulted in a large population of breast cancer survivors who require regular follow-up, probably exceeding 2 million women. A rational plan for breast cancer follow-up takes into consideration the natural history of the disease and the influence of various therapies. This plan should account for the likely sites and timing of recurrences as well as the ability of treatment to effectively influence disease outcome. Women with breast cancer also require regular follow-up to detect and manage complications and side effects of therapy, such as lymphedema and premature menopause and its consequences. This chapter reviews the pertinent data and explains the recent shift from intensive medical surveillance to a less aggressive approach.

What are the goals of breast cancer follow-up?

There are several goals of medical surveillance following primary breast cancer therapy. One reason for continued follow-up is contribution to research and accumulation of data.[2] Another is the detection of new primary breast cancers in the contralateral breast at an early stage. Studies have demonstrated that women with a history of invasive breast cancer have a greater risk for developing a contralateral breast cancer. Other goals include the detection of recurrent disease in patients who may benefit from therapy, patient rehabilitation and psychological support, evaluation of treatment effects, and risk counseling for the patient and family.[3] Because most women survive breast cancer, it is also important for them to continue routine primary care and preventive health practices and to maintain a relationship with their primary care providers.

FOLLOW-UP OF IN SITU BREAST DISEASE

How is the patient with in situ breast disease followed?

Before the widespread use of screening mammography, ductal carcinoma in situ (DCIS) was an infrequently encountered problem routinely treated with mastectomy. Thus, there is a limited amount of information regarding the natural history of this disease.[4] In recent years, coinciding with the use of screening mammography, there has been a marked increase in the incidence of DCIS in asymptomatic women. In one series, DCIS represented 20% of all screen-detected breast cancers, and the overall rate of DCIS detection by screening mammography was 0.78 per 1000 mammograms, with the rate increasing with age. Therefore, about 1 case of DCIS is detected for every 1300 mammograms performed.[5]

Depending on the individual circumstances, patients with DCIS generally undergo surgery (lumpectomy or mastectomy) and may also receive radiation therapy, tamoxifen, or both. Patients with DCIS are at a very low risk for systemic disease but have a substantial risk for developing recurrence in the conserved breast that may be invasive breast cancer or a recurrent in situ lesion, and they are also at risk for a contralateral breast cancer. The estimates of recurrence risk after breast conservation therapy vary across studies and are influenced by factors such as tumor grade, tumor size, margin width, patient age, and treatment. In one large clinical trial, after a mean follow-up of 90 months, the incidence of ipsilateral invasive breast cancer in patients treated with lumpectomy alone was 13.4%.[6] The addition of radiation to lumpectomy reduced the rate of invasive recurrence to 3.9% and the rate of recurrent DCIS to 8.2%. A more recent study cited high nuclear grade as the factor most strongly associated with recurrence in women treated with lumpectomy alone, although this variable was not able to predict an invasive versus noninvasive recurrence. Women with DCIS of high nuclear grade had high 5-year recurrence rates for invasive cancer of 11.8% and for DCIS of 17.1%, whereas women with low-nuclear-grade tumors had relatively low 5-year recurrence rates for invasive cancer of 4.8% and for DCIS of 4.8%.[7] Women with high-nuclear-grade DCIS or DCIS treated with lumpectomy alone had relatively high rates of invasive breast cancer recurrence when compared with patients diagnosed with DCIS of low nuclear grade and treated with radiotherapy.[7]

The National Surgical Adjuvant Breast and Bowel Project (NSABP) Protocol B-24 examined the role of tamoxifen in women treated for DCIS with breast-conserving surgery and radiation. After completing radiotherapy, women were randomized to placebo or tamoxifen. The women treated with tamoxifen had an 8.2% incidence of ipsilateral breast cancer (4.1% invasive and 4.2% noninvasive) compared with 13.4% of the placebo group (7.2 % invasive and 6.2% noninvasive) at

Table 31–1 Follow-up after Treatment for Ductal Carcinoma In Situ

- Interval history and physical exam every 6 mo for 5 yr, then annually
- Mammogram every 12 mo
- If tamoxifen is given:
  - Annual pelvic exam with Pap smear if appropriate
  - Ophthalmology exam if cataracts or vision problems
  - Consider monitoring for bone density loss if premenopausal

Data from Writing Committee. NCCN breast cancer clinical practice guidelines. JNCCN 2003;1:148–188.

Table 31–2 Follow-up after Treatment for LCIS

- Interval history and physical exam every 6–12 mo
- Mammogram every 12 mo unless after bilateral mastectomy
- If tamoxifen is given:
  - Annual pelvic exam with Pap smear if appropriate
  - Ophthalmology exam if cataracts or vision problems
  - Consider monitoring for bone density loss if premenopausal

Data from Writing Committee. NCCN breast cancer clinical practice guidelines. JNCCN 2003;1:148–188.

a median follow-up of 74 months.[8] In addition, tamoxifen reduced the risk for contralateral breast cancer.

The goal of follow-up after DCIS is therefore to screen for a new or recurrent cancer in the conserved breast or in the contralateral breast. Screening for distant metastases has no role. Follow-up for women with DCIS involves a history and physical examination every 6 to 12 months for 5 years. Postexcision mammogram should be performed after surgery, and before radiation, to ensure completeness of resection and is especially important for cancers manifested by microcalcifications. The first postradiation mammogram should be performed 6 months after the completion of radiation to record the new baseline breast appearance.[9] Mammograms performed before this 6-month interval may be suboptimal because of edema and skin changes. Mammography is then recommended annually and should be performed on both breasts (Table 31–1).

Although the incidence of DCIS continues to rise, the incidence of lobular carcinoma in situ (LCIS), which accounts for 13% of in situ breast carcinomas, has been stable since 1988.[10] The true incidence of LCIS in the general population is unknown because there are no specific clinical or mammographic signs. LCIS is thought to represent a transitional intraepithelial, or in situ, stage in the evolution of breast cancer, and it is assumed to be distributed throughout breast tissue, having close to a 100% incidence of bilaterality and multicentricity.[11] The presence of LCIS is a marker of future risk for breast cancer development. About 0.5% to 1% of women with LCIS develop invasive breast cancer annually.[12] The risk is bilateral and not limited to the breast in which LCIS was found.

The management of LCIS is conceptually different from the management of other breast cancers, reflecting the view that LCIS is a precancerous lesion and not a true cancer. The goal of treatment is prevention of an invasive lesion or early detection while the invasive lesion remains confined to the breast. Consensus now supports observation alone as the most appropriate treatment for LCIS.[13] Bilateral mastectomy, with or without reconstruction, is considered for women with a strong family history or genetic susceptibility, and for those who view their personal risk for breast cancer as unacceptably high.

Surgical excision to achieve negative margins is not needed at the initiation of surveillance. Similarly, radiation therapy has no currently established role in the treatment of this disease. Treatments that do not account for the bilaterality of this process (i.e., unilateral mastectomy) are not logical.

Tamoxifen decreases the risk for a subsequent invasive breast cancer in women with LCIS. The NSABP P-01 breast cancer prevention trial included 826 women with LCIS. Among women with LCIS who received no treatment, the average annual rate of invasive cancer was 12.99 per 1000 women. Tamoxifen decreased the annual rate per 1000 to 5.69, a risk reduction of 56%.[14]

Patients with LCIS treated with observation alone or bilateral mastectomy share a good prognosis. Consensus follow-up recommendations include history and physical examinations every 6 to 12 months for 5 years and annually thereafter in conjunction with yearly mammography for those being followed by observation (Table 31–2).

FOLLOW-UP OF INVASIVE BREAST CANCER

About one third of patients with a history of breast cancer will experience a recurrence and ultimately die of their disease. Recurrence rates increase with the size of the primary tumor and lymph node involvement, whereas adequate surgical treatment and adjuvant therapy are associated with lower recurrence rates.

Women with a history of breast cancer remain at risk for recurrence for the rest of their lives. As will be detailed, although most recurrences occur within 5 years of diagnosis, the hazard of recurrence decreases slowly through year 12, and very late recurrences are not uncommon.[15] However, most relapses occur during the first decade, with the rate of relapse peaking between years 2 and 5 after diagnosis. Late mortality estimates are less than 2% per year beginning 15 years after primary treatment.[16]

In women with a history of invasive breast cancer, a yearly mammogram of the remaining breast tissue is indicated. Mammography of the reconstructed breast or of the chest wall has a low yield and is not recommended.[17] As noted, for cases of mammographically detected breast cancer, a postexcision mammogram may be performed before radiation to ensure completeness of resection and is especially important for DCIS diagnosed by radiographic microcalcifications. The first postradiation mammogram should be performed 6 months after the completion of radiation to record the new baseline breast appearance.[9] Mammograms performed before this 6-month interval may be suboptimal owing to edema and skin changes. Mammography is then recommended annually and should be performed on both breasts.

Consensus recommendations for follow-up of invasive breast cancer include history and physical examinations every 3 to 6 months for the first 3 years, then every 6 to 12 months for 2 years, then annually. Pelvic examination and cervical cytology should be continued annually for patients with an intact uterus. Prompt evaluation of new signs and symptoms,

Table 31–3   Follow-up after Treatment for Invasive
Breast Cancer

- Interval history and physical every 4–6 mo for 5 yr, then every 12 mo
- Mammogram every 12 mo (and 6 mo after radiation if breast conservation is performed)
- Pelvic examination every 12 mo if uterus is present and patient is taking tamoxifen
- Prompt evaluation of new signs and symptoms
- Osteoporosis screening and appropriate treatment (see text) for high-risk women
  - All women older than 65 yr
  - Women aged 60–64 yr with:
    a. Family history
    b. Body weight > 70 kg
    c. Prior nontraumatic fracture
    d. Other risk factors
  - Postmenopausal women of any age receiving aromatase inhibitors
  - Premenopausal women with therapy-associated menopause

ongoing patient education, continued coordination of care, and psychosocial support should also be maintained (Table 31–3).

What is the timing of breast cancer recurrence?

The timing of breast cancer recurrence affects the frequency of follow-up examinations and testing. Because breast cancer may recur at any time following treatment, all patients must continue on surveillance throughout life. A large series from Milan examining the risk for locoregional and distant recurrence rates over 12 years of follow-up in 2233 patients following breast-conserving therapy consisting of quadrantectomy, axillary dissection, and radiotherapy was published in 1995.[18] This series reported 119 local recurrences, 32 new ipsilateral cancers, and 414 distant metastases as first events. Distant metastases occurred in up to 5% of patients per year for the first 2 years after therapy, after which the recurrence rates declined sharply. In contrast, locoregional recurrence rates did not show a peak of incidence, instead remaining constant for the 12-year follow-up period, at about 1% per year.

Another large study analyzing the clinical course of 3585 patients enrolled in seven Eastern Cooperative Oncology Group (ECOG) adjuvant trials was reported in 1996.[15] This study included both premenopausal and postmenopausal women in its analysis, and most women had positive lymph nodes at the time of diagnosis. Forty-five percent (1625) of patients experienced a recurrence during the median follow-up of 8.1 years. One hundred eighty-two patients (5%) died without recurrence and were censored for recurrence at the time of death. The hazard of recurrence was greatest between 1 and 2 years after surgery (13.3%), then decreased consistently from 2 to 5 years. Beyond 5 years, the hazard of recurrence decreased slowly. Between years 5 and 8, the hazard of recurrence was 4.7%, and between years 8 and 12, it was 3.4% ($P = .01$). Higher-risk subsets (patients with more than three positive nodes) had a higher hazard of recurrence at all time intervals but demonstrated the same temporal pattern of recurrence as the lower-risk subsets.

Estrogen receptor (ER) status affected the timing of recurrence in this study. Overall, the hazard of recurrence was increased for the ER-negative patients compared with the ER-positive patients. However, the increased hazard associated with ER negativity reflected the higher hazard of recurrence in years 0 to 5. Between years 3 and 4, the hazards for ER-negative and ER-positive patients crossed, and beyond 5 years, the hazard was greater for ER-positive patients. There is therefore no definable point at which a woman may be considered cured of her disease, nor free from risk for the development of a new primary breast tumor.

What is the rate of locoregional recurrence following mastectomy?

Local recurrence following mastectomy most commonly presents as nodularity in or under the skin of the chest wall, usually in or near the mastectomy scar. Regional recurrence presents as palpable adenopathy in the previously treated axilla or supraclavicular or infraclavicular nodes. The rate of isolated locoregional failure after mastectomy ranges from 2% to 20% depending on the tumor size, lymph node involvement, and length of follow-up.[3] Many of the data regarding locoregional recurrences in patients treated with mastectomy were generated from the time period before widespread use of adjuvant systemic therapy and regional radiation. However, 20-year follow-up of NSABP B-06 showed a local and regional recurrence rate of 14.8 % in patients treated with total mastectomy.[19] The size of the primary tumor, lymph node involvement, and use of adjuvant radiation all can influence the rate of locoregional recurrence following mastectomy. A meta-analysis of randomized trials conducted by the Early Breast Cancer Trialists' Collaborative Group demonstrated that adjuvant chest wall irradiation can decrease local recurrence but did not impact survival, likely reflecting the increased likelihood of occult distant disease in women presenting with locoregional failure after mastectomy.[20]

Almost all patients with an isolated local recurrence following mastectomy develop distant disease, despite local therapy. In one series of patients treated for local or regional recurrence after mastectomy from 1968 to 1978, the 5- and 10-year actuarial rates of freedom from distant metastasis were 30% and 7%, with overall survival only 26% at 10 years.[21] Because locoregional recurrence following mastectomy is frequently associated with distant disease, a metastatic assessment is indicated before any aggressive local therapy is employed.

What is the risk for locoregional recurrence following breast-conserving therapy?

Ipsilateral recurrence after lumpectomy and radiotherapy occurs at a rate of 0.5% to 1% per year and generally presents in a fashion similar to that of primary breast cancer.[22] Abnormalities on mammogram, palpable masses, and suspicious nipple discharge must be evaluated as potential signs of recurrent disease. The risk for locoregional recurrence increases with positive margins of resection, multifocal disease, young age at diagnosis, and the absence of radiotherapy. The rate of recurrent cancer in the ipsilateral breast among women with negative nodes treated with breast-conserving therapy, systemic therapy, and radiation is about 6% at 10 years of follow-up.[19] Trials with broader inclusion criteria have reported ipsilateral failure rates from 8.8% in the Milan trial, reported at 20 years,[23] to 22% in the National Cancer Institute study,[24] reported at a median follow-up of 18.4 years. In contrast to locoregional recurrence after mastectomy, an in-breast recurrence is associated with synchronous distant metastases in only 10% of cases, and most patients will be effectively treated and not experience further recurrence.[25] Therefore, the overall survival of patients after primary treatment with mastectomy or with breast-conserving therapy is equivalent at 20 years. When radiotherapy is omitted from breast-conserving therapy, the locoregional recurrence rate increases significantly (39.2% in the NSABP series) but without a corresponding decrement in overall survival. As already noted, it is essential to follow the conserved breast with periodic physical examinations and annual mammography.

What are the most common sites of distant disease relapse?

It is important to understand the pattern of distant breast cancer recurrence because this knowledge can be used to focus the history and physical examinations during surveillance visits. Distant recurrence rates in women with a history of invasive breast cancer vary from 5% to 80%, depending on stage and other prognostic factors.[3] Current data on the patterns of breast cancer recurrence reflect a period of time before the widespread use of breast conservation and systemic therapy; nonetheless, they are important to our understanding of the disease.

The skeletal system represents the most common site of distant relapse, followed by lung or pleura and liver. Kamby and colleagues reported a series of 415 patients with first recurrence and found the most common sites of distant metastatic disease were bone (31%), lung (19%), and liver (15%).[26] The central nervous system is the first distant site of metastasis in less than 5% of patients who develop distant metastasis.[27] Between 10% and 15% of patients have disease at multiple sites at the time of presentation with distant metastatic disease.

Should women with a history of breast cancer have routine chest radiographs or imaging studies?

Most patients with metastatic disease are diagnosed with distant disease following symptoms or abnormality detected on physical exam. A number of trials have examined the potential role of radiographic modalities to screen for asymptomatic breast cancer recurrence. Reflecting the fact that the skeleton is the most common site of initial distant relapse, most studies have examined the potential role of nuclear medicine bone scanning.

The NSABP performed a prospective study of 2697 women with a history of stage II breast cancer followed with routine bone scans. Only 0.6% of scans detected metastasis in asymptomatic patients.[28] In a trial reported by Pedrazzini and associates, routine bone scanning done at baseline and repeated at 1 year could provide early detection of a recurrence for 2.4%

of the population studied.[29] These clinical trials fail to support routine radionuclide scintigraphy in the follow-up of the asymptomatic patient.

The performance of routine chest radiographs as a method of detecting recurrence has also been examined. Intrathoracic recurrence can present as lung metastases, pleural recurrence with associated effusion, and mediastinal disease. A review of retrospective studies of chest radiographs as a method of detection reported that first recurrence was detected by chest films in 2.7%, with a range of 0% to 5.1%.[30] Another study followed 241 patients with routine chest radiographs and bone scans during the first 2 years after surgical treatment.[31] Twelve patients (5%) were discovered to have pulmonary metastasis on routine sequential chest radiography. Four of these 12 patients were symptomatic. Overall, 1091 chest radiographs in 241 patients were required to detect occult metastases in 8 cases. Based on these and similar studies, routine chest radiography is not recommended.

Computed tomography (CT), magnetic resonance imaging (MRI), and positron emission technology (PET) are newer imaging modalities potentially able to screen patients for asymptomatic first recurrence. Large prospective trials addressing the potential utility of these techniques have not been reported, and the routine use of these tests in the asymptomatic patient is not recommended.

Should routine blood work be performed during breast cancer follow-up?

There are insufficient data to suggest that patients should receive routine complete blood counts as part of a surveillance program. Similarly, chemistry profiles have not been found to be helpful in detecting recurrences in the asymptomatic patient. In one retrospective review, chemistry studies detected initial recurrence in only 5.9% of cases (range, 1.2% to 12.0%).[30] However, in a study of 6.3% of patients who did develop liver metastases, only 1.3% were asymptomatic.[32]

Are there data available to support the use of tumor markers in surveillance of the breast cancer patient?

The serial measurement of tumor markers represents a newer approach to screening for breast cancer recurrence. Carcinoembryonic antigen (CEA), CA-15-3, and CA-27.29 are three commonly measured markers. Compared with conventional disease assessment tools, biochemical markers assess the total-body burden of disease rather than the size of a single lesion, making them potentially more sensitive for early detection.

The serum markers CA-15-3 and CA-27.29 measure a class of glycoproteins secreted by breast cancer cells. CA-15-3 was the first available test. It can be measured in the sera radioimmunologically with the monoclonal antibodies DF3 and 115-D8. Multiple studies have reported that the incidence of CA-15-3 elevation increases with the stage of disease, with incidences of elevation from 5% to 30%, 15% to 50%, 60% to 70%, and 65% to 90% in stages I, II, III, and IV, respectively.[33] Large tumor burden correlates with high marker values.[34] Despite this correlation with extent of disease, low CA-15-3 levels do not exclude metastatic disease, and a given level does not predict stage of disease. In addition, CA-15-3 is elevated in 5% to 6% of healthy people, and more often in individuals with benign diseases of the liver and biliary system or with benign mastopathic disease of the breast.[34] There are few studies examining the value of CA-15-3 in prospective trials of the follow-up of breast cancer patients after primary treatment. A recently reported prospective trial by Kokko and associates of CA-15-3 levels measured regularly in 243 patients with primary breast cancer for a median follow-up of 4.3 years demonstrated a mean lead time to diagnosis of 3 months. Other studies have reported mean lead times varying from 9.5 months,[35] 4.2 months,[36] and 64 days.[37] Despite these findings, there is no evidence that lead time affects the benefit and outcome of treatment for metastatic disease. A large prospective randomized trial is required to examine this question.

CA-27.29 has been compared with CA-15-3 in a retrospective trial of 275 patients. This study found CA-27.29 to be more sensitive in the patient populations studied, with incidences of elevation of 29%, 36%, and 59% in stages I, II, and III, respectively. In contrast, CA-15-3 measured in the same samples was elevated 15%, 23%, and 54%, respectively.[38] Chan and coworkers conducted a study to determine the ability of CA-27.29 to predict relapse and lead time from the marker elevation to clinical evidence of disease.[39] The study reported a sensitivity of CA-27.29 positivity of 57.7% and a lead time of 5.3 months.

CEA belongs to a family of cell surface glycoproteins with increased expression in breast cancer as well as other malignancies. The level of CEA is elevated in 10% to 60% of patients with breast cancer, with the likelihood and degree of elevation related to the stage of disease.[3] The false-positive rate in patients without disease recurrence has varied from 0% to 11%, depending on the study. In patients in whom elevated CEA levels precede clinical evidence, the lead time varies between 3 and 7 months.[40]

The American Society of Clinical Oncology (ASCO) Tumor Markers Panel evaluated the available evidence to assess the value of using CEA, CA-27.29, and CA-15-3 as markers of asymptomatic recurrence. They found insufficient evidence to support the routine use of these markers in the screening, diagnosis, staging, or follow-up of breast cancer.[41] Although a rising marker can detect a recurrence after primary treatment, there is no established clinical benefit to this detection, and options for therapy remain essentially unchanged. The ASCO Guidelines state that "there has been no demonstrated impact on the most significant outcomes (improved disease-free or overall survival, better quality of life, lesser toxicity, or improved cost-effectiveness)."[41]

The overall strategy of intensive surveillance after breast cancer has been tested in controlled trials. Two large prospective randomized controlled trials involving more than 2500 early-stage breast cancer patients compared intensive surveillance (serial bone scans, liver ultrasounds, chest radiographs, and laboratory testing) with routine surveillance.[42,43] Both studies determined that most patients with metastatic disease presented with symptoms rather than findings on the screening examinations. Neither study was able to detect a survival benefit or improvement in quality of life related to intensive surveillance, concluding that such surveillance is not indicated in the follow-up of early-stage breast cancer patients. There are not randomized data of this quality to assess the value of

tumor markers in this setting, but the available uncontrolled data cited earlier do not suggest that the use of markers would lead to a survival benefit.

What is the risk for developing a second primary breast cancer?

Patients with breast cancer are at risk for a second primary breast cancer. Ten years after treatment, the risk for developing a new breast cancer is equal to or greater than the risk for developing a disease recurrence.[44] Patients who develop bilateral breast cancer, synchronously or asynchronously, may have a strong family history of breast cancer and are at risk for carrying a BRCA1 or BRCA2 mutation. Second primary breast cancers are curable, especially if detected early. Women with a history of invasive breast cancer have a greater risk for developing a contralateral breast cancer. The magnitude of this risk is about 0.5% to 1% per year of follow-up. In a large series of patients followed at Memorial Sloan-Kettering for a median of 18.2 years, the average annual incidence was 8 per 1000 per year of follow-up (0.8%). This risk was age dependent: women younger than 45 years at the time of diagnosis have an average annual rate of contralateral breast cancer of about 1%, whereas those older than 50 years at diagnosis face a risk of about 0.5% per year.[45] The incidence of contralateral breast cancer was about 9% at 20 years and 25 years in the NSABP B-06 and B-04 studies, respectively.[19,46] Other studies have demonstrated that contralateral breast cancer exhibits a prognosis similar to that of the first breast, making early detection and treatment valuable.[47] The primary source of overall mortality is largely determined by the risk for distant disease from the first primary cancer, although the risk for a new primary or recurrence is real.[45] These data provide further support for the need for annual mammography after breast cancer treatment.

COMPLICATIONS OF THERAPY

What complications of local therapy may be seen in follow-up?

The current therapy for breast cancer often includes one or more local treatments associated with complications. In general, women are treated with either mastectomy or breast-conserving therapy followed by radiation. Axillary lymph nodes are generally evaluated with a sentinel node biopsy, a level 1 and 2 axillary nodal dissection, or both. The risk for local complications can increase with systemic therapy and with the degree of local therapy required.[48]

Axillary surgery can result in persistent numbness or discomfort, swelling (lymphedema), and decreased range of motion of the arm. Mild symptoms are common and have been reported in about one third of women 2 to 5 years after axillary node dissection.[49] The increasing use of sentinel lymph node procedures is hoped to decrease the likelihood of local morbidity. One study by Schijven and colleagues compared morbidity in 213 patients treated with axillary lymph node dissection (ALND) with 180 patients treated with sentinel node biopsy (SNB) using a disease-specific quality-of-life questionnaire.[50] Patients having SNB had a 3.2-fold lower risk for pain, a 5-fold lower risk for lymphedema, a 7.7-fold lower risk for numbness, a 7.1-fold lower risk for loss of strength in the affected arm, and a 2.9-fold lower risk for impaired use of the arm. Axillary radiotherapy added to the risk for lymphedema by 2.4-fold and enhanced the impaired use of the arm by 2.6-fold.

Although most cases of lymphedema are mild, it can have a significant impact on a woman's quality of life. Identified risk factors include axillary radiation, extent of axillary surgery, obesity, and weight gain.[51] Before any treatment for lymphedema is started, a cancer recurrence involving the axilla or brachial plexus, axillary vein thrombosis, or infection should be considered and treated if present. Recommendations for treatment are limited by the lack of prospective randomized trials on therapy options but may include compression garments and comprehensive physical therapy (manual lymphatic drainage).[52] Surgery, diuretics, and compression pumps are ineffective.

What are the long-term side effects of chemotherapy?

An increasing number of women receive adjuvant systemic chemotherapy for breast cancer. These treatments may be associated with weight gain, infertility, chemotherapy-induced premature menopause, and neuropathy.[53] Women with chemotherapy-induced ovarian failure may be at increased risk for osteoporosis and should consider bone density monitoring. Less common side effects include cardiac dysfunction from anthracycline-based chemotherapy and leukemia-myelodysplastic syndromes. The potential for development of these complications should be considered during follow-up if a woman presents with concerning symptoms. As discussed earlier, there are no data to support the use of complete blood counts to screen for bone marrow relapse or myelodysplasia or serial echocardiography, or of multigated acquisition scanning to screen for cardiac dysfunction.[16]

How should women on hormonal therapy be followed?

Antiestrogen hormonal therapies are frequently used in the treatment of women with early-stage breast cancer and are highly effective for patients with hormone receptor–positive disease. Although they are generally well tolerated as compared with chemotherapy, hormonal treatments are associated with significant side effects, and because of the duration of treatment, these effects may persist for years.

Tamoxifen and anastrozole are the most commonly used agents in the adjuvant setting for early-stage breast cancer. Both are associated with vasomotor symptoms and vaginal atrophy and dryness. The major serious side effects of tamoxifen are rare and related to its weak estrogen agonist properties. These include thromboembolic disease (deep vein thrombosis, pulmonary embolism, and stroke), cataracts, and endometrial carcinoma. Uterine cancer occurs at a rate of 0.2% per year in women receiving adjuvant tamoxifen therapy.[14] Relative to tamoxifen, anastrozole has a better

Table 31–4 Incidence of Predefined Adverse Events at the First and Updated Analyses of the ATAC Trial

Adverse Event	Percentage of Patients		
	Anastrozole	Tamoxifen	P Value
Hot flashes	34.3	39.7	<.0001
Musculoskeletal disorder	27.8	21.3	<.0001
Fatigue	15.6	15.1	.5415
Fractures	5.9	3.7	<.0001
Vaginal bleeding	4.5	8.2	<.0001
Vaginal discharge	2.8	11.4	<.0001
Endometrial cancer	0.1	0.5	.0267
Cataracts	3.5	3.7	.5427
Venous thromboembolic events	2.1	3.5	.0006
Ischemic cerebrovascular events	1.0	2.1	.0006
Ischemic cardiovascular events	2.5	1.9	.1391

ATAC, Arimidex, Tamoxifen, Alone or in Combination.
Data from Winer EP, Hudis C, Burstein HJ, et al. American Society of Clinical Oncology Technology Assessment Working Group update: Use of aromatase inhibitors in the adjuvant setting. J Clin Oncol 2003;21:2597–2599.

side-effect profile in terms of hot flashes, vaginal bleeding, endometrial cancer, stroke, and thrombotic events; however, increases in musculoskeletal symptoms and fractures are reported.[54]

The best comparison of side effects of tamoxifen and anastrozole is the recently reported Arimidex, Tamoxifen, Alone or in Combination (ATAC) adjuvant breast cancer trial.[55] Selected side effects reported in this study are shown in Table 31–4.

Vasomotor symptoms (or hot flashes) are one of the most common complaints of breast cancer patients. In randomized placebo-controlled trials, a reduction of 20% to 30% in hot flash frequency and severity is noted with placebo alone, demonstrating the importance of well-designed trials to address treatment options for this bothersome complaint.[56] Scientifically designed clinical trials have reported that treatments such as black cohosh and vitamin E are not more effective than placebo.[57,58] Likewise, studies have also reported that soy products are only marginally or no more effective than placebo for treatment of menopausal symptoms.[59] Bothersome symptoms of hot flashes may be treated with serotonin-reuptake inhibitors such as venlafaxine; Loprinzi and associates reported a placebo-controlled study showing up to a 61% reduction in hot flash score in treated women.[60] Other possible agents include clonidine and gabapentin.

Two prospective trials have evaluated potential clinical benefit of screening for endometrial cancer in patients receiving adjuvant tamoxifen. Barakat and coworkers[61] examined the potential benefit of screening with endometrial biopsy. In this study of premenopausal and postmenopausal breast cancer patients with a median age of 50 years, 111 women had a total of 635 endometrial biopsies, with a mean number of 5.8 samplings per patient. Of the biopsies, 544 (86%) revealed benign endometrium and 82 (12.6%) were insufficient for diagnosis. In 9 (1.4%), biopsy results were abnormal, leading to further evaluation. In total, 14 patients underwent a dilation and curettage (D&C). Although 3 of the 111 patients (2.7%) were ultimately treated with hysterectomy, only 1 of the 111 (0.9%) had pathology detected by screening endometrial biopsy.

Gerber and colleagues[62] addressed the role of transvaginal sonography (TVS) in 247 postmenopausal women with breast cancer and compared them with 98 women with breast cancer not eligible for tamoxifen therapy. The mean age of the patients was 60 years in both groups. They performed TVS every 6 months for up to 5 years. Fifty-two asymptomatic women with morphologically suspect or thickened endometrium (10 mm) underwent hysteroscopy or D&C. This resulted in four uterine perforations. Histology demonstrated atrophy in 38 patients, polyps in 9, hyperplasia in 4, and endometrial cancer in 1. Twenty screened patients reported vaginal bleeding. Five had atrophy, 5 had polyps, and 4 had hyperplasia. Two women had endometrial cancer identified by bleeding only despite having screening TVS. Overall, 1265 TVS procedures detected 1 asymptomatic cancer.

These two studies and others support the guidelines that routine endometrial surveillance of women treated with adjuvant tamoxifen is not warranted.[63] Women receiving tamoxifen should have annual gynecologic examination. Endometrial biopsy, with or without transvaginal ultrasound, should be used in patients with abnormal vaginal bleeding or discharge. There is no current role for screening endometrial biopsy or transvaginal[64] ultrasound in asymptomatic women off a clinical trial, and such screening attempts may be associated with significant morbidity.

How should bone density be followed in women treated for breast cancer?

Osteopenia and osteoporosis are common and important issues in women with breast cancer. Most women with a newly diagnosed breast cancer are at risk related either to age or breast cancer therapy. One of the most common side effects of adjuvant chemotherapy is permanent ovarian failure, occurring in 63% to 85% of premenopausal patients treated with cyclophosphamide, methotrexate, and fluorouracil and in 50% or more of women treated with anthracyclines.[65] Age is an important determinant of ovarian failure, with women older than 40 years developing menopause more frequently and after a shorter duration of chemotherapy.[66] There is a growing interest in the United States in the use of ovarian suppression or ablation as an adjuvant breast cancer therapy in premenopausal women, and this has been an established practice in Europe.[67]

Ovarian suppression results in a decrease in estrogen levels and is associated with an increased risk for osteoporosis and fracture.[48] Chemotherapy-induced ovarian failure causes rapid and significant bone loss in the spine and femur, detectable within 6 months of starting chemotherapy. Shapiro and colleagues[65] reported highly significant bone loss in the lumbar spine by 6 months, with further increase at 12 months, in 35 women with chemotherapy-induced ovarian failure. The median decreases of bone mineral density (BMD) in the spine from 0 to 6 months and 6 to 12 months were −4.0% and −3.7%, respectively. Fourteen patients who retained ovarian

function had no significant decreases in BMD during the same time period.

Tamoxifen also has important effects on bone density. Tamoxifen acts as an estrogen agonist in bone. This results in a preservation of BMD in postmenopausal women; however, in premenopausal women, tamoxifen has been associated with bone loss.[68] The antiresorptive properties of tamoxifen are modest: Although tamoxifen preserves BMD in postmenopausal patients, there is no reduction in vertebral and femoral fractures in women receiving tamoxifen.[69]

Anastrozole recently received approval for the adjuvant treatment of postmenopausal women with early-stage ER-positive breast cancer based on the results of the ATAC trial.[70] Although the combination of drugs was not superior to tamoxifen alone, anastrozole alone improved disease-free survival and reduced contralateral breast cancers. The most serious adverse event was the fracture rate in the anastrozole group as compared with the tamoxifen group. In a recent update with a median follow-up of 37 months, the fracture rate in the anastrozole arm was 7.1%, as compared with 4.4% in the tamoxifen arm.[54] Indirect evidence suggests that roughly one third of the excess fracture risk seen with anastrozole is related to an absence of tamoxifen effect.[71] Data from three large studies show a consistent improvement in disease-free survival among postmenopausal women treated in the adjuvant setting with aromatase inhibitors. Optimal adjuvant hormonal therapy for a postmenopausal woman with hormone receptor–positive breast cancer includes an aromatase inhibitor as initial therapy or after treatment with tamoxifen.[72] Tamoxifen continues to be the optimal adjuvant hormonal therapy for premenopausal women with receptor-positive breast cancer.

In part reflecting the approval of anastrozole in the adjuvant setting and concern that this trend in adjuvant hormonal therapy would make osteoporosis a greater health problem in the future, an ASCO panel updated the recommendations on bone health in women with a history of breast cancer in 2003.[71] The panel recommended "in otherwise healthy women, a strong body of evidence supports a strategy of early detection and therapy of osteoporosis." Breast cancer patients determined to be at high risk (older than 65 years, 60 to 64 years of age with other risk factors, any woman taking aromatase inhibitors, and premenopausal women with therapy-induced menopause) should have annual bone densitometry, and as in women without breast cancer, subsequent treatments are guided by BMD result. Basic measures include adequate calcium intake (1200 mg/day) with vitamin D (400 to 800 IU), exercise, and smoking cessation. Breast cancer patients with osteoporosis (T score, −2.5 or lower) should initiate pharmacologic therapy (i.e., oral bisphosphonates) and continue annual BMD screening. Breast cancer patients with osteopenia (T score, −1 to −2.5) should have basic measures instituted in conjunction with annual BMD screening, but the panel concluded that current evidence does not support use of bisphosphonates for this group.

Who should conduct breast cancer surveillance?

The initial breast cancer surveillance guidelines stated, "Cancer patients should have the right to treatment by an oncologist indefinitely after a cancer diagnosis in accordance with ASCO policy."[73] Since the time the original guidelines were published, questions have been raised about the evidence available to support this statement.

Because breast cancer is a disease treated by multiple subspecialists, patients have often scheduled regular follow-up visits with surgeons, radiation oncologists, and medical oncologists. Coordination of care is important to avoid a burdensome and expensive redundancy of effort for the first 5 years following primary therapy. A randomized trial involving 296 breast cancer patients in England was reported in 1996.[74] The patients were randomized to follow-up with a general practitioner or in a multidisciplinary breast clinic. They were followed in both settings with regular scheduled history and physical examinations and yearly mammograms. This trial was designed to assess effects on time to diagnosis of recurrence and quality of life when responsibility of follow-up was shifted to the primary care provider. Although the follow-up period reported was short (18 months), the results did not detect a difference in time to diagnosis, increase in anxiety, or deterioration in health-related quality of life in women receiving care from generalists. Most recurrences detected by the patients occurred in the interval between follow-up exams, and almost half (7 of 16; 44%) of the recurrences in the specialist follow-up group presented first to a general practitioner. Although generalization of these data is limited in terms of sample size, follow-up time, and cultural factors, they suggest that effective follow-up may occur in various settings. It is recommended that follow-up of breast cancer patients be performed in a setting in which continuity of care is possible and in which an individual experienced in the care and examination of cancer patients performs the surveillance. These findings support the assertion that women should be well educated about symptoms of recurrence because most recurrences become symptomatic during the interval between follow-up visits.

The goals of breast cancer surveillance include medical assessment for disease recurrence, sharing information regarding advances in treatment, ensuring compliance with surveillance guidelines, providing psychological support, and managing side effects and complications of therapy. Patients are best served by a coordinated multidisciplinary follow-up effort between generalists and specialists. The development of a strong doctor–patient relationship and careful attention to history and physical examination deserve emphasis over diagnostic testing and best serve the unique health concerns of the breast cancer survivor.

REFERENCES

1. Jemal A, Murray T, Samuels A, et al. Cancer statistics, 2003. CA Cancer J Clin 2003;53:5–26.
2. Hughes L, Courtney S. Follow up of patients with breast cancer. BMJ 1985;290:1229–1230.
3. McKee M, Edge S. Breast cancer follow-up. Probl Gen Surg 2000;17:87–100.
4. Morrow M, Strom EA, Bassett LW, et al. Standard for the management of ductal carcinoma in situ of the breast (DCIS). CA Cancer J Clin 2002;52:256–276.
5. Ernster VL, Ballard-Barbash R, Barlow W, et al. Detection of ductal carcinoma in situ in women undergoing screening mammography. J Natl Cancer Inst 2002;94:1546–1554.
6. Fisher B, Dignam J, Wolmark N, et al. Lumpectomy and radiation therapy for the treatment of intraductal breast cancer: Findings from the National Surgical Adjuvant Breast and Bowel Project B-17. J Clin Oncol 1998;16:441–452.
7. Kerlikowske K, Molinaro A, Cha I, et al. Characteristics associated with recurrence among women with ductal carcinoma in situ treated with lumpectomy. J Natl Cancer Inst 2003;95:1692–1702.
8. Fisher B, Dignam J, Wolmark N, et al. Tamoxifen in treatment of intraductal breast cancer: National Surgical Adjuvant Breast and Bowel Project B-24 randomized controlled trial. Lancet 1999;353:1993–2000.
9. Sardi A, Eckholdt G, McKinnon WM, et al. The significance of mammographic findings after breast-conserving therapy for carcinoma of the breast. Surg Gynecol Obstet 1991;173:309–312.
10. Garfinkel L, Boring CC, Heath CW Jr. Changing trends: An overview of breast cancer incidence and mortality. Cancer 1994:74:222–227.
11. Frykberg ER. Lobular carcinoma in situ of the breast. Breast J 1999;5(5):296–303.
12. Haagensen CD, Bodian C, Haagensen DE. Breast carcinoma: Risk and detection. Philadelphia, WB Saunders, 1981.
13. Writing Committee. NCCN breast cancer clinical practice guidelines. JNCCN 2003;1:148–188.
14. Fisher B, Constantino JP, Wickerham DL, et al. Tamoxifen for prevention of breast cancer: Report of the National Surgical Adjuvant Breast and Bowel Project P-1 study. J Natl Cancer Inst 1998;90:1371.
15. Saphner T, Tormey DC, Gray R. Annual hazard rates of recurrence for breast cancer after primary therapy. J Clin Oncol 1996;14(10):2738–2746.
16. Langlands AO, Pocock SJ, Kerr GR, et al. Long-term survival of patients with breast cancer: A study of the curability of the disease. Br Med J 1979;2:1247–1251.
17. Mendelson EB. Evaluation of the postoperative breast. Radiol Clin North Am 1992;30:107–138.
18. Veronesi U, Marubini E, Del Vecchio M, et al. Local recurrences and distant metastases after conservative breast cancer treatments: partly independent events. J Natl Cancer Inst 1995;87:19–27.
19. Fisher B, Anderson S, Bryant J, et al. Twenty-year follow-up of a randomized trial comparing total mastectomy, lumpectomy, and lumpectomy plus irradiation for the treatment of invasive breast cancer. N Engl J Med 2002;347:1233–1241.
20. Early Breast Cancer Trialists' Collaborative Group. Effects of radiotherapy and surgery in early breast cancer. An overview of randomized trials. N Engl J Med 1995;333:1444–1451.
21. Aberizk WJ, Silver B, Henderson IC, et al. The use of radiotherapy for treatment of isolated locoregional recurrence of breast carcinoma after mastectomy. Cancer 1986;58:1214.
22. Recht A, Schnitt SJ Connolly JL. Prognosis following local or regional recurrence after conservative surgery and radiotherapy for early stage breast carcinoma. Int J Radiat Oncol Biol Phys 1989;16:3–9.
23. Veronesi U, Cascinelli N, Mariani L, et al. Twenty-year follow-up of a randomized study comparing breast-conserving surgery with radical mastectomy for early breast cancer. N Engl J Med 2002;347:1227–1232.
24. Poggi M, Danforth D, Sciuto, L, et al. Eighteen year results in the treatment of early breast carcinoma with mastectomy versus breast conservation therapy. Cancer 2003;98:697–702.
25. Fisher ER, Anderson S, Redmond C, et al. Ipsilateral breast tumor recurrence and survival following lumpectomy and radiation: Pathological findings from NSABP protocol B-06. Senim Surg Oncol 1992;8:161–166.
26. Kamby C, Vejborg I, Kristensen B, et al. Metastatic pattern in recurrent breast cancer. Cancer 1988;62:2226–2233.
27. Valagussa P, Tesoro-Tess J, Rossi A, et al. Adjuvant CMF effect on site of first recurrence and appropriate followup intervals, in operable breast cancer with positive axillary nodes. Breast Cancer Res Treat 1982;1:349.
28. Wickerham L, Fisher B, Cronin W, et al. The efficacy of bone scanning in the follow-up of patients with operable breast cancer. Breast Cancer Res Treat 1984;4:303–307.
29. Pedrazzini A, Gelber R, Isley M, et al. First repeated bone scan in the observation of patients with operable breast cancer. J Clin Oncol 1986;4:389–394.
30. Schapira DV, Urban N. A minimalist policy for breast cancer surveillance. JAMA 1991;265:380–382.
31. Chaudary MA, Maisey M, Shaw PJ, et al. Sequential bone scans and chest radiographs in the postoperative management of early breast cancer. Br J Surg 1983;70:517–520.

32. ASCO Breast Cancer Surveillance Expert Panel. Recommended Breast Cancer Surveillance Guidelines. J Clin Oncol 1997;15:2149–2156.

33. Hayes DF, Bast RC, Desch CE, et al. Tumor marker utility grading system: A framework to evaluate clinical utility of tumor markers. J Natl Cancer Inst 1996;88:1456–1466.

34. Kokko R, Holli K, Hakama M. Ca 15-3 in the follow-up of localized breast cancer: A prospective study. Eur J Cancer 2002;38:1189–1193.

35. Geraghty J, Coveney E, Sherry F, et al. Ca 15-3 in patients with locoregional and metastatic breast carcinoma. Cancer 1992;70:2831–2834.

36. Molina R, Zanon G, Filella X, et al. Use of serial carcinoembryonic antigen and Ca 15-3 assays in detecting relapses in breast cancer patients. Br Cancer Res Treat 1995;36:41–48.

37. Soletormos G, Nielsen D, Shioler V, et al. A novel method for monitoring high-risk breast cancer with tumor markers: Ca 15-3 compared to CEA and TPA. Ann Oncol 1993;36:861–869.

38. Gion M, Mione R, Leon AE, et al. Comparison of the diagnostic accuracy of CA 27.29 and CA 15-3 in primary breast cancer. Clin Chem 1999;45:630–637.

39. Chan DW, Beveridge RA, Muss H, et al. Use of Truquant BR radioimmunoassay for early detection of breast cancer recurrence in patients with stage II and stage III disease. J Clin Oncol 1997;15:2322–2328.

40. Hayes DF, Kaplan W. Evaluation of patients after primary therapy. In Harris JR, Lippmann ME, Morrow M, Hellman S (eds). Diseases of the Breast. Philadelphia, Lippincott-Raven, 1996, pp. 629–648.

41. Bast R, Ravdin P, Hayes D, et al. 2000 Update of recommendations for the use of tumor markers in breast and colorectal cancer: Clinical practice guidelines of the American Society of Clinical Oncology. J Clin Oncol 2001;19:1865–1878.

42. Rosselli Del Turco M, Palli D, Cariddi A, et al. Intensive diagnostic follow-up after treatment of primary breast cancer. A randomized trial. National Research Council Project on Breast Cancer Follow-up. JAMA 1994;271:1593–1597.

43. The GIVIO Investigators. Impact of follow-up testing on survival and health-related quality of life in breast cancer patients. A multicenter randomized controlled trial. JAMA 1994;271:1587–1592.

44. Edge SE, Levine EG, Arredondo MA, et al. Breast cancer. In Johnson FE, Virgo KS (eds). Cancer Patient Follow-up: Surveillance Strategies after Primary Treatment of Cancer. St. Louis, Mosby–Year Book, 1997, pp. 290–335.

45. Rosen P, Groshen S, Kinne D, Hellman S. Contralateral breast carcinoma: An assessment of risk and prognosis in stage I (T1N0) and stage II (T1N1) patients with 20 years follow-up. Surgery 1989;106:904.

46. Fisher B, Jeong JH, Anderson S, et al. Twenty-five year follow-up of a randomized trial comparing radical mastectomy, total mastectomy, and total mastectomy followed by irradiation. N Engl J Med 2002;347:5567–5575.

47. Khafagy M, Schottenfeld D, Robbins G. Prognosis of the second breast cancer. The role of previous exposure to the first primary. Cancer 1975;35:596–599.

48. Partridge AH, Winer EP, Burstein HJ. Follow-up care of breast cancer survivors. Semin Oncol 2003;30:817–825.

49. Warmuth MA, Bowen G, Prosnitz LR, et al. Complications of axillary lymph node dissection for carcinoma of the breast: A report based on patient survey. Cancer 1998;83:1362–1368.

50. Schijven MP, Vingerhoets AJ, Rutten HJ, et al. Comparison of morbidity between axillary lymph node dissection and sentinel node biopsy. Eur J Surg Oncol 2003;29:341–350.

51. Herd-Smith A, Russo A, Muraca MG, et al. Prognostic factors for lymphedema after primary treatment of breast carcinoma. Cancer 2001;92:1783–1787.

52. Harris SR, Hugi MR, Olivotto IA, et al. Clinical practice guidelines for the care and treatment of breast cancer: Lymphedema. CMAJ 2001;164:191–199.

53. Partridge AH, Burstein HJ, Winer EP. Side effects of chemotherapy and combined chemo-hormonal therapy in women with early stage breast cancer. J Natl Cancer Inst Monogr 2001;30:135–142.

54. Sainsbury JR. Beneficial side effect profile of anastrozole compared with tamoxifen confirmed by additional 7 months of exposure data: A safety update from the Arimidex Tamoxifen Alone or in Combination (ATAC) trial [abstract]. Breast Cancer Res Treat 2002;76(Suppl 1):A633.

55. ATAC Trialists' Group. Anastrozole alone or in combination with tamoxifen versus tamoxifen alone for adjuvant treatment of postmenopausal women with early breast cancer: First results of the ATAC randomized trial. Lancet 2002;359:2131–2139.

56. Sloan JA, Loprinzi CL, Novotny PJ, et al. Methodologic lessons learned from hot flash studies. J Clin Oncol 2001;19:4280–4290.

57. Barton DL, Loprinzi CL, Quella SK, et al. Prospective evaluation of vitamin E for hot flashes in breast cancer survivors. J Clin Oncol 1998;16:495–500.

58. Jacobson JS, Troxel AB, Evans J, et al. Randomized trial of black cohosh for the treatment of hot flashes among women with a history of breast cancer. J Clin Oncol 2001;19:2739–2745.

59. Stearns V, Hayes DF. Cooling off hot flashes. J Clin Oncol 2002;20:1436–1438.

60. Loprinzi CL, Kugler JW, Sloan JA, et al. Venlafaxine in management of hot flashes in survivors of breast cancer: A randomized controlled trial. Lancet 2000;356:2059–2063.

61. Barakat RR, Gilewski T, Almadrones L, et al. Effect of adjuvant tamoxifen on the endometrium in postmenopausal women with breast cancer: A prospective study using office endometrial biopsy. J Clin Oncol 2000;18:3459–3463.

62. Gerber B, Krause A, Muller H, et al. Effects of adjuvant tamoxifen on the endometrium in postmenopausal women with breast cancer: A prospective long term study using transvaginal ultrasound. J Clin Oncol 2000;18:3464–3470.

63. Committee on Gynecologic Practice, the American College of Obstetricians and Gynecologists. ACOG Committee Opinion: Tamoxifen and endometrial cancer. Int J Gynecol Obstet 2001;73:77–79.

64. Runowicz CD, Gynecologic surveillance of women on tamoxifen: First do no harm. J Clin Oncol 2000;18:3457–3458.

65. Shapiro CL, Manola J, Leboff M. Ovarian failure after adjuvant chemotherapy is associated with rapid bone loss in women with early stage breast cancer. J Clin Oncol 2001;19:3306–3311.

66. Goodwin PJ, Ennis M, Pritchard KI, et al. Adjuvant treatment and onset of menopause predict weight gain after breast cancer diagnosis. J Clin Oncol 1999;17:120–129.

67. Boccardo F, Rubagotti A, Amoroso M, et al. Cyclophosphamide, methotrexate, and fluorouracil versus tamoxifen plus ovarian suppression as adjuvant treatment of estrogen-receptor positive pre/perimenopausal breast cancer patients: results of the Italian breast cancer adjuvant study group 02 randomized trial. J Clin Oncol 2000;18:2718–2727.

68. Powles T, Hickish T, Kanis JA, et al. Effect of tamoxifen on bone mineral density measured by dual-energy x-ray absorptiometry in healthy premenopausal and postmenopausal women. J Clin Oncol 1996;14:78–84.

69. Ramaswamy B, Shapiro CL. Osteopenia and osteoporosis in women with breast cancer. Semin Oncol 2003;30:763–775.

70. Baum M, Buzdar AV, Cuzick J, et al. Anastrozole or in combination with tamoxifen versus tamoxifen alone for adjuvant treatment of postmenopausal women with early breast cancer: First results of the ATAC randomized trial. Lancet 2002;359:2131–2139.

71. Hillner B, Ingle JN, Chlebowski RT, et al. American Society of Clinical Oncology 2003 update on the role of bisphosphonates and bone health issues in women with breast cancer. J Clin Oncol 2003;21:4042–4057.

72. Winer EP, Hudis C, Burstein HJ, et al. American Society of Clinical Oncology Technology Assessment on the use of aromatase inhibitors as adjuvant therapy for women with hormone receptor-positive breast cancer: Status report 2004. J Clin Oncol 2005;23:619–629.

73. American Society of Clinical Oncology. Recommended breast cancer surveillance guidelines. J Clin Oncol 1997;15:2149–2156.

74. Grunfeld E, Mant D, Yudkin P, et al. Routine follow up of breast cancer in primary care: Randomized trial. BMJ 1996;313:665–669.

SECTION VI

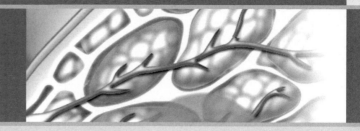

MANAGEMENT OF METASTATIC BREAST CANCER

CHAPTER 32

Management of Metastatic Breast Cancer

I

Introduction and Principles of Treatment

Ruth Oratz

What is the scope of the problem?

Despite advances in screening and early diagnosis of breast cancer, many women still develop and die from metastatic disease. Adjuvant systemic therapy has increased the survival of women who present with early-stage disease but has certainly not completely eradicated the risk for recurrence. Relapse rates following standard current adjuvant therapy for patients presenting at the various stages is as follows: stage I, 10% to 30%; stage II, 40% to 60%; and stage III, greater than 90%.[1]

The annual incidence of all newly diagnosed cases of breast cancer is greater than 200,000, and more than 50,000 women will die of breast cancer this year. Most women present with early-stage disease. Although fewer than 10% of patients in the United States present with stage IV disease, this represents a significant number of women: 10,000 to 15,000 with metastatic disease.[2]

At this time, metastatic breast cancer is rarely cured. Median survival after development of metastatic disease is 2 to 3 years.[3–5] Treatment may be effective for palliating symptoms, with responders enjoying not only an enhanced quality but also, in some cases, prolongation of life. Nonetheless, cure is not an expectation, and research efforts both at the basic science and at the clinical levels must be directed at defining better and more effective therapies that may offer the possibility of cure for patients with metastatic disease.

NATURAL HISTORY AND CLINICAL PATTERNS OF METASTASES

When do metastases appear?

Although up to 75% of recurrences occur within the first 5 years of diagnosis, metastatic disease continues to appear after this time and has been well documented as long as 25 or 30 years after first presentation.[5]

What are the sites of metastatic disease?

The most common sites of metastasis are bone, lungs, liver, chest wall, and central nervous system (CNS). Less common sites are the adrenals, ovaries, pericardium, thyroid, and bone marrow.[1] Factors that may determine the site of relapse include the disease-free interval, histologic subtype of the primary lesion, estrogen receptor (ER) status of the primary tumor, and possibly, the type of adjuvant therapy. In patients with short disease-free intervals, visceral disease predominates, whereas if the disease-free interval is longer, bone metastases are more likely. Invasive lobular carcinoma is more likely to spread to peritoneum, pleura, adrenal glands, uterus, and ovaries. Invasive ductal carcinoma is more likely to spread to liver, lung, and bone[6–9] (Table 32–1).

What are the important prognostic factors in metastatic breast cancer?

ER status is an important prognostic factor. Estrogen stimulates the growth of many breast tumors. About 30% of unselected breast cancers are ER positive. In general, patients with ER-positive tumors who are postmenopausal have a more favorable prognosis once recurrence develops. These patients are more likely to develop osseous metastases than visceral metastases, and there may be a longer disease-free interval from the time of primary diagnosis until the development of metastatic disease. Once metastatic disease is diagnosed, patients with ER-positive tumors may have a more indolent clinical course, with slower progression of disease and longer survival. Some patients have survived in excess of 10 years with ER-positive osseous metastases. In contrast, patients with ER-negative tumors may have more aggressive disease, with a

Table 32–1   Common Sites of Metastatic Breast Cancer

Bone
Liver
Lung
Central nervous system

Table 32–2   Important Prognostic Factors in Metastatic Breast Cancer

Disease-free interval—length of time from diagnosis of primary lesion until development of metastatic disease
Number of metastatic sites
Skeletal vs. visceral metastases
Estrogen/progesterone receptor expression
HER-2-neu expression

shorter disease-free interval, more rapid spread and growth of metastases, a higher incidence of visceral metastases, and shorter long-term survival.[10–12]

Postmenopausal patients are more likely than premenopausal patients to have ER-positive disease. In addition, expression of hormone receptors may correlate with other prognostic factors, including *HER-2/neu.* Tumors that overexpress *HER-2/neu* are more likely to be ER negative and to be associated with more aggressive disease. There are also data suggesting that the ER and *HER-2/neu* interact. Overexpression or amplification of *HER-2/neu* may be associated with relative tamoxifen resistance in tumors that are ER positive.[13–20] It has also been noted that hormone receptors may be less frequently expressed in tumors arising in patients with genetic mutations in *BRCA1.* This may affect prognosis as well.[21,22]

Survival from the time of diagnosis of recurrent disease may also depend on the site of metastasis. Patients with bone-only metastases may have a longer median survival than do those with extraskeletal metastases. In some studies, survival was almost twice as long if bone metastases rather than visceral metastases were present.[10–12] In one study, median survival of patients with skeletal involvement was 48 months, with one third of patients living longer than 5 years. Patients with visceral disease have a median survival of 6 months.[12] Also, in patients with local chest wall recurrence alone, survival is longer than in those with visceral disease.

Some preliminary data suggest that adjuvant therapy may have an impact on sites of recurrence. A retrospective review of adjuvant therapy clinical trials by the International Breast Cancer Study Group compared relapse rates and sites of relapse. Women who had received a full course of adjuvant chemotherapy were compared with those followed by observation alone after surgery or who had only one cycle of perioperative chemotherapy. Similar rates of relapse were observed in both groups, but there was a significant difference in locoregional and soft tissue relapse between the two groups. Those who had received the more effective chemotherapy had only an 18% relapse rate in soft tissue, compared with a 36% relapse rate in locoregional and soft tissue sites in women who had received the less effective adjuvant treatment. There were no differences in the incidence of visceral or bony metastases. This information is inconclusive as to the effect of adjuvant therapy on site of relapse and has not been confirmed in other large studies[23] (Table 32–2).

How does metastatic disease progress?

In some instances, metastatic disease follows a rather indolent course, with little in the way of symptoms or complications. This pattern of metastatic disease is most often associated with older age at diagnosis, postmenopausal status, longer disease-free interval, smaller tumor burden, ER-positive tumors, and bony rather than visceral sites of metastases.

In other instances, disease is rapidly progressive, causing a great deal of morbidity, pain, and discomfort. This pattern of metastasis is more commonly seen in patients who have widespread visceral disease, who are premenopausal, or who have multiple sites of involvement with greater tumor burden and ER-negative and *HER-2/neu*–positive tumors.

DIAGNOSIS AND WORKUP OF METASTATIC DISEASE

How is metastatic disease diagnosed?

Less than 10% of patients present with stage IV disease, but this is only a small fraction of all women who will ultimately develop advanced breast cancer. Most patients are diagnosed with metastatic breast cancer after having been treated for stage I, II, or III disease.

Patients should be followed after initial diagnosis for the possibilities of both local and distant recurrence. Careful history and physical examination should be performed at regular intervals. Mammographic surveillance is indicated for patients who have had breast-conserving surgery. Chest radiographs may detect asymptomatic pulmonary metastases and may be indicated for patients at risk. Although many patients will develop osseous metastases, routine use of nuclear bone scans or radiographic bone surveys has not proved cost-effective and is not routinely recommended for patients who present with early-stage disease. Serum chemistries (aspartate aminotransferase [AST], alanine aminotransferase [ALT], lactate dehydrogenase [LDH], and alkaline phosphatase) may be helpful in screening for liver or bone metastases. It is unclear, however, whether there is a survival advantage for regular, intensive testing.

Two large studies have addressed the impact of intensive surveillance on survival of patients following diagnosis of breast cancer. In both trials, women were randomly assigned to either intensive follow-up (defined as physician visits, blood tests, bone scans, and chest radiographs on a scheduled basis) or routine follow-up (defined as physician visits and testing only as clinically indicated). Screening mammography was conducted in both arms of each study. Once metastatic disease was diagnosed, therapy was initiated. The reported results were strikingly similar in the two studies. There was a small increase in the frequency of detection of metastases in the intensively followed group but no survival difference.[24,25]

Furthermore, the dollar cost of routine testing for the asymptomatic patient must be considered. One financial analysis published in 1990 found that the direct cost of intensive follow-up (with physician visits, blood tests, mammography, nuclear bone scans, and chest films) would be at least five times higher than for less intensive follow-up (physician visits, mammography). The range of cost was from about $1000 per patient over 5 years for the routine follow-up to more than $5000 per patient for the intensively followed group. Given the number of women to be followed, the estimated difference in cost for the two follow-up approaches over a 5-year period in the United States could exceed $800 million.[26]

Positron emission tomography (PET) scanning is a new diagnostic modality that offers several advantages over anatomically oriented imaging such as radiography, computed tomography (CT) scanning, ultrasoundy, and conventional nuclear imaging. PET most commonly uses the radiotracer ^{18}F-fluorodeoxyglucose (FDG), which is actively transported into cells through the glucose transport mechanism and then undergoes phosphorylation in the initial step of glycolysis. FDG-6P (phosphorylated FDG), however, is not a substrate for additional phosphorylation and is blocked from further metabolism. Most malignant cells lack the phosphatase enzymes necessary for dephosphorylation of FDG-6P, allowing high levels of this compound to accumulate. The amount of FDG uptake in the cells reflects the overall metabolic activity and identifies cells that are more active. This correlates with malignancy and with biologic behavior of certain tumor types. Higher-grade tumors tend to accumulate higher levels of FDG than lower-grade tumors. This may be helpful in detecting areas of involvement by metastatic tumor and in differentiating rapidly growing from more indolent tumors.[27–30]

PET scanning may be useful in staging and in serial evaluations after diagnosis of breast cancer. PET scanning has been used in breast cancer. It has been reported to detect metastases in axillary lymph nodes with high sensitivity and specificity. However, some series also report significant numbers of false-positive and false-negative results.[31–34] Distant sites of disease, including pulmonary, osseous, and distant nodal sites, are more reliably detected by PET.[35–36] There may be an increasing role for PET imaging in the early detection of metastatic disease and in monitoring response to therapy. PET is costly but may be a more efficient imaging method than more conventional anatomically based studies.

Serum cancer markers, such as carcinoembryonic antigen (CEA) and CA-15-3, may have some utility in detecting early metastases. CA-15-3 has been shown to have a high degree of both sensitivity (81.5%) and specificity (66%) and a high predictive value (92%) in the detection of osseous metastases.[37] CEA may be elevated in metastatic breast cancer but is also increased in a number of other malignancies, including lung cancer, gastrointestinal tract carcinomas (stomach, colon, rectum, pancreas), and ovarian cancer. In addition, patients who smoke cigarettes, have benign liver disease, or have inflammatory diseases of the breast or liver may also have elevated serum CEA. CA-15-3 may be somewhat more specific and may be predictive of recurrence.[38–42] The usefulness of monitoring these serum markers has not

yet been clearly established, and the financial cost is not insignificant.

It is clear that follow-up is necessary after the diagnosis of breast cancer, but the degree to which routine use of invasive or costly testing is indicated needs further definition. To date, no survival advantage has been demonstrated following the use of intensive follow-up screening for metastatic disease. Careful history and physical examination at regular intervals are recommended. Surveillance mammography is indicated, as discussed elsewhere. Until clearcut data defining the utility of other tests emerge, the routine use of screening radiographs, scans, and serum markers cannot be recommended. These tests may be helpful in detecting early recurrence, and their use will be determined by the treating physician, regional standards of care, and third-party payers.

What is the workup for a newly diagnosed stage IV patient?

Metastatic disease may be diagnosed because either the patient presents with a new clinical sign or symptom, or a routine screening test demonstrates an abnormality suspicious of recurrence. If a patient presents with a symptom indicative of metastatic involvement, an appropriately directed workup to confirm the diagnosis is indicated. For example, a complaint of pain may lead to a radiograph or bone scan; cough or shortness of breath may direct one to order a chest film or CT scan. On the other hand, an abnormality on a routine screening test may trigger other diagnostic interventions. For example, elevated serum markers and liver function tests in an asymptomatic patient may prompt a request for an abdominal CT scan looking for liver metastases, or a PET scan for a more generalized examination.

After a patient is identified as having metastatic disease, a complete staging workup to define the extent of disease should be undertaken. This begins with a thorough history and physical examination. Laboratory tests include a complete blood count (CBC) with differential; clinical chemistries including electrolytes, transaminases (ALT, AST), alkaline phosphatase, albumin, calcium, LDH, and possibly serum markers (CEA and CA-15-3). Imaging studies should be used as indicated to define the anatomic sites of involvement. It is important to know the full extent of disease when embarking on treatment in order to define optimal therapy, determine response, and define progression.

The first site of recurrent disease should be documented histologically, whenever technically feasible, given lesions that can undergo biopsy with acceptable risk. The differential diagnosis of a new lesion in a patient with a history of breast cancer includes metastases from primary breast cancer, benign lesions, and other primary or metastatic malignancies. It is imperative to confirm the histologic nature of the lesion as recurrent or metastatic breast cancer for diagnostic and prognostic purposes and before beginning toxic and costly therapies. Biopsy should be performed on the site that is most accessible and that would render an adequate tissue sample with the least morbidity for the patient. Often, a fine-needle aspiration biopsy with radiologic guidance can be performed on pulmonary, hepatic, soft tissue, or osseous sites. Sometimes, a surgical biopsy is required. Again, it must

demonstrated statistically significant higher response rates for letrozole, longer duration of responses, and longer time to treatment failure. The overall response rate for 2.5 mg/day of letrozole was 24% and that for 40 mg four times per day of megestrol acetate 40 was 16%. The median duration of response was 33 months versus 18 months.[76,77] Another large study comparing letrozole to megestrol acetate showed that these two agents were equivalent in clinical activity. The toxicity profile of letrozole was much more favorable than that of megestrol acetate.[71] There was less weight gain and fewer cardiovascular events, including thrombophlebitis, myocardial infarction, cerebrovascular accidents, and pulmonary emboli, in the patients treated with the aromatase inhibitor.

Letrozole has also been tested in the first-line metastatic setting. In a large international trial, women with locally advanced, locoregionally recurrent, or metastatic breast cancer were randomly assigned to treatment with either letrozole (2,5 mg/day) or tamoxifen (20 mg/day). In this study, letrozole treatment resulted in statistically significant higher response rates (30% vs. 20%) and greater overall clinical benefit (49% vs. 3 8%). Time to progression and time to treatment failure were longer in the letrozole group. The rate of adverse events was similar in both treatment arms, although the pattern of toxicity was somewhat different, consistent with observations in other studies.[78,79]

Fadrozole

Fadrozole is presently available only in Japan and is not used in the United States or Europe. It has also been studied as second-line therapy in postmenopausal women with advanced breast cancer compared with megestrol acetate. In two randomized, double-blind studies, there were no differences in response rates.[80] There was no definitive difference in median survival time. It was concluded that fadrozole and megestrol acetate were equivalent. The dose of fadrozole is 1 mg twice daily.

In the first-line metastatic setting, fadrozole (1 mg twice daily) has been compared in a phase III randomized study with tamoxifen (20 mg/day orally).[81] This study was not double-blind. Patients were crossed over when there was disease progression or toxicity. No significant differences in response rates were noted. The tamoxifen-treated patients had longer time to treatment failure (8.5 months) compared with the fadrozole-treated patients (6.1 months). Duration of response and overall survival were similar in both treatment arms.[81]

Vorozole

Vorozole is also a selective, nonsteroidal aromatase inhibitor. It has been shown to suppress aromatase enzyme activity in doses of 2.5 and 5 mg once daily.[82,83] In one study of patients with advanced breast cancer failing on tamoxifen, women were randomly assigned to treatment with either vorozole (2.5 mg once daily) or megestrol acetate (40 mg four times daily). This was not a double-blind study. There were no significant differences between the groups in overall response rate, clinical benefit, time to progression, or survival. Vorozole was determined to be equivalent in efficacy to megestrol acetate.[84] In two other open-label studies of patients with advanced breast cancer, vorozole was compared with aminoglutethimide.[85,86] In both studies, vorozole was superior to

aminoglutethimide in overall response rates and overall clinical benefit. However, duration of response, time to treatment failure, time to progression, and overall survival were similar for both agents. Therefore, it was concluded that vorozole offered no significant advantages over megestrol acetate or aminoglutethimide. It is no longer in clinical development or clinical use.

Exemestane

Exemestane (Aromasin) is a potent steroidal aromatase inhibitor that partially lacks cross-resistance with nonsteroidal aromatase inhibitors. Exemestane is a derivative of androstenedione and competes with this natural ligand for the binding site on the aromatase enzyme. Its binding with aromatase is irreversible; therefore, this agent is sometimes called a "suicide" inhibitor. The dose of exemestane is 25 mg/day, and the half-life of the drug is 24 hours.

Exemestane was first studied in the third-line setting in patients whose metastatic breast cancer progressed after two endocrine therapies. In these third-line studies, activity was seen with exemestane. Response rates ranged from 7% to 13%, and overall clinical benefit was seen in 24% to 30% of treated patients.[87,88] These studies demonstrated that women treated with nonsteroidal aromatase inhibitors may still derive benefit from further hormonal therapy with the steroidal agent exemestane. This observation has implications for sequencing of hormonal therapy.

In the second-line setting, exemestane (25 mg/day) was also compared with megestrol acetate (40 mg four times daily). A phase III randomized trial was conducted in women whose advanced breast cancer progressed while taking tamoxifen. Although not statistically significant, objective response rates were slightly better for exemestane than for megestrol acetate (15% and 12.4%, respectively). Statistically significant advantages in mediation duration of survival, overall survival, time to tumor progression, and time to treatment failure were noted in favor of exemestane.[89] Exemestane-related toxicity is similar to that of other aromatase inhibitors. All of these agents are better tolerated than megestrol acetate.

Exemestane has not yet been compared with tamoxifen as first-line therapy in a large randomized phase III trial, but phase III studies are ongoing. In a small randomized phase II trial of exemestane versus tamoxifen, there was a suggestion of superiority of exemestane in response rate, overall clinical benefit, and time to progression.[90] However, it may be reasonable to extrapolate from the experience with the other aromatase inhibitors that this agent will also be at least equivalent to if not superior to tamoxifen.

Formestane

Formestane, like exemestane, is a steroidal, noncompetitive aromatase inhibitor. Formestane suppresses serum estrogen concentrations significantly but is less effective than anastrozole in this regard.[91] Its antiaromatase activity is less consistent than other aromatase inhibitors.[91,92] It has been tested in second- and third-line therapy and in first-line therapy of advanced breast cancer. Unlike the other aromatase inhibitors, formestane is not available in oral formulation and is administered as an intramuscular injection, 250 mg every 14 days. In comparison with megestrol acetate, formestane showed no

11. Jaiyesimi IA, Buzdar AU... breast cancer: Twenty-eig... 529.
12. Cole MP, Jones CTA, Tod... breast cancer: An early cli... 1971;25:270.
13. Morgan LR, Schein PS, W... ifen in advanced breast ca... ters. Cancer Treat Rep 19...
14. Ward HWC. Anti-oestro... tamoxifen at two dose lev...
15. Tormey DC, Lippman MI... doses with and without... Ann Intern Med 1983;98:
16. Fisher B, Costantino J, R... evaluating tamoxifen in t... breast cancer who have... Med 1989;320:479.
17. Rutqvist LE, Mattson A... among postmenopausal... randomized trial of adj... 85:1398.
18. Saphner T, Tormey DC,... patients who received ad... 1991;9:286,
19. Kaiser-Kupfer MI, Lippn... Rep 1978;62:315.
20. Pavlidis NA, Petris C, B... term, low-dose tamoxi... Cancer 1992;69:2961.
21. Gerner EW. Ocular toxi... 420.
22. Diver JMJ, Jackson IM,... indications. Lancet 1986
23. Fentiman IS, Powles T... Lancet 1987;2:1070.
24. Turken S, Siris E, Seldin... density in women with l...
25. Pomander T, Rutqvist... tamoxifen in early brea... postmenopausal womer
26. Pomander T, Rutqvist... adjuvant tamoxifen in... 1993;29A:497.
27. Kristensen B, Ejlersten... metabolism in postmen... domized study. J Clin C
28. Powles TJ, Sickish T,... mineral density measu... healthy premenopausa... 1996;14:78–84.
29. Gotfriedsen A, Christia... bone mineral content... Cancer 1984;53:853–85
30. Fentiman IS, Caleffi I... women receiving tam... 262–264.
31. Schapira DV, Kumar... with tamoxifen. Breast
32. Love RR, Newcomb PA... on lipid and lipoprotei... negative breast cancer.
33. Bagade JD, Wolter J, Su... on plasma lipids and... Metab 1990;70:1132–1
34. McDonald CC, Stewar... adjuvant tamoxifen tr...
35. Killackey MA, Hakes... breast cancer patien... 1985;69:237–238.
36. Barakat RR. The effec... 1995;9:129–134, 139–
37. Pomander T, Rutqvist... early breast cancer:... 1989;21:117–120.

Response rate... tamoxifen ran... of response is...

Toxicities re... fluid retention... thromboembo... particularly u... more than 10... median weight... also be seen, ... a result of p... endometrium.

Recently, syn... PR have been... oped as an abo... France. The com... PR-positive bre... activity in a nur... 200 to 400 mg/... Response rates a... ally well tolerate... effects are hot fla... patients.

What is the r... treatment of...

Another category... treatment of meta... These drugs act to... blocking release... Complete endocri... amenorrheic. The... menopausal patie... menopausal women... Goserelin (Zolad... is administered by n... response rate is ab... hot flashes in 80%... patients. In postme... did demonstrate a r... possibility of other n... Leuprolide (Lupro... been clinically useful... rate in one study of p...

Are androgens e...

Androgens have also l... tion of breast cancer. T... apy after antiestrogens... LHRH agonists. The... androgens is as antipr... rates may approach 20%... them less useful than... with metastatic breast... cause hirsutism, deeper... increased libido in 60%... monly used agents in th... and fluoxymesterone.[133]

Table 32–13 Indirect Comparisons of Antiaromatase Agents versus Megestrol Acetate as Second-Line Therapy

	EXE, 25 mg	MA	ANA, 1 mg	MA*	LET, 2.5 mg	MA
No. of patients	366	403	263	253	174	189
CR + PR (%)	15	12.4	12.4	12.2	23.6	16.4
CR + PR + SD ≥ 24 wk (%)	37.4	34.6	42.2	40.3	34.5	31.7
Median TTP (mo)	4.7	3.9†	4.8	4.6	5.6	5.5
Median survival (mo)	NR	26.7†	26.7	22.5†	25.3	21.5

*Pooled data.
†Statistical significance.
ANA, anastrozole; CR, complete response; EXE, exemestane; LET, letrozole; MA, megestrol acetate; NR, not reported; PR, partial response; TTP, time to progression.
From Kaulmann M, et al. Proc Am Soc Clin Oncol 1999;18:109a; Buzdar A, et al. Cancer 1998;83:1142–1152; and Dombernowsky P, et al. J Clin Oncol 1998;16:453–461.

advantages in either time to treatment failure or overall survival. Formestane was considered equivalent to megestrol acetate in efficacy and safety and offered a suitable alternative to progestin for the treatment of women with metastatic breast cancer.[93,94] Formestane was also tested against tamoxifen in the first-line setting. It was found to be comparable to tamoxifen in efficacy and tolerability, with no statistically significant differences in response rates, duration of response, or survival. Tamoxifen was superior in time to treatment failure (9.7 months vs. 6.5 months) and time to progression (9.7 months vs. 7.0 months)[95] (Table 32–13).

Should aromatase inhibitors be first-line therapy?

Data from first-line trials comparing aromatase inhibitors to tamoxifen have established the efficacy of anastrozole and letrozole in this setting. Preliminary studies of exemestane in this setting indicate that this agent will also most likely have a role in first-line therapy. Data from large, randomized trials is pending. Compared with tamoxifen, antiaromatase agents result in fewer hot flashes; less vaginal bleeding, discharge, and endometrial abnormalities; and fewer thromboembolic events. However, a serious concern is the increased rate of bone mineral density loss with antiaromatase agents, associated with a higher rate of fractures and increased musculoskeletal complaints.

In summary, several aromatase inhibitors have been tested in the treatment of advanced breast cancer. Arimidex, letrozole, and exemestane have all demonstrated superiority over megestrol acetate in the second-line treatment of postmenopausal women with advanced breast cancer. All three of these agents are available in the United States and Europe and are approved for this indication. These agents have replaced megestrol acetate in the second-line setting. Fadrozole, vorozole, and formestane are active agents but not superior to megestrol acetate. Fadrozole is available in Japan. The other two agents are not in clinical use at this time. The antiaromatase agents are better tolerated than megestrol acetate. Major toxicities include hot flashes (5% to 13%); headache (<10%); and nausea (5% to 30%). There is significantly less weight gain, edema, thromboembolic events, and cardiovascular events compared with megestrol acetate.

Are there differences between the antiaromatase agents?

Although there are some differences in mechanism of action among these agents and therefore theoretically some potential differences in efficacy, clinical data do not demonstrate significant differences in response rates, duration of responses, or time to treatment failure. In vitro data point out some differences in suppression of aromatase activity, levels of aromatase protein, and levels of circulation serum estrogens. However, the clinical significance of these differences is not yet apparent.[96,97] These observations are drawn from similar but not identically designed studies comparing the single agents either to megestrol acetate or to tamoxifen. A recently completed randomized phase III head-to-head comparison of letrozole and anastrozole in the second-line setting has been published. This study demonstrated superiority of letrozole over anastrozole in objective response rate (19% vs. 12%, respectively). There were, however, no differences in time to progression, overall clinical benefit, duration of response, or overall survival. Adverse events were comparable for both drugs.[98] A head-to-head comparison of anastrozole and exemestane is ongoing.

How can these agents be used sequentially?

With several agents now available for endocrine therapy of metastatic breast cancer, the optimal sequence of administration is yet to be determined. Several trials have examined different sequences of antiaromatase agents. In one phase II trial, exemestane was administered to postmenopausal women with metastatic breast cancer that had progressed during treatment with a nonsteroidal aromatase inhibitor (including aminoglutethimide, anastrozole, letrozole, and vorozole). Objective responses were seen in 6% of patients, but overall clinical benefit was observed in 24% of patients. Furthermore, the median duration of response on exemestane was 58.4 weeks, and median duration of overall success was 37 weeks—a very meaningful and impressive observation. One fourth of patients derived a significant benefit from exemestane therapy after failing on a nonsteroidal aromatase inhibitor.[99]

Another smaller study examined two different sequences of therapy: (1) exemestane followed by either anastrozole or

letrozole, and (;
tane.[100] In this
treated initially
the other seque
resistance betw
matase agents.
sequence of use.

At the presen
regarding the p
They may be use
ing tamoxifen; cr
to another may r

What are the risks of arom

In general, the a
few side effects.
flashes, vaginal
ache. These are
with megestrol
inhibitors have si
vaginal bleeding,
phenomena.

Musculoskeletal
Aromatase inhibito
musculoskeletal sy
implications of the
sis and fractures, a
depends on estroge
action on bone and
postmenopausal wo
bone demineralizat
Concomitant use o
this side effect.[109] Ex
effect, may have few
aromatase inhibito
exemestane was sho
also noted in a shor
women, in which m
after estrogen supp

Cardiovascular Eff
The long-term cardi
agents are not well d
of aromatase inhibito
blood lipids. One stu
letrozole for breast c
cholesterol, apolipopr
for cardiovascular di
anastrozole and tamo
was shown to reduce
increase serum trigly
impact on the lipid pr
terol and LDL befor
anastrozole treatment
triglycerides and HDL.

Additional hormonal ma
duce meaningful clinical res
sensitive disease that is foll
The other agents discussed
glutethimide, LHRH agon
considered for these therap

After disease progresse:
hormonal treatments, che
Hypothetically, hormone
sensitive tumor cell popula
behind resistant ER- a
chemotherapy may produc

What is tumor flare to hormonal treatm

The syndrome of horm
uncommonly reported a
patients started on tamo
therapy.[138,139] Bone pain is
may be associated with
scan. Erythema of cuta
Hypercalcemia may occur
osseous metastases. The n
a reactive process to ho
increased osteoblastic ac
tases.[140] Patients should b
initially during the ear
Usually, the flare synd
requires no special inte
scribed for comfort. The
itored if there is clinical
treated appropriately if
predict a better outcome

Is there a role for hormonal therapi

Combination regimer
agents have definitely r
prolonged survival tha
therefore reasonable t
hormonal agents woul
than single-agent endo
have addressed this que

Two randomized tri
Institute (NCI) and t
Group (NCCTG), com
nation of tamoxifen p
there was a slightly hig
arm, but this was not s
survival difference. To
the combination and
voice changes, which
group.[142,143] In trials c
ifen plus medroxyproj
with tamoxifen plus
was seen for the co
of response, or ov
current recommenda

IV

Hypercalcemia from Metastatic Breast Cancer

Ruth Oratz

How is hypercalcemia defined, and what is its presentation in metastatic breast cancer?

Hypercalcemia is a common metabolic complication of malignancy. It is seen in breast cancer, lung cancer, and gastrointestinal and gynecologic malignancies. Up to one third of breast cancer patients may develop hypercalcemia at some point during the course of the illness. The mean survival following the development of hypercalcemia is 3 months.[1-3] Hypercalcemia is defined as elevation of the corrected serum calcium to greater than 10.5 mg/dL. Patients usually become symptomatic at levels greater than 14 mg/dL. The clinical presentation includes symptoms of fatigue, anorexia, constipation, and nausea. At first, these may be subtle and difficult to distinguish from the symptoms of advanced metastatic disease or the treatments used to palliate metastatic disease (chemotherapy and radiation therapy). As the hypercalcemia progresses, patients may become dehydrated, confused, lethargic, or stuporous. Seizures may occur. Slowed cardiac conduction may become evident on the electrocardiogram, and ultimately bradyarrhythmias and complete heart block may ensue. If left untreated, hypercalcemia is potentially fatal.[4]

The differential diagnosis of the clinical presentation of hypercalcemia includes central nervous system (CNS) metastases (particularly carcinomatous meningitis), other metabolic disorders (hyponatremia, hypernatremia, hypoglycemia, hyperglycemia), infection, subdural hematoma, subarachnoid hemorrhage, and oversedation from narcotic analgesics. The differential diagnosis of the finding of elevated serum calcium is primary hyperparathyroidism.

What is the cause of hypercalcemia in patients with metastatic breast cancer?

There are two physiologic explanations for the development of serum hypercalcemia in patients with metastatic breast cancer: (1) increased release of calcium into the serum by osteolytic bone destruction from metastatic lesions and (2) humorally mediated hypercalcemia by parathyroid hormone (PTH)-like factors. In metastatic breast cancer, bone destruction by osteolytic metastases is the more common cause of hypercalcemia. Bone destruction by tumor cells leads to activation of osteoclasts, and this may lead to hypercalcemia.[3] In

the absence of significant bone metastases, PTH-like factors secreted by the tumor mediate bone resorption and release of calcium.[5-7]

How is hypercalcemia treated?

Treatment of hypercalcemia is most effectively managed by reducing the underlying tumor burden. Other therapeutic measures include restoring adequate hydration and instituting antihypercalcemic agents. Vigorous hydration with normal saline helps to lower the serum calcium concentration, correct intravascular volume depletion, and enhance urinary calcium excretion. Hydration alone will not result in long-term remission of hypercalcemia, however.

The bisphosphonates are stable analogues of pyrophosphate and act by inhibiting osteoclast activity. A number of these agents are useful in the clinical setting.[8-12] Etidronate, pamidronate, and zoledronate are the most commonly used of these drugs and require intravenous infusion. Infusion time varies from 90 minutes to 24 hours depending on the agent. They are extremely effective in lowering serum calcium and are active in more than two thirds of patients. The bisphosphonates are generally well tolerated with few side effects, including fever, mild renal insufficiency, and hypophosphatemia or hyperphosphatemia. Dosing is adjusted for both the serum calcium concentration and serum creatinine. Electrolytes should be carefully monitored during administration. These agents should be considered as first-line therapy for hypercalcemia, particularly when multiple osseous metastases are present.

There are additional data that bisphosphonates may also contribute to bone healing in skeletal metastases and may help alleviate bone pain, reduce the incidence of pathologic fractures, and lower analgesic requirements.[7,11] The bisphosphonates are therefore indicated in the presence of bone disease as evidenced by radiographic imaging and as prophylactic therapy in women with extraskeletal metastases without evidence of bone metastases.

Gallium nitrate is another useful antihypercalcemic agent. Its mechanism of action is the inhibition of calcium resorption from bone. Randomized double-blind studies have shown that gallium nitrate is more effective in inducing normocalcemia and maintaining duration of response than calcitonin. The median duration of normocalcemia following treatment with gallium nitrate is 7.5 days, whereas it is 1 day after calcitonin treatment. Gallium nitrate is also given by continuous intravenous infusion and is administered over 5 days. It may be nephrotoxic and should not be administered with other nephrotoxic agents such as aminoglycosides.[13]

Calcitonin is normally secreted by the parafollicular cells of the thyroid gland and modulates serum calcium by inhibiting osteoclastic bone resorption and enhancing renal excretion of calcium in the distal tubule.[14] It is therefore useful as a treatment for malignant hypercalcemia. Although calcitonin will induce a hypocalcemic response in up to 80% of treated patients, the duration of response is short, and tachyphylaxis limits its usefulness. Salmon calcitonin is the most potent form of the hormone and is given by subcutaneous injection every 12 hours. Side effects include nausea, vomiting, and allergic reactions.[14]

Mithramycin has also been used to treat malignant hypercalcemia in patients with metastatic breast cancer. This antineoplastic agent was shown to cause hypocalcemia—possibly by its toxic effects on osteoclasts. It is administered by intravenous bolus and results in lowering of the serum calcium within 3 to 4 days after administration. Its duration of response is unpredictable, and the main side effects are nausea, myelosuppression, and nephrotoxicity. It is not recommended for first-line therapy.[15] Other agents, including glucocorticoids and loop diuretics, have been used in managing malignant hypercalcemia, but their effects are neither significant nor long lasting, and they should be reserved for use as adjunctive agents.[16]

REFERENCES

1. Galasko CSB, Bennett A. Hypercalcemia in patients with advanced mammary cancer. BMJ 1971;3:573.
2. Hickey RC, Samaan NA, Jackson GL. Hypercalcemia in patients with breast cancer. Arch Surg 1981;116:545.
3. Mundy GR. Hypercalcemia of malignancy revisited. J Clin Invest 1988;82:1.
4. Bajorunas DR. Clinical manifestations of cancer-related hypercalcemia. Semin Oncol 1990;17:16–25.
5. Broadus AD, Mangia M, Ikeda K, et al. Humoral hypercalcemia of cancer. Identification of a novel parathyroid hormone-like peptide. N Engl J Med 1988;319:556.
6. Burtis WJ, Brady TG, Orloff JJ, et al. Immunochemical characterization of circulating parathyroid hormone related protein in patients with humoral hypercalcemia of cancer. N Engl J Med 1990;322:1106.
7. Hortobagyi GN, Theriault RL, Porter L, et al. Efficacy of pamidronate in reducing skeletal complications in patients with breast cancer and lytic bone metastases. Protocol 19 Aredia Breast Cancer Study Group. N Engl J Med 1996;335:1785–1791.
8. Kanis JA, Urwin GH, Gray RES, et al. Effects of intravenous etidronate disodium on skeletal and calcium metabolism. Ann Intern Med 1987;82:55.
9. Mannix KA, Carmichael J, Harris AL, et al. Single high dose infusions of aminohydroxypropylidine diphosphonate for severe malignant hypercalcemia. Cancer 1989;64:1358.
10. Body JJ, Mancini I. Bisphosphonates for cancer patients: Why, how and when? Support Care Cancer 2002;10:399–407.
11. Berenson JR, Rosen LS, Howell A, et al. Zoledronic acid reduces skeletal-related events in patients with osteolytic metastases. Cancer 2001;91:1191–1200.
12. Hillner BE, Ingle JN, Chlebowski RT, et al. ASCO 2003 update on the role of bisphosphonates and bone health issues in women with breast cancer. J Clin Oncol 2003;21:4042–4057.
13. Warell RP, Israel R, Friscone M, et al. Gallium nitrate for acute treatment of cancer-related hypercalcemia: A randomized, double-blind comparison to calcitonin. Ann Intern Med 1988;108:669.
14. Mundy GR. Pathophysiology of cancer-associated hypercalcemia. Semin Oncol 1990;17:10.
15. Elias EG, Reynoso G, Mittleman A. Control of hypercalcemia with mithramycin. Ann Surg 1972;175:431.
16. Percival RC, Yates AJP, Gray RES, et al. Role of glucocorticoids in the management of hypercalcemia. BMJ 1984;289:287.

V

Brain Metastases from Breast Cancer

Erik C. Parker and
Patrick J. Kelly

What is the scope of the problem?

Even though metastases to organs other than the brain are more common, brain metastases are more debilitating and more rapidly fatal if untreated than metastases to other organ systems. Twenty-five percent (or 131,000) of the 527,000 cancer patients expected to die each year in the United States ultimately develop intracranial metastases.[1] Brain metastases from solid tumors are solitary in about 50% to 65% of the cases when the diagnosis is made during life.[2] In 9% of the patients, the brain metastasis may be the only apparent site of the cancer.[3] Statistics indicate that patients treated by operation and irradiation[4,5] survive longer with a higher quality of life than those who undergo radiation therapy alone.[4,6–8] Surprisingly, only a small percentage of these patients are ever offered a surgical procedure.

Other than lung cancer, breast cancer is the most common source of metastases to the central nervous system (CNS). In contrast to most other cancers, breast cancer more commonly tends to involve all intracranial and intraspinal compartments—bone, meninges, parenchyma—and can involve two or more compartments simultaneously. Breast cancer metastases are frequently more slowly growing and more sensitive to radiation and chemotherapy than metastatic cancers from other organ systems. The goal of surgical intervention is to decompress brain and spinal cord to preserve neurologic function and provide the time necessary for chemotherapy and radiation therapy to exert their efficacy.

The following paragraphs describe the patterns of breast cancer metastases to the CNS and the symptoms and signs associated with these lesions. The various elements of the diagnostic workup are outlined, and the therapeutic options for CNS metastases from breast cancer are discussed.

CLINICAL PRESENTATIONS

What are the anatomic patterns of central nervous system involvement?

Metastatic tumors in general, and tumors from the breast in particular, reach the CNS primarily by the intravascular route. Tumor cells from the primary site or from a non-CNS metastatic deposit, notably the lung, enter the bloodstream and are carried to capillary networks in the CNS. These blood-borne metastatic tumor cells are deposited there and continue to grow in this new location. In addition, tumor cells can enter the veins and be carried to other venous plexuses located within the vertebral bodies of the spine or within the spinal canal, where the deposited tumor cells can then grow as an enlarging solid mass.

Blood-borne metastatic tumors can reach and grow in any tissue supplied by blood vessels: bone, meninges (coverings of the brain), and within the substance of the brain itself or within the spinal cord. Breast metastases seem to exploit these opportunities more than most metastatic tumors. In general, breast cancer metastatic to the CNS is classified into three broad categories: (1) intra-axial (within the substance of the brain), (2) extra-axial (outside the substance of the brain), and (3) diffuse cerebrospinal fluid (CSF) dissemination.

What is the presentation of intra-axial lesions?

The most common site of metastatic tumor deposits is at the junction of the gray and white matter of the cerebral hemispheres. Thus, most of these lesions are just beneath the cortical layer on the "surface" of the brain. However, the cortical surface is made up of the hills and valleys of the gyri and convolutions and the sulci and fissures, respectively. A metastatic tumor located at the gray–white junction in the crown of a gyrus can seem very superficial and just beneath the skull on contrast-enhanced CT. In contrast, a metastatic tumor at the gray–white junction at the depths of a deep sulcus or fissure may appear to be 4 to 5 cm below the surface of the brain (Fig. 32–4).

Occasional breast metastatic tumors, however, can be found deep within the substance of the cerebral hemispheres in deep gray matter masses such as the basal ganglia or the thalamus. Metastases can also occur to the choroid plexus, which is located in the lateral, third, and fourth ventricles. Additionally, 15% of metastatic tumors can be found in the cerebellum.

Probably because the brain stem receives 10% of the blood supply to the CNS, about 10% of all metastatic tumors can be found in the brain stem.

What is the presentation of extra-axial metastases?

A small percentage of metastatic breast tumors target the dural covering of the brain or diploic layer of the skull. These usually grow intracranially and compress the surface of the brain (Fig. 32–5). Metastases to the dura or bone at the base of the skull compress the base of the brain or the cranial nerves located there. On occasion, skull metastases can grow outward as well as internally, causing a protrusion or deformity of the skull in this region. In these cases, patients will complain of a firm, enlarging "bump" on the head.

Dural metastases can grow along the surface of the brain and present as an extensive sheet of tumor covering a large portion of the cerebral cortex. More usually, however, the dural-based lesion grows as a defined mass and locally compresses the cerebral cortex. This pattern is similar to the growth pattern of meningiomas, benign primary tumors of the dura, which are not metastatic. Nevertheless, metastatic breast tumors growing in this fashion can occasionally be confused with meningiomas and will not infrequently invade the arachnoid sac and pial covering of the brain to invade and derive blood supply from the brain itself.

Metastatic tumors can grow into the spinal canal directly from a metastatic deposit to some element of the vertebra (usually the vertebral body), narrow the spinal canal, and compress the spinal cord. In addition, metastatic tumor cells carried to the spinal canal through the vertebral venous (Batson's) plexus and deposited in the epidural fat surrounding the spinal cord can grow, restrict the diameter of the spinal canal, and compress the spinal cord in the absence of any obvious bone involvement.

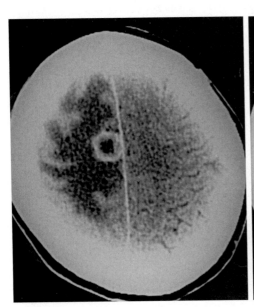
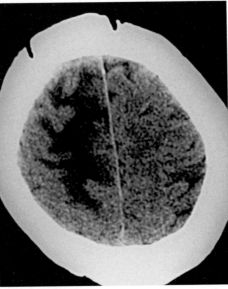

Figure 32–4 Preoperative (*left*) and postoperative (*right*) contrast-enhanced CT scans showing an intra-axial metastatic tumor from breast in a 48-year-old woman. Note the subcortical location, which appears deep below the surface of the brain but which is, in fact, just beneath the interhemispheric fissure. Note also the significant degree of white matter edema. The postoperative contrast-enhanced CT scan confirms complete excision of the tumor. The white matter edema may require weeks to resolve.

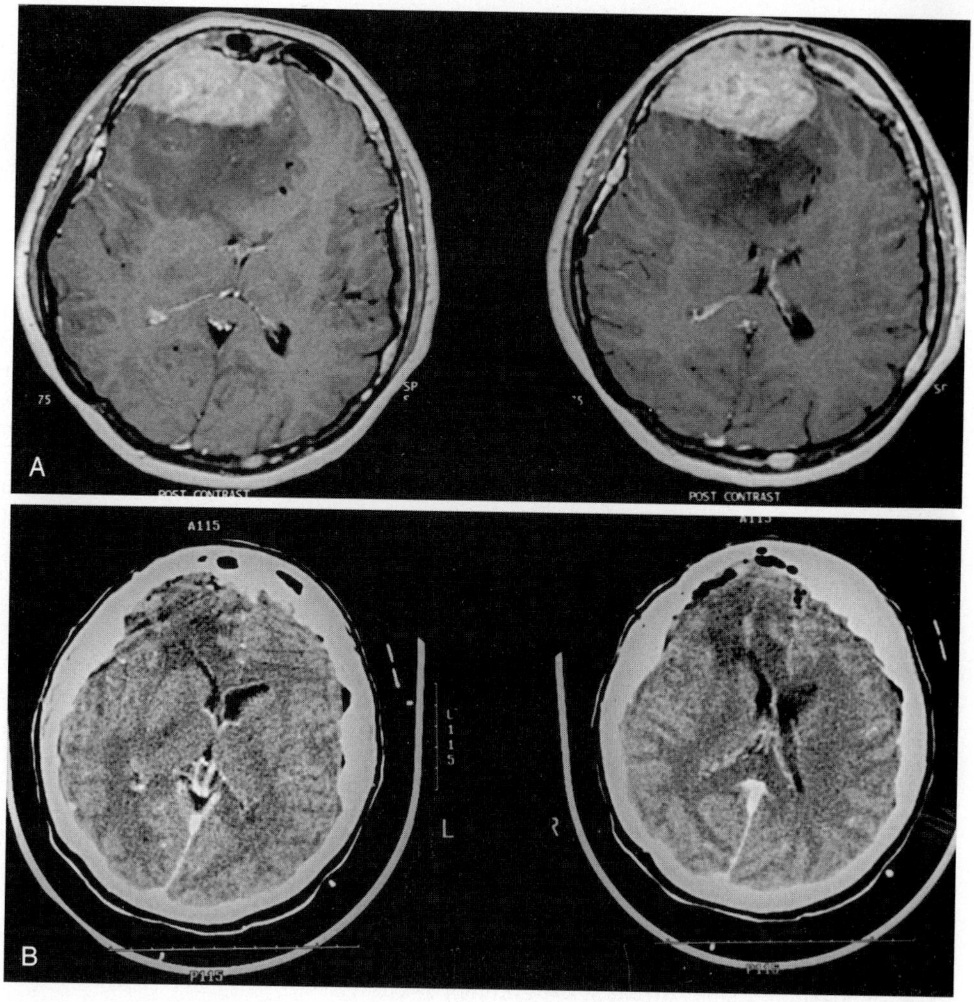

Figure 32–5 *A,* A preoperative gadolinium-enhanced MRI scan showing a breast carcinoma metastasis to the skull. This has eroded through the dura in the right frontal region and invaded the frontal lobe. Note the edema and mass effect in the brain as evidenced by the compression of the ventricular system. *B,* Postoperative contrast-enhanced CT scan after resection of the tumor and cranioplasty. Note the absence of mass effect and that the ventricular system has now resumed a normal configuration.

How does metastatic breast cancer disseminate through the cerebrospinal fluid?

Metastatic breast tumor cells can enter the CSF in three major ways. First, tumor cells transmitted to blood vessels that traverse the subarachnoid space or are located in the thin pial surface can rupture through the wall of the vessel and seed the CSF. Second, and more frequently, large or small tumor metastatic deposits can grow through the cortex and pial surface and thus be in contact with the CSF, which bathes the surface of the brain. These cells then break off the main tumor mass and are carried by the CSF to distant locations. Finally, tumor cells can be deposited and grow in tufts of choroid plexus, a structure composed of fine blood vessels that manufactures most of the CSF. Choroid plexus is located within each of the components of the ventricular system (cavities of the brain). Tumor cells can break off the metastatic tumor mass growing from the choroid plexus and seed the CSF.

CSF is produced in the ventricles and exits at the base of the brain. In its flow pattern, CSF then bathes the entire surface of the brain, spinal cord, cranial nerves, and spinal nerves; passes along the base of the brain; and then passes over the surface of the brain to absorption sites, most of which are located along the large dural sinuses (veins). Tumor cells that enter the CSF can survive and be transported to and deposited on any structure bathed by CSF. Tumor cells transported in this way frequently grow as a sheet of cells within the arachnoid space and cover the brain surface, surrounding and not infrequently invading cranial and spinal nerves.

What is the clinical presentation of carcinomatous meningitis?

Interference with the flow of CSF causing hydrocephalus is the most frequent result of CSF dissemination by most metastatic tumors. Occasionally, metastatic tumor cells disseminated through the CSF and subarachnoid space can induce an inflammatory reaction and produce symptoms similar to bacterial or viral meningitis; this is more commonly associated with metastatic breast cancer than with other solid metastatic tumors.

How do metastatic brain tumors cause symptoms?

In general, metastatic tumors produce symptoms in three ways: (1) by impairing the function of, or destroying, brain or cranial nerve tissue; (2) by producing seizures; and (3) by causing increased intracranial pressure (Table 32–14).

Table 32–14   Signs and Symptoms of Brain Metastases

Abnormal gait
Aphasia
Headache
Focal weakness
Mental status change
Seizure
Visual field deficit

Impaired Function or Destruction of Brain or Cranial Nerve Tissue

Breast tumors metastatic to the substance of the brain are growing masses that compress adjacent normal tissue. In addition, many of these tumors parasitize the blood supply to the brain and thus reduce the supply of oxygen and nutrients to brain tissue. Finally, some tumors cause chemical abnormalities around them that poison the surrounding normal cells and cause dysfunction of the neurons and swelling. These factors, alone or in combination, impair or inhibit the function of that part of the brain.

The symptoms that result depend on what part of the brain is involved. A metastatic tumor in the motor strip will cause weakness of the lower part of the face, arm, or leg, singly or severally, on the opposite side of the body. A tumor in the occipital lobe may cause loss of some or all of the visual field on the side opposite the tumor. Destruction of large parts of the dominant frontal lobe (the left frontal lobe in most persons) or of the connections between the frontal lobes may cause personality changes.

However, there are parts of the brain that can be destroyed with no noticeable change in the patient's neurologic function or behavior. Large regions of the right frontal lobe and some of the right temporal lobe can be destroyed without noticeable effects. Metastatic tumors in these "silent" regions produce symptoms by the mechanisms listed below.

At the base of the skull, metastatic tumors can compress cranial nerves such as the optic nerves and chiasm, the fifth cranial nerve (which transmits sensation from the face), or the lower cranial nerves (which control important functions such as swallowing).

Seizures

Tumors in functional brain regions can cause electrical dysfunction (irritation). This is due to chemical abnormalities produced by the tumor in the local environment of the neuronal elements. In addition, loss of oxygen and nutrients owing to the tumor's parasitizing the blood supply of the neurons can cause cortical irritation. Finally, destruction of inhibitory neurons by the tumor can "disinhibit" other neurons, allowing them to discharge with a higher frequency than usual. Any or all of these factors can result in abnormal brain electrical phenomena that clinically manifest as seizures (also called "fits," convulsions, or epilepsy). The actual clinical presentation of the seizures frequently depends on the region of the brain involved. Seizures can be focal or generalized.

Focal Seizures. Focal seizures are not associated with a loss of consciousness and can be sensory or motor. For example, metastatic tumors in or near the motor strip can produce focal motor seizures, which present as twitching of the face, arm, or leg, or all three. Tumors in the sensory areas of the brain can cause sensory seizures: episodic paresthesia (pins-and-needles sensations) on the opposite side of the body. Lesions located in the occipital regions in or near the visual areas can cause abnormal visual phenomena—formed or nonformed hallucinations such as flashing lights in the opposite (contralateral) visual field.

Generalized Seizures

Partial Complex Seizures. These are usually associated with lesions of the deep temporal area (mesial or hippocampal regions) or base (orbital surface) of the frontal lobe. Brief episodes in which the patient loses consciousness and will not respond to those around him or her (absence attacks) and episodes in which the patient in this brief unresponsive period exhibits a programmed and stereotypic movement (automatism) are referred to as *partial complex seizures.* In addition, an olfactory hallucination in which the patient experiences an unpleasant odor (frequently the smell of burning rubber) is called an *uncinate fit* and is characteristic of mesial temporal or basal frontal lesions.

Grand Mal Seizures. Grand mal seizures can occur with any intracranial tumor in any location. These generalized seizures are familiar to most medical practitioners and nonmedical people alike. In these spells, the patient loses consciousness, extends head, arms, and legs (tonic phase), and then "shakes" (clonic phase). The jaw muscles clamp shut, the tongue or the inside of the mouth is frequently bitten, and the patient's airway can become compromised. Patients may also lose bladder control. Occasionally, the seizure may be preceded by focal components, such as twitching of the face or arm or a loss of the ability to speak, before the electrical disturbance spreads to both sides of the brain to produce the grand mal seizure.

Increased Intracranial Pressure

The inside of the skull can be considered a nonexpandable closed box. There is room within for only the brain, its blood supply, and spinal fluid. The mass of a metastatic tumor within the cranial cavity takes up space. In addition, swelling of brain tissue around the tumor adds to the mass effect. As the mass grows, blood vessels and spinal fluid spaces can be compressed, which accommodates the growing mass for a time. The brain can re-form around the growing mass as water between the cells of the brain and within the cells is redistributed. Finally, no further shifts of blood or water are possible, and pressure inside the skull begins to increase.

There is another mechanism for increased intracranial pressure: hydrocephalus. As explained earlier, most of the CSF is produced by the choroid plexus located within each of the ventricles of the brain. It flows to the base of the brain and then around the surface of the brain, where it is finally absorbed. All elements of the ventricular system are normally in communication. Fluid produced in the two lateral ventricles passes to the midline third ventricle by means of the foramina of Monro. This fluid, as well as fluid produced by the choroid plexus of the third ventricle, passes through the narrow aqueduct of Sylvius to the fourth ventricle, located between the brain stem and the cerebellum, and from there to the basilar cisterns around the brain stem (cisterna magna and cerebellopontine angle cisterns).

A tumor mass that compresses any component of this fluid pathway can cause the buildup of fluid upstream from that obstruction. The ventricles of the brain enlarge, and this is called *obstructive hydrocephalus*. Obstructive hydrocephalus is most frequently noted in patients with metastatic lesions in the posterior fossa, brain stem, or cerebellum. Here the tumor mass and associated swelling (edema) deform and ultimately obliterate the fourth ventricle, the aqueduct of Sylvius, or both.

Hydrocephalus can also result from subarachnoid metastases that obstruct the flow of spinal fluid along the base or surface of the brain (communicating hydrocephalus). Obstructive and communicating hydrocephalus results in retention of an increased amount of CSF inside the "closed box" of the intracranial cavity. This results in increased intracranial pressure.

As increased intracranial pressure becomes symptomatic, patients initially complain of a dull headache. Characteristically, the headache occurs in the morning but persists throughout the day and night. It can awaken the patient from sleep; not infrequently it is associated with nausea and, in some instances, vomiting. As pressure increases, blood delivery to the brain decreases, and this results in nonspecific symptoms such as mental sluggishness and recent memory dysfunction.

The intracranial cavity is divided into three separate compartments by membranes formed by the dura mater. These include the supratentorial and infratentorial compartments separated from each other by the tentorium, and the right and left supratentorial compartments separated by the falx cerebri. The cerebral hemispheres occupy the right and left supratentorial compartments; the brain stem and cerebellum occupy the infratentorial compartment (posterior fossa). As intracranial pressure continues to increase, part of the brain itself is shifted into another compartment of the intracranial cavity. This is called *herniation*, which causes its own set of symptoms and signs.

What are the signs and symptoms of herniation?

In transfalcine herniation, a large mass in one hemisphere pushes the medial aspect of that hemisphere across the falx into the other supratentorial compartment. When this happens, patients can become confused, are occasionally disoriented, and lose control of bowel and bladder function.

Herniation of the medial temporal lobe across the tentorium into the infratentorial space results in compression of the midbrain—a component of the brain stem that controls consciousness and eye movements and transmits motor control from the cerebral hemispheres to the lower brain stem, spinal cord, and eventually the spinal nerves that activate the muscles of the face, arms, and legs. Compression of the midbrain results in papillary abnormalities, then paralysis and abnormal motor reflexes (decerebrate and decorticate posturing), and finally coma. The prognosis is very poor once this scenario has occurred, and the probability of useful survival is low, despite aggressive therapy delivered at this late stage.

The goal of our efforts in the management of CNS metastases from breast cancer is early diagnosis and treatment to prevent neurologic progression due to tumor mass effect and increased intracranial pressure. Treatment must be instituted long before herniation becomes a possibility.

How do calvarial metastases present?

These lesions frequently deform the skull as the inner and outer tables of the calvarium are pushed apart by the expanding mass in the diploë. The protruding outer table can result in a cosmetic deformity if located in front of the hairline or in a painful hard or firm protrusion of the skull beneath the scalp when located behind the hairline. Breast metastatic tumors that break through the inner table of the skull and grow intracranially frequently invade the dura and cross the arachnoid space to compress and usually invade the underlying brain tissue. In this case, and depending on the anatomic location of the lesion, patients can experience seizures or neurologic deficit similar to the situation noted with intra-axial tumor masses. A large mass growing from the skull intracranially will eventually raise intracranial pressure.

How does breast cancer affect the spinal cord?

Patients with metastatic lesions that compress the spinal cord usually present with localized pain that corresponds to the level of cord compression. Percussion over this area will evoke or worsen the pain. Patients with bone involvement may complain of pain for many weeks before the onset of neurologic deficit as a result of spinal cord compression.

As the spinal cord compression continues, neurologic deficit progresses over the next few hours or days. The patient complains of numbness of the body and legs below the region of cord compression and difficulty walking, due at first to a proprioceptive gait disturbance and then to weakness. Eventually, the weakness in the legs (for thoracic lesions) and arms and legs (for upper and mid-cervical regions) becomes noticeable and progresses to complete flaccid paralysis in hours or days if not treated. Not infrequently, when the expanding mass is located lateral to the spinal cord, the sensory loss to pain and temperature is noted on one side of the body, and the muscle weakness is noted on the opposite side. If untreated, the sensory and motor deficit will progress to bilateral involvement. Bowel and bladder control is lost as the neurologic deficit progresses.

Cauda equina (lumbar and sacral) metastases produce back pain and occasionally radicular pain in the legs. The neurologic deficit may involve only one nerve root initially but then progresses over the next several days to involve several nerve roots and then the entire cauda equina. Neurologic examination will reveal percussion tenderness, flaccid paraplegia, areflexia, and sensory loss below the level of the lesion involving the sacral dermatomes.

How does breast cancer affect the pituitary gland?

Metastases to the pituitary gland are not common in most cancers. However, in series of breast cancer patients, pituitary metastases can account for as much as 20% of all intracranial metastases.[8] A growing mass lesion in the pituitary fossa can cause endocrine dysfunction, headaches, and ultimately visual field impairment as the lesion enlarges.

What is carcinomatous meningitis?

The symptoms of carcinomatous meningitis are similar to those of any meningitis: headache, photophobia, stiff neck, and low-grade fever. Elevation of the supine patient's legs off the bed will frequently result in pain in the back and in a sciatic distribution. Sometimes, the pain is referred also to the occipital region. These patients are frequently lethargic and occasionally confused. Elevation of intracranial pressure can also be noted if the meningeal process impedes the flow of CSF.

How is central nervous system metastasis diagnosed?

A history of breast cancer months or even several years in the past should raise suspicion of a CNS metastasis in a patient presenting with headaches, diplopia, sensory abnormalities, focal weakness, neck or back pain, or seizures. In fact, the existence of any of these symptoms should prompt a CT or magnetic resonance imaging (MRI) examination of the head or spine, depending on the symptoms. The clinician should record the histologic subtype of the breast tumor and question the patient on how it was found as well as how and how soon it was treated. Was the tumor treated by biopsy and radiation, chemotherapy, or both; by lumpectomy; or by radical mastectomy? Were any lymph nodes positive for tumor? The patient should be questioned about symptoms that could reflect pulmonary, liver, or bone metastases. A nonaggressively treated primary tumor or the presence of positive nodes or distant metastases increases the likelihood of future CNS metastases. The clinician should carefully record the duration of the neurologic symptoms and their mode of onset. The clinical manifestations of seizures, especially focality of onset, can provide important information regarding the anatomic localization of the CNS lesion.

A general physical examination is important to investigating the presence of non-CNS disease, which may increase suspicion of the existence of CNS metastases, and assessing the risk-to-benefit ratio of any therapeutic interventions for CNS metastases, if found. Each breast should be examined for recurrent disease or metastases to the other breast. Auscultation of the lungs may reveal evidence of pulmonary metastases.

DIAGNOSTIC MODALITIES

What are the roles of computed tomography and magnetic resonance imaging?

The introduction of CT in the early 1970s revolutionized the evaluation of cancer patients for the existence of CNS metastatic disease. With CT, clinicians could actually see metastatic tumors directly instead of having to infer their presence and location indirectly from intracranial shifts of blood vessels and parts of the ventricular system from their normal positions on cerebral angiography and ventriculography. Additionally, CT scanning allowed the discovery of tumors before they became symptomatic. Because of these advantages, CT rapidly became the standard diagnostic procedure for the detection and localization of metastases.

Metastatic tumors produce swelling (edema) of the surrounding brain tissue. This is easily detected on CT because it is hypodense in comparison with normal brain tissue. More importantly, metastatic tumor masses in general, and breast cancer metastatic lesions in particular, accept contrast on the contrast-enhanced CT series and appear as a white circumscribed mass with hypodense (edematous) brain tissue surrounding the lesion. In addition, multiple metastatic lesions can be noted. This is important information if surgery is a consideration.

CT scanning also provides information on the degree of the mass effect produced by the lesion and surrounding edema. The midline of the brain, some of the more prominent sulci and fissures, and the ventricular system are usually seen very well on CT scanning. Enlargement of the ventricular system owing to hydrocephalus is easily detected.

MRI provides many of the same benefits of CT scanning while offering several advantages. MRI provides exquisite anatomic detail of the normal structures of the brain and spinal cord. It is also much more sensitive than CT and has become the imaging modality of choice in the detection of small intracranial metastases. These lesions are characterized by edema (prolonged signal on T2-weighted images) and by contrast enhancement, which shows the metastatic tumor deposit. The contrast agent used with MRI, gadolinium, has a much lower potential for toxicity than traditional contrast agents used during CT scanning. Recent studies have established the utility of triple-dose gadolinium administration in demonstrating smaller metastatic lesions, especially in patients with a single known metastasis or equivocal findings on previous MRI examination.[9,10] MRI also provides a safe, effective, and noninvasive method of evaluating the spinal cord when spinal metastases are suspected.

MRI can be used to provide additional diagnostic information about the characteristics of a lesion. Radiation-induced necrosis, an infrequent complication of brain irradiation, can be indistinguishable from tumor progression using conventional CT and MRI techniques. When the clinical situation warrants further investigation, magnetic resonance spectroscopy may be useful. This technique, which provides information on the relative concentration of various compounds in a given volume of tissue, can be used to differentiate between tumor progression and radiation necrosis as well as other lesions of similar appearance such as cerebral abscess and demyelinating disease.[11,12]

An area in which CT scanning remains the most useful modality is imaging of bony structures because it provides exquisite bone detail. This is an important consideration in the evaluation of metastatic breast cancer, which can metastasize to the skull. The clinician should request bone windows, which allow improved visualization of the bony structures including the skull base and calvarium. In addition, CT is also useful in the evaluation of spinal metastases, especially when the vertebrae are involved.

With MRI's ever-increasing availability and its inherent advantages, it has become the screening tool of choice for evaluating the CNS in patients with metastatic cancer (Fig. 32–6). CT scanning remains useful, however, because it is better tolerated by many patients, provides superior imaging of

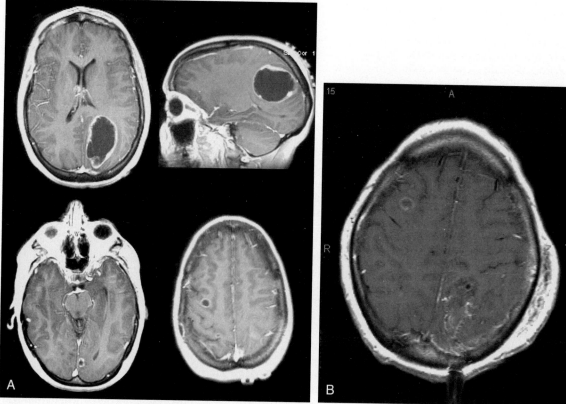

Figure 32–6. *A,* A preoperative gadolinium-enhanced MRI scan reveals multiple ring-enhancing lesions. The largest of these lesions is located in the left parietal lobe and is exerting mass effect on the ventricular system and surrounding brain parenchyma. Multiple smaller metastases are present and involve both hemispheres. The location of these lesions at the gray–white junction is typical of metastatic lesions. *B,* A postoperative MRI reveals complete excision of the left parietal lesion with resolution of mass effect. The remaining lesions will be treated with radiation therapy.

bony structures, and is quick and inexpensive. Additionally, it may be used with patients for whom MRI is contraindicated because of the presence of a pacemaker or some other implanted medical device.

When is lumbar puncture useful in diagnosing central nervous system metastases?

Examination of spinal fluid obtained by lumbar puncture, C1-2 puncture, or cisterna magna puncture is necessary to establish the presence of carcinomatous meningitis and in situations in which there is suspicion of tumor cell seeding of the CSF. Lumbar puncture should not be performed without CT or MRI to exclude an intracranial mass lesion. Lumbar puncture should not be done if there is evidence of increased intracranial pressure, a midline shift on CT or MRI, or evidence of other significant mass effect.

THERAPEUTIC OPTIONS

When is surgery indicated?

The decision to remove an intracranial metastasis depends on a careful analysis of the risks and benefits of the surgery.

Obviously, no surgeon is ever going to cure cancer by removing a distant metastasis. However, as a baseline, it is good to consider that the mean survival of a patient with metastatic disease to the CNS treated without surgery is about 3 months. Removing metastatic tumor masses from the brain prolongs survival. The degree of prolongation will depend on many factors, including the biology of the original tumor, the presence of extra-CNS metastases, and the age and general medical condition of the patient.

There is a great deal of benefit in resecting a solitary brain metastasis in a patient with a past history of breast cancer, no other evidence of disease, and a long tumor-free interval between the initial primary and the discovery of the CNS metastasis. In contrast, there is only modest benefit in resecting a metastasis in a patient recently diagnosed with breast cancer with multiple metastases in other organ systems.

Surgical risk relates to the anatomic location of the metastatic tumor and its depth below the surface of the brain. A metastasis can be removed from the nondominant frontal lobe with very low risk. The risk of removing a lesion in the brain stem is high and usually unacceptable. In the past, clinicians were pessimistic about the benefit derived from the surgical resection of a solitary metastatic brain tumor because the benefit of resection did not outweigh the risk of classic procedures to resect them. However, improvements in surgical techniques and perioperative management have resulted in significant reductions in surgical mortality and morbidity.[1,5,6,13,14] It has for some time been generally agreed that surgical excision is indicated in a medically stable patient harboring a "surgically accessible" solitary intracranial metastasis.[14,15] Randomized prospective trials have demonstrated significantly improved length of survival for patients undergoing resection of single metastases followed by whole-brain irradiation as compared with those receiving radiation alone. One such study demonstrated an increase in length of survival from 15 to 40 weeks and duration of functional independence from 8 to 38 weeks.[16] Another trial had similar findings, with survival increased from 24 to 40 weeks and independence from 14 to 30 weeks.[17]

Aggressive surgical treatment is becoming more accepted in the setting of multiple or recurrent metastatic brain tumors. A retrospective study compared the outcomes of matched patients with either single or multiple brain metastases. Patients with multiple lesions undergoing resection of all lesions displayed results similar to those undergoing resection of a solitary metastasis. Those with multiple tumors who underwent surgery in which all known lesions were not resected, however, had a significantly shorter median postoperative survival and lower rates of symptomatic improvement. Operative morbidity and mortality were not significantly different among the three groups. These findings led the authors of this study to conclude that patients with limited systemic disease and more than one accessible metastatic brain tumor should be considered for surgical resection of all such lesions.[18] Similarly, reoperation for recurrent intracranial metastases is becoming more frequently advocated. It has been demonstrated that in younger patients with controlled systemic disease and a high functional status, repeat resection of these lesions can improve outcome. When properly selected, patients undergoing second and even third operations may enjoy prolonged survival and improved quality of life.[19]

Many metastatic lesions lie close to the cortical surface, are macroscopically circumscribed, and can be resected by conventional craniotomy with acceptable levels of mortality and morbidity. Some neurosurgeons recommend not operating on more deeply seated tumors, however, especially in the dominant hemisphere, where the risk is higher and the benefit is not as clear.[5] The use of stereotaxis is often of benefit in cases involving surgically complex tumor locations.

What is nonstereotactic craniotomy?

Traditional approaches to the removal of any brain lesion (including metastatic tumors) involve opening the scalp, skull, and dural coverings of the brain. These techniques have evolved over the past 100 years. With the exception of stereotactic guidance and the operating microscope, they have changed little in the past 50 years. Classic craniotomy still has a place in the resection of skull- and dural-based lesions and skull-based metastases. There is rarely a problem in finding these superficial lesions and their borders. In addition, these lesions must be dissected away from invaded brain tissue in many cases, and adequate exposure is necessary.

Classic craniotomy for intra-axial metastatic tumors employed large scalp flaps and craniotomy openings that exposed much normal brain tissue to unnecessary injury. Localization methods for metastatic tumors were qualitative and imprecise, and in some cases surgeons could actually miss the metastatic tumor—especially when the lesions were small or deep below the surface of the brain. The incorporation of surgical ultrasonographic imaging increased the number of cases in which a surgeon could locate and completely resect the lesion.

What is stereotactic resection?

With the advent of CT and MRI, surgeons began rethinking their surgical approaches to common intracranial tumors. These computer-based imaging modalities provide precise information on the anatomic localization and extent of intracranial tumors. In addition, CT and MRI provide a three-dimensionally-precise database that can be transported to a stereotactically defined surgical field. Imaging-based stereotaxis improves the accuracy with which CT and MRI information can be used in surgical planning for the removal of metastatic tumors and also makes minimally invasive resection techniques for metastatic tumors possible.[15,20]

During the past 2 decades, we have developed and refined the technology of computer-assisted volumetric stereotactic removal of a wide variety of intra-axial lesions, including metastatic tumors.[15,20–22] The technique has proved especially useful in the safe resection of metastatic tumors from important subcortical areas. The technique provides a safe, minimally invasive method of removing solitary metastatic tumors. We are now evaluating the benefit of removing two or more lesions in selected cases.

When using frame-based stereotaxis, computer simulation of the operation is carried out from a preoperative database comprising stereotactic CT, MRI, and digital angiography (DA). This information is acquired with the patient's head held in a CT- or MRI-compatible stereotactic head frame, placed under local anesthesia. The tumor volume is reconstructed from the imaging studies.[15,23] The surgeon chooses a surgical approach, and the surgical procedure is simulated on a computer display terminal.

The actual procedure is done under general anesthesia. The stereotactic head frame is reapplied, and the surgery is done through a 2- to 3-inch incision and a circular bone opening. A computer display shows the relationship of the CT- and MRI-defined tumor volume to the three-dimensionally-defined surgical field. These computer-generated images allow the surgeon to find not only the tumor but also the interface between tumor and surrounding brain tissue (Fig. 32–7). Thus, the surgical approach is preplanned, is direct, and exposes no more brain tissue than absolutely necessary to remove the tumor.

A more recently developed technology, which has become very widespread over the past few years, is frameless stereotaxis. This system, although less precise and therefore less well suited to deeply located tumors, does not require the placement of a head frame during the data acquisition phase. Instead, fiducials, markers that are visible on CT and MRI scans, are placed on the patient's head before obtaining preoperative imaging studies. These fiducials remain in place until the time of the operation. When the patient is under general anesthesia and the head has been secured in place, the fiducials are used to register the patient's current position in space relative to some fixed reference point. A computer that has been loaded with the CT or MRI information then

Figure 32–7. Frame-based, computer-assisted stereotactic craniotomy with volumetric excision of a metastatic tumor. The reformatted CT- and MRI-defined limits of the tumor are presented to the surgeon on a computer display screen as well as into a heads-up display unit on the operating microscope (A). The surgeon exposes the tumor by a stereotactically placed circular bone opening. The computer display helps the surgeon know where the tumor stops and normal brain tissue begins. (From Kelly PJ, Kall BA, Goerss SJ, et al. Results of computer-assisted stereotactic laser resection of deep-seated intracranial lesions. Mayo Clin Proc 1986;61: 20–27.)

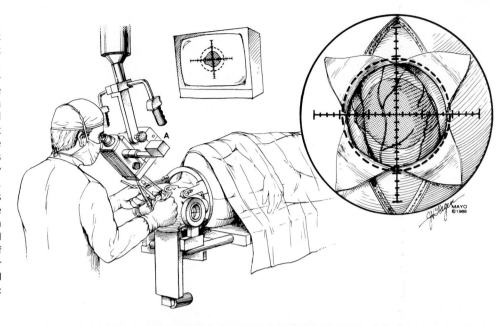

Figure 32–8. An example of use of a frameless stereotactic system. In this case, the Cygnus system (Compass International Inc., Rochester, MN) is being used in planning the resection of a metastatic tumor. Following registration of the system, the location of a pointer placed into the operative field is displayed in real time on the computer screen. This location is indicated by cross-hairs, which are superimposed over sagittal, coronal, and axial images as well as a three-dimensional reconstruction of the MRI data. Although not as precise as frame-based stereotaxis, this allows very accurate placement of scalp and bone flaps and can be used during the operation to aid in tumor resection and maintain spatial orientation.

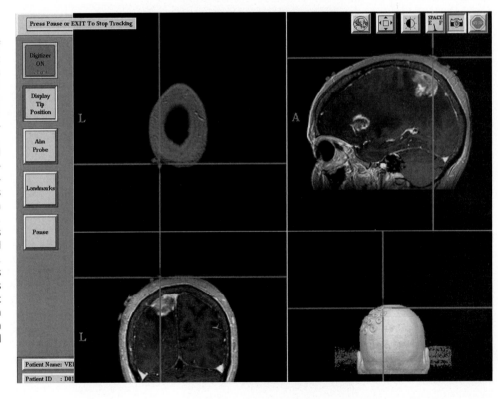

correlates the three-dimensional imaging data to the location and orientation of the patient's head. The system can then be used intraoperatively to view the location of a pointer or some other specialized surgical instrument on a three-dimensional representation of the imaging data. Although this type of stereotaxis is less well suited to cases in which a high degree of precision is required, it can be very useful for placing a skin incision and underlying bone flap for routine tumor resections (Fig. 32–8). This type of approach also has some advantages over frame-based stereotaxis. It avoids the need for a second procedure (placement of the head frame before obtaining the imaging studies), is better tolerated by most patients, and is cost-effective because the fiducials can be placed and studies can be obtained before the patient is admitted, allowing admission on the morning of surgery. Each case must be evaluated independently in order to select the most appropriate form of stereotaxis (if any) for the given resection.

What is stereotactic radiosurgery?

Stereotactic radiosurgery is based on many beams of radiation intersecting at a precise point. At this point, the radiation dose is additive so that the radiation delivered to the location is very high. The patient's head, held in a stereotactic frame, is positioned so that a target, often a metastatic tumor, is in the center of all of these intersecting beams of radiation; the tumor receives a lethal dose of radiation, while the surrounding brain tissue receives a much smaller dose of radiation. Typically, stereotactic radiosurgery is done in a single treatment session. If the therapy is effective, the tumor stops growing, and its cells die within several weeks or months. The dead tissue is eventually cleared from the brain tissue after an inflammatory reaction.

There are two general methods of delivering stereotactic radiosurgery: the Leksell gamma knife and a stereotactic linear accelerator. With the gamma knife, radiation from cobalt 201 sources arranged in a spherical pattern is collimated into narrow beams directed toward the center of the sphere[24] (Fig. 32–9). In stereotactic linear accelerator radiosurgery, a radiation generator tube is rotated around the patient's head, directing the constant beam toward a present center (isocenter) point.[25] Both of these modalities use gamma radiation. The gamma knife beams project toward the center of a sphere; the linear accelerator directs the beam toward a central target as the linear accelerator tube rotates.

There is an important appeal in using stereotactic radiosurgery: it is totally noninvasive. There is no skin incision or bone opening and no brain manipulation, and the procedure can be accomplished during a 1-day hospitalization. Indeed, many centers offer this form of treatment on an outpatient basis. These factors make radiosurgery a cost-effective alternative for the treatment of brain metastases.[26]

Radiosurgery is appropriate for small (<3 cm in diameter) tumors. Larger tumors and those associated with significant swelling around the tumor are not good candidates for stereotactic radiosurgery because more swelling of the surrounding brain parenchyma will occur after radiosurgery in the weeks

and months following treatment. This could result in increased intracranial pressure and mass effect, neurologic deficit, and risk for herniation.

Stereotactic radiosurgery may be useful when other forms of therapy are not appropriate or are of little benefit. An example is a metastatic tumor located in the brain stem. Such tumors are usually associated with a very poor prognosis. In these cases, surgical resection may be contraindicated because of excessive risk for neurologic deficit, and whole-brain radiation therapy is of questionable benefit. Radiosurgery has been shown to be an effective palliative treatment option for this group, with survival times approaching those of patients with metastatic tumors in other parts of the brain.[27] Radiosurgery may also be used to treat patients harboring multiple tumors with good results.[28]

When is radiation therapy indicated?

Even though an apparent gross total excision of metastatic tumor may have been achieved, local postoperative external-beam radiation therapy is usually recommended. This is because microscopic residual tumor may remain following surgical resection and will continue to grow if not treated. Whole-brain irradiation is more controversial. This practice is based on the assumption that other microscopic metastatic tumors, not yet visualized on CT or MRI, may exist throughout the brain. In cases in which surgery or radiosurgery is not an option and whole-brain radiation therapy is used as the primary treatment modality, its efficacy is well documented; median survival time is increased to 4 months, as compared with 1 month for patients treated with steroids alone.[29]

The utility of whole-brain radiation following successful removal of a single brain metastasis is less certain. A prospective trial examined patients who had undergone complete surgical resection of a solitary brain metastasis. Patients were randomized into groups receiving postoperative whole-brain radiotherapy and those receiving no further treatment. Not surprisingly, the patients treated with radiation had lower rates of tumor recurrence or appearance of new metastases. Likewise, they were less likely to die of neurologic causes than those who were not irradiated. However, when survival and length of functional independence were compared, there was no significant difference between the two groups.[30] Similarly, adjuvant whole-brain radiation conferred no improvement in length of survival in patients treated with stereotactic radiosurgery.[28]

Whole-brain radiation is not without complications; most notably, it has been found to be associated with a significant risk for the development of a progressive dementia.[31] Because of concerns about cognitive decline, there is a growing trend toward avoiding postoperative radiation in patients with completely resected tumors, particularly the elderly. With the widespread availability of high-resolution MRI, which is very sensitive for metastatic disease, the use of routine postoperative radiation is now being called into question, and there is ongoing investigation into its role in the treatment of CNS metastatic cancer.

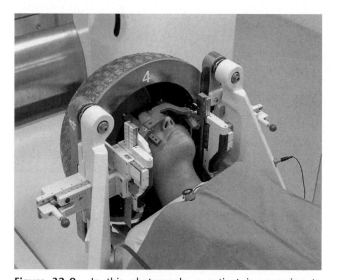

Figure 32–9. In this photograph, a patient is preparing to undergo gamma knife radiosurgery. The patient has been placed in a head frame that has then been attached to the collimator. This collimator directs 201 separate beams of radiation toward the target. This target has been defined during the planning stage of the procedure based on imaging data (usually MRI) obtained with the head frame in place. (Photo courtesy of Elekta, Stockholm, Sweden.)

When is intrathecal chemotherapy indicated?

Intrathecal chemotherapy is considered when there has been documented CSF seeding and in the treatment of carcinomatous meningitis. The chemotherapeutic agents can be administered by repeated lumbar punctures. A more tolerable alternative to many lumbar punctures, however, is the insertion of an Ommaya reservoir. The Ommaya reservoir consists of a medical-grade plastic bubble, which sits permanently under the scalp, connected to a catheter directed through a small hole in the skull into the lateral ventricle of the brain. The bubble (reservoir) may be tapped through the scalp with a thin needle. The chemotherapeutic agent is then instilled into the reservoir and on into the ventricular fluid, which then bathes the entire brain and spinal cord surface with the chemotherapeutic agent as the CSF circulates.

What are the expected results of treatment?

Average survival following resection of a solitary brain metastasis followed by radiation therapy is about 1 year when all types of cancer are considered as a group and for breast cancer in general. Postoperative mean survival in CNS metastatic breast cancer is 11.5 months, 2-year survival is 18%, and 3-year survival is 16%. However, there is wide variation in postoperative survival in breast cancer patients undergoing resection procedures for CNS metastases. This is usually related to the basic malignancy, its degree of local control at the primary site, and metastatic disease in other organ systems. A long tumor-free interval between initial diagnosis and CNS metastasis indicates prolonged survival following removal of the brain metastasis; shorter duration of survival is expected for older patients and those with a poorer preoperative functional status.

Comparison of results between definitive modalities of treatment of brain metastases can be difficult. In the absence of prospective randomized studies, selection bias and other factors can obscure differences in outcome. Although it is clear that most patients treated with either radiosurgery or surgical resection will live longer than those treated with radiation alone, there is a less dramatic difference between these two modes of therapy. Some studies have found that patients treated with surgery have better local control and longer survival than those treated with stereotactic radiosurgery.[32] Others, however, have suggested that there is no benefit to surgery over radiosurgery in selected patients.[33]

Surgical morbidity is directly related to the anatomic location of the lesion and the surgical approach employed. Stortenbecker,[2,34] in 1954, reported a 30-day operative mortality of 24%. Ransohoff,[5] in 1975, reported a 10% mortality (morbidity not available). Haar and Patterson,[13] in their 1972 series, found and 11% mortality and 24% morbidity. Kelly and colleagues,[14] in 1988, reporting on a series of stereotactically resected, centrally located, and deep-seated tumors, found no mortality and 9% morbidity. Postoperative results have improved: postoperative morbidity following stereotactic resection is now less than 6% (unpublished data).

What are the future directions for diagnosis and treatment of central nervous system metastases?

In the future, patient empowerment by information technology and cost consciousness will emphasize quality-of-life issues, reduction of length of hospital stays, and the avoidance of costly rehabilitation and nursing care made necessary by neurologic deficits. Physicians will therefore stress early detection of CNS metastases and low-morbidity, minimally invasive, cost-effective procedures to treat them.

In the past, brain surgery in patients with metastatic disease was considered risky and futile. Spatial errors in locating metastatic tumors by subcortical incision into important brain tissue and large craniotomies to resect large and symptomatic metastatic tumors could result in the disruption of more brain parenchyma than intended, causing postoperative neurologic deficit and an unacceptable quality of life.

Stereotactic techniques have greatly reduced the risk of metastatic tumor resection procedures. Oncologists, who once submitted their patients for brain surgery only as a last resort after radiation therapy had failed to control the CNS metastasis, are now considering surgical resection of the lesion as a first option. This course of action is now considered preferable to external-beam radiation therapy alone, in which a significant risk for dementia exists if survival is prolonged.

Modern, minimally invasive, low-risk surgical options that provide prolonged life expectancy and maintain quality of life from a neurologic standpoint now exist. A recently developed and much promoted method of tumor resection, the use of intraoperative MRI, may prove to be useful. As yet, however, the technology is cumbersome and expensive and has not been shown to provide improved outcomes or reduced morbidity in the treatment of metastatic brain tumors. Development of endoscopic or robotic techniques using frameless stereotactic control may reduce the risk and the cost of removing small CNS metastases.

The detection of CNS metastatic disease is now very straightforward with modern imaging methods such as high-resolution CT and MRI. Intracranial and intraspinal metastatic lesions are detected earlier than in the past and before the patient has developed neurologic deficit. Magnetic resonance perfusion scans and spectroscopy will further increase the sensitivity for the detection of intracranial brain metastases. It is clear that breast cancer patients with good local control of their primary disease can derive significant benefit from surgical resection of metastatic lesions. In the future, surgery will stress minimally invasive techniques that provide maximum tumor removal with much less risk than that associated with neurosurgery in the past. With early detection methods, we will be resecting smaller and smaller lesions from neurologically normal patients.

As the risk of resecting these lesions declines, the employment of surgical and radiosurgical procedures for the treatment of patients with multiple metastases is becoming more commonplace. In addition, as new metastatic lesions to the CNS are discovered, repeat minimally invasive and radiosurgical procedures may prolong quality of life. Future research should be directed toward defining strategies that direct the use of currently available treatment modalities to maximize survival while optimizing quality of life.

REFERENCES

1. Black P. Brain metastasis: Current status and recommended guidelines for management. Neurosurgery 1979;5:617–631.
2. Stortebecker TP. Metastatic tumors of the brain from a neurosurgical point of view; a follow-up study of 158 cases. J Neurosurg 1954;11:84–111.

3. Posner JB, Chernik NL. Intracranial metastases from systemic cancer. Adv Neurol 1978;19:579–592.
4. Galicich JH, Sundaresan N, Thaler HT. Surgical treatment of single brain metastasis. Evaluation of results by computerized tomography scanning. J Neurosurg 1980;53:63–67.
5. Ransohoff J. Surgical management of metastatic tumors. Semin Oncol 1975;2:21–27.
6. Lang EF, Slater J. Metastatic brain tumors. Results of surgical and non-surgical treatment. Surg Clin North Am 1964;44:865–872.
7. Order SE, Hellman S, Von Essen CF, Kligerman MM. Improvement in quality of survival following whole-brain irradiation for brain metastasis. Radiology 1968;91:149–153.
8. Takakura K, Sano K, Hirano A, Hojo S. Metastatic Tumors of the Central Nervous System. Tokyo, Ikagu-Shoin, 1982.
9. Sze G, Johnson C, Kawamura Y, et al. Comparison of single- and triple-dose contrast material in the MR screening of brain metastases. AJNR Am J Neuroradiol 1998;19:821–828.
10. Yuh WT, Tali ET, Nguyen HD, et al. The effect of contrast dose, imaging time, and lesion size in the MR detection of intracerebral metastasis. AJNR Am J Neuroradiol 1995;16:373–380.
11. Kimura T, Sako K, Tohyama Y, et al. Diagnosis and treatment of progressive space-occupying radiation necrosis following stereotactic radiosurgery for brain metastasis: Value of proton magnetic resonance spectroscopy. Acta Neurochir (Wien) 2003;145:557–564.
12. Kimura T, Sako K, Gotoh T, et al. In vivo single-voxel proton MR spectroscopy in brain lesions with ring-like enhancement. NMR Biomed 2001;14:339–349.
13. Haar F, Patterson RH Jr. Surgery for metastatic intracranial neoplasm. Cancer 1972;30:1241–1245.
14. Kelly PJ, Kall BA, Goerss SJ. Results of computed tomography-based computer-assisted stereotactic resection of metastatic intracranial tumors. Neurosurgery 1988;22:7–17.
15. Kelly PJ. Tumor Stereotaxis. Philadelphia, WB Saunders, 1991, pp 358–369.
16. Patchell RA, Tibbs PA, Walsh JW, et al. A randomized trial of surgery in the treatment of single metastases to the brain. N Engl J Med 1990;322:494–500.
17. Vecht CJ, Haaxma-Reiche H, Noordijk EM, et al. Treatment of single brain metastasis: Radiotherapy alone or combined with neurosurgery? Ann Neurol 1993;33:583–590.
18. Bindal RK, Sawaya R, Leavens ME, Lee JJ. Surgical treatment of multiple brain metastases. J Neurosurg 1993;79:210–216.
19. Bindal RK, Sawaya R, Leavens ME, et al. Reoperation for recurrent metastatic brain tumors. J Neurosurg 1995;83:600–604.
20. Kelly PJ, Alker GJ, Jr. A stereotactic approach to deep-seated central nervous system neoplasms using the carbon dioxide laser. Surg Neurol 1981;15:331–334.
21. Kelly PJ, Kall BA, Goerss S, Cascino TL. Results of computer-assisted stereotactic resection of deep-seated intracranial lesions. Mayo Clin Proc 1986;61:20–27.
22. Kelly PJ, Kall BA, Goerss S, Earnest FT. Computer-assisted stereotaxic laser resection of intra-axial brain neoplasms. J Neurosurg 1986;64:427–439.
23. Kelly PJ, Kall BA, Goerss S. Transposition of volumetric information derived from computed tomography scanning into stereotactic space. Surg Neurol 1984;21:465–471.
24. Lunsford LD, Flickinger J, Coffey RJ. Stereotactic gamma knife radiosurgery. Initial North American experience in 207 patients. Arch Neurol 1990;47:169–175.
25. Adler JR, Cox RS, Kaplan I, Martin DP. Stereotactic radiosurgical treatment of brain metastases. J Neurosurg 1992;76:444–449.
26. Rutigliano MJ, Lunsford LD, Kondziolka D, et al. The cost effectiveness of stereotactic radiosurgery versus surgical resection in the treatment of solitary metastatic brain tumors. Neurosurgery 1995;37:445–453; discussion, 453–455.
27. Huang CF, Kondziolka D, Flickinger JC, Lunsford LD. Stereotactic radiosurgery for brainstem metastases. J Neurosurg 1999;91:563–568.
28. Chen JC, O'Day S, Morton D, et al. Stereotactic radiosurgery in the treatment of metastatic disease to the brain. Stereotact Funct Neurosurg 1999;73:60–63.
29. Lagerwaard FJ, Levendag PC, Nowak PJ, et al. Identification of prognostic factors in patients with brain metastases: A review of 1292 patients. Int J Radiat Oncol Biol Phys 1999;43:795–803.
30. Patchell RA, Tibbs PA, Regine WF, et al. Postoperative radiotherapy in the treatment of single metastases to the brain: A randomized trial. JAMA 1998;280:1485–1489.
31. DeAngelis LM, Delattre JY, Posner JB. Radiation-induced dementia in patients cured of brain metastases. Neurology 1989;39:789–796.
32. Bindal AK, Bindal RK, Hess KR, et al. Surgery versus radiosurgery in the treatment of brain metastasis. J Neurosurg 1996;84:748–754.
33. Muacevic A, Kreth FW, Horstmann GA, et al. Surgery and radiotherapy compared with gamma knife radiosurgery in the treatment of solitary cerebral metastases of small diameter. J Neurosurg 1999;91:35–43.
34. Rand RW, Jacques DB, Melbye RW, et al. Gamma knife radiosurgery for metastatic brain tumors. Acta Neurochir Suppl (Wien) 1995;63:85–88.

VI

Spinal Column Metastases from Breast Cancer

Andrea F. Douglas and Paul R. Cooper

Carcinoma of the breast that metastasizes to the spine can adversely affect the patient's quality of life by producing intractable pain and motor, sensory, and sphincter deficits that prevent normal functioning. Prevention of paraplegia and sphincter deficit results in an improved quality of life. Restorative surgery may result in longer survival as well, but available data have failed to make this clear.[1–3]

Advances in imaging of the spine with MRI and high-resolution CT provide heretofore unobtainable information regarding the anatomy of bone involvement and neural compression. These improvements in imaging, along with technical and conceptual advances in surgical management, have resulted in improvement in neurologic outcome and quality of life for patients with metastatic breast tumors to the spine.

Nonetheless, there still exists a certain reluctance on the part of medical and radiation oncologists to integrate surgery into an overall management strategy. Frequently, when surgical therapy is considered, patients have a severe neurologic deficit that is unlikely to respond to treatment. It is worthwhile, then, to review the evolution in management of this entity that has occurred during the past 15 to 20 years.

What are the clinical presentations of breast cancer metastases to the spine?

Eighty-five to 90% of patients with breast cancer who present with spinal metastases already have a known primary lesion, and most already have documented metastatic disease in other locations.

Pain

Pain is the most common first symptom of spinal metastases; even in patients who present with neurologic deficit, careful questioning will reveal that pain preceded the onset of neurologic symptoms by days or weeks. The pain may be constant or exacerbated by changes in position. It may be localized to the site of the spinal metastasis, or it may be radicular and follow a dermatomal pattern from compression of a nerve root within the spinal canal or as it exits the spinal canal in one of the bony neural foramina.

In the cervical spine, pain will characteristically radiate from the neck to the shoulder, arm, or hand. Thoracic pain may be localized to the spine or follow a dermatomal pattern, unilaterally or bilaterally. In the lumbar region, metastases commonly produce lower back pain; when radicular pain is present, it involves the buttock, leg, and foot, and the patient's symptoms may be mistakenly ascribed to a lumbar disc herniation. This is particularly true when spinal involvement is the first presentation of metastatic disease.

Sensory Deficit

Loss or diminution of pinprick or light-touch perception in the trunk may provide a general idea of the level of spinal cord compression in the thoracic spine. Cervical spinal cord compression frequently does not produce upper extremity sensory loss and results in an upper thoracic sensory level. However, the presence of sensory loss or pain in a dermatomal distribution involving an upper extremity may provide reliable localization of the site of the lesion.

Motor Deficit

Motor deficit may result from compression of the spinal cord, nerve roots exiting from the spinal canal, or the nerves of the cauda equina within the spinal canal. When the spinal cord is compressed, the motor deficit will usually be bilateral, although it may be more pronounced on one side or the other. Weakness of the upper extremities is evidence of compression of the cervical spinal cord. Laterally placed cervical lesions may compress a single root and produce unilateral motor deficit confined to one or two muscle groups. Sphincteric dysfunction with urinary retention and loss of voluntary control of the rectal sphincter resulting from cervical or thoracic spinal cord compression is a late sign and is usually present only when motor deficit is profound. However, with compression of the conus medullaris at the T11 through L1 levels, bladder and bowel dysfunction tend to be among the first symptoms.

With metastases at the L1 level and below, motor deficit will result from compression of the peripheral nerves of the cauda equina, and weakness is more likely to be unilateral or more marked on one side than is the case when deficit results from spinal cord compression. When compression at these levels is severe or located centrally within the spinal canal, involvement of the sacral nerve roots will produce sphincter dysfunction. With compression at lower lumbar levels, sphincteric dysfunction may be severe, with simultaneous preservation of proximal motor function in the legs.

Reflex Changes

Compression of the upper motor neurons contained within the spinal cord may produce increased deep tendon reflexes. Lower motor neuron dysfunction caused by cauda equina involvement or compression of a single nerve root within a neural foramen will result in decreased deep tendon reflexes. For the most part, assessment of the deep tendon reflexes is not helpful in localizing a lesion unless the reflexes are clearly asymmetrical. However, the presence of a Babinski reflex is a generally reliable sign of spinal cord (or brain) dysfunction.

What are the components of an appropriate imaging evaluation of known or suspected spinal metastases?

The goal of the imaging evaluation of a patient with known or suspected metastatic disease of the spine is localization of the lesion, documentation of the presence of neural compression, evaluation of the three-dimensional anatomy of bony destruction, and determination of spinal alignment and stability. No single imaging modality is capable of achieving all of these goals. In patients with suspected metastatic spinal involvement, we routinely use a combination of plain films, MRI, and CT.

Plain Films

Plain films are an essential first study in all patients with known or suspected metastatic disease of the spine. The level to be examined is determined by the patient's signs and symptoms. Lateral plain films will show vertebral body destruction and are the best study for the assessment of spinal alignment. Films done in the frontal projection are useful for demonstration of destruction of the pedicles and delineation of paraspinal soft tissue masses (Fig. 32–10). Dynamic lateral views of the spine in flexion and extension are also useful in determining spinal instability that may result from bony destruction.[4]

Magnetic Resonance Imaging

MRI is the imaging modality of choice for the assessment of neural compression by bone or soft tissue. Sagittal and axial images will show the level and exact configuration of neoplastic involvement and compression. Sagittal images will also provide a useful assessment of alignment, in addition to showing displacement of the spinal cord by bone or metastases (Fig. 32–11). An altered signal within bone will define the presence and extent of metastases, although CT images provide superior definition of bony anatomy. Contrast enhancement of metastases using intravenous gadolinium is unnecessary because the contrast may alter the abnormal marrow signal typically observed with bony metastatic disease, causing the lesion to appear normal in comparison to other vertebral levels.

Because the presence of central nervous system metastases has such a profound effect on prognosis and therapeutic decision making, it is essential that the brain be studied with MRI with and without gadolinium enhancement at the same time that evaluation of the spine is being carried out.

Computed Tomography

Ideally, axial CT is performed after the metastatic lesion is localized by plain films or MRI. CT provides superior definition of bony anatomy and is a particularly valuable aid to the surgeon in determining spinal stability, the need for internal fixation, and the type of operative approach based on the

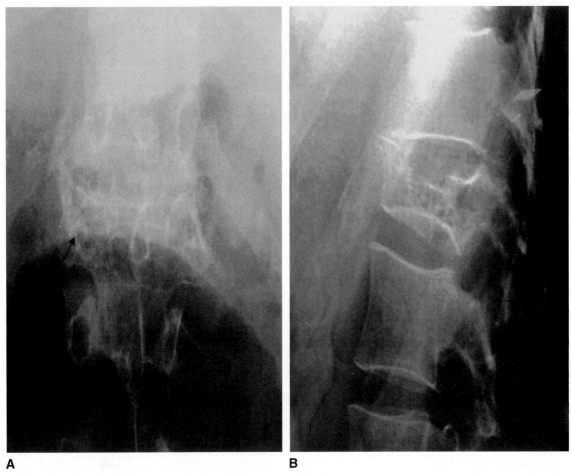

A   **B**

Figure 32–10   *A,* This anteroposterior projection plain film of the thoracolumbar junction shows loss of definition of the right pedicle of L1 (*arrow* points to destroyed pedicle). *B,* In the lateral projection of the same patient, loss in height of the involved spinal level second-ary to a pathologic compression fracture is notable. The relative preservation of the disc spaces adjacent to the metastatic lesion is an important finding distinguishing this entity from osteomyelitis of the spine.

exact extent and location of bone destruction. Axial images taken at 1-mm intervals can be reformatted in the sagittal and coronal planes to provide accurate delineation of the three-dimensional bony anatomy of the lesion and to assess spinal alignment (see Fig. 32–11C). This technique is particularly valuable at the cervicothoracic junction or other regions that are difficult to image on plain films.

In distinction to MRI, the intravenous administration of iodinated contrast agents in CT will result in enhancement of tumor and provide clearer definition of neural compression within the spinal canal. Contrast administration may be help-ful in defining the location of tumor when MRI is unavailable or cannot be performed because of patient refusal or the pres-ence of implanted cardiac pacemakers, or when metallic inter-nal fixation devices from prior spinal surgery are likely to preclude useful MRI examination.

Computed Tomographic Myelography
Myelography using iodinated contrast material placed in the subarachnoid space followed by CT scanning has been used infrequently since the advent of high-resolution MRI. Even when MRI is unavailable or cannot be used, plain CT after intravenous contrast administration is usually sufficient to define the presence and extent of metastases. Myelography is

probably most useful in patients with internal fixation devices who are suspected of having recurrent tumor. Because the metallic implants will produce extensive artifact on MRI, CT myelography may be the only imaging modality that can define the extent of neural compression.

Spinal Angiography and Embolization
In the past, spinal angiography was performed preoperatively in all patients before transthoracic or lumbar retroperitoneal resection of spinal tumors. Because these approaches necessi-tate ligation of radicular vessels supplying the vasculature to the spinal cord, it was formerly believed that definition of the arterial supply of the anterior spinal artery was essential to avoid spinal cord ischemia and infarction. In practice, unilat-eral ligation of three or even four adjacent radicular vessels is safe, and spinal angiography is unnecessary except in reoper-ations in which an approach is contemplated that is contralat-eral to previously ligated radicular vessels. Additional ligation of radicular vessels in this situation can result in spinal cord ischemia and exacerbation of neurologic deficit.

Embolization of tumor vessels may be carried out at the time of spinal arteriography. This technique may be helpful for tumors that are known to be highly vascular such as metastatic hypernephroma, melanoma, or thyroid tumors.

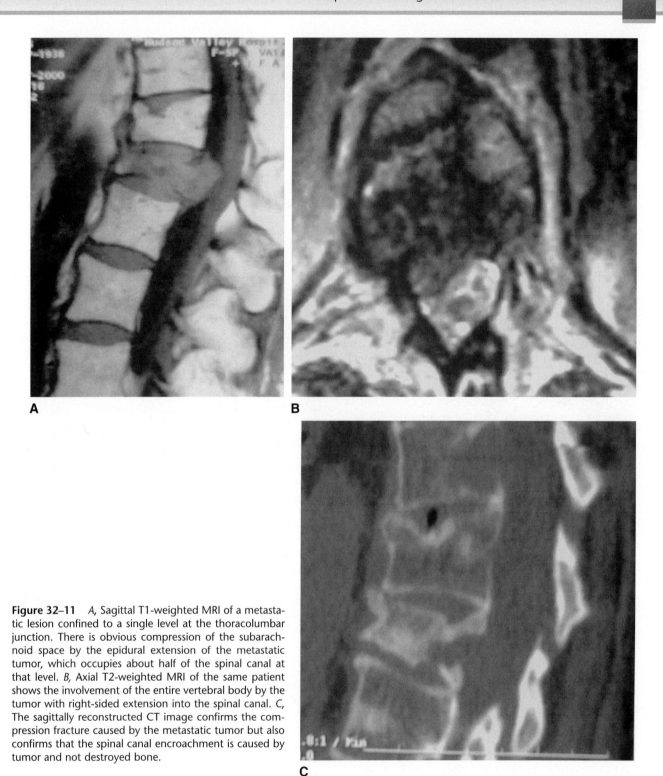

Figure 32–11 *A,* Sagittal T1-weighted MRI of a metastatic lesion confined to a single level at the thoracolumbar junction. There is obvious compression of the subarachnoid space by the epidural extension of the metastatic tumor, which occupies about half of the spinal canal at that level. *B,* Axial T2-weighted MRI of the same patient shows the involvement of the entire vertebral body by the tumor with right-sided extension into the spinal canal. *C,* The sagittally reconstructed CT image confirms the compression fracture caused by the metastatic tumor but also confirms that the spinal canal encroachment is caused by tumor and not destroyed bone.

Metastatic breast neoplasms are infrequently highly vascular and embolization is rarely necessary.

What considerations are most important in therapeutic decision making for spinal metastases?

Surgical resection of spinal metastases of carcinoma of the breast is an important treatment option for palliation of pain and prevention of irreversible neurologic deficit. Surgeons have become increasingly aggressive in selecting patients for operative resection and more radical in their choice of operative approaches.[5–12] However, there has been a reluctance on the part of some medical oncologists to refer their patients for resection of spinal metastases because operative resection is rarely curative, patients are frequently debilitated from their systemic disease and prior treatments, and historically the neurologic outcome after laminectomy was little or no better than radiation and chemotherapy.[6,13–18] It is now clear that

Table 32–15 Clinical Criteria Favoring Radiation Therapy as Primary Treatment Modality

Radiation-responsive tumor
Moderately radiation-responsive tumor in a patient with little or no neurologic deficit
Neural compression from soft tissue only
Expected survival less than 3–4 mo
Patient unlikely to tolerate surgical intervention
Complete neurologic deficit below the level of compression
Multiple vertebral body lesions at multiple spinal levels

Table 32–16 Clinical Criteria Favoring Surgical Intervention as Primary Treatment Modality

Neural compression secondary to retropulsed bone
Neural compression from spinal deformity
Spinal instability resulting from ligamentous and bony destruction by tumor
Rapid progression of neurologic deficit
Failure of radiation therapy (after prior therapy or progression of deficit during treatment)
Occult primary tumor

properly timed resection of spinal metastases in selected patients has an important role to play in their overall management.[19–25]

Indications for Nonoperative Management

The indications for radiation therapy and other forms of nonoperative management are listed in Table 32–15 and discussed in detail in this section.

Patients who are found to have small metastatic lesions of the vertebral bodies without extension into the spinal canal in the course of a routine evaluation for clinical staging are appropriate candidates for radiation therapy. Similarly, patients who present with spinal pain and are neurologically intact without imaging or clinical evidence of spinal cord or cauda equina compression by tumor or spinal instability and deformity may be managed initially with radiation therapy. Patients with an expected survival of less than 3 to 4 months are usually not candidates for spinal surgery, nor are those who are so debilitated that they are unlikely to tolerate surgical intervention. If any of these patients has any evidence of kyphotic deformity, then thoracolumbosacral orthotic bracing or rigid cervical collars should be used, and bedrest should be encouraged.

Patients with a complete neurologic deficit will not regain useful motor function even if decompressed; thus, operative decompression makes little sense. Even in patients with preservation of sensation but absent motor function, return of sufficient motor function to permit ambulation is exceptional, and operative decompression must be approached with a good deal of skepticism.

The patient with mild deficit (e.g., ambulatory but with less than normal strength) may be a candidate for radiation therapy provided that the total amount of tumor mass (and particularly that within the spinal canal) is small. Such patients must be examined at least twice daily, and surgical consultation must be obtained at the moment that there is progression of neurologic dysfunction. Patients with mild deficit should be placed on corticosteroids, which are useful for pain palliation and may ameliorate neurologic deficits while radiation therapy is being carried out.

Indications for Operative Management

The indications for operative management as the primary treatment modality are listed in Table 32–16 and are discussed in detail subsequently.

Patients who present with rapidly progressive neurologic deterioration are unlikely to have amelioration of their deficit with radiation or chemotherapy. Although administration of high-dose corticosteroids (methylprednisolone, 250 mg every 6 hours) may result in temporary improvement of neurologic function, recurrent deterioration is the rule, and such patients are best referred for early surgical consultation. Although patients who present with slowly progressive but severe deficit (nonambulatory but with movement of the lower extremities) may sometimes respond to radiation therapy, reversal of deficit is more rapid, more complete, and more certain with operative decompression. Moreover, operative intervention removes the risk for deterioration during or after radiation therapy.

In patients with neural compression, it is important to use imaging studies to determine whether compression is caused by a soft tissue tumor or partially destroyed vertebral body that has retropulsed into the spinal canal. This distinction is of great importance and frequently difficult to make on MRI alone. Axial or sagittal CT scans will readily distinguish bone from soft tissue tumor (see Fig. 32–11C). If there is bone in the spinal canal, surgical decompression is indicated; radiation therapy as the primary treatment in this situation is futile and will not prevent further neurologic deterioration. Similarly, surgical therapy is also indicated when compression is caused by spinal instability, subluxation, or kyphotic deformity resulting from bony destruction.

Neurologic deterioration in patients who have been managed with radiation therapy or chemotherapy as the primary treatment is an indication for surgery. It is inexcusable for patients who present intact or who have mildly impaired motor function to be observed, because they deteriorate while receiving radiation therapy. Although systemic chemotherapy may decrease the size or slow the growth of metastatic lesions, it has been our experience that chemotherapy is rarely effective in reversing neurologic deficit caused by spinal cord or cauda equina compression from metastatic carcinoma of the breast.

Patients with metastatic disease with a solitary spinal metastasis and pain alone or pain with neurologic deficit have received attention recently as a unique group with respect to the indications for surgery. This group of patients is thought to be among those who would reap the greatest benefit from en bloc surgical resection of their tumor; en bloc resection may be oncologically superior in reducing local tumor recurrence compared with traditional piecemeal resection.[7,11,12,24] Adjunctive postoperative radiation therapy is recommended in this group, but recent studies have suggested that preoperative radiation leads to higher surgical complication rates because of scarring and an increased incidence of wound breakdown and infection.[8,26,27,28] It must be emphasized, however, that a single metastasis to the spine without other systemic disease is an exceedingly unusual phenomenon. Even in patients without initial evidence of systemic metastases, diffuse disease is usually present and will become manifest with the passage of time.

What are the surgical approaches to spinal metastases?

More than 25 years ago, the reported results of surgical treatment of metastatic disease of the spine followed by radiation therapy were no better than radiation alone. In 1978, Gilbert and colleagues,[16] in a widely cited study, could find no difference in outcome when patients with metastatic spinal tumors who had been treated with radiation therapy or surgery were compared. Other authors who performed meta-analyses of results reported in the literature reached similar conclusions.[6,13,14] The failure of surgery to improve on the results of radiation therapy led Black[29] in 1979 to state that "radiotherapy alone should, in general, be the primary form of treatment for spinal metastasis. Radiotherapy seems to be superior to surgical decompression alone, and it is equally as effective as a combination of operation and radiotherapy."

In retrospect, the reasons for the unsatisfactory results of surgery are now clear. Surgical treatment at the time that Black and others did their reviews consisted almost exclusively of laminectomy, regardless of the location of the tumor, extent of bony destruction, or presence of spinal deformity.[6,30–35] Because most epidural metastatic lesions originate from the vertebral body, compression usually originates anterior to the spinal cord or cauda equina. Laminectomy with posterior decompression does little to relieve the ventral pressure on the spinal cord. Attempts to remove anterior tumor through a posterior approach usually result in manipulation of the spinal cord and failure to remove the large bulk of ventral tumor. In addition, the resected laminae are frequently the only bony elements providing stability, and their removal may lead to kyphosis with subsequent compression of the spinal cord as the spine deforms further following the operation.

The development of anterior approaches to the spine by a number of groups[23,36–40] revolutionized the ability of surgeons to prevent or reverse neurologic deficit. An understanding of spinal biomechanics and the application of internal fixation techniques have enabled spinal surgeons to perform radical resection of spinal tumors and vertebral elements while retaining stability, preventing spinal deformity, and minimizing local recurrence. Although quality of survival is clearly improved, it is not yet clear whether the length of survival is affected.[1,27,41,42]

A detailed description of the operative techniques currently used is beyond the scope of this discussion; however, the indications for various procedures and the general nature of the approaches and the techniques available are informative and aid the medical oncologist in understanding why particular operative treatments are chosen by the spinal surgeon.

Thoracic Spine

The thoracic region is the most common location for spinal metastases. Because the thoracic spine is stabilized by the rib cage, even extensive bony destruction by vertebral metastases may not compromise spinal stability or alignment. However, the thoracic spinal canal is small in relation to the size of the spinal cord, and relatively small volumes of intraspinal tumor may result in profound neurologic deficit.

Because most thoracic metastases originate in the vertebral body, decompression is most safely and effectively carried out through anterior or anterolateral approaches. We prefer to use a thoracotomy approach to the thoracic vertebral bodies.[43] The vertebral body is resected along with epidural tumor. The vertebral body is replaced with methylmethacrylate, which is molded to the contours of the bony defect.[44] The strength of the methylmethacrylate fixation may be enhanced by Steinmann pins or a stent of Silastic tubing filled with methylmethacrylate placed within the liquid cement before it hardens, or with the use of plates or rods secured to the adjacent vertebral bodies by intravertebral screws (Fig. 32–12). We usually avoid the use of bone grafts because of the limited life expectancy of most patients and the high incidence of failed fusion in patients who have been or will be treated with radiation therapy.

Above the T11 level, resection of a single vertebral body with acrylic vertebral body replacement will generally not result in spinal instability, and no further treatment is indicated provided that the posterior vertebral elements (laminae and facets) remain intact. If two or more contiguous vertebral bodies must be resected or if there is involvement of the posterior vertebral elements, a second posterior incision is made, and supplemental posterior fixation is used, usually during the same anesthetic period. At T11 and T12, the point of transition from the relatively stable thoracic spine to the more mobile lumbar spine junction, anterior instrumentation must be used or consideration given to the use of additional posterior fixation devices (Fig. 32–13).

The lateral parascapular approach has been described and may be used to achieve both anterior and posterior decompression of the spinal cord with one incision through an extrapleural approach.[45] It has the disadvantage of providing less direct access to the anterior aspect of the spinal cord; in addition, it is difficult to place anterior fixation devices using this technique. Other posterolateral approaches with resection of the pedicle have been described, but these have disadvantages similar to those of the lateral parascapular approach.

Although laminectomy is contraindicated in patients who have ventral compression of the spinal cord, its use is still appropriate and effective in certain circumstances.[42] In 15% to 20% of patients with spinal metastases, compression is located only dorsally and may be effectively relieved with laminectomy. If the vertebral body is not involved by tumor, no additional surgical treatment is required. If the vertebral body is involved but there is no anterior spinal cord compression, posterior fixation would be indicated.

If there is circumferential compression of the spinal cord, both anterior and posterior decompressive procedures may be used.[5,6,9,11,12,24,26] The anterior compressive lesion would usually be treated first. Combined anterior and posterior decompressive procedures (vertebral body resection and laminectomy) will usually require the use of posterior fixation.

Lumbar Spine

The lumbar region is the second most common site of spinal metastases. The spinal cord ends at about L1, and metastatic spinal lesions below this level will affect the lumbar and sacral nerve roots of the cauda equina. Anterior compression of neural elements in the lumbar spine may be treated with vertebral body resection through a retroperitoneal approach. Because of the greater mobility of the lumbar spine, anterior instrumentation is usually indicated after vertebral body resection

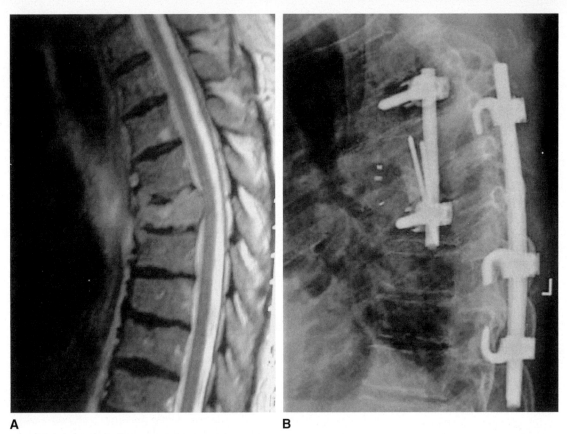

A   **B**

Figure 32–12   *A,* Preoperative T2-weighted sagittal MRI of a T6 metastatic lesion with epidural extension of the tumor with associated kyphotic deformity of the thoracic spine at that level secondary to pathologic compression fracture of the vertebral body. *B,* Lateral radiograph following transthoracic vertebral body resection, acrylic vertebral body replacement, and stabilization using Steinmann pins and anterior thoracic rod, with supplemental posterior stabilization with a hook-and-rod construct.

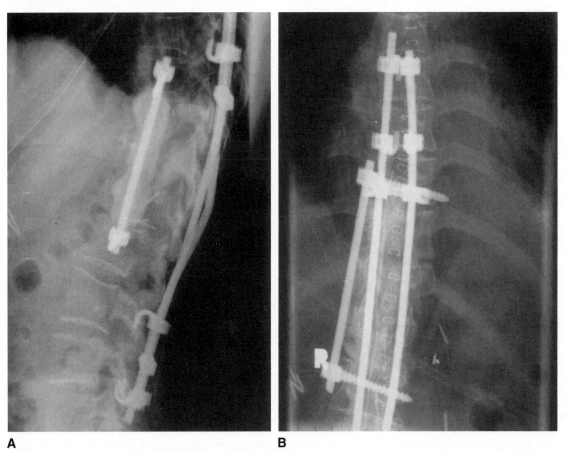

A   **B**

Figure 32–13   *A,* Postoperative lateral radiograph of a patient with a metastasis at the thoracolumbar junction. After resection of the T11-L1 vertebral bodies through an anterior thoracolumbar approach, the vertebral bodies were replaced with methylmethacrylate, and an anterior fixation device was placed. A second incision was then made to place a rod-and-hook construct posteriorly to provide additional stabilization. *B,* A postoperative anteroposterior radiograph of the same patient.

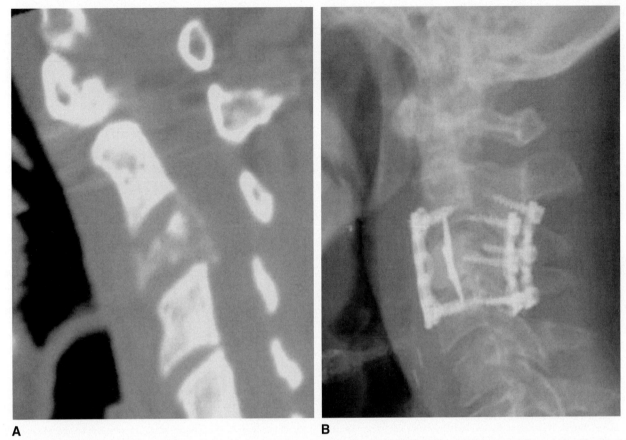

A   **B**

Figure 32–14   *A*, Preoperative sagittally reconstructed CT view of the cervical spine showing the destruction of the vertebral body of C3 by tumor with a notable kyphotic deformity. *B*, Postoperative lateral cervical radiograph showing radiopaque acrylic vertebral body replacement of C5 reinforced by an anterior cervical plate and supplemented by posterior cervical lateral mass plates spanning the level of the anterior fusion.

and replacement with methylmethacrylate. If there is involvement of the posterior vertebral elements or laminectomy is indicated, supplemental posterior fixation will be necessary.

As is the case for the thoracic spine, laminectomy is indicated when there is posterior compression of the dural tube. Because the nerve roots of the cauda equina are much more tolerant of manipulation than the spinal cord, laminectomy may sometimes be appropriate and effective below the L1 level to resect a tumor or tumor-involved vertebral body anterior to the spinal cord. If the vertebral body is involved, placement of posterior instrumentation will be necessary.

Cervical Spine
The cervical vertebrae are the least commonly affected region of the spine with metastatic disease. Compression almost always results from tumor extending out of an involved vertebral body or from the bone of a partially destroyed vertebral body retropulsed into the spinal canal. Because the cervical region is the most mobile segment of the spinal axis, vertebral body involvement commonly results in kyphotic deformity.

Anterior compression is managed from the same anterior approach used for spinal cord compression caused by cervical disc herniations or degenerative disease. The vertebral body is resected down to the dura, although extensive lateral resection of tumor is limited by the vertebral arteries. If kyphotic deformity is present, it may be corrected at the time of resection. Steinmann pins may be placed in the vertebral bodies above

and below the one resected to secure the methylmethacrylate. Alternatively, anterior cervical plates may be screwed to the vertebral bodies adjacent to the one resected, stabilizing the spine and preventing the acrylic from displacing. If there is a kyphotic deformity or if laminectomy is also necessary for decompression of posterior tumor, supplemental posterior instrumentation may be appropriate (Fig. 32–14).

What are the outcomes of spinal surgery for breast cancer metastases?

There have been no large series in which the results of spinal surgery for the treatment of breast metastases have been specifically examined; however, 94% of our own patients with a variety of metastatic tumors had improvement or stabilization of their motor deficits after operation, and more than 90% were ambulatory.[19] Other authors have reported similar satisfactory neurologic results.[3,11,22,25,28,46] Although the procedures necessary to relieve neural compression are often extensive, we had no mortality within 30 days of surgery in our series.[19]

With increased length of survival as a result of aggressive chemotherapy of systemic disease, a major problem has been recurrence of local spinal disease in patients whose systemic disease is otherwise well controlled. Although surgical resection of spinal metastases is not curative, it is now clear that aggressive reduction of tumor bulk will minimize the incidence of local recurrence in patients with extended survival. Our goal in patients with a single metastasis or well-controlled systemic disease is removal of all grossly visible tumor and all bone that is involved with tumor on imaging studies. This may frequently entail total resection of all vertebral elements (spondylectomy) using combined anterior and posterior surgery.[7,9–11] This has been generally well tolerated and appears to have minimized local recurrence.

Because neurologic outcome after surgery is closely related to the patient's preoperative deficit, it is essential that patients be decompressed early before severe neurologic dysfunction is present. It is therefore important that spinal surgeons share, along with medical and radiation oncologists, in the formulation of management strategies at the time of presentation.

REFERENCES

1. Helweg-Larsen S. Clinical outcome in metastatic spinal cord compression: A prospective study of 153 patients. Acta Neurol Scand 1996;94:269–275.
2. Tomita T, Galicich JH, Sundaresan N. Radiation therapy for spinal epidural metastases with complete block. Acta Radiol Oncol 1983;22:135–143.
3. Weigel B, Maghsudi M, Neumann C, et al. Surgical management of symptomatic spinal metastases. Postoperative outcome and quality of life. Spine 1999;24(21):2240–2246.
4. Denis F. Spinal instability as defined by the three-column concept in acute spinal trauma. Clin Orthop 1984;189:65–76.
5. Abe E, Sato K, Murai H, et al. Total spondylectomy for solitary spinal metastasis of the thoracolumbar spine: A preliminary report. Tohoku J Exp Med 2000;190(1):33–49.
6. Bilsky MH, Boland P, Lis E, et al. Single-stage posterolateral transpedicle approach for spondylectomy, epidural decompression, and circumferential fusion of spinal metastases. Spine 2000;25(17):2240–2249.
7. Boriani S, Biagini R, De Iure F, et al. En bloc resections of bone tumors of the thoracolumbar spine. A preliminary report on 29 patients. Spine 1996;21(16):1927–1931.
8. Fourney DR, Abi-Said D, Lang FF, et al. Use of pedicle screw fixation in the management of malignant spinal disease: Experience in 100 consecutive procedures. J Neurosurg 2001;94(1 Suppl):25–37.
9. Heary RF, Vaccaro AR, Benevenia J, Cotler JM. "En-bloc" vertebrectomy in the mobile lumbar spine. Surg Neurol 1998;50(6):548–556.
10. Sundaresan N, Digiacinto GV, Krol G, et al. Spondylectomy for malignant tumors of the spine. J Clin Oncol 1989;7:1485–1491.
11. Tomita K, Kawahara N, Baba H, et al. Total en bloc spondylectomy for solitary spinal metastases. Int Orthop 1994;18(5):291–298.
12. Tomita K, Kawahara N, Kobayashi T, et al. Surgical strategy for spinal metastases. Spine 2001;26(3):298–306.
13. Barcena A, Lobato RD, Rivas JJ, et al. Spinal metastatic disease: Analysis of factors determining functional prognosis and the choice of treatment. Neurosurgery 1984;15:820–827.
14. Fidler MW. Anterior decompression and stabilisation of metastatic spinal fractures. J Bone Joint Surg 1986;68B:83–90.
15. Findlay GFG. Adverse effects of the management of malignant spinal cord compression. J Neurol Neurosurg Psychiatry 1984;47:761–768.
16. Gilbert RW, Kim J-H, Posner JB. Epidural spinal cord compression from metastatic tumor: Diagnosis and treatment. Ann Neurol 1978;3:40–51.
17. Maranzano E, Latini P. Effectiveness of radiation therapy without surgery in metastatic spinal cord compression: Final results from a prospective trial. Int J Radiat Oncol Biol Phys 1995;32(4):959–967.
18. Young RF, Post EM, King GA. Treatment of spinal epidural metastases. Randomized prospective comparison of laminectomy and radiotherapy. J Neurosurg 1980;53:741–748.
19. Cooper PR, Errico TJ, Martin R, et al. A systematic approach to spinal reconstruction after anterior decompression for neoplastic disease of the thoracic and lumbar spine. Neurosurgery 1993;32:1–8.
20. Manabe S, Tateishi A, Abe M, Ohno T. Surgical treatment of metastatic tumors of the spine. Spine 1989;14:41–47.
21. Siegal T, Siegal T. Current considerations in the management of neoplastic spinal cord compression. Spine 1989;14:223–228.
22. Siegal T, Siegal T. Surgical decompression of anterior and posterior malignant epidural tumors compressing the spinal cord: A prospective study. Neurosurgery 1985;17:424–432.
23. Sundaresan N, Galicich JH, Bains MS, et al. Vertebral body resection in the treatment of cancer involving the spine. Cancer 1984;53:1393–1396.
24. Sundaresan N, Rothman A, Manhart K, Kelliher K. Surgery for solitary metastases of the spine. Rationale and results of treatment. Spine 2002;27(16):1802–1806.
25. Sundaresan N, Steinberger AA, Moore F, et al. Indications and results of combined anterior-posterior approaches for spine tumor surgery. J Neurosurg 1996;85:438–4467.
26. Fourney DR, Abi-Said D, Rhines LD, et al. Simultaneous anterior-posterior approach to the thoracic and lumbar spine for the radical resection of tumors followed by reconstruction and stabilization. J Neurosurg 2001;94(2 Suppl):232–244.
27. Ghogawala Z, Mansfield FL, Borges LF. Spinal radiation before surgical decompression adversely affects outcomes of surgery for symptomatic metastatic cord compression. Spine 2001;26:818–824.
28. Wise JJ, Fischgrund JS, Herkowitz HN, et al. Complication, survival rates, and risk factors of surgery for metastatic disease of the spine. Spine 1999;24(18):1943–1951.
29. Black P. Spinal metastasis: Current status and recommended guidelines for management. Neurosurgery 1979;5:726–746.
30. Hall AJ, McKay NNS. The results of laminectomy for compression of the cord and cauda equina by extradural malignant tumor. J Bone Joint Surg Br 1973;55:497–505.
31. Harrington KD. Metastatic disease of the spine. J Bone Joint Surg Am 1986;68:1110–1115.
32. Livingston KE, Perrin RG. The neurosurgical management of spinal metastases causing cord and cauda equina compression. J Neurosurg 1978;53:839–843.
33. Smith R. An evaluation of surgical treatment for spinal cord compression due to metastatic carcinoma. J Neurol Neurosurg Psychiatry 1965;28:152–158.
34. Wild WO, Porter RW. Metastatic tumor of the spine: A study of 45 cases. Arch Surg 1963;87:825–830.
35. Wright RL. Malignant tumors in the spinal extradural space. Results of surgical treatment. Ann Surg 1963;157:277–231.
36. Harrington KD. Anterior cord compression and spinal stabilization for patients with metastatic lesions of the spine. J Neurosurg 1984;61:107–117.
37. Harrington KD. The use of methylmethacrylate for vertebral-body replacement and anterior stabilization of pathological fracture-dislocations of the spine due to metastatic malignant disease. J Bone Joint Surg Am 1981;63:36–46.
38. Kostuik JP, Errico TJ, Gleason, Errico CC. Spinal stabilization of vertebral column tumors. Spine 1988;13:250–256.
39. Sundaresan N, Bains M, McCormack P. Surgical treatment of spinal cord compression in patients with lung cancer. Neurosurgery 1985;16:350–356.
40. Sundaresan N, Galicich JH, Lane JM, et al. Treatment of neoplastic epidural spinal cord compression by vertebral body resection and stabilization. J Neurosurg 1985;63:676–684.
41. Gokaslan ZL, York JE, Walsh G, et al. Transthoracic vertebrectomy for metastatic spinal tumors. J Neurosurg 1998;89(4):599–609.
42. Rompe JD, Hopf CG, Eysel P. Outcome after palliative posterior surgery for metastatic disease of the spine: Evaluation of 106 consecutive patients after decompression and stabilization with the Cotrel-Dubousset instrumentation. Arch Orthop Trauma Surg 1999;119:394–400.
43. Anderson TM, Mansour KA, Miller JI Jr. Thoracic approaches to anterior spinal operations: Anterior thoracic approaches. Ann Thoracic Surg 1993;55:1447–1451.
44. Errico TJ, Cooper PR. A new method for stabilizing the thoracic and lumbar spine with methylmethacrylate. Technical note. Neurosurgery 1993;32:678–679.
45. Fessler R. Lateral parascapular extrapleural approach to the upper thoracic spine. J Neurosurg 1991;75:349–355.
46. Sioutros PJ, Arbit E, Meshulam CF, Galicich JH. Spinal metastases from solid tumors. Analysis of factors affecting survival. Cancer 1995;76(8):1453–1459.

VII

Ocular Metastases from Breast Cancer

Carol L. Shields,
Hakan Demirci, and
Jerry A. Shields

How common are ocular metastases?

Historically, metastatic tumors to the eye were believed to be rare. A classic ophthalmic textbook in 1966 stated that few surgeons had observed more than one case of ocular metastasis.[1] It was later realized that ocular metastases were more common, and over the past 43 years there have been several reports on the incidence and prognosis of patients with metastatic tumors to the eye.[2–11] Albert and associates found that 2% of 213 patients with known systemic cancer and metastases had choroidal metastases.[3] Bloch and Gartner reported that 8% of eyes in 230 patients with autopsy-proven carcinomas had histologically confirmed uveal metastatic foci.[5] Nelson and coworkers found in an autopsy study that 4% of patients dying of carcinoma had ocular metastases.[8] They estimated that in the year 1983, 22,000 patients who died of cancer had ocular metastatic disease.[8] As the life expectancy of patients with cancer improves, it is expected that the number of patients with ocular metastases will rise accordingly.

Most reports on ocular metastases come from pathology laboratories or from general cancer centers where patients have had known primary cancers or metastatic disease and the eyes were subsequently examined. These studies have focused on the source of the primary tumor as well as on general clinical and histopathologic features of the tumor (derived from autopsy or pathology reports in some instances).[2–6,8] Ocular metastases on file at the Armed Forces Institute of Pathology were reviewed by Hart in 1962[2] and Ferry and Font in 1974.[6]

There are only a few comprehensive reports on the clinical features of ocular metastases from an ophthalmologic point of view. In 1979, Stephens and Shields reviewed 70 cases of uveal metastases and provided general details on the clinical findings of these tumors.[7] In 1997, Shields and coworkers reported extensive detail on the clinical features and management of uveal metastases in a large group of 420 consecutive patients.[11] Others have focused on the features of uveal metastases from specific primary sites such as breast,[12–16] prostate,[17] and skin[18–20] and carcinoid tumors.[21] In 1987, Freedman and Folk reported on the clinical aspects of metastatic tumors to the choroid in 61 patients, and they addressed specifically the factors affecting the median survival time after ocular diagnosis.[9] Later, Shields and Shields summarized their experience with clinical features, diagnostic techniques, and management of uveal metastases in a textbook and three atlases on ocular tumors.[22–26]

What are the most common sites of ocular metastasis?

Metastatic tumors generally spread to the ocular region through hematogenous dissemination. Metastases can occur in the intraocular structures such as the uvea, retina, optic disc, or vitreous cavity, and they can manifest in the adnexal structures like the eyelid, conjunctiva, or orbit.[11,27–33] Most ocular metastases are detected in the uvea. The uvea is a vascular bed located between the retina and sclera. It is composed of melanocytes, sensory nerves, and a high-flow network of blood vessels that provide nutrition to the outer layers of the retina. The uvea is divided into the iris, ciliary body, and choroid. In an analysis of 950 individual uveal metastases, metastatic tumors occurred most often in the choroid (88%) and less frequently in the iris (9%) or ciliary body (2%)[11] (Fig. 32–15). Occasionally, metastases are located in the orbit.[27–29] Rarely, ocular metastases are found in the eyelid, conjunctiva, optic disc, or other structures.[30–33]

Uveal metastases most commonly originate from primary cancers in the breast (47%), lung (21%), gastrointestinal tract (4%), kidney (2%), skin (melanoma) (2%), prostate gland (2%), and other sites (4%)[11] (Table 32–17; Fig. 32–16). In about 17% of all patients, the primary tumor site remains unknown. Orbital metastases most frequently originate from primary cancers in the breast (53%), prostate gland (12%), lung (8%), skin (melanoma) (6%), kidney (5%), gastrointestinal tract (5%), and others (4%).[27,28] In 7% of patients, the primary site remains unknown.

At the time of presentation with a uveal metastasis, about 30% of patients had no known history of primary cancer.[11] Subsequent evaluation of these patients revealed a primary tumor most commonly in the lung (35%) and less frequently in the breast (7%) and other sites (6%) (Figs. 32–17 and 32–18) Despite repeated evaluation, the primary site in these select patients who present without a history of cancer remains unknown in 51% of patients. Nearly half of such patients with no detectable primary site died of diffuse metastatic disease shortly after the ocular diagnosis.[11]

PATIENT FEATURES

Breast cancer is the most common malignancy to metastasize to the uvea, accounting for 39% to 49% of all uveal

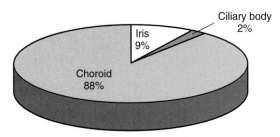

Figure 32–15 Anatomic location of 950 consecutive uveal metastases.

Table 32–17   Uveal Metastases Related to Site of Primary Cancer in 520 Eyes of 420 Patients

	Primary Site of Tumor							
	Breast	**Lung**	**Kidney**	**GI**	**Skin**	**Prostate**	**Other**	**Unknown**
Eyes (n = 520)	260	108	19	10	11	11	20	81
Patients (n = 420)	196	90	18	9	9	9	16	73
Age* (yr) (n = 420)	56	57	60	65	50	67	57	64
Race (n = 420)								
White	175	80	17	9	9	8	15	67
African American	17	10	1	0	0	0	1	5
Other	4	0	0	0	0	1	0	1
Sex (n = 420)								
Male	2	55	13	8	5	9	5	40
Female	194	35	5	1	4	0	11	33
Laterality (n = 420)								
Unilateral	132	72	17	8	7	7	12	65
Bilateral	64	18	1	1	2	2	4	8
Symptoms (n = 520)								
None	28	12	4	1	1	3	2	8
Blurred vision	192	68	14	5	4	7	12	59
Flashes, floaters	35	14	0	2	2	0	6	6
Pain	5	14	1	2	4	1	0	8
Other ocular metastases								
Eyelid	1	0	0	0	1	0	1	0
Orbit	2	1	0	1	0	1	0	2
Conjunctiva	2	1	0	0	2	0	1	2
Retina	2	1	0	0	0	0	0	2
Optic disc	10	1	1	0	0	0	2	10
Location of uveal metastases								
Iris (n = 43)	17	8	2	1	4	1	2	8
Ciliary body (n = 21)	4	2	2	1	3	1	1	7
Choroid (n = 479)	252	98	18	8	5	10	17	71
Number* of uveal metastases/location								
If iris	2	1	1	2	1	1	7	1
If ciliary body	1	1	1	1	1	1	1	1
If choroid	2	1	1	1	2	1	1	2
Choroidal metastasis								
Base (mm)*	8	9	9	8	7	9	10	8
Thickness (mm)*	2	3	4	4	1	3	2	3
Color (n = 479)								
Yellow	249	90	17	5	0	9	12	66
Brown/gray	2	1	1	0	5	0	5	3
Orange	1	7	0	3	0	1	0	2
Shape (n = 479)								
Plateau	197	55	7	1	3	5	12	45
Dome	55	43	11	7	2	5	5	24
Mushroom	0	0	0	0	0	0	0	2

*Mean.
GI, gastrointestinal.
Data from Shields CL, Shields JA, Gross NE, et al. Survey of 520 eyes with uveal metastases. Ophthalmology 1997;104:1265–1276.

metastasis.[3–11] In a review of 3802 breast cancer patients, Kamby and coworkers reported that the five most common sites of metastasis from breast cancer were the lung (71%), bone (71%), lymph nodes (67%), liver (62%), and pleura (50%).[34] Ocular metastasis from breast cancer occurs in 9% to 37% of patients, depending on the source of the study.[5,8,14] Uveal metastases represent the smallest detectable lesions of systemic dissemination of breast cancer and occur at a median of 3 years following diagnosis of the primary tumor.[14]

Uveal metastases are more commonly found in women, primarily owing to the high frequency of breast cancer metastatic to the eye. In an analysis of 450 patients with uveal metastases from all primary cancer sites, the tumor was found in men in 33% and women in 67%.[11] Uveal metastases in men originated from cancer of the lung (40%), gastrointestinal tract (9%), kidney (6%), skin (melanoma) (4%), prostate gland (6%), breast (1%), others (4%), and unknown primary site (29%). Single cases of breast cancer metastatic to the eye in men have been published.[35] Uveal metastases in women

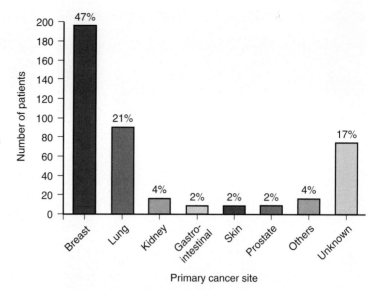

Figure 32–16 Location of primary cancer in 420 patients with uveal metastases.

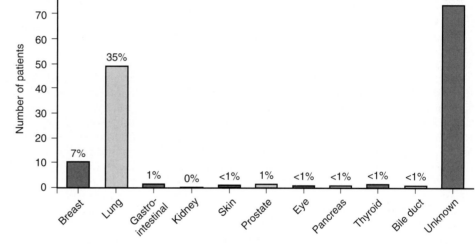

Figure 32–17 Eventual primary cancer site in 142 patients who presented with a uveal metastasis and no prior history of cancer.

were from cancer of the breast (68%), lung (12%), gastrointestinal tract (2%), kidney (<1%), skin (melanoma) (1%), prostate gland (0%), others (4%), and unknown (12%). In an analysis of 264 patients with uveal metastases from breast cancer, the primary tumor was found in women in 99% and men in 1%.[15]

What patient characteristics increase the risk for ocular metastases?

Ocular metastases from any primary site typically occur in the sixth to seventh decades of life at a mean age at 58 years (median, 58 years; range, 10 to 85 years).[11] For breast cancer metastasis, the mean age at diagnosis of the ocular metastasis was 56 years (median, 57 years; range, 23 to 84 years).[15]

Most patients with ocular metastases from breast cancer have a known history of breast cancer and previous nonocular metastases. Of 264 patients with uveal metastasis from breast cancer, the eye finding was the first manifestation of

breast cancer in 3%.[15] In 14% of patients, the ocular metastasis was the first metastatic site. The locations of systemic nonocular metastases before and after the detection of ocular metastasis are listed in Table 32–17.

Of those patients who develop ocular metastases, the mean age at diagnosis of the primary breast cancer was 56 years (median, 57 years; range, 23 to 84 years).[15] The initial treatment of breast cancer was radical or modified mastectomy (83%), systemic chemotherapy (42%), external-beam radiotherapy (27%), lumpectomy with or without lymph node dissection (14%), and hormone therapy (4%). The axillary lymph nodes were involved in 46% of patients who developed eventual uveal metastases. At the time of diagnosis of the ocular metastases, 52% of patients were on systemic therapy, including chemotherapeutic agents (36%), hormone therapy (20%), and immunotherapeutic agents (2%). Uveal metastases developed a mean of 65 months after the diagnosis of the primary breast cancer (median, 48 months; range, 0 to 300 months).[15]

Intraocular metastases show a strong tendency to involve the posterior uvea (choroid). Less commonly, the tumor

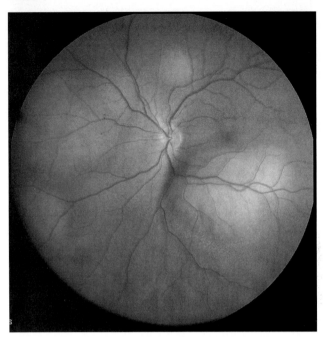

Figure 32–18   Choroidal metastasis from lung cancer. The amelanotic choroidal mass was discovered in a patient with no known cancer. Subsequent systemic evaluation revealed a primary lung cancer.

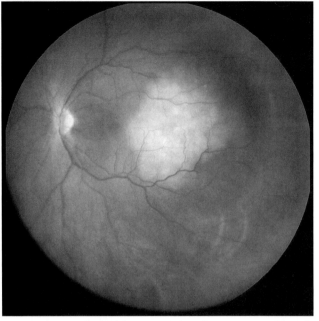

Figure 32–19   Choroidal metastasis from breast cancer. The well-circumscribed choroidal metastasis in the posterior pole of the eye was discovered in a patient with breast cancer.

affects the iris or ciliary body. Rarely do metastases involve the optic disc or retina. Of 361 eyes with uveal metastases, the tumor was located in the choroid in 349 eyes, iris in 23 eyes, and ciliary body in 2 eyes.[15] Some patients had metastatic tumors in more than one intraocular location.

In general, intraocular metastases commonly show multifocality, bilaterality, or both. In an analysis of 520 eyes with uveal metastases from all primary sites, the median number of metastatic tumors per eye was 1, and the mean was 1.6.[11] Furthermore, 370 eyes (71%) had 1 focus, 63 (12%) had 2 foci, and 87 (17%) had 3 or more foci, up to a maximum number of 13 metastatic foci in one eye.[11] The tumor was unilateral in 76% and bilateral in 24% of patients. With regard to ocular metastases from breast cancer, the tumor was unilateral in 62% and bilateral in 38%.[15] Of 99 patients (38%) with bilateral uveal metastases from breast cancer, 85 (32%) had bilateral involvement at the time of diagnosis, and 14 (5%) developed the second eye involvement after a mean follow-up of 10 months (median, 7 months; range, 2 to 33 months). The mean number of the uveal metastatic tumors (from breast cancer) per eye was 2 (median, 1; range, 1 to 19), and more than one metastatic focus was detected in 48%.[15]

What are the clinical features of ocular metastases?

The clinical features of metastatic tumors to the eye vary with the location of the ocular tumor.[23–26]

Choroidal Metastases

The patient with a metastatic tumor to the choroid may be asymptomatic or may experience painless blurred vision. In rare instances, pain caused by secondary glaucoma can be

the initial manifestation. Ophthalmoscopic examination of a choroidal metastasis characteristically reveals a homogeneous, creamy yellow placoid lesion in the posterior choroid (Fig. 32–19; see also Fig. 32–18). Tumors that are slightly more elevated can produce a serous detachment of the retina and alterations in the retinal pigment epithelium (RPE). The RPE changes can be marked, appearing as well-delineated clumps of golden-brown pigment on the surface of the tumor. In some instances, the tumor may appear multinodular.

In some cases, a choroidal metastasis can be highly elevated and have a dome shape, similar to a primary amelanotic melanoma.[36] The finding of multiple choroidal tumors in such a case, however, is strong evidence for a metastatic tumor rather than a primary melanoma, which is usually solitary.

Serous detachment of the sensory retina is associated with choroidal metastases from breast cancer in 64% of cases.[15] In some instances the detachment involves only the fovea adjacent to the tumor, whereas in other cases it may be bullous. When the detachment is extensive, dramatic shifting of the subretinal fluid can be demonstrated with movements of the patient's head.

Several conditions can clinically simulate a metastatic cancer to the choroid and should be considered in the differential diagnosis.[37] These include amelanotic nevus, amelanotic melanoma, hemangioma, osteoma, posterior scleritis, retinitis and choroiditis, rhegmatogenous retinal detachment, Harada's disease, uveal effusion syndrome, and central serous chorioretinopathy.[23–26,37–39] A detailed history is often helpful in making the differentiation, but the ophthalmoscopic differences are also very important. The specific clinical features of the various tumors and pseudotumors are illustrated in textbooks.[22–26] With some experience, the clinician can differentiate simulating lesions from metastatic tumors by their typical ophthalmoscopic features and by using ancillary diagnostic procedures, to be discussed subsequently.

A choroidal melanoma is the most important lesion to differentiate from a metastatic tumor.[36] The melanoma is characteristically pigmented but can be completely amelanotic and closely resemble the color of a metastasis. The melanoma is typically unilateral, solitary, and more elevated. An amelanotic melanoma frequently has large visible intrinsic blood vessels and often assumes a mushroom shape from herniation through Bruch's membrane; these findings rarely occur with a metastatic tumor.

A choroidal hemangioma can also resemble a metastatic tumor in size, shape, and location.[38] The distinct red-orange color of most hemangiomas differentiates them from the yellow color of a metastatic tumor. A choroidal hemangioma is classically unilateral and unifocal.

A choroidal osteoma characteristically appears as an amelanotic choroidal mass.[39] Like a metastatic tumor, it is more common in women. In contrast to a metastatic tumor, it has an irregular but well-defined border and can show subretinal neovascularization on the surface. We have seen one patient who underwent three breast biopsies elsewhere because a choroidal osteoma was suspected to be a metastatic cancer, before the correct diagnosis was eventually established. Ultrasonography and CT of a choroidal osteoma reveal echoes characteristic of a calcified plaque.

A number of inflammatory processes of the fundus can simulate a choroidal metastasis. Certain viral and mycotic infections are more commonly seen in patients with systemic cancer, thus making the differentiation even more difficult. Patients with cytomegalovirus (CMV) retinitis often have a history of cancer and are on chemotherapy. The yellow-white areas of retinal necrosis may be bilateral and multiple. In contrast to metastatic tumors, they involve the retina rather than the choroid, have an irregular border, and frequently show surrounding and overlying retinal hemorrhages. Mycotic retinitis or choroiditis also can resemble a choroidal metastasis but is more likely to be associated with inflammatory signs.

Ciliary Body Metastases

Ciliary body metastases are often difficult to detect clinically. They can masquerade as a chronic uveitis or secondary glaucoma, and the affected patient may be treated with topical or systemic corticosteroids or glaucoma medications, while the tumor remains undetected. Like primary ciliary body melanoma, a ciliary body metastasis can produce a shallow anterior chamber, subluxated lens, or cataract. Prominent episcleral blood vessels can occur in the quadrant of the lesion. In some cases, the ciliary body may be involved because of anterior extension of a diffuse tumor from the choroid. With time, some ciliary body metastases can extend through the iris root into the anterior chamber. The differential diagnosis of a ciliary body metastasis includes many of the same conditions that fall under the differential diagnosis of choroidal metastasis, except for those that affect only the posterior pole, such as central serous chorioretinopathy, choroidal hemangioma, and osteoma.

Iris Metastases

The clinical presentation of iris metastases can vary greatly.[11,33] Some patients with iris metastases are visually asymptomatic or have only mild symptoms. In some instances, however, pain caused by inflammation or secondary glaucoma can be the presenting manifestation. Occasionally, iris metastases are

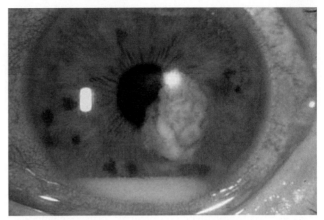

Figure 32–20 Iris metastasis. The amelanotic papillary margin metastasis on the iris originated from breast cancer and has shed cells into the anterior chamber angle, causing tumor-related hypopyon.

multiple and bilateral. Slit-lamp biomicroscopy reveals an iris mass that is usually pink or white, depending on the intrinsic vascularity. In some cases, iris metastases are friable, and loosely cohesive cells settle in the inferior portion of the anterior chamber angle, producing a pseudohypopyon, simulating endophthalmitis (Fig. 32–20). The differential diagnosis of metastatic tumors to the iris includes amelanotic melanoma, leiomyoma, granulomatous iritis, and endophthalmitis.

Retinal Metastases

Metastatic tumors to the retina are extremely rare. Retinal metastases are less cohesive than choroidal metastases and may seed tumor cells into the vitreous. They sometimes resemble a retinitis and can have associated exudation or hemorrhage.

Optic Disc Metastases

Metastatic tumors can develop in the optic disc, and both optic nerves can be involved simultaneously.[32] Optic disc metastases can clinically resemble papilledema, papillitis, or various types of pseudopapilledema.

Vitreous Metastases

Metastatic tumors to the vitreous are extremely rare and generally occur in patients who have retinal or ciliary body metastasis. Affected patients develop floaters, and vitreous examination reveals clumps of tumor cells. The differential diagnosis includes inflammatory vitritis, senile vitritis, endophthalmitis, vitreous hemorrhage, synchysis scintillans, asteroid hyalosis, and large cell lymphoma.

Conjunctival Metastases

Conjunctival metastases appear as a circumscribed or diffuse pink mass with prominent feeder vessels.[25,30,31] Most often, they are found on the bulbar conjunctiva near the limbus and can be multifocal. The differential diagnosis includes pinguecula, pterygium, conjunctivitis, squamous cell carcinoma, and amelanotic melanoma.

Eyelid Metastases

Isolated eyelid metastasis from systemic cancer is rare. In most instances, an eyelid metastasis is an anterior extension of an orbital metastasis. It appears as a noninflammatory mass and can resemble a chalazion, hordeolum, or basal cell carcinoma.

Orbital Metastases

Orbital metastasis from breast cancer usually presents with painless proptosis, ocular motility problems, or a palpable mass.[24,27-29] Enophthalmos, an uncommon finding, strongly suggests metastases from scirrhous breast carcinoma; however, orbital varix, congenital orbital asymmetry, and post-traumatic orbital fat atrophy can produce a similar picture.[40] Orbital metastases are best visualized by CT or MRI and appear most often as a diffuse, poorly circumscribed mass within the orbital soft tissues. It is rare to find bilateral simultaneous metastases. The differential diagnosis includes orbital inflammatory pseudotumor, cavernous hemangioma, neurilemoma, and lymphoma.

What are the clinical features of ocular paraneoplastic syndromes?

A paraneoplastic syndrome is defined as the malfunction of an organ system from cancer in a remote site of the body without the presence of metastases in that end organ. Neurologic paraneoplastic syndromes include peripheral neuropathy, cerebellar degeneration, myasthenia gravis, and motor neuron degeneration. Ocular paraneoplastic syndromes include optic neuritis, external ophthalmoplegia, and retinal disease.[41] Retinal paraneoplastic syndromes consist of carcinoma-associated retinopathy (CAR), melanoma-associated retinopathy (MAR), acquired cone dysfunction, bilateral diffuse uveal melanocytic proliferation (BDUMP), and Vogt-Koyanagi-Harada (VKH)-like syndrome. Breast cancer can produce CAR and BDUMP. In CAR, the patient notes night blindness, photopsia, transient obscuration of vision, ring scotoma, and photophobia. In BDUMP, multiple pigmented and nonpigmented uveal tumors develop along with dilated episcleral vessels, rapid-onset cataract, anterior uveitis, and serous retinal detachment.

Once an ocular metastasis is suspected, how is the diagnosis confirmed?

A number of ancillary ophthalmic procedures may aid in the diagnosis of metastatic tumors. These include a systemic evaluation, intravenous fluorescein angiography (IVFA), indocyanine green (ICG) angiography, ultrasonography, optical coherence tomography (OCT), CT, MRI, fine-needle aspiration biopsy (FNAB), and surgical biopsy.

Systemic Evaluation

Once a metastatic tumor to the intraocular structures is suspected on the basis of ophthalmic examination, a detailed systemic evaluation is mandatory. The patient's history may reveal a previous malignancy, which can be helpful in the diagnosis. As mentioned earlier, however, many patients seen by the ophthalmologist have no history of cancer. Initially, if a female patient has a suspected metastatic tumor, breast and lung examination with appropriate ancillary studies is indicated. In men, the evaluation should be directed initially toward a primary tumor in the lung; later, if the lung is normal, gastrointestinal tract, kidney, thyroid, pancreas, and other organs are evaluated.

Fluorescein Angiography

IVFA is a method of imaging the vascularity within a choroidal tumor and is sometimes helpful in the diagnosis of a choroidal metastasis.[11,22-26] In contrast to choroidal hemangioma and melanoma, most metastatic carcinomas are hypofluorescent in the arterial and early venous phases and show progressive hyperfluorescence in the subsequent phases. Pinpoint foci of hyperfluorescence appear over the tumor in the venous phase and persist into the late angiograms. There may be moderate late hyperfluorescence of serous subretinal fluid related to the metastatic tumor.

Indocyanine Green Angiography

ICG angiography provides detail of the choroidal vascular pattern. Imaging of choroidal metastases with this technique generally reveals mild hypofluorescence throughout the angiogram, whereas choroidal melanoma shows gradual hyperfluorescence over 5 to 10 minutes, and choroidal hemangioma shows bright hyperfluorescence within 1 minute.[42]

Ultrasonography

Ocular ultrasonography provides resolution within 1 mm and is useful in the diagnosis of intraocular metastasis. A-scan ultrasonography demonstrates a sharp initial spike and moderate internal reflectivity. This is in contrast to malignant melanoma, which usually shows relatively low internal reflectivity. B-scan ultrasonography typically shows a choroidal mass pattern with moderate to high acoustic solidity, overlying subretinal fluid, and no choroidal excavation. In contrast, melanoma shows relative acoustic hollowness.

Optical Coherence Tomography

OCT is a method of imaging the retina with high resolution of 8 mm. This technique allows for subclinical analysis of minor subretinal fluid, retinal edema, and retinal pigment epithelial changes associated with choroidal metastases. This can assist in deciphering the exact cause of visual loss.

Computed Tomography

CT is used most frequently in the evaluation of metastatic orbital tumors and less often for intraocular tumors. This technique can demonstrate the anatomic location and configuration of orbital metastases as well as surrounding periorbital changes. It is important to evaluate the brain in all patients with ocular metastasis from breast cancer because brain involvement occurs in nearly 30% of patients (Table 32–18).

Magnetic Resonance Imaging

MRI is useful in delineating the anatomic location, configuration, and internal tissue qualities of choroidal and orbital metastases. It is superior to CT for soft tissue resolution, especially when using fat-suppression technique, orbital surface coil, and gadolinium enhancement. In general, uveal metastases are slightly hyperintense compared to vitreous on T1-weighted images and hypointense compared to vitreous on

Table 32–18   Locations of Systemic Nonocular Metastases Before and After the Uveal Metastasis Was Established in 264 Consecutive Patients with Uveal Metastasis from Breast Cancer*

Location of Systemic Metastases	No. of Patients (%)
Diagnosed Before the Ocular Metastasis Was Established	
Lung	71 (27)
Long bone	68 (26)
Chest wall	19 (7)
Spine	17 (6)
Liver	14 (5)
Other breast	16 (6)
Brain	15 (6)
Skin	10 (4)
Skull	8 (3)
Others	6 (2)
None	116 (44)
Diagnosed After the Ocular Metastasis Was Established	
Brain	73 (28)
Lung	64 (24)
Long bone	64 (24)
Liver	37 (14)
Spine	22 (8)
Chest wall	18 (6)
Skull	10 (4)
Skin	5 (2)
Others	14 (5)

*Some patients had more than one treatment modality; some patients had systemic metastases in more than one location.
Data from Demirci H, Shields CL, Chao A, Shields JA. Uveal metastasis from breast cancer in 264 patients. Am J Ophthalmology 2003;136: 264–271.

T2-weighted images.[43] The associated retinal detachment is hyperintense compared to vitreous on T1-weighted images and isointense compared to vitreous on T2-weighted images. Metastatic carcinomas show mild enhancement with gadolinium. Orbital metastases show a hyperintense signal compared to the suppressed orbital fat on T1- and T2-weighted images and moderate gadolinium enhancement.

Fine-Needle Aspiration Biopsy

When the diagnosis of an ocular lesion is particularly difficult to establish, FNAB is appropriate.[23,44] This technique requires exceptional skill for lesions within the eye, using indirect ophthalmoscopy to guide the needle through the pars plana of the ciliary body into the solid mass. For orbital lesions, ultrasound or CT is employed for localization of deep lesions. An adequate cytologic sample is obtained in nearly 90% of cases.[44] This is especially useful for patients who present with no previous cancer and in whom systemic evaluation is nonrevealing.

Surgical Biopsy

Open surgical biopsy is commonly employed to diagnose orbital, conjunctival, and eyelid metastases and less commonly for intraocular metastases. In such instances, complete resection is performed if the tumor is circumscribed. For ill-defined lesions, incisional biopsy is performed. For intraocular metastases, the biopsy is performed microscopically through a scleral flap. Surgical biopsy obtains more tissue for the pathologist, but radiotherapy or chemotherapy

is generally indicated to eliminate tumor seeding at the biopsy site.

What are the pathologic characteristics of ocular metastases?

Because the intraocular structures and orbit have no lymphatic channels, metastatic tumors reach these sites by hematogenous routes. Probably because of its marked vascularity, the uvea is the location of most ocular metastases, especially the posterior portion of the choroids.

Gross examination of an eye with metastatic carcinoma usually reveals one or more diffuse or nodular amelanotic tumors in the uvea. In rare instances, the mass is highly elevated with a dome shape, similar to that of choroidal melanoma, but melanoma is generally pigmented.

Low-power magnification of a metastatic carcinoma reveals a placoid or diffuse mass, often with an overlying serous detachment of the sensory retina. Well-differentiated tumors may retain certain histologic or histochemical features of the primary tumor. Breast metastases typically appear histologically as solid epithelial nests or glandular structures. It is important to differentiate a primary adenocarcinoma of the retinal pigment epithelium, ciliary body epithelium, or iris pigment epithelium from a metastatic adenocarcinoma.

What are the treatment options for ocular metastases?

The preferred treatment for an ocular metastasis from breast cancer depends on the location, extent, activity, and symptoms related to the ocular tumor as well as the patient's systemic status.[22–26,45] Management may involve observation alone, chemotherapy, hormone therapy, laser treatment, irradiation, or surgical resection.

Observation

Some metastatic tumors to the eye are inactive and require no treatment. They may have regressed spontaneously, or they may have regressed following systemic treatment of the primary breast cancer months or years previously. With some experience, the ocular oncologist can recognize such inactive metastasis. When located in the choroid, they are generally flat tumors with pigment epithelial clumping on the tumor surface and without retinal detachment.

Chemotherapy and Hormone Therapy

Active tumors, characterized by a homogeneous mass with a secondary retinal detachment, usually require treatment. In general, if the patient is asymptomatic and the eye tumor appears to be controlled with the chemotherapy or hormone therapy that is being used to treat the systemic disease, then no specific ocular treatment is indicated. The patient should be followed at 2- to 4-month intervals for documentation of tumor and visual status.

Laser Photocoagulation and Thermotherapy

Rarely, choroidal metastases are treated with laser photocoagulation or thermotherapy. This is employed only for small tumors located outside the macular region. Methods of laser treatment using diode red, diode green, or argon laser can be applied to small choroidal metastases measuring less than 5 or 6 mm in base dimension.[46] Thermotherapy, using a large spot diode laser to heat the tumor to a subphotocoagulation level, is gaining some interest. These methods, however, are damaging to the normal retina and induce a dense scotoma. For this reason, most clinicians prefer focal treatment with radiotherapy rather than methods of laser or thermotherapy.

Radiotherapy

If the patient has an active choroidal metastasis, external-beam irradiation is generally effective in controlling the tumor.[47,48] The entire uvea or orbit is irradiated, with about 3000 cGy delivered in divided doses over 3 weeks.[47,48] Plaque brachytherapy is a method of focal radiotherapy using an implant with radioactive sources. The implant is surgically applied to the eye to deliver a radiation dose to a select region. This minimizes radiotherapy to surrounding normal structures. Plaque brachytherapy is employed for circumscribed tumors measuring less than 18 mm at the base and less than 10 mm in thickness.[49] The benefit of plaque brachytherapy is the speed of treatment—it takes only 2 to 4 days to deliver the dose. This is important for patients whose life expectancy is limited because it occupies less time of their remaining days than other methods of radiotherapy.[49]

After radiotherapy, choroidal metastases decrease in tumor thickness on ultrasonography, and secondary retinal detachment resolves, often with improved visual acuity. Rudoler and associates found that external-beam radiotherapy provides globe preservation in 98% of patients, with visual improvement or vision better than 20/200 in 57% of patients.[47,48] Ocular radiation complications were found in 12% of patients.[47,48]

Surgical Excision and Enucleation

In some instances, enucleation or local surgical excision of an intraocular metastasis may be justified. Uncontrollable large tumors occasionally require enucleation for intractable pain caused by secondary glaucoma. However, chemotherapy or radiotherapy, rather than enucleation, should generally be considered first. Local excision of a tumor that has metastasized to the eyelid, conjunctiva, orbit, and occasionally the intraocular structures is justified in certain instances. This technique is useful for both diagnostic and therapeutic reasons.

What is the prognosis of the patient with ocular metastases?

In general, the life prognosis is poor for patients with metastatic tumors to the ocular structures.[9,15] Patients with breast carcinoma metastatic to the uvea have a mean survival of 18 months, which is better survival than for patients with metastases from lung cancer (mean, 6 months) or cutaneous melanoma (mean, 1 month).[9] Data collected from our department showed Kaplan-Meier survival estimates for patients with uveal metastasis from breast cancer to be 65% at 1 year, 34% at 3 years, and 24% at 5 years.[15]

SUMMARY

Breast cancer metastatic to the eye most commonly is detected in the choroid and much less often in the orbit, conjunctiva, eyelid, ciliary body, iris, retina, and optic nerve. In 16% of patients, the ocular metastasis is the first metastatic site, and in 3% of patients, it is the initial manifestation of breast cancer. Survival is poor, at 24% by 5 years.

REFERENCES

1. Duke-Elder S. System of Ophthalmology, vol. 9: Diseases of the Uveal Tract. St. Louis, CV Mosby, 1966, p 917.
2. Hart WM. Metastatic carcinoma to the eye and orbit. Int Ophthalmol Clin 1962;212:465–482.
3. Albert DM, Rubenstein RA, Scheie HG. Tumors metastasis to the eye. I. Incidence in 213 adult patients with generalized malignancy. Am J Ophthalmol 1967;63:723–726.
4. Jensen OA. Metastatic tumors of the eye and orbit. A histopathological analysis of a Danish series. Acta Pathol Microbiol Scand Suppl 1970;212:201–214.
5. Bloch RS, Gartner S. The incidence of ocular metastatic carcinoma. Arch Ophthalmol 1971;85:673–675.
6. Ferry AP, Font RL. Carcinoma metastatic to the eye and orbit. I. A clinicopathologic study of 227 cases. Arch Ophthalmol 1974;92:276–286.
7. Stephens RF, Shields JA. Diagnosis and management of cancer metastatic to the uvea: A study of 70 cases. Ophthalmology 1979;86:1336–1349.
8. Nelson CC, Hertzberg BS, Klintworth GK. A histopathologic study of 716 unselected eyes in patients with cancer at the time of death. Am J Ophthalmol 1983;95:788–793.
9. Freedman MI, Folk JC. Metastatic tumors to the eye and orbit. Patient survival and clinical characteristics. Arch Ophthalmol 1987;105:1215–1219.
10. Eliassi-Rad B, Albert DM, Green WR. Frequency of ocular metastases in patients dying of cancer in eye bank populations. Br J Ophthalmol 1996;80:125–128.
11. Shields CL, Shields JA, Gross NE, et al. Survey of 520 eyes with uveal metastases. Ophthalmology 1997;104:1265–1276.
12. Bullock JD, Yanes B. Ophthalmic manifestations of metastatic breast cancer. Ophthalmology 1980;87:961–973.
13. Merrill CF, Kaufman DI, Dimitrov NV. Breast cancer metastatic to the eye is a common entity. Cancer 1991;68:623–627.
14. Mewis L, Young SE. Breast carcinoma metastatic to the choroid. Analysis of 67 patients. Ophthalmology 1982;89:147–151.
15. Demirci H, Shields CL, Chao A, Shields JA. Uveal metastasis from breast cancer in 264 patients. Am J Ophthalmol 2003;136:264–271.
16. Amichetti M, Caffo O, Minatel E, et al. Ocular metastases from breast carcinoma: A multicentric retrospective study. Oncol Rep 2000;7:761–765.
17. De Potter P, Shields CL, Shields JA, Tardio DJ. Uveal metastasis from prostate carcinoma. Cancer 1993;71:2791–2796.
18. Font RL, Naumann G, Zimmerman LE. Primary malignant melanoma of the skin metastatic to the eye and orbit. Report of ten cases and review of literature. Am J Ophthalmol 1967;63:438–554.
19. Fishman ML, Tomaszewski MM, Kuwabara T. Malignant melanoma of the skin metastatic to the eye. Frequency in autopsy series. Arch Ophthalmol 1976;94:1309–1311.
20. Debustros S, Augsburger JJ, Shields JA, et al. Intraocular metastases from cutaneous malignant melanoma. Arch Ophthalmol 1985;103:937–940.
21. Harbour JW, De Potter P, Shields CL, Shields JA. Uveal metastasis from carcinoid tumor: Clinical observations in nine cases. Ophthalmology 1994;101:1084–1090.
22. Shields JA, Shields CL. Metastatic tumors to the intraocular structures. In Intraocular Tumors: A Text and Atlas. Philadelphia, WB Saunders, 1992, pp 207–238.
23. Shields JA, Shields CL. Metastatic tumors to the uvea, retina, and optic disc. In Atlas of Intraocular Tumors. Philadelphia, Lippincott Williams & Wilkins, 1999, pp 151–169.

24. Shields JA, Shields CL. Metastatic tumors to the orbit. In Atlas of Orbital Tumors. Philadelphia, Lippincott Williams & Wilkins, 1999, pp 187–199.

25. Shields JA, Shields CL. Tumors and pseudotumors of the conjunctiva: Lymphoid, leukemic, and metastatic tumors. In Atlas of Eyelid and Conjunctival Tumors. Philadelphia, Lippincott Williams & Wilkins, 1999, pp 289–299.

26. Shields JA, Shields CL. Tumors and pseudotumors of the eyelid: Lymphoid, plasmacytic, and metastatic tumors. In Atlas of Eyelid and Conjunctival Tumors. Philadelphia, Lippincott Williams & Wilkins, 1999, pp 127–137.

27. Shields CL, Shields JA, Peggs M. Tumors metastatic to the orbit. J Ophthalm Plast Reconstr Surg 1988;4:73–80.

28. Shields JA, Shields CL, Brotman HK, et al. Cancer metastatic to the orbit. The 2000 Robert M. Curts Lecture. Ophthalmic Plast Reconstr Surg 2001;17: 346–354.

29. Shields JA, Shields CL, Scartozzi R. Survey of 1264 orbital tumors and pseudotumors. The 2002 Montgomery Lecture, part 1. Ophthalmology 2004;111:997–1008.

30. Shields CL, Demirci H, Karatza EC, Shields JA. Clinical survey of 1643 tumors and simulating lesions of the conjunctiva. Opthalmology 2004;111:1747–1754.

31. Kiratli H, Shields CL, Shields JA, De Potter P. Metastatic tumors to the conjunctiva. Report of ten cases. Br J Ophthalmol 1996;80:5–8.

32. Shields JA, Shields CL, Singh AD. Metastatic neoplasms in the optic disc: The 1999 Bjerrum Lecture—part 2. Arch Ophthalmol. 2000;118: 217–224.

33. Shields JA, Shields CL, Kiratli H, DePotter P. Metastatic tumors to the iris in 40 patients. Am J Ophthalmol 1995;119:422–430.

34. Kamby C, Ejlertsen B, Andersen J, et al. The pattern of metastases in human breast cancer. Influence of systemic adjuvant therapy and impact on survival. Acta Oncol 1988;27:715–719.

35. O'Brien J, Wieland M, Filer R. Breast cancer metastatic to the choroid in a male patient. Retina 2000;2:214–216.

36. Shields JA, Shields CL. Posterior uveal melanoma: Clinical and pathologic features. In Intraocular Tumors: A Text and Atlas. Philadelphia, WB Saunders, 1992, pp 117–136.

37. Michelson JB, Stephens RF, Shields JA. Clinical conditions mistaken for metastatic cancer to the choroid. Ann Ophthalmol 1979;11:149–153.

38. Shields CL, Honavar SG, Shields JA, et al. Circumscribed choroidal hemangioma. Clinical manifestations and factors predictive of visual outcome in 200 consecutive cases. Ophthalmology 2001;108:2237–2248.

39. Shields CL, Shields JA, Augsburger JJ. Review of choroidal osteomas. Surv Ophthalmol 1988;33:17–27.

40. Shields CL, Stopyra GA, Marr BP, et al. Enophthalmos as initial manifestation of occult mammogram-negative breast carcinoma. Ophthalmic Surg Lasers Imaging 2004;35:56–57.

41. Lim JI. Paraneoplastic syndromes. Ophthalmol Clin North Am 1999; 12:213–224.

42. Shields CL, Shields CL, De Potter P. Patterns of indocyanine green angiography of choroidal tumors. Br J Ophthalmol 1995;79:237–245.

43. De Potter P, Shields JA, Shields CL, et al. Metastatic carcinoma to the choroid and optic nerve: Unusual magnetic resonance imaging findings. Int Ophthalmol 1992;16:39–44.

44. Shields JA, Shields CL, Ehya H, et al. Fine needle aspiration biopsy of suspected intraocular tumors. The 1992 Urwick Lecture. Ophthalmology 1993;100:1677–1684.

45. Char DH. Treatment of choroidal metastasis. Arch Ophthalmol 1991; 18: 333.

46. Levinger S, Merin S, Seigal R, Pe'er J. Laser therapy in the management of choroidal breast tumor metastases. Ophthalmic Surg Lasers Imaging 2001;32:294–299.

47. Rudoler SB, Corn BW, Shields CL, et al. External beam irradiation for choroid metastases: Identification of factors predisposing to long-term sequelae. Int J Radiat Oncol Biol Phys 1997;(1)38:251–256.

48. Rudoler SB, Shields CL, Corn BW, et al. Functional vision is improved in the majority of patients treated with external-beam radiotherapy for choroid metastases: A multivariate analysis of 188 patients. J Clin Oncol 1997;15:1244–1251.

49. Shields CL, Shields JA, De Potter P, et al. Plaque radiotherapy in the management of uveal metastasis. Arch Ophthalmol 1997;115:203–209.

VIII

Thoracic Metastases from Breast Cancer

Jason P. Shaw and Lawrence R. Glassman

What is the role of surgery in the treatment of breast carcinoma metastatic to the lung?

The treatment algorithm for patients with breast cancer who are found to have pulmonary metastases remains controversial. Although most patients who develop breast cancer metastases die from complications of their disease,[1] new treatment options have increased median survival times in selected patients.[2] Furthermore, recent retrospective studies based on tumor registries,[3] as well as observational studies,[4,5] have described favorable outcomes for selected breast cancer patients with isolated pulmonary metastases who undergo surgical resection, compared with historical controls. These findings have made a valid case for surgical resection of isolated pulmonary metastases in selected breast cancer patients.

How is the diagnosis of lung metastasis made?

In the absence of endobronchial lesions or large malignant effusions, most patients with lung metastases are asymptomatic at the time of diagnosis. Pulmonary metastases tend to be peripherally located, often identified during pretreatment staging workup or post-treatment surveillance. Some patients may develop symptoms such as cough, shortness of breath, or hemoptysis, all of which merit further evaluation. Chest radiographs, frequently obtained as part of preoperative evaluation, should be part of the routine surveillance of patients with newly diagnosed breast cancer. If a patient develops symptoms or if a pulmonary nodule is discovered incidentally, further imaging studies, particularly a CT scan of the chest, ought to be pursued. Isolated involvement of the lung and pleural space occurs in 15% to 25% of women with metastatic breast cancer.[6] Before pursuing thoracic surgical intervention, evaluation should include CT scanning of the chest and abdomen and a bone scan to exclude widely disseminated disease.

Tissue biopsy may be obtained by transthoracic or transbronchial needle biopsy or surgical biopsy. Distinguishing breast carcinoma from primary lung carcinoma may be difficult without immunohistologic stains. Several antibodies indicative of breast cancer origin have been described, including estrogen and progesterone receptors, GCDFP-15, and S-100, whereas expression of thyroid transcription factor-1 (TTF-1) identifies lung adenocarcinomas.[7] If transbronchial or transthoracic needle biopsy is nondiagnostic, surgery is indicated to make a diagnosis.

What are the goals of metastasectomy?

Resection of a new pulmonary nodule in a patient with a history of breast cancer may be indicated to aid diagnosis and guide further therapy, and in selected cases to achieve possible curative resection. About 3% of all women with breast cancer develop a solitary pulmonary nodule detectable on chest radiograph[8,9]; however, only 30% to 40% of those nodules prove to be metastases; of nonmetastatic nodules, most represent primary lung tumors. All solitary lung nodules should be biopsied or resected because nearly half are a new primary lung cancer, especially among smokers.[10] The challenge for the clinician remains in selecting which patients would benefit most from surgical resection of lung metastasis and having clear treatment goals to justify the morbidity of surgery.

What palliative treatments may be beneficial?

Less commonly, resection of a metastatic lesion in a breast cancer patient may be considered for palliation. Patients may develop obstructive symptoms or hemoptysis secondary to tumor invasion of mainstem bronchi. Treatment of the endobronchial lesion may include external-beam radiation, endobronchial radiation (brachytherapy), laser therapy, or endobronchial resection and stenting of the obstructed airway to improve bronchial patency.

What factors must be considered in selecting operative candidates?

The same criteria that apply to patients undergoing pulmonary metastasectomy for other primary tumors apply to those with breast cancer:

- Controlled or controllable primary tumor
- Tumor completely resectable
- No extrapulmonary spread detectable
- No local recurrence
- Adequate cardiopulmonary reserve to tolerate the proposed lung resection

In addition, several other patient- and tumor-specific factors ought to be considered because of their prognostic significance. Positive postsurgical outcomes have been associated with a long disease-free interval (DFI),[3,11,12] complete resection of the tumor,[3,9,13] and positive ER status.[13] Although ER status and DFI may be easily obtainable, preoperative determination of whether pulmonary metastases are amenable to complete resection occasionally poses a formidable challenge to the surgeon. Complete surgical resection is predictive of a favorable outcome, whereas the number of metastases alone is not. Causes of incomplete resections include tumor involvement of lymph nodes, chest wall, or diaphragm and inadequate or short margins of resection.[3] For these reasons, preoperative imaging studies are crucial in patient selection and for planning operative strategy.

What is the best surgical approach?

Surgery may proceed after appropriate preoperative evaluation has been completed and the patient deemed a suitable surgical candidate. The surgical approach and extent of pulmonary resection must be individualized. For solitary or unilateral disease, the standard approach has been a small lateral thoracotomy that permits complete palpation of the lung to assess for metastases not seen on CT scan. Options for resection of bilateral disease include median sternotomy, staged or sequential lateral thoracotomies, or bilateral transsternal thoracotomy, also known as a "clamshell" approach.

More recently, video-assisted thoracic surgery (VATS) has become an important technique and may be used in certain circumstances, primarily to aid in diagnosis. The use of VATS for routine resection of pulmonary metastases remains controversial. The same principles that apply to an "open" case ought to apply to VATS in terms of obtaining complete resection. In a prospective trial evaluating the efficacy of VATS for metastasectomy, McCormack and colleagues found that 10 of 18 patients had additional malignant lesions found at thoracotomy after "complete resection" by VATS.[14] The study was set to accrue 50 patients but was closed early with a 56% incomplete resection rate of VATS. It should be noted, however, that this study pre-dates the use of spiral CT scans, which have been shown to be more sensitive in detecting additional pulmonary lesions that might otherwise be missed by traditional CT scans.[15]

An ideal case for the VATS technique would be the patient whose lesion has been followed for longer than 3 months in whom no additional lesions have developed; technically, the lesion should be solitary, peripheral, and easily resectable with a superficial wedge. Lesions deeper in the parenchyma or close to the hilum are less well suited to resection by VATS. As a rule, metastasectomy should include an adequate margin of normal surrounding tissue, whereas resection for a primary lung carcinoma requires a formal lobectomy. Conservative nonanatomic resections are ideal for metastasectomy because they preserve lung function and allow for complete resection with a minimal risk for local recurrence. Because many metastases are small and may not be detected by preoperative imaging studies, direct intraoperative palpation of the atelectatic lung may enable the detection of occult nodules. At this time, we generally favor an open approach, using VATS on a case-by-case basis.

What is the long-term survival after metastasectomy?

Long-term results of resection of pulmonary metastases vary and are largely based on retrospective and observational data from heterogeneous patient populations. Nonetheless, the data are encouraging. Retrospective data from a tumor registry of 467 patients undergoing metastasectomy for breast cancer revealed a 5-year survival rate that ranged from 13% to 50%, with cumulative 5- and 10-year survival rates of 35% and 20%, respectively.[3] A recent retrospective single-institution study[16] showed a 5-year survival rate of 45% with surgery. These results compare favorably with historical controls; however, there are no randomized trials published to date comparing surgery and adjuvant therapy to adjuvant therapy alone.

How often do pleural effusions develop in breast cancer patients? What causes them?

Breast carcinoma is the most common cause of malignant pleural effusions in women and the second most common cause in general. Over the course of their disease, 7% to 11% of breast carcinoma patients develop malignant pleural effusions.[17–19] Although autopsy studies show pleural disease in about half of all breast cancer cases,[20] many patients are asymptomatic. Pleural effusions may be caused by obstruction of lymphatic drainage by tumor.[21] Pleural implants, lymphangitic spread to mediastinal or internal mammary nodes, or tumor cell suspension in the pleural space may all result in increased pleural osmotic pressure. Additionally, the inflammatory response to any of the above may result in increased capillary permeability, resulting in an accumulation of pleural fluid. Malignant effusions need to be differentiated from other common causes of effusions, including infection, congestive heart failure, and hypoalbuminemia.

How are malignant effusions diagnosed?

A new pleural effusion in a patient with a history of breast carcinoma should be viewed as secondary to malignancy until proven otherwise. A malignant pleural effusion is defined by the presence of malignant cells within the pleura or pleural fluid. In most cases, a diagnosis can be established by pleural fluid cytology or percutaneous pleural biopsy. Fluid cytology has a diagnostic yield of 60% to 70%, is easily performed, and is often therapeutic as well as diagnostic.[19,21,22] Large-volume and repeat taps may increase the diagnostic yield. Percutaneous pleural biopsy has a diagnostic yield of about 45%, is more difficult to perform, and is less clinically applicable. Malignant pleural effusions are usually exudative, often bloody, with low glucose concentration. Specific markers, such as carcinoembryonic antigen levels, although not specific for breast carcinoma, may be elevated. If fluid cytology is nondiagnostic, thoracoscopic pleural biopsy should be considered because it has a sensitivity approaching 95%.[19] Once a diagnosis is made, further treatment is initiated.

How should malignant effusions be managed?

The algorithm for the evaluation and treatment of a breast cancer patient with a pleural effusion is similar to that for any patient with a suspected malignant effusion, keeping in mind a few important differences. In general, patients with malignant effusions secondary to breast cancer have a better prognosis than those with effusions secondary to lung, gastric, or ovarian cancer.[21] Some patients may have a good response to chemotherapy,[22,23] with documented cases of resolution after initiation of chemotherapy.[24,25] However, treatment remains palliative, with more aggressive or surgical approaches reserved for cases of recurrent effusions in symptomatic patients who have failed medical therapy or with trapped lungs.

The approach to managing malignant effusions should be individualized to each patient, taking into account the degree of symptoms, the patient's general condition and expected survival, and the response of the primary tumor to systemic therapy. If the patient is asymptomatic, observation is a valid option. For the symptomatic patient with limited survival and very poor performance status, repeat pleurocentesis is a satisfactory option. Insertion of an indwelling tunneled soft catheter such as the PleurX system (Denver Biomaterial, Denver) allows for chronic home drainage of the effusion and avoids unnecessary hospitalization. Freedom from recurrent effusion may be as good with such an approach as with sclerosants[22]; however, randomized trials are underway at the present time. Most malignant effusions recur after thoracentesis or tube thoracostomy alone. Standard practice combines drainage with pleurodesis unless the patient is too debilitated to tolerate the procedure. It is crucial to confirm good lung re-expansion following the initial drainage of pleural fluid before attempting pleurodesis. Pleurodesis with sclerosis using bleomycin[26] or sterile talc as a slurry is the current procedure of choice, with both treatments having efficacy rates in the range of 75%.[27]

What is the management of patients who have failed pleurodesis or have a trapped lung?

For patients with a trapped lung or in whom attempts at pleurodesis have failed, several options are available for palliation. Options include intermittent drainage using an indwelling pleural catheter or VATS to facilitate lung re-expansion by removal of the "visceral peel," with or without partial pleurectomy.[28]

Indwelling pleural drainage tubes can be inserted under local anesthesia and may be drained intermittently by the patient or caregiver at home when the patient is symptomatic. They have been shown to be safe and effective and are a good treatment option for patients with poor performance status.[28,29]

Pleuroperitoneal shunting is also an option. Pleuroperitoneal shunts are unidirectional catheters with a valved pumping chamber that facilitate passage of pleural fluid to the peritoneal cavity (Denver shunt, Codmen and Shurtleff, Randolph, MA). The shunts can be inserted using a modified Seldinger technique or through thoracoscopy or minithoracotomy. Although the catheters can be inserted with a low mortality and morbidity, they are easily obstructed by fibrinous debris.[30] Additionally, they require that a patient or caregiver actively compress the pump chamber at regular intervals. For these reasons, pleuroperitoneal shunts are a less attractive option.

VATS with or without partial decortication or pleurectomy is a highly effective method of achieving successful pleurodesis[31] as well as biopsy of the tumor. It also has the advantage of allowing concurrent drainage and pleurodesis. VATS pleurodesis also has the added benefit of ensuring that insufflated talc is uniformly delivered to the pleural surface and that chest tubes are optimally positioned under direct vision. It does require that the patient be able to tolerate general anesthesia and single-lung ventilation, and it may be associated with higher costs than pleurodesis through tube thoracostomy.[32]

Pleurectomy is the most effective form of ensuring successful pleurodesis and prevention of recurrence of a malignant effusion; however, it is associated with high morbidity and mortality rates and is not generally recommended.[11,33] Its use should be reserved for patients with trapped lung who have a long expected survival and who are in good general condition.

What is the best method for pleurodesis (timing, size of tube, sclerosing agent, patient rotation)?

Successful pleurodesis may be achieved through small-bore chest tubes.[34] Smaller chest tubes usually cause less discomfort and are better tolerated by the patient; however, they may become more easily occluded, requiring repeat chest tube insertion. For that reason, we prefer to use a medium-sized chest tube in the range of 20 to 28 French. In addition, the amount of daily pleural fluid drainage should be relatively low, in the range of 100 to 200 mL/day, before initiation of sclerosing therapy. Talc is the most effective agent for use under general anesthesia; other agents, including bleomycin, may be equally effective.[35] Talc has been shown to be superior to other agents, including tetracycline or bleomycin in several trials, including one that examined malignant effusions secondary to breast cancer.[36] Once the sclerosant is administered, the chest tube should be clamped or placed to water seal for 1 to 3 hours. Patient rotation has been proposed to facilitate distribution of medication throughout the pleural cavity. This practice has not been validated in clinical trials; nuclear tracers injected into the pleural cavity are distributed widely after a short interval. A prospective randomized trial suggested that patient rotation did not contribute to success of talc pleurodesis and was associated with increased patient discomfort.[37] There appears to be a similar success rate of pleurodesis using talc slurry through a chest tube, as through talc insufflation ("poudrage") with VATS. The decision for sclerosis under general anesthesia should be tailored to the needs of the patient.[32]

In which patients with breast cancer is chest wall reconstruction indicated?

Breast cancer patients may require chest wall resection and reconstruction for palliation of pain or for removal of an ulcerated mass that produces significant discomfort. This is best accomplished with a multidisciplinary approach, including thoracic and plastic surgeons, as well as medical or radiation oncologists to help provide the best chance of local control. There are primarily three scenarios in which breast cancer patients might require chest wall resection:

1. *Locally advanced disease.* Although most breast cancers are detected earlier with modern screening strategies, occasional patients may present with advanced local disease and direct chest wall invasion. Invasion of the ribs or intercostal musculature requires en bloc full-thickness chest wall resection. Recurrence with solitary disease in the internal mammary lymph node region may also be treated with chest wall resection and reconstruction.
2. *Radiation necrosis,* often seen 15 to 20 years after completion of therapy, results from ischemia and damage to soft tissues surrounding the irradiated field. The affected area of chest wall may frequently be infected or less often may harbor residual tumor, both of which situations pose particular challenges for the surgeon.
3. *Local recurrence* may involve tumor invasion of the musculoskeletal elements underlying the breast. Often, this occurs in the setting of prior irradiation or infection. Local recurrence may follow several patterns, including primary involvement of internal mammary chain nodes or direct invasion of ribs or chest wall musculature. Local recurrence may cause pain and produce a cosmetically displeasing ulcerated mass, both of which are indications for palliative resection. Some authors have advocated a disease-free interval of longer than 2 years as the criterion for selecting candidates for resection of the chest wall recurrence for local failure.[25]

What should the preoperative evaluation include?

A thorough history and examination may give clues as to the aggressiveness of the tumor and overall prognosis. A chest wall recurrence carries a worse prognosis in a patient who has undergone prior modified radical mastectomy than in a patient who has undergone prior breast-conserving therapy (i.e., lumpectomy and radiation). Physical examination may give clues to the extent of the disease. Short disease-free interval, rapid growth, overlying skin fixation, and pain may portend a worse prognosis. Preoperative radiologic evaluation should include a chest radiograph and either a CT scan or MRI of the chest to assess the extent of disease. Incisional or needle biopsies of the lesion may help confirm a diagnosis of suspected chest wall recurrence. Preoperative lung function testing should be obtained if a patient has known intrinsic lung disease or poor respiratory reserve, especially if there is a chance that the patient may require concomitant lung resection.

What are adequate margins of resection?

We advocate en bloc resection of all involved ribs and one additional rib cephalic and caudal to the lesion. A minithoracotomy enables manual inspection and palpation of the inner surface of the chest wall and assessment of underlying viscera. Involvement of the great vessels precludes resection. If feasible, a 5-cm margin of clinically normal-appearing tissue in all planes is advocated in the hope of obtaining 1- to 2-cm histologic margins. Although frozen sections of soft tissues may aid in confirming tumor-free margins, some tissues, such as bone, are not amenable to frozen section, and thus sound clinical judgment is paramount. Adequate resection of the diseased tissues is important to provide healthy, viable margins on which subsequent chest wall reconstruction relies.

What are the goals for reconstructing the chest wall?

Chest wall reconstruction must adequately remove all devitalized or tumor-involved tissue, restore rigidity to prevent a flail chest, and provide adequate soft tissue coverage to close the pleural space and protect the underlying viscera. Reconstruction should provide a tension-free closure with healthy tissue coverage. Careful preoperative planning with plastic surgery consultation should allow for a satisfactory result in all cases.

What are the surgical options for reconstruction?

Reconstruction of the chest wall must be individualized, taking into account the size and location of the defect, the presence or absence of associated infection, and the general condition of the patient. Options for reconstruction include autologous materials (e.g., muscle flaps) or prosthetic grafts including polytetrafluoroethylene (PTFE) or Prolene mesh with or without the use of methylmethacrylate to add structural rigidity. A retrospective study demonstrated no difference in outcomes between Prolene and PTFE for reconstruction, and both were shown to be safe.[38] Frequently used regional flaps include latissimus dorsi, pectoralis major, and rectus abdominis flaps. Occasionally, an omental flap can be used if regional myocutaneous flaps are not an option.[39] In the presence of significant potential infection, the need to avoid foreign materials should prompt consideration of reconstruction using completely autologous material. This may lack the structural support of the prosthetic materials but is less likely to be complicated by ongoing sepsis.

The choice of flap is based on the size of the defect as well as the region of chest wall affected. Each pedicled flap is tethered by its blood supply, although more complicated free myocutaneous flaps may overcome this obstacle and help in closing larger defects. Split-thickness skin grafts may be required for coverage of donor sites. Chest wall stabilization is required for most full-thickness breast resection defects, particularly if they are large, laterally located involving the curve of the ribs, or involving a significant part of the sternum, or if the patient has poor pulmonary function.

REFERENCES

1. Greenberg PA, Hortobagyi GN, Smith TL, et al. Long-term follow-up of patients with complete remission following combination chemotherapy for metastatic breast cancer. J Clin Oncol 1996;14(8):2197–2205.
2. Giordano SH, Buzdar AU, Smith TL, et al. Is breast cancer survival improving? Cancer 2004;100(1):44–52.
3. Friedel G, Pastorino U, Ginsberg RJ, et al. Results of lung metastasectomy from breast cancer: Prognostic criteria on the basis of 467 cases of the International Registry of Lung Metastases. Eur J Cardiothorac Surg 2002;22(3):335–344.
4. Staren ED, Salerno C, Rongione A, et al. Pulmonary resection for metastatic breast cancer. Arch Surg 1992;127(11):1282–1284.
5. Ludwig C, Stoelben E, Hasse J. Disease-free survival after resection of lung metastases in patients with breast cancer. Eur J Surg Oncol 2003;29(6):532–535.
6. Patanaphan V, Salazar OM, Risco R. Breast cancer: Metastatic patterns and their prognosis. South Med J 1988;81(9):1109–1112.
7. Raab SS, Berg LC, Swanson PE, Wick MR. Adenocarcinoma in the lung in patients with breast cancer. A prospective analysis of the discriminatory value of immunohistology. Am J Clin Pathol 1993;100(1):27–35.
8. Casey JJ, Stempel BG, Scanlon EF, Fry WA. The solitary pulmonary nodule in the patient with breast cancer. Surgery 1984;96(4):801–805.
9. McDonald ML, Deschamps C, Ilstrup DM, et al. Pulmonary resection for metastatic breast cancer. Ann Thorac Surg 1994;58(6):1599–1602.
10. Wilkins EW Jr, Head JM, Burke JF. Pulmonary resection for metastatic neoplasms in the lung. Experience at the Massachusetts General Hospital. Am J Surg 1978;135(4):480–483.
11. Lanza LA, Natarajan G, Roth JA, Putnam JB Jr. Long-term survival after resection of pulmonary metastases from carcinoma of the breast. Ann Thorac Surg 1992;54(2):244–247; discussion, 248.
12. Simpson R, Kennedy C, Carmalt H, et al. Pulmonary resection for metastatic breast cancer. Aust N Z J Surg 1997;67(10):717–719.
13. Livartowski A, Chapelier A, Beuzedoc P, et al. Surgery of lung metastases of breast cancer: Analysis of 40 cases. Bull Cancer 1998;85(9):800.
14. McCormack PM, Bains MS, Begg CB, et al. Role of video-assisted thoracic surgery in the treatment of pulmonary metastases: Results of a prospective trial. Ann Thorac Surg 1996;62(1):213–216; discussion, 216.
15. Remy-Jardin M, Remy J, Giraud F, Marquette CH. Pulmonary nodules: Detection with thick-section spiral CT versus conventional CT. Radiology 1993;187(2):513–520.
16. Planchard D, Soria JC, Michiels S, et al. Uncertain benefit from surgery in patients with lung metastases from breast carcinoma. Cancer 2004;100(1):28–35.
17. Apffelstaedt JP, Van Zyl JA, Muller AG. Breast cancer complicated by pleural effusion: Patient characteristics and results of surgical management. J Surg Oncol 1995;58(3):173–175.
18. Kreisman H, Wolkove N, Finkelstein HS, et al. Breast cancer and thoracic metastases: Review of 119 patients. Thorax 1983;38(3):175–179.
19. Weichselbaum R, Marck A, Hellman S. Pathogenesis of pleural effusion in carcinoma of the breast. Int J Radiat Oncol Biol Phys 1977;2(9–10):963–965.
20. Lee YT. Patterns of metastasis and natural courses of breast carcinoma. Cancer Metastasis Rev 1985;4(2):153–172.
21. Sahn SA, Good JT Jr. Pleural fluid pH in malignant effusions. Diagnostic, prognostic, and therapeutic implications. Ann Intern Med 1988;108(3):345–349.
22. Lynch TJ Jr. Management of malignant pleural effusions. Chest 1993;103(4 Suppl):385S–389S.
23. Jones SE, Durie BG, Salmon SA. Combination chemotherapy with Adriamycin and cyclophosphamide for advanced breast cancer. Cancer 1975;36(1):90–97.
24. Deslauriers J, Brisson J, Cartier R, et al. Carcinoma of the lung. Evaluation of satellite nodules as a factor influencing prognosis after resection. J Thorac Cardiovasc Surg 1989;97(4):504–512.
25. Reshad K, Inui K, Takeuchi Y, et al. Treatment of malignant pleural effusion. Chest 1985;88(3):393–397.
26. Moffett MJ, Ruckdeschel JC. Bleomycin and tetracycline in malignant pleural effusions: A review. Semin Oncol 1992;19(2 Suppl 5):59–62; discussion, 62–63.
27. Mager HJ, Maesen B, Verzijlbergen F, Schramel F. Distribution of talc suspension during treatment of malignant pleural effusion with talc pleurodesis. Lung Cancer 2002;36(1):77–81.
28. Putnam JB Jr, Walsh GL, Swisher SG, et al. Outpatient management of malignant pleural effusion by a chronic indwelling pleural catheter. Ann Thorac Surg 2000;69(2):369–375.
29. Walsh FW, Alberts WM, Solomon DA, Goldman AL. Malignant pleural effusions: Pleurodesis using a small-bore percutaneous catheter. South Med J 1989;82(8):963–965, 972.
30. Petrou M, Kaplan D, Goldstraw P, Management of recurrent malignant pleural effusions. The complementary role talc pleurodesis and pleuroperitoneal shunting. Cancer 1995;75(3):801–805.
31. de Campos JR, Vargas FS, de Campos Werebe E, et al. Thoracoscopy talc poudrage: A 15-year experience. Chest 2001;119(3):801–806.
32. Yim AP, Chan AT, Lee TW, et al. Thoracoscopic talc insufflation versus talc slurry for symptomatic malignant pleural effusion. Ann Thorac Surg 1996;62(6):1655–1658.
33. Martini N, Bains MS, Beattie EJ Jr. Indications for pleurectomy in malignant effusion. Cancer 1975;35(3):734–738.
34. Clementsen P, Evald T, Grode G, et al. Treatment of malignant pleural effusion: Pleurodesis using a small percutaneous catheter. A prospective randomized study. Respir Med 1998;92(3):593–596.
35. Ong KC, Indumathi V, Raghuram J, Ong YY. A comparative study of pleurodesis using talc slurry and bleomycin in the management of malignant pleural effusions. Respirology 2000;5(2):99–103.

36. Fentiman IS, Rubens RD, Hayward JL. A comparison of intracavitary talc and tetracycline for the control of pleural effusions secondary to breast cancer. Eur J Cancer Clin Oncol 1986;22(9):1079–1081.
37. Zimmer PW, Hill M, Casey K, et al. Prospective randomized trial of talc slurry vs bleomycin in pleurodesis for symptomatic malignant pleural effusions. Chest 1997;112(2):430–434.
38. Deschamps C, Tirnaksiz BM, Darbandi R, et al. Early and long-term results of prosthetic chest wall reconstruction. J Thorac Cardiovasc Surg 1999;117(3):588–591; discussion, 591–592.
39. Hultman CS, Carlson GW, Losken A, et al. Utility of the omentum in the reconstruction of complex extraperitoneal wounds and defects: Donor-site complications in 135 patients from 1975 to 2000. Ann Surg 2002;235(6):782–795.

IX

Bone Metastases from Breast Cancer

James C. Wittig and Justin G. Lamont

Breast cancer is the most common cause of skeletal metastases.[1,2] Bone is the second most common site to be involved by metastatic breast cancer, and it is the first site of metastatic disease in 26% of breast cancer patients.[3] It is also the most common site that clinically manifests. On autopsy studies, up to 90% of patients who die from breast cancer have bone metastases.[4] Patients who develop bone metastases survive an average of 2 years from the time of the first bone metastasis. Although most patients have organ involvement in addition to their bone metastases, there is a subgroup of women who solely develop skeletal metastases. Women who develop bone-only metastases have a more favorable prognosis than those with isolated organ metastases or combined skeletal and organ metastases.[5,6] In fact, in patients with a single bony metastasis and no organ involvement, proper treatment can in rare cases provide prolonged disease-free survival or even cure.

Skeletal metastases can result in significant complications that have a negative impact on the quality of life. Pain, pathologic fracture, neurologic complications, and hypercalcemia are all potential complications. Pain and pathologic fracture lead to forced immobilization and progressive deterioration. Hypercalcemia is the most common paraneoplastic syndrome and is discussed in Part IV of this chapter.[7] Neurologic complications, including paralysis from spine lesions, can occur. The axial skeleton and proximal ends of the long bones of the lower extremities are the most common sites of bone metastases. The pattern of skeletal metastatic sites follows the distribution of Batson's plexus or the vertebral vein system.[8] Batson's plexus is a low-pressure, high-volume, valveless venous system that bypasses caval, portal, and pulmonary systems and allows direct access of cells to the bone from distant anatomic sites.

Bone metastases stimulate bone resorption and osteolysis primarily through direct or indirect stimulation of osteoclasts. Cancer cells secrete cytokines that stimulate osteoclasts to resorb bone. Passive hyperemia that occurs secondary to the presence of neoplasm also results in stimulation of local osteoclasts. Less prominent mechanisms may include direct resorption of bone by the tumor cells through production and secretion of proteinases that degrade bony matrix.[9,10] In most instances of breast cancer metastases, the osteoblasts respond to the enhanced osteoclast activity by laying down new bone. This osteoblastic response appears as sclerosis on a plain radiograph.

TREATMENT GUIDELINES

What is the best diagnostic radiographic screening technique for bone metastases?

Early detection of skeletal metastases permits prompt intervention that may have a significant impact on the quality of life. Pain may be absent in up to 50% of patients with skeletal metastases.[11] Thus, early detection through periodic surveillance with bone scintigraphy may be justified.[12] ^{99m}Tc-scintigraphy is the best screening method for bony metastases. In the skeletal phase of the scan, lesions usually appear as localized areas of uptake owing to the osteoblastic response induced by the metastatic deposit. Lesions as small as 2 mm can be detected.[13] Bone scans demonstrate skeletal involvement much earlier than plain radiographs. In order for a lesion to be visualized on a plain radiograph, 30% to 50% of the bone must be destroyed. False-negative bone scans typically occur with tumors that do not evoke a significant osteoblastic response, such as myeloma. False-negative bone scans are unusual in breast cancer patients, however, because breast cancer metastases invariably evoke a mixed osteolytic and osteoblastic response.[14] Bone scintigraphy is an excellent tool for screening for occult metastases, determining multiple sites of disease throughout the body or in the same bone, and monitoring response to treatment. However, bone scan does not provide any information about the structural integrity of bone. Plain radiographs or CT or MRI scans must be correlated with the bone scan.

Plain radiography is often the first radiographic study performed on breast cancer patients who present with pain referable to a specific bone or joint. Plain radiography is also performed as a correlate to a positive bone scan during routine surveillance in an asymptomatic patient. Most metastatic lesions start in the medullary bone, although tumors can metastasize to the cortex and periosteum. Thirty to 50% of the medullary bone must be destroyed before a lesion becomes evident on a plain radiograph.[12] Subtle cortical destruction by a lesion or a cortical metastasis may be radiographically detectable at an earlier stage. Most breast cancer metastases radiographically demonstrate mixed areas of lysis and sclerosis; however, purely lytic and sclerotic lesions do occur. Lesions can be classified as permeative, moth-eaten, or geographic. Permeative and moth-eaten lesions are more common, consistent with their aggressive, often rapidly grow-ing, malignant nature. These lesions permeate the bone, which is unable to respond rapidly enough against the tumor to encapsulate it. Geographic lesions in which there is a sharp zone of transition between the tumor and adjacent normal bone are less common. This type of radiographic presentation denotes a slower growing, less aggressive neoplasm.

CT and MRI are useful for detecting and characterizing suspected bone metastases that are not visible on plain radiographs. About 50% of patients with bone scan–positive skeletal metastases and negative radiographs have lesions detectable on a CT scan.[15,16] MRI and CT are useful for deter-mining cortical involvement, extramedullary growth, and intramedullary extent of tumor, all of which are important for determining the indications for surgery as well as for planning a procedure. MRI and CT are also useful for detecting occult fractures through neoplasms and for identifying other causes

of pain, such as arthritic processes and tendinopathies. MRI is better than CT for evaluating the presence and size of any soft tissue component of the neoplasm as well as for determining the intramedullary extent of the lesion. In the evaluation of spine lesions, MRI is important for detecting epidural exten-sion, spinal cord compression, and extent of disease within individual vertebral bodies and throughout the entire spine. In patients who cannot undergo an MRI, CT myelography can be used to evaluate spinal cord compression. CT is especially efficacious for evaluating the presence and depth of subtle endosteal erosion or cortical involvement that may not be evident on plain radiographs. This information is often used when deciding whether a patient's bone should be prophylactically fixed for an impending pathologic fracture (Fig. 32–21).

It can be difficult to differentiate a new sclerotic lesion from a healing lesion on radiographs. In response to treatment,

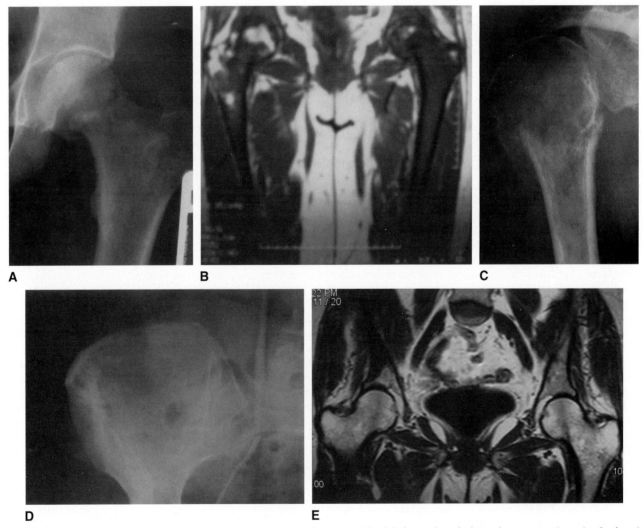

Figure 32–21   *A,* Plain radiograph demonstrating a pathologic fracture of the left femoral neck through a permeative mixed sclerotic breast cancer metastasis. Most breast cancer metastases to bone result in a mixed sclerotic and lytic lesion on plain radiographs. *B,* MRI of same patient demonstrates tumor involvement of the entire femoral shaft that was not accurately depicted on the plain radiograph. This information is important for surgical planning and for monitoring response to treatment. *C,* Plain radiograph demonstrating a mixed sclerotic and lytic lesion and pathologic fracture of the right proximal humerus. *D,* Example of a mixed sclerotic and lytic lesion of the right ilium secondary to breast cancer metastases. *E,* MRI accurately demonstrates the intramedullary extent of the lesion. The lesion is noted to encroach on the acetabulum. Close follow-up or treatment may be warranted to detect early involvement of the hip joint and prevent a potential complication.

most healing lesions become more sclerotic and calcified on plain radiographs. On bone scan, a flare phenomenon, in which the lesion demonstrates more intense uptake, may occur during the early stages of healing. This often signifies a more intense osteoblastic response during the healing phase. The activity on bone scan should become less intense once the lesion is completely healed. This may take several months.

Progression of disease appears as enlargement, increasing lysis, and loss of the osteoblastic response on plain radiographs. Bone scintigraphy is nonspecific in measuring disease progression from response to treatment of isolated metastases and must be correlated with plain radiographs. On bone scan, existing lesions may show increased uptake with disease progression, although rapidly growing lesions with little osteoblastic response and bone formation may show decreased uptake. In addition, the flare phenomenon may occur during the initial stages of healing. The role of MRI in assessing response to treatment is not well defined.

When is magnetic resonance imaging indicated in the assessment of possible bone metastases?

MRI is useful for determining the presence of a metastatic lesion that has not produced sufficient bone destruction to be evident on plain radiographs as well as the presence of lesions that do not demonstrate uptake on the bone scan (false-negative bone scan). The entire bone can be visualized in a single plane, thus enabling detection of additional occult lesions within the same bone. Coexisting lesions should be considered for fixation during the same surgical procedure. Skeletal metastases typically involve the metaphyseal regions of the long bones and therefore may exist in conjunction with arthritis at adjacent joints. Arthritic processes induce sclerosis and cyst formation that may obscure bone scan and plain radiographic results. MRI is especially useful in discerning the presence of a metastatic deposit in the presence of arthritis. Gadolinium contrast enhancement may be useful. MRI often identifies other mechanical abnormalities at adjacent joints that may contribute to or be the sole cause of pain. It is also useful for evaluating complications associated with chemotherapy and radiation such as avascular necrosis, radiation-induced necrosis, stress fractures, and radiation-induced neoplasms.

MRI is crucial for evaluating spine metastases. It is the test of choice for detecting spinal cord compression and can help differentiate among benign osteoporotic compression fractures, infections, and malignant vertebral lesions or fractures.

MRI is problematic in claustrophobic patients who cannot tolerate the study. It is also contraindicated in patients with devices such as cardiac pacemakers, intracranial aneurysm clips, and ferromagnetic fragments in or around the eye. In these instances, CT of the bone with reformatted coronal and sagittal reconstructions may be invaluable.

How do bone metastases affect prognosis?

There is no recognized method of assessing the prognosis of patients with breast cancer who have metastatic lesions restricted to bone. Patients who have only skeletal metastases at the time of initial diagnosis or who develop skeletal metastases without visceral metastases at a later date have better survival rates than patients who develop visceral metastases only or combined visceral and bony metastases.[5,6,17] The distribution of skeletal metastases on bone scans and the radiographic appearance of osteosclerosis can be of prognostic value for patients with breast cancer who have metastases confined to bone.[18] Patients whose bone metastases are all cranial to the lumbosacral junction have a significantly longer survival than those who have bone metastases caudal to the junction (36% vs. 16% 5-year survival). The presence of osteosclerosis is indicative of a more slowly growing neoplasm and hence provides a measure of the biologic aggressiveness. The presence of radiographic osteosclerosis in metastatic bone lesions at the time of initial presentation is associated with a more favorable prognosis (42% 5-year survival rate in patients with lesions that demonstrate osteosclerosis vs. 23% 5-year survival rate in patients whose lesions do not demonstrate sclerosis). Sherry and associates[19] found that survival did not correlate with the number of metastatic deposits in patients with metastases restricted to bone.

Patients who can be stratified into a more favorable prognostic category may benefit from more aggressive surgical treatment. Yamashita and coworkers found several variables associated with a more favorable prognosis in patients with breast cancer metastases confined to bone.[6] These included an absence of extraosseous metastases; cranial bone metastases; a solitary bone metastasis; presence of osteosclerosis on a plain radiograph; and absence evidence of hypercalcemia. In the study by Yamashita and coworkers, the median survival time after first diagnosis of a bone metastasis was 35 months. The median survival after visceral metastases was only 5 months. Perez and colleagues also reported a better prognosis for patients who develop skeletal metastases solely versus visceral metastases.[5] In their study, the median survival of patients with skeletal metastases was 28 months, and 25% of patients survived at least 5 years. Patients who developed visceral metastases had a median survival of 13 months, and less than 10% survived 5 years.

Pathologic fracture and spinal cord compression are common orthopedic complications that seriously compromise the quality of life of a patient. Yamashita and coworkers reported a 13% rate of pathologic fracture and 32% rate of spinal cord compression.[6] These rates are similar to those reported by Perez and colleagues.[5] The median survival after a long bone pathologic fracture was 14 months (range, 1 to 80 months), indicating that about 50% of patients survive longer than 1 year after developing a long bone pathologic fracture. The median survival after spinal cord compression was 8 months (range, 2 to 74 months), and 42% of patients survived longer than 2 years.

What are the indications for biopsy?

The indications for biopsy of metastatic bone lesions are as follows:

1. A known primary breast cancer with a bony lesion suspected to be a metastasis. This is important for staging, prognostic purposes, and planning treatment. The biopsy must confirm the presence of metastatic breast cancer in

bone and exclude primary bone tumors, infections, and metastatic lesions from primary sources other than breast before initiating treatment.

2. Suspected progression of disease or failure of treatment denoted by formation of new bony lesions.
3. Presence of one or more skeletal lesions with no known primary source. Biopsy is performed to establish a diagnosis and direct staging studies. One must not assume that a lesion is metastatic. It must be approached as if it were a primary sarcoma despite the metastatic appearance.
4. Assessment of the efficacy of treatment by the histologic response of a lesion.
5. Presence of localized bone pain with a lesion on bone scan and negative radiographs.[20]

What is the role of a closed biopsy?

A closed biopsy is performed percutaneously or through a small stab incision in the skin. A specific type of needle is subsequently inserted and directed under radiologic supervision (fluoroscopy or CT scan) down to the neoplasm. Two types of needles can be used, depending on the clinical-radiographic presentation: a fine needle (16 to 22 gauge) for fine-needle aspiration (FNA) or a core needle (trephine-type or Craig needle). This is in contrast to an open biopsy, in which a longer incision is carried directly down to the lesion and biopsy material is obtained under direct visualization.

During closed biopsy procedures, CT guidance is especially important for sampling lesions that are adjacent to critical structures. FNA is usually performed for cytogenetic analysis, most often to confirm the initial presentation of a bone metastasis in the setting of known metastatic breast cancer. Core needle samples are amenable to paraffin block processing and are useful when analysis of the architecture of the tissues and cells is pertinent. Core needle biopsy is indicated in a patient with a history of nonmetastatic breast cancer who develops one or more bony lesions. Adequate sampling with a core needle may be necessary to exclude the presence of a primary bone tumor, infection, or metastatic disease from a second primary neoplasm. Core needles are also used for sampling blastic metastases. It is often impossible to penetrate the sclerotic bone with a fine needle. Fine needles are more effective at sampling purely lytic lesions or lesions with a soft tissue component.

A closed needle biopsy offers several advantages over a formal open biopsy. These advantages include local anesthesia, less blood loss, quicker healing, fewer wound complications, and hence more rapid initiation of chemotherapy and radiation; less surrounding soft tissue contamination with reduced risk for local soft tissue recurrence; and fewer biopsy-related pathologic fractures. Disadvantages, which may include inadequacy of specimen size and sampling error, can be minimized by having the biopsy performed by an experienced radiologist or orthopedic oncologist and the specimen analyzed by experienced pathologists. Several aspirations or cores should be obtained. At experienced centers, the diagnostic accuracy rate of a closed biopsy is similar to that of an open biopsy, and there are far fewer complications than with an open biopsy.[21]

Contraindications to a biopsy may include skin conditions such as infection, bleeding diatheses coexisting with a hypervascular tumor, and any need for open surgery. In the case of a hypervascular tumor or a patient with a bleeding diathesis, needle biopsy offers obvious advantages over an open biopsy. On the other hand, when a patient develops a pathologic fracture in the presence of known metastatic breast cancer, intraoperative biopsy with frozen section pathologic analysis of the neoplasm is indicated to confirm the presence of metastatic carcinoma. Once the diagnosis is confirmed, fixation commences. In these instances, there is usually no need to perform a biopsy preoperatively.

What are the indications for alternative and adjunctive nonoperative treatments?

Alternative and adjunctive nonoperative treatments of bone metastases include radiation therapy, chemotherapy, hormonal therapy, and bisphosphonates. The indications for radiation therapy include pain relief and suppression of local tumor growth. Suppression of local tumor growth is important in the treatment of impending fractures, after surgical fracture fixation of metastatic lesions, and in the treatment of neural compression. Complications associated with radiation treatment of bone lesions include marrow fibrosis, which may preclude chemotherapy. Marrow fibrosis destroys the hematopoietic ability of bone marrow and therefore interferes with the body's ability to restore blood counts after chemotherapy.

In the management of an impending fracture—a potential fracture in a bone with weaked structural integrity owing to a metastatic lesion—occasionally a lesion will heal with radiation, especially if it is mechanically protected.[22] More than 80% of patients with a limited number of well-localized bone metastases can be treated effectively with external-beam radiation.[23–25] Radiation may render the patient asymptomatic and control the disease for an extended period. Patients with numerous areas of skeletal involvement may benefit more from a systemic approach consisting of chemotherapy with or without endocrine therapy, and with or without systemic radionucleotide therapy. Supplemental external-beam radiation may be used to target the most symptomatic areas.

Irradiation of a weight-bearing bone should be undertaken only after careful evaluation of the potential fracture risk produced by the underlying lesion. There is an increased risk for pathologic fracture in the peri-irradiation period owing to an induced hyperemic response at the periphery of the tumor. This weakens the bone and increases the risk for spontaneous fracture. Mechanical protection is important until the bone's structural integrity has been restored.

Radiation achieves at least partial pain relief in 80% to 90% of patients.[26] Most metastases begin to respond over the course of 10 to 14 days. Seventy percent of patients experience pain relief within 2 weeks of starting therapy. Within 3 months, 90% of patients achieve pain relief.[27] Fifty to 70% of patients achieve sustained pain relief for 1 year or more.[28] Patients with breast and prostate metastases who have a significant osteoblastic response derive better pain relief from radiation therapy than patients with long bone lesions from other primary tumors, such as kidney and lung, which are usually more lytic and compromise the mechanical integrity of the bone to a greater degree.[29] High doses of postoperative radiation (>3000 cGy) have been associated with poor healing of pathologic fractures. The optimal dose and fractionation regimen are debated. Generally, 2500 to 3000 cGy is administered over 10 to 15 fractions.

Bisphosphonates are stable analogues of inorganic pyrophosphate. They inhibit bone resorption through inhibition of osteoclast function and have been shown to decrease the rate of pathologic fractures and skeletal complications in patients with breast cancer and metastatic bone lesions. There are different generations of bisphosphonates with different potencies and effects. The bisphosphonates are generally safe compounds with few side effects. Several large randomized studies have been performed to analyze the efficacy of pamidronate in the management of metastatic bone lesions.[30]

The goals of chemotherapy and hormonal treatment in patients with metastatic disease involving bone are pain control, disease stabilization, and reduction in the risk for morbid skeletal events. Additionally, the use of chemotherapy and hormonal treatment in metastatic breast cancer has been shown to prolong survival.[31] In one study, there was an 18% complete response rate and a 65% partial response rate in patients with metastatic bone lesions treated with a multiagent chemotherapy regimen.[31]

Systemic radionucleotides can be very effective in treating symptomatic bone metastases. These agents treat all sites rapidly and selectively, thereby reducing toxicity and enhancing the therapeutic ratio.[26] Strontium 89 is the most commonly used radioisotope in bony metastatic disease.[32,33] It localizes in the mineral of bone by combining with the calcium component of hydroxyapatite. Actively calcifying areas concentrate most of the isotope, and therefore it has particular efficacy in treating breast cancer metastases. Degradation of the isotope in host bone administers local short-acting radiation to the adjacent tumor cells. Strontium 89 has very good response rates, ranging from 51% to 91%.[33] The only significant toxic effect of strontium 89 is myelotoxicity, which is usually temporary. Strontium 89 can be safely used in conjunction with external-beam radiation.

When and how should orthopedic surgical management be instituted?

The management of patients with skeletal metastases from breast cancer must be individualized. Important considerations include age, comorbidities, prognosis, pain, presence of an isolated skeletal metastasis or bone-only metastases, location of metastatic disease, presence of an impending or actual pathologic fracture, and the patient's overall activity level. Patients may present with asymptomatic bone metastases, painful metastatic disease, and pathologic fractures. Treatment of patients with asymptomatic skeletal disease is aimed at diagnosis through biopsy, systemic control of disease through chemotherapy, and hormonal treatment and observation of all bones involved with the disease. Referral should be made to an orthopedic surgeon for evaluation, biopsy, recommendations, and periodic observation of lesions. In general, asymptomatic lesions are at low risk for fracture. Serial observation for disease progression and further bony destruction is warranted so that any bone at risk for fracture can be identified and treated before actually fracturing. MRI is important in evaluating spine metastases. A baseline MRI is important to identify any epidural extension of tumor that can cause neurologic compromise. Systemic therapy,

radiation, braces, casts, and analgesics are effective methods for treating selected lesions. Surgery by means of internal fixation or prosthetic replacement offers the most effective and expedient means of pain control and restoration of function for patients with actual pathologic fractures.

Most pathologic fractures do not heal. In a study of 129 pathologic fractures, only 37% of pathologic fractures due to breast cancer healed.[22] High doses of postoperative radiation (>3000 cGy) are associated with poor healing. Rigid internal fixation supplemented with bone cement increases the probability of bony union. The surgeon must choose a form of fixation that does not ultimately rely on bony union.

Patients with skeletal metastases often are in poor medical condition and have a limited life expectancy. Surgical intervention must be undertaken with the intention of avoiding future surgery. Surgical principles of management of pathologic fractures or impending pathologic fractures are as follows:

1. Curettage to remove all gross disease
2. Use of immediate rigid fixation consisting of internal fixation with polymethylmethacrylate (PMMA or bone cement) or cemented prosthetic replacement
3. Filling defects with bone cement
4. Adjuvant radiation or chemotherapy

Painful lesions and pathologic fractures should be referred to an experienced orthopedic surgeon for evaluation and treatment. Many patients without an actual fracture do not require surgery. Symptomatic relief is usually satisfactory with a combination of radiation and medical therapy. Patients at low risk for fracture or those who are poor surgical candidates can often be effectively managed with conservative means, such as bracing, casting, non–weight bearing, and radiation. Anatomic site may play a role in selecting treatment. Lesions in weight-bearing bones are often treated more aggressively than upper extremity lesions.

Prophylactic fixation is warranted for impending fractures in the following circumstances:

1. Fixation eliminates the need for narcotic analgesics or reduces pain.
2. Equally effective nonoperative treatments are not available.
3. Surgical treatment for the impending fracture would be significantly safer or more effective than surgery for an actual fracture.
4. Surgery permits mobilization and early return to function.

Pathologic fractures are best treated by operative fixation. Even if fractures can heal with nonoperative treatment, the protracted treatment time required for closed management is inappropriate because this period generally is increased by the presence of tumor. Primary goals are to allow immediate weight bearing and return to activity, not to promote fracture healing. Prosthetic replacement and stabilization with polymethylmethacrylate (bone cement) are frequently used. These techniques would be avoided in the treatment of non-neoplastic fractures. Tumor removal and bone stabilization best meet the goals of diagnosis, functional stability, and pain relief. In general, the metastatic deposit should be excised. Treatment includes intralesional (marginal resection or curettage) and extralesional (wide) excision. Intralesional curettage is usually performed in or around a fracture site at the time of stabilization. Extralesional excision or resection is usually performed for a solitary metastatic deposit or for lesions that have destroyed a large segment of the bone with no cortices left for reconstructing with bone cement. It is the most effective way to achieve local tumor control. Cures are occasionally reported following resection of isolated bone metastases.

Surgical treatment of pathologic fractures is based on anatomic location, extent of the lesion, and condition of the patient. Surgery is indicated for most patients. Patients with a very short life expectancy (usually less than 2 weeks) or who are poor surgical candidates can be treated conservatively by stabilizing the bone with a cast or a brace and by providing sufficient medication for pain relief.

The surgical procedure is aimed at preventing the need for future surgeries. In general, one should choose a device (e.g., rods and nails, prosthetic replacements, and screws and plates) that will fix the entire bone and prevent complications should disease progression occur. Intramedullary devices are usually used for diaphyseal fractures or metadiaphyseal fractures in long bones. The bone proximal and distal to the lesion must be free of disease to allow secure fixation of the device in good bone. Adjunctive use of methylmethacrylate or bone cement enhances fixation, fills defects, enables immediate weight bearing and use of the extremity, and reduces the risk for hardware failure that requires reoperation. Amputation is rarely needed in the management of metastatic breast lesions to bone.

Whenever feasible, gross tumor should be removed so that tumor is not carried by the rod and implanted at a more distal site. Intramedullary rods can be placed through limited incisions with minimal blood loss and low risk for infection. Use of strong nails of wide diameter and supplementation with bone cement are preferred to prevent hardware failure for these types of fractures, which may require a prolonged time to heal or may never heal.

Cemented prosthetic replacement is indicated for pathologic lesions that affect the epiphyseal areas of the bone. They may also be used for select metaphyseal lesions, particularly those that extend into the epiphyses. Special prostheses with long stems permit fixation of the entire bone. Screws and plates have selected indications and in most instances are not recommended because they do not provide fixation for the entire bone.

Radiation therapy of bone metastases remains the principal surgical adjuvant. It should be delivered to the entire surgical field and along the length of any prosthesis or internal fixation device.[23,27] This addresses tumor cells that have been spread by the surgical procedure along the intramedullary canal and soft tissues. Local tumor control helps prevent destabilization of the implant by preventing local tumor progression from affecting the structural integrity of the bone in which the implant is fixed. Postoperative radiation prevents local tumor progression that could affect the structural integrity of the bone and lead to implant failure.

SPECIFIC ANATOMIC SITES

Spine Lesions

The spine is the most common site of skeletal metastases. In a study by Toma and colleagues, the survival time of patients with vertebral metastases was longer than that of patients with bone metastases to other sites.[34] Pain is the most common presenting symptom and may be secondary to intraosseous disease, spinal instability, vertebral compression fracture, epidural compression, or nerve root involvement. In about 5% of patients with widespread cancer, there is spinal cord or nerve root involvement. Neurologic involvement occurs in about 20% of patients with neoplastic involvement of the spine and may be the initial presenting symptom.[35,36] Between 30% and 50% of the vertebral body must be destroyed before the damage is visible on plain films. Lysis of a pedicle may be the only radiographic finding in the early stages of vertebral involvement. MRI is warranted to detect extraosseous growth of tumor and epidural compression.

Surgical intervention is usually not needed for asymptomatic lesions discovered on bone scan. The indications for operative intervention include progressive neurologic compromise, intractable pain, recurrence of cord compromise following local irradiation, fracture with spinal instability, need for tissue diagnosis, and an impending fracture not responsive to radiation. The surgical approach should be based on the location of instability or epidural compression. The spinal canal is decompressed, and the spine is stabilized. Bone graft and bone cement are used to augment internal fixation. Radiation is recommended postoperatively. Further details about specific methods of decompression and stabilization are discussed elsewhere in this chapter.

Hip Lesions

The hip is the most common site of a pathologic fracture. This is because of the high incidence of metastases to this area and the high magnitude of forces concentrated in the hip area. Metastatic disease to the hip can involve the pelvis and acetabulum and the proximal femur. Complications caused by lesions to the proximal femur may arise from metastatic involvement of the femoral head or neck, intertrochanteric region, subtrochanteric region, or any combination. Surgical treatment of femoral head or femoral neck fractures entails endoprosthetic replacement, usually with a long-stem femoral component or total hip replacement. Prostheses permit rapid mobilization and weight bearing. Lesions in this region are not treated with internal fixation because of the poor quality of the bone and because of the risk that progression of the lesion can result in loss of fixation. Adequate pain relief and return to prefracture ambulatory status are successful more than 90% of the time. Long-stem prostheses are recommended to fix the entire femoral shaft, especially if there is coexisting disease distally that may progress or if the patient is at risk for additional metastases to the same bone in the future. This is especially necessary for patients in whom a prolonged survival is expected. Cemented stems have less risk for loosening and a lower incidence of postoperative thigh pain than do porous ingrowth stems, especially when adjunctive measures are used. Significant acetabular disease should be addressed during the same surgery.

Management of intertrochanteric and subtrochanteric fractures varies. Plate and screw fixation augmented with bone cement or second-generation femoral rods with fixation extending across the femoral neck have been employed successfully. Lane and colleagues have recommended long-stem cemented prostheses for metastatic involvement in any area

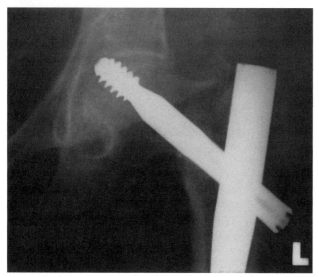

Figure 32–22 Plain radiograph demonstrating failure of fixation of a pathologic fracture of the left proximal femur. The patient presented 1 year earlier with a pathologic fracture of the proximal femur secondary to a breast cancer metastasis. Internal fixation was performed, and the patient underwent postoperative irradiation. The tumor progressed, and the fracture never healed. Ultimately, the hardware failed, and the screw penetrated the femoral head. This patient required a second surgery with placement of a long-stem cemented hemiarthroplasty. Whenever feasible, a curettage of the tumor, as well as fixation that does not rely on bony union, is recommended.

of the proximal femur.[37] This technique is reliable and avoids late failure of fixation from proximal progression of intertrochanteric and subtrochanteric lesions (Fig. 32–22). It also treats simultaneous lesions more distal in the shaft and permits early, rapid mobilization. In Lane's report, there were no instances of loosening or dislocation, and there were two infections (1.2%).[37] Long-stem cemented hemiarthroplasties are preferred (Fig. 32–23). A bipolar device lessens acetabular wear in cases in which metastases have not affected the acetabulum. Massive bone destruction is better addressed with a large special tumor prosthesis.

Lesions of the hemipelvis not directly involving the hip joint can generally be treated with modification of weight bearing and external-beam radiation. Avulsion fractures of the anterior superior and anterior inferior iliac spines, iliac crest, and superoinferior pubic rami are common and should be treated nonoperatively. Unstable pathologic fractures of the hemipelvis usually involve the periacetabular area. Periacetabular lesions are much more difficult to treat surgically. Surgical approaches are more complex and are associated with greater blood loss and a higher risk for complications. Most lesions in which the femoral head is not pushed into the pelvis can be treated with restricted weight bearing, medical treatment, and radiotherapy. Reconstructive techniques must transfer load-bearing stresses into structurally intact bone in the upper ilium and adjacent sacroiliac joint. This may be accomplished by use of multiple Steinmann pins, reinforced bone cement, and antiprotrusio devices (Fig. 32–24). When there is massive bone destruction, a saddle

prosthesis can be used. The saddle prosthesis articulates with the remaining ilium.[38]

Femoral Shaft

Pathologic fractures of the femoral shaft are stabilized with intramedullary nails. Cement is used to add stability, prevent shortening, and decrease the risk for hardware failure. Coexisting disease in the proximal femur region should be addressed by using a cephalomedullary nail that provides fixation across the femoral neck in addition to fixing the femoral shaft or a long-stem hemiarthroplasty. Plate and screw fixation combined with bone cement is not preferred because of the risk for fracture proximal and distal to the plate and increased operative time. Intramedullary rod fixation is generally done by the open method; that is, the tumor-fracture site is exposed, the tumor is curetted, bone cement is injected proximally and distally, and the intramedullary rod is inserted. Immediate ambulation with full weight bearing is permitted a few days after surgery. Small lesions responsive to radiation may be treated before fracture by the closed method if the cortices are intact and there is normal proximal bone. The rod is inserted through a small incision at the greater trochanter and placed in an antegrade manner across the lesion to obtain good distal fixation.

Humerus

The upper extremity is less commonly involved with metastatic disease than the spine, pelvis, and lower extremities. Humeral fractures can be severely disabling, preventing patients from feeding themselves, attending to hygiene, and transferring with the use of external aids. Surgical stabilization is recommended for patients at risk for fracture and to permit rapid use of a crutch or walker in patients with concomitant lower extremity lesions. Humeral shaft fractures are amenable to intramedullary nails that may be augmented with bone cement similar to femoral shaft fractures. Pathologic fractures involving the proximal humeral metaphyseal regions, humeral head, or neck are amenable to long-stem endoprosthetic replacement. Shoulder function is limited following endoprosthetic replacement because of the need for muscle reattachment and rehabilitation in the presence of postoperative radiation. Pain relief is reliable, however, and a stable shoulder is provided for good elbow and hand function. Severe bone destruction of the proximal humerus with significant extraosseous extension of tumor may necessitate replacement with a tumor prosthesis. When patients have had mastectomies on the same side of the humeral lesion, postoperative edema is much worse after fracture stabilization. Elastic sleeves and gloves can be fitted by occupational therapists for assistance with this problem. Lesions of the distal humerus may require plate and screw fixation augmented with bone cement, crossed flexible intramedullary rods, a long-stem humeral and ulnar constrained elbow arthroplasty, or a distal humerus replacement with a constrained total elbow. Choice of implant depends on the degree of bone destruction and presence of coexisting disease within the remaining humerus.

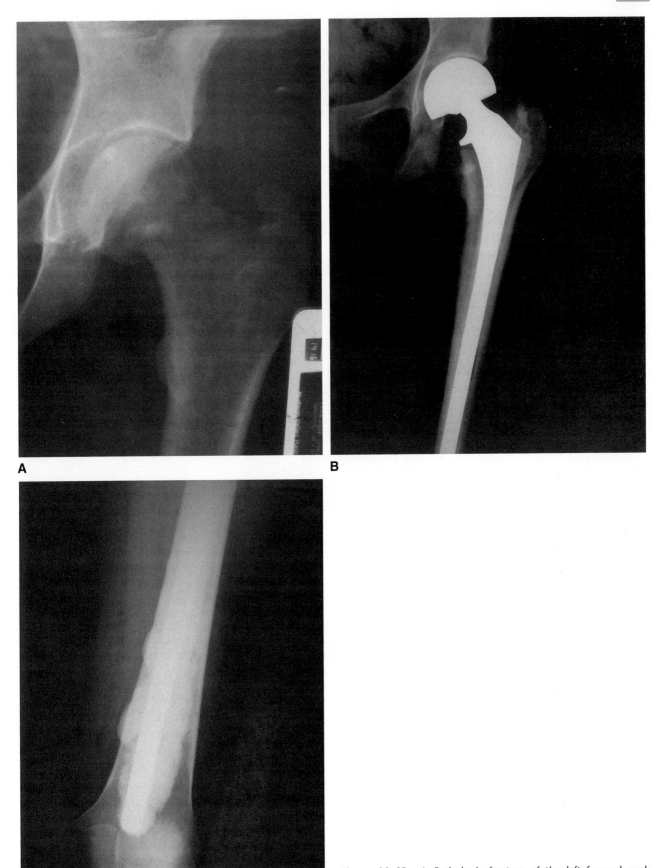

Figure 32–23 *A*, Pathologic fracture of the left femoral neck. *B*, Fixation with a long-stem cemented hemiarthroplasty. *C*, Distal end of the femur demonstrating fixation of the entire femoral shaft with the long-stem hemiarthroplasty.

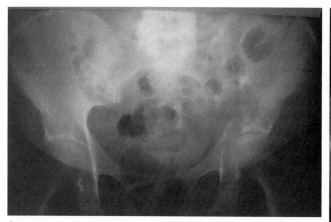

A

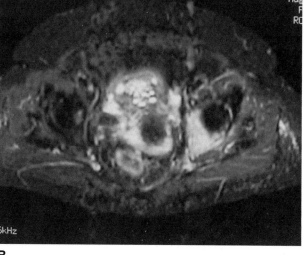

B

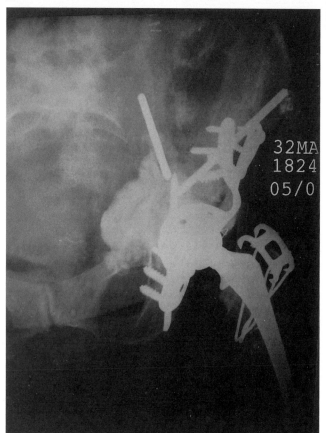

C

Figure 32–24 *A,* Plain radiograph demonstrating a pathologic fracture and destruction of almost the entire left acetabulum through an extensive breast cancer metastasis involving the pelvic bone. *B,* MRI of same patient demonstrating extensive involvement of the acetabulum. *C,* The patient underwent fixation with a long-stem total hip replacement, antiprotrusio cage, bone cement, and Steinmann pins. The Steinmann pins transfer the forces across the hip into remaining intact bone of the ilium. The long-stem femoral component provides fixation for the entire femur that was also involved by metastases.

PROPHYLAXIS AND REHABILITATION

When is prophylactic surgery needed?

Patients with known metastatic lesions in bone may be at risk for developing a fracture through the affected bone because of weakening of the structural integrity. This is referred to as an impending fracture. There is no specific definition of an impending fracture, and the indications for operative treatment continue to be controversial. One strong indication includes lesions that are still painful after radiation especially, those with functional pain.

Criteria have been developed to estimate the risk for fracturing through a metastatic bone lesion and hence for providing the surgeon with indications for prophylactic surgical stabilization of the bone. Although criteria have been developed to estimate the risk for a patient's developing a pathologic fracture, retrospective analysis has shown that radiographic criteria alone do not accurately predict fracture.

Three common indications are as follows:

1. Lesion larger than 2.5 cm
2. Greater than 50% cortical destruction
3. Intractable pain attributable to the bone lesion

In a study by Keene and colleagues,[39] it was not possible to use defect size to predict pathologic fractures. A scoring system for assessing the risk for pathologic fractures has been proposed by Mirels and associates.[40] It is based on the following variables: site, pain, lesion size. In Mirels' classification, almost all patients with functional pain ultimately developed a fracture. The fracture rate was 5% in patients with lesions less than one third of the bone diameter and was 81% in patients with lesions greater than two thirds of the diameter of bone. In the 1960s, Beals and coworkers[41] observed that 58% of breast cancer patients with well-defined lytic lesions larger than 2.5 cm involving the cortex of the femur developed pathologic fractures. Fidler[42] showed a significant difference in the risk for pathologic fracture when there is greater than 50% destruction of the cortex regardless of the size of the lesion.

Is there a safe role for rehabilitation treatment?

Rehabilitation is often indicated for patients with skeletal metastases. Patients with a limited life span benefit the most from rapid restoration of function after treatment of metastatic bone disease. The indications for rehabilitation and the specific type of rehabilitation are dictated by the clinical circumstances, sites of lesions, potential for fracture, overall medical condition, and postoperative status. Patients who are being treated with radiation for an impending fracture of a weight-bearing bone can be taught crutch ambulation with non–weight bearing on the affected extremity. Patients receiving radiation also benefit from gentle range-of-motion exercises of adjacent joints to prevent radiation-induced contractures and to control swelling and lymphedema. Postoperative rehabilitation is indicated to mobilize patients and restore them to presurgical functional status. Patients may be eligible for acute rehabilitation depending on their overall medical condition, presurgical functional status, and degree of deconditioning. Patients who were active preoperatively and who sustain a pathologic fracture may have a rehabilitation course similar to patients who sustain a nonpathologic fracture. Patients who are poor candidates for acute rehabilitation (severely deconditioned and compromised) may be candidates for a more prolonged, less intense rehabilitation program at a skilled nursing facility or at home. In a study by Blunting and colleagues, the risk for pathologic fracture resulting from rehabilitation was found to be low.[43]

REFERENCES

1. Abrams HL, Spiro R, Goldstein N. Metastases in carcinoma: Analysis of 1000 autopsied cases. Cancer 1950;23:74.
2. Toma S, Venturino A, Sogno G, et al. Metastatic bone tumors: Nonsurgical treatment, outcome and survival. Clin Orthop 1993;295:246.
3. Fisher B, Ravdin RG. Surgical adjuvant chemotherapy in cancer of the breast: Results of a decade of cooperative investigation. Ann Surg 1986;168:337.
4. Mundy GR, Yoneda T. Facilitation and suppression of bone metastases. Clin Orthop 1995;312:34.
5. Perez JE, Machiavelli M, Leone BA, et al. Bone-only versus visceral-only metastatic pattern in breast cancer: Analysis of 150 patients. Am J Clin Oncol 1990;13(4):294.
6. Yamashita K, Koyama H, Inaji H. Prognostic significance of bone metastases from breast cancer. Clin Orthop 1995;312:89.
7. Walls J, Bundred N, Howell A. Hypercalcemia and bone resorption in malignancy. Clin Orthop 1995;312:51.
8. Batson OV. The function of the vertebral veins and their role in the spread of metastasis. Arch Surg 1940;112:138.
9. Cockett MI, Murphy G, Birch ML, et al. Matrix metalloproteinases and metastatic cancer. Biochem Soc Symp 1998;63:295.
10. Sanchez-Sweatman OH, Lee J, Orr FW, et al. Direct osteolysis induced by metastatic murine melanoma cells: Role of matrix metalloproteinases. Eur J Cancer 1997;33:918.
11. Galasko CSB. Skeletal metastases and mammary cancer. Ann R Coll Surg Engl 1972;50:3.
12. Edelstyn GA, Gillespie PJ, Grebell FS. The radiological demonstration of osseous metastases: Experimental observations. Clin Radiol 1967;18:158.
13. Gosfield E, Alavi A, Kneeland B. Comparison of radionuclide bone scans and MRI in detecting spinal metastases. J Nucl Med 1993;34:2191.
14. Mehta RC, Wilson MA, Perlman SB. False negative bone scan in extensive metastatic disease: CT and MR findings. J Comput Assist Tomogr 1989;13:717.
15. Muindi J, Coombes RC, Golding S, et al. The role of computed tomography in the detection of bone metastases in breast cancer patients. Br J Radiol 1983;56:233.
16. Redmond J, Spring DB, Munderloh SH, et al. Spinal computed tomography scanning in the evaluation of metastatic disease. Cancer 1984;54:253.
17. Coleman RE, Rubens RD. The clinical course of bone metastases from breast cancer. Br J cancer. 1987;55:61.
18. Cutler SJ, Asire AJ, Taylor SG. Classification of patients with disseminated cancer of the breast. Cancer 1969;24:861.
19. Sherry MM, Greco FA, Johnson DH, et al. Metastatic breast cancer confined to the skeletal system: An indolent disease. Am J Med 1986;81:381.
20. Collins JD, Bassett L, Main GD, et al. Percutaneous biopsy following positive bone scans. Radiology 1979;132:439.
21. Welker JA, Henshaw RM, Jelinek J, et al. The percutaneous needle biopsy is safe and recommended in the diagnosis of musculoskeletal masses: Outcomes analysis of 155 patients treated at a sarcoma referral center. Cancer 2000;89:2677.
22. Gainor BJ, Buchert D. Fracture healing in metastatic bone disease. Clin Orthop 1983;178:297.
23. Takahashi I, Niibe H, Mitsuhashi N, et al. Palliative radiotherapy of bone metastases. Adv Exp Med Biol 1992;324:227.
24. Bates T, Yarnold JR, Blitzer P, et al. Bone metastasis consensus statement. Int J Radiat Oncol Biol Phys 1992;324:227.
25. Blitzer P. Reanalysis of the RTOG study of the palliation of symptomatic osseous metastasis. Cancer 1985;55:1468.
26. Porter AT, Fontanesi J. Palliative irradiation for bone metastasis: A new paradigm. Int J Radiat Oncol Biol Phys 1994;29:1199.
27. Allen KL, Johnson TW, Hibbs GG. Effective bone palliation as related to various treatment regimens. Cancer 1976;37:984.
28. Glibert HA, Kagan HR, Nussbaum H. Evaluation of radiation therapy of bone metastases: Pain relief and quality. AJR Am J Roentgenol 1977;129:1095.
29. Tong D, Gillick L, Hendrickson FR. The palliation of symptomatic osseous metastases: Final results of the study by the radiation therapy oncology group. Cancer 1982;50:893.
30. Fulfaro F, Casuccio A, Ticozzi C, et al. The role of bisphosphonates in the treatment of painful metastatic bone disease: A review of phase III trials. Pain 1998;78:157.
31. Harvey HA. Issues concerning the role of chemotherapy and hormonal therapy of bone metastases from breast carcinoma. Cancer 1997;80:1646.
32. Perez CA, Cosmatos D, Garcia DM, et al. Irradiation in relapsing carcinoma of the prostate. Cancer 1993;71:1110.
33. Porter AT, McEwan AJB, Powe JE. Results of a randomized phase III trial to evaluate the efficacy of strontium-89 adjuvant to local field external beam irradiation inn the management of endocrine resistant metastatic prostate cancer. Int J Radiat Oncol Biol Phys 1993;25:805.
34. Toma S, Venturino A, Sogno G, et al. Metastatic bone tumors: Nonsurgical treatment, outcome and survival. Clin Orthop 1993;295:246.

35. Siegel T, Siegel T. Current considerations in the management of neoplastic spinal cord compression. Spine 1989;14:223.
36. O'Connor MI, Currier BL. Metastatic disease of the spine. Orthopedics 1992;15:611.
37. Lane JM, Sculco TP, Zolan S. Treatment of pathological fractures of the hip by endoprosthetic replacement. J Bone Joint Surg Am 1980;62:954.
38. Aboulafia AJ, Buch R, Malawer MM. Reconstruction using the saddle prosthesis following excision of primary and metastatic periacetabular tumors. Clin Orthop 1995;314:203.
39. Keene JS, Sellinger DS, McBeath AA, et al. Metastatic breast cancer in the femur: A search for the lesion at risk of fracture. Clin Orthop 1986;203:282.
40. Mirels H. Metastatic disease in long bones: A proposed scoring system for diagnosing impending pathological fractures. Clin Orthop 1989; 249:256.
41. Beals RK, Lawton GD, Snell WE. Prophylactic internal fixation of the femur in metastatic breast cancer. Cancer 1971;28:1350.
42. Fidler M. Prophylactic internal fixation of secondary neoplastic deposits in long bones. BMJ 1973;1:341.
43. Blunting RW. Rehabilitation of cancer patients with skeletal metastases. Clin Orthop 1995;312:197.

X

Radiation Therapy for Metastatic Breast Cancer

John Rescigno and Anthony Berson

Breast cancer is the second leading cause of cancer death in women. About 39,800 women died of breast cancer in 2003, accounting for 15% of all cancer deaths.[1] Decisions about the use of localized therapy in the patient with advanced breast cancer can be complex. The primary goals of radiation therapy for metastatic breast cancer are alleviation of symptoms and improvement of functional status. Another benefit may be a modest improvement in survival in a small proportion of patients. Radiation often relieves localized symptoms such as pain. In other circumstances, although the patient is asymptomatic, impending problems, such as bronchial obstruction, cord compression, or bone fracture, can be prevented with radiotherapy. Decisions regarding the use of radiation therapy need to take into account the patient's prognosis, with the goal of obtaining durable control of symptoms within the patient's life span. Additionally, there is a subset of patients with minimal metastatic disease or chest wall recurrence in whom radiation might contribute to long-term durable control and possibly cure of the breast cancer.

What is the role of radiotherapy, and what are the optimal dose and fractionation for the palliation of bone metastases?

More than half of patients with metastatic breast cancer have bone as an initial site of metastasis. Two thirds of these patients present with metastatic disease limited to bone. Bone metastases tend to occur in patients with more well-differentiated, ER-positive tumors.[2] The relatively high frequency of bone metastases makes breast cancer the most common primary site in randomized studies of radiotherapy for the palliation of bone metastases.

Pain Relief

Long-term relief of pain is an important goal of radiation therapy, given the favorable prognosis of patients with metastatic disease to bone compared with other systemic sites. Radiation therapy is the mainstay of treatment for bone metastases. Local field radiotherapy is highly effective in relieving pain and preventing fractures and is typically associated with minimal side effects.

Mechanism of Pain Relief. The precise mechanism of relief of bone pain by radiotherapy is not known. The direct cytotoxic effects of radiation on tumor cells can provide shrinkage of tumor, decrease stretching of the periosteum, and allow for repair of bone with healing of microfractures and macrofractures. However, it is unknown whether tumor cell cytotoxicity is the primary factor in analgesia achieved with radiation. The fact that rapid pain relief may be seen at doses as low as 4 Gy (which is not expected to induce tumor shrinkage) suggests other mechanisms. It is likely that radiation also affects normal bone turnover through cytotoxic activity on osteoclasts and osteoblasts. In theory, cytotoxicity of radiotherapy on normal bone cells could lead to decreased production of cytokines that stimulate nociceptors, such as substance P, bradykinin, and prostaglandins, providing pain response at relatively low doses. In fact, radiotherapy pain response is correlated with suppression of osteoclast activity measured by urinary markers of bone degradation.[3] The mechanism of radiotherapeutic analgesia may therefore have parallels to the mechanism of action of bisphosphonates.

Optimal Dose and Fractionation for Pain Relief. Eighteen trials assessing fractionation and dose of radiotherapy for painful bone metastases have been published.[4,5] Randomized trials comparing a single fraction of 8 Gy with multiple-fraction radiotherapy regimens (20 to 30 Gy in 5 to 10 fractions) reveal similar overall response rates. Pain relief is typically achieved 1 to 4 weeks after treatment, and the duration of response is 12 to 24 weeks. In pooled analyses of patients with varied primary cancers, about one third of patients with metastasis to bone had complete pain relief, and an additional one third of patients had partial relief of pain, irrespective of the dose fractionation used.[4] Breast cancer is associated with higher response rates than non–breast cancer histologies. An important difference between an 8-Gy single-fraction treatment and higher dose fractionated treatment is that a significantly greater proportion of patients treated with the single fraction require retreatment (about 23% vs. 8%).[4] However, more than 80% of patients with persistent or recurrent pain secondary to breast cancer metastases respond to retreatment.[6] Individual studies have found that remineralization based on CT density measurements is significantly better after 30 Gy in 10 fractions compared with 8 Gy in 1 fraction[7] and that the actual pathologic fracture rate may be higher after 8 Gy in 1 fraction versus 24 Gy in 6 fractions (4% vs. 2%).[8] However, the Radiation Therapy Oncology Group (RTOG) trial 7402 found a higher pathologic fracture rate with 40 Gy in 15 fractions compared with 20 Gy in 4 fractions (18% vs. 4%),[9] suggesting that a dose of 40 Gy in 15 fractions may inhibit remineralization of bone and contribute to pathologic fracture risk and that the optimal total dose or dose per fraction should be less.

In summary, all trials of radiation fractionation for palliation of bone metastases suggest similar pain relief irrespective of the dose-fractionation schedule. However, radiation oncology communities throughout the world have been slow to adopt a single 8-Gy fraction approach. Reinterpretations of the randomized trial data taking into account analgesic use, need for retreatment, and complete response rates suggest that fractionated treatment to higher total dose leads to more complete and durable response.[10,11] Problems with available data, including heterogeneity of primary cancers, patients, and prognoses; differing length of follow-up and time to assessment of response; failure to take into account analgesic use in most studies; varied and insufficient methods of pain evaluation; variable definitions of response; and variable and unspecified actual target dose are all reasons for skepticism in accepting the null hypothesis from the randomized trials of total dose and fractionation. However, the arms of the larger trials that included hundreds of patients are likely to be evenly balanced for known and unknown factors that could affect the results, and despite differences in methodology and reporting, the results of the trials are strikingly consistent.

Additional randomized trials using careful assessment of analgesic consumption and validated quality-of-life tools in more well-defined patient populations and stratified by single or multiple painful bone sites are warranted. To this end, the RTOG trial 9714 included 452 women with breast cancer and 445 men with prostate cancer.[5] Pain response rates were similar with 8 Gy in 1 fraction compared with 30 Gy in 10 fractions. Overall response was 66% irrespective of the treatment regimen. The complete pain response was only 17%, without any difference between arms. In patients with one site of painful bone metastasis, the complete pain response rates were 18% with 8 Gy and 25% with 30 Gy ($P = .17$). One third of patients required no analgesic medication by 3 months after treatment. Response was the same irrespective of bisphosphonate use at the time of radiation. Acute grades 2, 3, and 4 toxicity were seen in 10%, 2.8%, and 0.2%, respectively. More patients experienced toxicity in the higher-dose arm (17% vs. 10%).

Should 8 Gy in 1 fraction be the standard treatment for women with painful bone metastasis from breast cancer? In patients with poor performance status and limited prognosis (e.g., less than 6 months), the convenience and relative ease of administration supports single-fraction treatment if the only goal of treatment is pain relief. For patients with a better prognosis, such as those with metastatic disease confined to bone, those with a long disease-free interval, or those naïve-responsive to systemic therapy, the frequent need for retreatment and indirect evidence suggesting improved complete response and duration of response support consideration of higher doses such as 30 Gy in 10 fractions. Such a fractionation scheme might also be appropriate for patients at risk for fracture of weight-bearing bones (see later). Sites that could be associated with unique toxicity, such as the skull or joint spaces, may be better treated with 3 Gy or lower dose per fraction. For patients with an isolated bone metastasis, biopsy proof of recurrent breast cancer is usually warranted. Such patients can be considered for higher-dose radiotherapy with the additional goal of long-term durable control of disease (e.g., 35 Gy in 14 fractions or 40 Gy in 20 fractions).

Prevention of Pathologic Fractures

In addition to pain relief, prevention of pathologic fracture is a major goal of therapy, and assessment by an orthopedic surgeon is warranted for selected patients with good performance status who are at risk for pathologic fracture. Prediction of the risk for pathologic fracture is extremely difficult. Factors such as involvement of more than 50% of the cortex of long bones, lesions larger than 2.5 cm in the weight-bearing regions of the proximal femur, or avulsion of the lesser trochanter are commonly cited criteria for consideration of orthopedic stabilization before radiotherapy.[12] Involvement of the subtrochanteric femur over even a small area places the patient at risk for fracture. However, in a study of risk factors for fracture in breast cancer patients with proximal femur lesions, no clearly definable criteria could be established.[13]

A scoring system was developed to predict risk for pathologic fracture based on four factors: cortical involvement (less than half, one half to two thirds, and more than two thirds), site (upper limb, lower limb, peritrochanter), presence of pain (mild, moderate, severe), and lesion characteristics (blastic, mixed, lytic).[14] For each factor, a score from 1 to 3 is given, and the scores are summed (minimum score, 4; maximum score, 12). Patients with a score of 7 or less have a low probability of fracture (5%) and can be treated with radiation alone. Patients with a score of 8 have a 15% fracture risk, and patients with a score of 9 or more have at least a 33% risk for fracture. Recent modification of the scoring system accounts for greater risk in patients with a lesion proximal to the lesser trochanter, a lesion in the proximal humerus, a breast cancer primary, lack of bisphosphonate therapy, and presence of osteoporosis.[15] For patients who require orthopedic stabilization, radiotherapy is recommended postoperatively to improve functional recovery and to minimize the risk for prosthesis failure. Doses should be limited to 30 Gy or less in patients who have experienced long bone fracture so that healing is not inhibited.

What is the role of radiotherapy in the setting of bisphosphonate use?

Bisphosphonates reduce osteoclast activity and inhibit bone resorption. Bisphosphonate therapy has been shown in randomized trials to reduce the incidence of fractures, hypercalcemia, and the need for radiotherapy. There is also a trend toward reduction in the need for orthopedic surgery and in the risk for spinal cord compression. In a pooled analysis of patients with primarily breast cancer and myeloma who received bisphosphonate therapy, the need for radiotherapy was reduced by one third (odds ratio, 0.67; 95% confidence interval, 0.57%–0.79%).[16] None of the trials prespecified the criteria for administration of radiation.

Reports of the incidence of radiotherapy in patients treated with bisphosphonate versus control patients not receiving bisphosphonate are available from five randomized trials including 1625 patients with breast cancer.[16] Combining these studies, radiotherapy to bone was used in 43% of control patients versus 33% of patients receiving bisphosphonate therapy. The continued significant rate of radiotherapy is a result of the complications from bone metastases for which bisphosphonate therapy is inadequate. The most common indication is pain before or during bisphosphonate therapy. Evidence is lacking to justify the use of bisphosphonates for rapid pain relief or as first-line therapy for bone pain. In a pooled analysis of studies that examined pain relief, fewer than 15% of patients achieved major pain relief after 12 weeks of therapy.[17] Other indications for radiation include associated soft tissue masses, nerve root compression, pathologic fracture, and epidural disease. It is appropriate to consider radiotherapy complementary to bisphosphonate therapy analogous to the paradigm of combined-modality therapy for localized solid tumors: systemic bisphosphonates are most effective in preventing complications from asymptomatic or occult metastatic bone disease, whereas radiotherapy is most appropriate for the treatment of clinically apparent disease.

Can widespread bone metastases be treated with radiotherapy?

Other means of systemic treatment of bone metastases besides bisphosphonates, hormonal therapy, and chemotherapy include the use of hemibody irradiation and bone-seeking radioisotopes. Most patients with diffuse bone pain experience response of pain with hemibody irradiation, and 20% have complete response.[18] Relief usually occurs within 1 week of treatment. Breast and prostate cancers respond better than other types of cancers. The treatment involves the administration of single-fraction or multiple-fraction radiotherapy to one half of the body, often followed about 2 to 4 weeks later (to allow for hematopoietic recovery) by treatment of the other half of the body. The body is typically demarcated at the level of the umbilicus, and the distal extremities and calvarium are excluded. A dose of 8 Gy has been used for the lower body, whereas a single-fraction dose of 6 Gy has been used for the upper body to limit the incidence of pneumonitis. Toxicity is less with customized shielding of nonosseous normal tissue. Treatment of the ribs can be accomplished with electrons, so that the normal underlying lung is not exposed. Treatment is associated with severe temporary hematologic toxicity in 10% of patients. Use of cytokine support is appropriate for patients with significant neutropenia after treatment. Vomiting is frequent, and premedication is indicated. Low-grade fever is common as well. Fractionated regimens are likely to improve the therapeutic ratio. For example, 17.5 Gy delivered in 2.5-Gy fractions has been used for treatment and prevention of bone metastasis complications with good effect and acceptable hematologic toxicity.[19]

Radionuclide therapy has also been used to treat widespread bone metastases and is the primary subject of a recent review.[20] A variety of systemically administered agents have been developed. The two most commonly used agents are strontium 89 and samarium 153. Strontium 89 has a half-life of 50 days, and samarium 153 has a half-life of 1.9 days. The shorter half-life of samarium translates into a higher dose rate, quicker pain relief, and more rapid hematologic toxicity and recovery. Meaningful response is seen in about 80% of patients. A minority of patients will have significant flare of pain, which may correlate with improved response. Pain relief is maintained for an average of 6 months. Nadir counts are usually more than half of the pretreatment counts. After administration of strontium 89, nadir occurs by 8 weeks, and recovery occurs by 4 months. The time course of myelosuppression is about twice as fast with samarium 153. Therapy with samarium 153 should not be administered on the same day as a bisphosphonate, which competes for the same binding sites. Treatment is not suitable for patients with purely lytic disease and minimal uptake on bone scan. For patients with recurrent pain, treatment can be safely repeated after hematologic recovery.

The role of hemibody irradiation and radionuclides in breast cancer may become more limited with the widespread use of bisphosphonates and the availability of more effective hormonal agents and chemotherapy. More effective systemic therapy may shift the pattern of symptomatic progression later in the natural history of the disease when visceral sites become the predominant problem. Hemibody irradiation and radionuclide therapy are most appropriate for patients with diffuse bone pain refractory to hormonal therapy and chemotherapy, with a life expectancy of at least 3 months and satisfactory hematologic reserve.

What is the role of whole-brain radiotherapy in the management of brain metastases?

Although the median survival of patients with breast cancer after diagnosis of bone metastasis is about 2 years, the median survival after brain metastasis is generally 4 months.[21] This is partly due to the direct effect of brain metastasis on function and survival. However, many patients develop brain metastases late in the course of their disease, when progressive extracranial disease dictates survival. Breast cancer is the second leading cause of brain metastasis, and about 15% of patients are diagnosed clinically. In randomized trials of therapy for brain metastases, typically more than half of patients have lung cancer, and less than one fourth of patients have breast cancer. Therefore, the specificity for breast cancer of brain metastases radiotherapy trials might be less than in trials of palliation of bone metastases.

Corticosteroids were first used in 1957 for the treatment of peritumoral edema associated with brain metastases from breast cancer.[22] Median survival of patients treated with steroids alone is 2 months. The addition of whole-brain radiotherapy (WBRT) extends this time to 4 months. Most symptomatic patients have a clinical response with WBRT. The clinical response rate, degree of response, and duration of response depend on the extent of tumor and the severity of initial neurologic deficits. Breast cancer responds better than other primary cancers.[23] The most common WBRT fractionation is 30 Gy in 10 fractions over 2 weeks. In two randomized RTOG trials of more than 1800 patients with a variety of primary cancers, fractionation schedules of 20 Gy in 1 week,

30 Gy in 2 weeks, 30 Gy in 3 weeks, 40 Gy in 3 weeks, and 40 Gy in 4 weeks were tested.[24] No significant differences between the fractionation regimens were seen. Overall improvement in neurologic function was seen in about half of patients and maintained in more than three fourths of these patients. Normal functionality was achieved in one third of patients that were partly bedridden. Brain metastasis was the cause of death in 40% of patients. Additional randomized trials from the RTOG have shown no significant differences in outcome based on dose-fractionation schemes, including 30 Gy in 2 weeks versus 50 Gy in 4 weeks,[25] or versus a hyperfractionated regimen of 54.4 Gy at 1.6 Gy twice daily.[26] All regimens were associated with response of neurologic symptoms in most patients and a median survival of about 4 months. This result may be partly due to the heterogeneity of the patients enrolled in the trials, including patients with variable performance status, different primary tumor histologies, and the shortened survival that is most frequently dictated by progressive extracranial metastases. Recursive partitioning analysis of patients treated with a variety of dose-fractionation regimens suggests that factors unrelated to radiotherapy treatment parameters best predict survival: patients with a Karnofsky performance score (KPS) of at least 70, controlled primary tumor, brain as the only site of metastases, and age younger than 65 years were found to have a median survival of 7.1 months.[27]

In patients who have undergone resection, the need for WBRT has been studied. Most patients have further failure in the brain at both the site of resection and remote sites in the brain. For example, in a randomized study of 95 patients who underwent MRI-defined complete resection of a solitary brain metastasis, 70% of patients had recurrence, including 46% who had relapse at the initial site of disease. Postoperative WBRT was associated with a three-fourths relative risk reduction in recurrence (resulting in an overall relapse rate of only 18%) and with decreased risk for death from neurologic causes.[28] Therefore, postoperative WBRT is recommended for patients who undergo resection of a solitary metastasis and who have controlled extracranial disease.

What is the role of stereotactic radiosurgery in the management of brain metastases?

The survival outcome with WBRT is poor, and up to half of patients will die from progressive brain metastases with the use of WBRT alone. Therefore, continued efforts to improve on the results of WBRT are needed. WBRT is increasingly being supplemented by more aggressive treatment directed at known sites of brain metastases using stereotactic single-fraction radiotherapy ("radiosurgery"), stereotactic multifraction radiotherapy, or surgical resection. Stereotactic radiosurgery delivers a focal high dose of radiation using three-dimensional treatment planning, often with MRI image fusion to contrast-enhanced CT image data, and a stereotactic localization device to aim multiple highly collimated beams. Sharp dose gradients near the edge of the tumor limit the dose to normal brain tissue. Therapy can be delivered with the Leksell gamma knife system, which consists of 201 small cobalt 60 sources all collimated to a single focal point. Another technology allows for linear accelerator–based treatment using a specialized cylindrical collimator placed onto the head

of the machine to aim a small radiation beam while the accelerator gantry moves in multiple arcs around a precisely localized target. Fractionated stereotactic radiotherapy can be done using mini-multileaf collimators and less invasive head immobilization and localization procedures.

Surgery or stereotactic radiation is likely to be associated with decreased risk for neurologic death and improved survival in appropriately selected patients. For example, surgically treated breast cancer patients with brain metastases have a median survival of about 16 months.[29,30] The value of more aggressive treatment for patients with brain metastasis is clearly shown by two of the three randomized trials of surgical resection of solitary metastasis plus WBRT versus WBRT alone in patients with a variety of primary tumor histologies.[31-33] Patchell and associates[31] found improved local control (20% brain failure vs. 52% brain failure) and median survival (40 weeks vs. 15 weeks) with the addition of surgery. In another trial, surgery improved median survival from 6 months to 10 months.[32] Another multicenter randomized trial of 84 patients did not reveal any advantage to surgical resection.[33] This may be due to the selection of patients with worse performance status or more extracranial disease, failure to achieve complete resection in some patients, and crossover of one fourth of patients receiving WBRT to surgery.

Selection criteria for radiosurgery are similar to those for surgical resection, that is—patients with solitary metastases, good performance status, and limited or responsive extracranial disease. Patients with surgically inaccessible lesions that are deep within the brain parenchyma or that involve Broca's area or the visual cortex can be safely treated with radiosurgery. Surgery is preferred for patients who are highly symptomatic and have accessible lesions because it provides more immediate relief of symptoms. Additionally, in the few patients with solitary brain metastases without extracranial disease, surgery is required for diagnostic purposes. About 10% of patients with good performance status and a solitary brain metastasis will have a diagnosis unrelated to the known primary cancer upon biopsy of the brain tumor.[31]

Radiosurgery may also be appropriate in patients with two or three brain metastases. In 68 women with metastatic breast cancer, Amendola and associates found that survival after radiosurgery was independent of the number of lesions (median survival, 7 months).[34] In a study of 248 patients with 421 brain lesions from a variety of primary cancers, there was only 11% progression within the radiosurgery volume at a median follow-up of 26 months. Surgery was required in 6% of patients for mass effect or steroid dependency secondary to radiation necrosis.[35] Mehta and colleagues reviewed more than 2100 lesions treated with radiosurgery to a median dose of 18 Gy and found that 86% of lesions were stable or responded.[36] A retrospective study of 122 patients who were eligible for surgical resection combined 37.5 Gy WBRT followed by a median radiosurgery boost of 17 Gy. An 86% brain tumor control rate was obtained, and the median survival was longer than 1 year, which compares favorably with results of trials of surgical resection and WBRT.[37] RTOG 95-08 randomized patients with one to three brain metastases to WBRT followed by a radiosurgery boost versus WBRT alone (37.5 Gy in 15 fractions). In patients with a single brain metastasis, survival was improved from a median of 4.9 months in the WBRT arm to 6.5 months in the WBRT plus radiosurgery arm.[38]

Outcome after radiosurgery is similar to outcome after surgical resection. Radiosurgery, however, is minimally invasive and can be done on a purely outpatient basis. Patients can return to work or resume normal daily activities the following day. This contrasts with surgical resection, which requires hospitalization and inpatient recovery times that can significantly delay postoperative WBRT. Patient preference and physician bias will likely preclude a successful randomized trial of radiosurgery versus surgical resection.

WBRT is generally recommended before or after radiosurgery. In a multi-institutional retrospective study of stereotactic radiosurgery in the treatment of single brain metastasis, of 71 patients who had newly diagnosed brain metastases, the brain control rate at 1 year was 53% with radiosurgery and WBRT, as compared with 18% for radiosurgery alone.[39] However, salvage therapy with WBRT is possible after radiosurgery, and survival appears uncompromised with a deferred treatment strategy.[40] Patients with metastasis larger than 3 cm are best treated with WBRT as initial treatment because tumor control may be inferior with radiosurgery alone. Patients who respond to WBRT can be considered for radiosurgery.

Is there a role for radiosensitizers in the treatment of brain metastases?

Early trials of radiosensitizers such as misonidazole[41] and bromodioxyuridine[42] yielded disappointing results. Temozolomide is an alkylating agent that is orally bioavailable and crosses the blood-brain barrier. It has been shown to yield higher response rates in combination with WBRT than does WBRT alone.[43] Whether this translates into improved quality of life and survival is yet to be determined. Motexafin gadolinium catalyzes the oxidation of intracellular ascorbate, glutathione, and protein thiols, depleting the cell of reducing metabolites. A randomized phase III study comparing motexafin gadolinium and WBRT versus WBRT alone found no difference in survival.[44] There was improved 6-month freedom from neurologic progression as judged by investigators but not by an independent events review committee. There did appear to be a benefit in time to neurologic progression in patients with lung cancer, who constituted most of the patients in this study.

The compound RSR13 is a synthetic allosteric modifier of hemoglobin that reduces the oxygen-binding affinity of hemoglobin and allows increased oxygen delivery to hypoxic cells. This agent was studied in combination with oxygen and WBRT versus oxygen and WBRT alone in 538 patients with multiple brain metastases (115 with metastatic breast cancer).[45] RSR13 was associated with improved survival for the entire study group ($P = .17$; $P = .01$ by Cox multivariate regression). In the subgroup of patients with metastatic breast cancer, survival was nearly doubled (4.6 months vs. 8.7 months). A study limited to metastatic breast cancer is planned to confirm these results.

In summary, no trials of a radiosensitizing agent have yielded improvement in survival over WBRT alone for a diverse population of patients with metastatic cancer to brain. Subsets of patients who might benefit have been retrospectively identified. Radiosensitizers remain an exciting area of research for patients with metastatic breast cancer to the brain. Measurements of quality of life and neurologic outcome will need to be incorporated into future trials.

What is the palliative role of radiotherapy for other common sites of metastases?

Spinal Cord Compression

Breast cancer is the most common cause of spinal cord compression in women. Breast cancer is the underlying cause in half of women with spinal cord compression. Radiation therapy alone has most commonly been used for the treatment of spinal cord compression. Corticosteroids are initiated immediately before radiation. A total dose of 30 Gy in 10 fractions is appropriate, although shorter dose schedules have been employed with similar outcome.[46]

Surgery is useful to establish a diagnosis if uncertain. Patients with acceptable performance status in whom bony retropulsion is likely to be the primary cause of neurologic deficit should also be treated with surgery. Patients with rapid deterioration of neurologic function or with high-grade cervical cord compression should also be considered for surgery. Patients with high cervical spine cord compression should be evaluated for atlantoaxial subluxation. If no or minimal subluxation is present, a stabilizing collar (e.g., Philadelphia collar) can be used before radiation therapy.

A prospective study of 275 consecutive patients with a variety of primary tumors found pain response in 82% of patients.[47] Three fourths of patients had preservation of ability to walk or recovery of function. Improvement in sphincter function was noted in 46% of patients with initial deficits. Patients with breast cancer and prostate cancer had better response than those with other solid tumors. Recovery of sensory or motor deficits is related to pretreatment neurologic status. Few patients with paraplegia or incontinence regain function with radiotherapy. In a study of 70 patients, two thirds of patients who were ambulatory at the time of radiotherapy remained ambulatory, whereas fewer than one third of patients who were initially nonambulatory regained function, and 16% of paraplegic patients regained the ability to walk.[48]

Laminectomy rarely removes the bulk of the tumor, it fails to relieve pain, and it can destabilize the spine. However, vertebral body resection and radical decompressive surgery with postoperative radiotherapy was recently reported to be superior to radiotherapy alone in the only randomized trial of spinal cord compression conducted to date.[49] Patients with a single site of cord compression and a minimum 3-month life expectancy were enrolled. The trial was stopped early after 101 patients were enrolled. Patients who received surgery plus radiation therapy retained the ability to walk significantly longer (126 days vs. 35 days with radiation therapy alone). In a total of 32 patients who could not walk at the time of enrollment, 56% of those who received surgery and radiation therapy recovered the ability to walk, compared with 19% who received radiation therapy alone. Functional scores, maintenance of continence, and decreased use of steroids and narcotics were all improved in patients undergoing decompressive surgery versus radiotherapy alone. Survival was slightly better in patients undergoing surgery (median, 4.2 months vs. 3.3 months; $P = .08$). The threshold for recommending surgery in patients with breast cancer may be higher because such patients generally respond better to radiation therapy. However, patients with neurologic deficit and life expectancy of at least 3 months should be considered for surgery based on the results of this phase III study.

Brachial Plexopathy

Extension of tumor from supraclavicular, infraclavicular, and axillary nodes into the brachial plexus can lead to devastating pain and loss of function of the upper extremity. Involvement of the lower plexus will affect the C7-T1 nerve roots and cause pain in the shoulder, arm, medial forearm, and fourth and fifth digits. Supraclavicular node involvement can cause upper plexus involvement and pain and numbness at the posterior arm, index finger, and thumb from involvement of C5 and C6 nerves. Occasionally, Horner's syndrome is present. The treatment of choice is local radiotherapy. Optimally, CT-based treatment planning is performed to target the full extent of disease and to avoid uninvolved tissue volumes such as the shoulder while providing adequate dose to the target. The rate of plexopathy secondary to radiation is expected to be less than 1% with a dose of 50 Gy using conventional fractionation. The response rate depends on the time from symptom onset to the initiation of radiation therapy, although most patients benefit from treatment, having reduction in pain and improvement in arm mobility. Re-irradiation is not possible after prior full-dose treatment because of the risk for brachial plexopathy from retreatment.

Choroidal Metastases

More than one third of intraocular metastases are due to breast cancer.[50] Uveal metastasis can be the initial manifestation of breast cancer metastasis in up to 16% of patients.[51] Bilateral metastases have been noted in 38% of patients; about half of these are synchronous. The most common presenting symptom is decreased or blurred vision. Other presenting signs or symptoms include floaters and photopsia. Occasionally, symptoms can include diplopia, pain, uveitis, or headache. Indirect funduscopic examination is used to establish the diagnosis. Findings include detachment of the retina, usually posteriorly. The surface of the tumor may have a mottled appearance. Occasionally, hemorrhage and pigmentary changes may occur over the involved area. For single lesions, the appearance is similar to that of a primary ocular melanoma. Ultrasonography is useful in distinguishing between melanoma and metastatic disease. CT and MRI have a limited role in the diagnosis of ocular metastasis. Nevertheless, brain imaging should be performed because of a significant diagnosis of concurrent central nervous system (CNS) metastases. A 22% incidence of concurrent CNS metastases has been reported, with an additional 19% of patients diagnosed at a subsequent date.[52] External-beam radiation therapy is usually recommended. Radiotherapy is indicated when there is secondary retinal detachment, impending or actual decrease in visual acuity, or rapidly enlarging tumor. In some situations, observation with close monitoring may be appropriate. The goal of radiation treatment is to encompass all of the choroid from the equator posteriorly, with a margin. Usually, radiation to the lens can be avoided by using a lateral field with a half-beam D-shaped block. For unilateral disease, a single lateral field is effective in delivering the dose to the eye while avoiding multiple pathways that could compromise subsequent palliative treatment in adjacent areas. Typical doses of radiation include 30 to 40 Gy over 2 to 4 weeks. External-beam radiation can provide local tumor control in up to 85% of cases. Initially, vision may deteriorate during or after radiation due to shifting subretinal fluid and retinal detachment.

Is there a role for definitive radiotherapy after locoregional recurrence or limited metastatic disease?

Locoregional recurrence of breast cancer after mastectomy remains a problem in more than 15% of patients undergoing mastectomy (Fig. 32–25). Risk factors for locoregional recurrence include lack of postoperative radiotherapy, large

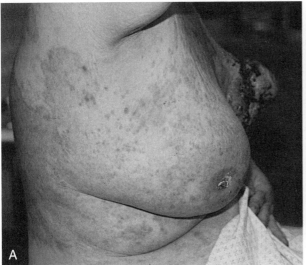
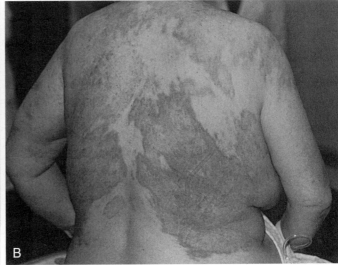

Figure 32–25 *A and B,* Locally advanced breast cancer en cuirasse. From Steinfeld AD. Treatment of metastatic breast cancer. In Roses DF (ed): Breast Cancer. Philadelphia, Churchill Livingstone, 1999, p. 573.

primary tumor, lymph node involvement, presence of extra-capsular extension, vascular or lymphatic invasion, involvement of the skin, and involved surgical margins. Patients usually present with an asymptomatic nodule or nodules in the skin or subcutaneously, often near the scar. Occasionally, recurrence has the appearance of an erythematous rash. Rarely, the skin and subcutaneous tissues are diffusely infiltrated and ulcerated (carcinoma en cuirasse; see Fig. 32–25). About half of patients have prior or synchronous presentation of distant metastases as a component of failure at the time of locoregional recurrence. For these patients, radiotherapy is generally directed toward palliation of symptoms. Morbidity from locoregional recurrence can be significant, with more than half of patients experiencing bleeding, ulceration, severe pain, upper extremity edema, or brachial plexopathy.[53] Therefore, local control of disease remains an important goal, and all symptomatic patients should be considered for radiotherapy. In patients who have not had prior radiotherapy, large fields encompassing the chest wall and regional nodes are necessary to avoid marginal failures. A dose of at least 50 Gy in standard fractionation is necessary to treat microscopic disease, and at least 60 Gy is needed for gross disease. Long-term local control can be achieved in more than 80% of patients who receive radiation therapy or surgical resection followed by radiation therapy.[54,55] Patients who have had prior chest wall radiotherapy may be eligible for palliative re-irradiation with electrons, interstitial brachytherapy, or surface brachytherapy. Hyperthermia and photodynamic therapy have also been used with some success.

The fact that most patients with isolated locoregional recurrence ultimately experience relapse at distant sites has been a justification for an approach that assumes that all such patients should be treated with palliative intent only; consequently, such patients are often labeled as having stage IV disease. A corollary is that chest wall recurrence is only a marker of a definitive risk for distant metastasis and not a potential source of metastasis. However, in the era of improved systemic adjuvant chemotherapy, patients who might otherwise have experienced relapse at distant sites may manifest locoregional failure as the only site of failure. A subset of these patients can enjoy long-term disease control and possibly cure with the use of salvage radiation therapy.

A prerequisite of cure is durable control of locally recurrent disease. In a study of 121 patients who received chemotherapy for isolated locoregional recurrence, the 5-year disease-free survival was 35% for patients initially rendered disease free with local therapy and 13% for patients who were not disease free by the start of chemotherapy.[56] Selected patients with minimum-volume chest wall relapse have better survival, with up to half of patients remaining relapse free at 10 years after treatment of the local recurrence.[57,58] Factors associated with long-term disease-free survival after chest wall recurrence include longer disease-free interval from mastectomy to local recurrence, negative nodes at initial diagnosis of breast cancer, resectable recurrence, and positive ER status.

Only one randomized trial has examined the use of systemic therapy after excision and radiation therapy for chest wall recurrence.[58] One hundred seventy-eight women with a disease-free interval of at least 1 year from initial diagnosis and low-volume isolated chest wall recurrence were randomized to receive tamoxifen versus observation after surgical resection and radiotherapy. Tamoxifen resulted in improved disease-free survival, which was limited to reducing the risk for another locoregional relapse by nearly half (31% vs. 16%). The use of cytotoxic chemotherapy as "secondary adjuvant" treatment after resection and radiation of isolated locoregional recurrence has led to improved 5-year survival compared with local therapy alone in single-institution studies.[56,59] The International Breast Cancer Study Group (IBCSG) 27-02 trial is testing whether systemic chemotherapy after surgical resection with or without radiation results in improved survival of patients who suffer isolated locoregional recurrence.

Advances in systemic therapy, including hormonal therapy, single-agent or combination chemotherapy, and molecular targeted therapy, are shifting the paradigm of treatment of metastatic breast cancer from palliation to long-term disease control. The radiation oncologist's distinction between curative therapy and palliative therapy becomes less clear if the end point is long-term disease remission. For example, a patient with a solitary metastasis who responds to initial systemic therapy will usually ultimately have cancer recurrence and progression at that site, and consolidative radiotherapy can forestall or prevent relapse. In rare cases, patients with metastatic disease can remain in complete remission for more than 20 years.[60,61] A study from the University of Texas M. D. Anderson Cancer Center of 134 patients with chest wall recurrence or isolated distant metastasis who were rendered disease free with surgery and, when possible, radiotherapy, were treated with systemic chemotherapy and achieved a 15-year disease-free survival rate of 24%.[62] A more recent cohort of patients from the same institution found a 5-year disease-free survival rate of 59% with the use of multimodal therapy.[59] Another study of 60 patients with minimal metastatic disease amenable to local therapy followed by high-dose chemotherapy resulted in a 5-year relapse-free survival of 52%.[63] Although a significant proportion of patients in these studies had chest wall failure only, long-term survivorship was seen in patients who presented with distant soft tissue or visceral metastases.

Although metastatic breast cancer to the liver is usually associated with advanced and incurable disease, patients with metastatic disease to the lung may experience long-term survival with localized therapy. Of 467 patients with breast cancer selected for lung metastasectomy in the International Registry of Lung Metastases, the 15-year survival rate was 20%.[64] Multimodality treatment for asymptomatic metastatic breast cancer should be limited to patients with good performance status and an extent and distribution of disease that is amenable to surgery or radiation with the intent of rendering the patient disease free. Strict attention to the morbidities of therapy is important because most patients ultimately experience relapse at sites away from the clinically apparent surgical-radiotherapeutic target. Newer modalities such as intensity-modulated radiotherapy and extracranial body stereotactic radiotherapy limit the morbidity of treatment by more precisely targeting the metastatic tumor. Such focused radiotherapy techniques can be given with more convenient accelerated treatment regimens that avoid delays in full-dose systemic therapy. Additionally, analogous to stereotactic treatment of intracranial disease, extracranial radiosurgery and intensity-modulated radiotherapy may be viable alternatives to surgery and, because postoperative morbidity is avoided, more widely applicable than surgery in efforts to maintain durable control of clinically apparent metastatic disease.

Improved imaging modalities, including functional imaging, have the potential to enhance selection of patients who might benefit from aggressive combined-modality treatment of metastatic disease. Improved imaging will also allow increased targeting accuracy when used in conjunction with radiation treatment planning systems. Advances in systemic chemotherapy, radiotherapy delivery, and patient selection are likely to provide the foundation for increased use of radiation metastasectomy in the combined modality management of metastatic breast cancer. Improvements in disease-free survival, quality of life, and possibly overall survival can be anticipated in selected good-prognosis patients with metastatic breast cancer.

REFERENCES

1. Jemal A, Murray T, Samuels A, et al. Cancer statistics, 2003. CA Cancer J Clin 2003;53:5–26.
2. James JJ, Evans AJ, Pinder SE, et al. Bone metastases from breast carcinoma: Histopathological-radiologic correlations and prognostic features. Br J Cancer 2003;89:660–665.
3. Hoskin PJ, Stratford MRL, Folkes LK, et al. Effect of local radiotherapy for bone pain on urinary markers of osteoclast activity. Lancet 2000; 355:1428–1429.
4. Wu JSY, Wong R, Johnston M, et al. Meta-analysis of dose-fractionation radiotherapy trials for the palliation of painful bone metastases. Int J Radiat Oncol Biol Phys 2003;55:594–605.
5. Hartsell WF, Scott C, Bruner DW, et al. Phase III randomized trial of 8Gy in 1 fraction vs. 30Gy in 10 fractions for palliation of painful bone metastases. Int J Radiat Oncol Biol Phys 2003;57(Suppl 2):S124.
6. vander Linden Y, Lok J, Steenland E, et al. Re-irradiation of painful bone metastases: A further analysis of the Dutch Bone Metastasis Study. Int J Radiat Oncol Biol Phys 2003;57(Suppl):S222.
7. Koswig S, Buchali A, Bohmer D, et al. Palliative radiotherapy of bone metastases. A retrospective analysis of 176 patients. Strahlenther Onkol 1999;175:509–514.
8. Wu J, Bezjak A, Chow E, et al. Primary treatment endpoint following palliative radiotherapy for painful bone metastases: Need for a consensus definition? Clin Oncol 2002;14:70–77.
9. Chander S, Sarin R. Single fraction radiotherapy for bone metastases: Are all questions answered? Radiother Oncol 1999;52:191–193.
10. Ratanatharathorn V, Powers WE, Moss WT, et al. Bone metastasis: Review and critical analysis of random allocation trials of local field treatment. Int J Radiat Oncol Biol Phys 1999;44:1–18.
11. Blitzer PH. Reanalysis of the RTOG study of palliation of symptomatic osseous metastasis. Cancer 1985;55:1468–1472.
12. Parrish F, Murray SJ. Surgical treatment for secondary neoplastic fractures. J Bone Joint Surg Am 1970;52:66–86.
13. Keene JS, Sellinger DS, McBeath AA, et al. Metastatic breast cancer in the femur: A search for the lesion at risk for fracture. Clin Orthop 1986; 203:282–288.
14. Mirels H. Metastatic disease in long bones: A proposed scoring system for diagnosing impending pathologic fractures. Clin Orthop 1989;249: 256–264.
15. Patel B, DeGroot H. Evaluation of the risk of pathologic fractures secondary to metastatic bone disease. Orthopaedics 2001;24:612–617.
16. Ross JR, Saunders Y, Edmonds PM, et al. Systematic review of role of bisphosphonates on skeletal morbidity in metastatic cancer. BMJ 2003;327:469–474.
17. Wong R, Wiffen PJ. Bisphosphonates for the relief of pain secondary to bone metastases (Cochrane Methodology Review). In The Cochrane Library, Issue 4, 2003. Chichester, UK, John Wiley & Sons.
18. Salazar OM, Rubin P, Hendrickson FR, et al. Single dose half-body irradiation for the palliation of multiple bone metastasis from solid tumors: Final Radiation Therapy Oncology Group Report. Cancer 1986;58:29–36.
19. Scarantino CW, Caplan R, Rotman M, et al. A phase I/II study to evaluate the effect of fractionated hemibody irradiation in the treatment of osseous metastases-RTOG 88-022. Int J Radiat Oncol Biol Phys 1996; 36:37–48.
20. Serafini AN. Therapy of metastatic bone pain. J Nucl Med 2001;42: 895–906.
21. Mahmoud-Ahmed AS, Suh JH, Lee SY, et al. Results of whole brain radiotherapy from breast cancer: A retrospective study. Int J Radiat Oncol Biol Phys 2002;54:810–817.
22. Kofman S, Garvin JS, Nagamani D, et al. Treatment of cerebral metastases from breast cancer with prednisone. JAMA 1957;163:1473–1476.
23. Nieder C, Berberich W, Schnabel K. Tumor-related prognostic factors for remission of brain metastases after radiotherapy. Int J Radiat Oncol Biol Phys 1997;39:25–30.
24. Borgelt B, Gelber R, Kramer S, et al. The palliation of brain metastases: Final results of the first two studies by the Radiation Therapy Oncology Group. Int J Radiat Oncol Biol Phys 1980;6:1–9.
25. Kurtz JM, Gelber R, Brady LW, et al. The palliation of brain metastases in a favorable patient population: A randomized clinical trial by the Radiation Therapy Oncology Group. Int J Radiat Oncol Biol Phys 1981;7:891–895.
26. Murray KJ, Scott C, Greenberg HM, et al. A randomized phase III study of accelerated hyperfractionation vs standard treatment in patients with unresected brain metastases. A report of the Radiation Therapy Oncology Group (RTOG) 9104. Int J Radiat Oncol Biol Phys 1997; 39:571–574.
27. Gaspar L, Scott C, Rotman M, et al. Recursive partitioning analysis (RPA) of prognostic factors in three Radiation Therapy Oncology Group (RTOG) brain metastases trials. Int J Radiat Oncol Biol Phys 1997;37:745–751.
28. Patchell RA, Tibbs PA, Regine WF, et al. Postoperative radiotherapy in the treatment of single metastases to the brain: A randomized trial. JAMA 1998;280:1485–1489.
29. Pieper DR, Hess KR, Sawaya RE. Role of surgery in the treatment of brain metastases in patients with breast cancer. Ann Surg Oncol 1997;4:481–490.
30. Wronski M, Arbit E, McCormick B. Surgical treatment of 70 patients with brain metastases from breast carcinoma. Cancer 1997;80:1746–1754.
31. Patchell RA, Tibbs PA, Walsh JW, et al. A randomized trial of surgery in the treatment of single metastases to the brain. N Engl J Med 1990;322:494–500.
32. Noordijk EM, Vecht CJ, Haaxma-Reich H, et al. The choice of treatment of single brain metastasis should be based on extracranial tumor activity and age. Int J Radiat Oncol Biol Phys 1994;29:711–717.
33. Mintz AH, Kestle J, Rathbone MP, et al. A randomized trial to assess the efficacy of surgery in addition to radiotherapy in patients with a single cerebral metastasis. Cancer 1996;78:1470–1476.
34. Amendola BE, Wolf AL, Coy SR, et al. Gamma knife radiosurgery in the treatment of patients with single and multiple brain metastases from carcinoma of the breast. Cancer J 2000;6:88–92.
35. Alexander E III, Moriarty TM, Davis RB, et al. Stereotactic radiosurgery for the definitive, noninvasive treatment of brain metastases. J Natl Cancer Inst 1995;87:34–40.
36. Mehta MP, Boyd TS, Sinha P. The status of stereotactic radiosurgery for cerebral metastases in 1998. J Radiosurg 1998;1:17–29.
37. Auchter RM, Lamond JP, Alexander E III, et al. A multiinstitutional outcome and prognostic factor analysis of radiosurgery for resectable single brain metastasis. Int J Radiat Oncol Biol Phys 1996;35:27–35.
38. Andrews DW, Scott CB, Sperduto PW, et al. Whole brain radiation therapy with or without stereotactic radiosurgery boost for patients with one to three brain metastases: Phase III results of RTOG 9508 randomized trial. Lancet 2004;363:1665–1672.
39. Flickinger JC, Kondziolka D, Lunsford LD, et al. A multiinstitutional experience with stereotactic radiosurgery for solitary brain metastasis. Int J Radiat Oncol Biol Phys 1994;28:797–802.
40. Sneed PK, Suh JH, Goetsch SJ, et al. A multi-institutional review of radiosurgery alone vs. radiosurgery with whole brain radiotherapy as the initial management of brain metastases. Int J Radiat Oncol Biol Phys 2002;53;519–526.
41. Komarnicky LT, Phillips TL, Martz K, et al. A randomized phase III protocol for the evaluation of misonidazole combined with radiation in the treatment of patients with brain metastases (RTOG-7916). Int J Radiat Oncol Biol Phys 1991;20:53–58.
42. Phillips TL, Scott CB, Leibel SA, et al. Results of a randomized comparison of radiotherapy and bromodeoxyuridine with radiotherapy alone for brain metastases: Report of RTOG trial 89-05. Int J Radiat Oncol Biol Phys 1995;33:339–348.

43. Antonadou D, Paraskevaidis M, Sarris G., et al. Phase II randomized trial of temozolomide and concurrent radiotherapy in patients with brain metastases. J Clin Oncol 2002;20:2644–3650.

44. Mehta MP, Rodrigus P, Terhaard CHJ, et al. Survival and neurologic outcomes in a randomized trial of motexafin gadolinium and whole-brain radiation therapy in brain metastases. J Clin Oncol 2003;21:2529–2536.

45. Suh J, Stea BD, Kresi JJ, et al. Results from a subgroup analysis of patients with metastatic breast cancer (MBC) in a phase 3, randomized, open-label, comparative study of standard whole brain radiation therapy (WBRT) with supplemental oxygen, with or without RSR13, in patients with brain metastases. San Antonio Breast Cancer Symposium Abstract 175, Dec 2003.

46. Hoskin PJ, Grover A, Bhana R. Metastatic spinal cord compression: Radiotherapy outcome and dose fractionation. Radiother Oncol 2003;68:175–189.

47. Maranzano E, Latini P. Effectiveness of radiation therapy without surgery in metastatic spinal cord compression: Final results of a prospective trial. Int J Radiat Oncol Biol Phys 1995;32:959–967.

48. Leviov M, Dale J, Stein M, et al. The management of metastatic spinal cord compression. Int J Radiat Oncol Biol Phys 1993;27:231–234.

49. Regine WF, Tibbs PA, Young A, et al. Metastatic spinal cord compression: A randomized trial of direct decompressive surgical resection plus radiotherapy vs. radiotherapy alone. Int J Radiat Oncol Biol Phys 2003;57(Suppl): S125.

50. Albert DM. Tumor metastasis to the eye: Tumor incidence in 213 patients with generalized malignancy. Am J Ophthalmol 1967;63:723–726.

51. Demirci H, Shields CL, Chao AN, Shields JA. Uveal metastasis from breast cancer in 264 patients. Am J Ophthalmol 2003;136:264–271.

52. Thatcher N, Thomas PRM. Choroidal metastases from breast carcinoma: A survey of 42 patients and the use of radiation therapy. Clin Radiol 1975;26:549–553.

53. Bedwinek JM, Fineberg B, Lee J, et al. Analysis of failures following local treatment of isolated local-regional recurrence of breast cancer. Int J Radiat Oncol Biol Phys 1981;7:581–585.

54. Hsi RA, Antell A, Schultz DJ, Solin LJ. Radiation therapy for chest wall recurrence of breast cancer after mastectomy in a favorable subgroup of patients. Int J Radiat Oncol Biol Phys 1998;42:495–499.

55. Halverson KJ, Perez CA, Kuske RP, et al. Locoregional recurrence of breast cancer: A retrospective comparison of irradiation alone versus irradiation and systemic therapy. Am J Clin Oncol 1992;15:93–101.

56. Beck TM, Hart NE, Woodard DA, et al. Local or regionally recurrent carcinoma of the breast: Results of therapy in 121 patients. J Clin Oncol 1983;1:400–405.

57. Kamby C, Sengelov L. Survival and pattern of failure following locoregional recurrence of breast cancer. Clin Oncol (R Coll Radiol) 1999;11:156–163.

58. Waeber M, Castiglione-Gertsch M, Dietrich D, et al. Adjuvant therapy after excision and radiation of isolated postmastectomy locoregional breast cancer recurrence: Definitive results of a phase III randomized trial (SAKK 23/82) comparing tamoxifen with observation. Ann Oncol 2003;14:1215–1221.

59. Rivera E, Holmes FA, Buzdar AU, et al. Fluorouracil, doxorubicin, and cyclophosphamide followed by tamoxifen as adjuvant treatment for patients with stage IV breast cancer with no evidence of disease. Breast J 2002;8:2–9.

60. Tomiak E, Piccart M, Mignolet F, et al. Characterisation of complete responders to combination chemotherapy for advanced breast cancer: A retrospective EORTC Breast Group study. Eur J Cancer 1996;32A:1876–1887.

61. Greenberg PA, Hortobagyi GN, Smith TL, et al. Long-term follow-up of patients with complete remission following combination chemotherapy for metastatic breast cancer. J Clin Oncol 1996;14:2197–2205.

62. Holmes FA, Buzdar AU, Kau SW, et al. Combined-modality approach for patients with isolated recurrences of breast cancer (IV-NED): The M.D. Anderson experience. Breast Dis 1994;7:7–20.

63. Nieto Y, Nawaz S, Jones RB, et al. Prognostic model for relapse after high-dose chemotherapy with autologous stem-cell transplantation for stage IV oligometastatic breast cancer. J Clin Oncol 2002;20:707–718.

64. Friedel G, Pastorino U, Ginsberg RJ, et al. Results of lung metastasectomy from breast cancer: Prognostic criteria on the basis of 467 cases from the International Registry of Lung Metastases. Eur J Cardiothorac Surg 2002;22:335–344.

XI

Management of Pain for Metastatic Breast Cancer and Management of the Terminal Patient

Joseph Lowy

BACKGROUND

About 40,000 deaths resulted from breast cancer in the United States in 2004. Most of these patients and many of the patients who survive breast cancer experience considerable suffering. The suffering has physical, psychological (emotional), social (practical), and spiritual components. There is ample evidence that these aspects of suffering are not being addressed adequately by the medical profession.[1] *Palliative care* is the total care of patients with progressive advanced disease. It is concerned with all of the aspects of suffering and focuses on both the quality of life of the patient and the support of the family and those close to the patient. Terminal care is instituted when it is extremely likely that death will occur within a short period of time.

In his book *The Nature of Suffering and the Goals of Medicine*, Eric Cassell discusses a case of a patient with breast cancer:

The obligation of physicians to relieve human suffering stretches back into antiquity. Despite this fact, little attention is explicitly given to the problem of suffering in medical education, research, or practice. . . . Even in the best settings and with the best physicians, it is not uncommon for suffering to occur not only during the course of a disease but as a result of its treatment.

A 35 year old sculptor with cancer of the breast that had spread widely was treated by competent physicians employing advanced knowledge and technology and acting out of kindness and true concern. At every stage, the treatment as well as disease was a source of suffering to her. She was frightened and uncertain about her future but could get little information from her physicians, and what she was told was not always the truth. She was unaware, for example, that the radiation therapy to the breast (in lieu of a mastectomy) could be so disfiguring. After her ovaries were removed and a regimen of medications that were masculinizing, she became obese, grew facial and body hair of a male type, and her libido disappeared. When tumor invaded the nerves near her shoulder, she lost strength in the hand she used in sculpting and became profoundly depressed. At one time she had watery diarrhea that would occur unexpectedly and often cause incontinence, sometimes when visitors were present. She could not get her physicians to give her medication to stop the diarrhea because they were afraid of possible disease-related side effects (although she was not told the reason). She had a pathological fracture of her thigh resulting from an area of cancer in the bone. Treatment was delayed while her physicians openly disagreed about pinning her hip.

She had come to believe that it was her desire to live that would end each remission, because every time her cancer would respond to treatment and her hope rekindle, a new manifestation would appear. Thus, when a new course of chemotherapy was started, she was torn between her desire to live and her fear that allowing hope to emerge again would merely expose her to misery if the treatment failed. . . . In common with most patients with similar illnesses, she was constantly tortured by fears of what tomorrow would bring. Each tomorrow was seen as worse than today, as heralding increased sickness, pain or disability—never as the beginning of better times.

This young woman had severe pain and other physical symptoms that caused her suffering. She also suffered from threats that were social and others that were personal and private. She suffered from the effects of the disease and its treatment on her appearance and her abilities. She also suffered unremittingly from her perception of a future.[2]

Good palliative care addresses suffering in all of its forms and throughout the trajectory of illness. It should not be reserved for the terminal phase but rather should be increased proportionately as curative or life-prolonging therapy is reduced. Physicians are understandably focused on the cure and treatment of the disease of cancer. Disproportionate emphasis on treating the disease may undermine the goals of care for a patient with advanced breast cancer: the relief of suffering, optimization of quality of life until death, and focus on comfort in the terminal phase.

How significant a problem is pain in breast cancer?

Most patients with advanced cancer have significant pain. Portenoy and colleagues reported that pain was present in 63% of 246 patients undergoing active treatment for breast, prostate, colon and ovarian cancer. The pain was rated moderate to severe in 43% of patients.[3] Despite the high incidence of pain in patients with cancer, this debilitating symptom remains underassessed and undertreated. Barriers to effective pain treatment, especially the use of opioids, must be overcome because up to 90% of cancer-related pain can be controlled with analgesic drug therapy in conjunction with nonpharmacologic methods.[4] Successful treatment of pain is dependent on thorough assessment, judicious investigation, comprehensive management, and frequent reassessment. Diagnosis-specific treatment may be instituted if a specific etiology for the pain is established; however, nonspecific treatment of pain should take place before or without a specific diagnosis, if necessary.

How should pain be assessed?

A complete history of the pain includes location, duration, quality, intensity, and response to treatment. Pain should be rated using a verbal (0 to 10) or written pain scale.

The assessment strategy should be appropriate for the patient's functional status and expected survival. CT and MRI are time-consuming and inappropriate for a bedridden patient with days to live. However, a sophisticated diagnostic workup is indicated if the patient wants it and the expected information obtained is likely to change the treatment approach.

Pain can be both acute and chronic. This categorization of pain is of more than academic interest. Although acute pain is usually self-limited and responds to medical treatment, chronic pain (defined as lasting more than 3 months) is much more than a temporal extension of acute pain. Changes occur in both central neural processing and peripheral nerves. The results may include a decrease in objective signs of pain as well as development of such generalized symptoms as anorexia, malaise, sleep disturbance, and irritability. Good management of these patients demands attention to the effects that chronic pain has on the person suffering from it[5] (Table 32–19).

Table 32–19 Common Causes of Pain in Breast Cancer

Acute Pain Syndromes
Acute pain associated with diagnostic and therapeutic interventions
Acute pain due to procedures and postmastectomy pain
Acute Pain Associated with Anti-Cancer Therapies
Pain associated with chemotherapy and infusion
Pain associated with chemotherapy toxicity
Mucositis and painful peripheral neuropathy
Pain associated with hormonal therapy (hormone-induced pain flare in breast cancer)
Pain associated with radiotherapy
Early-onset brachial plexopathy
Chronic Pain Syndromes
Bone Pain Syndromes
Pain syndrome of hip, base of skull, and multiple bony metastases
Back pain and epidural spinal cord compression
Visceral Pain Syndromes
Pleural, pericardial
Liver
Bowel obstruction
Peritoneum
Pain Syndromes Associated with Tumor Infiltration of Nerves
Tumor infiltration of peripheral nerves
Tumor infiltration of brachial plexus
Tumor infiltration of meninges
Chronic Pain Syndromes Associated with Cancer Therapy
Postchemotherapy pain syndromes
Chronic painful peripheral neuropathy
Avascular necrosis or osteoporosis
Postsurgical pain syndromes including postmastectomy pain syndrome
Phantom breast pain
Chronic postradiation pain syndrome
Radiation-induced brachial plexopathy

Table 32–20   Physiologic Types of Breast Cancer Pain

Type of Pain	Example	Character	Treatment
Somatic (nociceptive)	Bone metastasis	Dull, aching, focal	Nonopioid analgesics, opioids
Visceral	Intestinal obstruction	Dull, aching, throbbing	Nonopioid analgesics, opioids
Neuropathic	Brachial plexopathy	Burning, shooting, sharp	Nonopioid analgesics, opioids, adjuvants

From a physiologic standpoint, there are three types of pain: somatic (nociceptive), visceral, and neuropathic. Somatic pain develops once nociceptors in tissues are activated. Visceral pain results from involvement by tumor of thoracic and abdominal viscera and is not as well localized as somatic pain. Neuropathic pain results from injury to the peripheral or central nervous system and most commonly occurs as a result of tumor compression or infiltration of peripheral nerves, nerve roots, or the spinal cord. Surgical trauma and radiation-induced injury to nerves may also result in this type of pain. Neuropathic pain is often described as severe. Although there may be a constant dull ache or pressure, superimposed burning or shooting pains are often described (Table 32–20).

What is the approach to pain management in the patient with breast cancer?

The use of medications is predicated on the World Health Organization (WHO) analgesic ladder (Fig. 32–26). Mild to moderate pain may be treated with a nonopioid analgesic such as acetaminophen and nonsteroidal anti-inflammatory drugs (NSAIDs). Opioids, however, are the mainstay of cancer pain management and should be used for persistent or moderate to severe pain. Opioid treatment and titration should be initiated with immediate-release products, often combined with acetaminophen or aspirin (including codeine, hydrocodone, and oxycodone). Persistent or more severe pain warrants the use of higher doses of oxycodone or tramadol, morphine, hydromorphone, fentanyl, and methadone.

Patients with chronic or anticipated chronic pain should receive around-the-clock dosing with longer-acting or continuous medications such as sustained-release morphine, sustained-release oxycodone, transdermal fentanyl, or, when appropriate, continuous infusion through the intravenous or subcutaneous route.

Patients who receive an around-the-clock regimen should also have available to them a short-acting opioid given on an as-needed basis for breakthrough pain. When possible, the breakthrough drug is the short-acting form of the maintenance drug. Short-acting oral opioids may usually be given every hour, whereas parenteral forms can be offered up to every 15 to 30 minutes. The initial rescue dose is usually about 15% of the 24-hour baseline dose; however, doses must be individualized.

Drug selection and doses are dependent on such factors as pain intensity, prior opioid use and adverse effects, preferred route of administration, and coexisting disease. For example, buildup of the toxic metabolites of morphine in the setting of renal disease makes hydromorphone and fentanyl the preferred agents for maintenance therapy in this setting. Initial doses are selected, and doses are titrated until good analgesia

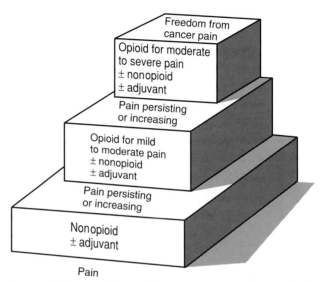

Figure 32–26 World Health Organization analgesic ladder. (From World Health Organization. Cancer Pain Relief, 2nd ed. Geneva, WHO, 1996.)

is reported or intolerable side effects occur. Dosing intervals may require adjustment. The total dose of opioid used over 24 hours is calculated, and the maintenance dose is changed accordingly so that patients require no more than several breakthrough doses daily.

Physicians should familiarize themselves with equianalgesic dosing guidelines and oral to parenteral relative potencies. Conversion of oral to parenteral doses and equianalgesic dosing for morphine and hydromorphone are illustrated in Figure 32–27.[6]

Transdermal fentanyl[7] is a popular alternative to oral and other parenteral opioids. However, familiarity of its pharmacokinetics is essential for its optimal use. It is recommended that patients be stabilized on an oral opioid regimen (or conversion from patient-controlled analgesia [PCA]) by calculating the 24-hour dose of the opioid used and converting this to the equianalgesic dose of fentanyl. For example, a 100-μg/hour fentanyl patch is about equianalgesic to 2 to 4 mg/hour of intravenous morphine. There is a delay of 8 to 12 hours in achieving effective analgesia the first time the patch is applied, so the prior form of analgesic should be continued for this period. Likewise, serum concentration falls slowly after the patch is removed. As a rule, dose changes should not be made more frequently than once every 72 hours, although some patients require a dosing interval of 48 hours. Given these limitations, transdermal fentanyl should be reserved for patients with stable pain, especially those unable to take oral medications. Short-acting rescue opioids must be available for breakthrough pain. Choices include oral short-acting opioids such

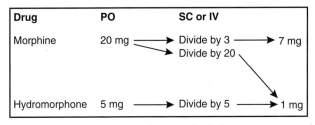

Drug	PO	SC or IV
Morphine	20 mg	Divide by 3 → 7 mg Divide by 20
Hydromorphone	5 mg	Divide by 5 → 1 mg

Figure 32–27 Conversion of oral opioid doses to parenteral doses. (Data from Pocket Guide to Hospice/Palliative Care Medicine. Glenview, IL, American Academy of Hospice and Palliative Medicine, 2003, p. 80.)

as morphine (pill or elixir) and oral transmucosal fentanyl citrate, which is absorbed across the buccal mucosa.

Opioid adverse effects are common. They are gastrointestinal (nausea, vomiting, constipation), autonomic (xerostomia, urinary retention, and postural hypotension), central nervous system (drowsiness, delirium, respiratory depression, and myoclonus), and cutaneous (pruritus, diaphoresis). The four approaches to these side effects are (1) dose reduction, (2) specific therapy, (3) opioid switch, and (4) change route of administration.[8] Constipation is the most common side effect of chronic opioid therapy. Patients should undergo routine prophylaxis with stool softeners and cathartics. Sedation may be counteracted with methylphenidate or dextroamphetamine. Small doses are initiated in the morning, usually with a second dose given at midday.

Which adjuvant analgesics are effective in cancer pain management?

Adjuvant analgesic drugs can be administered at any stage of the WHO ladder; however, severe pain warrants administration of a strong opioid immediately. Adjuvant analgesics may be used initially for mild pain or in addition to opioids for moderate to severe pain. Acetaminophen and NSAIDs are important first-line agents for mild to moderate pain control. The newer cyclo-oxygenase-2 (COX-2) NSAIDs are currently being studied, and there is some early evidence of their potential effectiveness in metastatic bone pain, as has been demonstrated with the older NSAIDs.[9,10] Unlike opioids, NSAIDs and acetaminophen have a ceiling effect to their efficacy, so that increasing doses beyond a certain level does not result in a greater therapeutic effect.

Corticosteroids may provide effective analgesia in such varied situations as metastatic bone pain, pain related to nerve compression, pain from epidural spinal cord compression, and painful liver metastases.

Adjuvant therapy can be particularly helpful in the treatment of neuropathic pain. The tricyclic antidepressants have been used in a variety of chronic neuropathic pain syndromes, including postherpetic neuralgia and painful diabetic neuropathy. There is a growing body of evidence supporting the use of anticonvulsant drugs for neuropathic pain. In particular, gabapentin has been shown to be effective as an adjuvant to opioid analgesia for neuropathic cancer pain.[11]

Other agents found to be effective as adjuvants include lidocaine and other antiarrythmic-anesthetic agents given systemically, such as clonidine, baclofen, and N-methyl-D-

aspartate (NMDA) antagonists. The latter group includes dextromethorphan and ketamine. The ketamine produces analgesia in doses much lower than those needed to produce anesthesia. Also, methadone has anti-NMDA receptor effects.

Bisphosphonate compounds should always be considered in the setting of bone metastases. Pamidronate, 60 to 90 mg intravenous infusion every 2 to 4 weeks, has been shown to decrease pain, slow the growth of tumor metastases, and prevent fractures.[12]

When are interventional strategies indicated for cancer pain?

Patients whose pain is not adequately controlled with systemic analgesics or in whom side effects of these medications are intolerable may be candidates for interventional anesthetic techniques including spinal anesthesia and peripheral neurolytic blockade. Opioids, local anesthetics, and clonidine may all be administered for spinal analgesia. The epidural dose of opioid required to manage pain is about 10% of the systemic dose. Subarachnoid administration of morphine doses are as low as 1% of the systemic dose. In cancer pain, spinal opioids are most effective for patients with deep, constant somatic pain.[13] Although effective, the use of spinal analgesia is invasive, highly technical, and costly because its delivery requires the use of indwelling catheters and pumps. This should be considered for use only in patients who have a prognosis of more than several months.

Neural blockade may be effective when pain is well localized. Local anesthetics can be injected in various locations, including the brachial plexus and pleural cavity. Newer techniques, such as radiofrequency ablation (RFA) therapy, are currently being studied for painful bone metastases[14] and painful soft tissue tumors. In extreme circumstances, neurosurgical intervention may be considered. Techniques available include intracranial and spinal ablative procedures.[15] The decision to employ any of these techniques is based on expected survival, pain location, and character and patient preferences.

Which nonpharmacologic methods of pain management are effective?

Good communication is the most important intervention for improved patient outcome. Patients must feel that they are being listened to. In addition to specific questions regarding pain assessment, they should be asked how else they may be suffering and what concerns they may have. To ensure true informed consent, the physician must discuss with the patient the important risks and benefits of, and alternatives to, all treatments (including chemotherapy) and procedures. The patients and caregivers should be educated about the high rate of effective pain control and the safety and effectiveness of opioids. Specialized cognitive-behavioral interventions may help patients develop skills to cope with pain and its secondary effects. These techniques include relaxation, imagery, hypnosis, reframing, distraction, structured support, and psychotherapy.[16] Such nonpharmacologic strategies should be used in conjunction with pharmacologic treatment. Cognitive-behavioral skills are more difficult to acquire once pain is severe or chronic. Physical methods such as massage,[17] ice, or heat may be used at any time. There is a growing body of literature supporting the use of music therapy as a means to reduce pain intensity and related distress associated with pain.[18] Other complementary therapies that have been demonstrated to be effective in cancer pain include acupuncture and transcutaneous electrical nerve stimulation (TENS). Pastoral and spiritual care, as well as group support, may be extremely effective complementary therapies and should be made available to all patients.

When is it appropriate to begin palliative and terminal care?

Palliative care is interdisciplinary and focuses on the management of physical, psychological, social, and spiritual issues. Terminal care begins when the patient is likely to die within days or weeks. Effective palliative care should be integrated into cancer care from the beginning, rather than reserved for the end of life. It is especially important that the oncologist inform patients whether the goal of treatment is cure or palliation. As with other cancers, patients with breast cancer overestimate the potential benefits of chemotherapy.[19] This misunderstanding of the value of chemotherapy may interfere significantly with appropriate decision making. A survey of medical oncologists revealed little hesitation in recommending second-line treatments for breast cancer despite their lack of enthusiasm for benefit. This is consistent with the fact that medical oncologists are more likely than nonmedical oncologists to continue aggressive treatments for potentially small benefits.[20] Chemotherapy is frequently given within weeks of death despite the fact that, through abundant clinical research, the oncologist has accurate data concerning survival in patients with terminal disease. The avoidance of ineffective chemotherapy and redefinition of goals of care from cure to quality of life require awareness of prognosis.

The physician's ability to predict terminally ill cancer patients' survival has been evaluated in several studies. Overall, estimates tend to be overly optimistic.[21,22] Multiple studies relate survival to performance status. The Karnofsky performance score (KPS) is the standard most often used. A KPS of less than 50% (patient requires considerable assistance and frequent medical care) suggests a life expectancy of fewer than 8 weeks.[23] This knowledge affords the treating physician the opportunity to help the patient modify goals of care to avoid futile attempts to prolong life with chemotherapy and focus on the alleviation of symptoms and distress and support for the patient and family. It is also a time to determine the patient's wishes with respect to advance directives and end-of-life care, if this has not yet been done.

Where do patients die, and when is referral to hospice appropriate?

When surveyed, 50% to 70% of cancer patients prefer to be cared for at home and to die at home, although as death approaches, some patients and relatives begin to express a preference for death in hospice.[24] In the United States, the Medicare hospice benefit was devised predominantly as home care for the terminally ill, with inpatient hospice available for respite care, when necessary. Despite the availability of this benefit and, more importantly, the palliative care administered through hospice, most cancer patients in the United States continue to die in hospitals or other long-term facilities. Between 1991 and 1996, only 20.7% of women older than 65 years dying of breast cancer were enrolled in hospice (although the ratio of hospice use increased over those years from 11.1% to 27.1%).[25]

What is expected during the terminal phase of a patient with breast cancer?

Common signs and symptoms in patients with advanced cancer include fatigue and generalized weakness, anorexia, pain, mental status changes, dyspnea, nausea, and vomiting. The proper management of these symptoms necessitates a thorough assessment and attention to physical and psychological factors. Cancer cachexia is a particularly troublesome symptom and, in breast cancer, has been shown to correlate with tumor bulk. Total parenteral nutrition does not improve cancer survival.[26] In the terminal breast cancer patient, the goals, risks, and benefits of artificial nutrition and hydration should be discussed with patient and family. Loss of appetite is natural and does not appear to contribute to patient suffering.

Most patients have their symptoms relieved by adhering to current palliative care guidelines for pain and other symptom control methods. Occasionally, refractory symptoms necessitate the use of induced sedation (also known as *palliative sedation* or *terminal sedation*). The three most common symptoms that result in the use of induced sedation are pain, agitation or delirium, and dyspnea. This extreme measure should be undertaken only for severe refractory symptoms in the setting of fully informed consent by the patient or health care proxy. Death is understood to be a possible side effect (double effect) because the primary goal is the relief of suffering.

When should advanced care planning take place?

All patients should be given the opportunity to express feelings about the type of care they would like to receive at the end of their lives. To do this properly, patients need to be informed of their status, prognosis, and range of available supportive measures. This information is often withheld or delayed for fear that the patient will lose hope. In general, however, patients want to know the truth about their diagnosis and prognosis. It has been shown that in the absence of prognostic information from their physicians, patients tend to overestimate their survival and express a preference for life-extending therapy. Patients who thought there was at least a 10% chance that they would not live for 6 months expressed a greater preference for comfort care.[27]

Physicians are responsible for initiating discussions with patients regarding advanced care planning as a matter of routine. The patients should assign a health care proxy or durable power of attorney for health care in case they lose capacity to make decisions. A living will or written advance directive is also advisable to help direct care. Goals of care must be established as the patient's status changes. Early in a patient's care, remission or cure may be the goal. With advanced disease progression, this goal may change to being home with family and ultimately to having a peaceful death.

REFERENCES

1. The SUPPORT Principal Investigators. A controlled trial to improve care for seriously ill hospitalized patients. JAMA 1995;274:1591–1598.
2. Cassell EJ. The Nature of Suffering and the Goals of Medicine. New York, Oxford University Press, 1991, pp 30–31.
3. Portenoy RK, Thaler HT, Kornblith AB, et al. The Memorial Symptom Assessment Scale: An instrument for the evaluation of symptom prevalence, characteristics and distress. Eur J Cancer 1994;30(a):1326–1336.
4. Jacox A, Carr DB, Payne R. New clinical-practice guidelines for the management of pain in patients with cancer. N Engl J Med 1994;330(9):651–655.
5. Payne R, Gonzales ER. Pathophysiology of pain in cancer and other terminal diseases. In Doyle D, Hanks G, Cherny N, Calman K (eds). Textbook of Palliative Medicine, 3rd ed. New York, Oxford University Press, 2004, pp 288–298.
6. Storey P, Knight CF, Schonwelter RX. Pocket Guide to Hospice/Palliative Medicine. Glenview, IL, American Academy of Hospice and Palliative Medicine, 2003, p 80.
7. Payne R, Chandler S, Einhaus M. Guidelines for the clinical use of transdermal fentanyl. Anti-Cancer Drugs 1995;6:50–53.
8. Hanks G, Cherny NI, Fallon M. Opioid analgesic therapy. In Doyle D, Hanks G, Cherny N, Calman K (eds). Textbook of Palliative Medicine, 3rd ed. New York, Oxford University Press, 2004, pp 316–341.
9. Sabino MA, Ghilardi JR, Jonger JL, et al. Simultaneous reduction in cancer pain, bone destruction and tumor growth by selective inhibition of cyclooxygenase-2. Cancer Res 2002;62(24):7343–7349.
10. Eisenberg E, Berkey CS, Carr DB, et al. Efficiency and safety of non-steroidal anti-inflammatory drugs for cancer pain: A meta-analysis. J Clin Oncol 1994;12:2756–2765.
11. Caraceni A, Zecca E, Martini C, et al. Gabapentin as an adjuvant to opioid analgesia for neuropathic cancer pain. J Pain Symptom Manage 1999;17:441–445.
12. Hortobagyi GN, Theriault RL, Porter L, et al. Efficacy of pamidronate in reducing skeletal complications in patients with breast cancer and lytic bone metastases. N Engl J Med 1996;335:1785–1781.
13. Swarm RA, Karanikolas M, Courius MJ. Anaesthetic techniques for pain control. In Doyle D, Hanks G, Cherny N, Calman K (eds). Textbook of Palliative Medicine, 3rd ed. New York, Oxford University Press, 2004, pp 378–396.
14. Dupuy DE, Safran H, Mayo-Smith WW, et al. Radiofrequency ablation of osseous metastatic disease. Radiology 1998;209:389.
15. Hassenbusch SJ, Cherney NI. Neurosurgical approaches in palliative medicine. In Doyle D, Hanks G, Cherny N, Calman K (eds). Textbook of Palliative Medicine, 3rd ed. New York, Oxford University Press, 2004, pp 396–404.
16. Syrjak KL, Roth-Roemer S. Nonpharmacologic management of pain. In Berger AM, Portnoy RK, Weissman DE (eds). Principles and Practice of Palliative Care and Supportive Oncology, 2nd ed. Philadelphia, Lippincott Williams & Wilkins, 2002, pp 98–115.
17. Weinrich SP, Weinrich MC. The effect of massage on pain in cancer patients. Appl Nurs Res 1990;3(4):140–145.
18. O'Callaghan C. Bringing music to life: Music therapy and palliative care experiences in a cancer hospital. J Palliat Care 2001;13(3):155–160.
19. Raudin PM, Siminoff IA, Harvey JA. Survey of breast cancer patients concerning their knowledge and expectations of adjuvant therapy. J Clin Oncol 1998;515:521.
20. Benner SE, Fetting JH, Brenner MH. A stopping rule for standard chemotherapy for metastatic breast cancer: Lessons from a survey of Maryland medical oncologists. Cancer Investigation 1994;12:451–455.
21. Parker EM. Accuracy of predictions of survival: Later stages of cancer. BMJ 1972;2:29–31.
22. Maltoni M, Nanni O, Derni S, et al. Clinical prediction of survival is more accurate than the Karnofsky performance status in estimating life span of terminally ill cancer patients. Eur J Cancer 1994;6:764–766.
23. Evans C, McCarthy M. Prognostic uncertainty in terminal care: Can the Karnofsky Index help? Lancet 1985;1:1204–1206.
24. Higginson IJ, Bruera E. Care of patients who are dying and their families. In Souhami RL, Tannock I, Hohenberger P, et al (eds). Oxford Textbook of Oncology, 2nd ed. New York, Oxford University Press, 2002, pp 1103–1120.
25. Lacken NA, Freeman JL. Hospice use by older women dying with breast cancer between 1991 and 1996. J Palliat Care 2003;19(1):49–53.
26. American College of Physicians. Parenteral nutrition in patients receiving cancer chemotherapy. Ann Intern Med 1989;110:734–736.
27. Weeks JC, Cook EF, O'Day SJ, et al. Relationship between cancer patients' predictions of survival and their treatment preferences. JAMA 1998;279:1709–1714.

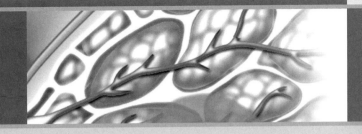

SECTION **VII**

SPECIAL ISSUES IN BREAST CANCER TREATMENT

CHAPTER 33

Surgical Treatment of Patients at High Risk of Breast Cancer

Freya R. Schnabel

DEFINITION OF RISK

All women have a baseline risk for developing breast cancer. There is no immunity from the disease. However, there are known factors that increase a woman's risk for developing breast cancer over the baseline level, and they have been discussed in detail elsewhere in this volume. Risk factors for breast cancer stem from a variety of sources, including family history, reproductive factors, and environmental exposures. The care of women at high risk for the development of breast cancer is challenging and requires careful risk assessment and discussion of strategies to manage that risk.

It is clear that most women overestimate their risk for developing breast cancer. Anxiety, apprehension, and misinformation may alter a woman's perception of her risk. Therefore, it is the job of the clinician to clarify an individual woman's risk for breast cancer as precisely as possible, communicate that risk clearly, and explore the various approaches to assessing breast cancer risk to arrive at a strategy that is appropriate in each case at that particular point in time.

How can we quantify breast cancer risk?

Quantifying breast cancer risk provides advantages for both the patient and the clinician. Many women possess multiple risk factors for breast cancer that interact and combine to produce the overall risk for that individual. Quantifying risk allows individuals to compare their risks with known benchmarks. As interventions to modify risk become available, risk–benefit analyses can help define levels of risk that justify particular interventions.

The initial medical history taken from a women being assessed for breast cancer risk should include detailed information concerning all established risk factors. Reproductive factors such as age at menarche, parity, age at first birth, and the use of hormone replacement therapy should be documented, along with breast-feeding history, because there may be some protective effect.[1] Prior history of benign breast disease should be explored, particularly a history of atypical hyperplasia or lobular carcinoma in situ. These conditions are associated with a significant increase in breast cancer risk[2] and should be carefully confirmed, including review of pathologic material if necessary. A history of other malignancies should be sought. A prior history of Hodgkin's disease treated with mantle irradiation (including the neck, supraclavicular, infraclavicular, axillary, mediastinal, and hilar regions in one field) confers an increased risk for breast cancer to the survivor.[3] Family history of breast cancer is an important aspect of breast cancer risk assessment. The patient should be queried carefully, and information regarding both maternal and paternal lines documented, including relatives' age at diagnosis, the presence of bilateral disease, and any incidence of ovarian cancer. In addition, some sense of the number of unaffected relatives may be helpful. A family history of breast cancer in a patient's single aunt is more significant than a history of breast cancer in one of six aunts. Similarly, a close relative who developed breast cancer at age 40 years has more significance than one who was diagnosed with the disease at age 90 years. A history of other cancers in the family, particularly ovarian cancer, is important. The combination of breast and ovarian cancer in a family is particularly predictive for an inherited susceptibility to these diseases. It may be helpful to draw out the pedigree to get a sense of the pattern of breast cancer in a family. This information should be updated periodically. Patients whose family history suggests an inherited genetic tendency for the disease should be referred for genetic counseling and testing because this will help clarify their risk more precisely.[4]

An individual woman may have multiple risk factors for breast cancer, and her overall risk will represent a complex combination of these factors. A variety of mathematical models have been used to quantify a woman's risk for breast cancer. The advantage of these models is the ability to use the risk estimate generated to facilitate communication with patients and present information in a manner that could be interpreted by the patient in a meaningful fashion.

The Gail model[5] is probably the most widely used model for estimating breast cancer risk. This model was used by the National Surgical Adjuvant Breast and Bowel Project (NSABP) as a criterion for inclusion in the P-1 trial, which established the use of tamoxifen as a chemopreventive agent for breast cancer.[6] The Gail model includes as variables the patient's present age, age at menarche, age at first live birth, number of first-degree relatives with breast cancer, and number of benign breast biopsies, with a factor included to weight for the presence of atypical hyperplasia. The Gail model produces both a lifetime estimate for the risk of developing breast cancer and an estimate of the risk of developing the disease in the next 5 years. When discussing the results of a Gail model assessment with a patient, the lifetime risk can be compared with the widely disseminated 1-in-9 population risk estimate. The estimate of 5-year risk is extremely helpful because most patients are able to better understand this shorter term possibility. The Gail model is limited by the exclusion of family history beyond first-degree relatives. Particularly when the disease is seen on the paternal side of the family, there may be no affected first-degree relatives, thus resulting in an underestimate of risk by the Gail model.

The Claus model[7] focuses on family history, includes both first- and second-degree relatives with the disease, and incorporates the age at which they developed breast cancer. The Claus model produces an estimate of the probability that a woman will develop breast cancer over a series of 10-year intervals. The Claus model provides a better estimate of breast cancer risk for women with extended family histories of the disease.

BRCAPRO[8] is a new model intended to help evaluate a woman whose family history suggests an inherited susceptibility to breast cancer. This model produces a probability estimate that the individual woman will be found to carry a mutation in the BRCA1 or BRCA2 genes. Use of this model may be helpful to women considering genetic testing. Other models using sophisticated mathematical methods such as bayesian networks and including a multitude of risk factors are being actively developed. These models may provide a better estimate for individuals whose background contains risk factors from multiple sources.

How is a patient with inherited susceptibility to breast cancer evaluated?

The first step in evaluating an individual with the inherited susceptibility to breast cancer is identifying that individual. There are a number of inherited syndromes that include an increased susceptibility to breast cancer; hence, a detailed family history of all neoplastic diseases should be documented in women being evaluated for breast cancer risk. The most common inherited syndromes involving an increased risk for breast cancer are listed in Table 33–1. Families in which there

is an inherited susceptibility to breast cancer are recognizable by the presence of multiple generations with affected individuals, with early age at onset, more bilateral cases than would be predicted, and an increased incidence of other cancers, particularly ovarian cancer. The frequency of BRCA1 and BRCA2 mutations is increased in the Ashkenazi (Eastern European) Jewish population as compared with other ethnic groups.[9] As a result, a lower threshold should be maintained for recommending genetic evaluation to women in this group.

When a pattern suggestive of inherited susceptibility to breast cancer is identified in a patient's family, genetic counseling should be offered.[10] The process of genetic counseling is particularly important to allow patients to understand the level of risk they face, the decisions they may face regarding the risk for other associated cancers (particularly ovarian cancer), and the psychosocial ramifications of a positive result. Genetic testing should always be performed in the context of pretest counseling to ensure that the patient understands the above concepts and is prepared to accept and act on the results. A patient who is not prepared to accept and act on the results of genetic testing should not be tested. At the present time, there is no indication to test minor children because the information obtained from the testing will not benefit the child in any meaningful way at the time the results are obtained.

A special consideration in genetic testing is a woman who is newly diagnosed with unilateral breast cancer and whose family history suggests she may be a mutation carrier. In this setting, genetic testing before definitive cancer surgery may be indicated. Women with BRCA1 and BRCA2 mutations are at higher risk for the development of contralateral disease, and consideration would therefore be given to the performance of bilateral mastectomy, for treatment and prophylaxis. Testing for BRCA1 and BRCA2, particularly in Ashkenazi Jewish individuals, can be done with a rapid turn-around and may affect the treatment of the newly diagnosed breast cancer in a woman whose family history suggests that she may be a mutation carrier.

Once the results of the genetic testing are available, a further discussion regarding the options for managing breast cancer risk should be conducted with the benefit of this updated information. In addition, the increased risk for other malignancies, particularly ovarian cancer, should be addressed. It is also critical that a patient understand that the failure to identify a mutation in the known genes does not imply a lower baseline risk and that there are almost certainly genes as yet undiscovered that play a role in a familial form of breast cancer.[11]

Table 33–1   Hereditary Breast Cancer Syndromes

Syndrome or Disease	Inheritance	Sites/Tumors	Genetic Mutation
Breast-ovarian syndrome	Autosomal dominant	Breast, ovarian, prostate	BRCA1
Male breast cancer	Autosomal dominant	Breast, ovarian, male breast, pancreatic	BRCA2
Li-Fraumeni	Autosomal dominant	Breast, soft tissue, bone, brain, hematologic, adrenal	p53
Ataxia-telangiectasia	Autosomal recessive	Lymphoma, breast, ovarian, leukemia, oral cavity, stomach, pancreas, bladder	chr 11q22
Cowden's (multiple hamartoma)	Autosomal dominant (variable expressivity)	Facial trichilemmomas, papillomatosis of lips and oral cavity, thyroid nodules, gastrointestinal polyps, breast fibroadenomas	chr 10q22-23

What is the significance of atypical hyperplasias in breast cancer risk?

In dealing with patients with a history of benign breast disease, it is important for the clinician to recognize that most subcategories of benign breast disease confer no clear increase in breast cancer risk. Commonly observed cyclic breast pain and symmetrical bilateral nodularity on clinical breast examination do not imply an increased risk for malignancy. Typical fibroadenomas of the breast not associated with proliferative benign disease in the adjacent breast tissue are generally thought to have no association with subsequent risk for breast cancer.[12] However, seminal work by Dupont and Page established the association between certain categories of benign breast disease and an increased risk for breast cancer.[2] Benign lesions containing atypical ductal or lobular hyperplasia as defined by histologic analysis are associated with a relative risk of 4 to 5 for the development of breast cancer. Lobular carcinoma in situ (LCIS), also called lobular neoplasia, has been associated with a 6- to 9-fold increase in breast cancer risk.[13] When atypical hyperplasia is combined with a family history of breast cancer, there is a synergistic effect, and there is an approximately 10-fold increase in breast cancer risk.[2] These data have been corroborated by other investigators, and it appears that when atypical hyperplasia is detected by cytologic analysis, the association with breast cancer risk is the same. Wrensch and colleagues analyzed nipple aspirate fluid for the presence of atypia and demonstrated a relative risk of breast cancer of approximately 5 in women with atypia diagnosed by this method.[14] Fabian and associates performed random four-quadrant fine-needle aspirations of the breast for cytology and also documented a 5 times relative risk for breast cancer in women with atypical cytology.[15] In this study, women with an elevated Gail model risk who had hyperplasia with atypia in their fine-needle aspiration samples had an observed breast cancer incidence of 15% at 3 years. Thus, it appears that cellular atypia in the breast is a meaningful marker for increased risk for breast cancer, particularly when combined with a background of elevated risk from other sources.

Ductal lavage represents an opportunity to evaluate for the presence of atypia in breast ductal cells and thereby help stratify an individual woman's risk for breast cancer.[16] This relatively new technique involves cannulating the orifices of nipple ducts that produce nipple aspirate fluid with a double-lumen microcatheter, then irrigating the ducts to collect ductal cells for cytologic analysis. Atypia can be identified by this minimally invasive office-based method, with that information incorporated into the patient's breast cancer risk assessment. For many women, this objective data point, which is cell based and obtained in real time, may be an important aid in quantifying their breast cancer risk as precisely as possible.[17] When added to a positive family history, these data may be the impetus needed for a patient to consider active risk modification interventions. It is particularly significant that in the NSABP P-1 trial, the subset of patients who benefited most from tamoxifen were those who entered the trial with a history of atypical hyperplasia.[5] Individual patients can be offered ductal lavage on a yearly basis and their results tracked over time. Ductal lavage is becoming increasingly integrated into the comprehensive assessment of high-risk women as a tool for improved breast cancer risk stratification.[18]

What are the management strategies available for high-risk women?

The product of a comprehensive breast cancer risk assessment should be some statistical quantification of a women's risk for developing breast cancer. This objective analysis may help to decrease the influence of anxiety and emotional factors on a woman's perception of her risk for breast cancer. However, it is important for the clinician to recognize that every woman will understand her risk for breast cancer in an individual manner, which may be governed by diverse issues such as the previous breast cancer experiences of friends and relatives and aspects of her own personality (e.g., qualities of being risk averse or risk taking in other aspects of her life). The discussion of breast cancer risk and risk management strategies is a dialogue, not a monologue, and the patient must participate. Breast cancer risk changes with time, and risk assessment should be periodically updated. There is no single strategy for managing breast cancer risk that is appropriate for every woman at any moment in time.

STRATEGIES

There are three major categories of strategies available to high-risk women: intensive surveillance, chemoprevention, and prophylactic mastectomy.

What is an appropriate surveillance strategy for high-risk patients?

Intensive surveillance should be offered to all high-risk patients, regardless of whether they undertake active risk reduction methods. The purpose of this strategy is to offer the patient every possible opportunity for the early detection of breast cancer. The benefits of such programs are not clearly established, although there are some data in the medical literature to support the effectiveness of this approach in early detection.[19]

Surveillance programs include the elements of breast self-examination, clinical breast examination, and breast imaging. Breast self-examination has become controversial, and the benefit to the patient has not been established in published studies. However, informing patients regarding the visible and obvious signs of breast disease (e.g. skin changes, change in breast contour) is good practice and prevents a patient from neglecting to bring an obvious sign to medical attention. Clinical breast examination is very important, particularly in young women, and we generally recommend clinical breast examinations every 6 months to our high-risk patients. Our approach to breast imaging for high-risk patients has evolved with time, as our understanding of the benefits and limitations of each technique has increased. Yearly mammography is recommended for all women after age 40 years. When caring for high-risk women, particularly those with a family history of breast cancer at a young age, the age at first mammography should be adjusted downward. Screening ultrasound may identify mammographically occult masses in high-risk women with dense breasts and has been increasingly integrated into clinical practice. There is also emerging evidence in the medical literature to support the use of screening breast magnetic resonance imaging (MRI) for high-risk women. Although it is expensive and inconvenient, it appears that a small percentage of lesions will be detected by this method without producing recognizable signs by other imaging modalities. A paper from investigators in the Netherlands reviewed their experience with screening MRI in women known to be *BRCA1* and *BRCA2* mutation carriers.[20] In their experience, MRI detected invasive cancer more accurately than mammography; however, mammography remained superior in the diagnosis of ductal carcinoma in situ (DCIS). Despite the expense and the potential for generating benign biopsies, it seems clear that MRI should be offered to very high-risk women for the increased ability to detect breast cancer using this method.

What is the role of chemoprevention for high-risk women?

The NSABP P-1 trial provided a landmark in the management of women at high risk for developing breast cancer.[5] This prospective randomized trial established the clear benefit of tamoxifen in reducing the risk for breast cancer development in high-risk women. Five years of treatment with tamoxifen provided an average of almost 50% reduction in breast cancer development (both DCIS and invasive disease) for women in the study. Of note, the subgroup that benefited most from tamoxifen was the group of women who entered the trial with atypical hyperplasia or LCIS. At this point, tamoxifen remains the one agent clearly demonstrated to reduce the risk for breast cancer in high-risk women.

The Study of Tamoxifen and Raloxifene (STAR) trial is a randomized prospective trial being conducted at present by the NSABP to evaluate the potential use of raloxifene in breast cancer risk reduction. Raloxifene, a selective estrogen receptor modulator like tamoxifen, is a Food and Drug Administration–approved treatment for osteoporosis. Early data support its efficacy in breast cancer risk reduction[21]; however, the results of the STAR trial will complete our understanding of the potential role of this agent in chemoprevention.

There is also ongoing research into other candidate agents for breast cancer chemoprevention. Aromatase inhibitors represent a promising category of agents under consideration for their effectiveness in breast cancer prevention.[22] A recent study associated aspirin use with a reduction in the incidence of breast cancer.[23] Cyclo-oxygenase-2 (COX-2) inhibitors are also being studied for their potential use in reducing breast cancer risk.[24] As our understanding of the basic science of breast cancer development advances, we may anticipate additional possible interventions to reduce the risk for breast cancer in high-risk women.

What is the role of prophylactic surgery in the management of high-risk women?

Certainly, bilateral prophylactic total mastectomy provides a high-risk patient with the greatest possible reduction in the risk for breast cancer development. Hartman and coworkers reviewed the experience of the Mayo Clinic in prophylactic

surgery for breast cancer prevention and demonstrated a 90% reduction in breast cancer risk with this technique as performed between 1963 and 1993.[25] Many procedures, however, were performed for indications that might not be considered appropriate at this time, and many of the operations were done as subcutaneous mastectomies, which differs from the current standard. We might expect a greater degree of risk reduction with total mastectomy as the approach because the technique of total mastectomy should provide greater extirpation of at-risk breast tissue.

In our time, bilateral prophylactic total mastectomy is almost exclusively the province of those women at highest risk for developing breast cancer: women who are known *BRCA1* and *BRCA2* carriers. In those cases, the exquisitely high level of risk would seem to justify this intervention. Patients undergoing this procedure should also be offered the option of immediate breast reconstruction.

What modifiable risk factors should be considered in high-risk patients?

Some risk factors for breast cancer are clearly beyond a woman's control—for example, age at menarche and menopause and family history of the disease. However, there are other potential risk factors that are subject to modification by an at-risk woman. These include obesity, diet and exercise, smoking, and alcohol consumption.[26] These lifestyle factors may represent relatively small risks, but positive interventions may provide an individual with health benefits beyond any potential impact on breast cancer risk. Avoidance of risk-taking behaviors is another potential advantage to high-risk patients. The Women's Health Initiative provided clarification of the increased risk for breast cancer associated with combined estrogen-progestin hormone replacement therapy given to postmenopausal women.[27] Although hormone replacement therapy affords symptomatic relief for women suffering from significant menopausal symptoms, it also increases the risk for breast cancer and appears to increase the risk of some types of cardiovascular disease and should thus be viewed as a short-term strategy. For women at high risk for developing breast cancer, any intervention that will increase that risk further should be viewed with caution.

What is an appropriate surveillance strategy for associated ovarian cancer risk?

Women at high risk for breast cancer on the basis of putative or documented inherited genetic syndromes are also at risk for a variety of other malignancies, and they should be appropriately informed and screened. Women at high risk for breast cancer because of inherited mutations in *BRCA1* and *BRCA2* are also at increased risk for the development of ovarian cancer.[28] The estimated cumulative risk for developing ovarian cancer in a woman with a *BRCA1* mutation is 30% by age 60 years. The management of increased risk for ovarian cancer differs greatly from our approach to the management of women at high risk for breast cancer. At present, there is no effective way to diagnose ovarian cancer at an early enough stage that survival from the disease is increased. Neither screening ultrasound nor CA-125 testing has been shown to reduce the mortality from ovarian cancer. Oral contraceptives afford some risk reduction and may provide an appealing option for younger women at risk for ovarian cancer.[29] However, there is some evidence that women who take oral contraceptives for long periods of time beginning at a young age may have an increased risk for breast cancer.[30] Women for whom fertility is not a concern most frequently opt for prophylactic bilateral oophorectomy, which may be performed laparoscopically. This procedure affords the patient dramatic risk reduction, but a small risk for primary peritoneal cancer remains.

REFERENCES

1. Newcomb PA, Storer BE, Longnecker MP, et al. Lactation and a reduced risk of premenopausal breast cancer. N Engl J Med 1994;330:81.
2. Dupont WD, Page DL. Risk factors for breast cancer in women with proliferative breast disease. N Engl J Med 1985;312:146–151.
3. Bhatia S, Robison LL, Oberlin O, et al. Breast cancer and other second neoplasms after childhood Hodgkin's disease. N Engl J Med 1996;334:745–751.
4. Newman B, Mu H, Butler LM, et al. Frequency of breast cancer attributable to BRCA1 in a population-based series of American women. JAMA 1998;279:915–921.
5. Costantino JP, Gail MH, Pee D, et al. Validation studies for models projecting the risk of invasive and total breast cancer incidence. J Natl Cancer Inst 1999;91:1541–1548.
6. Fisher B, Costantino JP, Wickerham DL, et al. Tamoxifen for prevention of breast cancer: Report of the National Surgical Adjuvant Breast and Bowel Project P-1 study. J Natl Cancer Inst 1998;90:1371–1388.
7. Claus EB, Risch N, Thompson WD. Autosomal dominant inheritance of early-onset breast cancer: Implications for risk prediction. Cancer 1994;73:643–651.
8. Euhus DM. Understanding mathematical models for breast cancer risk assessment and counseling. Breast J 2201;7:224–232.
9. Struewing JP, Hartge P, Wacholder S, et al. The risk of cancer associated with specific mutations of BRCA1 and BRCA2 among Ashkenazi Jews. N Engl J Med 1997;336:1401–1408.
10. Statement of the American Society of Human Genetics on genetic testing for breast and ovarian cancer predisposition. Am J Hum Genet 1994;55:i–iv.
11. Weber BL, Nathanson KL. Low penetrance genes associated with increased risk for breast cancer. Eur J Cancer 2000;36:1193–1199.
12. Dupont WD, Page DL, Parl FF, et al. Long-term risk of breast cancer in women with fibroadenoma. N Engl J Med 1994;331:10–15.
13. Page DL, Kidd TE Jr, Dupont WD, et al. Lobular neoplasia of the breast: Higher risk for subsequent invasive cancer predicted by more extensive disease. Hum Pathol 1991;22:1232.
14. Wrensch MR, Petrakis NL, King EB, et al. Breast cancer incidence in women with abnormal cytology in nipple aspirates of breast fluid. Am J Epidemiol 1992;135:130–141.
15. Fabian CJ, Kimler BF, Zalles CM, et al. Short-term breast cancer prediction by random periareolar fine-needle aspiration cytology and the Gail risk model. J Natl Cancer Inst 2000;92:1217–1227.
16. Dooley WC, Ljung B-M, Veronesi U, et al. Ductal lavage for detection of cellular atypia in women at high risk for breast cancer. J Natl Cancer Inst 2001;93:1624–1632.
17. Vogel VG. Atypia in the assessment of breast cancer risk: Implications for management. Diag Cytopathol 2004;30:151–157.
18. Hollingsworth AB, Singeltary SE, Morrow M, et al. Current comprehensive assessment and management of women at increased risk for breast cancer. Am J Surg 2004;187:349–362.
19. Mitra N, Schnabel FR, Neugut AI, Heitjan DF. Estimating the effect of an intensive surveillance program on stage of breast carcinoma at diagnosis: A propensity score analysis. Cancer 2001;91:1709–1715.
20. Kriege M, Brekelmans CTM, Boetes C, et al. Efficacy of MRI and mammography for breast cancer screening in women with a familial or genetic predisposition. N Engl J Med 2004;351:427–437.
21. Cummings SR, Eckert S, Krueger KA, et al. The effect of raloxifene on risk of breast cancer in postmenopausal women. Results from the MORE randomized trial. JAMA 1999;281:2189–2197.
22. Gross PE. Breast cancer prevention-clinical trials strategies involving aromatase inhibitors. J Steroid Biochem Mole Biol 2003;86:487–493.
23. Terry MB, Gammon MD, Zhang FF. Association of frequency and duration of aspirin use and hormone receptor status with breast cancer risk. JAMA 2004;291:2433–2440.
24. Davies GLS. Cyclooxygenase-2 and chemoprevention of breast cancer. J Steroid Biochem Mole Biol 2003;86:495–499.
25. Hartmann LC, Schaid DJ, Woods JE. Efficacy of bilateral prophylactic mastectomy in women with a family history of breast cancer. N Engl J Med 1999;340:77–85.
26. Lash TL, Aschengrau A. Active and passive cigarette smoking and the occurrence of breast cancer. Am J Epidemiol 1999;149:5–12.
27. Chlebowski RT, Hendrix SL, Langer RD, et al. Influence of estrogen plus progestin on breast cancer and mammography in healthy postmenopausal women. JAMA 2003;289:3243–3253.
28. Easton D, Ford D, Bishop DT, and the Breast Cancer Linkage Consortium. Cancer incidence in BRCA1 carriers. Am J Hum Genet 1995;56:265–271.
29. Narod SA, Risch H, Moslehi R, et al. Oral contraceptives and the risk of hereditary ovarian cancer. N Engl J Med 1998;339:424–428.
30. Brinton LA, Daling JR, Liff JM, et al. Oral contraceptives and breast cancer risk among younger women. J Natl Cancer Inst 1995;87:827–835.

CHAPTER 34

Treatment of Unusual Malignant Neoplasias and Clinical Presentations

Alison Estabrook and Gladys Giron

Breast cancer does not always present clinically as a palpable mass or thickening in the breast tissue. It may mimic an infection, as in inflammatory breast cancer, or present as an irritation of the nipple (Paget's disease). It may present as an axillary mass. Some breast cancers are partially cystic (intracystic papillary carcinoma) and require careful clinical examination after aspiration. The breast can also develop sarcomas or lymphomas and can be the site of metastatic carcinomas. This chapter describes these unusual presentations and uncommon sarcomas and primary lymphomas.

PAGET'S DISEASE

What is Paget's disease?

It was not until after his retirement from the practice of surgery that Sir James Paget first reported 15 cases of chronic nipple ulceration in 1874. He described "a florid intensely red raw surface . . . like the surface of very acute diffuse eczema."[1] He proposed that chronic irritation was the cause of the malignancies diagnosed in these women within 2 years of initial presentation.[2] This rare condition of the nipple–areolar complex was later given the eponym of *Paget's disease*. It is reported in most series to occur in 1% to 3% of all breast malignancies. The classic histologic finding is that of Paget's cells within the epidermis of the nipple and areola. The origin of these cells is controversial and has spawned two theories of histogenesis. The first is the epidermotropic theory, in which malignant cells in the terminal ducts migrate to the nipple.[3] The second is the transformation theory, in which epidermal cells of the nipple transform into Paget's cells. This latter theory assumes that Paget's cells are independent of the carcinomas found within the mammary gland in most cases.[4] Immunohistochemical studies favor the epidermotropic theory, which is in keeping with the observation that essentially all patients are found to have concomitant malignancies of ductal origin.[3,5,6]

How does Paget's disease present clinically?

Patients typically present with an erythematous, scaly or weeping eczematous lesion of the nipple (Figs. 34–1 and 34–2). This may be associated with bleeding. In later stages, there may be progression to erosion and ulceration with eventual effacement of the nipple–areolar complex. Subjectively, patients notice a change in sensation over the area such as burning and itching. Paget's disease involves the nipple first, before progressing to the areola. Sole involvement of the areola is not characteristic. The differential diagnosis includes inflammatory and malignant processes: eczema, psoriasis, other dermatologic conditions; florid papillomatosis; Bowen's disease; and amelanotic melanoma of the nipple.[7,8] A delay in diagnosis often results because patients are initially treated with topical steroids for variable periods. When eczematoid changes of the nipple do not respond to such treatment promptly, Paget's disease must be excluded.

The diagnosis may be made with a punch biopsy of a representative area performed in an office setting but may require a wedge biopsy. Some authors report cytologic analysis of smears of the weeping fluid or blood, but this is not always diagnostic.[9] Along with diagnosing the nipple-areolar lesion, attention must be paid to the remaining breast. Studies of mastectomy specimens have demonstrated that nearly 100% of patients with Paget's disease do have an underlying malignancy.[10–12] Less than half of these are palpable masses. The most common location for these carcinomas is central, but they have been reported in all quadrants. About 40% to 50% of patients with Paget's disease have no clinically detectable mammary mass.[13] Most palpable disease is invasive carcinoma, whereas most undetectable disease is carcinoma in situ. Focal changes in the nipple–areolar complex, such as thickening or a retroareolar mass, may be detected on mammography, but typically this modality is most helpful in identifying concomitant tumors.[14] Ultrasonography offers no further diagnostic advantage.[15]

What are the histologic features of Paget's disease?

The characteristic Paget's cells are identified in the keratinizing epithelium of the nipple epidermis (Fig. 34–3). Paget's cells are large round cells with abundant pale or clear cytoplasm, pleomorphic nuclei, and large nucleoli. They occur singly in the superficial epidermal layers and may form clusters in the basal layers.[7] Associated invasive carcinoma is overwhelmingly of ductal origin. Accompanying intraductal carcinoma is characterized by comedo or solid growth patterns. Because comedocarcinoma is often associated with calcifications, this may be detected mammographically.[7]

Histochemical characteristics suggesting a mammary origin for these cells include the distribution of carcinoembryonic antigen, cytokeratins, estrogen receptors, and *HER-2/neu* receptors.[7]

How has the treatment of Paget's disease of the breast evolved?

Traditionally, the treatment of Paget's disease has been mastectomy. In patients undergoing mastectomy for Paget's disease with an associated invasive carcinoma, postoperative prognosis and survival are directly related to the stage of the carcinoma. When associated with intraductal carcinoma, the 10-year survival rate after mastectomy has been reported as 100%.[16]

For patients with Paget's disease and extensive underlying carcinoma, total mastectomy with operative assessment of the axilla remains the standard approach. The axilla may be addressed with a sentinel lymph node biopsy followed by

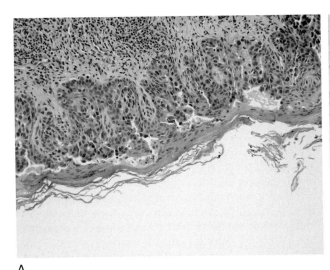

Figure 34–1 Patient with biopsy-proven Paget's disease of the nipple, refusing standard treatment.

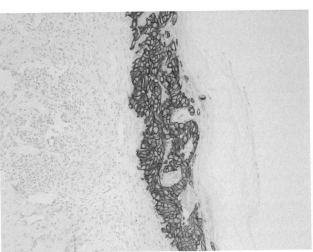

Figure 34–2 Same patient as in Figure 34–2 about 6 months later, with visible progression of disease.

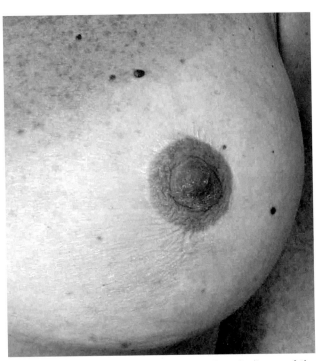

A

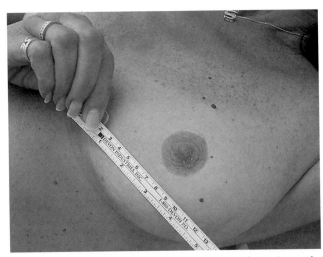

B

Figure 34–3 Paget's disease. *A*, H&E stain. *B*, E-cadherin stain.

Table 34–1   Results of Breast-Conserving Surgery in Paget's Disease

Study	Treatment Modality	No. of Patients	Follow-up	Local Recurrence	Mortality
Paone & Baker (1981)[18]	WLE	6	5–10 yr	0	0
Lagios et al. (1989)[19]	WLE	5	50 mo	1 (20%)	0
Fourquet et al. (1987)[20]	RT RT + WLE	17 3	90 mo	3 (15%)	0
Stockdale et al. (1989)[21]	RT	19	63 mo	3 (15.8%)	1 (5.3%)
Bulens et al. (1990)[22]	RT	13	52 mo	0	0
el Sharkawi et al. (1992)[23]	RT	3	60 mo	0	0
Dixon et al. (1991)[11]	WLE	10	56 mo	4 (40%)	0
Pierce et al. (1997)[4]	RT RT + WLE	22 6	62 mo	3 (10%)	0
Bijker et al. (2001)[24]	RT + WLE	61	76.8 mo	4 (6.5%)	1 (1.6%)
Marshall et al. (2003)[17]	RT RT + WLE RT+ PE	2 25 9	113 mo	4 (11%)	2 (5.5%)

*This is the 10- to 15-year update for Pierce et al. (1997).
RT, radiation therapy; PE, partial excision; WLE, wide local excision.

axillary node dissection for positive metastatic lymph node involvement. Increasingly, patients are presenting with early-stage breast cancers and cancers that are nonpalpable and only detected radiographically. This has led to the acceptance of breast-conserving surgery for both invasive and in situ breast cancer. The use of conservation is being explored in appropriate cases of Paget's disease.

Breast conservation approaches in the management of Paget's disease include excision of the nipple–areolar complex with central segmentectomy, with or without radiation therapy. Table 34–1 summarizes current available reports of breast conservation approaches to Paget's disease.[4,11,17–24] Although numbers are small, the observed local recurrence rates are lower in more recent series, and mortality remains low.

Is breast-conserving treatment appropriate for Paget's disease?

The application of breast-conserving surgery for Paget's disease is similar to that for patients without this special clinical presentation. One obvious exception is the almost universal need for excision of the nipple–areolar complex, with its cosmetic implications. The foremost surgical goal is that of achieving negative margins. In most cases, an elliptic incision encompassing the entire nipple–areolar complex is necessary. A central cone of tissue is dissected out to a depth of at least 2 cm, or down to the chest wall. All margins must be inked and histologically evaluated. Emphasis again is placed on preoperative assessment for a concomitant breast cancer that must be treated accordingly. Kothari and colleagues illustrated this point in a study of 70 women with Paget's disease treated with mastectomy.[25] Only one third presented with a palpable mass, and of these masses, only 25% were confined to the retroareolar region. They then extrapolated that cone excision of the nipple alone would have resulted in incomplete excision in 75% of the cases. Complete nipple resection with partial areolar excision may be possible in cases in which the areola is large and the extent of disease is small. The axilla should be evaluated surgically in patients with underlying carcinoma and extensive ductal carcinoma in situ (DCIS) with microinvasion. This may start with a sentinel lymph node biopsy.

Is radiation therapy required after breast-conserving therapy?

The decision to proceed with adjuvant radiation therapy depends on the extent of disease as determined by pathologic examination of the surgical specimen. Radiation therapists advocate postoperative mammography to rule out residual microcalcifications before proceeding with definitive radiation treatment, the standard in treatment of in situ and invasive breast cancer without Paget's disease.[17] In the subgroup of patients presenting with Paget's disease of the nipple and no identifiable mammary malignancy, treatment should proceed as though there were underlying DCIS—that is, breast-conserving surgery followed by radiation therapy.

Cosmetic reconstruction of the nipple–areolar complex is delayed until all treatment is completed. A plastic surgeon should then be consulted to review the options available. Reconstruction most often entails a local "skate" flap with skin graft and subsequent tattooing. Other options include tattooing alone and composite graft from the contralateral nipple.[26]

In our review of the treatment of Paget's disease of the breast at Columbia-Presbyterian Medical Center between 1990 and 1997, 24 patients underwent breast-conserving therapy and 21 patients underwent modified radical mastectomy. Most of the patients treated conservatively presented without an underlying mass and had unifocal areas of DCIS. They were treated with a wide local excision performed through an elliptic incision including the entire nipple–areolar complex. Histologically negative margins were obtained in all cases. At a mean follow-up of 82.5 months, three patients (16.67%) in the breast conservation group had developed a local recurrence within a median time of 24 months. At a mean follow-up of 90 months, three patients in the mastectomy group (14.3%) had recurrence within a median time of 23 months. The mortality rate was 16.67% for the conservation group and 22.2% for the mastectomy group. This long-term follow-up demonstrates that in carefully chosen cases, breast conservation with particular attention to negative margins results in local recurrence rates and overall survival rates equivalent to those of modified radical mastectomy.

UNUSUAL PRESENTATIONS

Inflammatory Carcinoma of the Breast

What is inflammatory carcinoma of the breast?

Haagensen described this presentation as "the most malignant type of breast cancer."[27] The term *inflammatory carcinoma of the breast* was coined by Lee and Tannenbaum in their historic paper in 1924.[28] This term describes a constellation of signs and symptoms without any specific pathologic or radiologic features. Thus, it is primarily a clinical diagnosis. In a description of cases of inflammatory breast cancer (IBC) at Barnes Hospital, Ellis and Teitelbaum suggested that demonstration of dermal lymphatic invasion by tumor cells was necessary for the diagnosis to be made.[29] In the latest revision of the American Joint Committee on Cancer (AJCC) Staging Manual, IBC is defined as a T4d tumor corresponding to at least stage III disease. A patient must meet the clinical criteria for inflammatory cancer and have biopsy-proven cancer within either the dermal lymphatics or the breast parenchyma.[30]

How does inflammatory carcinoma of the breast present clinically?

The frequency of IBC ranges from 1% to 10% in published series.[31] Mean age at diagnosis of women with IBC is comparable to that of women with noninflammatory breast cancer. However, women with IBC present at a younger age than those with locally advanced cancer without inflammatory features.[31] Patients often complain of pain or tenderness as a first symptom. The breast becomes enlarged, indurated, and erythematous.[27] Following presentation, the disease progresses rapidly. In his personal series, Haagensen noted an interval from onset of symptoms to diagnosis and treatment of 4 weeks, compared with 6.8 weeks for other types for breast cancer.[27]

In general, the clinical diagnosis of IBC is made when a patient presents with sudden enlargement of the breast, erythema, and edema of the skin overlying the breast and chest wall with advancing disease (Fig. 34–4). The term *peau d'orange* is used to describe the orange peel–like appearance of the breast with enlarged pores in mostly dependent areas. The skin color may range from pink in the early stages to deep

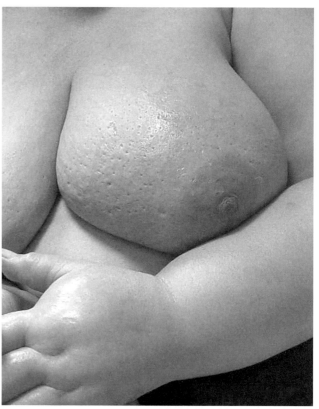

Figure 34–4 Patient presenting with inflammatory carcinoma and painful upper extremity lymphedema.

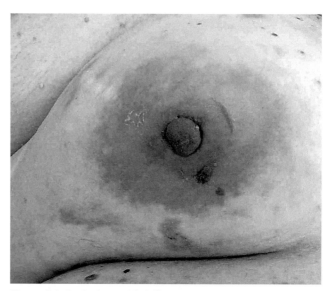

Figure 34–5 Patient with inflammatory carcinoma manifesting with pink to violaceous hue predominantly centrally in the breast.

red-purple (Fig. 34–5). Haagensen believed only redness affecting more than one third of the skin of the breast could be regarded as significant in making the diagnosis.[27] We now know that a certain extent of skin involvement is not needed in diagnosing inflammatory cancer. There may be nipple retraction, and the nipple epithelium may become reddened and crusted with disease progression.[27] Most patients present

Table 34–2 Signs and Symptoms of Inflammatory Cancer

Arm edema
Arm pain or tenderness
Breast enlargement
Breast pain or tenderness
Clinically positive axillary exam
Erythema (pink to purple)
Nipple retraction
Rapid progression of symptoms
Skin edema (peau d'orange)
Warmth of skin

Table 34–3 Differential Diagnosis of Inflammatory Cancer

Abscess
Mastitis
Duct ectasia
Locally advanced breast cancer with skin involvement
Necrotic tumors of the breast
Carcinoma en cuirasse
Leukemic involvement of the breast
Lymphosarcomatous involvement of the breast
Secondary inflammatory carcinoma of the breast

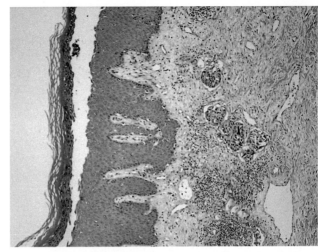

Figure 34–6 Inflammatory breast cancer. Tumoral emboli are seen in the dermal lymphatics.

with a clinically positive axilla. About 50% have an associated palpable mass, but one commonly encounters diffuse induration with no obvious localized tumor. Table 34–2 summarizes the possible signs and symptoms encountered.

The differential diagnoses are numerous and are listed in Table 34–3. The most common misdiagnosis is of an abscess or mastitis and often leads to a delay in proper treatment. The average age of a patient with IBC is 52 years, and breast infections in this age group are rare. Therefore, a short course of antibiotics may be initiated, but only with close follow-up as the workup continues. Of note, this section deals with primary inflammatory carcinoma, which should be differentiated from secondary inflammatory carcinoma of the breast. The latter is recurrent carcinoma with inflammatory features not observed with the initial malignancy.[31]

Workup includes a thorough physical examination. A punch biopsy of the skin performed in the office under local anesthesia may confirm the presence of tumor emboli within dermal lymphatics. If a tumor is palpable, a core biopsy in the office setting, preferably through the same punch biopsy incision, will yield valuable information to guide therapy. If a mass is not palpable, ultrasonography may reveal a discrete mass, and an image-guided core biopsy can then be obtained. Ultrasonography will also show marked skin thickening, thickened Cooper's ligaments, edema of the subcutaneous space, pectoral muscle invasion, or axillary involvement.[14,32] Although there are no pathognomic mammographic signs, ultrasonography can reveal skin thickening as well as thickening of the subcutaneous tissues, parenchyma, and retromammary fat.[14] In a recent series from University of Texas M. D. Anderson Cancer Center, the mammograms of 26 women with primary inflammatory breast cancer were reviewed.[33] A mammographic mass was seen in only 4 patients (15%), and malignant-appearing calcifications were seen in 6 patients (23%). The authors then concluded that common mammographic findings for this presentation of breast cancer

include skin thickening, diffusely increased density, trabecular thickening, and axillary adenopathy. Masses and malignant-appearing calcifications were uncommonly seen. Mammography will aid in ruling out contralateral disease. Magnetic resonance imaging (MRI) of the breast has not been shown to offer additional benefit.[34]

What are the pathologic features of inflammatory carcinoma of the breast?

It must be emphasized that the IBC does not constitute a separate histologic subtype of breast cancer. The clinically observed features thus described are the basis for the diagnosis and can be associated with any of the histologic subtypes of invasive breast cancer.

The gross pathologic features include large tumors or such diffuse involvement of the breast tissue that precise measurement is nearly impossible. Skin thickening is observed on specimen examination. In a 1978 review of IBC by Lucas and Perez-Mesa, the skin measurements averaged 2 to 8 mm, whereas normal breast skin thickness is 1 ± 0.2 mm.[35]

Dermal lymphatic invasion by tumor cells may be seen microscopically but is not necessary for diagnosis (Fig. 34–6). Often, distinguishing between vascular and lymphatic emboli is difficult.[31] There is no direct correlation between the extent of dermal emboli identified and clinical presentation or prognosis.[31] Absence of dermal emboli has been reported in 50% to 60% of patients presenting with IBC.[36,37] Most tumors in patients with IBC are estrogen and progesterone receptor negative with *HER-2/neu* amplification.[31,38]

What are the current treatment recommendations for inflammatory carcinoma of the breast?

In 1943, Haagensen and Stout reported on the Columbia Presbyterian Hospital experience with IBC between 1915 and 1942, concluding that most patients had died of their disease within a 2-year period.[27] Years later, Haagensen would comment that this collective experience and his own personal series taught him that IBC was incurable by radical mastectomy and that "limited irradiation and chemotherapy can be tried."[27] This is still an aggressive form of breast cancer, with about 40% of cases presenting with metastatic disease and a median disease-free survival of less than 2.5 years.[38] After it became clear that mechanical and localized treatment alone could not eradicate metastatic tumor cells, treatment strategies changed, with radiation and chemotherapy combined with surgery becoming standard for these patients. The use of primary systemic therapy was first instituted in the 1970s and was soon followed by the demonstration of high tumor regression rates in patients with inoperable locally advanced cancer or IBC.[39]

The current treatment approach involves establishment of a diagnosis and a thorough survey for metastatic disease, followed by the use of induction chemotherapy, surgery, and radiotherapy. The first report describing primary systemic therapy was published by the Milan group in 1978, wherein overall disease-free survival was 53% at 3 years, compared with 41% for a group treated with radiation alone.[40] An international expert panel recently described its collective experience in treating patients with locally advanced breast cancer, including IBC.[41] They concluded that primary systemic therapy is indeed the standard treatment. A period of in vivo testing of response should last a minimum of three or four cycles. Patients whose cancers do not respond or who experience cancer progression during that time may be offered second-line neoadjuvant chemotherapy or immediate modified radical mastectomy. The authors point out that it is more appropriate to administer maximum chemotherapy before surgery and that it is unknown whether additional postoperative chemotherapy improves or worsens results. The international group looks to the future results of the National Surgical Adjuvant Breast and Bowel Project Trial B-27 and the European Cooperative Trial in Operable Breast Cancer for answers.

What is the extent of surgery for inflammatory breast cancer?

The surgical treatment is a modified radical mastectomy, with operative treatment being offered in all but the most advanced of cases. A topic of great concern and controversy is that of pathologic axillary staging. Clearly, the pathologic extent of lymph node disease cannot be assessed without an axillary node dissection before instituting chemotherapy. Such information can be useful for planning postoperative radiation therapy, although it is less of an issue for IBC than for locally advanced breast cancer. The use of pretreatment sentinel lymph node biopsy in this group is not established because most cases present with rather advanced clinical nodal status. A pretreatment pathologic assessment can usually be made easily with a fine-needle aspiration (FNA) of palpable nodes demonstrating malignant cells. Although there are published reports of breast conservation after preoperative chemotherapy and radiation therapy, this approach cannot be currently recommended.[42-44] Reconstruction using autogenous tissue to either reconstruct the breast and missing skin or resurface the chest wall is often performed.

When is radiation appropriate in the treatment of inflammatory breast cancer?

Radiotherapy has been shown to provide improvement in locoregional disease control in patients with IBC.[45] Postoperative radiotherapy is an integral part of the standard treatment of IBC.[46,47] Preoperative radiation therapy combined with neoadjuvant chemotherapy has not been established as standard at this time.[41] Postoperative radiotherapy is administered to the chest wall and regional lymph node basins. Overall survival, relapse-free survival, and local recurrence rate were not affected by treatment sequence.[46]

Future developments to improve the survival in patients with IBC will likely result from intensive chemotherapy and autologous hematopoietic stem cell transplantation.[48-50] Additionally, future interventions may result from ongoing research on genetic determinants of IBC.[38]

Breast Cancer Presenting with Axillary Metastases and Occult Primary Site

One of the most difficult clinical scenarios facing the clinician caring for breast cancer patients is that of the patient presenting with disease metastatic to the axilla without an identifiable primary site. The management of such a patient includes a careful, exhaustive workup to identify the primary site and recognition of the importance of locoregional control to the patient's ultimate course.

How is a patient with isolated axillary metastasis evaluated?

The incidence of breast cancer presenting with axillary metastasis and an occult primary is reportedly between 0.3% and 5% of all breast malignancies.[51,52] In general, these patients present with one or more painless, enlarged axillary lymph nodes in the absence of a palpable breast mass. The differential diagnosis includes lymphoma, other primary site malignancies such as lung cancer, and an occult primary breast cancer. FNA biopsy can identify malignant cells and may rule out a lymphoma but may not rule out a nonbreast primary. A thorough history, physical examination, and chest radiograph are usually sufficient to exclude most other primary sources.[53] Further imaging studies and colonoscopy may be necessary. Contrast-enhanced computed tomography (CT) scans of the chest can be successful in identification of occult breast primaries.[54] A core biopsy or an open biopsy of the enlarged axillary lymph nodes is necessary to effectively rule out lymphoproliferative disorders, provide evidence of breast origin, and obtain hormone receptor status. FNA does not yield a sufficient amount of tissue.

A careful search for the primary lesion in the breast is required. Clearly, a carcinoma that has metastasized to the axilla without an obvious primary site may be aggressive in its biology despite a small size. Most of the classic studies of this clinical presentation were published before the current era of advanced breast imaging, and it behooves the clinician to take advantage of presently available techniques. Bilateral mammography, with particular attention to the ipsilateral breast, and comparison with previous studies is the initial step. A sensitivity of 29% and specificity of 73% for mammography have been reported in this setting.[52] Ultrasonography is the appropriate next step to try to identify masses not seen by mammography owing to tissue density. Kolb and associates reported that screening ultrasound found 17% more cancers than mammography alone in women with dense breast tissue.[55] The use of MRI in this setting was evaluated by Olson and colleagues.[56] Forty women with biopsy-proven axillary metastatic adenocarcinoma without evidence of a breast primary underwent breast MRI imaging with and without gadolinium enhancement. MRI identified the primary breast lesion in 70% of patients (28 of 40) and allowed breast conservation in 47% (16 of 40) in suitable cases. This modality has gained popularity and should be employed when radiologists experienced with the technique are part of the multidisciplinary team. Positron emission tomography (PET) scanning is another modality currently being used to help identify occult primaries.[57] Qualified radiologists should be available to interpret these results.

What is the appropriate management of the patient with an axillary metastasis and a clinically occult primary lesion?

If a primary lesion is identified, the management scheme reverts to the typical pattern for any patient of similar stage disease. Despite a comprehensive workup and exhaustive pathologic examination of a mastectomy specimen, the primary tumor may not be found in up to one third of cases.[58] Even if a primary lesion is not identified, the breast must be treated in some way. Failure to treat the ipsilateral breast leads to a rate of clinical tumor occurrence approaching 40% in some small series and 56% in a series reported from University of Texas M. D. Anderson Cancer Center.[53,56,59] In the past, modified radical mastectomy was the standard therapy. The tumor yield of pathologic analysis of these mastectomy specimens reported in the literature varies from 30% to 70%.[53,56,59] Axillary node dissection will reveal metastatic disease in lymph nodes. Most studies report a median of three to five involved lymph nodes found in removed axillary contents.[53,60] Patients with four or more involved axillary lymph nodes are usually treated with chest wall irradiation after mastectomy.

Another treatment option is complete axillary node dissection followed by whole-breast irradiation to control local disease although the primary is occult. The report from M. D. Anderson cited earlier documented a 12% ipsilateral tumor recurrence rate in 25 patients treated with breast irradiation and no difference in survival than in patients who had undergone mastectomy.[59] The experience of Fourquet and coworkers at the Institut Curie in Paris was similar.[53] Of 44 patients treated with whole-breast irradiation between 1960 and 1993, 9 had local disease recurrence. All of these were treated with mastectomy. A retrospective series of 35 patients from Memorial Sloan-Kettering Cancer Center also documented equivalent 5-year survival rates in patients treated with mastectomy and those treated with breast irradiation.[51] In summary, the available data suggest that primary breast irradiation following axillary dissection provides survival equivalent to that of modified radical mastectomy.[58]

Patients with occult primary breast cancer and positive axillary disease are candidates for adjuvant chemotherapy and

radiation.[58] Prognosis has been reported as equivalent to or even better than prognosis for same-stage nonoccult breast cancers.[58]

Radiation-Associated Breast Cancer

Who is at risk for radiation-associated breast cancer?

A variety of soft tissue neoplasms, including breast cancers, are known to be associated with radiation exposure. This has been demonstrated in women exposed through multiple chest radiographic examinations for follow-up of pulmonary tuberculosis, through spine films for scoliosis, or as treatment for acne, postpartum mastitis, neonatal thymic enlargement, and skin hemangiomas.[61] Perhaps the most well-known association between breast cancer risk and nontherapeutic radiation is that of the atomic bomb explosions at Hiroshima and Nagasaki. Long-term follow-up of survivors has shown a proportional increase in risk with increasing dose of radiation exposure. This is illustrated by the 25% lower risk observed in Nagasaki, where the exposure was lower, than in Hiroshima.[61]

The improved survival of patients diagnosed with and treated for Hodgkin's disease has been accompanied by the development of second neoplasms as a long-term consequence.[62-64] The cumulative risk for such a second malignancy is reportedly 10% to 20% at 20 years of follow-up.[62,64] The most common solid tumor encountered in women in this setting is breast cancer.[62-64] Affected patients likely received mantle irradiation. This is defined as including the neck, supraclavicular, infraclavicular, axillary, mediastinal, and hilar regions in one field[64] (Fig. 34-7). With mantle irradiation, the largest doses are delivered to the unshielded upper outer quadrants.[63]

Travis and colleagues recently published the results of a series of 3817 female survivors of Hodgkin's disease diagnosed at or younger than age 30 years.[63] There were 105 cases of breast cancer. A radiation dose of at least 4 Gy to the breast was associated with a 3.2-fold increase in risk compared with those receiving lower doses. If the dose was increased to greater than 40 Gy, the risk increased eightfold. The increased risk was observed for at least 25 years after treatment. The use of alkylating chemotherapy agents decreased the risk for breast cancer when delivered alone or in combination with radiation therapy. This reduction appears to be related to

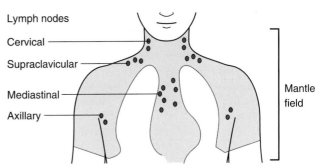

Figure 34-7 The field of radiation (including the mantle field) for Hodgkin's disease.

ovarian dysfunction and the resultant diminished hormonal stimulation of breast tissue. Van Leeuwen and colleagues similarly demonstrated a relationship between early menopause and a reduced risk for breast cancer in survivors of Hodgkin's disease.[65]

There is evidence that patients with known *BRCA1* or *BRCA2* mutations are at increased risk for developing late second primary breast cancers following breast conservation and radiation. Haffty and colleagues obtained complete sequencing results of *BRCA1* and *BRCA2* genes in 127 women with breast cancer diagnosed at or younger than age 42 years who had undergone breast-conserving surgery and postoperative radiation therapy.[66] They identified 22 women with mutations in *BRCA1* or *BRCA2*. At 12 years of follow-up, the rate of ipsilateral breast cancer (49%) and contralateral breast cancer (42%) was statistically significantly higher than in the remaining 105 women with sporadic breast cancer (21% rate of ipsilateral breast cancer and 9% rate of contralateral breast cancer). Haffty also concluded that there is no increased risk for radiation-induced contralateral breast cancer in *BRCA1* and *BRCA2* patients because the rate of contralateral breast cancer was the same in mutation carriers undergoing mastectomy as in those undergoing lumpectomy and radiation.

What are the clinical features of radiation-associated breast cancer?

The risk for radiation-associated breast cancer is inversely related to the age at the time of exposure. Yahalom and associates reported that the highest risk is observed in patients treated between the ages of 10 and 20 years and manifests later in life.[64] Carmichael and colleagues reported that the age-related excess risk does not become manifest until 10 years after the exposure.[61] These age-related effects support the theory that breast tissue is most susceptible to radiation damage during the early phases of breast development.[61,63]

Most of these breast cancers arise within the field of radiation therapy.[62] Although bilateral breast cancers have been reported, this is not the norm.[61,62] Bhatia and coworkers reported that of 17 women who underwent irradiation, 5 had bilateral breast cancer.[62] A report from Irvine Medical Center described a male with synchronous bilateral breast cancer following mantle irradiation for Hodgkin's disease and suggested that conditions associated with relative hyperestrogenism may further increase the risk in males.[67]

What are the pathologic features and treatment of radiation-associated breast cancer?

There are no pathognomonic features of radiation-induced breast cancer. Most series do not address the pathology of these tumors. In their series of 16 patients treated for Hodgkin's disease, Bhatia and colleagues found that the majority of tumors were infiltrating ductal and lobular in histology.[62] In their series of *BRCA1* and *BRCAA2* carriers with breast cancer after lumpectomy and radiation therapy, Haffty and associates reported that most of the tumors were infiltrating ductal cancers.[66]

Treatment is dependent on the characteristics of the breast cancer. Most clinicians would not advocate breast conservation because re-irradiation is often not possible. Deutsch and colleagues, however, reported the use of lumpectomy and breast irradiation for breast cancer in 12 women previously treated with radiation for Hodgkin's disease.[68] They reached the conclusion that such treatment is not contraindicated. There is presently no evidence that these tumors behave more aggressively or present at more advanced stages.

Certainly, long-term follow-up of patients who have been exposed to ionizing radiation is of utmost importance. Regular breast self-examinations and yearly clinical breast examinations are recommended. Although there is no consensus, current recommendations include baseline mammography 5 to 8 years after exposure and every 18 months thereafter.[61,63] Ultrasonography and MRI may play a role in surveillance of these patients. The use of chemopreventive agents (tamoxifen or other selective estrogen receptor modulators [SERMs]) or oophorectomy may be indicated, especially in those with known genetic susceptibility.[63,66] Bilateral mastectomy may also be offered in appropriate cases.

UNUSUAL NEOPLASMS

Intracystic Papillary Carcinoma

What is an intracystic papillary carcinoma?

In general, papillary breast lesions present a challenge to the clinician in terms of diagnosis, implications, and management. These lesions run the gamut from benign to invasive cancer. Solorzano and associates divide papillary carcinomas into noninvasive and invasive forms.[69] The noninvasive group is further subdivided into a diffuse form corresponding to the papillary variant of DCIS and a localized form corresponding to intracystic papillary carcinomas (IPC).[69,70] IPC can be found in isolation or with intraductal carcinoma (DCIS) or frankly invasive disease.[72]

How do intracystic papillary carcinomas present?

Most patients present with a palpable mass, although nipple discharge has been reported in 15% in one series.[69] The mean age of affected patients is reported to be in the sixth decade.[69,71,72] Most are therefore postmenopausal.[69,72] Imaging studies can provide some aid, although there are no pathognomonic findings. Mammography may show a cystic lesion with well-defined borders and an irregular contour, which may be obliterated in areas of invasion into surrounding breast tissue.[72–74] Sonography can demonstrate a well-defined cystic mass with a shaggy, irregular growth arising from the cyst wall.[73] Although rarely used, pneumocystography may differentiate an IPC from a simple cyst by outlining inner wall irregularities.[73,74]

The differential diagnosis includes benign cystic masses, carcinoma invading adjacent breast parenchyma containing cystic disease, or a high-grade solid carcinoma that has undergone central necrosis.[72] Benign cysts are common and are seen in perimenopausal women. Thus, when a cystic lesion is found in a postmenopausal woman who is not on hormone replacement therapy, suspicion for a malignancy is high.

The first step in diagnosing a cystic lesion is aspiration, because the fluid obtained may provide diagnostic clues. A cystic lesion is more likely to harbor a malignancy if frank blood or blood-tinged fluid is aspirated.[72,75] Markopoulos and colleagues caution, however, that blood does not definitively make a cancer diagnosis, nor does its absence exclude one.[72] In addition, simple cysts that recur repeatedly after aspiration of typical serous fluid should be investigated for possible intraluminal growths. Although cytology may reinforce the suspicion of a papillary neoplasm, the information gained is generally not adequate for complete characterization of the lesion and planning of definitive treatment. Core biopsy was inconclusive in about 30% in one series.[69] Levine and colleagues suggest using radiographic guidance to ensure adequate tissue sampling from any solid areas seen within or associated with cystic masses.[76] Recent reports suggest abnormal cytology of nipple aspirate fluid, and ductoscopy demonstrating irregular, friable areas corresponding to IPC may be useful for diagnosis.[77,78] An excisional biopsy is usually needed for definitive diagnosis of an IPC. Frozen sections are also not definitive because these lesions may contain a spectrum of malignant change, and permanent histologic sections should be used to direct definitive surgical management.

What are the pathologic features of intracystic papillary carcinomas?

IPC has long been thought to develop from the epithelial lining of cysts. This theory has been challenged by those who believe that these tumors develop from the growth of ductal epithelium eventually obstructing the ductal lumen. The resulting cystic dilation then results in the formation of an IPC.[79] The gross appearance of these tumors varies according to the relative contributions by the cystic and solid components.[80] Larger tumors may contain clotted blood and floating papillary fragments.[80] Similarly, the microscopic appearance is varied. High nuclear grade and tumor necrosis are seen in aggressive tumors.[69] Associated DCIS or invasive cancer can be identified up to 40% of the time.[69] A high rate of estrogen receptor positivity is reported.[69]

What is the treatment of intracystic papillary carcinoma?

There is no standard treatment regimen for IPC. Treatment must be individualized according to histologic findings and extent of disease. Carter and colleagues reported on 41 patients with IPC and found that IPC without associated DCIS or invasive carcinoma had an excellent prognosis.[70] Before this observation, all subtypes of IPC were lumped together, and thus most authors concluded that these lesions carried a poor prognosis and were best managed with modified radical mastectomies.[69] Although some have recommended local excision alone for IPC, others have demonstrated that these lesions have a potential for axillary nodal involvement and may lead to metastatic disease.[73,81] For pure

IPC, there is a low likelihood of axillary lymph node metastases; hence, operative axillary staging is not recommended.[69] A retrospective review of 41 patients with IPC treated at M. D. Anderson Cancer Center reported no influence on recurrence or survival by the use of radiation therapy. There is no consensus regarding the use of chemotherapy, radiation therapy, or hormonal therapy.

Cystosarcoma Phyllodes

What is a cystosarcoma phyllodes tumor?

Cystosarcoma phyllodes (CSP) is an unusual fibroepithelial tumor of the breast, accounting for about 0.5% of all breast tumors and 2.5% of all fibroepithelial lesions.[82] The tumor was given its name by Johannes Müller in the 19th century because of its gross fleshy appearance, resembling a sarcoma.[83] Some authors advocate the use of the term *phyllodes tumor* to include both the benign and malignant variants encountered.[83] The criteria for diagnosis, prediction of natural history, and appropriate management all evoke controversy.

How does cystosarcoma phyllodes present clinically?

Clinically, CSP can be difficult to distinguish from the more common fibroadenoma (FAD) of the breast. The average patient with CSP is in her 40s at the time of diagnosis, which is a later presentation than seen with FAD. Nonetheless, there is a well-described incidence of CSP in adolescents.[84] These tumors have been reported in males.[85] On physical examination, CSP most often presents as a painless, mobile, fleshy mass of the breast. A subset of patients will report the recent, rapid growth of a previously stable mass. This specific presentation may reflect the possible origin from a preexisting FAD in up to 25% of cases, as evidenced by histologic remnants of FAD.[86] CSP can attain very large sizes, with tumors up to 20 cm reported in the literature.[87] Any benign-appearing mass larger than 2 cm in diameter should have CSP included in its differential diagnosis. The presence of a rapidly growing, large breast mass in the absence of axillary nodal involvement raises the suspicion of this diagnosis.

On mammography, CSPs resemble benign lesions. They often have the appearance of FAD and may be associated with large, coarse calcifications.[88,89] On ultrasonography, CSPs also resemble benign lesions. The presence of indistinct borders, heterogeneous internal echoes, and cystic spaces within a solid mass may be diagnostic of CSP.[89] MRI offers no advantage over ultrasonography other than providing the surgeon with information regarding possible chest wall involvement by the largest of tumors.[89]

FNA may be helpful in suggesting the diagnosis but cannot definitively distinguish between CSP and FAD in all cases.[90] This modality is helpful in ruling out a breast carcinoma. Core needle biopsy can reliably provide a tissue diagnosis favoring a phyllodes tumor, thereby allowing better planned surgical management.[91] If these modalities fail to distinguish CSP from FAD, a carefully planned incisional biopsy can provide the needed information.

What are the pathologic features of cystosarcoma phyllodes?

The gross appearance of this tumor is that of a single or multinodular, well-circumscribed mass lacking a capsule.[87] The tissue is gray to tan and may include areas of hemorrhage and necrosis.[87] Microscopically, a stromal component with expansion and increased cellularity is observed.[87] These tumors are further classified according to histologic characteristics into benign, low-grade malignant (borderline), or high-grade malignant.[87] The precise pathologic classification of a given tumor can be quite complex and is beyond the scope of this chapter.

What are the treatment and prognosis of cystosarcoma phyllodes?

Most CSPs behave in a benign fashion. The main feature distinguishing their behavior from other benign lesions is their propensity for local recurrence. Table 34–4 summarizes collected series of CSPs in the literature with observed rates of local recurrence following excision.[92–98] The local recurrence rate is quite variable, partly owing to differences in extent of surgical resection undertaken. The cornerstone of the surgical approach to CSP is wide local excision with histologically negative margins. Locally recurrent CSP may show degeneration into more sarcomatous histology (resembling fibrosarcoma), resulting in a poor prognosis. In cases in which CSP and FAD cannot be pathologically distinguished preoperatively, the surgeon may choose to take a margin of normal tissue surrounding the lesion in an effort to avoid reoperation. Although this approach may overtreat the FAD, it is problematic only in that it may create a cosmetic deformity for the treatment of a benign lesion. When the diagnosis of CSP is made postoperatively, re-excision to obtain negative margins should be considered after discussion with the patient. The risk for local recurrence and the required surveillance is balanced against the need for further operation and potentially reduced cosmesis. Bulky disease may require simple mastectomy to achieve local control. Axillary node dissection is not

indicated unless the tumor is associated with carcinomatous elements.

The risk for metastatic disease is confined to CSP classified histologically as malignant. The criteria for such a designation, as defined by Kessinger and associates, include assessment of the tumor margin, stromal overgrowth, cellular atypia, and number of mitoses per high-power field.[99] Although the histologic appearance of CSP does not clearly predict the clinical behavior, reported cases of metastatic CSP arose in lesions classified histologically as malignant.[86,92,94,95] As with other sarcomas, metastases are hematogenous to the lung, liver, and bone as the most frequent sites of involvement. There is no consistently effective systemic therapy; therefore, metastatic malignant CSP is a uniformly fatal illness.[99]

Primary Sarcomas of the Breast

What are primary sarcomas of the breast?

Primary soft tissue sarcomas of the breast represent less than 1% of all breast malignancies, with an estimated annual incidence of 44.8 new cases per 10 million women.[100–103] A variety of subtypes are encountered. The most common are malignant fibrous histiocytomas, fibrosarcomas, stromal sarcomas, liposarcomas, and angiosarcomas. These tumors behave as sarcomas do elsewhere in the body. They are locally aggressive, and when they metastasize, it is through a hematogenous route. Because of their rarity, we must rely on retrospective case series. The result is a lack of comprehensive data regarding their optimal management.

How do primary sarcomas of the breast present?

Most primary breast sarcomas (PBSs) present as painless masses, often exhibiting rapid growth. The masses can be round or lobulated and may be fixed to the underlying chest wall. The mean tumor size in the literature is 4 to 5 cm, although tumors as large as 30 cm have been reported.[100–103] Palpable axillary adenopathy is uncommon and when encountered usually represents reactive lymph nodes uninvolved by metastatic disease. A clinically negative axilla in the presence of a large tumor may be indicative of a breast sarcoma. Although uncommon, cases of involved lymph nodes have been reported in patients with distant disease at the time of presentation.[104] The differential diagnosis is age dependent. In young patients, giant FADs and unilateral macromastia are to be considered. In older patients, locally advanced breast carcinoma and phyllodes tumors are included in the list of possible diagnoses. The definitive diagnosis can only be made histologically.

On mammography, these lesions appear as round or lobulated nodular masses with smooth or indistinct borders, and they may have coarse calcifications associated with necrotic or vascular areas.[89] A liposarcoma might be considered in the case of a rapidly growing tumor with a fatty component as seen on mammography.[89] On sonography, these tumors may appear as hypoechoic nodular masses with smooth or indistinct borders, although a large variability is encountered.[89]

Table 34–4   Risk for Local Recurrence in Cystosarcoma Phyllodes (CSP)

Study	Incidence of Local Recurrence	
	Benign CSP (%)	Malignant CSP (%)
Treves & Sunderland (1951)[86]	4/37 (11)	0/18 (0)
Pietruszka & Barnes (1978)[92]	4/16 (25)	1/17 (6)
Hajdu et al. (1976)[93]	28/150 (19)	4/49 (8)
Contarini et al. (1982)[94]	3/22 (14)	3/16 (19)
Hines et al. (1987)[95]	4/15 (27)	6/10 (60)
Salvadori et al. (1989)[96]	1/24 (4)	13/30 (43)
Bennett et al. (1992)[97]	3/14 (21)	2/11 (18)
Christensen et al. (1993)[98]	7/36 (19)	2/18 (11)

Further experience is needed to determine the characteristics of these tumors on MRI.

What are the histologic features of primary breast sarcomas?

These tumors arise from the interlobular mesenchymal elements of the breast stroma.[105] Grossly, they are pale and fleshy and may contain hemorrhagic and necrotic areas.[105] The diagnosis of PBS can be made only after the specimen is adequately sampled to rule out the presence of in situ or invasive carcinoma.[105] Invasive carcinoma would lead to the classification of the tumor as a metaplastic carcinoma and not a case of PBS. The histologic classification of the sarcoma depends on the subtype.

What is the treatment of primary breast sarcomas?

A needle biopsy may not yield a specific diagnosis but may be suggestive of mesenchymal elements. As with extremity sarcomas, a well-planned incisional biopsy may be necessary to clarify the diagnosis. Once PBS is diagnosed, surgical intervention is the first and most important step in treatment.[104,106] Many consider simple mastectomy the gold standard, but others reserve this for very large tumors.[103] In a retrospective series of 53 cases of PBS, Blanchard and associates noted no improvement in disease-free survival in patients undergoing mastectomy.[104] Because most primary breast sarcomas are unicentric, wide local excision with negative margins is considered appropriate treatment.[104,107,108] Zelek and colleagues consider breast conservation acceptable in patients with low-grade tumors and in tumors smaller than 5 cm, as long as negative surgical margins are achieved.[103] These patients have the option of salvage mastectomy in the case of local recurrence, although this can be accompanied by distant disease.[103] Axillary lymph node dissection is not indicated because the nodes are rarely involved.

There is no consensus regarding the use of radiation therapy and chemotherapy. Postoperative radiation may be used in patients undergoing mastectomy because chest wall recurrences are observed.[103] In patients electing breast conservation, postoperative radiation therapy may be considered, especially in patients with microscopically close or positive margins refusing further surgery, those with high-grade tumors, and those with large tumors.[103] A small series from the National Institutes of Health (NIH) suggests a possible beneficial effect of postoperative radiation therapy in achieving local control.[109]

It is not known whether postoperative chemotherapy affects long-term survival in patients with PBS.[103] As with sarcomas elsewhere in the body, PBS is thought to be poorly chemosensitive, with response rates on the order of 20% to 40%.[103,108] There are studies indicating increased disease-free and overall survival rates with regimens using doxorubicin and epirubicin for sarcomas in general.[110,111] How these regimens apply to breast sarcomas requires further investigation. Trent and coworkers recommend considering neoadjuvant therapy for tumors larger than 5 cm, followed by surgical resection, but most agree this requires further investigation as well.[112]

Size, histologic subtype, and grade have the greatest impact on overall prognosis.[103,108,112] A report of 60 cases of PBS from the M. D. Anderson Cancer Center suggests that tumors smaller than 5 cm have a better prognosis, regardless of other tumor characteristics.[108] Many of the earlier series of PBS reported a very poor prognosis. This is attributable in part to the inclusion of angiosarcomas, which have a well-known poor outcome. Once angiosarcomas are removed from the overall group, the natural history of PBS is comparable to that of sarcomas elsewhere in the body.[103] Disease recurrence is observed as a local event or as distant lung metastases in most cases.[103] In most series, the 5-year disease-free survival rate is about 50%.[103]

Angiosarcomas

What defines an angiosarcoma of the breast?

As discussed earlier, sarcomas are rare breast malignancies. Of this varied group of tumors, 0.04% is represented by angiosarcomas.[113] Angiosarcomas of the breast are classified as primary or secondary. Secondary angiosarcomas are diagnosed in patients with a history of lymphedema or local radiation therapy. All other angiosarcomas are primary.

How do angiosarcomas of the breast present?

Primary angiosarcomas affect women in the second to fourth decades of life.[114,115] Secondary angiosarcomas are diagnosed in patients with breast carcinoma treated with radiotherapy or followed by the development of lymphedema. Those affected are more commonly older than 50 years.[114]

A rare but well-known example of a secondary angiosarcoma is that of the lymphangiosarcoma arising in the lymphedematous, ipsilateral arm of women treated with radical mastectomy. This was first described by Stewart and Treves in 1948.[116] More recently, secondary angiosarcomas are reported in irradiated mastectomy scars and after breast conservation.[103,104,113–115,117] Although breast conservation, including postoperative irradiation, is increasingly popular, these tumors are uncommon, with about 100 cases reported in the literature.[115] The latency period for secondary angiosarcomas is between 4 and 7 years.[115] Although rare, secondary angiosarcomas have been described after segmental mastectomy alone and after breast irradiation alone or accompanied by chemotherapy without surgical intervention.[114]

There are no clinical features to distinguish primary from secondary angiosarcomas. Patients usually present with a superficial, painless, palpable mass or masses associated with a bluish discoloration. Patients may complain of ecchymosis of the breast in the absence of recent trauma. However, patients may present with no skin changes. Diffuse breast enlargement is also observed. As with other sarcomas, those in the breast spread through a hematogenous route, making axillary nodal involvement rare. The differential diagnosis includes benign lesions, postradiation telangiectases, and traumatic ecchymosis.[105] The diagnosis may be made with FNA, but an open biopsy is generally needed.[114]

Liberman and associates reviewed the radiologic findings of 29 women with biopsy-proven angiosarcomas of the breast.[118] Mammographic findings included a solitary uncalcified mass in 52% of patients, with the remainder presenting with calcified masses, skin thickening, or no findings. Sonography was performed on five patients and showed single or multiple solid masses in four, with no findings in the other patient. MRI was performed in one patient and revealed low signal intensity on T1-weighted images but higher signal intensity on T2-weighted images. At this time, the MRI appearance of breast sarcomas is limited to a few case reports.[89]

What are the pathologic features of breast angiosarcomas?

The violaceous skin color observed with angiosarcomas reflects the hemorrhage and vascularity associated with these tumors when located superficially.[105] Rosen describes the gross appearance as that of a friable, firm or spongy, hemorrhagic tumor.[105] Low-grade tumors have the appearance of normal endothelium. High-grade tumors are characterized by nuclear atypia and mitoses accompanied by hemorrhagic areas.[115]

What are the treatment and prognosis of breast angiosarcomas?

Once diagnosed, the treatment of angiosarcomas is complete surgical resection of the tumor with negative margins. In the case of postmastectomy angiosarcomas, this may require chest wall resection. For lymphangiosarcomas of Stewart-Treves syndrome, patients have been treated by forequarter amputation. Simple mastectomy and occasionally wide local excision are used to treat patients with secondary angiosarcomas after breast conservation.[113] Axillary lymph node dissection is not indicated.

In a review of the English literature, Monroe and colleagues found that 55 of 75 patients experienced a local recurrence, most within 1 year following surgical resection.[115] The surgical resection in these patients varied from wide local excision to extended radical mastectomy. Salvage procedures (ranging from mastectomy to chest wall resection) may be indicated because most distant metastases occur after local recurrence.[115] The most common site of distant failure is the contralateral breast, followed by the lung.[115]

Radiation oncologists at the University of Florida recommend hyperfractionated postoperative radiation therapy with wide fields to achieve improved local control.[119] In the case of angiosarcomas arising in previously irradiated areas, they recommend preoperative radiation therapy to allow removal of tissue at risk for radiation-associated complications and to allow for tissue flap coverage as needed. There is no consensus regarding the use of chemotherapy in the treatment of these tumors. Short-lived responses have been reported.[119] Application of vascular-targeting agents may have a role in the future.[115]

These aggressive tumors have an overall poor prognosis. Higher tumor grade is associated with worse outcome. In a review of 118,115 breast cancer cases in patients treated with breast conservation, Marchal and colleagues found 9 angiosarcomas of the breast.[114] At 32 months of follow-up,

only 1 patient was still alive. In the literature, the median survival from the time of diagnosis is a little more than 1 year. For a woman who has undergone breast-conserving therapy for the treatment of primary breast cancer, any new mass in the irradiated field, especially if pigmented and enlarging, must be viewed with extreme suspicion and excised for biopsy promptly.

Breast Lymphomas

What defines a breast lymphoma?

Breast lymphomas make up less than 0.5% of all breast malignancies.[120] This group of tumors is broken down into cases of primary breast lymphoma (PBL) and secondary breast lymphoma (SBL). The criteria used to make the diagnosis of PBL were introduced by Wiseman and Liao in 1972[121] and are as follows:

1. The submitted specimen is adequate for analysis.
2. Both mammary tissue and lymphomatous infiltrate are present in the specimen.
3. There is no evidence of widespread disease or previous history of extramammary lymphoma.
4. Axillary nodal or bone marrow involvement is acceptable. All other lymphomas fall under the category of SBL.

How do breast lymphomas present?

The most common clinical presentation of a breast lymphoma is that of a painless palpable mass. Less common findings may include skin thickening and pain.[122] The masses are larger than most breast carcinomas at the time of diagnosis.[123] Enlarged ipsilateral axillary lymph nodes are reported in 13% to 50% of cases.[122,124] Associated B symptoms (fever > 38°C, weight loss > 10% total body weight over previous 6 months, and drenching night sweats) are unusual but have been reported in some series.[123,125] Unexplained right-sided predominance is observed.[123,124,126] Synchronous bilateral breast involvement is seen in 5% to 25% of cases.[127] When bilateral disease presents with rapid, diffuse enlargement in pregnant or puerperal women, the associated histology is that of a Burkitt's lymphoma with its attendant poor prognosis and rapid disease progression.[127] As with breast carcinoma, PBL is a disease of women, although cases in male patients have been reported.[128,129]

The clinical presentation is nonspecific, and similarly, there are no pathognomonic mammographic features to distinguish breast lymphomas from other benign or malignant breast masses. Liberman and colleagues reviewed a series of 29 patients with breast lymphoma and found that only three cases had been detected only by mammography.[124] These three cases were identified as solitary masses. When discovered by mammography, breast lymphomas are solitary uncalcified masses, and observed axillary lymph node involvement is nonspecific.[124] Ultrasonography provides further nonspecific evidence of a solid mass. Other radiologic modalities, such as technetium scintigraphy and MRI, may be useful in making the diagnosis, but further experience is needed.[123,130]

The diagnosis of SBL is made more easily because of concurrent widespread disease. The diagnosis of PBL is rarely made preoperatively, and most patients are thought to have breast carcinoma instead. FNA may be performed, and cytologic analysis can confirm the diagnosis, especially if coupled with flow cytometry.[127] Caution must employed with this technique because the cytologic appearance of the lymphomatous cells may mimic lobular carcinoma.[122] Excisional biopsy is required for precise histologic diagnosis, which can be aided by the use of cytokeratin staining.

What are the pathologic features of breast lymphomas?

There are no histologic features that serve to distinguish primary breast lymphomas from those found elsewhere. Most PBLs are of B-cell origin and are believed to arise from the breast equivalent of mucosa-associated lymphoid tissue (MALT). PBLs are further classified as diffuse large cell tumors predominantly, and SBLs are more commonly diffuse small cell tumors.[120,122] Although rare, Hodgkin's lymphoma and T-cell lymphomas of the breast have been described.[122,131]

What is the treatment of breast lymphoma?

After a breast mass has been proved to be a lymphoma, an evaluation of extent of disease is mandatory. This generally includes a chest radiograph; CT scan of the chest, abdomen, and pelvis; and bone marrow biopsy. For those found to have disseminated disease, the diagnosis of SBL is made, and systemic treatment proceeds accordingly.

For those found to have disease limited to the breast, treatment is dictated by histologic grade of tumor and stage of disease. For low-grade, early-stage tumors, treatment consists of local excision with or without radiation therapy.[122,128] Chemotherapy is added in patients with high-grade, early-stage tumors because the rate of distant relapse can be as high as 70%.[123,132]

Historically, PBL was associated with a poor prognosis and was treated by mastectomy with or without axillary node dissection followed by radiation therapy.[122,133] Currently, we know that stage for stage, the prognosis is comparable to that of lymphomas at other sites, and radical surgery offers no advantage.[133] Five-year survival rates in the literature vary widely from as low as 9% to as high as 90% with appropriate treatment.[122] The variation stems from differences in histologic subtypes, staging, and treatment in the retrospective series reported. Certainly, we must rely on such series because this is a rare breast malignancy.

Breast as the Site of Metastatic Lesions

Which neoplasms metastasize to the breast?

An estimated 211,240 new cases of breast cancer will be diagnosed in 2005, making this the most common site of primary malignancy in women.[134] In contrast, the breast is an unusual site of metastatic involvement. In the largest series to date, review of records from the Pathology Department at the Royal London Hospital from 1907 to 1999 revealed 60 patients with secondary, nonmammary neoplasms of the breast constituting 3% of all breast tumors.[135] The most common tumors that metastasize to the breast are lymphomas, lung cancers, melanomas, renal cell carcinomas, and ovarian cancers. In childhood, rhabdomyosarcoma predominates.[136] Metastatic prostate cancer to the male breast has been described; however, in men with metastatic carcinoma to the breast, the lung is the most frequent primary site.[137]

How do metastatic lesions to the breast present clinically?

The differential diagnosis clearly involves benign and malignant breast lesions. A degree of suspicion should be maintained in patients with even a remote history of nonmammary neoplasms because these lesions have been diagnosed simultaneously with the primary tumor and also up to 15 years after the initial diagnosis.[138] Most frequently, patients present with known disseminated disease, but the metastatic breast lesion may be the first manifestation of an occult primary tumor prompting further investigation.[136,138,139] A well-defined, palpable mass is most common and can be associated with rapid growth.[136,140] Multiple and bilateral masses have been described.[140] Some authors have noted inflammatory metastatic lesions from ovarian and gastric signet-ring cell cancers.[138,141,142]

There are no pathognomonic radiologic features to distinguish this group of varied lesions from primary breast lesions. Mammography can reveal single or multiple discrete nodules. In the case of hematologic primaries, the metastases may appear as ill-defined nodules.[143] Sonographic findings similarly include single or multiple solid nodules with varied echotextures and margin definition.[144]

What are the pathologic features of metastatic lesions?

FNA and core needle biopsy can provide accurate diagnosis of these metastatic lesions.[139,145,146] Although the diagnosis depends on the primary site, Vergier and colleagues noted some histologic findings that might be helpful in recognizing metastatic lesions to the breast in general: (1) features atypical to primary breast carcinoma, (2) well-circumscribed tumors with multiple satellite nodules, (3) no intraductal component, and (4) numerous lymphatic emboli.[136]

The type of primary tumors reported in the literature are varied and include papillary thyroid cancer, leiomyosarcoma, neuroblastoma, rectal cancer, gastroesophageal cancer, cervical and vaginal cancer, pancreatic cancer, and skin cancer. Melanoma is a common tumor encountered. A 30-year-old woman presented to our office with a painful, palpable mass of her left axillary tail. Noninvasive tests were not diagnostic, and after excision, the mass proved consistent with metastatic melanoma of unknown primary (Fig. 34–8). Arora and Robinson described 15 patients with cutaneous melanoma metastatic to the breast.[147] As with our patient, their patients were mostly in their 30s and premenopausal,

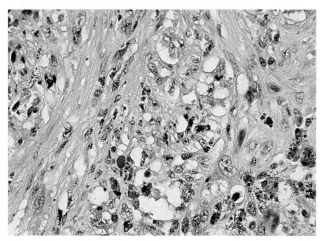

Figure 34–8 Metastatic melanoma composed of pleomorphic spindled and epithelioid cells with prominent nucleoli and cytoplasmic melanin pigment.

but in contrast, most had primary lesions identified in the upper extremity.

What is the treatment of metastatic lesions to the breast?

As mentioned earlier, FNA or core biopsy may suggest a non-breast primary.[148] Excisional biopsy may be required for confirmation. Extensive surgery is rarely indicated and should be reserved for appropriate patients in need of palliation of painful, bulky disease. Treatment is determined according to the primary tumor. Although patients with secondary breast lymphoma may have a fair prognosis, patients with metastatic disease to the breast have a generally poor outcome because this is invariably a manifestation of widespread disease. Certainly, cancers with effective systemic treatment have a more favorable course.

REFERENCES

1. Paget J. On disease of the mammary areola preceding cancer of the mammary gland. St Bartholomew's Hosp Rep 1874;10:87–89.
2. Coppes-Zantiga AR, Coppes MJ. Sir James Paget (1814–1889): A great academic Victorian. J Am Coll Surg 2000;191(1):70–74.
3. Cohen C, Guarner J, DeRose PB. Mammary Paget's disease and associated carcinoma. An immunohistochemical study. Arch Pathol Lab Med 1993;117(3):291–294.
4. Pierce LJ, Haffty BG, Solin LJ, et al. The conservative management of Paget's disease of the breast with radiotherapy. Cancer 1997;80(6):1065–1072.
5. Fu W, Lobocki CA, Silberberg BK, et al. Molecular markers in Paget disease of the breast. J Surg Oncol 2001;77(3):171–178.
6. Schelfhout VR, Coene ED, Delaey B, et al. Pathogenesis of Paget's disease: Epidermal heregulin-alpha, motility factor, and the HER receptor family. J Natl Cancer Inst 2000;92(8):622–628.
7. Rosen PP. Paget's disease of the nipple. In Rosen PP (ed). Rosen's Breast Pathology. Philadelphia, Lippincott Williams & Wilkins, 2001.
8. Stretch JR, Denton KJ, Millard PR, Horak E. Paget's disease of the male breast clinically and histopathologically mimicking melanoma. Histopathology 1991;19(5):470–472.
9. Sakorafas GH, Blanchard K, Sarr MG, Farley DR. Paget's disease of the breast. Cancer Treat Rev 2001;27(1):9–18.
10. Ashikari R, Park K, Huvos AG, Urban JA. Paget's disease of the breast. Cancer 1970;26(3):680–685.
11. Chaudary MA, Millis RR, Lane EB, Miller NA. Paget's disease of the nipple: A ten year review including clinical, pathological, and immunohistochemical findings. Breast Cancer Res Treat 1986;8(2):139–146.
12. Dixon AR, Galea MH, Ellis IO, et al. Paget's disease of the nipple. Br J Surg 1991;78(6):722–723.
13. Pierce LJ, Haffty BG, Solin LJ, et al. The conservative management of Paget's disease of the breast with radiotherapy. Cancer 1997;80(6):1065–1072.
14. Heywang-Kobrunner SH, Dershaw DD, Schreer I. Diagnostic Breast Imaging. Mammography, Sonography, Magnetic Resonance Imaging, and Interventional Procedures. New York, Thieme Stuttgart, 2001, p 292.
15. Cardenosa G. Breast Imaging Companion. New York, Lippincott Williams & Wilkins, 2001, p 212.
16. Kinne DW, Petrek JA, Osborne MP, et al. Breast carcinoma in situ. Arch Surg 1989;124(1):33–36.
17. Marshall JK, Griffith KA, Haffty BG, et al. Conservative management of Paget disease of the breast with radiotherapy: 10- and 15-year results. Cancer 2003;97(9):2142–2149.
18. Paone JF, Baker RR. Pathogenesis and treatment of Paget's disease of the breast. Cancer 1981;48(3):825–829.
19. Lagios MD, Margolin FR, Westdahl PR, Rose MR. Mammographically detected duct carcinoma in situ. Frequency of local recurrence following tylectomy and prognostic effect of nuclear grade on local recurrence. Cancer 1989;63(4):618–624.
20. Fourquet A, Campana F, Vielh P, et al. Paget's disease of the nipple without detectable breast tumor: Conservative management with radiation therapy. Int J Radiat Oncol Biol Phys 1987;13(10):1463–1465.
21. Stockdale AD, Brierley JD, White WF, et al. Radiotherapy for Paget's disease of the nipple: A conservative alternative. Lancet 1989;2(8664):664–666.
22. Bulens P, Vanuytsel L, Rijnders A, van der SE. Breast conserving treatment of Paget's disease. Radiother Oncol 1990;17(4):305–309.
23. el Sharkawi A, Waters JS. The place for conservative treatment in the management of Paget's disease of the nipple. Eur J Surg Oncol 1992;18(3):301–303.
24. Bijker N, Rutgers EJ, Duchateau L, et al. Breast-conserving therapy for Paget disease of the nipple: A prospective European Organization for Research and Treatment of Cancer study of 61 patients. Cancer 2001;91(3):472–477.
25. Kothari AS, Beechey-Newman N, Hamed H, et al. Paget disease of the nipple: A multifocal manifestation of higher-risk disease. Cancer 2002;95(1):1–7.
26. Maxwell GP, Hammond DC. Breast reconstruction following mastectomy and surgical management of the patient with high risk breast disease. In Grabb and Smith's Plastic Surgery. Philadelphia, Lippincott-Raven, 1997, pp 763–788.
27. Haagensen CD. Inflammatory carcinoma. In Haagensen CD (ed). Diseases of the Breast. Philadelphia, WB Saunders, 1986, pp 808–814.
28. Lee BJ, Tannenbaum NE. Inflammatory carcinoma of the breast. Surg Gynecol Obstet 1924;39:580.
29. Ellis DL, Teitelbaum SL. Inflammatory carcinoma of the breast. A pathologic definition. Cancer 1974;33:1045–1047.
30. Morrow M. Inflammatory breast cancer. In Greene FL, Page DL, Fleming ID, et al (eds). AJCC Cancer Staging Manual. New York, Springer, 2002, pp 221–240.
31. Rosen PP. Inflammatory carcinoma. In Rosen PP (ed). Rosen's Breast Pathology. Philadelphia, Lippincott Williams & Wilkins, 2001, pp 676–683.
32. Gunhan-Bilgen I, Ustun EE, Memis A. Inflammatory breast carcinoma: Mammographic, ultrasonographic, clinical, and pathologic findings in 142 cases. Radiology 2002;223(3):829–838.
33. Kushwaha AC, Whitman GJ, Stelling CB, et al. Primary inflammatory carcinoma of the breast: Retrospective review of mammographic findings. AJR Am J Roentgenol 2000;174(2):535–538.
34. Belli P, Constantini M, Romani M, Pastore G. Role of magnetic resonance imaging in inflammatory carcinoma of the breast. Rays 2002;27(4):299–305.
35. Lucas FV, Perez-Mesa C. Inflammatory carcinoma of the breast. Cancer 1978;41(4):1595–1605.

36. Bonnier P, Charpin C, Lejeune C, et al. Inflammatory carcinomas of the breast: A clinical, pathological, or a clinical and pathological definition? Int J Cancer 1995;62(4):382–385.

37. Droulias CA, Sewell CW, McSweeney MB, et al. Inflammatory carcinoma of the breast. A correlation of clinical radiologic and pathologic findings. Ann Surg 1976;184:217–222.

38. Kleer CG, van Golen KL, Merajver SD. Molecular biology of breast cancer metastasis. Inflammatory breast cancer: Clinical syndrome and molecular determinants. Breast Cancer Res 2000;2(6):423–429.

39. Hortobagyi G, Buzdar AU. Locally advanced breast cancer. In Bonadonna G, Hortobagyi GN, Gianni AM (eds). Textbook of Breast Cancer: A Clinical Guide to Therapy. London, Martin Dunitz, 1997, pp 155–168.

40. De Lenam, Zuoali R, Viganotti G. Combined chemotherapy-radiotherapy approach in locally advanced (T3b-T4) breast cancer. Cancer Chemother Pharmacol 1978, pp 53–59.

41. Kaufmann M, Von Minckwitz G, Smith R, et al. International expert panel on the use of primary (preoperative) systemic treatment of operable breast cancer: Review and recommendations. J Clin Oncol 2003;21(13):2600–2608.

42. Arthur DW, Schmidt-Ullrich RK, Friedman RB, et al. Accelerated superfractionated radiotherapy for inflammatory breast carcinoma: Complete response predicts outcome and allows for breast conservation. Int J Radiat Oncol Biol Phys 1999;44(2):289–296.

43. Brun B, Otmezguine Y, Feuilhade F, et al. Treatment of inflammatory breast cancer with combination chemotherapy and mastectomy versus breast conservation. Cancer 1988;61(6):1096–1103.

44. Cance WG, Carey LA, Calvo BF, et al. Long-term outcome of neoadjuvant therapy for locally advanced breast carcinoma: Effective clinical downstaging allows breast preservation and predicts outstanding local control and survival. Ann Surg 2002;236(3):295–302.

45. Sener SF, Imperato JP, Khandekar JD, et al. Achieving local control for inflammatory carcinoma of the breast. Surg Gynecol Obstet 1992;175:141–144.

46. Harris EE, Schultz D, Bertsch H, et al. Ten-year outcome after combined modality therapy for inflammatory breast cancer. Int J Radiat Oncol Biol Phys 2003;55(5):1200–1208.

47. Victor SJ, Horwitz EM, Kini VR, et al. Impact of clinical, pathologic, and treatment-related factors on outcome in patients with locally advanced breast cancer treated with multimodality therapy. Am J Clin Oncol 1999;22(2):119–125.

48. Arun B, Slack R, Gehan E, et al. Survival after autologous hematopoietic stem cell transplantation for patients with inflammatory breast carcinoma. Cancer 1999;85(1):93–99.

49. Jaiyesimi IA, Buzdar AU, Hortobagyi G. Inflammatory breast cancer: A review. J Clin Oncol 1992;10(6):1014–1024.

50. Schwartzberg L, Weaver C, Lewkow L, et al. High-dose chemotherapy with peripheral blood stem cell support for stage IIIB inflammatory carcinoma of the breast. Bone Marrow Transplant 1999;24(9):981–987.

51. Baron PL, Moore MP, Kinne DW, et al. Occult breast cancer presenting with axillary metastases. Updated management. Arch Surg 1990;125(2):210–214.

52. Scoggins CR, Vitola JV, Sandler MP, et al. Occult breast carcinoma presenting as an axillary mass. Am Surg 1999;65(1):1–5.

53. Fourquet A, de la Rouchfordiere A, Campana F. Occult primary cancer with axillary metastases. In Harris JR, Lippman ME, Morrow M, et al. (eds). Diseases of the Breast. Philadelphia, Lippincott-Raven, 1996, pp 892–896.

54. Akashi-Tanaka S, Fukutomi T, Miyakawa K, et al. Contrast-enhanced computed tomography for diagnosing the intraductal component and small invasive foci of breast cancer. Breast Cancer 2001;8(1):10–15.

55. Kolb TM, Lichy J, Newhouse JH. Occult cancer in women with dense breasts: Detection with screening US—diagnostic yield and tumor characteristics. Radiology 1998;207:191–199.

56. Olson JA, Jr., Morris EA, Van Zee KJ, et al. Magnetic resonance imaging facilitates breast conservation for occult breast cancer. Ann Surg Oncol 2000;7(6):411–415.

57. Adler LP, Crowe JP, al Kaisi NK, Sunshine JL. Evaluation of breast masses and axillary lymph nodes with [F-18] 2-deoxy-2-fluoro-D-glucose PET. Radiology 1993;187(3):743–750.

58. Brill KL, Brenin DR. Occult breast cancer and axillary mass. Curr Treat Options Oncol 2001;2(2):149–155.

59. Ellerbroek N, Holmes F, Singletary E, et al. Treatment of patients with isolated axillary nodal metastases from an occult primary carcinoma consistent with breast origin. Cancer 1990;66(7):1461–1467.

60. Rosen PP, Kimmel M. Occult breast carcinoma presenting with axillary lymph node metastases: A follow-up study of 48 patients. Hum Pathol 1990;21(5):518–523.

61. Carmichael A, Sami AS, Dixon JM. Breast cancer risk among the survivors of atomic bomb and patients exposed to therapeutic ionising radiation. Eur J Surg Oncol 2003;29(5):475–479.

62. Bhatia S, Robison LL, Oberlin O, et al. Breast cancer and other second neoplasms after childhood Hodgkin's disease. N Engl J Med 1996;334(12):745–751.

63. Travis LB, Hill DA, Dores GM, et al. Breast cancer following radiotherapy and chemotherapy among young women with Hodgkin disease. JAMA 2003;290(4):465–475.

64. Yahalom J, Petrek JA, Biddinger PW, et al. Breast cancer in patients irradiated for Hodgkin's disease: A clinical and pathologic analysis of 45 events in 37 patients. J Clin Oncol 1992;10(11):1674–1681.

65. van Leeuwen FE, Klokman WJ, Stovall M, et al. Roles of radiation dose, chemotherapy, and hormonal factors in breast cancer following Hodgkin's disease. J Natl Cancer Inst 2003;95(13):971–980.

66. Haffty BG, Harrold E, Khan AJ, et al. Outcome of conservatively managed early-onset breast cancer by BRCA1/2 status. Lancet 2002;359(9316):1471–1477.

67. Young GS, Wong JYC, Pezner RD. Bilateral breast cancer and other second neoplasms after childhood Hodgkin's disease. Breast Dis 1995;8:185–191.

68. Deutsch M, Gerszten K, Bloomer WD, Avisar E. Lumpectomy and breast irradiation for breast cancer arising after previous radiotherapy for Hodgkin's disease or lymphoma. Am J Clin Oncol 2001;24(1):33–34.

69. Solorzano CC, Middleton LP, Hunt KK, et al. Treatment and outcome of patients with intracystic papillary carcinoma of the breast. Am J Surg 2002;184(4):364–368.

70. Carter D, Orr SL, Merino MJ. Intracystic papillary carcinoma of the breast. After mastectomy, radiotherapy or excisional biopsy alone. Cancer 1983;52(1):14–19.

71. Harris KP, Faliakou EC, Exon DJ, et al. Treatment and outcome of intracystic papillary carcinoma of the breast. Br J Surg 1999;86(10):1274.

72. Markopoulos C, Kouskos E, Gogas H, et al. Diagnosis and treatment of intracystic breast carcinomas. Am Surg 2002;68(9):783–786.

73. Estabrook A, Asch T, Gump F, et al. Mammographic features of intracystic papillary lesions. Surg Gynecol Obstet 1990;170(2):113–116.

74. Ravichandran D, Carty NJ, al Talib RK, et al. Cystic carcinoma of the breast: A trap for the unwary. Ann R Coll Surg Engl 1995;77(2):123–126.

75. Ciatto S, Cariaggi P, Bulgaresi P. The value of routine cytologic examination of breast cyst fluids. Acta Cytol 1987;31(3):301–304.

76. Levine PH, Waisman J, Yang GC. Aspiration cytology of cystic carcinoma of the breast. Diagn Cytopathol 2003;28(1):39–44.

77. Krishnamurthy S, Sneige N, Thompson PA, et al. Nipple aspirate fluid cytology in breast carcinoma. Cancer 2003;99(2):97–104.

78. Yamamoto D, Ueda S, Senzaki H, et al. New diagnostic approach to intracystic lesions of the breast by fiberoptic ductoscopy. Anticancer Res 2001;21(6A):4113–4116.

79. Lefkowitz M, Lefkowitz W, Wargotz ES. Intraductal (intracystic) papillary carcinoma of the breast and its variants: A clinicopathological study of 77 cases. Hum Pathol 1994;25(8):802–809.

80. Rosen PP. Papillary carcinoma. In Rosen PP (ed). Rosen's Breast Pathology. Philadelphia, Lippincott Williams & Wilkins, 2001, pp 381–404.

81. Czernobilsky B. Intracystic carcinoma of the female breast. Surg Gynecol Obstet 1967;124(1):93–98.

82. Lester J, Stout AP. Cystosarcoma phyllodes. Cancer 1954;7(2):335–353.

83. Petrek JA. Phyllodes tumors. In Harris JR, Lippman ME, Morrow M, Osborne CK (eds). Diseases of the Breast. Philadelphia, Lippincott Williams & Wilkins, 2000, pp 669–675.

84. Andersson A, Bergdahl L. Cystosarcoma phyllodes in young women. Arch Surg 1978;113(6):742–744.

85. Konstantakos AK, Graham DJ. Cystosarcoma phyllodes tumors in men. Am Surg 2003;69(9):808–811.

86. Treves N, Sunderland DA. Cystosarcoma phyllodes of the breast: A malignant and a benign tumor. Cancer 1951;4:1286.

87. Rosen PP. Fibroepithelial neoplasms. In Rosen PP (ed). Rosen's Breast Pathology. Philadelphia, Lippincott Williams & Wilkins, 2001, pp 163–200.

88. Cole-Beuglet C, Soriano R, Kurtz AB, et al. Ultrasound, x-ray mammography, and histopathology of cystosarcoma phylloides. Radiology 1983;146(2):481–486.

89. Heywang-Kobrunner, Dershaw DD, Schreer I. Other semi-malignant and malignant tumors. In Diagnostic Breast Imaging. New York, Thieme Stuttgart, 2001, pp 325–338.

90. Simi U, Moretti D, Iacconi P, et al. Fine needle aspiration cytopathology of phyllodes tumor. Differential diagnosis with fibroadenoma. Acta Cytol 1988;32(1):63–66.

91. Komenaka IK, El Tamer M, Pile-Spellman E, Hibshoosh H. Core needle biopsy as a diagnostic tool to differentiate phyllodes tumor from fibroadenoma. Arch Surg 2003;138(9):987–990.

92. Pietruszka M, Barnes L. Cystosarcoma phylloides: A clinicopathologic analysis of 42 cases. Cancer 1978;41(5):1974–1983.

93. Hajdu SI, Espinosa MH, Robbins GF. Recurrent cystosarcoma phyllodes: A clinicopathologic study of 32 cases. Cancer 1976;38(3):1402–1406.

94. Contarini O, Urdaneta LF, Hagan W, Stephenson SE Jr. Cystosarcoma phylloides of the breast: A new therapeutic proposal. Am Surg 1982;48(4):157–166.

95. Hines JR, Murad TM, Beal JM. Prognostic indicators in cystosarcoma phylloides. Am J Surg 1987;153(3):276–280.

96. Salvadori B, Cusumano F, Del Bo R, et al. Surgical treatment of phyllodes tumors of the breast. Cancer 1989;63(12):2532–2536.

97. Bennett IC, Khan A, De Freitas R, et al. Phyllodes tumours: A clinicopathological review of 30 cases. Aust N Z J Surg 1992;62(8):628–633.

98. Christensen L, Schiodt T, Blichert-Toft M. Sarcomatoid tumours of the breast in Denmark from 1977 to 1987. A clinicopathological and immunohistochemical study of 100 cases. Eur J Cancer 1993;29A(13):1824–1831.

99. Kessinger A, Foley JF, Lemon HM, Miller DM. Metastatic cystosarcoma phyllodes: A case report and review of the literature. J Surg Oncol 1972;4(2):131–147.

100. Bardwil JM, Mocega EE, Butler JJ, Russin DJ. Angiosarcomas of the head and neck region. Am J Surg 1968;116(4):548–553.

101. Kennedy T, Biggart JD. Sarcoma of the breast. Br J Cancer 1967;21(4):635–644.

102. Norris HJ, Taylor HB. Sarcomas and related mesenchymal tumors of the breast. Cancer 1968;22(1):22–28.

103. Zelek L, Llombart-Cussac A, Terrier P, et al. Prognostic factors in primary breast sarcomas: A series of patients with long-term follow-up. J Clin Oncol 2003;21(13):2583–2588.

104. Blanchard DK, Reynolds CA, Grant CS, Donohue JH. Primary nonphylloides breast sarcomas. Am J Surg 2003;186(4):359–361.

105. Rosen PP. Sarcoma. In Rosen PP (ed). Rosen's Breast Pathology. Philadelphia, Lippincott Williams & Wilkins, 2001, pp 815–861.

106. Barrow BJ, Janjan NA, Gutman H, et al. Role of radiotherapy in sarcoma of the breast—a retrospective review of the M. D. Anderson experience. Radiother Oncol 1999;52(2):173–178.

107. Chaney AW, Pollack A, McNeese MD, et al. Primary treatment of cystosarcoma phylloides of the breast. Cancer 2000;89(7):1502–1511.

108. Gutman H, Pollock RE, Ross MI, et al. Sarcoma of the breast: Implications for extent of therapy. The M. D. Anderson experience. Surgery 1994;116(3):505–509.

109. Johnstone PA, Pierce LJ, Merino MJ, et al. Primary soft tissue sarcomas of the breast: Local-regional control with post-operative radiotherapy. Int J Radiat Oncol Biol Phys 1993;27(3):671–675.

110. Frustaci S, Gherlinzoni F, De Paoli A, et al. Adjuvant chemotherapy for adult soft tissue sarcomas of the extremities and girdles: Results of the Italian randomized cooperative trial. J Clin Oncol 2001;19(5):1238–1247.

111. Sarcoma Meta-Analysis Collaboration. Adjuvant chemotherapy for localised resectable soft-tissue sarcoma of adults: Meta-analysis of individual data. Lancet 1997;350:1647–1654.

112. Trent II JC, Benjamin RS, Valero V. Primary soft tissue sarcoma of the breast. Curr Treat Options Oncol 2001;2(2):169–176.

113. Williams EV, Banerjee D, Dallimore N, Monypenny IJ. Angiosarcoma of the breast following radiation therapy. Eur J Surg Oncol 1999;25(2):221–222.

114. Marchal C, Weber B, de Lafontan B, et al. Nine breast angiosarcomas after conservative treatment for breast carcinoma: A survey from French comprehensive Cancer Centers. Int J Radiat Oncol Biol Phys 1999;44(1):113–119.

115. Monroe AT, Feigenberg SJ, Mendenhall NP. Angiosarcoma after breast-conserving therapy. Cancer 2003;97(8):1832–1840.

116. Cozen W, Bernstein L, Wang F, et al. The risk of angiosarcoma following primary breast cancer. Br J Cancer 1999;81(3):532–536.

117. Body G, Sauvanet E, Calais G, et al. [Cutaneous angiosarcoma of the breast following surgery and irradiation of breast adenocarcinoma.] J Gynecol Obstet Biol Reprod (Paris) 1987;16(4):479–483.

118. Liberman L, Dershaw DD, Kaufman RJ, Rosen PP. Angiosarcoma of the breast. Radiology 1992;183(3):649–654.

119. Feigenberg SJ, Mendenhall NP, Reith JD, et al. Angiosarcoma after breast-conserving therapy: Experience with hyperfractionated radiotherapy. Int J Radiat Oncol Biol Phys 2002;52(3):620–626.

120. Shapiro CM, Mansur D. Bilateral primary breast lymphoma. Am J Clin Oncol 2001;24(1):85–86.

121. Wiseman C, Liao KT. Primary lymphoma of the breast. Cancer 1972;29(6):1705–1712.

122. Sabate JM, Gomez A, Torrubia S, et al. Lymphoma of the breast: Clinical and radiologic features with pathologic correlation in 28 patients. Breast J 2002;8(5):294–304.

123. Barista I, Baltali E, Tekuzman G, et al. Primary breast lymphomas—a retrospective analysis of twelve cases. Acta Oncol 2000;39(2):135–139.

124. Liberman L, Giess CS, Dershaw DD, et al. Non-Hodgkin lymphoma of the breast: Imaging characteristics and correlation with histopathologic findings. Radiology 1994;192(1):157–160.

125. Ha CS, Dubey P, Goyal LK, et al. Localized primary non-Hodgkin lymphoma of the breast. Am J Clin Oncol 1998;21(4):376–380.

126. Topalovski M, Crisan D, Mattson JC. Lymphoma of the breast. A clinicopathologic study of primary and secondary cases. Arch Pathol Lab Med 1999;123(12):1208–1218.

127. Brogi E, Harris NL. Lymphomas of the breast: Pathology and clinical behavior. Semin Oncol 1999;26(3):357–364.

128. Kim SH, Ezekiel MP, Kim RY. Primary lymphoma of the breast: Breast mass as an initial symptom. Am J Clin Oncol 1999;22(4):381–383.

129. Mattia AR, Ferry JA, Harris NL. Breast lymphoma. A B-cell spectrum including the low grade B-cell lymphoma of mucosa associated lymphoid tissue. Am J Surg Pathol 1993;17(6):574–587.

130. Hashimoto T, Kuwashima S, Sawada H, et al. Primary breast lymphoma detected with Tc-99m tetrofosmin scintigraphy. Clin Nucl Med 2001;26(5):463–465.

131. Aguilera NS, Tavassoli FA, Chu WS, Abbondanzo SL. T-cell lymphoma presenting in the breast: A histologic, immunophenotypic and molecular genetic study of four cases. Mod Pathol 2000;13(6):599–605.

132. Farinha P, Andre S, Cabecadas J, Soares J. High frequency of MALT lymphoma in a series of 14 cases of primary breast lymphoma. Appl Immunohistochem Mol Morphol 2002;10(2):115–120.

133. Domchek SM, Hecht JL, Fleming MD, et al. Lymphomas of the breast: Primary and secondary involvement. Cancer 2002;94(1):6–13.

134. Jemal A, Murray T, Ward E, et al. Cancer statistics, 2005. CA Cancer J Clin. 2005;55(1):10–30.

135. Georgiannos SN, Chin J, Goode AW, Sheaff M. Secondary neoplasms of the breast: A survey of the 20th century. Cancer 2001;92(9):2259–2266.

136. Vergier B, Trojani M, Coindre JM, Le Treut A. Metastases to the breast: Differential diagnosis from primary breast carcinoma. J Surg Oncol 1991;48(2):112–116.

137. Allen FJ, Van Velden DJ. Prostate carcinoma metastatic to the male breast. Br J Urol 1991;67(4):434–435.

138. Chaignaud B, Hall TJ, Powers C, et al. Diagnosis and natural history of extramammary tumors metastatic to the breast. J Am Coll Surg 1994;179(1):49–53.

139. Domanski HA. Metastases to the breast from extramammary neoplasms. A report of six cases with diagnosis by fine needle aspiration cytology. Acta Cytol 1996;40(6):1293–1300.

140. Moore DH, Wilson DK, Hurteau JA, et al. Gynecologic cancers metastatic to the breast. J Am Coll Surg 1998;187(2):178–181.

141. Briest S, Horn LC, Haupt R, et al. Metastasizing signet ring cell carcinoma of the stomach-mimicking bilateral inflammatory breast cancer. Gynecol Oncol 1999;74(3):491–494.

142. Ozguroglu M, Ersavasti G, Ilvan S, et al. Bilateral inflammatory breast metastases of epithelial ovarian cancer. Am J Clin Oncol 1999;22(4):408–410.

143. Paulus DD, Libshitz HI. Metastasis to the breast. Radiol Clin North Am 1982;20(3):561–568.

144. Derchi LE, Rizzatto G, Giuseppetti GM, et al. Metastatic tumors in the breast: Sonographic findings. J Ultrasound Med 1985;4(2):69–74.

145. Silverman JF, Feldman PS, Covell JL, Frable WJ. Fine needle aspiration cytology of neoplasms metastatic to the breast. Acta Cytol 1987;31(3): 291–300.

146. Sneige N, Zachariah S, Fanning TV, et al. Fine-needle aspiration cytology of metastatic neoplasms in the breast. Am J Clin Pathol 1989; 92(1):27–35.

147. Arora R, Robinson WA. Breast metastases from malignant melanoma. J Surg Oncol 1992;50(1):27–29.

148. Vazquez MF, Mitnick JS, Roses DF. Diagnosis of metastatic melanoma of the breast by aspiration biopsy. Breast Dis 1995;8:387–390.

CHAPTER 35

Treatment of the Pregnant Patient with Breast Cancer

Carol E. H. Scott-Conner, Peter R. Jochimsen, and Joel I. Sorosky

Two patients, not one, are involved when the clinician treats a pregnant or lactating patient with breast cancer. Concerns about individual mortality and the effect of treatment on the unborn or breast-feeding child lend a special poignancy and immediacy to the clinical decision-making process. This chapter defines the scope of the problem of breast cancer during pregnancy and lactation, discusses diagnosis and treatment, and summarizes current theories about the effects of pregnancy and lactation on mammary carcinogenesis. Benign breast lesions unique to pregnancy and the puerperium that can mimic breast cancer are described. Separate sections at the end of the chapter discuss the closely related issues of pregnancy after treatment for breast cancer and lactation after breast surgery.

SCOPE OF THE PROBLEM

How has pregnancy been regarded in the evolution of modern breast cancer treatment?

In 1896, Halsted reported performing a radical mastectomy on a lactating woman who subsequently survived for 30 years.[1] Harrington, in 1939, reported a 40% 10-year survival in a small series of node-negative women treated by radical mastectomy during pregnancy or lactation and stated that "the situation is by no means hopeless."[1] These early successes, however, were eclipsed by the experience of Haagensen at Columbia-Presbyterian Hospital, who wrote, in 1943, that "carcinoma of the breast developing during pregnancy or lactation is so malignant that surgery cannot cure this often enough to justify this method of treatment."[1] He reiterated this statement in subsequent publications until 1967, when he modified it to explain that although results were not as good as in nonpregnant patients, he no longer regarded pregnancy as an absolute contraindication to surgical therapy.[2–5] By that time, several authors had reported small series of patients that suggested that although the disease tended to be more advanced at presentation, the prognosis in women with negative lymph nodes was similar to that in women who were not pregnant.[1,6] Holleb and Farrow, reviewing the Memorial Hospital experience from 1920 to 1953, noted that there was a poor prognosis when the axillary nodes were involved but that "one cannot state dogmatically that it is the pregnancy per se which accounts for the unfavorable results of treatment since the stage of disease is usually advanced."[1] More recent data suggest a worse prognosis, but this crucial question remains unsettled and will be discussed later in the chapter.

Similarly, over the past several decades, scattered reports indicated that women who had been successfully treated for breast cancer could safely be allowed to become pregnant.[1] Each of these issues are discussed in detail in subsequent sections.

What is the definition of pregnancy-associated breast cancer?

Cancer of the breast diagnosed during pregnancy or within the first year after delivery is considered to be pregnancy-associated breast cancer (PABC). Some authors distinguish between cancer occurring during pregnancy and that occurring during lactation. However, because the period of lactation varies in length, 1 year after delivery has been accepted as the standard definition in most recent series.[7]

What is the incidence of pregnancy-associated breast cancer?

Carcinoma of the uterine cervix and breast cancer are the two most common malignancies diagnosed during pregnancy, each accounting for 25% of all malignancies so diagnosed.[8,9] Because cervical cancer is the only malignancy for which routine screening is done during pregnancy, it is the most prevalent cancer in most series. In the United States, breast cancer complicates 1 in 3000 deliveries.[8,10] The average obstetrician, if he or she attended 250 deliveries per year, would need to accumulate 40 years of clinical experience to encounter two or three cases of PABC.[11] This may lead to the perception that PABC is rare. When the subset of patients with breast cancer who are of childbearing age is considered, the incidence of PABC is about what would be predicted by chance, and the association no longer appears rare. If one assumes that the average woman has two pregnancies between the ages of 25 and 40 years, she is pregnant for a total of 18 out of 180 months. She would thus be pregnant 10% of that time. The calculated incidence correlates quite well with the observed co-incidence of pregnancy with breast cancer in women of that age group in series from the United States, the United Kingdom, and other western European countries.[1,4,12]

Similarly, if one estimates that 15% of women with breast cancer are of childbearing age, one would predict that 2% would have concurrent pregnancies.[10] Once again, the prediction is fairly close to what is seen clinically. In a series from Finland, 0.9% of all carcinoma of the breast occurred during pregnancy, and PABC constituted 1.1% of a similar series from Canada.[1] In Nigeria, where breast cancer is a disease of primarily premenopausal and perimenopausal (rather than older) women, the incidence of PABC is accordingly higher, ranging from 10% to 19% of all patients with breast cancer.[13] In contrast, breast cancer is considerably less common in India, and PABC is observed less frequently. Clinicians there suggest that breast cancer grows more rapidly when it occurs during the second and third trimesters or during lactation, compared with that seen in women who are not pregnant.[1] Similarly, in Japan, PABC makes up 0.76% of all breast cancer cases, with a suggestion of poorer survival and more advanced disease at presentation.[14]

When the probable latent or preclinical period of breast cancer is taken into account, it becomes likely that even larger numbers of young women with breast cancer have been pregnant at some time during the course of the disease, although they may not strictly meet the criteria for PABC. As early as 1956, T. T. and W. C. White wrote, "We believe that one-third of patients who develop breast cancer during the childbearing period will have pregnancy as a complication."[6] Finally, as women in developed countries delay childbearing into their 30s and 40s, the incidence of PABC is predicted to increase.[7] Birth rates among American women older than 35 years are the highest observed in 3 decades, at 41 births per 1000 for women between 35 and 39 years, and 8 per 1000 for those aged 40 to 44 years.

Are women with pregnancy-associated breast cancer more likely to have a positive family history?

In the Japanese series, a positive family history was three times more common among patients with PABC than in the general breast cancer population.[14] To establish this association, however, the "third degree of relationship by blood" was required, whereas most series limit the association to first-degree relatives. Studies have reported no difference in rate of positive family history when compared with age-matched controls.[2,6]

What are the implications of mutations of BRCA1 and BRCA2?

Although the influence of family history on PABC has been difficult to establish, reports are beginning to appear detailing the possible implications of BRCA1 and BRCA2 mutations for pregnancy and mammary carcinogenesis, including

PABC. Johannsson and colleagues[15] reported 10 pregnancy-associated breast cancers among BRCA1 or BRCA2 carriers, whereas only 2.7 would have been expected in the general population, for an odds ratio of 4.46. Subsequently, Shen and associates reported an excess proportion of allelic deletion at the BRCA2 locus in 88% of patients with PABC, compared with 20% of controls.[16]

Early pregnancy has also been reported to *increase* the risk for breast cancer in BRCA1 and BRCA2 mutation carriers, compared with nulliparous carriers, providing a possible mechanism for this observation.[17–19] This is thought to be consistent with other data showing that the wild form of these genes serves to regulate growth under conditions of hormonally induced proliferation. Women with mutations in either of these genes, lacking this growth-regulatory mechanism, may thus be uniquely vulnerable to the proliferative stimulation of pregnancy.

Although pregnancy appears to increase the risk for breast cancer among women who carry mutations of BRCA1 or BRCA2, breast-feeding decreases the risk, at least in women with mutations of BRCA2.[18] Again, the number of observations at the time of this writing is small.

Is there a higher risk for bilateral breast cancer?

Haagensen emphasized the need for careful follow-up of the contralateral breast and believed that women with PABC were at especially high risk for bilateral cancer.[4] The incidence in the Columbia-Presbyterian series from 1915 to 1953 was 7.3%, but these were metachronous rather than synchronous bilateral lesions. Haagensen's statements, based on observations in a limited number of patients, were subsequently cited by numerous authors. Several other early uncontrolled series reported similar findings.[1] It appears likely that a strong effect among women who have mutations of BRCA1 or BRCA2 is obscured by the large numbers who do not. There are virtually no statistical data.

What physiologic changes occur in the breast during pregnancy and lactation?

Pregnancy induces both proliferation and differentiation of the mammary epithelium. Both lobular and alveolar growth occur.[20] Differentiation of the alveoli into mature milk-producing cells requires the stimulus of cortisol, insulin, and prolactin.[21] Prolactin is the major stimulus to galactopoiesis, and levels of this hormone are markedly elevated during the later stages of pregnancy and lactation.[20,21] Steroidogenesis in the fetal-placental unit does not follow the conventional mechanisms of hormone production within a single organ. Rather, the final products result from interactions and interdependence of fetal, placental, and maternal components that individually do not possess the requisite enzymatic capabilities. During pregnancy, prolactin is secreted by fetal pituitary, maternal pituitary, and uterus. The weight of the breasts approximately doubles. Blood flow increases 180%.[20] The increases in size, weight, vascularity, and density make detection of mass lesions difficult, both clinically and mammographically. The normal physiologic changes become pathologically exaggerated in the gigantism that is extremely rarely associated with pregnancy.

EFFECTS OF PREGNANCY AND LACTATION ON MAMMARY CARCINOGENESIS

What physiologic changes occur during pregnancy that might favor tumor growth or induction?

Compounding the difficulties in assessment associated with the physiologic changes in the breast, an altered systemic milieu may play a role as well. Such a milieu might be potentially favorable to breast cancer growth. These factors include elevated hormone levels, changes in the breast that might render it more susceptible to carcinogens or to the spread of established malignancy, and the immunosuppressive effects of pregnancy itself.[22]

Pure concentrations of all three major estrogen fractions (estrone, estradiol, and estriol) rise significantly during pregnancy. Estriol secretion is 1000 times normal, and estradiol and estrone are increased about 10-fold.[20] The steroid hormones cortisol and growth hormone are elevated by two to three times as well.[22] Elevated cortisol levels may be responsible for some of the decreased cell-mediated immunity noted during pregnancy. Thymus-dependent lymphocyte levels are decreased in early pregnancy, in part due to increased cortisol. These levels recover after the 20th week of gestation. Human chorionic gonadotropin (hCG) is secreted by the syncytiotrophoblast. Despite reports concerning the suppressive effects of hCG and estrogens on cellular immunity, there is no increased incidence of malignancy in pregnant women. hCG exerts a dose-dependent protective effect on mammary carcinogenesis in animal models, and one case-control study showed that nulliparous women who had received hCG injections for weight control had a lower incidence of breast cancer than control women.[23]

The complex interactions between the pregnant woman, the fetus, and the cancer are poorly understood from the immunologic standpoint. The fetus is an F1 hybrid that is tolerated by an intact immune system. Whether the immune system is, in fact, intact during pregnancy, is debatable. Both T-cell function and cell-mediated immunity are depressed during pregnancy. Germinal centers in pelvic lymph nodes are depleted. The acceptance by the mother of the fetus (which is indeed a foreign graft with paternal antigens) depends in part on a state of partial immunologic tolerance. There is no demonstrable deficiency in immunity to other foreign antigens such as those carried by tumor cells. Breast cancer is also a condition in which antigenic tissue is tolerated by the host. Although there is evidence that pregnancy depresses cell-mediated immunity through hormonal changes such as increased production of glucocorticoids, there is no clinical evidence that these changes result in more rapid tumor growth and metastasis.[24] This is in contrast to patients in the same age group receiving immunosuppressive therapy to promote acceptance of renal allografts, who have an incidence of malignancy 100 to 1000 times greater than age-matched controls.[25]

Prolactin is significantly elevated. Although prolactin, when administered after a carcinogen, can promote tumor induction and growth in animal models of breast cancer, there is no evidence that it acts in a similar fashion in women with PABC.[26-28] The clinical observation that women with bone pain from metastatic cancer occasionally obtain relief from prolactin suppression implicates prolactin as a possible promoter.[27,28] In addition to hCG, the syncytiotrophoblast also secretes the glycoprotein human placental lactogen (hPL). hPL stimulates insulin growth factor I and induces insulin resistance and carbohydrate intolerance. Epidermal growth factor (EGF), a well-established mitogen, is also synthesized by the syncytiotrophoblast. Other growth factors produced by the human placenta include platelet-derived growth factor and transforming growth factor.

The murine homologue of BRCA1 is expressed at its highest levels in rapidly proliferating cells, such as breast tissue during puberty and pregnancy. Similarly, the expression of BRCA2 is induced in the mammary gland during puberty and pregnancy. Reduction of BRCA1 expression in vitro leads to accelerated growth, and overexpression leads to depressed growth, supporting a conceptual model in which this tumor suppressor gene negatively regulates proliferation.[19]

What is known from studies of experimental mammary cancer and pregnancy?

In a rat model, pregnancy enhances both tumor induction and growth, particularly when the animal is exposed to the carcinogen during the first half of pregnancy, when proliferation of breast tissue is maximum. Tumor expression is inhibited during the latter half of pregnancy, however, possibly by inducing differentiation in tumor cells.[1] Prolactin plays a significant role in tumor initiation and promotes the growth of diethylene anthracine–induced mammary tumors in mice. Its role in human breast tumorigenesis remains to be determined.[26,28,29] Chinese boat women who nursed their infants only from the right breast (according to traditional practice) demonstrated a two to three times lower risk for cancer in the breast used for nursing than in the contralateral breast.[27] Additional information about hormonal factors is included in the subsequent discussion of pregnancy termination.

BENIGN LESIONS IN PREGNANCY THAT CAN MIMIC BREAST CANCER

What benign lesions are unique to pregnancy and lactation?

Although most of the benign breast tumors seen in pregnancy are the same ones seen in women who are not pregnant (e.g., fibroadenomas, lipomas, papillomas), they may be altered in size or consistency as well as histologic appearance by the hormonal stimulation of pregnancy and lactation. About 30% of the breast masses in one series were lesions unique to pregnancy and lactation (lactating adenomas, galactoceles, mastitis, infarcts).[30]

The lactating adenoma (also called nodular lactational hyperplasia or lactating nodule) is a benign breast lesion unique to pregnancy and lactation.[20,30–34] These histologic changes overlap and may include lactating changes in preexisting fibroadenomas.[30] The terminology varies, and it is difficult to compare older series or to get an accurate picture of the incidence. In one series of breast biopsies in pregnant women, 13 of 17 were lactating adenomas (with three fibroadenomas and one carcinoma).[35] Histologically, lactating adenomas are characterized by florid lactational changes with a tubuloalveolar appearance to the glands. There is considerable variability in size, which can range from 1 cm up to more than 5 cm.[31] Some have suggested that the term should be reserved for lesions that closely resemble focal exaggerated changes similar to the physiologic hyperplasia of pregnancy and lactation.[32] Microscopic foci of lactating adenomas and the less common tubular adenomas have been identified within fibroadenomas, raising the possibility that these lesions arise within preexisting fibroadenomas.[31,36] Similar nodules have been described arising from ectopic breast tissue in the axilla and other extramammary sites, sometimes in association with drug administration (particularly hormones and antipsychotic or antihypertensive agents) rather than pregnancy.[31,32] The histologic appearance of florid lactational changes is shown in Figures 35–1 and 35–2, with comparison to in situ and invasive carcinomas of the breast.

Infarction of a fibroadenoma, a lactating adenoma, or hypertrophied breast tissue can occur during pregnancy.[20,37–44] The typical lesion presents with an increase in size and tenderness of a preexisting mass, or simply as a new tender mass where none was noted previously. Typically, the lesion remains mobile, but it may become fixed to the overlying skin. Generally, these lesions are small, about 2 to 3 cm in diameter, and may be multiple.[20,37] It is hypothesized that infarction occurs because of the increased metabolic demand associated with the hyperplasia of pregnancy.[37] The large "popcorn" calcifications, calcified fibroadenomas, seen on mammograms of older women may be the remnants of clinically unrecognized infarcts.[20] Histologic examination with conventional hematoxylin and eosin (H&E) stain may reveal only extensive necrosis with few or no residual glandular elements, leading the unwary to consider breast cancer as a possible diagnosis, especially on frozen section.[38,39] Masson's trichrome or reticulin stain may be helpful in demonstrating residual

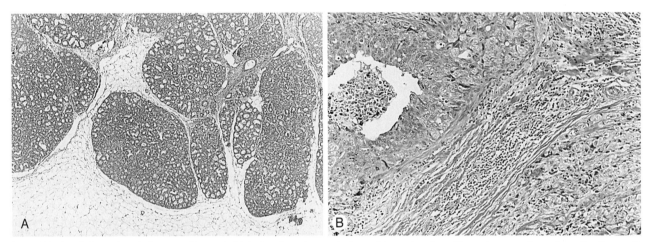

Figure 35–1 *A,* Lactational changes. Expanded lobules show hyperplasia and hypertrophy with an increased number of acinar units. (H&E, ×33.) *B,* In situ and invasive carcinoma of the breast. (H&E, ×33.) (Courtesy of Dr. Patricia Thomas.)

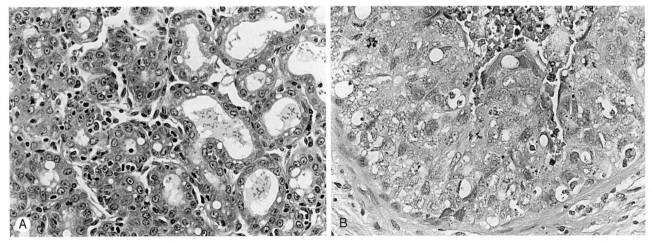

Figure 35–2 *A,* Lactational changes. High-power view demonstrates secretory vacuoles. (H&E, ×100.) *B,* In situ carcinoma of the breast. High-power view demonstrates high-grade cytology and multiple mitotic figures. (H&E, ×100.) (Courtesy of Dr. Patricia Thomas.)

fibroadenoma architecture when only extensive necrosis is seen on H&E.[38,39]

The main difficulty with these solid masses is the need to exclude malignancy. Large masses that do not regress after cessation of lactation may shrink with bromocriptine and may even require excision.[40–42]

Galactoceles are single or multiple nodules that contain retained milk (liquid if recent in formation, thickened if older). These palpable lesions are usually located peripherally in the breast. Sometimes fluctuance is elicited on palpation, and firm pressure on the mass occasionally expresses milk from the nipple.[45] Aspiration is both diagnostic and curative; if the lesion disappears totally and does not recur after aspiration of milky fluid, no further treatment is necessary.[35,45,46] A typical mammographic appearance, owing to the mixed water and fat densities (with a fat–water level seen best with a horizontally directed lateral beam with magnification), has been described,[45,46] but mammography is rarely necessary because the clinical picture is characteristic. The mammogram shown in Figure 35–3 demonstrates both a galactocele and a fibroadenoma in a lactating breast. Anything that obstructs the ductal system during lactation may cause a galactocele. Typically, these lesions occur at the cessation of lactation when milk is allowed to stagnate and inspissate in the ducts. The presentation may be delayed up to 6 to 10 months after cessation of nursing. Occasionally, a benign or malignant tumor is the cause of ductal obstruction, and this is why excision is advised if the lesion recurs after aspiration or if a mass persists.[34]

Lactational mastitis may rarely progress to breast abscess. Although inflammatory carcinoma of the breast is no more common in PABC than in the general population of breast cancer patients, it is a sufficiently frequent occurrence that one should always biopsy the wall when draining a breast abscess.[47–49]

What is the significance of bloody nipple discharge during pregnancy and lactation?

Bloody nipple discharge is common during the latter stages of pregnancy and lactation and does not necessarily portend serious consequences. Classic studies by Kline and Lash[50,51] included examination of nipple secretions of 50 women in the third trimester of pregnancy (4 of whom had a spontaneous hemorrhagic discharge). The authors demonstrated desquamated epithelial cells, similar to those seen with intraductal papillomas, and believed that pregnancy-induced changes in the ducts that led to the formation of delicate intraductal epithelial spurs, easily traumatized and shed, resulting in bleeding.[50,51] These persisted for up to 2 months (and rarely, longer) after delivery.[51]

Nipple discharge cytology is unlikely to be helpful in this situation because the proliferative changes associated with pregnancy may be mistaken for those of a neoplastic process.[34,43,50–54] There are no data available on use of ductal endoscopy, lavage, or ductography in this setting. If the bloody discharge persists more than 2 months after delivery, localizes to one duct, or is associated with a palpable mass, mammography and biopsy may be indicated to exclude breast cancer.[55] The presence of blood in the milk does not contraindicate breast-feeding. Typically, the bloody discharge ceases once breast-feeding is established.[54]

DIAGNOSIS AND TREATMENT

How does pregnancy-associated breast cancer present?

Most cases of PABC present as painless masses, and up to 90% of these masses (as is true of the population as a whole) are found by the patient herself.[55] Occasionally, an infant will inexplicably refuse to nurse from a breast that is subsequently demonstrated to harbor a breast cancer, the so-called milk-rejection sign.[55,56] Clearly, any breast mass warrants prompt attention, especially in a patient who is pregnant or lactating. Every effort must be made to reduce the delay between symptoms and diagnosis in PABC. A thorough breast examination should be an integral part of the initial prenatal physical examination. This should be done before the development of the physiologic breast changes enumerated earlier, which may conceal abnormalities. Delay in diagnosis may be minimized if both physician and patient are aware that breast changes may be manifestations of an underlying malignancy as well as normal alterations related to pregnancy and lactation. An enlarging mass that persists without regression, and other primary or secondary signs of malignancy (nipple retraction; fixation of mass to skin with or without skin thickening, dimpling, or fixation to underlying tissues; development of axillary lymphadenopathy) should be taken as indications of possible malignancy, and the diagnostic workup must be prompt given any of these findings. As in the nonpregnant patient, an occasional woman with PABC has extensive metastatic disease at initial presentation (sometimes with an occult breast primary).[57,58]

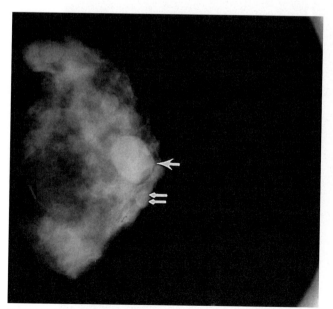

Figure 35–3 Craniocaudal mammogram of lactating breast showing two benign lesions: a subareolar lactating adenoma (*single arrow*) and a galactocele (*double arrow*). (Courtesy of Dr. Donald Young.)

availability of ultrasound (for diagnosis of placenta previa), there is considerable clinical experience with its use in late pregnancy. Adequate hydration before and during the scan facilitates rapid washout of the isotope from the blood. Foley catheter drainage of the bladder during the scan and for 8 to 12 hours after the scan avoids accumulation of isotope in the pelvis and hence minimizes fetal exposure. Using these precautions, the fetal dose was reduced from 194 to 76 mrem in one study (calculated using phantoms).[102] Once again, extreme selectivity is advocated.

What considerations govern the use of radiation therapy during pregnancy?

The fetus is extremely sensitive to both chemotherapy and radiation therapy. These effects are influenced by gestational age and dose and duration of therapy. A dose that produces fetal damage may not have perceptible effects on the mother. Death in utero can be manifested by fetal resorptions, spontaneous abortions, or stillbirths with or without malformations. Intrauterine growth retardation and prematurity are additional risks. Drug- or radiation-induced structural malformations may affect physical and mental growth and development as well as long-term viability.[103–107] Subtle point mutations may occur in the developing fetus, producing altered coding for proteins and manifesting as disease only years later. An irradiated fetus may develop recessive traits (leukemia or Hodgkin's disease) that may only appear in the second or third generation of life. The embryo is the most radiosensitive stage of human life, and there are varying sensitivities within the tissues of the human embryo. Any irradiation of gonadal tissue involves genetic damage with no threshold below which mutations do not occur. The fetus is most sensitive to radiation in early gestation during organogenesis. It has been estimated that 1 cGy produces five mutations in every 1 million genes exposed. As previously stated, the maximal permissible fetal dose of radiation is considered to be 5 cGy.[108]

In the preimplantation period, radiation produces an all-or-none effect in that it either destroys the fertilized egg or does not alter it significantly. The fetus is most sensitive to radiation at 18 to 38 days. During this period, doses of 10 to 40 cGy may cause visceral organ or somatic damage. Microcephaly, anencephaly, eye damage, growth deficiency, spina bifida, and foot damage have been reported with doses of 4 cGy or less, but cause and effect have not been reported with these lower doses. Knowledge of the effects of radiation therapy during human pregnancy comes from observations on the survivors of the blasts at Hiroshima and Nagasaki (dose difficult to quantitate) and from series of patients receiving head and neck irradiation for Hodgkin's disease (the dose used is about three fourths of the dose required for breast cancer, and the field is farther from the fetus), as well as very limited numbers of patients who have received breast irradiation during pregnancy.[47,62,72,98,104–110] The risks include fetal demise, teratogenesis or mutagenesis, and mental retardation, and are dependent on total dose and trimester. To put these risks into perspective, it is useful to recall that between 30% and 50% of human embryos abort spontaneously, and there is an average incidence of 2.75% of major malformations at birth, which increases to 6% to 10% overall once all malformations and genetic disorders become manifest.[100] Therapeutic abortion

may be considered if the fetal dose exceeds 10 cGy during the first trimester. The risk for abnormalities is low for exposure less than 5 cGy and rises with dose as 10 cGy is exceeded.[107,111] Population data obtained from atomic bomb survivors suggest that exposure at 8 to 15 weeks' gestation of 1 to 2 cGy doubles the frequency of severe mental retardation. From 4 to 17 weeks, the greater the dose, the smaller the brain and head size; beginning at a dose of 50 cGy, mental retardation increases in frequency with increasing dose.[106] The risk for teratogenesis or mutagenesis has been estimated at 1 in 1000 per 1 cGy of exposure. Exposure during later stages of pregnancy is less likely to cause abnormalities (because organogenesis is complete) but may result in more subtle problems such as sterility and subsequent development of malignancy in offspring.[107]

Much of the data concerning consequences of in utero irradiation in the medical setting come from Dekaban,[108] who studied 26 women. The children with severe congenital malformations had been irradiated between 3 and 10 weeks' gestation. More than half of the children developed anomalies (microcephaly, retinal degeneration, skeletal and genital abnormalities, and cataracts) at 250 cGy. This dose, administered before 2 or 3 weeks' gestation, increased spontaneous abortions but did not lead to severe congenital malformations. At 10 to 20 weeks' gestation, the effects were less severe than at 3 to 10 weeks, but there were children born with microcephaly, mental retardation, and small size. After 20 to 25 weeks, there were no severe abnormalities, with anemia, pigmentary changes, and dermal changes being the only toxic effects. These data support the recommendation that abdominal radiation should be avoided during the first half of pregnancy.[108]

An external radiation dose of 5000 cGy to the breast area exposes the fetus to at least 10 to 15 cGy and delivers several hundred cGy to the part of the fetus immediately below the diaphragm late in pregnancy.[62,105] Because much of this dose comes from internal scatter of radiation within the body of the woman, abdominal shielding is only partially effective. The fetal dose depends in part on the total dose administered, the distance of the fetus from the field source, the field size, and the energy source.[30,72] The fetal dose varies and must be individually calculated for each case.[105] Following a general guideline to limit the total fetal dose to 10 cGy, it becomes obvious that radiation therapy during pregnancy should be rarely employed if alternatives exist.[100]

Older series and scattered case reports describe use of radiation therapy in addition to radical or modified radical mastectomy, without evidence of adverse fetal sequelae or palliation of large, fixed, technically inoperable breast cancers, or the inadvertent exposure of a woman not known to be pregnant at the time of therapy.[47,104,107,109,110] Current practice emphasizes the use of chemotherapy rather than radiation therapy during pregnancy and reserves radiation therapy for special cases.

Can breast-conserving therapy be used during pregnancy?

As previously discussed, radiation therapy during pregnancy inevitably results in significant fetal radiation exposure, and its use is discouraged.[62,72,100] However, breast-conserving therapy has been reported during pregnancy, most commonly based on one of two strategies. In the first, wide local excision is performed at the time of diagnosis, with radiation therapy after delivery. Chemotherapy may be given in the interval between surgery and the initiation of radiation therapy. The little that is known about the long-term results is predicated on extrapolating the results from therapy in women who are not pregnant. In an alternative strategy, neoadjuvant chemotherapy is given and lumpectomy performed later. Concern has been raised that the risk for local failure may be increased in these women, because of the altered anatomy and physiology of the pregnant breast, with vascular engorgement and an active intercommunicating ductal system.[67,72,107,112] Data are not available to support this concern, and an increasing number of small series support the use of breast-conserving surgery in pregnancy.[113–116] Kuerer and colleagues reported on four patients who underwent breast-conserving surgery during pregnancy between 1995 and 1997.[115] These women were treated initially either with lumpectomy and level I or II axillary node dissection, followed by CAF chemotherapy every 21 to 28 days during the latter part of pregnancy, or with chemotherapy followed by surgery. Radiation therapy was given after delivery.[115] All women were alive with no evidence of disease at follow-up ranging from 33 to 55 months, and all pregnancies had normal outcomes. In a previous study, nine patients with PABC treated by BCS were compared with similar PABC patients treated by modified radical mastectomy, and outcomes were similar in stages I and II.[114]

There is additional evidence that selected patients who undergo breast-conserving therapy may benefit from chemotherapy before radiation therapy because long-term survival is predicated on distant disease failure rather than local failure.[113–116] As this becomes more widely accepted therapy, the issue of timing of radiation therapy may become less crucial for most patients.[112] At present, it is judicious to limit the use of breast-conserving therapy to those women who want to preserve the breast and are otherwise suitable candidates, and to those who are diagnosed late in pregnancy (so that the delay in initiation of radiation therapy is minimized).[72]

Can sentinel lymph node biopsy be used during pregnancy?

Isolated case reports document use of sentinel node biopsy during pregnancy. Little is known about whether the lymphatic pathways are altered during pregnancy. The radioisotope that is commonly used is approved for use during pregnancy, and fetal dose is acceptable. Lymphazurin (isosulfan blue) dye has not been approved for use in pregnancy, however. There are no large series documenting the predictive value of the technique.[113]

What considerations govern the use of chemotherapy during pregnancy?

General principles have been derived from experience treating primarily hematologic malignancies during pregnancy, with a more limited experience with solid tumors including breast cancer. Little is known about the use of chemotherapy for breast cancer during pregnancy, but some general principles can be laid down based on experience treating other malignancies (primarily hematologic).[112–120] All chemotherapeutic agents are theoretically teratogenic and mutagenic. Their use can result in fetal growth retardation, malformations, miscarriage, or fetal death. It is important to differentiate teratogenic and mutagenic effects from those related to an adverse uterine environment[121] or to transmission of maternal toxicity (e.g., hematopoietic depression, infection, hemorrhagic diathesis, myocardial toxicity). There is also the potential for effects on future fertility, recessive mutations, and impaired neurologic development. Long-term effects on the fetus are generally unknown, and there exists a need for long-term observation.[122] Material in the older literature is of limited relevance because lower doses of single agents were generally used, in contrast to modern practice.[123] Drugs used in combination, or chemotherapy combined with radiation therapy, may significantly increase the risk for fetal abnormalities.[119]

The physiologic changes associated with pregnancy directly affect the dosing and toxicity of chemotherapeutic agents. The usual increase in renal blood flow, glomerular filtration rate, and creatinine clearance may increase the clearance of drugs excreted by the kidneys. Amniotic fluid may act as a physiologic third space, effectively increasing the toxicity of certain agents (e.g., methotrexate) by delaying elimination. The physiologic increase in body water with the increase in plasma volume changes the volume of drug distribution. No human data on transplacental passage of antineoplastic agents are available,[124] but it is assumed to occur (especially with low-molecular-weight, highly lipid-soluble, nonionized, loosely bound drugs).[8]

The effect on the fetus is related to the particular drug, drug dosage, gestational age, and potential synergism if used with other drugs or with radiation therapy.[7,125] The National Cancer Institute (NCI) maintains a registry of patients who receive chemotherapy during pregnancy and is tracking outcomes.[8] Premature birth and low birth weight for gestational age are the most common complications and are probably underreported.[7,8,122] In a manner similar to radiation, the effects during the first few weeks are mainly teratogenic; during the second and third trimesters, intrauterine growth retardation becomes dominant.[60,98] The relative ease of identifying the sequelae of first-trimester exposure may have led to the perception that chemotherapy is safer during the later trimesters. More subtle effects, such as growth retardation, future development of neoplasms, or subtle abnormalities in neurologic development that might result from chemotherapy later in gestation, are not only more difficult to detect without careful long-term follow-up but also much harder to infer from animal studies.[122] With that caveat, some general observations about timing and specific agents follow.

The risk for spontaneous abortion is high when chemotherapy is given during the first trimester. Similarly, there is a significant trend toward greater fetal abnormalities at this time. Thirteen women who received chemotherapy for breast cancer during the first trimester were followed to term. Of the five whose pregnancies continued to term, two had major malformations in the infants, four suffered spontaneous abortions, and four had therapeutic abortions.[126] Registry data support the concept that chemotherapy given before implantation has no effect on the developing fetus.[125] The blastocyst is resistant to teratogens in the first 2 weeks of life; if not destroyed, a surviving blastocyst will not manifest any abnormalities from the teratogen. From the third to the eighth week of development (5 to 10 weeks' gestational age), there is maximal susceptibility to teratogenic agents. With the exception of brain and gonadal tissue, organogenesis ends by 13 weeks' gestation.

Most available data concerning chemotherapeutic teratogenicity and mutagenicity have been derived from laboratory animals.[124] Some generalities about specific agents that may be used in the treatment of PABC follow:

The risk of *alkylating agents* administered during pregnancy appears to be small, with no increased risk for congenital anomalies if given after the first trimester.

The *folate antagonists* aminopterin and methotrexate cause a high incidence of spontaneous abortion or fetal abnormality when administered during the first trimester. The effects vary with the dosage and the gestational age at time of administration. Limited data suggest that these agents are not harmful after the first trimester.

Although most *other chemotherapeutic agents*, including 6-mercaptopurine, azathioprine, 5-fluorouracil, alkylating agents, vinca alkaloids, doxorubicin (Adriamycin), and cisplatin, are known to be teratogenic in animals, there have been surprisingly few case reports of human fetal abnormalities resulting from the use of these drugs in the first trimester. Doxorubicin has been used in the later stages of pregnancy without reports of abnormalities.

Treatment with large doses of *corticosteroids* and cytotoxic agents, particularly during the last trimester of pregnancy, may produce neonatal bone marrow and adrenal gland suppression. Corticosteroids may be associated with cleft lip and palate.

Despite ample evidence of teratogenic effects and the potential for fetal wastage, there are many case reports of apparently healthy term neonates delivered despite administration of chemotherapy to the mother, even during the first trimester. The potential for teratogenesis exists but may be less than anticipated. It is obviously safer to avoid potential teratogenic exposure, but the decision to terminate a pregnancy must incorporate the social, religious, and ethical considerations of the patient and her family.[124]

In addition to concerns about the effect on the fetus, administration of chemotherapy during pregnancy is fraught with hazard owing to risk for sepsis, bleeding during unplanned labor and delivery, and other complications.[62] Delivery or cesarean section should be timed to avoid the chemotherapy nadirs, when bone marrow suppression is at a maximum. Timing of delivery may also affect the neonate because the placenta acts not only as a vehicle for drug delivery but also as the major route of drug excretion. Chemotherapy given shortly before delivery may not have been eliminated from the fetus by the time of delivery; the result may be prolonged drug presence in the neonate, who lacks the placental route of excretion.[124]

With respect to the specific treatment of breast cancer, it is advisable to avoid agents that have been associated with a high frequency of anomalies, particularly when alternative regimens exist.[125] Concurrent radiation therapy increases the risk.[123] During the first trimester, cyclophosphamide, methotrexate, and 5-fluorouracil (CMF) cannot be used,

owing to the toxicity of folate antagonists such as methotrexate. One series used the alternative cyclophosphamide, doxorubicin, and fluorouracil (CAF) regimen.[127] Because most women today are acutely aware of the damaging effect any drug may have on their unborn child, extensive counseling is needed. Such counseling must provide as much objective, scientific information as possible and avoid emotional bias.[120] The clinician may find it helpful to distinguish between the use of chemotherapy with curative intent and that for pure palliation. When cure is possible and the odds may be improved by adjuvant chemotherapy, modification or delay should be minimized. When cure is not possible, the goal should shift to the protection of the fetus.[127] Delaying chemotherapy until after delivery would seem to be the safest strategy and certainly provides the best protection for the unborn child, but it may do so at the expense of control of maternal disease because the greatest permissible time lapse before instituting adjuvant chemotherapy remains unknown.[72] Data on the use of combination chemotherapy for breast cancer during pregnancy consist mainly of isolated case reports; information from a registry of such cases is sorely needed.[109,123,128] A large retrospective French national survey identified 20 women who received chemotherapy during pregnancy.[129] 5-Fluorouracil, epirubicin, and cyclophosphamide were the agents most commonly used. One pregnancy resulted in a stillborn infant, and a second infant experienced intrauterine growth retardation, but overall, 95% of pregnancies resulted in live births with little related morbidity.

There are no data about newer chemotherapeutic agents such as taxol derivatives and trastuzumab (Herceptin). Tamoxifen may cause vaginal bleeding, spontaneous abortion, birth defects, and fetal deaths and should not be used during pregnancy.[113] The aromatase inhibitors are similarly precluded from use in pregnancy.

How should breast cancer be managed when diagnosed during lactation?

"Breast cancer arising during lactation is just as emotional but management is less complicated as there is no fetus to consider."[47] After delivery, the full range of therapeutic modalities is again available. The issues related to breast surgery during lactation have been discussed previously.

Breast-feeding during chemotherapy is contraindicated because antineoplastic agents may reach significant concentrations in breast milk.[22] Although little is known about excretion of drugs in milk, it is assumed that small molecules pass freely.[20] Case reports document that chemotherapeutic agents such as methotrexate and cyclophosphamide are excreted in the milk and can produce neonatal neutropenia.[55]

What is known about the hormone receptor status of pregnancy-associated breast cancer?

Older series of PABC that report ER and PR status indicate that a high percentage (up to 80%) of patients, studied with the older ligand-based receptor assays, were ER and PR negative.[7,14,30,130,131] Two general hypotheses have been advanced to account for these observations: first, that ER levels are falsely depressed or undetectable with standard assays in PABC; and second, that PABC tumors are truly ER negative because they fall into the subset of aggressive, largely ER-negative, tumors found in young women (whether or not they are pregnant).[131] Difficulties with ER and PR assays during pregnancy are discussed here. The more general question of whether these represent a subset of more biologically aggressive tumors (and that ER and PR negativity is simply another manifestation of this biologic behavior) is considered later in this chapter. Indirect evidence favoring this second hypothesis comes from old data in which oophorectomy failed to improve survival in PABC.[1] These data are difficult to interpret owing to inadequate information concerning stage of disease, deficiencies inherent in the old ligand-binding assays, and the common practice of therapeutic abortion.

Older ligand-binding assays measured ER in the cytosol. High levels of endogenous estrogen not only may have saturated the ER-binding sites but also may have triggered migration of the bound ER to the nucleus. It is thus generally suspected that the high levels of circulating estrogens in PABC contribute to false-negative ER assays.[1] In addition, high levels of circulating estrogen and progesterone down-regulate ER levels and could physiologically suppress these below the levels detectable by the standard ligand-binding assay.[131]

PR is inducible by high levels of estrogen and less easily saturated by circulating progesterone. It has been suggested that the finding of a tumor that is PR positive but ER negative, particularly in a patient younger than 51 years, indicates that the ER determination is probably falsely negative. In the latter stages of pregnancy, when progesterone levels are at their maximum, PR may be masked, and it may be necessary to remove free progesterone from the plasma before assay. This appears to be less of a problem with PR because of the relatively low affinity of PR for progesterone.[1]

Immunohistochemical testing has largely supplanted the ligand-binding assays. Middleton and coworkers reported the results of immunohistochemical testing on 39 patients with PABC (all invasive ductal carcinoma). ER was positive in 28%, PR was positive in 24%, and ER and PR were positive in 16%; these rates are similar to those of age-matched controls. HER-2/neu was positive in 28%, p53 was positive in 48%, and a high Ki-67 was noted in 60%; again, all these rates are similar to those of age-matched controls.[79] Although prolactin receptors have been demonstrated in some ER-deficient tumors in rats,[132] little is known about prolactin receptors during human pregnancy, and there is no evidence that the elevated prolactin levels associated with pregnancy stimulate tumor growth.

What is the prognosis of pregnancy-associated breast cancer?

The initial pessimism expressed by Haagensen has given way to the philosophy of treatment detailed above. Numerous studies over the past several decades have suggested that PABC tends to be more advanced at initial presentation but that it has an equivalent prognosis when patients are matched, by age and stage at diagnosis, with nonpregnant patients treated for breast cancer in the same institution at the same time period.[5,7,8,10,11,13–19,47,133–136] Older series, with inconsistent staging and inadequate control groups, showed fairly consistently that patients with PABC presented with more advanced

disease, suggesting that this was the reason for a significantly worse observed survival. Subsequent series of patients reported over the next decade reiterated the message that stage for stage, survival was equivalent, but that patients with PABC tend to present with larger tumors and more advanced disease.[7,11,91,134] This tendency to present with more advanced disease was largely ascribed to delay, as previously discussed. However, several studies published more recently suggest that this assumption may not be altogether correct. In 1991, Clark[134] reviewed his experience at Princess Margaret Hospital and noted that only 10% of patients presented with tumors less than 2 cm in diameter and that the 5-year survival of patients diagnosed during pregnancy was only 32% (regardless of nodal status; that is, node-negative patients had survival no better than node-positive patients). In several additional studies, poorer survival was shown in young PABC patients.[135,137] In a careful review of the Memorial Hospital experience, Anderson and associates[138] matched young women with operable breast cancer according to pregnancy status and demonstrated that in the subset of patients younger than 30 years with stage IIIa cancer, survival was decreased compared with nonpregnant controls. The extent to which this poor prognosis represents treatment delay, a more aggressive biologic behavior, or another manifestation of the poor outcome experienced by young women who develop breast cancer is unknown.

Kroman and colleagues, in a retrospective cohort analysis of 5652 women with breast cancer who were age 45 years or younger at the time of diagnosis, found the prognosis to be worse when the woman had been pregnant within 2 years of diagnosis.[139] This adverse affect was not affected by age, nodal status, tumor size, or whether the woman received adjuvant chemotherapy.[140]

Finally, in one careful study of pregnancy outcomes, there was a greater number of stillbirths, and live children were more likely to be born preterm or of low birth weight, suggesting a poor intrauterine environment.[126]

Can breast cancer metastasize to the products of conception?

Concern that the breast cancer may spread to the unborn child has been termed one of the myths of PABC and is cited as a major patient concern.[141,142] Metastatic spread to the placenta has been reported but is extremely rare, and spread to the fetus has never been reported (although such spread *has* been reported for melanoma, hematopoietic malignancies, hepatoma, and choriocarcinoma).[143–145] At least 55 cases of placental metastases have been reported in the literature. Melanoma is the most common, accounting for about one third, followed by hematopoietic malignancies. Breast cancer accounted for 13% of cases, and the remainder were divided among lung, sarcomas, and various gastrointestinal malignancies.[143] Occasionally, placental metastasis is the only sign of metastatic disease and has been associated with a poor maternal prognosis in other malignancies.[62] There are insufficient data to determine whether this is the case with breast cancer in particular.

Careful examination of the placenta is required, with histologic sections, even if the placenta appears grossly normal. It has been suggested that the actual incidence of placental metastases is underestimated because the gross appearance is normal in up to 50% of cases with histologic evidence of spread.[146–148] If metastases are found, the pathologist should document the extent of intervillous, intravillous, or fetal capillary involvement. Placental metastasis is generally found in conjunction with widespread metastatic disease. Fetal metastasis of other malignancies is usually associated with evidence of villous invasion or malignant cells within the fetal villous vessels.[143] Despite the lack of documented fetal transmission of breast cancer, close follow-up of the neonate has been suggested when these histologic findings are present.[143] Maternal breast cancer metastatic to the fetus has not yet been reported.

What are the ethical, psychosocial, and legal aspects of pregnancy-associated breast cancer?

At a time when the attention of both the woman and her family are focused on the future and on the prospect of bringing new life into the world, the woman and her loved ones must confront her own mortality. The diagnosis is unexpected and frightening, particularly since most patients with PABC are young and fall outside of the stereotypic "cancer patient" age range. There is a clear need for moral, emotional, and psychosocial support. The complexities of treatment of necessity involve multiple physicians from various specialties (obstetrics, surgery, and medical oncology, to name a few), and the team must develop a strategy that allows clear communication with the patient, ideally through a single professional.[149,150]

In the treatment of PABC, there may be occasions in which the best interests of the patient and fetus are perceived as being contradictory. The clear legal trend in support of patient decision-making autonomy in virtually all other aspects of care stands in contrast to certain notable cases in which courts have been inclined toward "criminalization of maternal conduct" when actions are taken during pregnancy that might harm the fetus.[146] So far, these cases have been limited to lifestyle choices in which the actions of the pregnant woman were arguably analogous to actions giving rise to charges of abuse and neglect. The opposite is more often expressed by patients with PABC, who overwhelmingly seem to put the welfare of their unborn child first. Major concerns articulated by patients in one study included "living to see my child grow up," receiving proper treatment for breast cancer, pregnancy making breast cancer worse, the possible effects of chemotherapy on the baby, and the "risk of not being there for my other children if I continue this pregnancy."[151] Women who become pregnant after treatment for breast cancer face additional worry about disease recurrence, ability to breastfeed, and health of the child.[148] Extensive needs for emotional support, reliable information, and patient advocacy may provide a special role for the nurse, allowing physicians to concentrate on medical aspects of care.[112,128]

A separate set of ethical and legal issues arises when cancer therapy is anticipated to destroy ovarian function. Experimental therapies such as oocyte cryopreservation for subsequent reimplantation are being offered to women, without sufficient data to show success of the procedure in humans.

The American Society for Reproductive Medicine, citing the "desperate feelings of cancer patients and the special status of ovarian tissue containing oocytes," noted the requirement that research in such areas adhere to the highest level of ethical and social sensitivity. When treatment can result in loss of ovarian function, it is essential that the risks and benefits of the treatment be fully explained to the patient to ensure that she had been given an adequate informed consent.[152]

PREGNANCY AFTER TREATMENT FOR BREAST CANCER AND LACTATION AFTER BREAST SURGERY

Is it safe or advisable for a woman to become pregnant after treatment for breast cancer?

When Cheek[83] surveyed the opinions of 47 nationally prominent surgeons in 1953 (choosing this method because little was available in the literature on which to base an opinion), there was no clear consensus about the advisability of pregnancy after treatment for breast cancer. In 1960, in a series of 20 women who became pregnant after treatment for breast cancer, neither termination of the pregnancy nor allowing it to go to term could be shown to affect outcome. By the early 1970s, a consensus was beginning to emerge in the literature that the woman who had survived for 2 or more years without evidence of disease could become pregnant without adverse sequelae, and this has been documented in numerous studies.[7,30,43,151–166]

As a general rule, cancer identified before conception should be adequately treated with appropriate follow-up before attempting pregnancy. Once successfully treated, few if any malignant diseases (other than those that require extirpation of the reproductive organs) absolutely preclude future pregnancy.

There are no prospective studies evaluating the effects of subsequent pregnancy on breast cancer patients. Although most recurrences occur within 2 years, many occur later. No studies have shown an adverse effect of a subsequent pregnancy even in patients with positive axillary nodes or patients whose pregnancy occurred earlier than 2 years after treatment.[164–166] Two large retrospective studies address this issue and have concluded that subsequent pregnancy does not negatively influence breast cancer survival and may have a beneficial effect. In a retrospective review of the Swedish Inpatient Care Registry, there was no untoward effect of pregnancy on the outcome of invasive breast cancer. Women who became pregnant after treatment for breast cancer demonstrated a trend toward improved prognosis compared with women not subsequently pregnant.[164–166] Sankila and colleagues[160] retrospectively reviewed data from Finland and concluded that survival rates of women who deliver liveborn children subsequent to the diagnosis of breast cancer are better than those who do not deliver. They speculated that this may be due to a "healthy mother effect" (i.e., that only women who feel well get pregnant) and that selection bias may play a significant role. However, the large number of patients (91) matched with 471 controls and the long follow-up are reassuring that subsequent pregnancy does not have an untoward effect on survival. Abortion does not improve survival, and termination of pregnancy for medical reasons is therefore considered only in women with recurrent disease.[20]

One review demonstrated that of women who are fertile after breast cancer, about 7% subsequently have children, and that the prognosis in this subset of patients was better than in the group as a whole.[73] Selection bias, the healthy mother effect, or sociologic factors may be at work.[6,73] This is another area in which data obtained from a registry could provide information of inestimable value. Petrek[161] has pointed out the difficulties in accumulating outcome data in these patients in the absence of such a registry and cautions that it is too soon to categorically pronounce it safe. There remains concern that the hormonal changes of pregnancy may stimulate dormant micrometastases.[161]

Adjuvant chemotherapy for operable breast cancer has a significant effect on subsequent fertility. Levels of follicle-stimulating hormone (FSH) and chronologic age predict ovulation reserve and reproductive potential. The risks for premature ovarian failure induced by chemotherapy can be estimated from a woman's age, the agent used, and the total dose.[123,150] Alkylating agents such as cyclophosphamide cause direct amenorrhea through direct ovarian depression. The severity of the follicular depletion seems to be a function of the number and activity of follicles present at the initiation of chemotherapy. Prepubertal ovaries not yet under cyclic hormonal control seem protected against destruction from chemotherapy. The younger the patient, the larger the reserve of oocytes that are available after chemotherapy. Thus, return of menses and ovulation are largely a function of age, dose, and duration of therapy, rather than the particular agent.[124] Whereas cyclophosphamide is a major cause of ovarian failure, methotrexate and 5-fluorouracil in adjuvant ranges were not associated with ovarian failure. There are little data concerning doxorubicin.[123,159] Adjuvant chemotherapy for breast cancer causes significant changes in ovarian function. Ovarian damage is the most significant long-term sequela of adjuvant chemotherapy in premenopausal women. The average rate of chemotherapy-related amenorrhea with CMF is 68%.[117] About 50% of women younger than 35 years resumed menses after a full course of adjuvant chemotherapy in one study.[123]

Why would a woman choose to become pregnant after treatment of breast cancer? The four major reasons cited by women in one survey were (1) desire for fulfillment of a cherished but interrupted goal (especially women who developed breast cancer after postponing childbearing or who were trying to become pregnant when they were diagnosed with breast cancer), (2) desire to regain a sense of normalcy, (3) as a way to reconnect, and (4) finally—why not? (i.e., that there are no data in the literature to suggest that it is a bad idea). Pregnancy subsequent to breast cancer treatment is a powerful stimulus to get well again.[151] Balanced against a woman's natural desire to get well again, to go on with her life, and to accomplish a cherished goal is the desire to provide maximum assurance of an uncomplicated pregnancy and of continued health. Because most recurrences occur early, many advise delaying pregnancy for 2 to 3 years. There are no hard data to support this position, which seems to be based on common sense as much as anything else.[20] A series of 32 women who became pregnant after breast conservation (including radiation

therapy) has been reported; 30 live births resulted (with one low-birth-weight infant, but no other adverse outcomes).[168] In the absence of evidence of recurrent disease, women who become pregnant after breast cancer should be managed like any other pregnant women.[20]

What are the options for hormonal control of fertility after breast cancer?

Little data are available concerning the safety of oral contraceptive use after breast cancer. Common sense would dictate that low-dose oral contraceptives might be a safe alternative for the woman who could be regarded as definitively cured.[162] The U.S. Food and Drug Administration (FDA) cites estrogen-dependent neoplasia as a contraindication. Medroxyprogesterone acetate suspension by injection every 3 months may be an attractive alternative to estrogen therapy (oral megestrol acetate [progestin] is approved for metastatic breast cancer). The FDA, however, cites a previous history of breast cancer as a contraindication.

The roles of in vitro fertilization (IVF) and oocyte donation in women rendered sterile but cured of breast cancer are totally unknown.[159] One patient underwent successful IVF 6 years after treatment for node-negative breast cancer,[152] and a second case report documented good outcome in a pregnancy produced from a donated oocyte.[164] Cryopreservation of autogenous oocytes for subsequent implantation is not currently advised in these cases.[153]

Is breast-feeding possible after breast surgery or radiation therapy?

Prior breast surgery may influence the ability of a woman to breast-feed. Circumareolar incisions may disrupt the innervation of the nipple–areolar complex, and excision of breast parenchyma in the central regions disrupts terminal ducts.[167] If a woman becomes pregnant and attempts to breast-feed several months after biopsy of a central lesion (particularly a ductal excision), the breast will become engorged and may become infected.[20] It is important that women with prior breast surgery or radiation therapy be identified prenatally as being at potential risk for problems during lactation. Early intervention includes assessment of lactation potential and a carefully individualized plan of care to allow breast-feeding while ensuring that the infant's nutritional needs are met.[167]

Radiation therapy results in diffuse tissue damage, including ductal shrinkage and lobular atrophy.[164,167] The treated breast generally does not swell as pregnancy develops. Although breast-feeding from the contralateral breast is feasible, many women have been advised not to attempt subsequent breast-feeding because of concerns about possible mastitis. In a survey of 52 pregnancies after radiation therapy, 18 (35%) reported lactation from the treated breast, and 24.5% successfully breast-fed.[163,168] Milk production is generally poor, and success rates have generally been lower in other series.[163,164] There are no data to suggest that breast-feeding after treatment for breast cancer is in any way injurious to the infant if precautions are taken to ensure that the baby derives adequate nutritional intake.[169,170]

Acknowledgments

Portions of the manuscript were reviewed by William Hesson and Sheldon Kurtz, JD.

REFERENCES

1. DiFronzo LA, O'Connell TX. Breast cancer in pregnancy and lactation. Surg Clin North Am 1996;76:267–278.
2. Haagensen CD. The treatment and results in cancer of the breast at the Presbyterian Hospital, New York. AJR Am J Roentgenol 1949;62:328–340.
3. Haagensen CD. Carcinoma of the breast; criteria for operability. Ann Surg 1943;118:859–870.
4. Haagensen CD. Cancer of the breast in pregnancy and during lactation. Am J Obstet Gynecol 1967;98:141–149.
5. Haagensen CD. Carcinoma of the breast in pregnancy. In Haagensen CD (ed). Diseases of the Breast, 2nd ed. Philadelphia, WB Saunders, 1971.
6. White TT, White WC. Breast cancer and pregnancy. Ann Surg 1956; 144:384–393.
7. Gemignani ML, Petrek JA, Borgen PL. Breast cancer and pregnancy Surg Clin North Am 1999;79:1157–1169.
8. Schwartz PE. Cancer in pregnancy. In Reece AE, Hobbins JC, Mahoney MJ, et al (eds). Medicine of the Fetus and Mother. Philadelphia, JB Lippincott, 1992, pp 1257–1281.
9. Bottles K. Pitfalls in cytology. In Koss LG, Linder J (eds). Errors and Pitfalls in Diagnostic Cytology. Baltimore, Williams & Wilkins, 1997, pp 134–146.
10. Barnavon Y, Wallack MK. Management of the pregnant patient with carcinoma of the breast. Surg Gynecol Obstet 1990;171:347–352.
11. Marchant DJ. Breast cancer in pregnancy. Clin Obstet Gynecol 1994; 37:993–997.
12. Saunders CM, Baum M. Breast cancer and pregnancy: A review. J R Soc Med 1993;86:162–165.
13. Chiedozo LC, Iweze FI, Aboh IF, et al. Breast cancer in pregnancy and lactation. Trop Geogr Med 1988;40:26–30.
14. Ishida T, Yokoe T, Kasumi F, et al. Clinicopathologic characteristics and prognosis of breast cancer patients associated with pregnancy and lactation: Analysis of case-control study in Japan. Jpn J Cancer Res 1992;83:1143–1149.
15. Johannsson O, Loman N, Borg D, Olsson H. Pregnancy-associated breast cancer in BRCA-1 and BRCA-2 germline mutation carriers. Lancet 1998;352(9137):1359–1360.
16. Shen T, Vortmeyer AO, Zhuang Z, Tavassoli FA. High frequency of allelic loss of BRCA-2 gene in pregnancy-associated breast carcinoma. J Natl Cancer Inst 1999;91:1686–1687.
17. Jernstrom H, Lerman C, Ghadirian P, et al. Pregnancy and risk of early breast cancer in carriers of BRCA-1 and BRCA-2. Lancet 1999; 354(9193):1846–1850.
18. Narod SA. Hormonal prevention of hereditary breast cancer. Ann N Y Acad Sci 2001;952:36–43.
19. Rajan JV, Marquis ST, Gardner HP, Chodosh LA. Developmental expression of BRCA2 colocalizes with BRCA1 and is associated with proliferation and differentiation in multiple tissues. Dev Biol 1997;184:385–401.
20. Hughes LE, Manset RE, Webster DJT. Benign Disorders and Diseases of the Breast: Concepts and Clinical Management. London, Balliere Tindall, 1989.
21. Danforth DN Jr. How subsequent pregnancy affects outcome in women with a prior breast cancer. Oncology 1991;5:23–30.
22. Fiorica JV. Special problems. Breast cancer and pregnancy. Obstet Gynecol Clin North Am 1994;21:721–732.
23. Bernstein L, Hanisch R, Sullivan-Halley J, et al. Treatment with human chorionic gonadotropin and risk of breast cancer. Cancer Epidemiol Biomarkers Prev 1995;4:437–440.
24. Hoover HC. Breast cancer during pregnancy and lactation. Surg Clin North Am 1990;70:1151–1162.
25. Penn I, Halgrimson CG, Starzl TE. De novo malignant tumors in organ transplant recipients. Transplant Proc 1971;3:773–783.
26. Welsch CW, Nagasawa H. Prolactin and murine mammary tumorigenesis: A review. Cancer Res 1977;37:951–963.
27. Petrakis NL. Breast secretory activity in nonlactating women, postpartum breast involution, and the epidemiology of breast cancer. Monogr Natl Cancer Inst 1977;47:161–164.
28. Foecking MK, Kibbey WE, Abou-Issa H, et al. Hormone-dependence of 7,12-dimethyl benz[a]anthracene-induced mammary tumor growth: Correlation with prostaglandin E2 content. J Natl Cancer Inst 1982;69:443–446.
29. Foecking MK, Abou-Issa H, Webb TE, et al. Concurrent changes in growth-related biochemical parameters during regression of hormone dependent rat mammary tumors. J Natl Cancer Inst 1983;71:773–778.
30. Harris JR, Hellman S, Henderson IC, et al. Breast Diseases. Philadelphia, JB Lippincott, 1987.
31. O'Hara MF, Page DL. Adenomas of the breast and ectopic breast under lactational influences. Hum Pathol 1985;16:707–712.
32. Slavin JL, Billson VR, Ostor AG. Nodular breast lesions during pregnancy and lactation. Histopathology 1993;22:481–485.
33. Tavassoli FA, Yet IT. Lactational and clear cell changes of the breast in nonlactating, nonpregnant women. Am J Clin Pathol 1987;87:23–29.
34. Canter JW, Oliver GC, Zalovdek CJ. Surgical diseases of the breast during pregnancy. Clin Obstet Gynecol 1983;26:853–864.
35. Collins JC, Liao S, Wile AG. Surgical management of breast masses in pregnant women. J Reprod Med 1995;40:785–788.
36. Novotny DB, Maygarden SJ, Shermer RW, et al. Fine needle aspiration of benign and malignant breast masses associated with pregnancy. Acta Cytol 1991;35:676–686.
37. Jimenez JF, Ryals RO, Cohen C. Spontaneous breast infarction associated with pregnancy presenting as a palpable mass. J Surg Oncol 1986; 32:174–178.
38. Majmudar B, Rosales-Quintana S. Infarction of breast fibroadenomas during pregnancy. JAMA 1975;231:963–964.
39. Rickert RR, Rajan S. Localized breast infarcts associated with pregnancy. Arch Pathol 1974;97:159–162.
40. Sumkin JH, Perroue AM, Harris KM, et al. Lactating adenoma: US features and literature review. Radiology 1998;206(1):271–274.
41. Behrendt VS, Barbakoff D, Askiu FB, Brem FR. Infarcted lactating adenoma presenting as a rapidly enlarging breast mass. AJR Am J Roentgenol 1999;173(4):944–945.
42. Reeves, ME, Tabuenca A. Lactating adenoma presenting as a giant breast mass. Surgery 2000;127(5):586–588.
43. Bland KI, Copeland EM. The Breast: Comprehensive Management of Benign and Malignant Diseases. Philadelphia, WB Saunders, 1991.
44. Robitaille Y, Seemayer TA, Thelmo WL, et al. Infarction of the mammary region mimicking carcinoma of the breast. Cancer 1974;33: 1183–1189.
45. Gomez A, Mata JM, Donoso L, et al. Galactocele: Three distinctive radiographic appearances. Radiology 1986;158:43–44.
46. Hall FM. Galactocele: Three distinctive radiographic appearances [letter]. Radiology 1986;160:852–853.
47. Clark RM, Chua T. Breast cancer and pregnancy: The ultimate challenge. Clin Oncol 1989;1:11–18.
48. Olsen CG, Gordon RE Jr. Breast disorders in nursing mothers. Am Fam Physician 1990;41:1509–1516.
49. Souadka A, Zouhal A, Souadka F, et al. Cancers du sein et grossesse. À propos de quarante-trois cas colliges à l'Institut National d'Oncologie entre 1985 et 1988. Rev Fr Gynecol Obstet 1994;89:67–72.
50. Kline TS, Lash S. Nipple secretion in pregnancy: A cytologic and histologic study. Am J Clin Pathol 1962;37:626–632.
51. Kline TS, Lash SR. The bleeding nipple of pregnancy and postpartum. A cytologic and histologic study. Acta Cytol 1984;8:336–340.
52. Dewitt JE. Management of nipple discharge by clinical findings. Am J Surg 1985;149:789–792.
53. Lafreniere R. Bloody nipple discharge during pregnancy: A rationale for conservative treatment. J Surg Oncol 1990;43:228–230.
54. O'Callaghan MA. Atypical discharge from the breast during pregnancy and/or lactation. Aust N Z J Obstet Gynecol 1981;21:214–216.
55. Gallenberg MM, Loprinzi CL. Breast cancer and pregnancy. Semin Oncol 1989;16:369–376.
56. Goldsmith HS. Milk-rejection sign of breast cancer. Am J Surg 1974; 127:280–281.
57. Evans RT, Stein RC, Ford HT, et al. Lactic acidosis. A presentation of metastatic breast cancer arising in pregnancy. Cancer 1992;69:453–456.
58. Torne A, Martinez-Roman S, Pahisa J, et al. Massive metastases from a lobular breast carcinoma from an unknown primary during pregnancy. A case report. J Reprod Med 1995;40:676–680.

59. Daly PA, Donnellan P. Breast cancer and pregnancy. Ir Med J 1992; 85:128–130.

60. Nettleton J, Long J, Kuban D, et al. Breast cancer during pregnancy: Quantifying the risk of treatment delay. Obstet Gynecol 1996;87:414–418.

61. Bottles K, Taylor R. Diagnosis of breast masses in pregnant and lactating women by aspiration cytology. Obstet Gynecol 1985;66:76S–78S.

62. Petrek JA. Breast cancer and pregnancy. Monogr Natl Cancer Inst 1994;16:113–121.

63. Liberman L, Giess CS, Dershaw DD, et al. Imaging of pregnancy-associated breast cancer. Radiology 1994;191:245–248.

64. Swinford AE, Adler DD, Garver KA. Mammographic appearance of the breasts during pregnancy and lactation: False assumptions. Acad Radiol 1998;5:467–472.

65. Parente JT, Amsel M, Lerner R, et al. Breast cancer associated with pregnancy. Obstet Gynecol 1988;71:861–864.

66. Finley JL, Silverman JF, Lannin DR. Fine needle aspiration cytology of breast masses in pregnant and lactating women. Diagn Cytopathol 1989;5:255–259.

67. Grenko RT, Lee KP, Lee KR. Fine needle aspiration cytology of lactating adenoma of the breast. Acta Cytol 1990;34:21–29.

68. Gupta RK, Wakefield SJ, Lallu S, et al. Aspiration cytodiagnosis of breast carcinoma in pregnancy and lactation with immunohistochemical and electron microscopic study of an unusual mammary malignancy with pleomorphic giant cells. Diagn Cytopathol 1992;8:352–356.

69. Gupta RK, McHutchison AG, Dowle CS, et al. Fine-needle aspiration cytodiagnosis of breast masses in pregnant and lactating women and its impact on management. Diagn Cytopathol 1993;9:156–159.

70. James K, Bridges J, Anthony PP. Breast tumour of pregnancy ("lactating adenoma"). J Pathol 1988;156:37–44.

71. Baron W. The pregnant surgical patient. Medical evaluation and management. Ann Intern Med 1984;101:683–691.

72. Petrek JA. Breast cancer during pregnancy. Cancer 1994;74:518–527.

73. Isaacs JH. Cancer of the breast in pregnancy. Surg Clin North Am 1995;75:47–51.

74. Middleton LP, Amin M, Gwyn K, et al. Breast carcinoma in pregnant women: Assessment of clinicopathologic and immunohistochemical features. Cancer 2003;98(5):1055–1060.

75. Ishida T, Yokoe T, Kasumi F, et al. Clinicopathologic characteristics and prognosis of breast cancer patients associated with pregnancy and lactation: Analysis of case control study in Japan. Jpn J Cancer Res 1992;83:1143–1149.

76. Shousha S. Breast carcinoma presenting during or shortly after pregnancy and lactation. Arch Pathol Lab Med 2000;124:1053–1060.

77. Bonnier P, Roman S, Dilheydy JM, et al. The influence of pregnancy on the outcome of breast cancer. A case-control study. Int J Cancer 1997; 72:720–727.

78. O'Donnell JR, Farrell MA. Acute myelogenous leukemia with bilateral mammary gland involvement. J Clin Pathol 1980;33:547–551.

79. Jones DED, d'Avignon MB, Lawrence R, et al. Burkitt's lymphoma: Obstetrics and gynecologic aspects. Obstet Gynecol 1980;56:533–536.

80. Barrenetzea G, Schneider J, Tanago JC, et al. Angiosarcoma of the breast and pregnancy: A new therapeutic approach. Eur J Obstet Gynecol Reprod Biol 1995;60:87–89.

81. Aghadiuno PU, Ibeziako PA. Clinicopathologic study of breast carcinoma occurring during pregnancy and lactation. Int J Gynaecol Obstet 1983;21:17–26.

82. Durodola JI. Burkitt's lymphoma presenting during lactation. Int J Gynaecol Obstet 1976;14:225–231.

83. Cheek JH. Survey of current opinions concerning carcinoma of the breast occurring during pregnancy. Arch Surg 1953;66:664–672.

84. Petrek JA, Dukoff R, Rogatko A. Prognosis of pregnancy-associated breast cancer. Cancer 1991;67:869–872.

85. Colditz GA, Rosner BA, Speizer FE. Risk factors for breast cancer according to family history of breast cancer. J Natl Cancer Inst 1996; 88:365–371.

86. Daling JR, Malone KE, Voigt LF, et al. Risk of breast cancer among young women: Relationship to induced abortion. J Natl Cancer Inst 1994;86:1584–1592.

87. Woods KL, Smith SR, Morrison JM. Parity and breast cancer: Evidence of a dual effect. BMJ 1980;281:419–421.

88. Sinha DK, Pazik JE. Tumorigenesis of mammary gland by 7,12-dimethylbenz(A)antracene during pregnancy: Relationship with DNA synthesis. Int J Cancer 1981;27:807–810.

89. Grubbs CJ, Hill DL, McDonough KC, et al. *N*-Nitroso-*N*-methylurea-induced mammary carcinogenesis: Effect of pregnancy on preneoplastic cells. J Natl Cancer Inst 1983;71:625–628.

90. Newcomb PA, Storer BE, Longnecker MP, et al. Pregnancy termination in relation to risk of breast cancer. JAMA 1996;275:282–288.

91. Lambe M, Hsieh C, Trichopoulos D, et al. Transient increase in the risk of breast cancer after giving birth. N Engl J Med 1994;331:5–9.

92. Lehrer S, Garey J, Shank B. Nomograms for determining the probability of axillary node involvement in women with breast cancer. J Cancer Res Clin Oncol 1995;121:123–125.

93. Hornstein E, Skornick Y, Rozin R. The management of breast carcinoma in pregnancy and lactation. J Surg Oncol 1982;21:179–182.

94. Kuczkowski KM: Nonobstetric surgery during pregnancy: What are the risks of anesthesia? Obstet Gynecol Surv 2004;59:52–56.

95. Mazze RI, Kallen B. Reproductive outcome after anesthesia and operation during pregnancy: A registry study of 5405 cases. Am J Obstet Gynecol 1989;161:1178–1185.

96. Kim Y, Pomper J, Goldberg ME. Anesthetic management of the pregnant patient with carcinoma of the breast. J Clin Anesth 1993;5:76–78.

97. D'Ercole FJ, Scott D, Bell E, et al. Paravertebral blockade for modified radical mastectomy in a pregnant patient. Anesth Analg 1999;88: 1351–1353.

98. Waalen J. Pregnancy poses tough questions for cancer treatment. J Natl Cancer Inst 1991;83:900–902.

99. Duncan PG, Pope WD, Cohen MM, et al. Fetal risk of anesthesia and surgery during pregnancy. Anesthesiology 1986;64:790–794.

100. Ngu SL, Duval P, Collins C. Foetal radiation dose in radiotherapy for breast cancer. Australas Radiol 1992;36:321–322.

101. Mattison DR, Angtuaco T. Magnetic resonance imaging in prenatal diagnosis. Clin Obstet Gynecol 1988;31:353–389.

102. Baker J, Ali A, Groch MW, et al. Bone scanning in pregnant patients with breast carcinoma. Clin Nucl Med 1987;12:519–524.

103. Brent RL. The effects of embryonic and fetal exposure to x-rays, microwaves, and ultrasound. Clin Perinatol 1986;13:615–648.

104. Willemese PHS, vd Sijde R, Sleijfer DT. Combination chemotherapy and radiation for stage IV breast cancer during pregnancy. Gynecol Oncol 1990;36:281.

105. Miller RW. Intrauterine radiation exposure and mental retardation. Health Phys 1988;55:295–298.

106. Brent R. The effect of embryonic and fetal exposure to xray, microwaves, and ultrasound: Counselling the pregnant and non-pregnant patient about these risks. Semin Oncol 1989;16:347–368.

107. Recht A, Come SE, Gelman RS, et al. Integration of conservative surgery, radiotherapy, and chemotherapy for the treatment of early state, node positive breast cancer: Sequencing, timing, and outcome. J Clin Oncol 1991;9:1662–1667.

108. Dekaban A. Abnormalities in children exposed to x-irradiation during various stages of gestation: Tentative timetable of radiation injury to the human fetus I. J Nucl Med 1968;9:471–477.

109. Murray CL, Reichert JA, Anderson J, et al. Multimodal cancer therapy for breast cancer in the first trimester of pregnancy. JAMA 1984;252: 2607–2608.

110. Kouvaris JR, Antypas CE, Sandilos PH, et al. Postoperative tailored radiotherapy for locally advanced breast cancer during pregnancy: A therapeutic dilemma. Am J Obstr Gynecol 2000;183:498–4999.

111. Mossman KL, Hill LT. Radiation risks in pregnancy. Obstet Gynecol 1982;60:237–242.

112. Recht A, Come SE, Henderson IC, et al. The sequencing of chemotherapy and radiation therapy after conservative surgery for early-stage breast cancer. N Engl J Med 1996;334:1356–1361.

113. Keleher AJ, Theriault RL, Gwyn KM, et al. Multidisciplinary management of breast cancer coincident with pregnancy. J Am Cancer Soc 2002;194:54–64.

114. Kuerer HM, Cunningham JD, Bleiweiss IJ, et al. Conservative surgery for breast cancer associated with pregnancy. Breast J 1998;4:171–176.

115. Kuerer HM, Gwyn K, Arnes FC, Theriault RL. Conservative surgery and chemotherapy for breast carcinoma during pregnancy. Surgery 2002;131:108–110.

116. Gemignani ML, Petrek JA. Pregnancy-associated breast cancer: Diagnosis and treatment. Breast J 2000;6:68–73.

117. Schapira DV, Chudley AE. Successful pregnancy following continuous treatment with combination chemotherapy before conception and throughout pregnancy. Cancer 1984;54:800–803.

118. Aviles A, Niz J. Long-term follow-up of children born to mothers with acute leukemia during pregnancy. Med Pediatr Oncol 1988;16:3–6.

119. Barber HRK. Fetal and neonatal effects of cytotoxic agents. Obstet Gynecol 1981;58:41–47.
120. Gililland J, Weinstein L. The effects of cancer chemotherapeutic agents on the developing fetus. Obstet Gynecol Surv 1983;38:6–12.
121. Mulvihill JJ, McKeen EA, Rosner F, et al. Pregnancy outcome in cancer patients. Cancer 1987;60:1143–1150.
122. Garber JE. Long-term follow-up of children exposed in utero to antineoplastic agents. Semin Oncol 1989;16:437–444.
123. Reichman BS, Green KB. Breast cancer in young women: Effect of chemotherapy on ovarian function, fertility, and birth defects. Monogr Natl Cancer Inst 1994;16:125–129.
124. Doll DC, Ringenberg QS, Yarbro JW. Antineoplastic agents and pregnancy. Semin Oncol 1989;16:337–346.
125. Blatt J, Mulvihill JJ, Ziegler JL, et al. Pregnancy outcome following cancer chemotherapy. Am J Med 1980;69:828–832.
126. Zemlickis D, Lishner M, Degendorker P, et al. Maternal and fetal outcome after breast cancer in pregnancy. Am J Obstet Gynecol 1992;166:781–787.
127. Doll DC, Ringenberg QS, Yarbro JW. Management of cancer during pregnancy. Arch Intern Med 1988;148:2058–2064.
128. Barni S, Ardizzoia A, Zanetta G, et al. Weekly doxorubicin chemotherapy for breast cancer in pregnancy. A case report. Tumori 1992;78:349–350.
129. Giacalone PL, Laffargue F, Benos P. Chemotherapy for breast carcinoma during pregnancy: A French national survey. Cancer 1999;86:2266–2272.
130. Holdaway IM, Mason BH, Kay RG. Steroid hormone receptors in breast tumors presenting during pregnancy and lactation. J Surg Oncol 1984;25:38–41.
131. Elledge RM, Ciocca DR, Langone G, et al. Estrogen receptor, progesterone receptor, and HER-2/neu protein in breast cancers from pregnant patients. Cancer 1993;71:2499–2506.
132. Costlow ME, Buschow RA, McGuire WL. Prolactin receptors in estrogen-receptor deficient mammary carcinoma. Science 1974;184:85–86.
133. Jones SE. Management of breast cancer in the pregnant patient. Contemp Oncol 1992;19–24.
134. Clark RM. Prognosis of breast cancer associated with pregnancy [letter]. BMJ 1991;302:1401.
135. Tretli S, Kvalheim G, Thoreson S, et al. Survival of breast cancer patients diagnosed during pregnancy or lactation. Br J Cancer 1988;58:382–384.
136. Barrat J, Marpeau L, Demuynck B. Cancer du sein et grossesse. Rev Fr Gynecol Obstet 1993;88:544–549.
137. Guinee VF, Olsson H, Moller T, et al. Effect of pregnancy on prognosis for young women with breast cancer. Lancet 1994;343:1587–1589.
138. Anderson BO, Petrek JA, Byrd DR, et al. Pregnancy influences breast cancer stage and diagnosis in women 30 years of age and younger. Ann Surg Oncol 1996;3:204–211.
139. Kroman N, Wohlfahrt J, Andersen KW, et al. Time since childbirth and prognosis in primary breast cancer: Population based study. BMJ 1997;315:851–855.
140. Reed W, Hannisdal E, Skovlund E, et al. Pregnancy and breast cancer: A population-based study. Virchows Arch 2003;443:44–50.
141. Baron RH. Dispelling the myths of pregnancy-associated breast cancer. Oncol Nurs Forum 1994;21:507–512.
142. Bandyk EA, Gilmore MA. Perceived concerns of pregnant women with breast cancer treated with chemotherapy. Oncol Nurs Forum 1995;22:975–977.
143. Eltorky M, Khare VK, Osborne P, et al. Placental metastasis from maternal carcinoma. A report of three cases. J Reprod Med 1995;40:339–403.
144. Potter JF, Schoeneman M. Metastasis of maternal cancer to the placenta and fetus. Cancer 1970;25:380–389.
145. Dunn JS Jr, Anderson CD, Brost BC. Breast cancer metastatic to the placenta. Obstet Gynecol 199;94(5 Pt 2):846.
146. Theriault RL, Stallings CB, Buzdar AU. Pregnancy and breast cancer: Clinical and legal issues. Am J Clin Oncol 1992;15:535–539.
147. Sedgely MG, Ostor AG, Fortune DW. Angiosarcoma of breast metastatic to ovary and placenta. Aust N Z J Obstet Gynaecol 1985;25:299–302.
148. Salamon MA, Sherer DM, Saller DN Jr, et al. Placental metastases in a patient with recurrent breast carcinoma. Am J Obstet Gynecol 1994;171:573–574.
149. Dow KH. Having children after breast cancer. Cancer Pract 1994;2:407–413.
150. Harris BG. Issues in nursing care of pregnant patients with cancer. Clin Issues Perinat Wom Health Nurs 1990;1:423–436.
151. Velentgas P, Daling JR, Malonek E, et al. Pregnancy after breast carcinoma: Outcomes and influence on mortality. Cancer 1999;85:2424–2432.
152. el Hussein E, Tan SL. Successful in vitro fertilization and embryo transfer after treatment of invasive carcinoma of the breast. Fertil Steril 1992;58:194–196.
153. Preftakes DK. Breast cancer and pregnancy: Implications for perinatal care and fetal outcomes. J Perinat Neonat Nurs 1994;7:31–41.
154. von Schoultz E, Johansson H, Wilking N, et al. Influence of prior and subsequent pregnancy on breast cancer prognosis. J Clin Oncol 1995;13:430–434.
155. Surbone D, Petrek JA. Childbearing issues in breast carcinoma survivors. Cancer 1997;79:1271–1278.
156. Kroman N, Jensen MB, Melbye M, et al. Should women be advised against pregnancy after breast cancer treatment? Lancet 1997;350:319–322.
157. Mueller BA, Simon MS, Deapen D, et al. Childbearing and survival with breast cancer in young women. Cancer 2003;98:1131–1140.
158. Blakely LJ, Buzdar AU, Lozada JA, et al. Effects of pregnancy after treatment for breast carcinoma on survival and risk of recurrence. Cancer 2004;100:465–469.
159. Sutton R, Buzdar AU, Hortobagyi GN. Pregnancy and offspring after adjuvant chemotherapy in breast cancer patients. Cancer 1990;65:847–850.
160. Sankila R, Heinavaara S, Hakulinen T. Survival of breast cancer patients after subsequent term pregnancy: "Healthy mother effect." Am J Obstet Gynecol 1994;170:818–823.
161. Petrek JA. Pregnancy safety after breast cancer. Cancer 1994;74:528–531.
162. Paridaens R. Sexual life and pregnancy before and after breast cancer. Acta Clin Belg Suppl 1993;15:51–55.
163. Dow KH, Harris JR, Roy C. Pregnancy after breast-conserving surgery and radiation therapy for breast cancer. Monogr Natl Cancer Inst 1994;16:131–137.
164. Sauer MV, Paulson RJ, Lobo RA. Successful pre-embryo donation in ovarian failure after treatment for breast cancer. Lancet 1990;335:723.
165. Averette HE, Mirhashemi R, Moffat FL. Pregnancy after breast carcinoma: The ultimate medical challenge. Cancer 1999;85:2301–2304.
166. Surbone A, Petrek JA. Childbearing issues in breast carcinoma survivors. Cancer 1997;79:1271–1278.
167. Neifert M. Breastfeeding after breast surgical procedure or breast cancer. Clin Issues Perinat Wom Health Nurs 1992;3:673–682.
168. Tralins AH. Lactation after conservative breast surgery combined with radiation therapy. Am J Clin Oncol 1995;18:40–43.
169. Higgins S, Haffty BG. Pregnancy and lactation after breast-conserving therapy for early stage breast cancer. Cancer 1994;73:2175–2180.
170. Varsos G, Yahalom J. Lactation following conservation surgery and radiotherapy for breast cancer. J Surg Oncol 1991;46:141–144.

CHAPTER 36

Treatment of Male Breast Cancer

Colleen D. Murphy and Patrick I. Borgen

Male breast cancer is an uncommon disease, accounting for 1% of all breast cancers and representing less than 1% of all malignancies in men. In 2005, the American Cancer Society estimated 1690 new cases of male breast cancer in the United States, with an estimated 460 deaths from the disease. By comparison, in the same year, there were an estimated 40,410 deaths in women.[1]

Male breast cancer was first recognized in ancient Egypt.[2] J. M. Wainwright[3] first documented the lethality of male breast cancer in 1927. The first documented case of male breast cancer belongs to the 14th-century British physician John of Arderne,[4] who discovered an enlarging mass beneath the right nipple of a priest in Colstone.

Before the 1990s, the incidence of male breast cancer remained stable.[5–8] Since 1991, however, there has been an unexplained rise in incidence.[9,10] By contrast, the incidence of female breast cancer has continued to increase across decades.[6] The geographic distribution of male breast cancer correlates with that of female breast cancer, with the highest incidence in North America and northern Europe, and the lowest incidence in Finland and Japan. Most countries report an incidence of less than 1 per 100,000.[11]

Like other rare conditions, discerning the epidemiology and pathogenesis of male breast cancer is challenging because of the limited data. In this chapter, we review the current literature to understand risk factors, presentation, diagnosis, and treatment options currently available for male breast cancer.

What are risk factors for male breast cancer?

Understanding the risk factors for male breast cancer is difficult because only small case-control studies have been performed and consensus data are lacking. The strongest and most consistently associated risk factors are age, family history, exposure to exogenous estrogens, abnormal testicular function, Klinefelter's syndrome, and radiation exposure[11–34] (Table 36–1).

The incidence of male breast cancer increases exponentially with age[5,7] but without the midlife decline in incidence characteristic of female breast cancer corresponding to the menopausal period.[11]

Family history is a significant risk factor for male breast cancer.[11,19,23] Several series have reported a family history of breast or ovarian cancer in first-degree relatives of up to 22% of men with breast carcinoma who have not undergone prior genetic screeening.[35–43] In addition, data from the Surveillance, Epidemiology and End Results program have shown that men with a first-degree relative with breast cancer have nearly a fourfold risk for male breast cancer.[44]

Male breast carcinomas are predominantly hormone sensitive, and it is believed that estrogen may play an etiologic role. Unfortunately, the actions of estrogen in the setting of breast carcinoma are not well understood.[45–48] The strongest evidence for a causal role of estrogen in male breast cancer is suggested by the development of breast cancer in three transsexual men with histories of chronic oral estrogen intake.[28] Anecdotal cases of male breast cancer have also been reported in men treated with estrogenic hormones for prostate carcinoma.[4,29,30,31] In addition, therapeutic treatment with digitalis, an estrogen-like drug, has been associated with male breast cancer.[19,23]

Several case-control studies have suggested that testicular abnormalities are a risk factor for male breast cancer. It is hypothesized that testicular insufficiency leads to increased endogenous estrogen levels and, therefore, increased risk. Significant correlations have been made between male breast cancer and patients with a history of mumps orchitis,[12] gonadal injury,[26] inguinal hernia repair,[26] and undescended testes.[13]

One of the strongest risk factors for breast cancer in men is Klinefelter's syndrome, a condition resulting from the inheritance of an extra X chromosome. This condition is associated with testicular insufficiency, gynecomastia, and increased excretion of follicle-stimulating hormone. These individuals have low levels of androsterone, resulting in a high estrogen-to-androgen ratio. The frequency of this disorder has been estimated to be 1 to 2 per 1000 men.[49] About 4% of men with breast cancer have been reported to have this syndrome.[50] When compared with the frequency of breast cancer in the general population, it appears that breast cancer may be 20 to 66 times more common in patients with Klinefelter's syndrome.[11,24,25]

Radiation exposure is a known risk factor for female breast cancer.[29,51,52] There is similar evidence to suggest a link between male breast cancer and radiation exposure.[32–34] Men with a history of childhood radiation treatments for thymic enlargement or pubertal gynecomastia are especially at risk.[29,51]

Table 36–4 Histopathologically Confirmed Diagnoses of Breast Masses in 187 Men

Diagnosis	Frequency (%)
Benign	
Gynecomastia	54
Lipoma	10
Proliferative fibrocystic changes	8
Cyst	5
Rosai-Dorfman disease	1
Malignant	
Infiltrating ductal carcinoma	11
Ductal carcinoma in situ	3
Metastatic disease	9

Data from Siddiqui MT, Zakowski MF, Ashfaq R, et al. Breast masses in males: Multi-institutional experience on fine-needle aspiration. Diagn Cytopathol 2002;26:87–91.

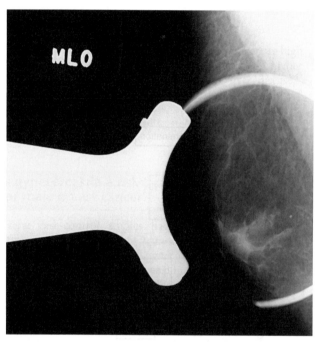

Figure 36–2 Central subareolar carcinoma seen on a mediolateral oblique mammographic view (magnified) in a male.

necrosis,[86] abscess,[86] juvenile papillomatosis,[87] papilloma,[88] neurilemoma,[89] cavernous hemangioma,[90] fibroadenoma,[91] spindle cell tumor,[92] granular cell tumor,[93] leiomyoma,[94] and carcinoid tumor.[95] Malignant conditions other than infiltrating ductal carcinoma and ductal carcinoma in situ include multiple myeloma,[86] malignant lymphoma,[86] metastatic lung adenocarcinoma,[86] metastatic prostate carcinoma,[96] and metastatic melanoma.[86]

Are radiology studies of value in diagnosis?

Recent studies suggest that mammography is both a useful tool to distinguish between malignant and benign male breast disease and an effective screening tool for the detection of contralateral cancer in patients with prior breast carcinoma (Fig. 36–2). A series of 104 prebiopsy mammograms of the male breast read by two independent radiologists blinded to histopathologic diagnosis showed sensitivity of 92% and specificity of 90%.[97] For benign conditions, sensitivity was 90% and specificity 92%. In a retrospective review of 236 male patients who underwent imaging for male breast disease, mammography correctly identified 13 of 14 cancers.[98]

These studies report the following frequencies of specific mammographic findings of male breast cancer: calcifications, 7% to 25%; retroareolar mass, 30% to 46%; eccentric mass, 54% to 60%; well-circumscribed mass, 23% to 60%; mass with irregular contour, 50% to 69%; nipple retraction, 43% to 58%; skin thickening, 21% to 58%; mass partially or completely obscured by gynecomastia, 21% to 50%.[97,98]

On the mammogram, gynecomastia is classically identified by a flame-shaped glandular proliferation extending from the nipple into the fatty tissue of the breast.[99] This finding is pathognomonic of gynecomastia.

Ultrasound evaluation of the male breast is infrequently described. In a study by Yang and colleagues,[100] ultrasound examination of 8 patients with male breast cancer revealed that 50% of the carcinomas were complex cystic masses. In a study by Gunhan-Bilgen and colleagues,[98] ultrasound correctly identified 15 cancers in 14 patients; two of these cancers had small cystic components, whereas mammography missed one cancer in these patients. Their report also suggested that ultrasound is useful for determining the extent of skin and muscle invasion and axillary lymph node involvement. These studies suggest that the use of ultrasound and mammography together may increase the sensitivity for breast cancer detection over the use of either modality alone.

What is the role of fine-needle aspiration cytology?

Recent studies suggest that fine-needle aspiration cytology (FNAC) of the male breast is an important and reliable technique to distinguish between benign and malignant conditions. A combined series of diagnostic breast aspirations from 520 male patients performed at the Johns Hopkins Hospital, Memorial Sloan-Kettering Cancer Center, or University of Texas Southwestern Medical Center demonstrated overall sensitivity and specificity of 95.3% and 100%, respectively, with a diagnostic accuracy of 98%.[86] Similar results have been obtained from large studies performed at other institutions with dedicated cytopathologists.[101,102]

What are the pathologic features of male breast cancer?

The pathologic features of male and female breast cancer are largely similar. Multiple series from the United States have shown that invasive ductal carcinoma accounts for 34% to 85% of male breast cancers, whereas tumors with a combination of invasive ductal cell and ductal carcinoma in situ constitute 18% to 48%.[36,37,55,78] Intraductal carcinoma was the only diagnosis in 5% to 17% of cases.[36,37,55,78] Medullary and tubular subtypes were identified in 1% to 2% of cases and inflammatory carcinoma in less than 1%.[36,37,55,78,79] Lobular carcinoma is a rare diagnosis in male breast cancer because the male breast lacks the hormonal influences required to undergo lobular differentiation; however, anecdotal cases of lobular carcinoma have been described in patients with Klinefelter's syndrome.[103] Case reports of male breast cancer with lobular carcinoma or lobular carcinoma in situ as a pathologic diagnosis should be questioned.

The presence of steroid hormone receptors is more common in male breast cancer than in female breast cancer. In most series, estrogen receptor positivity is as high as 80% to 85%, whereas progesterone receptor positivity approximates 75%.[36–40,79,104,105] Although *HER-2/neu* is normally overexpressed in 20% of female breast cancers,[106] reports of its overexpression in male breast cancer are highly variable. HER-2/neu protein overexpression has been reported in 9% to 56% of male breast cancer cases in studies relying on immunohistochemical staining of the cellular membrane.[107,108] Only one case of *HER-2/neu* gene amplification has been identified in studies using fluorescent in situ hybridization.[109]

What is the surgical treatment of male breast cancer?

Radical mastectomy was the earliest performed surgical procedure for male breast cancer, and as with female breast cancer there is no difference in survival between modified radical mastectomy and the more morbid Halsted mastectomy.[78,83,84,110] There are data to suggest that modified radical mastectomy offers no survival advantage over simple mastectomy, even in the setting of postoperative chemoradiation.[77] A role for radical mastectomy does exist when the tumor is fixed to the chest wall. Salvage mastectomy may be performed for locally advanced disease in medically unfit patients. Breast conservation is generally not applicable to males, owing to the small size of the breast.

The techniques of mastectomy and axillary dissection are essentially identical to those applied to female patients. Skin flaps should be developed to the same boundaries and should be of similar thickness in males and females. Axillary dissection should include levels I and II lymph nodes and is performed en bloc with the mastectomy.

Sentinel lymph node biopsy (SLNB) has been shown to be a successful technique for evaluating the axilla in male breast cancer patients. A study by Port and colleagues[111] showed successful identification of one or more sentinel lymph nodes in 15 of 16 male patients. SLNB is highly reliable in the hands of an experienced surgeon and is considered the standard of care for axillary evaluation of early-stage breast cancer in both male and female patients.

What is the role of adjuvant radiation therapy?

In female breast cancer patients, the goal of adjuvant radiation therapy is to improve locoregional control and overall survival in selected patients.[112] In female breast cancer, radiation therapy is typically given in the setting of breast-conserving therapy and to those patients considered at high risk for locoregional failure after mastectomy. The rationale behind adjuvant radiation therapy is the same in male breast cancer patients.

Studies examining the indications for radiation therapy in male breast cancer patients are limited. Anecdotal evidence

suggests a survival advantage in patients considered at high risk for relapse.[113–115] Some data, however, suggest that the risk for local recurrence in early-stage disease is not reduced by the addition of radiation therapy.[113] Until larger and better controlled studies are undertaken, the indications for adjuvant radiation therapy in male breast cancer patients remain uncertain.

What is the role of hormonal manipulation?

Orchiectomy is the oldest form of hormone therapy for disseminated male breast cancer.[116] Orchiectomy has been reported to have a 75% to 80% response rate,[117] stalling the progression of disease from 4 to 46 months.[118] Other forms of surgical ablative hormone therapy, including adrenalectomy and hypophysectomy, are of historical interest only because of their associated morbidities.

Tamoxifen has become the most widely used hormonal therapy in male breast cancer.[119] The earliest experience with tamoxifen was in the setting of disseminated disease, and there are data supporting its use as an adjuvant treatment in estrogen receptor–positive, node-positive patients. In a non-randomized trial of stage II and operable stage III patients, Ribeiro and Swindell[120] showed a 61% actuarial 5-year survival rate in tamoxifen-treated patients, compared with 44% for historical controls. In this same study, disease-free survival was 56% in tamoxifen-treated men, compared with 28% in the control group. Tamoxifen therapy may be used before or after orchiectomy, and failure to respond to one does not preclude a response to the other.[121] Common side effects of tamoxifen include diminished libido in 29%, weight gain in 25%, and hot flashes in 20%. The effects produce an attrition rate of nearly 20% in male patients.[122]

The selective aromatase inhibitor, anastrozole, is approved for first- and second-line treatment of female metastatic breast cancer. The first published case series of anastrozole therapy in five male breast cancer patients with metastatic disease showed disease stabilization without disease regression in three patients. This small series suggests that tamoxifen or orchiectomy is superior to anastrozole as first-line therapy for metastatic male breast cancer.[123]

Other hormonal agents that have been used to treat male breast cancer include estrogen, cyproterone acetate (an antiandrogen with progestational properties), androgens, progestins, aminoglutethimide, and luteinizing hormone–releasing hormone analogues. All have been shown to have response rates ranging from 30% to 62%.[117,124–126] Although data are lacking, these agents may be useful sequentially or in combination in patients who initially fail hormone therapy or in patients who experience relapse.[126]

What is the role of adjuvant chemotherapy?

Owing to the low incidence of male breast cancer, only retrospective studies are available to determine the treatment benefit gained from adjuvant chemotherapy. The earliest studies of stage II and stage III patients receiving either (1) cyclophosphamide, methotrexate, and 5-fluorouracil (CMF) or (2) 5-fluorouracil, doxorubicin, and cyclophosphamide (FAC) regimens showed a 5-year survival rate of 80% to 85%, which

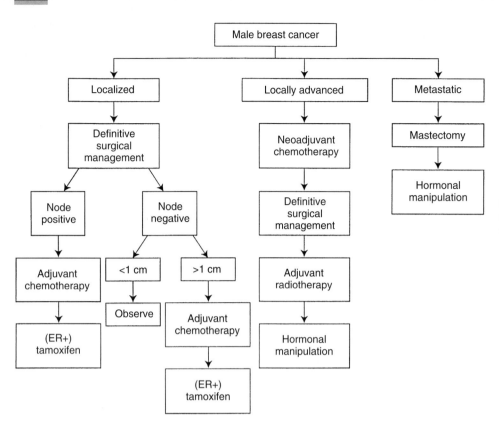

Figure 36-3 Algorithm for management of male breast cancer. ER, estrogen receptor.

is considerably higher than that of historical controls.[127,128] In a study by Yildirim and Berberoglu,[77] both CMF and FAC chemotherapy provided a survival advantage in patients with operable disease. Other case series have failed to show a survival benefit from adjuvant chemotherapy,[53,78] but the beneficial effects of chemotherapy in these patients may have been obscured by the high number of deaths due to comorbid conditions.

Trastuzumab, the monoclonal antibody against the epidermal growth factor receptor *HER-2/neu*, has been shown to improve survival beyond chemotherapy alone in female patients with breast cancers with *HER-2/neu* gene amplification. There is a single case report of a 52-year-old man who underwent radical mastectomy for pT4b breast cancer. He later developed a mastectomy scar recurrence and concomitant lung and thoracic spinal metastases that demonstrated *HER-2/neu* gene amplification. After receiving 9 months of trastuzumab therapy, he had partial clinical remission, including regression of pulmonary disease and stabilization of spinal metastasis.[109]

There are currently no prospective randomized trials evaluating adjuvant chemotherapy in male breast cancer. Because male and female breast cancers are biologically similar, it is reasonable to follow treatment guidelines for female breast cancer until further data are available. Our approach to the management of male breast cancer is outlined in Figure 36-3.

What is the prognosis for male breast cancer?

Data from the largest and most recent retrospective studies of male breast cancer show overall 5- and 10-year survival rates

of 51% to 86% and 24% to 64%, respectively.[36,37,39,53,78,109,129] Lymph node status is the strongest predictor of survival in all series: 5-year overall survival of lymph node–negative patients is 68% to 100%, compared with 47% to 73% for lymph node–positive patients.[36,37,39,53,55,129] At 10 years, survival for node-positive patients is grimmer: 11% to 38%, compared with 46% to 79% for node-negative patients. Overall 5-year survival stratified by stage has been reported as 100% for stage 0, 83% to 100% for stage I, 63% to 83% for stage II, 45% to 74% for stage III, and 0% to 25% for stage IV.[37,55,130]

Older literature reported a worse prognosis for male than female patients with breast cancer, which was attributed to the more advanced stage of disease at presentation.[74] Heller and colleagues[55] reported a markedly lower 10-year survival rate in node-positive males compared with node-positive females (11% vs. 43%), suggesting that when adjusted for stage, male breast cancer has a worse prognosis; however, in a study stratifying 130 node-positive patients by number of positive lymph nodes, male and female patients with breast cancer had similar prognoses.[85] Other studies have since supported this finding by suggesting that male and female breast cancers have similar disease-specific survival when compared by stage.[37,39,40,131]

The most common sites of distant relapse in male breast cancer are bone, lung, brain, liver, lymph nodes, and skin.[37,127] Reported distant relapse rates are 18% to 40%, whereas locoregional relapse rates are 5% to 19%.[37–40] The mean time from initial diagnosis to distant relapse is about 26 months,[74,132] and the average time from the diagnosis of metastasis to death is 8 to 26 months.[74,132] About one third of patients develop metastatic disease.[74]

What are prognostic factors?

The most important prognostic factors in male breast cancer are axillary lymph node involvement,[36,37,53,77–79] tumor size,[38,39,77,79,85,129] and hormone receptor status.[53,78,103] Multiple studies have shown a survival advantage for patients with no involved axillary lymph nodes compared with those with positive nodes. In addition, a significant survival difference has been reported between patients with one to three positive lymph nodes and those with four or more.[78] Larger tumors and a delay in diagnosis of longer than 6 months from the onset of symptoms confer a survival disadvantage,[37] whereas hormone receptor–positive tumors confer a survival advantage.

Anelli and associates[133] analyzed 36 male breast cancers for *p53* mutations and detected mutations in 42%. This is similar to the incidence of *p53* mutations in female breast cancer. They did not show a significant correlation between *p53* mutation and survival. A study by Pich and colleagues[108] demonstrated that the combination of *c-erbB-2* and *p53* immunoreactivity significantly decreases survival in male breast cancer patients.

FUTURE DIRECTIONS

Male breast cancer is a rare disease. Creation of a national male breast cancer database could facilitate clinical observation of a large number of patients to evaluate adjuvant chemotherapy, radiation therapy, and hormonal therapies. Access to large numbers of patients with male breast cancer would also provide the biologic samples required for the identification of genes associated with familial and sporadic male breast cancer. This knowledge, along with the advances in radiographic imaging, could provide a better understanding of this rare disease.

REFERENCES

1. American Cancer Society. What are the key statistics for breast cancer in men? Available at www.cancer.org. Accessed April 20, 2005.
2. Lewison EF. The surgical treatment of breast cancer: An historical and collective review. Surgery 1953;34:904–953.
3. Wainwright J. Carcinoma of the male breast: Clinical and pathologic study. Arch Surg 1927;14:836–859.
4. Holleb AI, Freeman HP, Farrow JH. Cancer of male breast. II. N Y State J Med 1968;68:656–663.
5. Ewertz M, Holmberg L, Karjalainen S, et al. Incidence of male breast cancer in Scandinavia, 1943–1982. Int J Cancer 1989;43:27–31.
6. Devesa SS, Silverman DT, Young JL, Jr., et al. Cancer incidence and mortality trends among whites in the United States, 1947–84. J Natl Cancer Inst 1987;79:701–770.
7. Moolgavkar SH, Lee JA, Hade RD. Comparison of age-specific mortality from breast cancer in males in the United States and Japan. J Natl Cancer Inst 1978;60:1223–1225.
8. La Vecchia C, Levi F, Lucchini F. Descriptive epidemiology of male breast cancer in Europe. Int J Cancer 1992;51:62–66.
9. Boring CC, Squires TS, Tong T. Cancer statistics, 1991. CA Cancer J Clin 1991;41:19–36.
10. Boring CC, Squires TS, Tong T. Cancer statistics, 1994. CA Cancer J Clin 1994;44:7–26.
11. Sasco AJ, Lowenfels AB, Pasker-de Jong P. Review article: Epidemiology of male breast cancer. A meta-analysis of published case-control studies and discussion of selected aetiological factors. Int J Cancer 1993;53:538–549.
12. Mabuchi K, Bross DS, Kessler, II. Risk factors for male breast cancer. J Natl Cancer Inst 1985;74:371–375.
13. Thomas DB, Jimenez LM, McTiernan A, et al. Breast cancer in men: Risk factors with hormonal implications. Am J Epidemiol 1992;135:734–748.
14. Hsing AW, McLaughlin JK, Cocco P, et al. Risk factors for male breast cancer (United States). Cancer Causes Control 1998;9:269–275.
15. Muir C, Waterhouse J, Mack T, et al. Cancer Incidence in Five Continents, vol 5. Lyon, France, International Agency for Research on Cancer, 1987, pp 882–883.
16. D'Avanzo B, La Vecchia C. Risk factors for male breast cancer. Br J Cancer 1995;71:1359–1362.
17. Steinitz R, Katz L, Ben-Hur M. Male breast cancer in Israel: Selected epidemiological aspects. Isr J Med Sci 1981;17:816–821.
18. Schottenfeld D, Lilienfeld AM, Diamond H. Some observations on the epidemiology of breast cancer among males. Am J Public Health 1963;53:890–897.
19. Ewertz M, Holmberg L, Tretli S, et al. Risk factors for male breast cancer—a case-control study from Scandinavia. Acta Oncol 2001;40:467–471.
20. Casagrande JT. A case-control study of male breast cancer. Cancer Res 1988;48:1326–1330.
21. Matanoski GM, Breysse PN, Elliott EA. Electromagnetic field exposure and male breast cancer. Lancet 1991;337:737.
22. Demers PA, Thomas DB, Rosenblatt KA, et al. Occupational exposure to electromagnetic fields and breast cancer in men. Am J Epidemiol 1991;134:340–347.
23. Lenfant-Pejovic MH, Mlika-Cabanne N, Bouchardy C, et al. Risk factors for male breast cancer: A Franco-Swiss case-control study. Int J Cancer 1990;45:661–665.
24. Hultborn R, Hanson C, Kopf I, et al. Prevalence of Klinefelter's syndrome in male breast cancer patients. Anticancer Res 1997;17:4293–4297.
25. Jackson AW, Muldal S, Ockey CH, et al. Carcinoma of male breast in association with the Klinefelter syndrome. BMJ 1965;5429:223–225.
26. Olsson H, Ranstam J. Head trauma and exposure to prolactin-elevating drugs as risk factors for male breast cancer. J Natl Cancer Inst 1988;80:679–683.
27. El-Gazayerli MM, Abdel-Aziz AS. On bilharziasis and male breast cancer in Egypt: A preliminary report and review of the literature. Br J Cancer 1963;17:566–571.
28. Pritchard TJ, Pankowsky DA, Crowe JP, et al. Breast cancer in a male-to-female transsexual. A case report. JAMA 1988;259:2278–2280.
29. Crichlow RW. Carcinoma of the male breast. Surg Gynecol Obstet 1972;134:1011–1019.
30. Liechty RD, Davis J, Gleysteen J. Cancer of the male breast: Forty cases. Cancer 1967;20:1617–1624.
31. Campbell JH, Cummins SD. Metastases, simulating mammary cancer, in prostatic carcinoma under estrogen therapy. Cancer 1951;4:303.
32. Greene MH, Goedert JJ, Bech-Hansen NT, et al. Radiogenic male breast cancer with in vitro sensitivity to ionizing radiation and bleomycin. Cancer Invest 1983;1:379–386.
33. Thomas DB, Rosenblatt K, Jimenez LM, et al. Ionizing radiation and breast cancer in men (United States). Cancer Causes Control. 1994;5:9–14.
34. Thompson DK, Li FP, Cassady JR. Breast cancer in a man 30 years after radiation for metastatic osteogenic sarcoma. Cancer 1979;44:2362–2365.
35. Storm HH, Olsen J. Risk of breast cancer in offspring of male breast-cancer patients. Lancet 1999;353:209.
36. Hill A, Yagmur Y, Tran KN, et al. Localized male breast carcinoma and family history. An analysis of 142 patients. Cancer 1999;86:821–825.
37. Borgen PI, Wong GY, Vlamis V, et al. Current management of male breast cancer. A review of 104 cases. Ann Surg 1992;215:451–457; discussion, 57–59.
38. Salvadori B, Saccozzi R, Manzari A, et al. Prognosis of breast cancer in males: An analysis of 170 cases. Eur J Cancer 1994;30A:930–935.
39. Cutuli B, Lacroze M, Dilhuydy JM, et al. Male breast cancer: Results of the treatments and prognostic factors in 397 cases. Eur J Cancer 1995;31A:1960–1964.
40. Stierer M, Rosen H, Weitensfelder W, et al. Male breast cancer: Austrian experience. World J Surg 1995;19:687–692; discussion, 92–93.

41. Basham VM, Lipscombe JM, Ward JM, et al. BRCA1 and BRCA2 mutations in a population-based study of male breast cancer. Breast Cancer Res 2002;4:R2.
42. Veeramasuneni R, Wagner M, Riley L, et al. Male breast cancer: A marker for secondary and familial neoplasms. Breast J 2002;8:258–259.
43. Hemminki K, Vaittinen P. Male breast cancer: Risk to daughters. Lancet 1999;353:1186–1187.
44. Rosenblatt KA, Thomas DB, McTiernan A, et al. Breast cancer in men: Aspects of familial aggregation. J Natl Cancer Inst 1991;83:849–854.
45. Zumoff B, Fishman J, Cassouto J, et al. Estradiol transformation in men with breast cancer. J Clin Endocrinol Metab 1966;26:960–966.
46. Dao TL, Morreal C, Nemoto T. Urinary estrogen excretion in men with breast cancer. N Engl J Med 1973;289:138–140.
47. Scheike O, Svenstrup B, Frandsen VA. Male breast cancer. II. Metabolism of oestradiol-17 beta in men with breast cancer. J Steroid Biochem 1973;4:489–501.
48. Ballerini P, Recchione C, Cavalleri A, et al. Hormones in male breast cancer. Tumori 1990;76:26–28.
49. Evans DB, Crichlow RW. Carcinoma of the male breast and Klinefelter's syndrome: Is there an association? CA Cancer J Clin 1987;37:246–251.
50. Scheike O, Visfeldt J, Petersen B. Male breast cancer. 3. Breast carcinoma in association with the Klinefelter syndrome. Acta Pathol Microbiol Scand [A] 1973;81:352–358.
51. Kelsey JL. A review of the epidemiology of human breast cancer. Epidemiol Rev 1979;1:74–109.
52. Wanebo CK, Johnson KG, Sato K, et al. Breast cancer after exposure to the atomic bombings of Hiroshima and Nagasaki. N Engl J Med 1968;279:667–671.
53. Goss PE, Reid C, Pintilie M, et al. Male breast carcinoma: A review of 229 patients who presented to the Princess Margaret Hospital during 40 years: 1955–1996. Cancer 1999;85:629–639.
54. Daniels IR, Layer GT. Gynaecomastia. Eur J Surg 2001;167:885–892.
55. Heller KS, Rosen PP, Schottenfeld D, et al. Male breast cancer: A clinicopathologic study of 97 cases. Ann Surg 1978;188:60–65.
56. Scheike O, Visfeldt J. Male breast cancer. 4. Gynecomastia in patients with breast cancer. Acta Pathol Microbiol Scand [A] 1973;81:359–365.
57. Olsson H, Bladstrom A, Alm P. Male gynecomastia and risk for malignant tumours—a cohort study. BMC Cancer 2002;2:26.
58. Lilleng R, Paksoy N, Vural G, et al. Assessment of fine needle aspiration cytology and histopathology for diagnosing male breast masses. Acta Cytol 1995;39:877–881.
59. Tirkkonen M, Kainu T, Loman N, et al. Somatic genetic alterations in BRCA2-associated and sporadic male breast cancer. Genes Chromosomes Cancer 1999;24:56–61.
60. Ojopi EP, Cavalli LR, Cavalieri LM, et al. Comparative genomic hybridization analysis of benign and invasive male breast neoplasms. Cancer Genet Cytogenet 2002;134:123–126.
61. Serra Diaz C, Vizoso F, Rodriguez JC, et al. Expression of pepsinogen C in gynecomastias and male breast carcinomas. World J Surg 1999;23:439–445.
62. Serra Diaz C, Vizoso F, Lamelas ML, et al. Expression and clinical significance of apolipoprotein D in male breast cancer and gynaecomastia. Br J Surg 1999;86:1190–1197.
63. Miki Y, Swensen J, Shattuck-Eidens D, et al. A strong candidate for the breast and ovarian cancer susceptibility gene BRCA1. Science 1994;266:66–71.
64. Wooster R, Bignell G, Lancaster J, et al. Identification of the breast cancer susceptibility gene BRCA2. Nature 1995;378:789–792.
65. Ottini L, Masala G, D'Amico C, et al. BRCA1 and BRCA2 mutation status and tumor characteristics in male breast cancer: A population-based study in Italy. Cancer Res 2003;63:342–347.
66. Frank TS, Deffenbaugh AM, Reid JE, et al. Clinical characteristics of individuals with germline mutations in BRCA1 and BRCA2: Analysis of 10,000 individuals. J Clin Oncol 2002;20:1480–1490.
67. Lynch HT, Watson P, Narod SA. The genetic epidemiology of male breast carcinoma. Cancer 1999;86:744–746.
68. Meijers-Heijboer H, van den Ouweland A, Klijn J, et al. Low-penetrance susceptibility to breast cancer due to CHEK2(*)1100delC in noncarriers of BRCA1 or BRCA2 mutations. Nat Genet 2002;31:55–59.
69. Wooster R, Mangion J, Eeles R, et al. A germline mutation in the androgen receptor gene in two brothers with breast cancer and Reifenstein syndrome. Nat Genet 1992;2:132–134.
70. Lobaccaro JM, Lumbroso S, Belon C, et al. Male breast cancer and the androgen receptor gene. Nat Genet 1993;5:109–110.
71. Young IE, Kurian KM, Annink C, et al. A polymorphism in the CYP17 gene is associated with male breast cancer. Br J Cancer 1999;81:141–143.
72. Boyd J, Rhei E, Federici MG, et al. Male breast cancer in the hereditary nonpolyposis colorectal cancer syndrome. Breast Cancer Res Treat 1999;53:87–91.
73. Fackenthal JD, Marsh DJ, Richardson AL, et al. Male breast cancer in Cowden syndrome patients with germline PTEN mutations. J Med Genet 2001;38:159–164.
74. Lefor AT, Numann PJ. Carcinoma of the breast in men. N Y State J Med 1988;88:293–296.
75. Siddiqui T, Weiner R, Moreb J, et al. Cancer of the male breast with prolonged survival. Cancer 1988;62:1632–1636.
76. Joshi MG, Lee AK, Loda M, et al. Male breast carcinoma: An evaluation of prognostic factors contributing to a poorer outcome. Cancer 1996;77:490–498.
77. Yildirim E, Berberoglu U. Male breast cancer: A 22-year experience. Eur J Surg Oncol 1998;24:548–552.
78. Donegan WL, Redlich PN, Lang PJ, et al. Carcinoma of the breast in males: A multiinstitutional survey. Cancer 1998;83:498–509.
79. Vetto J, Jun SY, Paduch D, et al. Stages at presentation, prognostic factors, and outcome of breast cancer in males. Am J Surg 1999;177:379–383.
80. Izquierdo MA, Alonso C, De Andres L, et al. Male breast cancer. Report of a series of 50 cases. Acta Oncol 1994;33:767–771.
81. El Omari-Alaoui H, Lahdiri I, Nejjar I, et al. Male breast cancer. A report of 71 cases. Cancer Radiother 2002;6:349–351.
82. Gupta S, Khanna NN, Khanna S. Paget's disease of the male breast: A clinicopathologic study and a collective review. J Surg Oncol 1983;22:151–156.
83. Ouriel K, Lotze MT, Hinshaw JR. Prognostic factors of carcinoma of the male breast. Surg Gynecol Obstet 1984;159:373–376.
84. Spence RA, MacKenzie G, Anderson JR, et al. Long-term survival following cancer of the male breast in Northern Ireland. A report of 81 cases. Cancer 1985;55:648–652.
85. Guinee VF, Olsson H, Moller T, et al. The prognosis of breast cancer in males. A report of 335 cases. Cancer 1993;71:154–161.
86. Siddiqui MT, Zakowski MF, Ashfaq R, et al. Breast masses in males: Multi-institutional experience on fine-needle aspiration. Diagn Cytopathol 2002;26:87–91.
87. Sund BS, Topstad TK, Nesland JM. A case of juvenile papillomatosis of the male breast. Cancer 1992;70:126–128.
88. Sara AS, Gottfried MR. Benign papilloma of the male breast following chronic phenothiazine therapy. Am J Clin Pathol 1987;87:649–650.
89. Martinez-Onsurbe P, Fuentes-Vaamonde E, Gonzalez-Estecha A, et al. Neurilemoma of the breast in a man. A case report. Acta Cytol 1992;36:511–513.
90. Shousha S, Theodorou NA, Bull TB. Cavernous haemangioma of breast in a man with contralateral gynaecomastia and a family history of breast carcinoma. Histopathology 1988;13:221–223.
91. Ansah-Boateng Y, Tavassoli FA. Fibroadenoma and cystosarcoma phyllodes of the male breast. Mod Pathol 1992;5:114–116.
92. Boger A. Benign spindle cell tumor of the male breast. Pathol Res Pract 1984;178:395–399.
93. Mariscal A, Perea RJ, Castella E, et al. Granular cell tumor of the breast in a male patient. AJR Am J Roentgenol 1995;165:63–64.
94. Allison JG, Dodds HM. Leiomyoma of the male nipple. A case report and literature review. Am Surg 1989;55:501–502.
95. Gill IS. Carcinoid tumour of the male breast. J R Soc Med 1990;83:401.
96. Allen FJ, Van Velden DJ. Prostate carcinoma metastatic to the male breast. Br J Urol 1991;67:434–435.
97. Evans GF, Anthony T, Turnage RH, et al. The diagnostic accuracy of mammography in the evaluation of male breast disease. Am J Surg 2001;181:96–100.
98. Gunhan-Bilgen I, Bozkaya H, Ustun EE, Memis A. Male breast disease: Clinical, mammographic, and ultrasonographic features. Eur J Radiol 2002;43:246–255.
99. Dershaw DD. Male mammography. AJR Am J Roentgenol 1986;146:127–131.
100. Yang WT, Whitman GJ, Yuen EH, et al. Sonographic features of primary breast cancer in men. AJR Am J Roentgenol 2001;176:413–416.
101. Westenend PJ, Jobse C. Evaluation of fine-needle aspiration cytology of breast masses in males. Cancer 2002;96:101–104.

102. Joshi A, Kapila K, Verma K. Fine needle aspiration cytology in the management of male breast masses. Nineteen years of experience. Acta Cytol 1999;43:334–338.

103. Sanchez AG, Villanueva AG, Redondo C. Lobular carcinoma of the breast in a patient with Klinefelter's syndrome. A case with bilateral, synchronous, histologically different breast tumors. Cancer 1986;57:1181–1183.

104. Friedman MA, Hoffman PG Jr, Dandolos EM, et al. Estrogen receptors in male breast cancer: Clinical and pathologic correlations. Cancer 1981;47:134–137.

105. Sandler B, Carman C, Perry RR. Cancer of the male breast. Am Surg 1994;60:816–820.

106. Slamon DJ, Clark GM, Wong SG, et al. Human breast cancer: Correlation of relapse and survival with amplification of the HER-2/neu oncogene. Science 1987;235:177–182.

107. Wang-Rodriguez J, Cross K, Gallagher S, et al. Male breast carcinoma: Correlation of ER, PR, Ki-67, Her2-Neu, and p53 with treatment and survival, a study of 65 cases. Mod Pathol 2002;15:853–861.

108. Pich A, Margaria E, Chiusa L. Oncogenes and male breast carcinoma: c-erbB-2 and p53 coexpression predicts a poor survival. J Clin Oncol 2000;18:2948–2956.

109. Rudlowski C, Rath W, Becker AJ, et al. Trastuzumab and breast cancer. N Engl J Med 2001;345:997–998.

110. Gough DB, Donohue JH, Evans MM, et al. A 50-year experience of male breast cancer: Is outcome changing? Surg Oncol 1993;2:325–333.

111. Port ER, Fey JV, Cody HS 3rd, et al. Sentinel lymph node biopsy in patients with male breast carcinoma. Cancer 2001;91:319–323.

112. Overgaard M, Hansen PS, Overgaard J, et al. Postoperative radiotherapy in high-risk premenopausal women with breast cancer who receive adjuvant chemotherapy. Danish Breast Cancer Cooperative Group 82b Trial. N Engl J Med 1997;337:949–955.

113. Chakravarthy A, Kim CR. Post-mastectomy radiation in male breast cancer. Radiother Oncol 2002;65:99–103.

114. Stranzl H, Mayer R, Quehenberger F, et al. Adjuvant radiotherapy in male breast cancer. Radiother Oncol 1999;53:29–35.

115. Schuchardt U, Seegenschmiedt MH, Kirschner MJ, et al. Adjuvant radiotherapy for breast carcinoma in men: A 20-year clinical experience. Am J Clin Oncol 1996;19:330–336.

116. Farrow JH AF. Effect of orchidectomy on skeletal metastases from cancer of the male breast. Science 1942;95:654.

117. Griffith H MF. Male breast cancer: Update on systemic therapy. Rev Endocr Related Cancer 1989;31:5–11.

118. Patel JK, Nemoto T, Dao TL. Metastatic breast cancer in males. Assessment of endocrine therapy. Cancer 1984;53:1344–1346.

119. Osborne CK. Tamoxifen in the treatment of breast cancer. N Engl J Med 1998;339:1609–1618.

120. Ribeiro G, Swindell R. Adjuvant tamoxifen for male breast cancer (MBC). Br J Cancer 1992;65:252–254.

121. Tirelli U, Tumolo S, Talamini R, et al. Tamoxifen before and after orchiectomy in advanced male breast cancer. Cancer Treat Rep 1982;66:1882–1883.

122. Anelli TF, Anelli A, Tran KN, et al. Tamoxifen administration is associated with a high rate of treatment-limiting symptoms in male breast cancer patients. Cancer 1994;74:74–77.

123. Giordano SH, Valero V, Buzdar AU, et al. Efficacy of anastrozole in male breast cancer. Am J Clin Oncol 2002;25:235–237.

124. Doberauer C, Niederle N, Schmidt CG. Advanced male breast cancer treatment with the LH-RH analogue buserelin alone or in combination with the antiandrogen flutamide. Cancer 1988;62:474–478.

125. Lopez M. Cyproterone acetate in the treatment of metastatic cancer of the male breast. Cancer 1985;55:2334–2336.

126. Lopez M, Di Lauro L, Lazzaro B, et al. Hormonal treatment of disseminated male breast cancer. Oncology 1985;42:345–349.

127. Bagley CS, Wesley MN, Young RC, et al. Adjuvant chemotherapy in males with cancer of the breast. Am J Clin Oncol 1987;10:55–60.

128. Patel HZ 2nd, Buzdar AU, Hortobagyi GN. Role of adjuvant chemotherapy in male breast cancer. Cancer 1989;64:1583–1585.

129. Ciatto S, Iossa A, Bonardi R, et al. Male breast carcinoma: Review of a multicenter series of 150 cases. Coordinating Center and Writing Committee of FONCAM (National Task Force for Breast Cancer), Italy. Tumori 1990;76:555–558.

130. Donegan WL, Redlich PN. Breast cancer in men. Surg Clin North Am 1996;76:343–363.

131. Willsher PC, Leach IH, Ellis IO, et al. A comparison outcome of male breast cancer with female breast cancer. Am J Surg 1997;173:185–188.

132. Digenis AG, Ross CB, Morrison JG, et al. Carcinoma of the male breast: A review of 41 cases. South Med J 1990;83:1162–1167.

133. Anelli A, Anelli TF, Youngson B, et al. Mutations of the p53 gene in male breast cancer. Cancer 1995;75:2233–2238.

CHAPTER 37

Gynecologic Management of the Woman with Breast Cancer

John P. Curtin and Steven R. Goldstein

For many women, their gynecologist acts as the primary care physician and as such may be directly involved in the screening, diagnosis, and follow-up of women with breast cancer. The current residency competencies expectations include both didactic and clinical training in the teaching of breast self-examination, the principles of breast examination, workup of an abnormal breast examination, and knowledge of breast cancer treatment options. As discussed in the section of this chapter on selective estrogen receptor modulators (SERMs), gynecologists may also play a critical role in identification and management of preventive medications designed to reduce the overall incidence of breast cancer. This role has been embraced and promoted by the American College of Obstetricians and Gynecologists (ACOG). The ACOG committee opinion[1] emphasizes the following:

· Performance of breast examination, which is an integral part of the complete gynecologic examination
· Instructing patients in the technique of breast self-examination
· Ordering screening mammography
· Recognition that certain patients may be at higher risk because of family history
· Performance of breast diagnostic procedures when indicated

An ever-increasing role for the gynecologists is to provide expertise in the follow-up of women who have been diagnosed with breast cancer. As discussed in previous chapters, the number of cases of breast cancer has increased dramatically over the past 2 decades. With more than 200,000 new cases of breast cancer diagnosed in the United States annually and the majority of new cases now involving smaller lesions owing to increased awareness and improved screening, the number of women who report a history of breast cancer will continue to increase. These patients often have specific gynecologic problems and concerns related to their history of breast cancer or the treatment effects, and there is the continued need for routine gynecologic care.

GYNECOLOGIC CARE FOR THE PATIENT WITH BREAST CANCER

When should a patient consult with her gynecologist?

Patients should maintain their routine schedule for gynecologic examination during and after the diagnosis of breast cancer. A yearly gynecologic examination that includes at a minimum a review of medical history and focused examination should be done. The gynecologist must be sure to include a discussion of any acute changes following the treatment, including issues related to menopause, sexuality, and depression.[2] Young patients who continue to menstruate should be asked about future pregnancy plans and current contraception plans.[3] For postmenopausal women or for those women who become menopausal during treatment, the most common questions involve issues of depression, sexuality, and management of menopausal symptoms. Although many young premenopausal women become amenorrheic during cytotoxic chemotherapy, the patient and physician should not assume that the patient will not regain her fertility potential after completion of chemotherapy. It is critical that patients continue to use contraception if pregnancy is possible.

What are the options for contraception after diagnosis of breast cancer?

Except for rare cases, hormonal contraceptives are contraindicated for women with a history of breast cancer. This includes oral contraceptives and injectable agents such as medroxyprogesterone acetate (Depo-Provera). In discussions with the patient, the gynecologist should determine whether the patient is interested in permanent sterilization or temporary contraception. If the patient desires permanent sterilization, two options are available for the woman (vasectomy can also be considered for the partner of a patient in a monogamous relationship). The first option for the patient is tubal ligation. This method is extremely successful (fewer than 5 to 10 failures per 1000 women sterilized) and can be accomplished on an outpatient basis. An added advantage for women with a history of breast cancer is the reduction in overall risk for ovarian cancer. The risk reduction associated with tubal ligation is about a 50% reduction in breast cancer incidence, equivalent to use of oral contraceptives for 5 years or longer.[4]

Barrier contraception with condoms and spermicide or diaphragm and spermicide is the most reliable option for the patient who is not ready to commit to permanent sterilization. The success rate for barrier methods approaches that of either an intrauterine device (IUD) or oral contraceptives, provided that the patient is highly motivated and regularly uses the chosen method of contraception regularly. An IUD may be considered as an alternative to barrier contraception; the efficacy rate is excellent. Before placement of an IUD, the patient must have recovered from any chemotherapy because chemotherapy-associated neutropenia may increase the risk for an IUD-associated infection.

For those patients who are closer to menopause or have a known *BRCA* gene mutation, a second option for permanent sterilization is a risk-reducing bilateral salpingo-oophorectomy (discussed later). This procedure reduces not only the overall incidence of gynecologic cancers but also the risk for a second breast cancer.

How are menopausal symptoms managed?

The standard treatment of menopausal symptoms remains use of estrogen replacement therapy (ERT). However, this therapeutic option is often contraindicated for women who have been diagnosed with breast cancer. In the past decade, there was an increase in the number of centers that proposed ERT (either alone or in combination with a progestin) for selected individuals.[5] Studies that reviewed large population databases or small prospective trials were initiated to test the hypothesis that ERT could be safely administered to women after a diagnosis of breast cancer. However, in the past 2 years, several significant studies have been published that question the role of ERT in many women, especially those with breast cancer history. The Women's Health Initiative (WHI) has published a series of reports that have challenged the benefits and safety of ERT usage.[6] More recently, a prospective study of hormonal replacement therapy in women with a history of breast cancer (HABITS) was stopped by the data safety monitoring committee because of a higher than acceptable rate of breast cancer recurrence or new primaries in the group of patients who were randomized to hormonal replacement therapy.[7] The findings of these two studies taken together suggest that except for a rare patient who fails to respond to non-hormonal therapy, systemic ERT should not be prescribed for patients who have been diagnosed with breast cancer.

Patients who have significant hot flashes either from tamoxifen therapy or from menopause may be managed by other methods. Venlafaxine (Effexor) has been prescribed with reported success in lowering the intensity and frequency of hot flashes. The side effects can often outweigh the benefits.[8] Many patients have tried nutritional or alternative medicine remedies with relief of symptoms. Generally, the use of alternative or complementary medications is safe, although some have raised the issue of the estrogenic effect of plant estrogens or phytoestrogens. Patients should always consult

with their treating physician before embarking on regular use of these agents.

Another common quality-of-life issue for menopausal women is vaginal atrophy; the most common complaints include vaginal dryness, lack of lubrication, and discomfort with intercourse. A number of nonprescription products have been marketed for the potential relief of these symptoms. Water-soluble lubricants have been reported to improve lubrication and decrease discomfort during intercourse. Vaginal moisturizers may also reduce the complaints related to dryness.

As described, the use of systemic estrogen is contraindicated in women with a history of breast cancer; however, in selected cases, topical estrogen may be used. Newer products, such as low-dose intravaginal estradiol delivery using a Silastic vaginal ring (Estring), have been studied in patients with prior diagnosis of breast cancer and significant symptoms of vaginal atrophy.[9] These agents deliver a continuous dosage of estradiol to the vaginal epithelium. Although there is a small amount of absorption, the serum estradiol levels do not increase above the normal postmenopausal serum estradiol levels.

How does family history affect the gynecologic care of women with history of breast cancer?

As discussed in other chapters, about 5% of all breast cancers may be due to an inherited factor; in the United States, therefore, there will be about 10,000 cases of breast cancer annually owing to a hereditary syndrome.[10] The importance of early identification of patients at risk is becoming increasingly important as new prevention and screening strategies are developed. Routine genetic testing for the most common genetic mutations is not warranted for the general population. The current recommendation is that a family history of breast or gynecologic cancer in one or more first-degree relatives should trigger a more thorough evaluation. First-degree relatives include sisters or mother. Multiple cancer cases in second-degree relatives (i.e., grandmothers, aunts, uncles, and cousins) should also raise suspicion, especially when all are linked to either the maternal or paternal side of the patient's family. There are several resources available that aid the clinician in assessing whether a patient may be at higher than average risk for carrying a gene mutation commonly linked to increased susceptibility to breast or ovarian cancer.

In the general population, the prevalence of identifiable gene mutations that will place the patient at increased risk for breast cancer is small. It is estimated that only 0.1% to 0.2% of the general population carries these genetic mutations. Routine testing of all patients has not been proposed; the patient who is referred for genetic testing is usually identified by family history or when newly diagnosed with a cancer. Some authors have suggested that if there is a 5% or greater chance of a woman's being a gene mutation carrier, testing to determine the presence or absence of known gene mutations is indicated. Estimates of prevalence of gene mutations based on family and personal disease characteristics are provided in Table 37–1.

The most common gene mutations associated with an increase risk of breast cancer are *BRCA1* and *BRCA2*; less

Table 37–1 Risk of *BRCA1* and *BRCA2* Mutations in Selected Populations

Family and Personal Disease Characteristics	Prevalence of Positive Test for *BRCA1* or *BRCA2* (%)
General population	0.1–0.2
Ashkenazi Jewish	2.0–2.5
Breast cancer at age < 36 yr	10
Breast cancer at age < 50 yr	6
Breast cancer, bilateral	15
Family history of breast cancer	5–15
Family history of breast and/or ovarian cancer	10–40

commonly, mutations of mismatch repair genes associated with hereditary nonpolyposis colon cancer (HNPCC) syndrome place the patient at increased risk. Individual practitioners have the option of providing the counseling and ordering the genetic tests directly or referring the patient thought to be at risk to a genetic counselor.

Patients with a more than 10% risk for a *BRCA1* or *BRCA2* mutation include those with breast and ovarian cancer within the same family at any age, particularly if within the same woman; a history of male breast cancer within the same family; multiple cases of early-onset breast cancer disease (age < 50 years) in the same family; and the presence of bilateral breast cancers.[11]

How are patients followed once they are identified as being at risk?

Patients have three general options if they are at an increased risk for developing gynecologic cancer due to either known genetic mutation or suggestive family history.

Normal Gynecologic Care

The first option is to maintain normal gynecologic care and follow-up with no added screening studies or testing. For some women, this is acceptable and desirable. For most women, however, some additional testing or risk-reducing surgery is recommended.

Additional Screening Studies

If the patient elects to be followed and wants additional screening studies, the patient must be advised that currently there are no proven screening methods to detect early ovarian, tubal, or peritoneal cancers. Some studies have suggested that regular screening transvaginal ultrasound (TVUS) examination may detect earlier-stage ovarian cancer. Other studies have examined the utility of serum tumor markers. In the absence of a proven method, it has been recommended that patients at risk for gynecologic cancer be examined twice yearly and have TVUS one or two times per year combined with serum CA-125 determinations.

The evaluation of the patient with an abnormal imaging study should include a repeat physical examination. If the serum tumor markers were normal, a repeat and possibly expanded panel of tumor markers should be obtained. In general, there should be a lower threshold for surgical intervention when the patient has a prior diagnosis of *BRCA* mutation. Although patients with *BRCA* mutation are at risk for developing metastatic disease involving the ovaries, in retrospective series of patients undergoing surgery for newly discovered ovarian mass, new gynecologic primary cancers are more common than metastatic disease.[12]

Given the lack of established screening methods, patients should be encouraged to enroll in prospective screening studies. These ongoing screening studies will hopefully clarify the emerging role of new serum testing as well as study the role of ultrasound evaluation.[13]

Risk-Reducing Surgery

Another option for patients at risk is to have a surgical procedure to remove the organs at risk. Because patients with *BRCA1* or *BRCA2* mutation are at risk for ovarian, tubal, and peritoneal primary cancer, surgery can reduce but not eliminate the potential for future *BRCA1*- or *BRCA2*-associated cancer.[14] This recognition has resulted in a change in terminology that more accurately conveys the intent of the surgical procedure. Instead of a "prophylactic" bilateral salpingo-oophorectomy, the preferred term should be "risk-reducing." The decrease in risk is difficult to calculate exactly, but data from clinical reports as well as from risk modeling suggest that the reduction in risk is greater than 90%[15] (Fig. 37–1). This can be translated for the *BRCA1*-positive patient into the reduction from a 30% lifetime risk for ovarian, tubal, or peritoneal cancer to a less than 3% risk for peritoneal cancer after risk-reducing salpingo-oophorectomy.

When the decision is made to proceed with a risk-reducing salpingo-oophorectomy (RRSO), this can usually be performed as a laparoscopic procedure. The laparoscopic approach has the advantage of minimal discomfort and can be performed as an outpatient procedure. There is some debate as to whether removal of the uterus is indicated as part of the risk-reducing surgery. It is our practice not to perform routine hysterectomy at the time of the RRSO unless there is specific uterine pathology. Others have advocated for inclusion of hysterectomy at the time of RRSO because of the potential association of papillary serous endometrial carcinoma of the uterus with *BRCA1* and *BRCA2*.[16] Other authors have postulated that any laparoscopic procedure removing only the tubes and ovaries would leave behind a small portion of the fallopian tube where the tube traverses the cornual region of the uterus.

Before the RRSO, the patient should be examined and have a recent TVUS and serum CA-125. Even if these tests are normal, there is still a small chance that at the time of the laparoscopic procedure, a small, clinically occult ovarian cancer will be discovered. A critical part of the consent process should include a discussion of the extent of surgery that the patient agrees to as well as the surgical capability of the surgeon. Processing of the specimen by the pathologist is also important, and the surgeon should communicate directly with the pathologist regarding the indications for RRSO.

The procedure is performed using a three- or four-trocar approach. The patient is placed under general anesthesia and laparoscopy initiated. It is our preference to use an open laparoscopic approach in all cases. After establishment of the pneumoperitoneum, a thorough inspection of the entire

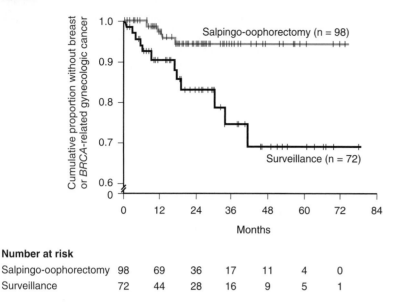

Figure 37–1   Prospective study of two cohorts of women at risk for breast cancers or gynecologic cancers related to *BCRA*. The number of women diagnosed with either gynecologic or breast cancer was significantly reduced for those patients who elected to undergo a risk-reducing salpingo-oophorectomy.   (Data from Kauff ND, Satagopan JM, Robson ME, et al. Risk-reducing salpingo-oophorectomy in women with a BRCA1 or BRCA2 mutation. N Engl J Med 2002;23;346:1609–1615.)

Number at risk

Salpingo-oophorectomy	98	69	36	17	11	4	0
Surveillance	72	44	28	16	9	5	1

abdomen is performed. This includes the peritoneal surfaces of the diaphragm and liver as well as the pelvis.

Rather than the typical pathologic examination of bilateral salpingo-oophorectomy specimens, the RRSO should be submitted to the pathologist in its entirety, with multiple sections obtained. Protocols for processing of these specimens have been published.[17]

Surveillance after RRSO is uncertain. Several reports have estimated that primary peritoneal papillary serous (PPPS) carcinoma following RRSO may be as high as 1 in 20 patients (5%). There are no accepted screening tests for these cancers; current ongoing studies are following patients with serial serum CA-125 determinations. There is no role for routine imaging studies such as ultrasound or computed tomography (CT) scans. As would be expected, most have a clinical presentation similar to that of epithelial ovarian carcinoma (EOC). The majority are stage III at the time of diagnosis. When the diagnosis is suspected, the workup should include CT scan imaging. Treatment is similar to that for EOC. The standard treatment includes initial surgical staging and debulking, followed by combination chemotherapy with carboplatin and paclitaxel.

Are additional gynecologic tests necessary when a patient has a history of breast cancer?

Unless the patient has specific complaints, the annual physical examination is sufficient. Patients should be followed with regular cervical cytology according to their own history and risk profile. The ACOG and the American Cancer Society have updated the cervical cytology screening recommendations. After age 30 years, patients who have had normal yearly Papanicolaou (Pap) smears can be followed with Pap smears every 2 to 3 years. Combining human papillomavirus testing with a Pap smear may allow for longer intervals between Pap smears, provided that both of the tests are normal. Patients do not appear to benefit from routine ultrasound examination or endometrial biopsy if on tamoxifen therapy.[18]

When do patients need to be concerned about tamoxifen-associated cancer?

In nearly all cases, endometrial cancer is associated with early warning signs. The most common sign is abnormal bleeding. For younger women, who may be menstruating normally, concerning changes could include periods that are heavier than usual or bleeding between periods. For postmenopausal patients, any vaginal bleeding should be a signal to both the patient and the physician that further evaluation is indicated. In addition, a persistent discharge should also be evaluated.

The most common reported cancer in patients taking tamoxifen is adenocarcinoma of the endometrium. This cancer is commonly associated with hyperestrogen states, including obesity, and unopposed estrogen replacement therapy. The risk for a tamoxifen-associated cancer depends on length of treatment.[19] After 5 years of tamoxifen therapy, the risk for endometrial cancer is about 6 cases per 1000 women. Although this is an increase in the expected rate of endometrial cancer, it is important to remember the significant role of tamoxifen in reducing the chance of a second breast cancer or a recurrence of breast cancer. Most studies have shown that the cancers associated with tamoxifen are similar to other estrogen-associated cancers in that the cancers tend to be low-grade, early-stage cancers confined to the uterus.[20] These types of tumors are generally cured by surgery alone.

Less commonly, tamoxifen is associated with rare uterine tumors known as *uterine sarcoma*. Based on a series of case reports in the literature, in 2002, the U.S. Food and Drug Administration (FDA) added information to the tamoxifen label advising patients and their physicians that tamoxifen usage can be associated with an increased risk for uterine sarcoma. In a trial of more than 8000 women with an intact uterus who were randomized to either tamoxifen or a placebo, there were a total of 70 cases of endometrial adenocarcinoma; 53 cases of endometrial cancer occurred in the tamoxifen-treated patients, and 17 cases occurred in the placebo group. There were 4 cases of uterine sarcoma in the group of more than 8000 women; however, all 4 cases occurred in women who received tamoxifen.[21] It is important to remember that these tumors are rare and that the increased risk associated with tamoxifen, although significant, is still quite low. The symptoms of uterine sarcoma are similar to those of the more common adenocarcinoma. Unfortunately, uterine sarcomas can be more difficult to treat. Uterine sarcomas are more commonly spread beyond the uterus at the time of diagnosis, and the overall mortality rate is higher for uterine sarcomas than for adenocarcinomas of the uterus.

How should abnormal vaginal bleeding be evaluated?

The patient is usually examined in the office. If the patient has not had cervical cytology testing within the past year, a specimen is obtained. Any cervical abnormalities should be noted; if noted, a biopsy can be performed if necessary. In most patients, an endometrial biopsy is performed in the office. The preferred instrument is a small flexible suction biopsy instrument similar to the Pipelle device. For most patients, this procedure is associated with mild cramping, which can be minimized by giving the patient a nonsteroidal anti-inflammatory drug (NSAID) just before the procedure. When the biopsy is performed, the size of the uterus as well as the amount of tissue obtained (i.e., minimal versus abundant) should be noted. An endocervical biopsy may be omitted during the initial evaluation, but in the patient with persistent bleeding, this should be performed to rule out an endocervical lesion.

When the endometrial biopsy cannot be obtained in the office, consideration should be given to performing a dilation and curettage (D&C) under anesthesia. Indications for a D&C would include persistent bleeding or progressive growth in the thickness of the endometrium. The D&C is considered to be the best diagnostic procedure for patients with either persistent abnormal bleeding or postmenopausal bleeding. Many practitioners will also perform a hysteroscopy at the same time to better visualize the endometrium.

Ultrasound may be helpful in triaging patients, especially postmenopausal patients. If ultrasound demonstrates a thin endometrium with no areas of thickening or polyps, then close follow-up may be an alternative to D&C. As discussed later, sonohysterography may be an important diagnostic aid in the evaluation of the patient taking tamoxifen who is symptomatic. The interval for follow-up should be about 3 months.

GYNECOLOGIC EFFECTS OF SELECTIVE ESTROGEN RECEPTOR MODULATORS (SERMs)

SERMs are synthetic compounds that bind to estrogen receptors and exert estrogen-agonistic effects in some tissues (i.e., bone, lipid) while being estrogen antagonists in other tissues (i.e., breast). Currently, two SERMs, tamoxifen and toremifene, are employed for treatment of breast cancer; tamoxifen is also FDA approved for prevention of breast cancer in high-risk women. Raloxifene is a SERM approved for

prevention and treatment of osteoporosis in postmenopausal women. However, it sharply reduced invasive and noninvasive breast cancer in women with osteoporosis during 4 years of therapy compared with placebo[22] and is currently being studied in a head-to-head comparison with tamoxifen in high-risk women (the Study of Tamoxifen and Raloxifene [STAR] trial). Other SERMs have had phase III trials suspended because of an increase in urinary incontinence and uterine prolapse.[23] Still other SERMs are in various stages of development. It appears that the gynecologic effects of SERMs are variable but obviously important in determining their utility for treatment or prevention of breast cancer.

Tamoxifen

Tamoxifen was the first clinically available SERM. Originally, it was referred to as "antiestrogen" because of its properties in the breast. Like other SERMs, it also exerts an antiresorptive effect on bone, thus improving bone mineral density in postmenopausal women as well as lowering total and low-density-lipoprotein cholesterol. It was developed in 1966 and FDA approved in 1978. It is the most widely prescribed anticancer drug in the world, currently with more than 12,000,000 woman-years of experience. It results in significant improvement in recurrence-free and overall survival rates in postmenopausal women with breast cancer.[24] In the middle to late 1980s, a series of letters to the editor and case reports started to suggest an association between endometrial carcinoma and breast cancer patients receiving tamoxifen.[25,26]

What is the evidence that tamoxifen causes endometrial abnormalities?

The first prospective study was published in 1990 by Neven and colleagues.[27] They reported on 16 patients followed prospectively with hysteroscopy for 36 months. Eight of these postmenopausal patients maintained the atrophic, inactive endometrium that one would expect in such postmenopausal patients. Seven developed proliferation, including four polyps, and one developed adenocarcinoma.

Gal and associates[28] reported on 38 patients who were followed prospectively for just 12 months. Eighteen percent (7 patients) developed hyperplasia, causing the authors to recommend "periodic blind endometrial sampling."

What is the role of transvaginal ultrasound?

At about the same time, TVUS had been introduced. The vaginal probe was employed in a variety of clinical settings. One early publication[29] described the use of TVUS before endometrial sampling in patients with postmenopausal bleeding. The maintenance of a thin distinct endometrial echo thinner than 5 mm was uniformly associated with lack of significant tissue (Fig. 37–2). Screening with TVUS has become the mainstay of current therapy in postmenopausal women with bleeding. A thin distinct endometrial echo has an extremely high negative predictive value (99%), and such patients can avoid endometrial sampling and its expense, discomfort, and risk.[30]

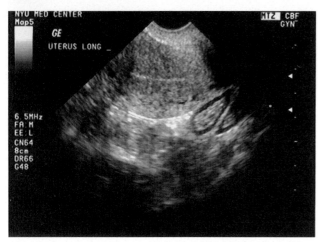

Figure 37–2   Long-axis transvaginal ultrasound view of a post-menopausal patient with bleeding. This thin distinct endometrial echo has a 99% negative predictive value in excluding significant tissue.

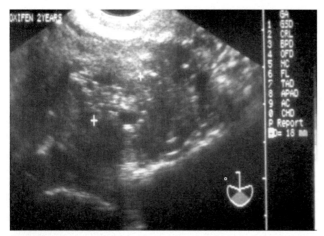

Figure 37–3   Transvaginal long-axis ultrasound view of a tamoxifen-treated patient. The central uterine echo measures 18 mm. Previously, a picture like this was misinterpreted as "endometrial" thickening.

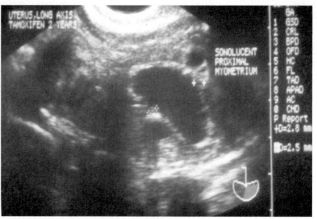

Figure 37–4   Same patient as in Figure 37–3 when viewed with saline infusion sonohysterography. The sonolucent (*black*) area centrally located is the fluid that has been instilled. The endometrium surrounding the fluid is thin, compatible with inactive atrophic change. The small sonolucencies under the surface epithelium represent microcystic change and are dilated atrophic cystic glands in the basalis of the endometrium and the proximal myometrium. The endometrium is outlined by calipers and is thin, measuring 2.8- and 2.5-mm, respectively.

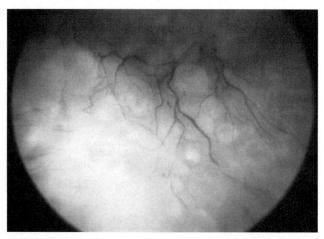

Figure 37–5   Hysteroscopy of the patient whose transvaginal ultrasound is pictured in Figure 37–4. Notice that the surface functionalis of the endometrium is thin and pale, compatible with atrophy. Coarse vessels are also typical of atrophic changes. There are noticeable blebs compatible with the microcystic change seen on ultrasound.

As a result of the newly discovered association of endometrial carcinoma and tamoxifen therapy, many tamoxifen patients were examined with TVUS. An unusual ultrasonographic appearance of the uterus in patients receiving tamoxifen was first reported in 1994.[31] Some patients displayed bizarre heterogenous echo patterns centrally located in the uterus, which represent a loss of the normal junctional zone between the basalis of the endometrium and the proximal myometrium. This was being misinterpreted as endometrial thickening on ultrasound. When viewed with saline infusion sonohysterography, such changes are often shown to be microcysts, which represent dilated cystic atrophic glands that can be located in the basalis of the endometrium, in the proximal myometrium, or even within polyps (Figs. 37–3 to 37–5).

A collective experience with tamoxifen was published by Schwartz and colleagues in 1998,[32] who found a 27% incidence of polyp formation, a 4% incidence of carcinoma, and a 9% incidence of proliferation or hyperplasia. Only 25% of tamoxifen patients maintained a thin endometrial echo 5 mm or smaller, although ultimately 59% of patients demonstrated atrophic endometrium but often required sonohysterography to prove it. In that report, a surveillance algorithm of patients receiving tamoxifen therapy was proposed. Unenhanced TVUS was performed. If the endometrial echo remained thin and distinct, measuring 5 mm or less, inactive atrophic endometrium was assumed, and follow-up was undertaken at appropriate intervals. If the central uterine echoes were thickened, the patient was interrogated with saline infusion sonohysterography. If there was thin endometrium surrounding the fluid and less than 3-mm single-layer measurements, with or without microcystic change, the patient was deemed to have inactive atrophic endometrium and followed at appropriate intervals, whereas any abnormal endometrial findings,

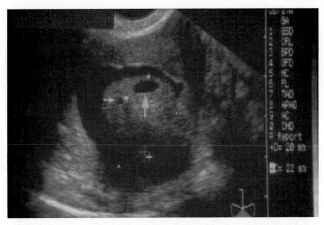

Figure 37–6   Saline infusion sonohysterogram of a tamoxifen-treated patient. A large centrally located polyp is seen. Small areas of microcystic change are seen within the polyp (*arrows*). The endometrium surrounding the fluid is thin, compatible with atrophy.

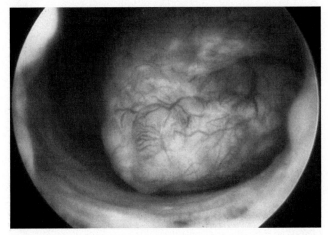

Figure 37–7   Operative hysteroscopy of the patient in Figure 37–6. Notice that the large tamoxifen-induced polyp has a similar surface appearance to that in the patient depicted in Figure 37–5.

more than 3-mm single-layer endometrial thickness, or focal lesions such as polyps were evaluated under direct vision by hysterography (Figs. 37–6 and 37–7).

Should tamoxifen patients have ongoing endometrial surveillance?

In 1996, the Gynecologic Practice Committee of the ACOG issued an opinion relative to tamoxifen and endometrial cancer,[33] in which they stated,

Women with breast cancer should have annual gynecologic examinations, including Pap test and bimanual rectal vaginal examinations. Any abnormal bleeding, including bloody discharge, spotting, or any other gynecologic symptoms should be evaluated thoroughly. Any bleeding or spotting should be investigated. Practitioners should be alert to the increased incidence of endometrial malignancy. Screening procedures or diagnostic test should be performed at the discretion of the individual gynecologist.

However, in April 2000, the same gynecologic practice committee altered its opinion.[34] At that point, they stated that

. . . because screening tests have not been effective in increasing the early detection of endometrial cancer in women using tamoxifen and may lead to more invasive and costly diagnostic procedures they are not recommended.

Is there a role for pretreatment screening?

This controversy about appropriate endometrial monitoring and surveillance of breast cancer patients treated with tamoxifen needs to be reexamined in light of research published by Berliere and coworkers.[35] Their initial publication involved 264 postmenopausal women with newly diagnosed breast cancer. They all had baseline TVUS. If the endometrial echo was larger than 4 mm, outpatient hysteroscopy with biopsy was performed. Seventeen percent of these asymptomatic postmenopausal women had baseline lesions (almost entirely polyps). All polyps were removed, and all patients were treated with tamoxifen. The incidence of atypical hyperplasia was significantly higher in the group that was abnormal initially and then treated ($P = .009$). Berliere's group updated their data several years later.[36] At that point, 575 patients with breast cancer had been studied up to 5 years, and 16.6% had endometrial polyps before tamoxifen therapy. In the group with no initial polyps, which is referred to as "squeaky clean," 12.9% developed polyps, and 0.7% developed atypical hyperplasia. In the group that had initial polyps removed and then were treated with tamoxifen, 17.6% developed benign polyps, and 11.7% developed atypical hyperplasia. Thus, there appear to be two distinct groups of women newly diagnosed with breast cancer in the postmenopausal state: those with initial polyps and those without initial polyps. The group with initial polyps represents a high-risk group, with 18 times the risk for developing atypical hyperplasia of the endometrium on tamoxifen therapy and with 1.5 times the risk for developing benign endometrial polyps subsequently. Such systematic pretreatment screening can identify the high-risk group. These patients may require ongoing surveillance, whereas the low-risk group may not and can be followed according to the ACOG Gynecologic Practice Committee Opinion.

What about SERMs and breast cancer prevention?

Breast Cancer Prevention Trial

In 1992, the National Surgical Adjuvant Breast and Bowel Project (NSABP) launched a prevention trial using tamoxifen. A total of 13,388 women aged 35 years or older who were deemed at high risk for breast cancers were enrolled at numerous sites throughout the United States and Canada. The overall incidence of breast cancer in the tamoxifen group was 3.4 cases per 1000, compared with a breast cancer incidence in the placebo group of 6.8 cases per 1000.[37] The trial was stopped 14 months before its planned completion because the Data and Safety Monitoring Board felt it was unethical to continue to allow one half of the participants, deemed to be at high risk for developing breast cancer, to continue to take placebo in view of the dramatic reduction of both invasive and noninvasive breast cancer in the tamoxifen-treated group.

Table 37–2   Black Box Warning Added to the Labeling for Tamoxifen by the FDA in 2002

NEW TAMOXIFEN LABELING: HEALTHY PATIENTS ADVERSE EVENTS				
	Tamoxifen	*Placebo*	*RR*	*CI*
Endometrial adenocarcinoma	2.2/1000 pt years	0.71/1000 pt years	Not given	
Uterine sarcoma	0.17/1000 pt years	0.00/100 pt years	Not given	
Stroke	1.43/1000 pt years	1.00/1000 pt years	1.42	(0.82–2.51)
Pulmonary embolism	0.75/1000 pt years	0.25/1000 pt years	3.01	(1.15–9.27)
BENEFICIAL EFFECTS				
Breast cancer	6.49/11000 pt years	3.38/1000 pt years	0.49	*P* < .00001

CI, confidence interval; RR, relative risk.

The trial, however, made available for the first time large-scale information about the effects of tamoxifen on healthy women. Previously, all studies of tamoxifen had been in women with breast cancer. The overall relative risk (RR) for endometrial cancer associated with tamoxifen therapy in healthy women was 2.53 (95% confidence interval [CI], 1.35%–4.97%). However, when further analyzed by age, the RR in women older than 50 years was 4.01 (95% CI, 1.70%–10.90%), whereas the RR in women aged 49 years or younger was 1.21 (95% CI, 0.41%–3.60%). Although menopausal status was not reported, this arbitrary breakdown into women younger than 50 years and older than 50 years is the closest thing to a premenopausal and postmenopausal group because the average age of menopause is 51.4 years.

In October 1998, based on these trial results, the FDA approved tamoxifen for the primary prevention of breast cancer in women at high risk for the disease. They recommended that the use of tamoxifen be limited to high-risk women because of the potentially serious side effects seen in the clinical trials, especially in women older than 50 years. The FDA did not actually determine high risk, but it made the recommendation that the decision to use tamoxifen as a prophylactic chemopreventive therapy needed to depend on a thorough evaluation of a woman's personal, family, and medical history; her age; and her understanding of the assessment of the risks and benefits of treatment.

What are the uterine effects of tamoxifen in women who do not have breast cancer?

In the NSABP's prevention trial, there were 15 cases of endometrial cancer in the placebo group.[37] Fourteen of these were revealed to be International Federation of Gynecology and Obstetrics (FIGO) stage I, and one was revealed to be FIGO stage 4. All 36 cases of endometrial carcinoma in the tamoxifen group were FIGO stage I. In May 2002, updated data from the trial were presented on 8306 women with an intact uterus with a median follow-up of 6.9 years and on all those who used tamoxifen for at least 2 years.[38] It revealed adenocarcinoma in 53 cases of tamoxifen therapy (52 FIGO stage I, 1 FIGO stage III), compared with 17 cases in the placebo group (16 FIGO stage I, 1 FIGO stage IV). Furthermore, there were 4 cases of uterine sarcoma in the tamoxifen group and no cases in the placebo group. Therefore, in 2002, the FDA added a "black box warning" to the label of tamoxifen that was directed at the use of breast cancer prevention and not treatment. This warning is summarized in Table 37–2.

Raloxifene

Like tamoxifen, raloxifene is also a SERM. It is a benzothiophene derivative, unlike the triphenylethylene family from which tamoxifen is derived. Raloxifene, not unlike tamoxifen, was originally investigated as a treatment for advanced breast cancer. Preclinical studies as summarized by Hol and associates indicated that raloxifene had an antiproliferative effect on both estrogen receptor–positive mammary tumors and estrogen receptor–positive human breast cancer cell lines.[39] In the 1980s, however, a small phase II trial revealed that raloxifene had no further antitumor effects in postmenopausal women with advanced breast cancer in whom tamoxifen therapy had failed.[40] After information had surfaced about the neoplasia-inducing capabilities of tamoxifen on the uterus of postmenopausal women,[27] there was renewed interest in raloxifene.

What are the effects of raloxifene?

Raloxifene has SERM-like properties in that it has estrogen agonistic activity on bone remodeling and lipid metabolism. It was FDA approved for prevention of osteoporosis in postmenopausal women in December 1997. Its indication was extended to treatment of osteoporosis in October 1999. In terms of its effect on the endometrium of postmenopausal women when compared with placebo,[41] there were no differences in endometrial thickness, endoluminal masses, proliferation, or hyperplasia. Raloxifene did not cause endometrial hyperplasia or cancer and was not associated with vaginal bleeding or increased endometrial thickness as measured by TVUS. However, in this, the only study of raloxifene with the uterus as the primary end point, women with any endometrial abnormality were excluded from the study. The study was a

1-year trial whose objective was to "analyze uterine effects of raloxifene in a general population of postmenopausal women with a normal endometrial at baseline." By excluding women with any endometrial abnormality, this becomes a study of low-risk women. Thus, a 5% incidence of polyps in 1 year in the group taking 60 mg of raloxifene must be compared with a 12.9% incidence of polyps in Berliere's low-risk tamoxifen group,[36] which had an average follow-up of more than 2 years (range, 1 to 5 years). The lack of any hyperplasia in the raloxifene group and the 2% incidence in the placebo group in this raloxifene uterine safety study needs to be compared with the 0.7% hyperplasia in the Berliere data. Thus, the utility of this uterine safety study with raloxifene may be diminished. Still, at 1 year in those women with a clean endometrium to begin with, there was no estrogen-like effect, and raloxifene did not behave significantly differently from placebo.

The published results from the Multiple Outcomes of Raloxifene Evaluation (MORE) trial provide a "real-world" experience with raloxifene in the endometrium.[42] There was no pretreatment selection. After 4 years, the RR of endometrial carcinoma with raloxifene compared with placebo was 0.91 (95% CI, 0.31%–2.70%). The only comparator for tamoxifen in women not already diagnosed with breast cancer was the RR of 4.01 (95% CI, 1.7%–10.90%) in the women older than 50 years in the NSABP prevention trial. Thus, any concerns about raloxifene in the endometrium brought by the uterine safety study, excluding the seemingly high-risk patients, are easily quelled by the real-world data comparing the MORE trial and the NSABP prevention trial.

What are other gynecologic effects of SERMs?

Pelvic Organ Prolapse and Urinary Incontinence

Levormeloxifene was a SERM developed by Novo Nordisk (Princeton, NJ) for the purpose of treatment and prevention of postmenopausal osteoporosis. Structurally, it is related to ormeloxifene used in India as an oral contraceptive under the name Centhroman since the 1980s. In 1998, levormeloxifene was in phase III trials that were suspended after 10 months because of adverse events that were mainly gynecologic but also gastrointestinal and genitourinary.[23] The RR for uterovaginal prolapse with levormeloxifene compared with placebo was 3.44 (95% CI, 2.13%–5.56%). The RR for urinary incontinence was 4.99 (95% CI, 3.55%–7.00%). Furthermore, the RR for having an unusual ultrasound appearance, discussed above with tamoxifen, was 14.96 (95% CI, 8.60%–26.00%). Those patients reporting leukorrhea as an adverse event had a RR of 14.30 (95% CI, 9.60%–21.51%). Postmenopausal atrophy of support elements is a precipitating factor in the development of genital prolapse. It is unclear whether this is simply an aging phenomenon or related to estrogen deprivation. No randomized trials exist. The pathogenesis of pelvic organ prolapse and urinary incontinence are poorly understood. Associated factors include increased age, increased parity, smoking, obesity, and chronic obstructive pulmonary disease. Connective tissue is weakened in aging as a result of decreases in collagen content.

Neither tamoxifen nor raloxifene has been associated with pelvic floor relaxation. In a post hoc analysis based on about 7000 postmenopausal women who had an intact uterus when they entered the study, 3 years of raloxifene therapy was associated with a significant reduction in the risk for pelvic floor surgery (50%).[43] The mechanism by which SERMs affect pelvic floor relaxation is not clear. The presence of estrogen receptors in pelvic floor tissues indicates that this region is a target for estrogen and may respond to SERMs. Similar to the known effects on collagen metabolism in bone tissue, SERMs may also affect tissue remodeling in the pelvic floor.

Genital Tract

Several studies suggest that tamoxifen has estrogenic effects in the vagina. In a study comparing postmenopausal women who had breast cancer with healthy, age-matched controls, the vaginal pH in the tamoxifen-treated group was significantly lower and was comparable with the pH levels in fertile women. Two thirds of tamoxifen-treated women had well-estrogenized vaginal smears, compared with none in the control group.[44] In the NSABP prevention trial, tamoxifen was associated with an increase in vaginal discharge that caused leukorrhea that was "moderately bothersome or worse" in 29% of patients, compared with 13% in the placebo group.[37] Although the effects of raloxifene on the vaginal mucosa have not been studied directly in clinical trials, raloxifene has not been associated with symptoms related to vaginal atrophy, including vaginitis, leukorrhea, or dyspareunia.[45] Droloxifene, another triphenylethylene derivative in the tamoxifen family, has also been associated with an increase in vaginal discharge.[46]

Unusual Ultrasound Appearance

The unusual ultrasound appearance mistaken for endometrial thickness was also found in a phase II trial of levormeloxifene. In that study, 65% of all women treated with levormeloxifene had an endometrial thickness above 8 mm after 12 months, compared with 0% in the placebo group. Endometrial biopsy at 12 months, however, revealed no cancers or hyperplasias, 18% "weakly proliferative," and 59% inactive or atrophic endometrium.

Idoxifene was also found to produce a dose-related "thickening" on TVUS, although 99% of endometrial biopsy results were benign or atrophic.[47]

It is most likely that these reported increases in endometrial thickness with levormeloxifene and idoxifene are similar sonographically to the tamoxifen effect discussed earlier, although in those trials, no sonohysterography was performed.

Vasomotor Symptoms

A higher incidence of hot flashes has been reported with tamoxifen therapy than with placebo. Among postmenopausal women taking tamoxifen, 16% sought treatment for vasomotor symptoms.[48] Extremely bothersome hot flashes also were common in the tamoxifen-treated group of the NSABP trial.[37]

In an integrated analysis of five randomized placebo-controlled trials, younger, healthy postmenopausal women receiving raloxifene has a significantly higher incidence of hot flashes (25%) than those receiving placebo (18%); however, that trial excluded women with severe vasomotor symptoms.[49] Furthermore, there was no therapy difference for the severity of hot flashes or for the discontinuation of therapy because of the hot flashes. Increased incidence of hot flashes in the raloxifene treatment group was observed only during the first 6 months of therapy. In older postmenopausal women with osteoporosis, the overall incidence of hot flashes was lower but still significantly different between raloxifene (9.7%) and placebo (6.4%).[50] Hot flashes also had been associated with toremifene, idoxifene, and raloxifene, all triphenylethylene derivatives.[51-53]

Summary

SERMs have played an important role in breast cancer treatment and more recently chemoprevention. In the future, existing as well as newly developed SERMs can be expected to be important pharmacologic agents in breast cancer prevention and treatment. The gynecologic effects of such SERMs vary from compound to compound and differ in premenopausal and postmenopausal patients. Decisions for use of such agents must take into account a patient's menopausal status, presence or absence of a uterus, and risk for developing new-onset breast cancer or breast cancer recurrence.

REFERENCES

1. ACOG committee opinion. Role of the obstetrician-gynecologist in the diagnosis and treatment of breast disease. Number 186, September 1997 (replaces no. 140, June 1994). Committee on Gynecologic Practice. American College of Obstetricians and Gynecologists. Int J Gynaecol Obstet 1997;59:162–163.
2. Ganz PA, Rowland JH, Desmond K, et al. Life after breast cancer: Understanding women's health-related quality of life and sexual functioning. J Clin Oncol 1998;16:501–514.
3. Avis NE, Crawford S, Manuel J. Psychosocial problems among younger women with breast cancer. Psychooncology 2004;13:295–308.
4. Ness RB, Grisso JA, Cottreau C, et al. Factors related to inflammation of the ovarian epithelium and risk of ovarian cancer. Epidemiology 2000; 11:111–117.
5. DiSaia PJ, Brewster W. Hormone replacement therapy for survivors of breast and endometrial cancer. Curr Oncol Rep 2002;4:152–158.
6. Warren MP. A comparative review of the risks and benefits of hormone replacement therapy regimens. Am J Obstet Gynecol 2004;190:1141–1167.
7. Holmberg L, Anderson H. HABITS steering and data monitoring committees. HABITS (hormonal replacement therapy after breast cancer—is it safe?), a randomised comparison: Trial stopped. Lancet 2004;7:363:453–455.
8. Loprinzi CL, Kugler JW, Sloan JA, et al. Venlafaxine in management of hot flashes in survivors of breast cancer: A randomised controlled trial. Lancet 2000;16:356:2059–2063.
9. Pritchard KI. The role of hormone replacement therapy in women with a previous diagnosis of breast cancer and a review of possible alternatives. Ann Oncol 2001;12:301–310.
10. Lynch HT, Snyder CL, Lynch JF, et al. Hereditary breast-ovarian cancer at the bedside: Role of the medical oncologist. J Clin Oncol 2003; 21:740–753.
11. Statement of the American Society of Clinical Oncology: Genetic testing for cancer susceptibility. Adopted on February 20, 1996. J Clin Oncol 1996;14(5):1730–176; discussion, 1737–1740.
12. Curtin JP, Barakat RR, Hoskins WJ. Ovarian disease in women with breast cancer. Obstet Gynecol 1994;84:449–452.
13. Fishman DA, Bozorgi K. The scientific basis of early detection of epithelial ovarian cancer: The National Ovarian Cancer Early Detection Program (NOCEDP). Cancer Treat Res 2002;107:3–28.
14. Meijers-Heijboer H, Brekelmans C, Menke-Pluymers M, et al. Use of genetic testing and prophylactic mastectomy and oophorectomy in women with breast or ovarian cancer from families with a BRCA1 or BRCA2 mutation. J Clin Oncol 2003;21:1675–1681.

15. Kauff ND, Satagopan JM, Robson ME, et al. Risk-reducing salpingo-oophorectomy in women with a BRCA1 or BRCA2 mutation. N Engl J Med 2002;23:1609–1615.
16. Goldman NA, Restivo A, Goldberg G. Screening and primary and secondary interventions for patients at high risk for ovarian cancer. Womens Oncol Rev 2003;4:269–274.
17. Colgan TJ. Challenges in the early diagnosis and staging of fallopian-tube carcinomas associated with BRCA mutations. Int Gynecol Pathol 2003;22:109–120.
18. Barakat RR, Gilewski TA, Almadrones L. Effect of adjuvant tamoxifen on the endometrium in women with breast cancer: A prospective study using office endometrial biopsy. J Clin Oncol 2000;18:3459–3463.
19. Wickerham DL, Fisher B, Wolmark N, et al. Association of tamoxifen and uterine sarcoma. J Clin Oncol 2002;20:2758–2760.
20. Barakat RR, Wong G, Curtin JP, et al. Tamoxifen use in breast cancer patients who subsequently develop corpus cancer is not associated with a higher incidence of adverse histologic features. Gynecol Oncol 1994;55:164–168.
21. Twombly R. FDA issues warning about "new" tamoxifen risk. J Natl Cancer Inst 2002;7:1122.
22. Cauley JA, Norton L, Lippman ME, et al. Continued breast cancer risk reduction in postmenopausal women treated with raloxifene: 4-Year results from the MORE trial. Breast Cancer Res Treat 2001;65:125–124.
23. Goldstein SR, Nanavati N. Adverse events that are associated with the selective estrogen receptor modulator levormeloxifene in an aborted phase III osteoporosis treatment study. Am J Obstet Gynecol 2002;187:521–527.
24. Early Breast Cancer Trialists' Collaborative Group. Effects of tamoxifen and of cytotoxic therapy on mortality in early breast cancer: An overview of 61 randomized trials among 28,896. N Engl J Med 1988;319:1681–1692.
25. Killachy MA, Hakes TB, Pierce VK. Endometrial adenocarcinoma in breast cancer patients receiving antiestrogens. Cancer Treat Rep 1885;69:237–238.
26. Jordon VC. Tamoxifen and endometrial cancer [letter]. Lancet 1989;2:117–120.
27. Neven P, De Muylder X, Van Belle Y, et al. Hysteroscopic follow-up during tamoxifen treatment. Eur J Obstet Gynecol Reprod Biol 1990;35:235–238.
28. Gal D, Kopel S, Bashevkin M, et al. Oncogenic potential of tamoxifen on endometria of postmenopausal women with breast cancer: preliminary report. Gynecol Oncol 1991;42:120–123.
29. Goldstein SR, Nachtigall M, Snyder JR, Nachtigall L. Endometrial assessment by vaginal ultrasonography before endometrial sampling in patients with postmenopausal bleeding. Am J Obstet Gynecol 1990;163:119–123.
30. Langer RD, Pierce JJ, O'Hanlan KA, et al. Transvaginal ultrasonography compared with endometrial biopsy for the detection of endometrial disease. Postmenopausal Estrogen/Progestin Interventions Trial. N Engl J Med 1997;337(25):1792–1798.
31. Goldstein SR. Unusual ultrasonographic appearance of the uterus in patients receiving tamoxifen. Am J Obstet Gynecol 1994;170:447–451.
32. Schwartz LB, Snyder J, Horan C, et al. The use of transvaginal ultrasound and saline infusion sonohysterography for the evaluation of asymptomatic postmenopausal breast cancer patients on tamoxifen. Ultrasound Obstet Gynecol 1997;10:1–6.
33. American College of Obstetricians and Gynecologists. Tamoxifen and endometrial cancer. ACOG Committee Opinion 169. ACOG, Washington, DC, 1996.
34. American College of Obstetricians and Gynecologists. Tamoxifen and endometrial cancer. ACOG Committee Opinion 232. ACOG, Washington, DC, 2000.
35. Berliere M, Charles A, Galant C, Donnex J. Uterine side effects of tamoxifen: A need for systematic pretreatment screening. Obstet Gynecol 1998;91:40–44.
36. Berliere M, Charles A, Galant C, et al. Identification of women at high risk of developing endometrial cancer on tamoxifen. Eur J Cancer 2000;36:S35–S36
37. Fisher B, Constantino JP, Wickerham DL, et al. Tamoxifen for prevention of breast cancer: Report of the National Surgical Adjuvant Breast and Bowel Project P-1 study. J Natl Cancer Inst 1998;90:1371–1388.
38. Wickerham DL, Fisher B, Wolmark N, et al. Association of tamoxifen and uterine sarcoma. J Clin Oncol 2002;20:2758–2760.

39. Hol T, Cox MB, Bryant HU, Draper MW. Selective estrogen receptor modulators and postmenopausal women's health. J Womens Health 1997;6:523–531.
40. Buzdar AU, Marcus C, Holmes F, et al. Phase II evaluation of LY156758 in metastatic breast cancer. Oncology 1988;45:344–345.
41. Goldstein SR, Scheele WH, Rajagopalan SK, et al. A 12-month comparative study of raloxifene, estrogen, and placebo on the postmenopausal endometrium. Obstet Gynecol 2000;95:95–103.
42. Cummings SR, Eckert S, Kruger KA, et al. The effect of raloxifene on risk of breast cancer in postmenopausal women: Results from the MORE randomized trial. JAMA 1999;281:2189–2197.
43. Goldstein SR, Neven P, Zhou L, et al. Raloxifene effect on frequency of surgery for pelvic floor relaxation. Obstet Gynecol 2001;98:91–96.
44. Miodrag A, Ekelund P, Burton R, Castleden CM. Tamoxifen and partial oestrogen agonism in postmenopausal women. Age Ageing 19912;20:52–54.
45. Davies GC, Huster WJ, Lu Y, et al. Adverse events reported by postmenopausal women in controlled trials with raloxifene. Obstet Gynecol 1999;93:558–565.˙
46. Bruning PF. Droloxifene, a new anti-oestrogen in postmenopausal advanced breast cancer: Preliminary results of a double-blind dose-finding phase II trial. Eur J Cancer 1992;28A:1404–1407.
47. Fleischer AC, Wheeler JE, Yeh IT, et al. Sonographic assessment of the endometrium in osteopenic postmenopausal women treated with idoxifene. J Ultrasound Med 1999;18:503–512.
48. Loprinzi CL, Zahasky KM, Sloan JA, et al. Tamoxifen induced hot flashes. Clin Breast Cancer 2000;1:52–56.
49. Davies GC, Huster WJ, Lu Y, et al. Adverse events reported by postmenopausal women in controlled trials with raloxifene. Obstet Gynecol 1999;93:558–565.
50. Ettinger B, Black DM, Mitlak BH, et al. Reduction of vertebral fracture risk in postmenopausal women with osteoporosis treated with raloxifene: Results from a 3-year randomized clinical trial. Multiple Outcomes of Raloxifene Evaluation (MORE) Investigators. JAMA 1999;282:637.
51. Dowsett M, Dixon JM, Horgan K, et al. Antiproliferative effects of idoxifene in a placebo-controlled trial in primary human breast cancer. Clin Cancer Res 2000;6:2260–2267.
52. Haarstad H, Lonning PE, Gundersen S, et al. Influence of droloxifene on metastatic breast cancer as first-line endocrine treatment. Acta Oncol 1998;37:65–68.
53. Gershanovich M, Garin A, Baltina D, et al. A phase III comparison of two toremifene doses to tamoxifen in postmenopausal women with advanced breast cancer. Eastern European Study Group. Breast Cancer Res Treat 1997;45:251–262.

SECTION VIII

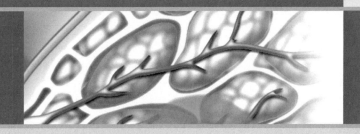

PSYCHOLOGICAL, NURSING, AND SOCIAL ISSUES

CHAPTER 38

Needs of Breast Cancer Patients and Their Families: Psychosocial Adaptation

Karen L. Weihs, Kelsey Menehan, Mary Politi, and Jane Lincoln

Care of the breast cancer patient involves preserving her quality of life as well as providing good medical care. Each health care professional contributes to the breast cancer patient's personal experience of illness and return to health through the quality of her or his relationship with the patient. When a woman with breast cancer is treated as a unique individual who can participate actively in her own care, the stage is set for an outcome that satisfies both the patient and her treatment team.

Relationships are fundamental to the patient's quality of life with breast cancer. We use the biopsychosocial model to organize our thinking about the multiple levels of relationships that influence the patient. This model presumes that the patient is part of a dynamic system through which pressures and changes reverberate and in which there are many resources for handling threats and solving problems. Awareness of the stresses and resources that emanate from each level of the system will help optimize patient care along with improving the quality of life for the patient and her family. Professional care providers are likely to enjoy making a difference in patients' overall well-being.

In this chapter, we discuss four levels within the biopsychosocial model.[1] These are the patient's relationships to (1) her body, (2) her self, (3) her family members and close significant friends, and (4) her community. Experiences at each of these levels affect the other levels and call up responses to stabilize the system. For example, the distress of the patient when she discovers that she has breast cancer and must have surgery calls up comforting and protective responses from her family members. A husband who is pained by his wife's distress might accuse her surgeon of acting too slowly or of giving incomplete information. If the surgeon understands that this is not primarily a response to himself or herself, but a misguided attempt by the husband to protect his wife, the surgeon will feel less distressed and more able to offer comfort to the husband, who may, in turn, be able to comfort his wife.

The relationships between levels of the biopsychosocial system are easily identified. Breast cancer, a change at the level of the patient's body, provokes emotional distress and alienation from her body, a change at the level of the patient's self. These changes reverberate to the level of the family, with the husband feeling a deep need to protect his wife and to vent his anger that the surgery will "damage" his wife and their sexual relationship. His reactions cannot be stabilized in the usual way within the family because of his wife's distress; therefore, the stress is directed to the next level up, the surgeon and the medical community. Clearly, the surgeon who takes the husband's attacks personally has fewer options for action than the surgeon who sees the husband as part of a powerful system, which is reacting to protect itself from threat.

More than for men, women's identity and self-esteem depend on the well-being of their family members and close friends. Conversely, changes in the family resulting from the breast cancer's impact on the patient are a major source of stress for patients. Among three measures of a patient's social support, family interaction was the strongest predictor of patients' psychological well-being in a prospective study of 661 early-stage breast cancer patients by Bloom.[2] Studies indicate that husbands also experience distress when their wives are diagnosed with breast cancer, sometimes more than their wives themselves.[3,4] When the breast cancer recurs, this phenomenon is even more salient.[3] Spousal distress can greatly affect the patient's response to breast cancer.

Thinking in terms of a cancer-related system rather than simply considering one individual with cancer allows clinicians to identify both risk factors and resources at each level of the system. For example, at the most basic cellular level, a cancer in an advanced stage with limited treatment options or a cancer with an unpredictable course is associated with higher risk to the psychological and social adjustment of the individual, and by extension her family and her broader community. However, it is not a one-way effect. The systems model presumes that high-risk characteristics at each of the other levels can also have an impact on the cellular level, perhaps accelerating the progression of the cancer or hindering recovery.

PERSONAL CONSIDERATIONS

Do psychosocial differences affect breast cancer progression?

Any formulation of cancer as a systems phenomenon necessarily raises the long-debated issue of connections between psychosocial characteristics and disease outcome. Most research on this topic has examined risk and protective factors in prospective longitudinal trials. Associations can be determined by such studies, but causal attributions cannot be made unless intervention trials demonstrate that changes in these risk and protective factors predict improved disease outcome.

The strongest evidence of a psychosocial risk factor for breast cancer progression is the patient's perception of dependable emotional support. However, results from studies that explore the role of "social support" during the year after breast cancer diagnosis as a protective factor against recurrence or mortality have been inconsistent, probably owing to variation in the definition of social support.

Studies that focus on the size of the patient's "social network," without consideration of her actual reliance on these individuals, have not found that it predicts future disease status.[5–7] In one of the strongest of these studies by Reynolds and colleagues[8] of 1011 women with newly diagnosed breast cancer, the researchers failed to find a significant effect for a measure of total contact with friends and relatives in predicting survival.

Other studies focus on functional social support, defined by the way support is used and how its recipient perceives it.[9–11] There is some evidence of improved disease outcome in association with breast cancer patients' satisfaction with support, but results of these studies are inconsistent.

Finally, some studies focus on dependable relationships, measured as the number of friends and relatives on whom the patient feels she can rely for support or help.[5,12,13] The study by Reynolds and colleagues[8] also measured the number of reliable supportive relationships by asking women about family members, friends, or other individuals with whom they could talk about the illness or about other personal problems. They found that women reporting fewer reliable supportive relationships were significantly more likely to die of breast cancer.

Dependable support from one's spouse or intimate partner has recently been shown to predict improved survival in breast cancer patients.[14] Marital status, however, is not a reliable predictor of disease outcome.[11,15]

The preponderance of evidence from studies of social support and breast cancer suggests that any protective benefit from social support is likely to be related to the patient's sense that she has dependable supportive relationships. A precise definition of social support is needed to allow an accurate assessment of its role in breast cancer progression

Very severe depressive symptoms, occurring in about 2% of breast cancer patients who meet criteria for the diagnosis of major depressive disorder, have also been linked to decreased survival.[16,17] In contrast, numerous studies find no association between normative elevations in emotional distress during the early stages of breast cancer and disease progression.[9,11,12,18–21] However, differences in the way women *process* this distress are related to differences in its duration[22] and in disease

outcome. For example, Weihs and coworkers[14] studied 79 breast cancer patients and found that coping through acceptance of emotions leads to decreasing distress between 12 and 36 months after diagnosis, and this pattern predicted longer survival after 7 years of follow-up. Healthy adaptation to breast cancer involves initially elevated distress followed by declines in distress over time. Such adaptation appears to be influenced by patients' coping processes and is likely related to disease outcome.

There is some evidence to support a "type C" biobehavioral cancer risk pattern,[23] with behavioral features including the repression or suppression of emotions (particularly anger), avoidance of conflict, overcooperation, unassertiveness, compliance with external authorities, high social desirability, and self-sacrificing. Weihs and associates[24] have documented a relationship between shortened survival after breast cancer recurrence and excessive emotional restraint as well as intense psychological distress.

Hurny[25] has postulated that reliance on a linear cause-and-effect model may be an inappropriate method of investigation because it does not take into consideration the complexity and circularity of mind-body-environment interactions. Even so, the fact that many of the so-called type C behavioral risk factors correlate with an outdated, but still enduring, societal norm in regard to women's submissive roles and self-negating behavior should be of concern to, and perhaps a focus of intervention for, health care practitioners in oncology. Clinical intervention research, although still in its infancy, is beginning to show not only behavioral changes but also changes in immune functions, at least of a temporary nature, related to psychological interventions.

Cancer is a very complex disease, and its multifaceted nature—along with the associated fear—tends to invite oversimplification. One way to counter unhelpful reductionism is to think of "risk factors" and "protective factors" rather than "causes." Risk factors can be genetic, environmental, psychological, or behavioral. Helping patients and their families build up their protective factors, while limiting known risk factors, may in the long run contribute more to their health than searching for singular causes of illness. A physician using the biopsychosocial model would certainly do no harm in "prescribing" such things as the appropriate expression of emotions, stress management, and the activation of patient's support networks alongside biomedical interventions such as surgery, chemotherapy and radiation therapy.

How does the diagnosis of breast cancer affect a woman's relationship to her body?

Cancer poses a threat to the woman's sense of bodily integrity and her conceptions of body image and sexuality. It is not uncommon for women with breast cancer to report that they feel betrayed by their bodies. For some, this translates into feeling unsafe in the world—strange, alone, odd, suddenly unlike everyone around them. Some women develop panic-like symptoms in the body—constriction in the chest, difficulty breathing, heightened startle response, a sense of dissociation from the body. These symptoms usually diminish as the woman adjusts to the diagnosis and mobilizes to receive treatment,[19,26] but the immediate impact on her relationship to her body, to her self, and to others can be profound.

Research has shown that women undergoing breast-conserving surgery might maintain a slightly healthier body image than those undergoing mastectomy,[27,28] but findings are conflicting. Some researchers have shown the opposite.[29,30] Age might contribute to a more positive body image following a mastectomy because studies have found that older women who undergo mastectomy can cope well psychologically.[31] It also may be true that women who identify as lesbians do not feel the distress about body image that heterosexual women do. One study, which compared coping issues, found less distress about body image, but an equivalent number of issues regarding sexuality, in lesbians as in heterosexual women.[32]

How is a woman's sexuality and sexual functioning affected by breast cancer?

Research on the impact of breast cancer on women's sexuality is in an early stage, although recent literature has begun to explore the issue.[28,32–35] Moreover, the subject of sexual adaptation is often not addressed in the oncologist's office. Breast cancer surgery and treatment remain an invasive and physiologically distressing sequence of events, although the emergence of breast-conserving techniques has ameliorated some of the effects on body image and sexuality.[27,28] The study by Kemeny and colleagues[36] of 83 patients randomized to mastectomy versus breast-conserving surgery showed that breast-conserving surgery, to a greater extent than mastectomy, preserved body image and integrity, protected feelings of sexual attractiveness and desirability, and contributed positively to the woman's perceptions that her sexual partner's reactions are unchanged as a result of treatment. These findings were consistent with those in Steinberg and associates' earlier study of 46 patients who underwent modified radical mastectomy compared with 21 patients who underwent lumpectomy and radiation,[37] and with a study of 99 Scandinavian breast cancer patients.[38] Breast reconstruction techniques have succeeded in returning to the woman a tangible sense of bodily integrity. Even so, patients report that lack of sensation in the new breast can be distressing. For example, one woman, after having bilateral mastectomies and reconstructions, described her chest, not without some humor, as having "two grapefruits attached." Chemotherapy and radiation treatment also affect the body's physiology in a way that can result in sexual morbidity. Most chemotherapeutic agents cause premature menopause, with its associated hot flashes, vaginal dryness, and loss of libido. Women attending several support groups at George Washington University reported mixed responses to vaginal lubrication products; for some, sexual activity was still painful. This disincentive, added to a lack of desire, discouraged them and their partners from renewing sexual relations.

One recent study suggests that problems with body image and sexual functioning may persist for many breast cancer survivors months or even years after treatment has ended. Of 784 breast cancer survivors from the greater Washington, DC, and the Los Angeles areas who responded to a mailed survey about their sexual attitudes, practices, relationships, and general well-being, 35% reported that breast cancer had a negative impact on their sex lives. Twenty-four percent were uncomfortable with the changes in their bodies; 26% no longer felt sexually attractive; 70% reported problems with lubrication; and 25% reported pain with intercourse more than half the time. The women who experience negative body image, premature menopause, and symptoms of emotional distress following treatment may be at particular risk for sexual dysfunction.[39]

In a follow-up study by the same researchers, of 472 patients from Los Angeles and 662 patients from Washington, DC, the most important predictors of sexual health were vaginal lubrication, emotional well-being, positive body image, quality of the partnered relationship, and absence of prior sexual problems with the partner.[33]

How does a partner's response to changes in sexuality affect the breast cancer patient?

The woman's adaptation to breast cancer is influenced not only by her own conceptions and beliefs about her body and her sexuality but also by the beliefs of her significant others and the greater society. Perceptions of body image correlate with sexual adaptation.[40] Traditional views of women in our society have tended to focus on certain ideals of attractiveness, often focusing on the breasts as a prime asset and object of desire. Although many women and men have eschewed such ideals, the cultural overlay remains strong. If a woman's emotional investment in her breasts is essential to her self-esteem, her feelings of loss and reduced self-worth will be disproportionately experienced. A minority of men—primarily those who receive a sense of reflected self-approval from a "beautiful" woman—may have disproportionately negative reactions to the loss of or disease in their partners' breast.[41]

Even men who adapt well to the changes wrought by breast cancer and who give their partners support may struggle with overwhelming fears about losing the woman they love. In a study of spouses 18 months after their wives' breast cancer diagnosis, 27% of men reported distress characterized by fear of disease recurrence, difficulty communicating their feelings about breast cancer, or changes in their sexual relationship with their wives.[42] A similar longitudinal study of 143 pairs of patients and their significant others documented significant psychological distress in a substantial minority of significant others up to 1 year after the patient's initial diagnosis.[43] Feelings of depression and dependency and the belief that such feelings should not be shared with their partners can result in the man's unconscious withdrawal both physically and emotionally as a means of self-protection. A member of a support group for spouses of breast cancer patients at George Washington University Cancer Center confessed that he was afraid to talk to his wife about his fears because he didn't want to upset her. "I'm supposed to be strong for her. I can't let her see how scary this is." With the group's help, he was able to articulate his concerns and eventually told his wife how he felt. The wife confessed that she too had been holding back, for fear of upsetting her husband. Being able to "practice" talking with his wife in the group enabled this husband to reestablish comfortable communication and intimacy.

Which patients are at risk for experiencing significant diminished sexuality?

Not all women experience changes in their sexual self-concept or behavior as a result of the cancer experience. Schain's[41] review of the literature suggests that women at extremely high risk for difficulties and in need of early intervention are women who (1) are young and have high emotional investment in their breasts, (2) have not had the children they hoped for or consider having children a major life goal, (3) may have been sexually abused, (4) did not get the treatment of their choice, (5) have few areas of gratification and sources of self-esteem outside of intimate interaction, (6) have a history of substance abuse, (7) have a history of psychiatric morbidity, and (8) have had multimodal therapy.[40,41] Infertility is often induced by chemotherapy, although patients of younger age and those who do not receive chemotherapy may escape treatment-related premature menopause.[44] The threat of infertility looms until treatment is complete, however, and creates distress.

The sexual issues of single women with breast cancer are receiving more attention as the age at which women marry increases and the age at which women are diagnosed with breast cancer decreases. The impact of the cancer on single women's sexuality and sexual activity differs according to their life goals and expectations. Some single women report intense grief at the loss of fertility and the ability to have children. Other issues involve whether and how to tell potential sexual partners or significant others about the diagnosis and its implications. The demise of significant relationships seems to occur more frequently with unmarried women, although it is true that some marriages break up in the aftermath of a cancer diagnosis. Single women face a difficult challenge in maintaining a secure emotional attachment or initiating emotional attachment. The sexual and relational issues of lesbian or bisexual women with breast cancer have not been explored adequately. Only recently have national studies of women's health begun to incorporate information on sexual orientation.[32,45]

What are the psychological stresses on the patient before a definitive diagnosis?

The period of uncertainty after finding a lump and before diagnosis can be the most stressful period of the entire cancer experience. Northouse and colleagues[46] found significant emotional distress in more than 200 women awaiting breast biopsy. Some studies suggest that fear of cancer itself is the primary stressor; others report the focus of concern to be the possible loss of the breast. Whatever the reason, women experience tremendous anxiety in this anticipatory phase. The danger here is that the fear will become so overwhelming that women will defend against it through denial, suppression, or avoidance and delay consulting a doctor.

Some researchers use the term *neglected breast cancer syndrome* to refer to this pattern of ignoring or denying breast cancer.[47] The researchers found that women with this syndrome often seek treatment because of symptoms of locally advanced disease, rather than self-discovered lumps or abnormal mammograms. When they do seek treatment, they behave in erratic, unpredictable ways, often denying or delaying treatment recommended by their physicians. It is important for these patients to be followed by a mental health professional in order to address issues such as fear, denial, and distrust that arise in breast cancer treatment.

What are the most common responses when a woman is told she has breast cancer?

The woman's response to hearing the words "You have cancer" vary according to the perceived nature of the cancer, the manner in which she is told the news,[48] her earlier experience with cancer, her defense mechanisms, the social support provided by those close to her, and her philosophy of life. Some patients respond with shock and disbelief and may later report that they heard no other information after getting the bad news, so overwhelming was their emotional reaction. Others display an almost stoic reaction, as if the diagnosis were inevitable. Health practitioners often experience anxiety when telling the news and are concerned about giving a proper response to whatever the patient's reaction.

Fallowfield and colleagues[29] studied 101 women with early breast cancer (T0–2, N0–1, M0) who were randomly assigned to mastectomy or breast conservation. They found that patients who perceived that the information they were given about diagnosis and treatment was inadequate were more likely to become anxious or depressed. In this study, contrary to some others, anxiety states and depressive illness, or both, were high in women who underwent mastectomy (33%), but not as high as in women with breast conservation followed by radiation therapy (38%). The authors concluded that radiation therapy itself carries considerable psychological morbidity.

Being told the diagnosis in the absence of a close friend or family member increases the psychological morbidity. For this reason, many oncologists make it a point to deliver information about the illness and treatment options over the course of several office visits, so that their patients have time to assimilate it. Patients are encouraged to bring a spouse, partner, family member, or friend to appointments—for emotional support, but also for another set of ears to hear important information. Some patients take notes or ask their doctor for permission to tape-record their conversations so that they can review later. More and more, patients are finding the information they need through the Internet, the American Cancer Society, or the National Cancer Institute. It is important for health care professionals to understand that the patient's efforts to overcome anxiety may manifest in incessant information gathering on one end of the spectrum, or in psychic numbing that can impede the necessary assimilation of data important for treatment decision making on the other.

How does defensiveness affect a patient's adaptation to a breast cancer diagnosis?

The adaptation process may include a number of defensive postures that have been traditionally characterized as pathologic in the psychoanalytic literature, including suppression, repression, and denial. We have noted how denial can be destructive if it hinders a person from receiving treatment in a timely manner. But denial, and the related defense mechanisms that alter the perception of reality, can serve very important functions as well. "[Denial] is positive and an advantage to the person to the degree that it allows the reality to be integrated without too much disturbance to an individual's psychic equilibrium. It is also positive to the degree it contributes to an individual's potential to counter maladaptive tendencies to give up, and not fight to live and do well".[49]

Rather than trying to confront what appear at first glance to be maladaptive defensive patterns, the clinician can attempt to expand the range of coping mechanisms open to the patient.[50] He or she can encourage patients to seek information, to take direct action in gaining control of their situation, and to activate their support networks, among other coping strategies.[51]

How does the woman's relationship with her physician and other health care professionals affect her adaptation to the breast cancer experience?

In adapting to the cancer experience, the woman's relationship with her surgeon, oncologist, and others on the health team is of critical importance. Benson[52] wrote that the interaction between physician and patient was one of the crucial elements in the placebo effect, or the body's ability to heal itself. Harris and Templeton[53] also discuss that positive interactions between physicians and patients can facilitate improved physical and mental health.

One potential barrier to a patient securing a workable attachment to a surgeon or medical oncologist is a perceived societal power differential between patients and physicians—and more particularly between women and men. A certain godlike mythology still attaches itself to the role of physician, despite the changes in the health care system wrought by managed care and the increased activism of patients as medical consumers. Women patients may inadvertently accept a more passive, subordinate role, allowing the oncologist, who is usually a man, to make important treatment decisions. This can be an adaptive arrangement for some patients, eliminating anxiety and simplifying the decision-making process, and a comfortable role for some doctors who perceive themselves as parental figures. But most patients today prefer a more active role in their health care, and most physicians look forward to having the patient act as a partner.

Lesbian women face significant barriers in communicating honestly with their physicians. Many lesbian women are not comfortable disclosing their sexual orientation, and the standard medical history taking questions presumes heterosexuality and often corners the responder, as in "Are you sexually active?" and the follow-up question, "Which form of birth control do you use?" Health care providers' reactions to disclosure of a homosexual orientation ranged from "embarrassment and discomfort to patronizing attitudes, outright hostility, and refusal to treat."[45] Some lesbian women may not be getting the routine care they need, including regular breast examinations and Papanicolaou smears, because of these barriers. It is not difficult to establish a comfortable setting for any sexual orientation. Helpful traits for clinicians included showing a willingness to listen; appearing to be accessible, attentive, and open; treating the patient respectfully; using neutral language (such as "partner" or "mate" rather than "boyfriend" or "husband"); taking time

during the visit; and showing gentleness during the physical examination.[45]

How can the physician enhance the physician–patient relationship?

Although there are no definitive models for the ideal physician–patient relationship, several guiding principles can be gleaned from a review of the literature. Patients' main communication issues revolve around maintaining a sense of control, seeking information, disclosing feelings, and searching for meaning.[54] Because the disease is so frightening and unpredictable, patients need interpersonal and environmental contexts that allow them to regain a sense of communication competence and therefore control.[55,56] For the physician, establishing consistent patterns of interaction with patients may be one of the means of enhancing their patients' sense of control. If patients are communicated with and treated in predictable ways, they will feel they are handling their illness more competently.

A moderate level of self-disclosure of feelings is key to healthy adjustment of cancer patients. It is important for physicians to remember that self-disclosure serves several important purposes: (1) it allows for catharsis, or draining of the tension and anxiety, (2) it allows people to receive feedback from others that normalizes the cancer experience, and (3) it enhances problem solving. The most effective response to patients' self-disclosure is simply "listening" or "being there."[54] In a qualitative study of 15 women living with breast cancer, Harris and Templeton[53] found that active listening was the most helpful characteristic for physicians to demonstrate when communicating with their patients. Further disclosure can be prescribed by referral to a support group.

On the health professional's side of the transactional process, literature points to three areas of communication that are important: (1) imparting information, (2) communicating hope, and (3) sharing control. Health care professionals struggle with what and how much to say to patients about their condition as well as how to say it in a way that is both honest and hope enhancing. In addition, they must deal with the growing complexity of a health care system in which various "players" have input and influence in the treatment process. No longer is the physician in complete control of health care decisions. Fortunately, sharing of control benefits the patient, allowing for the distribution of power in provider–patient relationships and the regaining of a sense of personal control.

In the end, the physician–patient relationship often defies easy formulation. It is as unique as the two individuals involved. What is important is that it be grounded in mutual trust and respect.

What are the most common diagnosable mental disorders among breast cancer patients and what are the warning signs?

Adjustment disorders are the most common psychiatric diagnoses in breast cancer patients, followed by depression and anxiety. Studies suggest that about 25% of patients with breast cancer experience depressed feelings significant enough to affect their daily functioning.[21,57] For most patients, these feelings lessen in a few weeks as their coping skills become activated and as they reconnect with people who care about them. It is important not to downplay severe depressed feelings, however, especially if they persist. Women who have had a premorbid clinical depression are more susceptible to the stress of a cancer diagnosis and treatment and are at greater risk for a depressive episode.[21]

A study of 205 newly diagnosed breast cancer patients assessed at 3 months after diagnosis found that 15% of patients experienced marked distress with a wide range of possible symptoms, including anxiety, depressed mood, social withdrawal, or unexplained physical complaints. Women with stressful life events in addition to breast cancer were found to have a greater likelihood of high emotional distress, ranging from 17% to 37% of patients, depending on the magnitude of their other stressors.[12] A history of depression or suicidality and regrets regarding the past are also associated with high vulnerability to psychiatric disorders and require early mental health interventions.[12,58] Mental health treatment is indicated if the patient's social, occupational, or academic functioning is impaired, or if the distress is not alleviated by supportive interactions with family, friends, or a breast cancer support group. Women who are isolated and who anticipate little emotional support from others in response to their breast cancer are more vulnerable to mental illness.[43] Women who are unhappily married, divorced, or widowed are particularly vulnerable.[38] Therefore, patients who cannot name a confidant or who say they have little personal support should always be strongly encouraged to participate in a support group and should be referred for mental health care as soon as psychological distress is reported.

Although most women have adequate inner resources and family and social supports to take them through this most devastating of life experiences, some are at higher risk for depression because of social isolation. A prospective study of 458 working-class women[59] found that women without a confidante were 30% more likely to suffer a major depression within 2 years after a severely stressful life event. Furthermore, studies report that depression in chronic illness is associated with increased morbidity and greater overall disability.[60]

Some women find themselves preoccupied with thoughts of death after receiving a breast cancer diagnosis. This is an expected response when one is confronted with a potentially life-threatening illness. Cancer is still associated with death for the general public, although today nearly half of people with cancer are cured or live with the disease for many years. Thoughts of death should be carefully differentiated from suicidal ideas or plans, which are much less common but require direct action. Physicians need to ask directly about suicidality when their patients mention thoughts of death. A statement such as "Some people feel so bad that they think they'd be better off dead. Have you been feeling that way?" can be used to avoid insulting the patient with such inquiries. Women with a plan for suicide should not leave the physician's office but should be seen directly by a psychiatrist to ensure safety and to begin appropriate treatment.

Supportive, problem-focused psychotherapy is indicated for adjustment disorders.[61] Psychotherapists with a range of backgrounds including psychiatry, psychology, social work,

and mental health nursing can provide this treatment. It is preferable to refer patients to mental health providers with some experience in medical settings who can integrate the patient's illness experience with her psychiatric treatment. Physicians should develop a collaborative relationship with a mental health professional or group, which allows a smooth referral to be made. Such referral practices make it more likely that the patient's emotional problems will be adequately addressed. When a woman's surgeon, oncologist, or other medical treatment provider recommends that she see a specific mental health professional, the patient is much more likely to follow the suggestion than she would be if only a general recommendation of psychotherapy or psychotropic medication is made.

When are antidepressant medications indicated for breast cancer patients?

Depressive disorders and anxiety disorders in breast cancer patients should be treated with antidepressant medications as well as psychotherapeutic interventions. Moderate to severe symptoms of anxiety or depression that persist for more than 2 weeks require a thorough review of psychiatric symptoms to determine their breadth and severity. If persistent depressed mood or loss of pleasure in all life activities is accompanied by thoughts of suicide, diminished ability to think or concentrate, or feelings of worthlessness or excessive guilt nearly every day, the patient may be suffering from a major depressive disorder. It is important to make this diagnosis because treatment can markedly reduce suffering and associated work, social, and family problems. Depressive disorders left untreated can result in hospitalization or even suicide. Fatigue, changes in weight or appetite, and trouble getting to sleep or staying asleep are also signs of major depressive disorder, but surgery, chemotherapy, and radiation therapy can induce these symptoms in many breast cancer patients. When they are combined with moderately severe sadness or lack of interest in life, however, they are also indicators of the need for treatment of a depressive disorder.

Some nonpsychiatric physicians elect to provide pharmacologic treatment without psychiatric consultation for depressive and anxiety disorders in their patients. Such pharmacologic intervention needs to continue for at least 6 months in order to prevent psychiatric morbidity. A physician who treats depressive disorders must maintain a close relationship with the patient in order to monitor symptom response to treatment, to interpret side effects, and to help patients to tolerate side effects until the full therapeutic antidepressant effect occurs. After the initial treatment response, patients should be seen at least monthly to monitor ongoing effectiveness and to strongly encourage continued medication compliance. Some patients believe that their symptom relief indicates that they can stop the treatment. However, just as stopping antibiotics for a severe wound infection after 5 days of treatment would undermine the full resolution of the infection, so too does stopping antidepressant treatment undermine the full resolution of a depressive disorder.

Bupropion is the preferred medication for starting treatment of depression in women who are sexually active. Although the serotonin-reuptake inhibitors fluoxetine, sertraline, paroxetine, citalopram, and escitalopram are often the first-line antidepressants used by general physicians and can reduce depressive symptoms, as many as one third of patients who take them experience changes in libido or anorgasmia as a side effect.[61] The *Handbook of Psychiatric Drug Therapy, 4th Edition,*[62] is a very good reference for the pharmacologic treatment of patients with psychiatric disorders.

When is anxiety a symptom warranting psychiatric intervention?

Patients who describe re-experiencing a highly traumatic event, such as being told they have breast cancer, may be suffering from an acute stress disorder. Re-experiencing involves feeling as if or dreaming that the trauma is happening again, some time after the actual occurrence. More than one third of breast cancer patients experience some of the symptoms of a stress disorder, including intrusive thoughts and symptoms of increased arousal. Trouble sleeping was found in 36%, and easy startling and hypervigilance were found in 27% of patients in a recent study of 160 patients with stage I breast cancer diagnosed 4 to 12 months before assessment.[63] Stress disorders of a more chronic nature are often related to past experiences of violence or sexual abuse. Women with such histories may be more vulnerable to psychiatric symptoms at the time of a breast cancer diagnosis. Persistence of intrusive thoughts, hyperarousal, sleep disturbance, and avoidance of medical care facilities for more than 8 weeks indicate that psychiatric evaluation and treatment are needed.

Women with anxious temperaments that predate the breast cancer and involve chronic worry, muscle tension, fatigue, chest tightness, or pain are at risk for flooding with these symptoms when they receive the cancer diagnosis. Such symptoms can be effectively treated with antidepressants. These drugs are preferable to benzodiazepines because they are equally effective while free of the risk for drug tolerance or dependence. Short-term benzodiazepine use for 1 to 2 weeks, however, can be very helpful while antidepressant medications are becoming effective. Alcohol abuse and dependence are prevalent in women with anxiety disorders and should be considered at the same time as any diagnostic assessment for anxiety disorders.

What is the role of support groups?

The ultimate challenge to a person's sense of place in the world is to know that she will die "before her time." Support groups can enhance patients' sense of control over their lives despite loss of control over the cancer. They can help women recognize and become more tolerant of strong, painful feelings, at the same time revealing and discarding unhelpful beliefs about not complaining and "toughing it out alone." Many patients believe it is unacceptable to speak of one's possible death from cancer because such talk might indicate loss of hope and a morbid preoccupation with negative outcomes. If they do speak of their fears, they are often silenced or pathologized by those they open up to, including health care providers and virtually everyone in their social networks. As Spiegel[64] wrote: "Paradoxically, we observed that when patients openly discussed the most serious issues [in group], such as dying and death, their fears were detoxified. They

came to realize that they feared the process of dying more than death itself. They were able to parse the fear into a series of problems: pain control, participation in medical decision-making, [and] making the best possible use of remaining time." A belief system that rigidly dictates positive thinking at all costs gives way to an empowering sharing of common fears in a group context that enhances coping and strengthens the patients' hold on the time remaining.

Some oncology clinicians routinely prescribe participation in a support group for women with breast cancer, regardless of the patient's degree of social support. The importance of support groups for maintaining one's quality of life has been documented. One study, for instance, found that participation in a breast cancer support group contributed to an improvement in psychological well-being, and this improvement continued 1 year after participating in the group.[26]

A more startling finding was a correlation between participation in weekly group therapy and increased longevity for women with advanced breast cancer. In a study that began at the time of their onset of metastatic breast cancer, 88 women were randomly assigned to either a professionally led, weekly group therapy or to no systematic psychosocial care. At follow-up 7 years later, the women in the intervention group had an average survival time of 36 months, compared with 18 months' average survival for the controls.[65] A study by Cunningham and coworkers[66] also found that women with metastatic breast cancer who "worked through" their feelings during supportive expressive group therapy benefited with better psychological well-being *and* longer survival.

A more recent study by Goodwin and colleagues[67] involved 235 women with metastatic breast cancer who were randomly assigned to supportive-expressive group therapy or no systematic psychosocial care. Adherence to the intervention methods used by Spiegel and associates[65] was rigorously enforced. Women assigned to supportive-expressive therapy had greater improvement in psychological symptoms and reported less pain than women in the control group. The psychological intervention did not prolong survival.

What can be concluded, then, about the effect of supportive expressive group therapy? It clearly benefits women who are distressed and in pain by reducing these symptoms. Whether it increases longevity will not be determined until further research is available.[68]

What is the impact of confronting death for the breast cancer patient?

Thinking excessively about death can contribute to depression and despair, but an honest confrontation with the reality of one's mortality can also have positive benefits. The sociologist Ernest Becker[69] postulated that our scientific society's insistence on "denying" the reality of death has led to a kind of psychic numbing. The "heroic" individual, according to Becker, is one who embraces more of the ambiguities and pain of life, not less. "Taking life seriously means that whatever man [or woman] does on this planet has to be done in the lived truth of the terror of creation, of the grotesque, of the rumble of panic underneath everything. Manipulative, utopian science, by deadening human sensitivity. . . falsifies our struggle by emptying us, by preventing us from incorporating the maximum of experience."

Numerous cancer patients have reported that a brush with death helped give meaning to their lives. They feel motivated to live life more fully, to appreciate each moment, to do now what they might have put off until tomorrow, to confront old hurts and resolve them. In short, their lives are enriched by the cancer experience.[70] On the other hand, there are some women who resent the suggestion that they must have a life-altering spiritual experience as a result of having breast cancer. As one breast cancer survivor aptly put it, "Cancer is a growth, not a growth experience."

What are the particular challenges faced by women who experience a recurrence of their cancer?

A recurrence forces the woman and her close significant friends and relations to revisit previous stages and renegotiate the psychological landscape. The return of cancer shatters hopes that the initial cancer was cured and heightens fears that this time the cancer will be fatal.[71] The recurrent phase of cancer has been reported as one of the most stressful phases over the entire course of illness.[72] Patients report shock and depression, anxiety and powerlessness, fears about death, disability, and pain, and a sense of injustice at the renewed assault of the cancer.[73] On the other hand, women bring to the experience of a recurrence the knowledge gained from their previous cancer journey. They know the intricacies of the health care system and how to marshal their inner resources and social supports to meet the new challenge.

Breast cancer recurrence affects the functioning of relationships between patients and their partners.[74] Women's adjustments are affected by the amount of symptom distress, hopelessness, and emotional support they perceive in themselves as well as the amount of emotional distress they perceive in their partners. Husbands' adjustments are affected by their own health problems and by feelings of hopelessness as well as by the symptom distress they observed in their wives.[71] Other family members can also experience a reduced quality of life in response to a recurrence, which can be influenced by the degree of hardiness in the family.[75] A family-focused approach to the care of women with recurrent disease that includes their partners and their family is recommended as each member in some way influences the adjustment of the others.

What is the impact on the breast cancer patient of contemplating a recurrence?

The possibility of recurrence is an ongoing mental health concern for most breast cancer patients regardless of prognosis. After treatment ends, many patients report feeling vulnerable because they are no longer actively "doing something" about their illness. Trigger points for anxiety about recurrence seem to intensify in relation to anniversary events (date of original diagnosis, date or surgery, date of completion of treatment), suspicious symptoms (particularly those that mimic feelings at the time of the original illness), any illness or change in health (particularly weight loss or fatigue), illness in a family member, recurrence or death of a fellow survivor, or times of particular life stress. To combat anxiety related to recurrence, patients can employ behavioral actions such as connecting with support systems, planning pleasurable activities, seeking professional counseling when needed, providing support to others, and learning and using relaxation techniques. Cognitive-emotional approaches include recognizing that trigger points exist and that anxiety fluctuates, enjoying life one day at a time, reframing feelings, and reflecting on positive changes that have resulted from the illness.[76]

How do people's belief systems affect their ability to handle the psychosocial impact of cancer?

Cancer challenges people's assumptions about life and their place in it. A breast cancer patient brings her beliefs about the world and her place in it to her experience of cancer and uses those beliefs to shape its meaning to her life.[77] Belief systems can assist the patient to weave the changes brought by cancer into the tapestry of her life, strengthening her identity, helping her to affirm: "I am a survivor, therefore I can overcome this." Conversely, belief systems can impair the patient's ability to cope with each aspect of cancer, sapping hope from a woman who believes "once more, I am a victim of a cruel world." The concept of meaning derives from a person's unique perception of her place in the world; these perceptions give a sense of coherence to life in the face of loss, change, and personal upheaval.[78] The search for meaning is a powerful component of coping and a method of reasserting cognitive control;[79] for example, a patient might decide that "I did not need this experience, and did not cause it, but I can and will learn from it." One study found that positive meaning ascribed to the pain of cancer, such as viewing it as a challenge, was associated with lower levels of depression.[80] Other studies found that a belief that control of the illness experience was within the control of the individual patient herself was associated with a positive "fighting spirit," an attitude associated in previous studies with longer survival, whereas the belief that external factors were in control of the illness was associated with anxious preoccupation about cancer.[81,82]

Can a patient's beliefs about life and about cancer hinder the adaptation process?

Misguided beliefs about cancer causation can be damaging to patient adjustment. A cancer diagnosis challenges people's assumptions about "the way life ought to be." One such assumption is that doing the "right" things—eating right, doing good deeds, believing correctly—will shield them from negative life events. These beliefs have deep roots in religion and in every culture, with more recent offshoots found in some of the popular writings about the mind–body connection. The news of a breast cancer diagnosis can often set patients on a life review in search of a deficiency that caused the cancer. They are encouraged by much of the cancer self-help literature, such as Siegel's[83] million-selling *Love, Medicine and Miracles*, and sometimes by well-meaning friends or family. The most common concern voiced by patients seems to be that an inability to deal well with stress might result in impaired immunity against cancer, and yet the relationship between stress and cancer is far from clear. A related belief states that cancer is, on some level, a psychological event. Writer Susan Sontag[84] wrote a polemic against such ideas, protesting that "People are encouraged to believe that they get sick because they (unconsciously) want to, and that they can cure themselves by the mobilization of will. . . . Psychological theories of illness are a powerful means of placing blame on the ill."

It is helpful to inform patients that our very human natures yearn for theories of causation. Finding "reasons why" provides a buffer against the random danger we all face. However, the search for the cause of a particular woman's breast cancer may divert emotional energy away from constructive coping with the urgent treatment decisions and tasks at hand. Patients can be encouraged to shift their focus toward reducing the negative impact of cancer in the present. There is evidence that social support from family, friends, or support groups counteracts the effects of stress, buffering people against negative life events and contributing to improved health and disease resistance.[16] Health care providers can reassure patients that the connections between mind and body are extremely complex indeed.

Breast cancer patients can use the mind–body literature for health-strengthening techniques, while setting aside self-blaming messages. Emotional well-being can be enhanced through new and old techniques such as yoga, biofeedback, meditation, and visualization, and from support groups. A patient can always use the cancer event as a catalyst for changing the things about her life that she already wanted to change. This "wake-up call" phenomenon, often remarked on by cancer survivors, is one of the ways in which positive meaning and purpose can derive from the cancer experience and serves to enhance rather than undermine personal power and life coherence.

The Danish writer Isak Dinesen said, "All sorrows can be borne if you can put them into a story or tell a story about them."[85] Health care providers can assist patients in integrating their cancer experience into their life story in a positive, creative way, and listening to the statements patients make during clinic or hospital encounters is an important first step.

Are there long-term psychological consequences of having had breast cancer?

The psychological impact of the illness may continue well beyond the end of treatment. A study of 127 women with breast cancer[86] found that the illness not only added to ongoing life stress but also increased the negative events or difficulties in other areas such as relationships with family and external stressors (e.g., education, work, housing, money, crime). The women continued to experience a higher level of perceived "threat" to their well-being in these "nonhealth" categories in each of the 3 years after their cancer diagnosis than they had reported before the diagnosis. However, it is important to keep in mind that most women cope well with the disorder, and factors such as emotional expression, social support, and psychosocial interventions can help minimize the negative effects of breast cancer.[87]

FAMILY CONSIDERATIONS

How does the diagnosis of breast cancer affect the patient's family?

Different families feel the reverberations of a woman's cancer very differently. Carter and McGoldrick[88] suggested that the individual, the family, and the illness each have a "life cycle," and how and at what stage these intertwine will determine the overall impact on the psychosocial system. The degree of disruption to the family system is affected by a number of factors, the most significant of which are (1) the timing of the illness in the life cycle, (2) the nature of the illness, (3) the openness of the family system, and (4) the family position of the ill family member. More recently, Veach and Nicholas[89] discussed a similar view of family development. They highlighted the unique stressors faced by families, depending on the clinical course of the cancer as well as the stage of the family life cycle. Using these views, a woman in her early 40s with breast cancer is out of sync with the expected natural process of illness and possible death. At this phase in the life cycle, the woman is at her peak in terms of family responsibilities and productivity; all things being equal, her illness leaves a gap in family functioning that is difficult, if not impossible, to fill. At the same time, the woman's adolescent daughter is at the life stage of moving away from the cocoon of family. The unique course of the illness can add additional stress to the individual and the family system, particularly if there are unexpected complications, debilitation, or an increased possibility of death. The significance of the ill person in the family constellation will contribute to the degree of distress. Understood in terms of functional role and the degree of emotional dependence of the family on the individual, the woman's significance is practically beyond measure.

Most families mount a resilient response, despite the suffering that is universal for those living with cancer.[90] They report feeling closer to one another after marshaling resources to fight the disease.[56,91] Although many families report this positive response, the physical and emotional pressures during the different stages of cancer can strain family relationships, even among families who cope well with cancer.[3,90] Multiple investigators have reported that about one third of adult cancer patients, their spouses, and their children have clinically significant distress and psychosocial dysfunction.[92,93] Some families of cancer patients express psychological distress as much as, if not more than, the patients themselves.[94,95]

The quality of the family environment affects the outcome of its members. Family environments experienced as cohesive and low in conflict include family members who are less distressed and have better coping than patients, partners, and children whose families are detached or high in conflict.[42,90,96] The latter family characteristics have also been linked to behavioral disorders in children whose parents have cancer.[96] The importance of family function for the psychological adjustment of its members becomes evident when it is assessed along with physical disability in the same patient population. Family function has a much greater effect than physical disability on the patient's mental health.[97]

Families whose members have the best mental health are likely to perceive their family environments to be cohesive and expressive, without the burden of excessive conflict. Research has shown that high emotional expressiveness and cohesion in family relationships predict better psychological adjustment to cancer in all family members.[98–100] Correlations of depression and anxiety among family members suggest that something shared by members of the same family influences the mental health of its members. Some attributes of the family may also influence the course of the biologic disease process. It is not yet clear whether the latter attributes are the same as those that correlate with psychological adjustment.

Cancer poses the risk for separations and losses that can best be contained in relationships that are secure. Psychological adjustment depends on adaptation of family relational processes in response to these threatened separations and losses that are related to cancer. The specific nature of the cancer threat, because of its potential for loss and separation, can set in motion either constructive or destructive transformations of family relationships. These transformations occur through the activation of attachment and care-giving relationships, which give rise to new forms of communication, joint problem solving, mutuality, and, at times, intimacy.[101]

How do family beliefs about illness affect patients' and family members' adjustment?

Family beliefs about illness may help or hinder adjustment. A family's belief system may need to expand during the time of acute illness; for example, if the patient has always been the children's primary parent, and she is profoundly debilitated by chemotherapy, the father/husband will need to expand his underutilized competencies for parenting, and the mother/wife/patient will need to let go of some control over this area in their family life.[102] Ideally, a renegotiation of roles should occur so that flexibility can replace time-worn routine in the household. The cycles of treatment require families to make ever-changing adjustments to the energy level of the patient, which should be made without denying the reality of fatigue at one extreme, or infantilizing the recovering patient at the other. These changes pose challenges to the most supportive and communicative of families.

The research of Reiss and colleagues[103] on chronic illness in families has shown that long-term accommodation of the family to illness can endanger other family priorities and lead to a neglect of normative family developmental issues. Particularly for the family of a woman with recurrent, advanced, or "chronic" breast cancer, belief systems may need to be examined so that the needs of both the well and the ill are validated, thus sparing the family the additional burdens of guilt, resentment, and truncated development. A working metaphor that Reiss' team found useful in removing guilt from the family dynamic was to view the illness as a 2-year-old tyrant who disrupts family life with excessive demands and threatens catastrophe if demands are not met. They[103] found it important to "separate the patient from the illness and to place all family members, including the patient, on the same team, a team whose joint task it is to evaluate current coping strategies and to experiment with more equitable and satisfying coping responses." In this era of outpatient mastectomies and home hospice care, families will assume more of the responsibility for medical care; programs to support family coping are needed to produce good medical outcomes with the use of fewer traditional medical resources.

How should information about the cancer be conveyed to children and other family members?

Children can sense when something is not right in their family environment. A child has a right to know about anything that affects the family as cancer does. The question is, how and at what level of detail should children be told? Knowledge of children's normal growth and development can be a guide in this regard. Very young children are dependent, are present oriented, and have a limited grasp of concepts. Breast cancer in the mother threatens their sense of predictability and consistency of nurturance. Thus, a seemingly selfish response of "Who will fix my breakfast?" when told of his mother's illness is normal for a 4-year-old. School-aged children, with their growing understanding of concepts and language, have the capacity to see their mother's illness as separate from them and may be curious about it. Children at this age also can engage in the magical thinking that may lead them to believe that they did something to cause the illness. Older school-aged children view death as a natural biologic process and have concerns about its effect on their own lives. Young teens and adolescents generally feel that they are not vulnerable to their mother's death. They will be challenged by the conflicting drives to pull away from the family toward independence and draw closer as they accept more responsibility for care giving.[89]

At the most basic level, children of all ages need to know (1) what has happened, (2) what will happen next, (3) that they did not cause the cancer, (4) that there is hope, even though they are upset now, and (5) that they are and will be loved and cared for.[104] Parents should feel free to communicate feelings as well as facts because that gives permission for children to acknowledge their own scary feelings. The first explanation can be as simple as the following:

I have a sickness. It is called cancer. The doctor is giving me medicine to help me get well. Sometimes I will feel sick or tired and sometimes I will be just fine. Dad will help me take care of you until I feel better.

Being sick makes me feel sad. You are a help. But it's OK for you to feel sad or angry or happy or whatever. Our feelings change but love is always there.

Listening to children's responses to the initial explanation will let parents know what the children can handle. Then parents can follow up with further explanation or ask their children if they're worried or have other questions.

One study showed that some children are not told about their mother's breast cancer until after surgery, if they are told at all.[105] The study also found that older children are often told about their mother's breast cancer earlier, and are provided with more information, than younger children.[105] It is important for health care professionals to support mothers in communicating with their children in the early phases of breast cancer, in age-appropriate ways.

As for telling other family members, the woman should not feel compelled to tell everyone right away. She may begin by telling the people with whom she feels most safe. Women report that concern about how people will react often delays their disclosure: "I'm having a hard enough time with this. I don't want to have to comfort someone else." In reality, family members react very differently to bad news. Some do get upset. Some people react in fear. Others, in their compulsion to help, offer unwanted advice or "war stories" from others' cancer experience, unintentionally increasing distress. The woman can be reassured that she need not feel responsible for people's reactions and assume the caretaker role. Recruiting her partner or a close friend to help in giving the news can be a significant buffer.

What are the particular psychosocial risks for children of breast cancer patients?

In most cases, mother–child relationships tend to stay strong or grow stronger following breast cancer. In interviews with 78 breast cancer patients, Lichtman and colleagues[106] found deterioration in only 12% of the relationships. Problems with children were more likely when the patients had a poor prognosis, more severe surgery, poorer psychological adjustment, and to a lesser extent, more difficulty with radiation therapy or chemotherapy. Interestingly, the mothers' relationships with their daughters were at a significantly greater risk than were their relationships with their sons. Seventeen percent of the patients reported that their daughters were fearful, withdrawn, hostile, or rejecting; only 8% reported having problems with their sons. Their fear of inheriting breast cancer and the mother's demands on the daughter for support were judged to be major contributing factors to the difficulties with adolescent and preadolescent daughters.

In another study of daughters of breast cancer patients, Wellisch and colleagues[107] reported that daughters who were adolescents at the time of their mother's illness had greater adjustment problems later on than daughters who were either latency age or young adults. Girls of this age group had greater feelings of discomfort about their mother's illness and more often changed their long-range life plans as a result of the experience. They also reported less sexual satisfaction later on in adult life.

How does the experience of breast cancer shape a woman's definition of self and her role within her family?

Many women are socialized to care for others, and caring for oneself can seem like a disavowal of an appropriate concern for other people. Requesting time and specific kinds of attention from others may represent for the woman with breast cancer a loss of role, such as manager in the family and provider of emotional sustenance.

A woman's struggle to see herself as a unique individual in the presence of breast cancer is shaped by ongoing changes in self-image for women in contemporary Western cultures. Carol Gilligan[108] described dilemmas in women's perceptions of themselves as they move toward defining themselves in their own terms. Gilligan and Belensky[109] found that women

who cope well with illness defined self-care as one of the aspects of their ability to be a caring person. In this schema, caring for others and caring for oneself are no longer in conflict but instead become an integrated part of one's core identity. Gilligan and Belensky[110] describe this critical step in women's adult development to be the transition from a conventional feminine role in which "goodness" is self-sacrifice, toward a truthful acknowledgment of oneself as deserving of the consideration one grants others. They call this evolution a movement from goodness to truth.

The urgent need for self-care often brings women with breast cancer to an awareness of the deception inherent in the feminine role of selflessness. They become aware of the destructiveness to self and other which that deception breeds. "The incongruity between the experience of self and the demands of role generates the movement from an understanding of self and other through roles, to an understanding of self and other beyond roles."[111] Weingarten,[102] a family therapist who has had breast cancer, described growth beyond the traditional parental role. In her book, *The Mother's Voice: Strengthening Intimacy in Family Relationships*, she described how breast cancer stimulated her realization that her children have strength to care for her and that she can be closer to them by being more genuine in disclosing her own needs along with attending to theirs.

What impact does the diagnosis of breast cancer have on a woman's relationship to the community?

Breast cancer patients and family members draw their perceptions of cancer from the attitudes of the larger society, their own ethnic group, their religious-spiritual community, their work community, and their own families of origin. The experience of illness cannot be adequately understood without understanding the larger cultural context. At the societal level, for example, a diagnosis of cancer still engenders fear and stigma, despite advances in the understanding of the disease, and this can be a hindrance in seeking and receiving treatment. McGoldrick and colleagues[112] wrote that the medical model's emphasis on diagnosing and curing disease often renders it inattentive to the patient's or family's perception of what is wrong and that this inattention accounts for at least some of the noncompliance, dissatisfaction with clinical care, and treatment failure experienced.

A woman's social network provides many positive resources as well. It acts as a buffer during times of crisis, protecting her from potential declines in physical and emotional well-being.[9,10,98,99] Weihs and associates[13] identified the provisions of social integration, nurturance, reassurance of worth, a sense of relative alliance, and guidance. No relationship can adequately furnish all provisions, but a network of relationships can. Social support is multifaceted and serves multiple functions, yet the underlying thread is that support reinforces the individual's sense of worth and being loved.

Of what influence are ethnic factors in the detection and treatment of breast cancer?

Certain ethnic groups suffer disproportionately from breast cancer. For example, the incidence is lower but mortality rates are higher for breast cancer in African American women than in women of other ethnic groups.[113] Studies that establish risk factors for breast cancer often do not include minority groups, however, making it difficult to determine the causes for these group differences. Many researchers believe that ethnicity is not an independently significant risk factor for breast cancer survival; factors such as age, socioeconomic status, stage of disease, and treatment are more important to consider in all ethnic groups.[114]

Attitudes toward health and illness are also influenced by ethnic factors. Zborowski's classic study[115] of 146 Jewish, Italian, Irish, and white Anglo-Saxon Protestant veterans hospitalized with painful physical illnesses found marked differences among the ethnic groups in response to pain and in their expectations of treatment. Through the use of structured interviews, the research demonstrated that Jewish and Italian patients tended to complain about their pain, whereas the Irish and white Anglo-Saxon Protestants did not. The Italians worried about the effects of their pain on their immediate situation, but once the pain was relieved, they easily forgot their suffering. The Jewish patients feared anything that stopped the pain, such as a pill, because they felt it would not deal with the real source of the problem. The Irish patients did not expect a cure, were fatalistic, and did not complain or even mention their pain.

African Americans tend to use more emotional restraint than their European American counterparts, a factor that may be associated with decreased survival time in women with recurrent breast cancer.[24] Higher emotional constraint in African Americans than in European Americans has been attributed to their predicament as members of a nondominant social group. This negative effect of racial discrimination on health has begun to be documented for other medical conditions.[116] African Americans enter a medical establishment designed by and for European Americans, for which they are sometimes not socialized. However, they must perceive the nuances of that system, of themselves, and of other people in it, in order to obtain medical treatment. In this context, intense effort to control oneself and to determine and meet others' expectations is understandable and probably advantageous.

Discussion of cancer is considered taboo in some African American southern communities. This taboo is based on a view of cancer as a minion of fate, which is active, powerful, and impossible to stop.[117] As a result, family and friends who might discuss the patient's cancer with her may consider such behavior to be tempting fate.

Further study of emotional constraint and control is needed to clarify the ways in which African American women may be emotionally overtaxed in obtaining social support and medical care when they have cancer.

What are the socioeconomic and class issues related to breast cancer?

Poverty has been associated with late diagnosis of cancer, barriers to treatment, and lower survival rates.[118] Studies show women from more deprived areas are less likely to get breast cancer but experience poorer survival than women from less-deprived areas.[119] Several barriers prevent poorer women from receiving mammograms and participating in breast cancer

early-detection programs, including high costs, limited availability to screening, physician referral requirements, fear of breast cancer detection, fear that detection will necessitate mastectomy, mammogram-related pain, and fear of radiation, which can affect their survival rates. One study showed that screen-detected cases of breast cancer had a better prognosis at diagnosis, regardless of the socioeconomic status of the patient.[119] Thus, increasing access to screening, helping poorer people to finance breast cancer care, and providing culturally sensitive cancer education programs might improve the survival rates for lower income groups.

Health care professionals also report numerous obstacles in providing cancer care to poor people: (1) fatalistic beliefs and attitudes among their peers regarding the prevention, control, and curability of cancer, (2) processes and systems that discourage providers from making referrals, and (3) limited access to resources to serve the needs of the disadvantaged. Strategies to enhance the delivery of care and services include greater involvement in community cancer control efforts, more focus on issues of poverty in medical training, more public advocacy for access to health care for all people, and the creation of delivery systems that better accommodate the needs of the disadvantaged. As one health care provider testified: "Our clinics could be of major assistance in screening patients for prevention and early detection of disease. These facilities need to be more accessible, and they need to require a minimal amount of their time per visit."[120]

In what ways does religious affiliation affect the woman's experience of breast cancer?

Religious beliefs and affiliation can play a key role in how a woman understands and copes with breast cancer. We have examined earlier how belief systems both are challenged by the cancer experience and provide needed succor. For African Americans, in particular, concepts of health and religion are closely meshed. Spirituality has been found to be a major resource for managing illness and stressful life events.[121] One study found that African Americans use prayer and spirituality as the primary source of support in coping with breast cancer.[122,123]

In other ethnic groups, religion and spirituality can also play a role in coping with breast cancer. One study of 39 women living in or near Ottawa, Canada, found that religion and spirituality can help patients to understand their illness, to strengthen their relationships, and to foster their support networks.[124]

An exploratory study found that women with metastatic breast cancer who rated spiritual expression as important had greater numbers of circulating white blood cells and total lymphocyte counts (both helper and cytotoxic T-cell counts) than those who were not as spiritually expressive, even after controlling for demographic, disease status, and treatment variables.[125] Although the mechanism for this relationship is not clear, the study indicates that there may be both physical and mental health benefits of spirituality in breast cancer patients.

Clinicians must work to understand their patients' religious beliefs and the role of their religious community in their experience of cancer. The community aspect of religious belief offers an important social and spiritual "holding space" for many in coping with their illness. The relationship of social support to overall health and well-being has been well established in the literature, and religious communities are key sources of that support. Churches and synagogues also can be important centers for community education about cancer. Some African American churches have nurse auxiliaries that can provide education about the importance of cancer prevention and early detection. These "insiders" have been quite successful in recruiting members to screening programs.[126]

WORKPLACE CONSIDERATIONS

What are the most important workplace issues for women with breast cancer who work outside the home?

Most women who enter the cancer clinic for treatment will have at least a part-time job outside the home. The workplace is an important component of most women's social network and provides resources, both emotional and financial, for weathering the cancer experience. The world of work is also a significant stressor for many women who are balancing the demands of home and career. The most important workplace issues for women with breast cancer are preserving income and access to health insurance benefits and setting a realistic pace at work during the acute phase of treatment.

Many people, both patients and employers, remain ignorant of the reality of breast cancer treatment, from the overall good prognosis to the odd rhythm of treatment side effects that leave many patients too ill to work for several days out of each chemotherapy cycle. Ignorance can translate into discrimination by employers based on expectations of negative outcome and, conversely, unrealistic expectations for normal productivity by the patients themselves. *Working Woman*[127] conducted a survey of 500 patients who continued to work while receiving treatment. Twenty five percent of the patients said that their job responsibilities were cut or that they were demoted, denied promotion, or passed over for a raise. Seven percent said they were fired as a result of their cancer. This survey also polled managers and colleagues and found a far more pessimistic view of the impact of cancer on job performance than the patients had.

People who have no first-hand knowledge of the improvements in breast cancer treatment and prognosis will not understand that most patients in active treatment can still perform adequately on the job and will resume previous performance ability following treatment. This survey revealed that 60% of the cancer patients undergoing treatment were able to maintain their regular hours during treatment. The challenge for society is to minimize the job stressors of those 60% as they undergo treatment and to protect the jobs and health insurance benefits of the sicker 40%.

How much and to whom should breast cancer patients reveal details of their medical condition?

Legal experts recommend that patients tell their supervisor soon after learning their diagnosis, thus setting the tone for open communication.[128] This period just after diagnosis is often the most anxiety provoking as women begin to gather opinions and make decisions about treatment. Once a course is chosen, patients need to learn about the likely side effects of treatment from their oncologists, and again inform supervisors of what may happen. In breast cancer support groups, women have learned that some patients are unable to work for 4 or 5 days after an infusion of doxorubicin despite antiemetics and rehydration therapy, whereas other women feel a slight nausea and miss only 1 day. Once patients have experienced their first treatment, they will have a better sense of how to pace their work lives (and home lives) around the dictates of side effects and fatigue.

Even when fully informed about the physical toll of treatment, patients may have unrealistic expectations of their ability to perform at work. Breast cancer is a blow to self-esteem, and although women may try to minimize the impact, certain biologic realities will intrude on their best intentions to maintain as "normal" a schedule as possible. Conscientious working women will experience the dilemma of not wanting to be excluded by coworkers from important tasks, yet not feeling "totally there" either. Well-meaning advice to "take it easy" does not validate the importance of women's jobs to their self-esteem and ignores the pressure to minimize cancer treatment's impact on household income. A woman's self-esteem may be tied to a social role of being the reliable one in both family and workplace. To preserve health and minimize guilt, roles and expectations in general need to be flexible during treatment and renegotiated during recovery.

What legal or legislative measures protect breast cancer patients' rights in the workplace?

Four laws protect breast cancer patients in the workplace: the Americans with Disabilities Act (ADA) of 1990, the Family and Medical Leave Act (FMLA) of 1993, the Health Insurance Portability and Accountability Act of 1996, and the related Consolidated Budget Reconciliation Act of 1985 (COBRA). Under the ADA, cancer is considered a disability and requires that employers who have 15 or more employees provide "reasonable accommodation" of the disability, which may include flexible work hours or leave policies, unless the accommodation would impose "undue hardship" on the employer. The Family and Medical Leave Act handles temporary, serious health conditions like cancer (or cancer in a spouse or child) for employees who have completed 1 year of service for at least 25 hours per week and who work for employers with 50 or more employees. The FMLA allows up to 12 weeks of unpaid leave in a 12-month period. The FMLA allows leave to be taken intermittently, which is particularly useful for breast cancer patients who may need to stay home for a few days out of every month during chemotherapy. The FMLA allows for up to 1 week absence per month for 12 months and allows a shorter workday; if medically required, a worker can reduce the workday from 8 hours by increments of 1 hour (a useful strategy for accommodating weeks of daily radiation therapy after lumpectomy).

The Health Insurance Portability and Accountability Act (HIPAA) of 1996 is most relevant to breast cancer survivors who are making a job change. It protects workers who have been covered under a group policy for a minimum of 18 months from losing health insurance, ensuring "portability" without waiting periods or preexisting condition limitations. This law should help with the "job lock" many cancer survivors experience. If the breast cancer survivor moves to a job that does not offer group health insurance, the law gives the right to purchase individual coverage; however, it does not protect against unreasonably high premiums for individuals outside of groups. The COBRA requirements (passed in the Consolidated Budget Reconciliation Act of 1985) allow individuals to keep their coverage after leaving an employer group for 18 months and protect against high premiums during that period.

Individual states are passing health insurance reforms, and survivors may want to consider a move to a state in which access to health insurance is facilitated, especially if they cannot find coverage in their current situation. Supporting advocacy groups like the National Coalition for Cancer Survivorship are also an important option for expanding breast cancer survivors' rights.

CONCLUSION

The cancer experience challenges not only the individual woman but also her entire network of affiliations, relationships, and support. Yet even as the experience reverberates through the system, numerous resources can emerge to help her mount a resilient response. Clinicians who are alert to the many levels of relationships that affect the woman's life will be able to accompany her more fully and helpfully as she fills gaps and calls forth resources in a successful adaptation to breast cancer.

REFERENCES

1. Engel G. Psychological Development in Health and Disease. Philadelphia, WB Saunders, 1962.
2. Bloom JR. Social support of the cancer patient. In Baider L, Kaplan-DeNour A, Cooper C (eds). Cancer and the Family. New York, John Wiley, 1996.
3. Carlson LE, Bultz BD, Speca M, St.-Pierre M. Partners of cancer patients. Part II. Current psychosocial interventions and suggestions for improvements. J Psychosoc Oncol 2000;18(3):33–43.
4. Kagawa-Singer M, Wellisch DK. Breast cancer patients' perceptions of their husbands' support in a cross-cultural context. Psychooncology 2003;12:24–37.
5. Waxler-Morrison N, Hislop GT, Mears B, Kan L. Effects of social relationships on survival for women with breast cancer: A prospective study. Social Sci Med 1991;33(2):177–183.
6. Cassileth BR, Walsh WP, Lusk EJ. Psychosocial correlates of cancer survival: A subsequent report 3 to 8 years after cancer diagnosis. J Clin Oncol 1988;6(11):1753–1759.
7. Funch DP, Marshall J. The role of stress, social support and age in survival from breast cancer. J Psychosom Res 1983;27(1):77–83.
8. Reynolds P, Boyd PT, Blacklow RS, et al. The National Cancer Institute Black/White Cancer Survival Study Group. Relationship between social ties and survival in black and white breast cancer patients. Cancer Epidemiol Biomarkers Prev 1994;3:253–259.
9. Ell K, Nishimoto R, Mediansky L, et al. Social relations, social support and survival among patients with cancer. J Psychosom Res 1992; 36(6):531–541.
10. Levy SM, Herberman RB, Lippman M, et al. Immunological and psychosocial predictors of disease recurrence in patients with early stage breast cancer. Behav Med 1991;17(2):67–75.
11. Giraldi T, Rodani MG, Cartei G, Grassi L. Psychosocial factors and breast cancer: A 6-year Italian follow-up study. Psychother Psychosom 1997;66(5):229–236.
12. Maunsell E, Brisson J, Deschenes L. Psychological distress after initial treatment of breast cancer. Cancer 1992;70(1):120–125.
13. Weihs KL, Simmens S, Mizrahi J, et al. Number of dependable social relationships predicts overall survival in stage II and III breast cancer patients. In press, J Psychosom Res.
14. Weihs KL, Enright T, Simmens S. Acceptance of emotion, resolution of distress and survival in breast cancer patients. Manuscript under review.
15. Reynolds P, Kaplan GA. Social connections and risk for cancer: Prospective evidence from the Alameda County Study. Behav Med 1990;16:101–110.
16. Watson M, Haviland JS, Greer S, et al. Influence of psychological response on survival in breast cancer: A population-based cohort study. Lancet 1999;354:1331–1336.
17. Hjerl K, Andersen EW, Keiding N, et al.. Depression as a prognostic factor for breast cancer mortality. Psychosomatics 2003;44(1):24–30.
18. Gallagher J, Parle M, Cairns D. Appraisal and psychological distress six months after diagnosis of breast cancer. Br J Health Psychol 2002; 7(3):365–376.
19. Nosarti C, Roberts JV, Crayford T, et al. Early psychological adjustment in breast cancer patients: A prospective study. J Psychosom Res 2002;53(6):1123–1130.
20. Northouse L. A longitudinal study of the adjustment of patients and husbands to breast cancer. Oncol Nurs Forum 1989;16(4):511–516.
21. Irvine D, Brown B, Crooks D, et al. Psychosocial adjustment of women with breast cancer. Cancer 1991;67(4):1097–1117.
22. Stanton AL, Danoff-Burg SM, Huggins ME. The first year after breast cancer diagnosis: Hope and coping strategies as predictors of adjustment. Psychooncology 2002;11(2):93–102.
23. Baltrusch HJF, Stangel W, Titze I. Stress, cancer and immunity: New developments in biopsychosocial and psychoneuroimmunologic research. Acta Neurol 1991;13(4):315–327.
24. Weiss K, Enright T, Simmens S, Reiss D. Negative affectivity, restriction of emotions, and site of metastases predict mortality in recurrent breast cancer. J Psychosom Res 2000;49:59–68.
25. Hurny C. Psyche and cancer. Ann Oncol 1990;1:6–8.
26. Montazeri A, Jarvandi S, Haghighat S, et al. Anxiety and depression in breast cancer patients before and after participation in a cancer support group. Patient Education Counseling 2001;45(3):195–198.
27. Moyer A. Psychosocial outcomes of breast-conserving surgery versus mastectomy: A meta-analytic review. Health Psychol 1997;16: 284–293.
28. Schover LR. The impact of breast cancer on sexuality, body image, and intimate relationships. CA Cancer J Clinicians 1991;41(2):112–120.
29. Fallowfield LJ, Baum M, Maguire GP. Effects of breast conservation on psychological morbidity associated with diagnosis and treatment of early breast cancer. BMJ1986;293:1331–1334.
30. Levy SM, Herberman RB, Lee JK, et al. Breast conservation versus mastectomy: Distress sequelae as a function of choice. J Clin Oncol 1989;7(3):367–375.
31. Cohen L, Hack TF, de Moor C, et al. The effects of type of surgery and time on psychological adjustment in women after breast cancer treatment. Ann Surg Oncol 2000;7(6):427–434.
32. Fobair P, O'Hanlan K, Koopman C, et al. Comparison of lesbian and heterosexual women's response to newly diagnosed breast cancer. Psychooncology 2001;10(1):40–51.
33. Ganz PA, Desmond KA, Belin TR, et al. Predictors of sexual health in women after a breast cancer diagnosis. J Clin Oncol 1999; 17(8):2371–2380.
34. Meyerowitz BE, Desmond KA, Rowland JH, et al. Sexuality following breast cancer. J Sex Marital Ther 1999;25(3):237–250.
35. Stead ML. Sexual dysfunction after treatment for gynaecologic and breast malignancies. Curr Opin Obstet Gynecol 2003;15(1):57–61.
36. Kemeny MM, Wellisch DK, Schain WS. Psychosocial outcome in a randomized surgical trial for treatment of primary breast cancer. Cancer 1988;62(6):1231–1237.
37. Steinberg MD, Juliano MA, Wise L. Psychological outcome of lumpectomy versus mastectomy in the treatment of breast cancer. Am J Psychiatry 1985;142:32–39.
38. Omne-Ponten M, Holmberg L, Burns T, et al. Determinants of the psycho-social outcome after operation for breast cancer. Results of a

prospective comparative interview study following mastectomy and breast conservation. Eur J Cancer 1992;28A(6/7):1062–1067.

39. Ganz PA, Rowland JH, Desmond K, et al. Life after breast cancer: Understanding women's health-related quality of life and sexual functioning. J Clin Oncol 1998;(2):501–514.

40. Schover LR. Sexuality and body image in younger women with breast cancer. J Natl Cancer Inst Monogr 1994;16:177–182.

41. Schain WS. The sexual and intimate consequences of breast cancer treatment. CA Cancer J Clinicians 1988;38(3):154–161.

42. Zahlis EH, Shands ME. The impact of breast cancer on the partner 18 months after diagnosis. Semin Oncol Nurs 1993;9(2):83–87.

43. Ell K, Nishimoto R, Mantell J, Hamovitch M. A longitudinal analysis of psychological adaptation among family members of patients with cancer. J Psychosom Res 1988;32(4/5):429–438.

44. Collicio FA, Agnello R, Staltzer J. Pregnancy after breast cancer: From psychosocial issues through conception. Oncology 1998;12(5):759–769.

45. Stevens PE, Tatum NO, White JC. Optimal care for lesbian patients. Patient Care 1996;15:121–140.

46. Northouse LL, Jeffs M, Cracchiolo-Caraway A, et al. Emotional distress reported by women and husbands prior to a breast biopsy. Nurs Res 1995;44(4):196–201.

47. Goffman TE, Lowe JR, Weiss D, Laronga C. Neglected breast cancer syndrome. Surgical Rounds, November issue, 2003;538–544.

48. Fogarty L, Curbow B, Wingard J, Mc Donnell K. The role of physician compassion in breast cancer treatment decision making. Presented at A Women's Health Conference. American Psychological Association, Washington, DC, Sept 19–21, 1996.

49. Slabey AE. Response to the diagnosis of cancer. In Slabey AE (ed). Adapting to Life-Threatening Illness. New York, Praeger, 1985

50. Wool MS, Goldberg RJ. Assessment of denial in cancer patients: Implications for intervention. J Psychosoc Oncol 1986;4(3):1–14.

51. Burckhart CS. Coping strategies of the chronically ill. Nurs Clin North Am 1987;22(3):543–550.

52. Benson H. The placebo effect. Harvard Med School Health Lett August 1980;3–4.

53. Harris SR, Templeton E. Who's listening? Experiences of women with breast cancer in communicating with physicians. Breast J 2001;7(6):444–449.

54. Northouse PG, Northouse LL. Communication and cancer: Issues confronting patients, health professionals, and family members. J Psychosoc Oncol 1987;5(3):17–46.

55. Taylor S. Adjustment to threatening events: A theory of cognitive adaptation. Am Psychologist 1983;38(11):116–117.

56. Taylor S, Brown J. Illusion and well-being: A social psychological perspective on mental health. Psychol Bull 1988;103(2):193–210.

57. Aapro M, Cull A. Depression in breast cancer patients: The need for treatment. Ann Oncol 1999;10:1–10.

58. Weisman A. Early diagnosis of vulnerability in cancer patients. Am J Med Sci 1976;271:187–196.

59. Brown G, Harris T. Social Origins of Depression: A Study of Psychiatric Disorder in Women. New York, Free Press, 1978.

60. Wells KB, Golding JM, Burnam MA. Psychiatric disorder in a sample of the general population with and without chronic medical conditions. Am J Psychiatry 1988;145:976–981.

61. Kaplan HI, Sadock BJ. Synopsis of Psychiatry: Behavioral Sciences, Clinical Psychiatry, 8th ed. New York, Lippincott Williams & Wilkins, 1998.

62. Hyman SE, Arana GW, Rosenbaum JF. Handbook of Psychiatric Drug Therapy, 4th ed. Boston, Little, Brown, 2000.

63. Green B, Rowland J, Krupnick J, et al. Life-threatening illness and posttraumatic stress disorder (PTSD). In Psychosocial and Behavioral Factors in Women's Health: Research, Prevention, Treatment, and Service Delivery in Clinical and Community Settings. Washington, DC, American Psychological Association, 1996.

64. Spiegel D. Effects of psychosocial support on patients with metastatic breast cancer. J Psychosoc Oncol 1992;10(2):113–120.

65. Spiegel D, Bloom JR, Kraemer HC, Gottheil E. Effect of psychosocial treatment on survival of patients with metastatic breast cancer. Lancet 1989;2:888–891.

66. Cunningham AJ, Edmonds CV, Jenkins GP, et al. A randomized controlled trial of the effects of group psychological therapy on survival in women with metastatic breast cancer. Psychooncology 1998;7:508–517.

67. Goodwin PJ, Leszcz M, Ennis M, et al. The effect of group psychosocial support on survival in metastatic breast cancer. N Engl J Med 2001;345(24):1719–1726.

68. Spiegel D. Mind matters—group therapy and survival in breast cancer. N Engl J Med 2001;345(24):1767–1768.

69. Becker E. The Denial of Death. New York, Free Press, 1973.

70. Becvar DS. I am a woman first: A message about breast cancer. Families Systems Health 1996;14(1):83–93.

71. Northouse LL, Dorris G, Charron-Moore C. Factors affecting couples adjustment to recurrent breast cancer. Social Sci Med 1995;41(1):69–76.

72. Silberfarb PM, Maurer LH, Crouthamel CS. Psychosocial aspects of neoplastic disease. I. Functional status of breast cancer patients during different treatment regimens. Am J Psychiatry 1980;137(4):450–455.

73. Vickberg SMJ. Fears about breast cancer recurrence: Interviews with a diverse sample. Cancer Pract 2001;9(5):237–243.

74. Baider L, Kaplan De-Nour A. Adjustment to cancer: Who is the patient—the husband or the wife? Isr J Med Sci 1988;24:631–636.

75. Northouse LL, Mood D, Kershaw T, et al. Quality of life of women with recurrent breast cancer and their family members. J Clin Oncol 2002;20(19):4050–4064.

76. Rowland JH. Back to the future: Dealing with the fear of recurrence. Presented at the Ninth Annual Assembly of the National Coalition for Cancer Survivorship, Washington, DC, November 2–6, 1994.

77. Fife BL. The conceptualization of meaning in illness. Social Sci Med 1994;38(2):309–316.

78. Frankl VE. Man's Search for Meaning: An Introduction to Logotherapy. Boston, Beacon, 1959.

79. Lewis FM. Attributions of control, experienced meaning, and psychosocial well-being in patients with advanced cancer. J Psychosoc Oncol 1989;7:105.

80. Barkwell DP. Ascribed meaning: A critical factor in coping and pain attenuation in patients with cancer related pain. J Palliat Care 1991;7(3):5–14.

81. Pettingale KW, Morris T, Greer S, Haybittle JL. Mental attitudes to cancer: An additional prognostic factor. Lancet 1985;1:750.

82. Watson M, Greer S, Pruyn J, van den Borne B. Locus of control and adjustment to cancer. Psychol Rep 1990;66:39–48.

83. Siegel B. Love, Medicine and Miracles. New York, Harper and Row, 1998.

84. Sontag S. Illness as Metaphor and AIDS and its Metaphors. New York, Anchor Books, 1990.

85. Arendt H. The Human Condition. Chicago, University of Chicago Press, 1958.

86. Weihs K. Escalation and persistence of stress after breast cancer: A systems view. Presented at A Women's Health Conference, American Psychological Association, Washington, DC, Sept 19–21, 1996.

87. Shapiro SL, Lopez AM, Schwartz GE, et al. Quality of life and breast cancer: Relationship to psychosocial variables. J Clin Psychol 2001;54(4):501–519.

88. Carter EA, McGoldrick M. The Family Life Cycle. New York, Gardner Press, 1980.

89. Veach TA, Nicholas DR. Understanding families of adults with cancer: Combining the clinical course of cancer and stages of family development. J Counseling Dev 1998;76:144–156.

90. Arpin K, Fitch M, Browne GB, Corey P. Prevalence and correlates of family dysfunction and poor adjustment to chronic illness in specialty clinics. J Clin Epidemiol 1990;43(4):373–383.

91. Skerett K. Couple adjustment to the experience of breast cancer. Families Systems Health 1998;16(3):281–298.

92. Derogatis LR, Morrow GR, Fetting J, et al. The prevalence of psychiatric disorders among cancer patients. JAMA 1983;249(6):751–757.

93. Grassi L, Rosti G. Psychosocial morbidity and adjustment to illness among long-term cancer survivors: A six-year-follow-up study. Psychosomatics 1996;37(6):523–532.

94. Ferrell B, Ervin K, Smith S, et al. Family perspectives of ovarian cancer. Cancer Pract 2002;10(6):269–276.

95. Omne-Ponten M, Holmberg L, Bergstrom R, et al. Psychosocial adjustment among husbands of women treated for breast cancer: Mastectomy vs. breast-conserving surgery. Eur J Cancer 1993;29A:1393–1397.

96. Lewis FM, Woods NF, Hough EE, Bensley LS. The family's functioning with chronic illness in the mother: The spouse's perspective. Social Sci Med 1989;29(11):1261–1269.

97. Vinokur AD, Threatt B, Caplan R, Zimmerman B. Physical and psychosocial functioning and adjustment to breast cancer. Cancer 1989;63:394–405.

98. Giese-Davis J, Hermanson K, Koopman C, et al. Quality of couples' relationship and adjustment to metastatic breast cancer. J Fam Psychol 2000;14(2):251–266.

99. Kayser K, Sormanti M, Strainchamps E. Women coping with cancer: The influence of relationship factors on psychosocial adjustment. Psychol Women Q 1999;23:725–730.

100. Trask PC, Paterson AG, Trask CL, et al. Parent and adolescent adjustment to pediatric cancer: Associations with coping, social support, and family function. J Pediatr Oncol Nurs 2003;20(1):36–47.

101. Weihs K, Politi M. Family systems in response to cancer: Optimizing family development in the face of cancer. In Crane DR, Marshall ES (eds). Handbook of Families and Health: Interdisciplinary Perspectives. Sage Publications, Thousand Oaks, CA, 2005.

102. Weingarten K. The Mother's Voice: Strengthening Intimacy in Family Relationships. New York, Harcourt Brace, 1994.

103. Reiss D, Gonzalez S, Steinglass P. Putting the illness in its place: Discussion groups for families with chronic medical illness. Family Process 1989;28:69–87.

104. American Cancer Society. Helping your child deal with a cancer diagnosis in the family [online]. Available at *www.cancer.org*. Accessed November 3, 2003.

105. Barnes J, Kroll L, Lee J, et al. Factors predicting communication about the diagnosis of maternal breast cancer to children. J Psychosom Res 2002;52(4):209–214.

106. Lichtman RR, Taylor SE, Wood JV, et al. Relations with children after breast cancer: The mother-daughter relationship at risk. J Psychosoc Oncol 1985;2(3/4):1–19.

107. Wellisch D, Gritz E, Schain W, et al. Psychological functioning of daughters of breast cancer patients: Part I. Psychosomatics 1991; 32(3):324–336.

108. Gilligan C. In a different voice: Women's conceptions of the self and morality. Harvard Educ Rev 1977;47:481–517.

109. Gilligan C, Belensky M. A naturalistic study of abortion decisions. New Directions Child Dev 1980;7:69–90.

110. Gilligan C, Belensky M. In a Different Voice: Psychological Theory and Women's Development. Cambridge, MA, Harvard University Press, 1982.

111. Attanucci J. In whose terms: A new perspective on self, role and relationship. In Gilligan C, Ward JV, McLean Taylor J, Bardige B (eds). Mapping the Moral Domain. Cambridge, MA, Harvard University Press, 1988.

112. McGoldrick M, Pearce JK, Giordano J. Ethnicity and Family Therapy. New York, Guilford Press, 1982.

113. Bernstein L, Teal CR, Joslyn S, Wilson J. Ethnicity-related variation in breast cancer risk factors. Cancer 2003;97(1 Suppl):222–229.

114. Perkins P, Cooksley CD, Cox JD. Breast cancer. Is ethnicity an independent prognostic factor for survival? Cancer 1996;78(6):1241–1247.

115. Zborowski M. People in Pain. San Francisco, Jossey-Bass, 1969, pp 236–250.

116. Krieger N, sidney S. Racial discrimination and blood pressure: The CARDIA study of young black and white adults. Am J Public Health 1996;86(10):1370–1378.

117. Mathews HF, Lannin DR, Mitchell JP. Coming to terms with advanced breast cancer: Black women's narratives from eastern North Carolina. Social Sci Med 1994;38(6):789–800.

118. Carnon AG, Ssemwogerere A, Lamont DW, et al. Relation between socioeconomic deprivation and pathological prognostic factors in women with breast cancer. BMJ 1994;309(6961):1054–1057.

119. Garvican L, Littlejohns P. Comparison of prognostic and socio-economic factors in screen-detected and symptomatic cases of breast cancer. Public Health1998;112(1):15–20.

120. American Cancer Society. Transcripts of the Public Hearings of the American Cancer Society on Cancer and the Poor. Atlanta, American Cancer Society, 1989.

121. Belgrave FZ. Psychosocial Aspects of Chronic Illness and Disability among African-Americans. Westport, CT, Auburn House, 1998.

122. Ashing-Giwa K, Ganz PA. Understanding the breast cancer experience of African-American women. J Psychosoc Oncol 1997;15(2):19–35.

123. Lannin DR, Matthews HF, Mitchell J, Swanson MS: Imparting cultural attitudes in African American women to decrease breast cancer mortality. Am J Surg 2002;184:418–423.

124. Gall TL, Cornblat MW. Breast cancer survivors give voice: A qualitative analysis of spiritual factors in long-term adjustment. Psychooncology 2002;11(6):524–535.

125. Sephton SE, Koopman C, Schaal M, et al. Spiritual expression and immune status in women with metastatic breast cancer: An exploratory study. Breast J 2001;7(5):345–353.

126. Robinson KD, Kimmel EA, Yasko JM. Reaching out to the African American community through innovative strategies. Oncol Nurs Forum 1995;22:1383–1391.

127. Chambliss L. The cancer reality gap. Working Woman 1996; Oct:46–48.

128. Boyle G. Legal barriers against employment discrimination for the breast cancer patient. Innovations Breast Cancer Care 1996;2(1): 13–16.

CHAPTER 39

Rehabilitation and Nursing Care

Jean Lynn

Nurses in a collaborative multidisciplinary setting are the indispensable members of breast health teams that develop supportive strategies to meet the growing demand for comprehensive, service-oriented care. The nurse's involvement includes, but is not limited to, patient triage, patient and family education, psychosocial support, administrative responsibilities that include financial and clinical management, and ultimately, patient advocacy.[1]

The nurse can also have an impact on breast cancer awareness in the community. She or he can offer lectures to increase awareness about early detection, screening guidelines, and risk factors and can promote the legislative and political agenda as a breast cancer advocate. Involvement with professional organizations and breast cancer advocacy groups complements the nurse's clinical skills, which, in turn, enhance the care of the breast cancer patient. This role expansion is an asset to the nurse and hence to the other members of the breast health team.

Nursing and patient advocacy go hand in hand. The continued increase in rates of breast cancer has become a very political issue, and consequently, nurses have become involved not only as participants in the breast cancer advocacy movement but also as partners in research, both as scientific reviewers and as a resource to investigators.

The period between the diagnosis of breast cancer and the selection of definitive surgery is an extremely stressful time for the patient. Because breast cancer treatment is highly complex and is a paradigm for multidisciplinary care, the nurse is instrumental in providing emotional and physical support for the woman and her family. Furthermore, nurses can play an essential role in providing continuity of care and individualized treatment plans for each patient. Ideally, the nurse becomes the *patient's navigator*. The nurse helps to educate the patient and her family about all aspects of treatment, follow-up, and subsequent therapy. Preoperative teaching is an integral component of the patient's preparation for and recovery from surgery.

The following text describes how the nurse can effectively care for the newly diagnosed breast cancer patient.

ADDRESSING PATIENT CONCERNS

How can a nurse reassure a patient who has just been diagnosed with breast cancer?

Most often, women want to get treatment started as soon as possible. The nurse can help to reassure the patient that breast cancer is *not* an emergency. Breast cancer may be present for 5 to 8 years before a tumor becomes clinically apparent, either by physical examination or by mammography. A woman with a new diagnosis of breast cancer should explore all her options before making decisions about her therapy. In most cases, waiting several weeks for definitive treatment will not compromise the long-term prognosis.

The nurse should explain that there is no known cause of breast cancer. Although there are many factors associated with an increased risk for developing the disease, about 75% of women who are diagnosed with breast cancer have no known risk factors. When breast cancer is detected early (<1 cm in size), long-term survival is greater than 90%. In fact, even though the incidence continues to rise in the United States, the mortality rate from breast cancer remains steady, and this rate experienced the first decline in 50 years in the early 1990s.[2] The nurse should promote positive thinking, guide the patient to gather information, and help her process the information.

What should nurses tell patients who seek to learn more about their disease?

The nurse should encourage the patient to incorporate her family or support network into the information-gathering phase of her treatment. Breast cancer is often a family issue. Encourage the patient to have another person with her when she visits with the physician. If that is not possible, a tape recorder might be helpful for information gathering. The patient should realize that breast cancer encompasses a broad spectrum of lesions with varying patterns of behavior. Therefore, there is no "one way" to treat breast cancer, and the patient should not compare her treatment with that of other women. Each breast cancer behaves differently, and the physician and nurse should provide the patient with information about the specific type of breast cancer she has and explain in detail the rationale behind her personalized treatment plan.

If the patient has access to a computer, there is a myriad of information on the Internet. (See "Internet Resources for Breast Cancer.") In addition to the informational pamphlets provided by the American Cancer Society and the National Cancer Institute, many books are available for the patient with a new diagnosis.

How should the nurse explain the various treatment options to the patient?

The nurse should emphasize that women are encouraged to become empowered with information that will help them participate in the decision-making process. Evidence-based decisions are the standard of care. The nurse should have up-to-date knowledge about the *evidence* supporting the choices that are being presented to patients. If there is no evidence to support a recommendation, the nurse should be able to discuss clinical trials that the physician feels may be appropriate for the patient.

Most often, women are not sure what type of questions to ask. The Susan G. Komen Foundation has provided a very useful pamphlet entitled "Questions to Ask the Doctor about Breast Cancer."[3] The Susan G. Komen website (*www.komen.org*) also has an interactive video titled *Anatomy of Breast Cancer*, available in English and Spanish, that the patient can refer to for additional information. The nurse should be prepared to discuss the answers to the questions in the pamphlet, which will complement the information already provided by the surgeon. Several of these questions are addressed in the following list:

1. *What are my treatment options? What is the surgeon recommending for me and why?*
2. *What are the potential risks and benefits of these procedures?*
3. *Will the tumor be analyzed for estrogen and progesterone receptors?* This is important information because it will help the oncologist who prescribes the definitive systemic therapy. When a tumor is estrogen or progesterone receptor positive, the tumor cells are binding to estrogen, progesterone, or both, and these hormones are promoting tumor activity.
4. *Will other special tests for HER-2/neu and proliferation rate be done on the tissue?* How this test is performed is as important as the information it provides. The most accurate method is the fluorescence in situ hybridization (FISH) test to determine *HER-2/neu* status. If the tumor is *HER-2/neu* positive, the oncologist will recommend an anthracycline-based chemotherapy regimen with or without trastuzumab (Herceptin) therapy.
5. *In addition to the radiation therapy, will I need additional treatment with drugs if I have breast-conserving surgery?* The surgeon will most likely not be able to give a definitive answer until the immunohistochemistry analysis (which detects molecular markers [proteins] in breast

tumors) is performed on the sentinel lymph node or the axillary node dissection, and the complete pathologic examination of the tumor is completed.[4,5]
6. *Is breast reconstruction something I should consider?* There is no time limit on this decision; hence, the woman should not feel pressured into making this decision until she is ready to do so.
7. *Should I consider a prophylactic mastectomy?* Most surgeons do not recommend this procedure, except in unusual circumstances. For many women the peace of mind that comes with not having to worry about breast cancer recurrence is very comforting, but the patient should understand that prophylactic mastectomy does not provide a 100% guarantee. In many cases, not all of the glandular tissue is removed. In most cases, however, mastectomy does reduce the risk for a second primary tumor.
8. *Is it necessary to evaluate the lymph nodes when treating breast cancer?* Most often, yes, if it is an invasive cancer. The nurse should explain that if the patient has a preinvasive cancer, there is no need to perform an axillary node dissection. However, if the preinvasive cancer is extensive, a sentinal lymph node biopsy may be performed. When lymph node dissection is performed, instruction about care of the affected arm will need to be incorporated into the preoperative teaching (Table 39–1).
9. *How long will I need to stay in the hospital? Will I need nursing care at home?* Generally speaking, most patients are in the hospital for a period of 6 to 23 hours. Ideally,

Table 39–1 Precautions for Patients Who Undergo an Axillary Node Dissection

If the sentinal lymph nodes are positive for cancer cells, the surgeon will proceed with an axillary node dissection to determine whether the nodes have any cancer cells.

Lymph nodes are located throughout the body. They filter fluids, proteins, and bacteria that are in our bodies. Occasionally, the removal of lymph nodes causes an ineffective filtering of this fluid, which sometimes results in edema (fluid accumulation) in the arm. This happens in a very small percentage of patients. The following guidelines have been established to help prevent lymphedema from occurring. It is important to review these guidelines and to incorporate them into your daily life:

1. Practice good skin hygiene; use lotion after bathing. When drying the arm, be gentle but thorough.
2. Avoid venipuncture, injections, and infusions into the affected arm.
3. Wear protective gloves when working outside or with water or cleaning products and during all activities that might result in injury to the affected arm.
4. Wear sunscreen to protect against sunburn, and use insect repellent to protect against bites and stings.
5. Do not cut hangnails or cut nails too short; do not push cuticles back to the nail bed.
6. Exercise and use the affected arm; full range of motion and return of strength should return within 2 months.

If a cut, insect bite, or other break in the skin occurs, wash the area with soap and water, use an antiseptic, and cover with a sterile dressing. Watch for any signs of infections, warmth, redness, pain, and/or tenderness.

Contact a physician immediately if an infection develops in the affected arm. She or he will most likely prescribe an antibiotic.

From Precautions for Patients Who Have an Axillary Node Dissection [pamphlet]. Washington, DC, The George Washington University Breast Care Center.

the nurse should see the patient for preoperative teaching a few days before the scheduled procedure. If this is not possible, the nurse should be sure that the patient receives written information about the proposed procedure, and the nurse should have a telephone consultation with the patient. Alternatively, patients may wish to correspond by e-mail. A written documentation of this correspondence is then placed in the patient's chart. Unless the patient has specific physical limitations, home nursing care is not necessary.

10. *Are there any special precautions or side effects from the axillary node dissection in addition to the lymphedema precautions?* Although special care is taken to prevent damage to the intercostobrachial nerve of the affected arm, many patients experience numbness in the armpit and inner arm down to the elbow. Sensation usually returns to the affected arm within several months, or perhaps even up to a year. Some patients indicate that the numbness never diminishes completely. When the numbness starts to dissipate, many patients experience a "pins and needles" sensation in the arm. This is quite common and reflects nerve regeneration. The nurse should instruct the patient to refrain from shaving with a razor in the affected armpit, because of the lack of feeling in that area; she should instead be instructed to use an electric razor to prevent cutting herself.

11. *What is radiation therapy?* The nurse can explain that radiation therapy is the use of high-intensity x-rays directed at the breast tissue to kill off any microscopic cells in the breast. This is given to prevent local recurrence of the breast cancer in the affected breast. The treatment is spaced over a period of 5 to 7 weeks. The nurse can also explain that before the treatment begins, the patient is "simulated." This procedure entails having the patient lie down on a hard table, with the affected arm hyperextended, which may be uncomfortable if it has been only a few weeks since surgery. This procedure takes about an hour; the technologists place markings on the breast surface to serve as landmarks for the daily treatments. These markings may be tattoos, which are permanent. The patient may request a nonpermanent marker, in which case the markings may fade and will require reapplication or touch-up during the treatment process. The simulation procedure is the longest session of radiation therapy. The actual time in treatment generally lasts only 20 minutes. An extra "boost" of radiation may be given to the area of the breast where the primary tumor originated. As detailed in Chapter 26, the usual dose of radiation is 5000 cGy, with a daily dose of 180 to 200 cGy/day. The nurse can suggest that the patient bring a book or portable music source to pass the time and should reassure the patient that the technologist is always within hearing distance and she is never alone.

12. *How soon will I begin radiation treatments?* This will depend on what the medical team decides is best. In any event, radiotherapy will not begin until the patient is completely healed from surgery.

13. *How many treatments will I receive?* The nurse can explain that the patient will be receiving treatments on a daily basis for about 20 minutes a day over a period of 5 to 7 weeks. Although this is an interruption of the patient's daily schedule, it is a relatively short period of time in the major treatment plan. Most women work full-time while receiving their therapy and schedule their appointments early in the morning, on their lunch hour, or after work. Once treatment is begun on a particular machine, the patient will have to stay with that machine for the duration of her therapy.

14. *What are the side effects of radiation therapy?* Although many women tolerate radiation therapy to the breast without any significant side effects, the nurse should inform the patient that one side effect from radiation may be fatigue due to the cumulative effect of radiation toward the third to fourth week of therapy. This usually subsides several weeks after radiation therapy is completed. Other side effects may be some breast tenderness and soreness, which gradually disappear over time; however, the irradiated breast may never feel completely normal compared with the other breast. Some women also describe "shooting pains" within the breast after receiving radiation that may or may not disappear. Another common side effect is skin redness, the "sunburn" effect. This side effect is more pronounced in fair-skinned people and usually subsides with time. As the redness goes away, there may be a darkening of the skin, and the pores can become enlarged and more noticeable. Fibrosis (thickening) of the breast tissue is a significant long-term effect. If the axilla has been irradiated, the patient may be prone to the subsequent appearance of lymphedema because the radiation compounds the scarring from surgery. The patient will also be unable to lactate from the irradiated breast.

15. *What should I do for my skin when receiving radiation therapy?* The nurse should advise the patient to follow these guidelines:
    a. Wash with mild soap (e.g., Dove, Neutrogena, Basis).
    b. Do not wear deodorant on the affected side because deodorants usually contain aluminum, which can interact with the radiation. Use cornstarch or talc-free baby powder as an alternative to deodorant. Health food stores may also have deodorant alternatives.
    c. Shave only with an electric razor. There will be no feeling or sensation in the armpit area because of nerve manipulation, and you might cut yourself without realizing it. This could increase the incidence of lymphedema or infection.
    d. Do not use any over-the-counter creams or lotions without checking with the nurse or physician in radiation therapy. Avoid direct sunlight to the area, and use sunscreen (SPF 15 or higher).
    e. Avoid tight bras or underwire bras. Wear a sports bra if possible.
    f. Use only unscented hydrophilic creams such as Aquaphor, Biafine Unscented, 99% to 100% pure aloe vera gel (with no added perfumes or dyes), or Radiacare gel or gel pads.

Although radiation therapy is generally used for women who choose breast-conserving therapy, some women may require it after a mastectomy to help prevent local recurrence.

What other information should patients receive preoperatively?

Before surgery, the physician may order several radiographs or blood tests to evaluate for metastatic disease. Routine laboratory tests include a complete blood count, which measures hemoglobin and hematocrit (red blood cell production). Other tests include liver chemistries and perhaps tumor marker studies as a baseline. A chest radiograph will be done, and the physician may order a bone scan and a computed tomography (CT) scan of the abdomen, depending on the clinical stage of presentation of disease. These are done to evaluate the lung, liver, and bones, which are the most common sites for breast cancer to spread. These tests may provoke some tension and anxiety, but they are performed to get a thorough overall picture of the patient and to have an established baseline from which to prescribe the most appropriate therapy.

The patient should be instructed before surgery that she will meet with the anesthesiologist. Encourage the patient to share any concerns she may have and to inform the anesthesiologist of any over-the-counter medicines, especially herbal medicines, that she may be taking.

Patients are admitted to the hospital on the day of surgery and usually stay in the hospital from 6 to 23 hours, depending on the type of surgery performed. On the day of surgery, the patient should wear a loose-fitting blouse that buttons down the front for the trip home. This will facilitate dressing because she should not need to raise her arm over her head owing to the incision in or near the axilla. She should also be instructed not to wear jewelry or contact lenses or to take any valuables with her to the hospital. If she is taking medications, advise her to check with the anesthesiologist to see if they must be taken on the morning of surgery. Also, if patients have dentures, hearing aids, canes, or walkers, these items should be labeled with the patient's name and placed in a secure area during the surgery.

How should nurses instruct patients during the postoperative period and adjuvant therapy?

It is unlikely that any side effects will occur, but patients should be made aware that there is potential for the following problems.

Seromas: These are fluid collections beneath the surgical site.

Fluid leakage from the drain: If the drain is not functioning properly—that is, if the suction device is malfunctioning—fluid may accumulate beneath the incision. If the patient notices that fluid accumulation has ceased in the drainage bulb or canister, the nurse may assess whether the tube is blocked with a clot and may then gently "milk" the tubing to clear the blockage.

Infection: If there is any fever or swelling (edema) around the drain site or incision, the patient should contact the physician immediately.

What care is required during the postoperative period?

Pain should be controlled before patient discharge. The nurse can explain to the patient that there will be some discomfort in the axilla. A prescribed pain medication or over-the-counter analgesic should be used. The nurse should encourage the patient to take rest periods, pace herself, and seek the support of friends and family during the first 2 weeks after the operation. Usually, many people are willing to help out. Suggest that a friend organize dinner meals for the next couple of weeks.

Exercises are commonly advised following breast surgery, usually beginning 24 hours after the drain has been removed. Exercising may be uncomfortable, and ibuprofen or acetaminophen may be taken before commencing exercise.

Most women are so busy that they do not "have time" for breast cancer. Obviously, there is no good time to have breast cancer, but it is also unrealistic to think that patients' schedules can be resumed as if nothing has happened. Encourage patients to allow time for processing this event. Support groups are very helpful. If a patient does not have access to a support group, the nurse may suggest an online support group provided through the Wellness Community by a licensed social worker (*www.thewellnesscommunity.org*). It is comforting for many women to talk to others who are undergoing the same experience.

What might nurses convey to patients about systemic treatments?

After surgery is completed and all the information has been obtained from the breast tumor, a consultation with a medical oncologist will be scheduled to discuss the possibility of adjuvant hormonal therapy, chemotherapy, or a combination of the two. The following questions are similar to ones that may be asked of the nurse.

Will I receive hormonal therapy?

The nurse should explain that if the tumor is estrogen or progesterone receptor positive, hormonal therapy may be prescribed by itself or in addition to chemotherapy and radiation. Hormonal therapy is used to prevent recurrence of the tumor and to reduce the patient's risk for developing a contralateral or ipsilateral breast tumor. Tamoxifen blocks tumor cells from binding with estrogen and stops tumor growth. Tamoxifen has been the gold standard for decades, but newer studies show that for postmenopausal women, aromatase inhibitors such as Arimidex are becoming the treatment of choice.[6] Although tamoxifen is well tolerated, it has side effects: hot flashes, decrease in libido, depression, vaginal dryness, and irregularity in the menstrual cycle. Patients, especially postmenopausal women, may also be at increased risk of thromboembolytic events. Women taking tamoxifen may also be at a slightly increased risk for developing cataracts. Other eye problems that have been reported are corneal scarring and retinal changes. Some benefits of using tamoxifen are that it increases bone augmentation and has a beneficial effect on coronary heart disease. Even though tamoxifen is an anti-estrogen drug, patients can still become pregnant while taking it. The nurse should instruct patients to use birth control while taking tamoxifen. There is also a risk for developing endometrial cancer. Therefore, annual gynecologic examinations should be performed.

In premenopausal women, tamoxifen stimulates the ovaries, which in turn increases estrogen and progesterone levels and may increase the incidence of ovarian cysts and stimulate ovulation while blocking estrogen in the breast. Side effects of aromatase inhibitors include hot flashes, arthralgias, fatigue, and occasional nausea. Women taking aromatase inhibitors are also more prone to fractures. The nurse should inform the patient about appropriate calcium intake (1200–1500 mg/day), and a DEXA (dual energy x-ray absortiometry) scan should be obtained prior to initiating treatment with an aromatase inhibitor. Vaginal dryness is a side effect of both of these therapies. Over-the-counter vaginal lubricants (e.g., Replens, Astroglide) can be used to alleviate this symptom. The usual course of therapy for tamoxifen and aromatase inhibitors is 5 years.

Will I have chemotherapy?

To many patients, chemotherapy sounds frightening, and questions about it are usually asked in the preoperative stage. To treat breast cancer aggressively and effectively and to decrease the possibility of a recurrence of the breast cancer or of a second primary cancer, chemotherapy is the most effective treatment we have at this time, in addition to surgery and radiation. The patient probably knows someone who has had chemotherapy in the past and whose memory of this experience is unpleasant. The side effects of chemotherapy are more manageable now than they were in years past. New medications minimize nausea and vomiting, and most women are able to work full-time while they are receiving chemotherapy.

How does chemotherapy work?

The nurse may explain that cancer cells proliferate at an uncontrolled rate. The cell division process is interrupted by chemotherapy, so that the cells cannot continue to multiply and divide. The drugs chosen to treat breast cancer have been shown to be effective against breast tumors through previous clinical trials. These drugs interfere with the cell division at different points in the cell cycle. This is why a combination of two or three drugs may be chosen as part of the treatment regimen.

Most women who undergo adjuvant chemotherapy tolerate it quite well. Because the chemotherapy affects fast-growing cells (i.e., tumor cells), it often affects other healthy, fast-growing cells in the body. These include the hair, the lining of the mouth, the lining of the gastrointestinal tract, and the blood cells in the bone marrow. The most devastating side effect for many women is hair loss.

Hair loss does not occur all at once. It is a gradual process that begins most often about 2 to 3 weeks after chemotherapy is administered. Many of my patients have shared that the hair loss occurs first in the pubic area and then on the head. Of course, this process depends on the drugs that are prescribed. Assurances that the hair will grow back do not necessarily diminish the patient's sense of loss. Some women have stated that they would endure more of the other side effects to avoid this one. When the hair does resume its growth, it takes about 3 months to grow in; most often, the hair is fine and is initially curly or wavy.

If the patient is likely to receive a drug that will definitely cause hair loss, the nurse should tell the patient where she can purchase a wig. It is very important to purchase a wig before the onset of hair loss. If the patient is receiving chemotherapy, the Look Good Feel Better Program of the American Cancer Society can help her with cosmetics application and styling of her wig. It is a half-day of pampering, and many women enjoy it.

How are chemotherapy side effects managed?

Although the nurse can facilitate access to resources and education, educating the patient to advocate for herself is just as important. Patients should be encouraged to ask questions. As the patient begins treatment, the nurse can teach her about the following:

1. *Keeping track of blood counts.* Blood counts are monitored on a weekly basis to evaluate the impact the chemotherapy has had on the bone marrow. The goal of chemotherapy is to give the maximum amount of drug in the shortest period of time, but at the same time, not to compromise the patient so that she will be susceptible to infection. If white blood cell counts fall below a certain point, patients can be more susceptible to infection. Therefore, the physician may prescribe filgrastim or pegfilgrastim to be used with chemotherapy. Filgrastim or pegfilgrastim is administered to stimulate the bone marrow to produce white blood cells.

2. *Eating a well-balanced diet.* Patients who are undergoing treatment always ask questions about food. The patient should avoid foods that are high in fat. This may be difficult to do on some days because the medications may cause patients to be hungry. Patients may experience waves of nausea and find that snacking on crackers or other light foods helps to alleviate this feeling. It is not uncommon for patients to gain weight while they are on chemotherapy. Other side effects that are not unusual include alterations in taste. Certain odors or food aromas may precipitate a wave of nausea. It is hard to predict just who will experience these symptoms, but patients who do should keep a record of the symptoms so they can avoid these foods in the future.

4. *Avoiding alcohol.* It is best not to drink alcohol. The drugs being given to the patient are metabolized in the liver, which is where alcohol is also metabolized. Liver enzyme values will also be monitored.

5. *Learning the dosage of drugs.* The drug dosage is determined by the patient's height and weight (body surface area). If the patient should gain or lose weight while on chemotherapy, the dosage may be changed. When chemotherapy is started, the patient should ask what her body surface area is, and what is the dosage of each drug being prescribed. Each time she receives chemotherapy, she should check the dose with the nurse.

6. *Chemotherapy-induced menopause.* If the patient is premenopausal, the chemotherapy may precipitate an early menopause. This depends on the patient's age at diagnosis. In some women, menstruation becomes irregular during chemotherapy. When chemotherapy is finished, the menstrual cycle may return to normal. Menopausal symptoms include hot flashes, vaginal dryness, sleep disturbances, mood swings, and decreased libido. The decrease in libido is also experienced while patients are undergoing chemotherapy because of alteration in body image, fatigue, and nausea. Because it is not advisable to use estrogen replacement therapy for these symptoms, other alternatives including vitamin E (400 IU daily) and the use of selective serotonin reuptake inhibitors (SSRIs; paroxetine and fluoxetine), venlafaxine, or gabapentin may also be prescribed.[7] As mentioned previously, the nurse should instruct the patient about using calcium supplements to help prevent

osteoporosis. The recommended dose of calcium for post-menopausal women is 1500 mg per day. The body can absorb only 500 μg at a time, so the supplements should be spaced out throughout the day. Low-dose vaginal estrogen is also used to help with vaginal dryness. Vagifem 25-μg tablets and an estradiol vaginal ring (Estring) are the most commonly prescribed medications that provide a local estrogenic effect. Vagifem tablets are inserted 1 tablet intravaginally each day for 14 days, then 1 tablet twice weekly thereafter. Estring is inserted into the upper third of the vaginal vault and is worn continously for 3 months. Estring releases estradiol, approximately 7.5 μg over 24 hours. Side efffects from both of these medications may include headache, vaginal spotting or discharge, allergic reaction, and skin rash.

The above therapies should be combined with an exercise routine such as walking or swimming to achieve maximum benefit.

How might breast cancer affect sexuality and intimacy?

Many women at the time of diagnosis may have a strong need for intimacy; others, conversely, may withdraw from their partner. As mentioned earlier, breast cancer is a life-changing event in a woman's life. Sexual arousal may take longer because of the side effects from medications and other treatments. Libido may not be very strong because of physical and emotional stress. Women may feel that they have become unattractive to their partners if they have had a mastectomy or have alopecia. However, the sexual health of the woman is important to the process of recovery. Some women may not feel comfortable initiating the discussion of side effects and what other women undergoing therapy have experienced. Chances are that if the nurse initiates the discussion, the patient will be relieved to be asked.

How is a prosthesis selected?

A Reach to Recovery referral should be made preoperatively. This allows more time for the American Cancer Society to match the woman with a volunteer who has had a similar experience. These volunteers are often able to offer their perspective on the healing process. They will also bring a temporary (cotton) prosthesis and a mastectomy bra for the woman who has not had reconstruction. The surgical healing process takes about 6 weeks, after which the patient can be fitted for a permanent prosthesis. Permanent prostheses vary in size, weight, texture, and—most significantly—price. The physician will provide a prescription for a breast prosthesis. Most health insurance plans cover from 50% to 80% of the total cost. If the patient needs financial assistance in procuring a prosthesis, the American Cancer Society has resources to assist the patient. The Reach to Recovery program will also provide a list of stores that sell prostheses.

When the woman is ready to have a fitting for a permanent prosthesis, she should make an appointment. The fitting takes about an hour, and she should not feel rushed. The breast tissue needs to be matched in weight to give a good body alignment. Mastectomy bras will also be needed. These, too, may be covered by insurance.

The nurse should become familiar with the shops in the area and visit them before making referrals. If the nurse can establish relationships with the fitters, it facilitates streamlining the care for women needing prostheses.

What are the interventions for menopausal symptoms?

As more young women are diagnosed with breast cancer, premature menopause is becoming more common. These symptoms affect the woman's quality of life and can be very uncomfortable.

Hot Flashes
Hot flashes are the most common side effect. The physiologic mechanism responsible for menopause is poorly understood. Some scientists postulate a pulsatile release of luteinizing hormone secreted from the ovary. This accompanies the decreasing levels of estrogen just before menopause. This release of luteinizing hormone may cause an alteration in sympathetic tone, causing vasodilatation, perspiration, and changes in blood flow, temperature, and heart rate. Hot flashes usually begin as a feeling of pressure in the head, neck, and upper chest and back that spreads to the entire body. The range and duration of hot flashes may vary; a woman may experience as few as one a day or as many as three an hour. Hot flashes interrupt sleep, causing irritability and insomnia. The good news is that hot flashes usually decrease with time as onset of menopause approaches.

To manage hot flashes, the nurse should provide the following suggestions:

- Wear absorbent cotton clothing.
- Dress in layers that can be removed as needed.
- Lower the thermostat.
- Avoid caffeine, spicy foods, and alcohol.
- Exercise regularly.
- Learn relaxation techniques.
- Record the number of hot flashes each day, and report this to the nurse or physician.

Nonhormonal interventions may include the following:

- Vitamin E, 400 IU twice a day (no side effects at this dosage)
- Black cohosh (over the counter in capsule form)
- SSRIs (paroxetine and fluoxetine)
- Antihypertensives (transdermal clonidine)

Atrophic Vaginitis
A drop in estrogen levels results in decreased elasticity of the vaginal wall. The vaginal lining becomes thinner and more fragile, and the pH becomes more alkaline, causing a woman to be at risk for vaginal or urinary tract infections. There is also decreased vaginal lubrication, which leads to dryness and dyspareunia.

Interventions for vaginal dryness include warm baths to alleviate vaginal itching and discomfort. Douches, feminine hygiene sprays, perfumed soaps, and perfumed toilet paper should be avoided. Over-the-counter agents are available to

Table 39–2 Drain Care after Surgery: Instructions for the Patient

After your surgery, you will notice a bulblike drain connected to tubing coming from your incision. This device suctions and collects fluid from the incisional area. The drain promotes healing and reduces the chance of infection.

The drain will be in place for 5 to 10 days after surgery. (The time varies from surgeon to surgeon.) You will most likely be discharged from the hospital with the drain in place. Your nurse will review the care of the drain with you. Remember to empty the drainage bottle every 12 hours or as often as directed. Refer to these instructions as needed:

1. Obtain a measuring cup to collect the fluid, and then wash your hands thoroughly.
2. Unpin the bottle from your dressing or your shirt.
3. Remove the rubber stopper from the bottle. Turn the bottle upside down, and squeeze the contents into the measuring cup. Empty the bottle completely, and keep a record of the amount of fluid in the measuring cup. *Note:* To prevent infection, do not let the rubber stopper or top of the bottle touch the measuring cup or any other surface.
4. Use one hand to squeeze all the air from the bottle. With the bottle still compressed, use your other hand to replace the rubber stopper. Do this to make sure the drain suction works well.
5. Pin the bottle back on your dressing or your shirt to avoid pulling it out accidentally. Wash your hands again (see Fig. 39–1).

From Drain Care after Surgery: Directions and Information [pamphlet]. Washington, DC, George Washington University Breast Care Center.

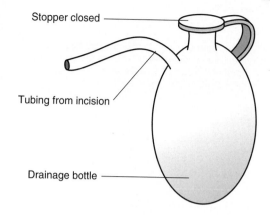

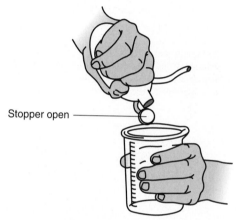

Figure 39–1 Postoperative drainage bulb. (From Drain Care after Surgery: Directions and Information [pamphlet]. Washington, DC, George Washington University Breast Care Center.)

counteract vaginal dryness. For everyday dryness, Replens, Gyne-Moistrin, Lubrin vaginal suppositories, Astroglide, or K-Y Jelly (or other water-soluble lubricant) may be used. Pharmacologic interventions include Estring and Vagifem tablets.

Vaginal Discharge and Yeast Infections

Vaginal discharge most often represents a yeast infection. It is exacerbated by factors that normally increase vaginal discharge, such as diabetes, antibiotic therapy, and extreme stress. Interventions include the use of Monistat, Femstat, or Diflucan.

Breast Self-Examination

After the acute phase of treatment is over, most women may benefit from individualized instruction in breast self-examination. The MammaCare method is a highly effective step-by-step program using the vertical strip technique. Certification to teach this technique can be obtained from the Mammatech Corporation (Gainesville, FL). Nurses can call 1-800-626-2273 for more information.

What are the long-term rehabilitation issues?

Although the diagnosis of breast cancer may pose adjustment issues later in life, it is important for women to try to find an appropriate balance. As breast cancer survivors, patients can become advocates for other women like themselves, either by volunteering for the Reach to Recovery program of the American Cancer Society or by becoming involved with other breast cancer support organizations. The National Breast Cancer Coalition, a grassroots advocacy effort, is a good example of how survivors have become advocates for themselves and other women. It has been very successful in securing money for breast cancer research and is influential on Capitol Hill, where breast cancer policy and legislation are initiated.

The nurse's role in the surgical setting is quite challenging, but it can be very rewarding. Roles continue to evolve as new treatment strategies become available. Promoting quality cancer care is the best gift nurses can provide to their patients. In addition to the Quality of Care Standards position by the Oncology Nursing Society, the National Breast Cancer Coalition Fund released the *Guide to Quality Breast Cancer Care* in 2002.[8] This is a comprehensive guide that provides excellent information for the breast cancer patient. This guide can be obtained free of charge by calling 1-866-624-5307 or through their website, *www.natlbcc.org*.

How should patients be instructed in drain care after surgery?

See Table 39–2 and Figure 39–1 for patient instructions on drain care after surgery.

Pendulum Exercises

While standing, bend forward at the hips, and allow the affected shoulder to hang loosely in front of the body. Place the uninvolved hand on a table or chair for support.

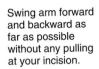

Swing arm forward and backward as far as possible without any pulling at your incision.

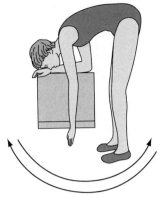

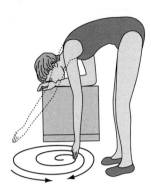

Swing the arm in a clockwise circle, beginning with small circles and gradually increasing the size. Make 10 circles, then make 10 circles in a counterclockwise direction.

Wall Climbing with the Fingertips

Stand facing the wall, and extend the affected arm directly in front of you so that your fingertips touch the wall (at arm's length from the wall). Creep up the side of the wall with your fingertips, taking a step toward the wall as you reach higher and higher up the wall. Repeat the procedure going down the wall, but taking a step backward this time.

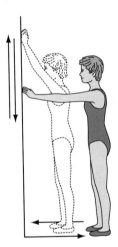

Repeat the above procedure, but this time position yourself perpendicular (at a right angle) to the wall so that the affected arm extends sideways up the wall. Keep your trunk straight, not leaning toward the wall or shrugging your shoulders. Place a pencil mark on the wall each day, and try to go a bit farther every day.

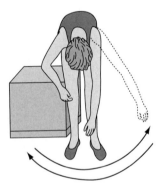

Swing the affected arm side to side across the chest 10 times in each direction.

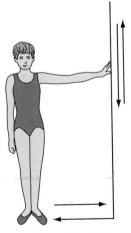

Figure 39–2   Patient exercises to be performed after breast-conserving surgery or mastectomy.   (From Breast Care Center. Washington, DC, George Washington University Medical Faculty Associates.)

What postoperative exercises should patients perform after breast-conserving surgery or mastectomy?

See Figure 39–2 for patient exercises to be performed after breast-conserving surgery or mastectomy. Patients should be advised not to start active range-of-motion exercises until they have been instructed to do so by their surgeon.

INTERNET RESOURCES FOR BREAST CANCER

- American Cancer Society: *www.cancer.org*
- National Institutes of Health: *www.nci.nih.gov*
- Breast Cancer Education Network: *www.healthtalk.com*
- Breast Cancer.Net: *www.breastcancer.net*
- Breast Health Network: *www.breasthealthnetwork.com*
- Breast Cancer Research Foundation: *www.bcrfcure.org*
- Cancer Care, Inc.: *www.cancercare.org*
- National Breast Cancer Coalition: *www.stopbreastcancer.org*
- National Coalition for Cancer Survivorship: *www.cancer advocacy.org*
- People Living With Cancer: *www.plwc.org*
- Susan G. Komen Foundation: *www.komen.org*
- Women's Cancer Network *www.wcn.org*
- Y-Me National Breast Cancer Organization: *www.y-me.org*

REFERENCES

1. Langer A, Hassey Dow K. The breast cancer advocacy movement and nursing. Oncol Nurs 1994;1:3.
2. American Cancer Society. Facts and Figures. Atlanta, American Cancer Society, 2004.
3. Komen Foundation. Questions to ask the doctor about breast cancer [online]. Available at www.komen.org. 2004.
4. Cserni G. Axillary staging of breast cancer and sentinel node. J Clin Pathol 2000;53:733–741.
5. Kellar SJ. Sentinel lymph node for breast cancer. AORN J 2001;74(2):197–201.
6. Baum M, Budzar AU, Cuzick J, et al. ATAC Trialists' Group. Anastrozole alone or in combination with tamoxifen versus tamoxifen alone for adjuvant treatment of postmenopausal women with early breast cancer: first results of the ATAC randomised trial. Lancet 2002;359:2131–2139 (erratum in Lancet 2002;360:1520).
7. Barton D, Loprinzi CL. Making sense of the evidence regarding nonhormonal treatments for hot flashes. Clin J Oncol Nurs 2004;8(1):39–41.
8. Guide to quality breast cancer care. 2002. National Breast Cancer Coalition Fund. www.natlbcc.org/nbccf

CHAPTER 40

Medicolegal Issues in Breast Cancer Diagnosis and Treatment

Jay A. Rappaport and Andrew I. Kaplan

OPENING STATEMENT

According to the last Annual Report of the National Practitioner Data Bank (NPDB), the central repository of information regarding malpractice payments made on behalf of physicians nationally, during calendar year 2002, 80.6% of new reports concerning malpractice payments were physician related, with the median and mean malpractice payment amounts totaling $150,000 and $275,094, respectively.[1] Significantly, diagnosis-related payments were the most frequently reported (36.7% of all payments).[1]

Although there is no comprehensive database tracking the basis, theory, and result of all medical malpractice claims in the United States, the Physician Insurers Association of America (PIAA), an association of more than 50 medical malpractice insurance carriers, regularly compiles malpractice claims data from more than 20 member companies to publish reports on national trends involving malpractice claims, particularly those involving breast cancer. According to the PIAA's *2000 Research Notes*, the average indemnity paid on breast cancer claims has consistently increased over the past 15 years. The average indemnity paid on breast cancer claims from 1990 to 1994 was $224,509, whereas the average indemnity from 1995 to 1999 was $231,596. Of note is the fact that the average indemnity paid for breast cancer claims over the entire 15 years from 1985 to 1999 was $251,505, well above the average indemnity of $163,743 for *all other malpractice claims made during that time period*.[2]

In fact, the most recent data accumulated by the PIAA suggest that the allegation of an error in the diagnosis of breast cancer has become the most prevalent condition precipitating medical malpractice lawsuits against all physicians. More than 41% of all claims involving breast cancer result in an indemnity payment to the claimant/patient. The latest figures released by the PIAA indicate that overall indemnification for all breast cancer malpractice litigation averaged $438,000 in 2002, *a 45% increase in the corresponding figure from 1995*.[3] Quite obviously, the public perception that earlier diagnosis virtually guarantees a cure, combined with the belief that clinical evaluation and mammography should be 100% accurate, has led to a deluge of claims for failure to diagnose breast cancer and a concomitant willingness by juries to compensate patients for those perceived failures.

Medical professionals are certainly familiar with a wide variety of stressors, uncertainties, and hurdles inherent to the practice of medicine, and the practitioner has learned and developed methods and algorithms to deal with them. When physicians are named as defendants in a lawsuit, however, it is akin to entering a foreign land without a passport or an appreciation of the language. It drags practitioners outside the medical arena and subjects them to forces over which they have little, if any, control and often even less knowledge.

The patients who bring such suits, particularly in the realm of breast cancer litigation, have their own significant stressors and anxieties. Both sides going forward must understand this fact. It serves no one to engage in characterizations of those who sue, or those who are sued.

This chapter seeks to raise questions and, whenever possible, to suggest answers as to why the national court system has seen such a steady influx of claims alleging practitioners' failure to diagnose and treat breast cancer in a timely fashion and the manner in which that influx has caused, and should cause, physicians to take stock in and accommodate their methods of practicing medicine in an increasingly litigious environment. Through our own experiences as medical malpractice litigators and through the analysis of jury verdicts and insurance claims made and paid in lawsuits arising from claims of failure to diagnose and treat breast cancer in a timely manner, we aim to enlighten the reader as to the legal theories and hurdles applicable to such claims and the medical theories most often elucidated and litigated by the patients who bring them. Although it is neither our intent nor our desire to offer suggestions as to the clinical management of patients, at the conclusion of this chapter, we offer suggestions as to the manner in which the practitioner may be proactive in both preventing and defending exposure to malpractice litigation.

What is malpractice?

We have always found it instructive, whether discussing the matter with physicians or laypersons, to educate the listener (or, in this case, reader) as to the charge delivered by the court to the average jury member sitting in judgment in a medical malpractice action, just before commencing deliberation. The *Pattern Jury Instructions* define malpractice as follows:

Malpractice is professional negligence and medical malpractice is the negligence of a doctor. Negligence is the failure to use reasonable care under the circumstances, doing something that a reasonably prudent doctor would not do under the circumstances, or failing to do something that a reasonably prudent doctor would do under the circumstances. It is a deviation or departure from accepted practice.[4]

A doctor who renders medical service to a patient is obligated to have that reasonable degree of knowledge and skill that is expected of an average specialist who performs or provides that medical service in the medical community in which the doctor practices.

The law recognizes that there are differences in the abilities of doctors, just as there are differences in the abilities of people engaged in other activities. To practice medicine, a doctor is not required to have the extraordinary knowledge and ability that belongs to a few doctors of exceptional ability. However, every doctor is required to keep reasonably informed of new developments in his or her field and to practice medicine or surgery in accordance with approved methods and means of treatment in general use. A doctor must also use his or her best judgment and whatever superior knowledge and skill he or she possesses, even if the knowledge and skill exceed that possessed by the average specialist in the medical community where the doctor practices.

By undertaking to perform a medical service, a doctor does not guarantee a good result. The fact that there was a bad result to the patient, by itself, does not make the doctor liable. The doctor is liable only if he or she was negligent. Whether the doctor was negligent is to be decided on the basis of the facts and conditions existing at the time of the claimed negligence.

A doctor is not liable for an error in judgment if he or she does what he or she decides is best after careful evaluation, if it is a judgment that a reasonably prudent doctor could have made under the circumstances.

If the doctor is negligent—that is, lacks the skill or knowledge required of him or her in providing a medical service, or fails to use reasonable care in providing the service, or fails to exercise his or her best judgment, and such failure is a substantial factor in causing harm to the patient—then the doctor is responsible for the injury or harm caused.

Breast cancer litigation is a form of tort litigation wherein a patient, termed the *plaintiff,* brings the action accusing a physician, the *defendant,* of a civil wrong. That civil wrong is negligence—failure to act as a "reasonable person," or to adhere to a particular standard of care. Negligence by a professional is termed *malpractice;* by a physician or hospital, *medical malpractice.* The burden of proving every essential element that constitutes malpractice in any given case remains with the patient from institution of the proceeding until the verdict is rendered and judgment entered.

In medical malpractice litigation, the standard of care arises from the physician's responsibility to possess and apply that reasonable degree of skill, learning, and ability ordinarily possessed by physicians within the community in which he or she practices. The standard of care within the community in which the defendant practices changes on a case-by-case basis; prior trial court decisions in similar actions have no precedential or binding effect. Thus, there is no set "standard of care" adherent to the management of patients with breast disease, nor could there be one. In each individual situation, it is the duty of the fact-finder—the jury (and occasionally of the appellate courts, in situations in which the jury's decision is inconsistent with the facts or the law presented)—to determine just what the applicable standard of care is in any given situation and to determine whether the defendant physician met that standard.

To establish a claim for civil negligence, there must first be proof of a duty owed (a physician–patient relationship). That relationship arises any time a physician undertakes to diagnose or treat conditions of the patient's breast, whether it be during examination within the confines of the office, in rendering advice over the telephone while "on call" for a colleague, or even in the performance and interpretation of mammography, despite the rarity of the interpreting radiologist's actually meeting the patient at all. In fact, according to the most recent PIAA statistics, radiologists are the specialists most frequently named as defendants in malpractice litigation, accounting for 33% of all claims. Obstetrician-gynecologists are second at 22.8%, and surgeons are third at 10.6%.[5]

Once it has been established that a duty to render appropriate care exists, the next prong in establishing a claim for medical malpractice lies in proving a *breach of duty* (commonly defined as a departure or deviation from good and accepted practice or care). Whether the physician breached is a determination made by the jury based on the medical evidence in the case and the testimony of the witnesses. More often than not, it is the testimony and the credibility of the expert witnesses in the case on the subjects of standard of care in the community and whether the particular practitioner on trial adhered to or departed from that standard that influence a jury's decision. Those experts are subject to cross-examination by opposing counsel, not only on the medical testimony given on the stand but also on their qualifications and credibility, and in the face of inconsistent sworn testimony they may have given previously on similar topics in other courts of law.

Medical treatises or guidelines applicable to the period of treatment at issue, as well as the defendant's own prior testimony, publications, and office protocols, may also come into play in the jury's analysis. Most courts adhere to the common rule that a text or treatise must first be acknowledged as authoritative in the field before it may be read to the jury, but once acknowledged as such, it may be used to establish that the defendant practitioner deviated from the authoritative standards as set forth within the publication and thus committed malpractice.

Most attorneys who select juries on behalf of patients will tell those juries that they are not claiming that the practitioner acted, or failed to act, intentionally, or that they are "bad" doctors. Instead, they allege one act, or series of acts, of malpractice as isolated incidents of breach of care in a longer history of good practice. Without a "bad result," meaning without injury, there is no case, but every jury is charged that a bad result, in and of itself, is not evidence of malpractice. It is not the result that legally determines whether there was negligence. Practically speaking, however, a jury faced with a bad result will undoubtedly consider that result in the exercise of deliberation.

An error in medical judgment is not evidence of malpractice, either. In context, the use of the word *judgment* here has a specific meaning. Judgment comes into play in the arena of malpractice litigation where, and only where, there are two (or more) ways for a physician to approach a situation. If there are two ways to deal with the situation, each acceptable in the medical community, the choice by the physician of the one over the other is the exercise of judgment, and if exercised appropriately, the physician can be defended, even if the chosen treatment failed.

Many a practitioner has attempted to defend an allegation of malpractice by asserting that an exercise of judgment cannot constitute negligence, and many a tribunal has allowed the pursuit of just such a defense. In reality, however, almost every action involving a physician's decision making as it pertained to a patient could conceivably be defended as such, and so the courts have attempted to limit the defense of judgment to those situations in which the practitioner had two very real and very acceptable treatment options available and chose one over the other to the unfortunate but unpredictable detriment of the patient.

In that regard, jurors are cautioned against casting *their* judgment on the defendant physician based on outcome, but rather are directed to consider what the physician had in front of him or her at the time care was rendered and decisions made. The reason for this directive, as would appear to be obvious, is that in hindsight we are almost all correct. Even claims brought against radiologists for the misreading of mammograms, which come as close as any case can to a question of accurate interpretation, are not immune from hindsight analysis because of the unique nature of breast imaging. The difficulty of getting the exact same view twice, the nature of the image, particularly of dense breasts, and the requirement of significant experience and ability can place these cases in the realm of hindsight as well. Any radiologist can tell you it is easier to spot a cancer on mammography once you know it is there.

The third, and most essential, prong in establishing medical malpractice—particularly in the realm of breast cancer litigation—is causation. It must be shown that the practitioner's action or inaction was the competent producing cause of injury to the patient. In other words, the burden is on the patient to prove that, *more likely than not,* earlier or alternative diagnosis or treatment would have positively affected outcome. Thus, it is not the patient's burden to establish that appropriate care would have resulted in cure (though in some situations that is the very allegation made); rather, it is enough to establish that it would have affected the quality and duration of life to the patient's benefit. So significant is the subject of causation that it maintains its own Pattern Jury Instruction. Proximate cause is defined in the *Pattern Jury Instructions* as follows:

An act or omission is regarded as a cause of an injury if it was a substantial factor in bringing about the injury, that is, if it had such an effect in producing the injury that reasonable people would regard it as a cause of the injury. There may be more than one cause of an injury, but to be substantial, it cannot be slight or trivial. You may, however, decide that a cause is substantial even if you assign a relatively small percentage to it.[6]

Acknowledging, then, that a delay in diagnosis, even a negligent delay, may not affect the patient's ultimate outcome, the law interposes the evidentiary requirement of "proximate cause" on plaintiffs seeking monetary damages in medical malpractice cases. Technically, if a physician's negligence did not cause harm, as it were, the patient should be unable to make out what is known as a *prima facie*, or sufficient on its face, case of medical malpractice that will survive dismissal at the close of plaintiff's evidence rather than reach the deliberation of the jury. In reality, however, rare is the action in which medical negligence is proven yet the claim dismissed by court or jury. As will be discussed further, the public perceives that earlier and accurate diagnosis alters outcome, and the public is often unwilling to forgive the practitioner who has breached the standard of care or accept that "it didn't make a difference."

The final prong in establishing a claim of medical malpractice, and perhaps the most obvious one, is that the patient must have sustained an actual injury as a result of the practitioner's malpractice in order to obtain reward for financial damages. Although punitive or punishment damage awards are rare, juries are instructed that under the appropriate circumstances, they can award noneconomic damages for pain and suffering as well as loss of consortium or society (an award made for harm to a close relationship, such as with a spouse or child). Indeed, it is common for a patient's spouse to be named as co-plaintiff in a malpractice action, to seek redress for loss of society, comfort, and companionship due to the injuries alleged, and to obtain remuneration in significant amounts in those cases in which a jury determines that plaintiffs have proven their claims.

Economic damages such as loss of earnings incurred to date and in the future, medical costs, rehabilitation and therapy costs, and out-of-pocket expenses for goods and services can be granted as well, and often constitute a hefty portion of the fees awarded. The fact is that cases involving allegations of negligence in the diagnosis and treatment of patients with breast cancer often involve devastating injuries, both emotionally and financially, to those who bring suit. In fact, according to the PIAA, the average award in medical malpractice actions involving breast cancer is second only to those cases involving brain damage suffered by infants at or around the time of delivery.[5]

As a caveat, although the burden of proof in all cases rests on the party asserting the claim, the defense, alternatively, must prove those issues raised by the defense, which are deemed *affirmative defenses*, and which must be set forth in the initial answer to the complaint. Perhaps the most significant of these affirmative defenses in the realm of breast cancer litigation is termed *culpable conduct*, or more correctly, *comparative negligence*, which is conduct by the patient that caused or contributed to her own damages and may reduce the ultimate verdict by the percentage of that culpability. In the area of breast cancer litigation, this usually means that the patient did not follow an instruction, which, if followed, would have improved her outcome or prognosis. Because in many instances in this area of litigation, the patient has died from her disease or likely will, this defense is one approached with care and trepidation. The patient's attorney will no doubt attempt to portray the defense and the doctor as "blaming the patient." Thus, to be effective, not only must such a defense be medically valid, but, as will be discussed further in this chapter, the basis for the defense must be well documented in the defendant physician's records and, preferably, supported by the records of the other nonparty treating practitioners.

Who sues whom and why?

Statistical analysis reveals that although most breast cancer occurs in women older than 50 years, most malpractice suits regarding breast cancer are brought by women younger than 50 years. In fact, according to the PIAA's *2002 Breast Cancer Study*—a data-sharing study of 450 paid malpractice cases in which the central allegation cited a delay in the diagnosis of breast cancer—the average age of claimants in breast cancer litigation is 45 years, with 68% of claimants younger than 50 years and 33% younger than 40 years.[5] Patients younger than 40 years accounted for 47.5% of the claims in which wrongful death as a result of missed diagnosis was pled.

By the same token, research reveals that the average indemnity payment for younger plaintiffs was significantly higher than that for older patients. Patients younger than 40 years accounted for 33% of claims made and 42.9% of indemnity reported. The average indemnity for patients younger than 30 years was $603,537, and younger than 40 years, $508,606, compared with an average award of just under $300,000 for patients between the ages of 50 and 70 years.[5] Almost one third of patients (31.3%) had a family history of breast cancer, and most patients—55.1%—were premenopausal.[5]

That younger patients bring the majority of claims and recover the largest awards for those claims stands to reason, particularly given the nature of malpractice litigation. In terms of awards, juries are given wide latitude, within certain established parameters, in determining damages, both economic and noneconomic. Life expectancy *had timely diagnosis been made* is a significant factor in the determination of compensation, not only for future loss of earnings but also for deriving the almost incalculable compensation for the loss of months, days, or weeks with loved ones left behind. Patients with young children inevitably garner more significant indemnity for the potential loss of parental guidance occasioned on their offspring.

The overwhelming majority of malpractice claims related to breast cancer involve failure to timely diagnose, as opposed to less frequently seen claims such as iatrogenic injury, unnecessary mastectomy, or burns related to radiation oncology. We undertook a simple Lexis/Nexis analysis, which revealed that of the 20 judicial decisions rendered in breast cancer matters at both the state and federal levels since January 2003 (not only jury verdicts but also decisions rendered on pretrial discovery issues), the underlying facts reflected that 16 of the 20, or 80% of the cases reviewed, revolved around allegations of a failure to timely diagnose and treat breast cancer. Two cases involved injuries secondary to radiation, and the other two alleged the unnecessary performance of mastectomy.[7]

Of the 17 jury verdicts or settlements in breast cancer litigation reached and reported to the *National Jury Verdict Reporter* in 2004, over the preceding 2-year period, 15 of the 17—or 88%—were matters involving radiologists or surgeons, and only one involved anything other than a failure to diagnose breast cancer in a timely manner.[7] Five of the 17 matters resulted in jury verdicts between $1.5 and $5.25 million, with an average jury verdict of $2,144,375. Only 3 of the

17 cases reported resulted in verdicts in favor of the defendant at the conclusion of trial. Ten of the 17 plaintiffs, or nearly 60%, were younger than 50 years, and two women younger than 50 years accounted for the two highest reported verdicts of $5.25 million and $4 million. The overwhelming majority of cases reported involved misread mammograms, and more than 50% also involved patients whose self-detected lumps had been diagnosed as benign or fibrocystic.[7] Given the difficulty in defending against public perception and intrinsic sympathy for the patient and her family, it is not difficult to understand why most breast cancer claims settle before a jury can price them.

Increased awareness of breast health, particularly the encouragement of earlier and more regular self-breast examinations, has led to not only earlier diagnosis of suspicious lesions but also increased awareness of their presence. Nonetheless, statistics seem to support that practitioners are often unimpressed with the presence of a painless, self-discovered mass in patients younger than 50 years, particularly those that have had a negative or equivocal mammogram. According to PIAA's report, in 58.9% of breast cancer claims, the patient found the lesion herself. In 38.7% of the cases, the patient's presenting symptom at the first physician visit was a lump in the breast, yet 24.4% of all patients in the study—110 of the 174 claims for which the patient presented with a specific complaint of a breast lump—were initially diagnosed with a benign condition such as a cyst, fibrocystic disease, or benign lump.[5] By way of comparison, the second most prevalent physical finding on examination in the cases cited, after palpable mass, was "pain in breast," and this appeared in only 16.2% of cases.[5] As will be discussed in the ensuing section, the practitioner must do more, particularly in the younger patient, to ensure the benignity of any palpable lesion appreciated by the physician or patient.

Accordingly, the specialists most often named as defendants in the cases cited (both by PIAA and in the informal survey by the authors) were radiologists, followed by obstetrician-gynecologists and surgeons.[5] Obviously, the most common allegation against radiologists was the failure to properly interpret mammography—at first blush, perhaps, somewhat surprising given the continued advancement and sensitivity of the technology. This may, however, also be reflective of the increased use of screening mammograms that, when used in hindsight, may be deemed by a plaintiff's expert to depict an undiagnosed mass, suspicious microcalcifications, or quality too poor to merit accurate and reliable interpretation.

For surgeons, obstetrician-gynecologists, and general practitioners, the most common theme in breast cancer litigation continues to be *physical findings failed to impress*, which PIAA found in 44% of claims, followed by *failure to refer to specialist for biopsy* in 40.5% of cases involving obstetrician-gynecologists or general practitioners.[5] Medically, this is equally unsurprising.

As mentioned, younger patients have lower indicia of suspicion for breast cancer from the moment they walk into the examination room. Doctors are less likely to order a biopsy or strict follow-up for younger patients, who are statistically less likely to have breast cancer. In addition, younger patients have denser breast tissue, which can obscure or obstruct the performance of physical examination as well as mammography. Pregnancy, breast-feeding, and hormonal changes can also cause changes in breast tissue, and—absent a family history of breast disease—younger patients are often poorer historians of breast health and less likely to seek medical attention expeditiously on the first potential signs of concern or irregularity.

Public perception cannot be discounted in its impact on breast cancer claims and verdicts. In this context, we would point out that even though there are extant studies that seem to indicate that delay, at times, does not affect outcome, this is a "hard sell" to jurors, indoctrinated as they are by campaigns that indicate that early detection saves lives. Once a patient or a potential juror accepts such a theory as truth, then, by definition, any delay is "bad," meaning that the delay in diagnosis is a compensable item of damages.

Clearly, survival is not the same as cure, but once a patient and a juror hear "survival" rates discussed in the examining room or the courtroom, the natural inclination is to tune out the pessimistic evidence of the natural biology of cancer and tune into the optimism of early detection and timely treatment in effectuating "cure." Well-publicized advances in technology benefit the practitioner and patient alike but also indoctrinate the mindset that failure is unacceptable. Accuracy at all times becomes mandatory and is, of course, impossible to achieve, particularly in those situations in which the patient maintains a level of responsibility for failure to heed the clinician's recommendations or warnings.

A patient's attorney will almost always argue that the response of the practitioner—radiologist, surgeon, gynecologist, or general practitioner—to complaints or findings was not nearly aggressive enough in the face of a potentially deadly yet curable disease. The mammography warranted magnification; the cyst warranted aspiration; the lump warranted biopsy, the pain required referral; her complaints necessitated follow-up in 3 months, not 6 months or a year. As long as the public perceives or misperceives that earlier diagnosis of breast cancer virtually guarantees a cure and that any delay in diagnosis is a death sentence—even in the face of objective medical expert testimony to the contrary—the number of malpractice claims related to the failure to diagnose breast cancer in a timely way will continue to rise, as will the rate of compensation for those claims, accordingly.

What is a physician to do?

Fortunately, many of the issues of the actual practice of breast care are, and should be, designed to avoid delay, and although it is an issue more for the practitioner than for the lawyers who represent them, the concept of "delay avoidance" ultimately inures to the benefit of the practitioner in the courtroom as well as the examination room.

At the outset, it is imperative for all physicians to be aware that the most important requirement of effective defense in litigation is documentation. If a fact, finding, or recommendation is not documented, the issue of its existence becomes almost purely one of credibility, a contest between the healthy physician or institution against the individual, frequently ill, patient. In context, it is important to realize that the physician will have many patients and will have seen many of them between the incidents complained of and the lawsuit. The patient, however, will have only one thing to recall: her own treatment.

This is not to say that the patient's recall will be at all times accurate or that the physician's will not be. However, common sense dictates that in this area the patient has an advantage, which can be reduced or removed by appropriate, thorough documentation. It is not really enough to say, "I always do it." If "it" is important enough to "always do," it is important enough to *always document.*

Documentation of a pertinent finding or recommendation and the fact that it has been conveyed to the patient or appropriate physician serves not only to contemporaneously establish the nature and purpose of treatment recommended and given but also to aid in the practitioner's legal defense months or years down the road, when memories have faded or have become biased by health problems and when credibility between the parties is at issue. Documentation of pertinent family histories, all breast complaints, and tactful notification of the risks of undiagnosed breast cancer for patients who do not follow up is mandatory in maintaining a complete chart.

Jurors have a natural inclination to accept what is written in a medical record as truth, or to at least provide the documented medical chart with the preferential inference of accuracy. In this way, communication and documentation truly go hand in hand. The passage of time, the backdrop of litigation, the sympathy afforded an ill patient or her family, and the suspicion of a physician's presumed self-interest can all be countered by a medical record replete with pertinent findings and recommendations entered contemporaneously with treatment, long before the prospect of litigation was ever entertained.

Insofar as charting is concerned, as time has passed, the charting requirements of the various insurance programs, both private and government, have increased to the point at which computer assistance has become available and may well become standard. It is not our purpose to deal in depth with this issue, but some observations are in order.

The practitioner and counsel are always advantaged by the maintenance of a complete chart. By *complete,* we mean one that contains all notes by the physician, all reports received, and, importantly, all memoranda that have to do with follow-up. Given the prevalence of claims against radiologists, documentation of the receipt and comparison of prior studies and inclusion of copies of those reports in the chart are extremely helpful. Telephone messages received should be acknowledged in the chart (stapled to a page is always good), and the response to them documented.

In addition to documenting all recommendations, documentation of the physician's thought process, including the diagnoses and tests considered and ruled out, as well as why, provides credible explanations of the judgment applied to potential jurors down the road. Documenting follow-up on any and all recommendations is imperative. A physician might recommend mammography, a mammographer might recommend sonography, a sonographer might recommend biopsy, and all three (or two, if the mammographer also performs sonography) might recommend a breast surgeon be consulted. On the next visit, a follow-up note can, and should, be generated. Did the patient comply? If not, why not? If so, when? Again, the testimony that "I always ask" is not as effective as a note documenting that the question was asked and a response received.

Some patients do not return after a recommendation for treatment or consult is made. Because most of these recommendations are or should be timed (mammogram "next week," for example), a follow-up system that accounts for the receipt of an appropriate report or consult note is helpful in countering the subtle, and sometimes not so subtle, indication by the patient's attorney that the physician in question did not care or, worse, abandoned the patient. These allegations are based on the unspoken but real supposition that in medical matters patients have given up the skills and knowledge they use in their everyday lives and have become dependent on the special skills of others. Because most jurors are patients as well, this argument holds weight and can sway opinion. Accurate documentation of a patient's reluctance to follow recommendations, pursue treatment, or keep appointments can help to counter the allegation that any delay was necessarily occasioned by the physician.

We believe that documentation of findings is an area with which most physicians are familiar. It is in the area of absence of findings where we find cases that are sometimes difficult to defend. Although the patient might complain of a mass or other abnormal finding, that finding at times cannot be, or is not, replicated on the physician's examination. Because there would be no suit without a later finding of a mass, a lesion, or the like, the inevitable allegation is that the malignancy was, in fact, the previously "missed" mass.

Here is where documentation can be of great assistance. A clear and accurate picture (literally, a drawing) of the area indicated by the patient will do much to assist in the defense of these cases, presuming, of course, that the malignancy is not where the patient initially felt a mass. To defend cases such as this, however, more is needed than good documentation. Appropriate referral (to a mammographer, sonographer, breast surgeon) is the best defense for the primary care physician, whether obstetrician-gynecologist or internist. If there is one lesson to be learned from the PIAA study, it is that a breast mass should always be resolved, whether it be by aspiration, biopsy, or appropriate referral. For the physician who receives the referral, the above rules for documentation apply, presuming nothing is found.

As an aside, we may be asked why we suggest that a physician go through these steps for something not clinically felt or appreciated. The answer lies in the reality that many jurors will believe that a patient is more familiar with her body than the physician is and, concurrently, that we are dealing with a common (an often-cited statistic is that one out of nine woman will suffer breast cancer) disease. If a disease is "common" and life threatening, an attorney will argue that its mortality demands that any and all steps be taken to rule it out, and this argument is a telling one.

In terms of mental approach, despite cliché, the courtroom is not a theater or a sports arena. There are, indeed, both theatrical and sports analogies used in the description and practice of the litigation process, but these analogies are often suspect. Using them, however, is helpful in developing the concept of breast cancer litigation and the appropriate litigation mindset.

Language is important to all of us, and in the courtroom it is particularly important. In the context of litigation, however, it takes a back seat to attitude. This is why physicians are directed to consider themselves as fact witnesses, not "defendants," and that they are not to "defend" their case, which is the responsibility and province of counsel. The reasons for this are multifactorial. First, once words such as defense are being used, we are in the realm of the lawyer, not the realm of the doctor. The simple reality is that the defense of a breast cancer case is the attorney's job, whereas the careful and truthful rendition of the facts and circumstances surrounding the incidents in question is the witness' job, be that witness another treating physician or the defendant.

It must be understood that sympathy is the unacknowledged, impermissible (the court will advise the jury not to use sympathy in its determinations) factor that must be recognized and controlled when possible. The physician defendant will not engender sympathy in the presence of the usual breast cancer sufferer or in the presence of the grieving family. Thus, any attitude other than professional commitment and concern works against the physician as a witness.

This does not mean that true sincerity, or caring, cannot be shown. It is antagonism toward the process, or the participants, that must be avoided. Thus, whereas the sporting arena analogy with its theme of two sides in competition is comparable, it is often, ultimately, counterproductive. Similarly, the "courtroom as theater" analogy distracts. Jurors, increasingly more sophisticated and litigation savvy, will detect actors and disregard them. Conversely, they will respond to a knowledgeable professional who presents without obvious ego, calmly indicating facts and opinions that bolster the reality of the defense.

Communication is the key element in establishing credibility and rapport with a patient and in gaining a patient's trust. In the breast cancer cases that we have litigated, invariably, either at the time of her deposition or at trial, the patient sets forth the basis for bringing suit: "He didn't tell me a thing." "She ignored my complaints." "He showed no compassion." "She never told me I needed a follow-up appointment." "No one ever suggested mammography," or "ultrasound," or "aspiration," or "biopsy." The list is endless, but it always centers on the patient's underlying mistrust of the physician for failing to simply and accurately convey pertinent findings and recommendations in a professional and timely manner.

As clichéd as it may seem, the "relationship" between physician and patient is often a key determining factor in whether a patient chooses to pursue legal remedy against a physician, irrespective of whether a cancer was "missed" or a departure from appropriate care occurred. The way the patient views her relationship with the physician matters.

By the same token, we often encounter, in the course of litigation, prior, contemporaneous, and subsequent treating physicians who we believe would be appropriate parties to the action, but for the patient's refusal to sue them. Our ability to implead these physicians, where applicable, is irrelevant for the purposes of this discussion, but, ultimately, it is our experience that the patient's rationale for excluding these physicians as party defendants is directly related to the basis for suing the party defendants: "He was the only one who was straight with me," or "I love Dr. Brown. She really listened to what I had to say." Rare is the patient who will pursue litigation against a physician with whom she has developed a relationship of mutual trust, courtesy, and respect.

It is certainly not the rule, but quite often a physician's honesty and ability to "connect" with the patient can overcome the inclination to sue for even the most damaging of medical errors. In fact, from the perspective of trial preparation, a physician's ability to build a rapport with his or her patients—and, specifically, what types of people or patients an individual physician best connects with—can assist counsel in determining what types of people would be preferential jurors.

SUMMATION

It has been neither the purpose nor the intent of this chapter to presume to advise physicians on practicing "good medicine," because that is the responsibility of the practitioner. Rather, it is our desire to address the recurrent themes in this area of litigation and to alert the reader to the pitfalls and potential perils that exist in the hopes of avoiding them. Although practicing with "litigation in mind" is distasteful to most physicians, the fact is that the prevention and the defense of a potential malpractice suit begin long before the patient retains an attorney and files a complaint.

In a society obsessed with litigation and saturated by the legal news media, physicians can no longer afford to remain ignorant of the legal ramifications of their actions or inactions. National financial constraints render malpractice insurance coverage and potential health maintenance inclusion or exclusion for individual physicians or physician groups precarious at best and often dependent solely on the number of malpractice claims *instituted* against the physician or entity, irrespective of the merits of those claims.

Just as preventive medicine affords the patient optimal opportunity to avoid disease, so too does the practice of preventive medicine afford the physician optimal odds for avoiding litigation. Quite simply, the best way to avoid litigation is to consistently render care that is in accord with good and accepted standards and to render care that is consistently care-ful; to communicate and to document; and to update not only one's medical education but also one's knowledge of the law as it applies to one's specialty and the practice of medicine as a whole. It is not necessary that the physician practice with litigation in mind, but it is imperative that the physician not ignore the prospect of litigation entirely.

In terms of preventing litigation, the role of physician as compassionate caregiver should not be underestimated. Reality informs us, however, that even thoughtful physicians who communicate well can be and are sued. As verdict awards increase, even the most conscientious of practitioners may ultimately find themselves in the role of defendant.

REFERENCES

1. National Practitioner Data Bank. 2002 Annual Report. NPDB, U.S. Department of Health and Human Services, Bureau of Health Professions, Rockville, MD, 2002, p 19.
2. Brott L. Breast cancer malpractice claims encouraging data [online]. Available at *http://www.pronational.com/news/advisor/breastcancer 3Q2001.htm.*
3. Quoted by Berlin L. U.S. Senate Committee on Health, Education, Labor, and Pensions. Re: Mammography Quality Standards Act Reauthorization. April 8, 2003, p 2.
4. 1 New York Pattern Jury Instruction NYP JI3d 2:150, Thomasan/West, Unified Court System, p 785 (2005).
5. Physician Insurers Association of America. Breast Cancer Study, 3rd ed. Rockville, MD, PIAA, 2002, pp 5–13.
6. 1 New York Pattern Jury Instruction NYP JI3d 2:70, Thomasan/West, Unified Court System, p 357 (2005).
7. [online]. Available at *http://www.Verdictsearch.com.* Accessed August 2004.

Index

Note: Page numbers followed by f and t refer to figures and tables, respectively.